Altchek's Diagnosis and Management of Ovarian Disorders

Third Edition

Altchek's Diagnosis and Management of Ovarian Disorders

Third Edition

Edited by

Liane Deligdisch, MD
Professor of Pathology and Obstetrics-Gynecology and Reproductive Science,
The Mount Sinai Medical Center and School of Medicine,
New York, NY, USA

Nathan G. Kase, MD
Professor in Obstetrics-Gynecology and Reproductive Sciences;
Professor of Endocrinology and Dean Emeritus,
The Mount Sinai School of Medicine,
New York, NY, USA

Carmel J. Cohen, MD
Professor of Obstetrics, Gynecology and Reproductive Science;
Professor of Gynecologic Oncology,
Ruttenberg Cancer Center,
The Mount Sinai School of Medicine,
New York, NY, USA

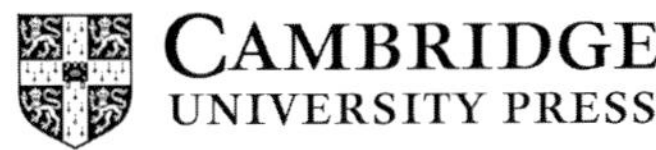

CAMBRIDGE
UNIVERSITY PRESS

CAMBRIDGE
UNIVERSITY PRESS

University Printing House, Cambridge CB2 8BS, United Kingdom

Published in the United States of America by Cambridge University Press, New York

Cambridge University Press is part of the University of Cambridge.

It furthers the University's mission by disseminating knowledge in the pursuit of education, learning and research at the highest international levels of excellence.

www.cambridge.org
Information on this title: www.cambridge.org/9781107012813

First edition first published 1996
Second edition first published 2003
Third edition first published 2013

Printed in Spain by Grafos SA, Arte sobre papel

A catalog record for this publication is available from the British Library

Library of Congress Cataloging in Publication data
Diagnosis and management of ovarian disorders.
Altchek's diagnosis and management of ovarian disorders / edited by Liane Deligdisch, MD, professor of pathology and obstetrics-gynecology and reproductive science, The Mount Sinai Medical Center and School of Medicine, New York, NY, USA, Nathan G. Kase, MD, professor in obstetrics, gynecology, and reproductive sciences, professor of endocrinology and dean emeritus, The Mount Sinai School of Medicine, New York, NY, USA, Carmel J. Cohen, MD, professor of obstetrics, gynecology, and reproductive science, professor of gynecologic oncology, Ruttenberg Cancer Center, The Mount Sinai School of Medicine, New York, NY, USA. – Third edition.
pages cm
Previous title: Diagnosis and management of ovarian disorders, edited by Albert Altchek and Liane Deligdisch.
Includes bibliographical references and index.
ISBN 978-1-107-01281-3
1. Ovaries – Diseases. I. Deligdisch, Liane, editor of compilation. II. Kase, Nathan G., 1930– editor of compilation. III. Cohen, Carmel J., editor of compilation. IV. Title. V. Title: Ovarian disorders.
RG441.D53 2013
618.1′1–dc23

2012043537

ISBN 978-1-107-01281-3 Hardback

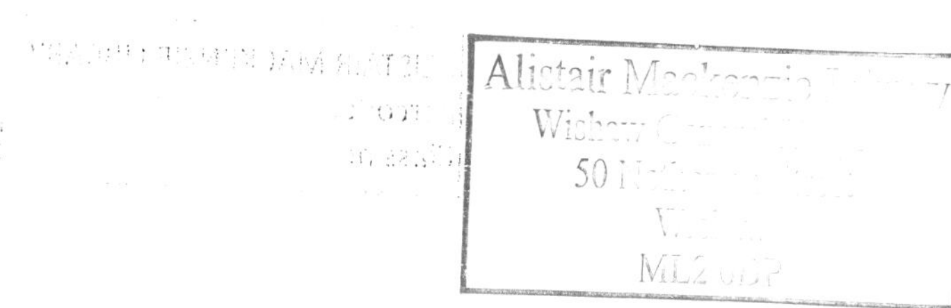

Contents

Contributors

The Late Albert Altchek, MD, FACS, FACOG
Formerly Clinical Professor of Obstetrics, Gynecology, and Reproductive Science, The Mount Sinai Medical Center and School of Medicine, New York, NY, USA

David H. Barad, MD, MS, FACOG
Director of Clinical ART and Senior Scientist, Center for Human Reproduction, New York, NY, USA

Katharine Batt, MD
Clinical Fellow, Division of Hematology/Medical Oncology, Tisch Cancer Institute, Brookdale Department of Geriatrics and Palliative Medicine, Mount Sinai School of Medicine, New York, NY, USA

Yuval Bdolah, MD, MSc
Senior Physician, Reproductive Endocrinology Division, Department of Obstetrics and Gynecology, Hebrew University-Hadassah Medical Center, Mount Scopus, Jerusalem, Israel

Revaz Botchorishvili, MD
Department of Gynecologic Surgery, CHU Clermont Ferrand, France

Nicolas Bourdel, MD
Department of Gynecologic Surgery, CHU Clermont Ferrand, France

Michael S. Broder, MD, MSHS
Adjunct Professor, Case Western Reserve University School of Medicine, Cleveland, OH, and President, Partnership for Health Analytic Research, LLC, Beverly Hills, CA, USA

Douglas N. Brown, MD, FACOG
Director, Division of Minimally Invasive Gynecologic Surgery, Department of Obstetrics and Gynecology, Walter Reed National Military Medical Center, Washington, DC, USA

Jubilee Brown, MD
Department Chair, Department of Gynecologic Oncology, The University of Texas MD Anderson Cancer Center, Houston, TX, USA

Antoine Maurice Bruhat, MD
Department of Gynecologic Surgery, CHU Clermont Ferrand, France

Michel Canis, MD
Department of Gynecologic Surgery, CHU Clermont Ferrand, France

Mine S. Cicek, PhD
Assistant Professor of Laboratory Medicine and Pathology, Department of Health Sciences Research, Mayo Clinic College of Medicine, Rochester MN, USA

Carmel J. Cohen, MD
Professor of Obstetrics, Gynecology and Reproductive Science; Professor of Gynecologic Oncology, Ruttenberg Cancer Center, The Mount Sinai School of Medicine, New York, NY, USA

Christopher P. Crum, MD
Professor, Department of Pathology, Harvard Medical School; Director, Division of Women's and Perinatal Pathology, Brigham and Women's Hospital, Boston, MA, USA

Christina E. Curtin
Department of Obstetrics, Gynecology, and Reproductive Sciences, Mount Sinai School of Medicine, New York, NY, USA

Liane Deligdisch, MD
Professor of Pathology and Obstetrics-Gynecology and Reproductive Science, The Mount Sinai Medical Center and School of Medicine, New York, NY, USA

Philip J. Di Saia, MD
The Dorothy Marsh Chair in Reproductive Biology; Professor, Department of Obstetrics and Gynecology, Division of Gynecologic Oncology University of California – Irvine, CA, USA

Ramez N. Eskander, MD
Clinical Instructor and Fellow, Department of Obstetrics and Gynecology, Division of Gynecologic Oncology, University of California – Irvine, CA, USA

Tamara Finger, MD
Fellow in Minimally Invasive Surgery, Division of Gynecologic Oncology, St Luke's-Roosevelt Hospital Center, New York, NY, USA

David Fishman, MD
Professor of Obstetrics, Gynecology, and Reproductive Science, Mount Sinai School of Medicine, New York, NY, USA

Brooke L. Fridley, PhD
Associate Professor of Biostatistics, Department of Health Sciences Research, Mayo Clinic College of Medicine, Rochester, MN, USA

David M. Gershenson, MD
Department Chair, Department of Gynecologic Oncology, The University of Texas MD Anderson Cancer Center, Houston, TX, USA

Norbert Gleicher, MD, FACOG, FACS
Medical Director and Chief Scientist, Centre for Human Reproduction, New York, NY, USA

Ellen L. Goode, PhD, MPH
Associate Professor of Epidemiology, Department of Health Sciences Research, Mayo Clinic College of Medicine, Rochester, MN, USA

Pierre S. Gordon, MD
Department of Obstetrics and Gynecology, Howard University Hospital, Washington, DC, USA

Ioannis Gryparis, MD
Gynecologist, Piraeus, Greece

Jonathan Hecht, MD, PhD
Associate Professor, Department of Pathology, Harvard Medical School; Associate Professor, Department of Pathology, Brigham and Women's Hospital, Boston, MA, USA

Wendy C. Hsiao, BS
Research Assistant, Partnership for Health Analytic Research, LLC, Beverly Hills, CA, USA

Eric C. Huang, MD, PhD
Division of Women's and Perinatal Pathology, Department of Pathology, Brigham and Women's Hospital, Harvard Medical School, Boston, MA, USA

Nathan G. Kase, MD
Professor in Obstetrics-Gynecology and Reproductive Sciences; Professor of Endocrinology and Dean Emeritus, The Mount Sinai School of Medicine, New York, NY, USA

Valentin Kolev, MD
Adjunct Assistant Clinical Professor, Department of Obstetrics, Gynecology, and Reproductive Sciences, The Mount Sinai School of Medicine, New York, NY, USA

Lale Kostakoglu, MD, MPH
Professor of Radiology, The Mount Sinai Hospital, New York, NY, USA

Neri Laufer, MD
Chairman and Professor, Department of Obstetrics and Gynecology, Hebrew University-Hadassah Medical Center, Ein Kerem, Jerusalem, Israel

Anna Laury, MD
Division of Women's and Perinatal Pathology, Department of Pathology, Brigham and Women's Hospital, Harvard Medical School, Boston, MA, USA

Gerard Mage, MD
Department of Gynecologic Surgery, CHU Clermont Ferrand, France

Angelica Mareş, MD
The Mount Sinai Medical Center and School of Medicine, New York, NY, USA

Maurie Markman, MD
Senior Vice President of Clinical Affairs and National Director for Medical Oncology, Cancer Treatment Centers of America, Eastern Regional Medical Center, Philadelphia, PA, USA

Luciano G. Nardo, MD, MRCOG
Consultant Gynaecologist, Manchester UK; Director, Gynehealth, Conceive International, and GM Imaging

Farr R. Nezhat, MD, FACOG, FACS
Professor of Clinical Obstetrics and Gynecology, Columbia University College of Physicians and Surgeons; Director of Minimally Invasive Surgery and Gynecologic Robotics; Director, MISGR Fellowship Program, Division of Gynecologic Oncology, St Luke's-Roosevelt Hospital Center, New York, NY, USA

Sree Durga Patchava, MD, MRCOG
Krishna Institute of Medical Sciences, Hyderabad, India

Tanja Pejovic, MD, PhD
Division Chief, Gynecologic Oncology, Department of Obstetrics and Gynecology, Oregon Health & Science University, Portland, OR, USA

Catherine M. Phelan, PhD, MD, MMS
Department of Cancer Epidemiology, H. Lee Moffitt Cancer Center & Research Institute, Tampa, FL, USA

Benoit Rabischong, MD
Department of Gynecologic Surgery, CHU Clermont Ferrand, France

Jamal Rahaman, MD, DGO, FACS, FACOG
Associate
Clinical Professor, Department of Obstetrics, Gynecology, and Reproductive Medicine, The Mount Sinai School of Medicine, New York, NY, USA

David Rodriguez-Buritica, MD
Department of Pediatrics, Division of Pediatric Endocrinology, Winthrop University Hospital, Mineola, NY, USA

Paul Saenger, MD
Department of Pediatrics, Division of Pediatric Endocrinology, Winthrop University Hospital, Mineola, NY, USA

Peter Schlosshauer, MD
Medical Director, Gynecor, Bostwick Laboratories, Uniondale, NY, USA

William L. Simpson Jr., MD
Associate Professor of Radiology, Mount Sinai School of Medicine, New York, NY, USA

Cardinale B. Smith, MD, MSCR
Assistant Professor, Division of Hematology/Medical Oncology, Tisch Cancer Institute, Brookdale Department of Geriatrics and Palliative Medicine, Mount Sinai School of Medicine, New York, NY, USA

Jason Sternchos, MD
Fellow in Minimally Invasive Surgery, Division of Gynecologic Oncology, St Luke's-Roosevelt Hospital Center, New York, NY, USA

Preface

The second edition of "Diagnosis and Management of Ovarian Disorders" was published in 2003, inspired by the widely enthusiastic reception of the first edition and the many advances in discovery and altered clinical practice during the 7 years following the publication of the first edition. In keeping with his purpose of providing the most current information, and presenting the views of not only credentialed but authoritative and respected contributors, the late Dr Albert Altchek organized a third edition of this book with his fellow editors. Unfortunately, he was not able to enjoy the final submissions by the selected contributors, and we, the current editors, dedicate this new edition, now entitled *Altchek's Diagnosis and Management of Ovarian Disorders*, to him. We celebrate his long career as a clinician, a curious and imaginative clinical investigator, and an informative and prolific author. We thank him for this, and we miss him.

While not dividing this new edition formally into various sections, we have preserved the approach of inviting experts in the fields of physiology, pathology, and basic science; authorities in the newest diagnostic procedures, and new approaches which translate molecular discovery to applied clinical techniques; and finally experienced clinicians who present contemporary management. While we have encouraged the authors to present data and opinions which are "evidence based," we have also required them to rely on "best evidence." This, of course, will occasionally result in differing templates for clinical management, and we encourage the reader to select from the menu of options when offered, benefitting from international perspectives.

Based on the critical acclaim for the second edition's modernity and contemporary relevance, the third edition (and therefore the reader) profits from the very elegant early chapters describing the remarkable new observations further explaining normal ovarian function, how steroid hormones work, and the subsequent departures from normal resulting in subsequent chapters discussing accidents in embryologic or gene mediated development resulting in clinical syndromes or benign neoplasia, both functional or simply morphologic. Chapters on menopause and the senescent ovary with considerations for management are essential for any clinician dealing with the aging female.

Chapters devoted to pathology discuss the spectrum of transformation from normal presentation to cancer both borderline and virulent, with a full discussion of the origin of "ovarian" cancers, the role of other Mullerian tissues, and the panoply of neoplasms now characterized by systems other than unique histology. The role of endometriosis as an important and prevalent disease in women of all ages, both as a "benign" disorder and as a cancer precursor has been updated with international contributions. All chapters dealing with infertility announce newly modified concepts, including formulas for management.

Finally, there are new chapters on epidemiology of ovarian cancer, risk assessment, screening, early detection, prevention, risk reducing interventions, and the latest techniques using minimally invasive surgery, staging, cytoreduction, chemotherapy, and a new chapter on palliative care.

We have attempted to assemble a readable single volume which can be an easily accessible resource for anyone interested in the marvelous and sometimes mysterious function of the human ovary in all of its states of health and age, with a vetted bibliography. We are most appreciative of the tireless and generous effort of our authors who have responded so well to our challenge. We are also very grateful for the patient, tolerant, and imaginative support of Cambridge University Press, especially represented by Mr. Nicholas Dunton, Senior Commissioning Editor; Mrs. Joanna Chamberlin, Editor, Medicine; and Mrs. Jane Seakins, Assistant Editor/Publishing Assistant, Medicine.

Carmel J. Cohen, MD
Liane Deligdisch, MD
Nathan G. Kase, MD

The normal human ovary part I: reproductive and endocrine functions

Nathan G. Kase, MD

Introduction

The major functions of the human ovary are the development, nurture, and release of a mature oocyte ready for fertilization and successful propagation of the species. In support of these processes, the ovary secretes steroid hormones which stimulate growth and development of organs of reproduction; are critically involved in the elaborate endocrine interchange which directs orderly, repetitive cyclic ovulations; and finally supports successful uterine implantation, placentation, and the corpus luteum-dependent phase of pregnancy. A description of how the ovary and its secretions achieve these reproductive functions is the focus of the first two chapters of this volume.

In addition, it is now clear from observations in prolonged physiologic (menopause) and non-physiologic (gonadal failure) hypogonadal states that ovarian steroid secretions have important influences on a variety of non-reproductive organ systems which determine the quality of life and the life expectancy of women. A more complete treatment of these issues is dealt with in Chapter 2, How Steroid Hormones Work, and Chapter 20, Menopause.

General principles

The physiologic responsibilities of the ovary are the periodic release of gametes (oocytes) and the timely sequential secretion of the hormones estradiol (E2), progesterone (P), and the inhibins A and B. These endocrine signals integrate the hypothalamus, anterior pituitary, and ovaries in a continuous repetitive process of follicle recruitment, rescue, maturation, selection, ovulation, corpus luteum formation, function, and regression. But the ovary cannot be viewed as a static, purely endocrine organ whose size and function waxes and wanes, depending on the stimulatory input of tropic hormones. Rather, the female gonad is a heterogeneous, constantly changing organ with cyclicity measured in days and weeks, with each phase governed by a specific anatomic subunit. The ovary is an envelope, the function of which in any month in adult menstrual life is defined by a single dominant follicle, and after ovulation its transformation into a corpus luteum (Fig. 1.1) [1,2].

Gonadotropin (endocrine) and follicle-dependent (intracrine) factors determine follicle "destiny"

The fate of each follicle is controlled by endocrine as well as intra-follicular factors (Fig. 1.2) [3,4]. In the human, regulation of the continuous process of activation and preliminary growth up to the small antral stage occurs independently of gonadotropin stimulation. Only at advanced antral stages do follicles unequivocally become dependent on follicle-stimulating hormone (FSH) for avoidance of apoptosis (atresia) and receipt of the impetus to further development. Whereas initial recruitment is cycle- and gonadotropin-independent, rescue and further development (cyclic recruitment) depends on the increase in circulating FSH during the transitional and early follicle phases of the menstrual cycle.

In simplest form, the development of follicles is divided into gonadotropin-independent (from gonadogenesis to pubescence), gonadotropin-"sensitive" (pubertal transition), and gonadotropin-dependent stages (adulthood). Gonadotropin involvement in adult follicle development can be refined further into gonadotropin and intra-follicular *survival factor* (antiatretic) dependence and gonadotropin plus intra-follicle *growth factor* follicle responsive (dominant follicle selection) stages. The lead follicle is selected from the rescued cohort of antral follicles by a combination of extrinsic (endocrine) and intrinsic (autocrine, paracrine) mechanisms. For example, by secreting increasingly high levels of estradiol and inhibin B, the selected follicle suppresses FSH availability. The result is a negative selection influence on the remaining follicle cohort, which lapse into atresia due to diminished availability of anti-apoptotic FSH. On the other hand, through intrinsic processes such as increased FSH receptors, local growth factors, and thecal vascular enhancement, the lead follicle maximizes usage of dwindling FSH, which fosters not only survival/positive selection, but stimulation of further growth, differentiation, and ultimately, ovulation [1,3,4].

The complex intra-ovarian mechanisms (intra-follicle), which in concert with systemic endocrine signals coordinate the "life cycle" of the follicle from formation to dominant follicle, ovulation, and corpus luteum function has been

Altchek's Diagnosis and Management of Ovarian Disorders, ed. Liane Deligdisch, Nathan G. Kase, and Carmel J. Cohen. Published by Cambridge University Press.

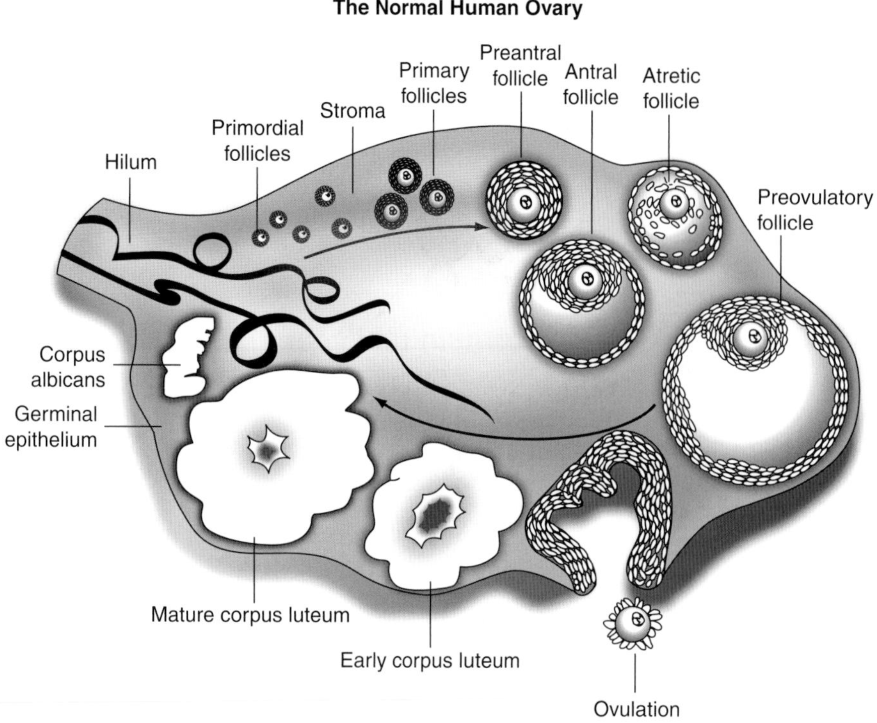

Fig. 1.1. The ovary is a heterogeneous constantly changing organ. Each phase of its function is governed by the development, differentiation and activity of a single specific anatomic subunit, either the dominant follicle or its post-ovulatory transmutation to the corpus luteum. These represent the end stage results of folliculogenesis beginning with emergence from a resting pool of primordial follicles, follicle recruitment, selection (rescue or atresia) and finally the dominant Graafian follicle.

intensively investigated. In particular, the intrinsic factors responsible for gonadal gender specification, maintenance, and nurture of the arrested follicle (somatic cells and oocytes), emergence from arrest and pre-FSH-dependent growth and differentiation (from primordial to preantral stages) are now better understood [5]. A plethora of growth factors, many belonging to the transforming growth factor-beta (TGF-β) superfamily, are expressed by ovarian somatic cells (granulosa and theca) as well as the germ cell (oocyte) in a developmental stage-related manner. Each element functions as intrafollicular integrators and regulators of folliculogenesis. As will be described, progression through successive stages of follicle development requires the continued bidirectional communication between oocyte and granulosa cells and granulosa and theca cells. Cross-talk between these intrafollicle constituents is conducted by cell-specific factors throughout the biologic "life" of the ovary, which in adult cyclic stages of follicle development interact with and are dependent on appropriately timed endocrine (gonadotropin) and metabolic input. In summary, coordination and control by both intrinsic and extrinsic elements determine the ultimate "destiny" of the follicle.

The ovarian processes that develop, store, protect, and support follicle "readiness" throughout life and the timely stimulatory events that yield an oocyte for fertilization involve practically every regulatory mechanism in human biology. These include classic endocrine signals, intracrine, autocrine, paracrine regulation, possibly neuronal input, and immune system contributions. With the single exception of FSH, none of these systems alone is sufficient to achieve reproduction competence by final growth and ovulation. Rather, these should be looked upon as participants in a collective, synergistic mutually facilitating response mechanism, which prepare for and maximize FSH and luteinizing hormone (LH) instructions (Fig. 1.3) [6].

These interactive mechanisms will be reviewed in detail in this chapter. The discussion will be organized in this sequence: (1) the molecular "players," (2) gonadal formation and folliculogenesis, (3) follicle development from arrest to pubescence and initiation of cyclic ovarian function, (4) antral follicle "selection" and ovulation, (5) the corpus luteum phase, and (6) the transitional (inter-cycle) phase.

"The molecular players": extrinsic and intrinsic factors in ovarian cycle functions

In the classic view, ovarian follicle development is regulated by the hypothalamic–pituitary–ovarian (H-P-O) axis, in which gonadotropin-releasing hormone (GnRH) controls the release of the gonadotropic hormones FSH and luteinizing hormone (LH), and that ovarian steroids exert both negative and positive regulatory effects on GnRH secretion [1,2,4]. While these endocrine aspects remain essentially accurate, intrinsic factors are now viewed as solely responsible for follicle development up to the preantral stage when some FSH sensitivity appears. Thereafter, intrinsic factors act to enhance, modify, and/or inhibit gonadotropin instructions [5].

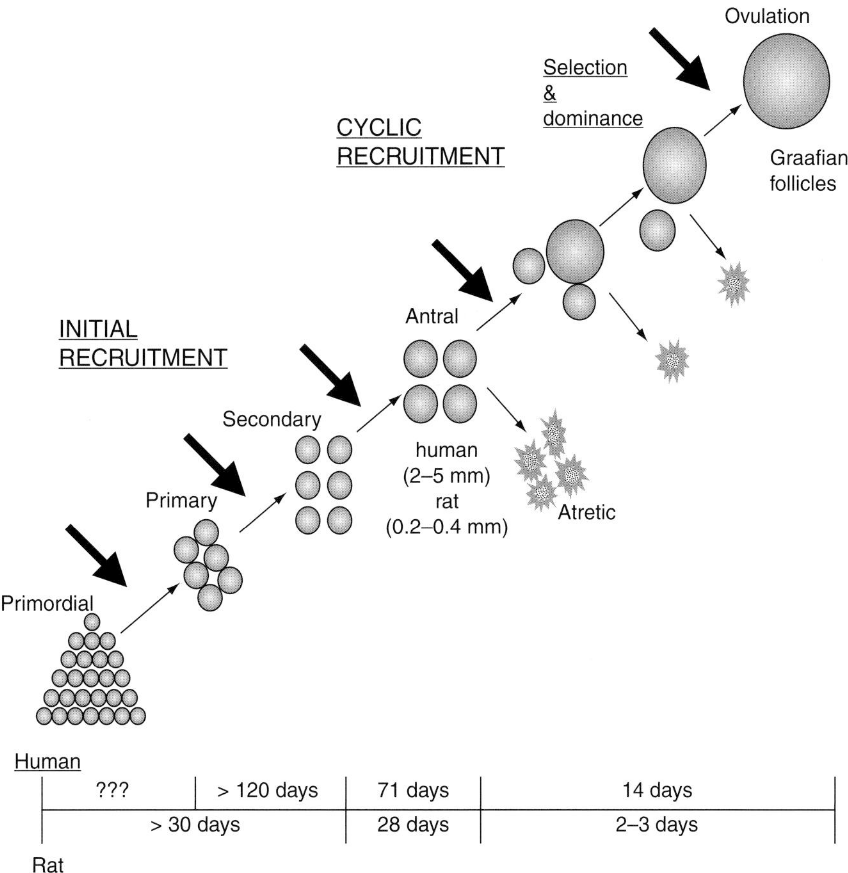

Fig. 1.2. The estimated "timelines" of activation of primordial follicle pool through initial recruitment, cyclic recruitment, selection, dominance and ovulation. Note loss (atresia) of follicle number at each stage of progression.

Consideration of the microenvironment factors and events involved in the control and promotion of follicle function begins with a review of the properties of the individual classes of molecules involved and their functional interactions.

Whereas in the classic endocrine pathways regulatory molecules (hormones) are secreted into the blood stream and transported to distant target tissues whose function they modify, at least three modes of local action are understood.

1. *Paracrine* modality: Regulatory molecules are secreted by one cell and influence functions of contiguous neighboring cells by means of gap junction connecting channels or interaction with cognate receptors
2. *Autocrine* modality: A cell regulates its own function by secreting factors which then interact with receptors on its own plasma membrane
3. *Intracrine* (or ultracrine) modality: A cell regulates its own function without secretion. Rather, unsecreted factors bind with intracellular receptors or participate in other modulating mechanisms, such as inclusion in transcriptomes or signalsomes.

The major "intrinsic" follicle regulators (Fig. 1.3)

The TGF-β superfamily

The TGF-β superfamily represents a functionally diverse group of proteins with at least 35 members in vertebrates; these proteins are widely distributed throughout the body and function as extracellular ligands involved in numerous physiological processes during both pre- and postnatal life (for superb reviews of this material on which much of the following has been drawn, see [2,5]). On the basis of structural characteristics, members of the superfamily have been classified into at least six groups:

1. The prototypic TGF-β subfamily
2. An extensive bone morphogenetic protein (BMP) subfamily
3. Growth and differentiation factor (GDF) subfamily
4. Activin/inhibin subfamily
5. Glial cell-derived, neurotrophic factor (GDNF) subfamily
6. As well as several additional members such as the emerging importance of anti-Mullerian hormone (AMH).

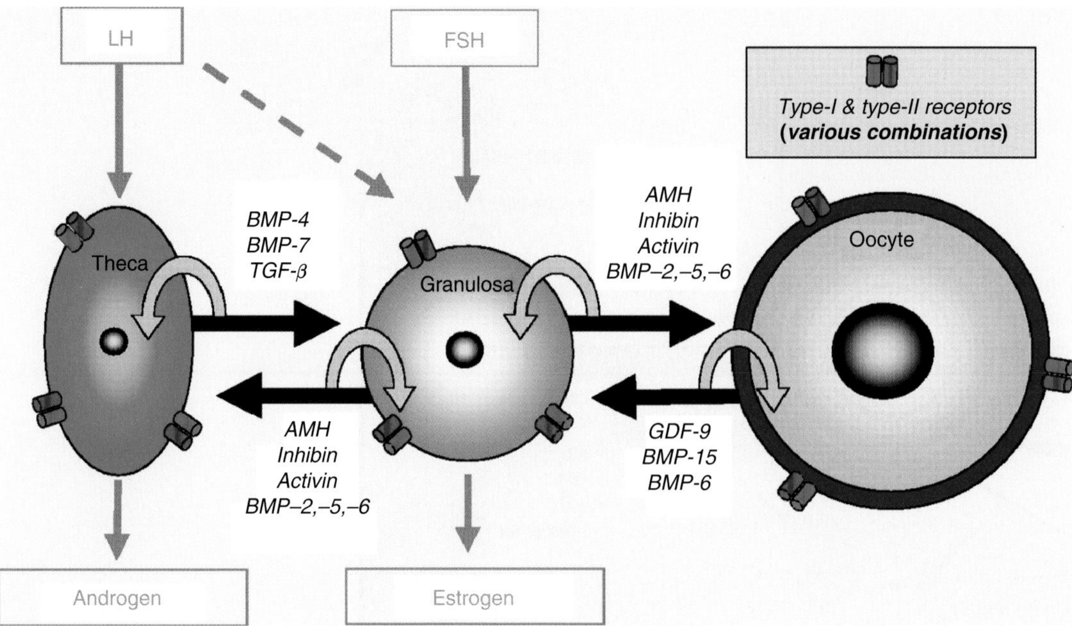

Fig. 1.3. Intercellular communication in the mammalian follicle. Bi-directional communication among oocyte and its companion somatic cells – the granulosa and theca. Note the interactions depicted involve autocrine and paracrine messages by members of the TGF-β superfamily proteins and their gonadotropin independent and dependent functions essential to follicle development, readiness for ovulation and endocrine secretory output. AMH, anti-Mullerian hormone; BMP, bone morphogenic protein; GD, growth differentiation factor. Reproduced from reference [5], with permission.

Intra-ovarian roles of TGF-β superfamily members

Studies in several mammalian species, principally rodents, indicate that several ligands, receptors, signaling intermediaries, and binding proteins associated with the TGF-β superfamily are expressed by oocytes and ovarian somatic cells in a developmental stage-related manner [7]. These play key roles in multiple aspects of follicle recruitment, granulosa and theca cell proliferation, steroidogenesis, gonadotropin receptor expression, oocyte maturation, ovulation, luteinization, and corpus luteum (CL) formation. In short, these elements function not solely in follicle development but throughout the entire lifespan of the follicle.

Although all known elements involved in the stepwise progression of follicle genesis, development, and function will be dealt with in detail in subsequent sections, a preliminary overview of the functions of prominent intrinsic factors will set the stage for the comprehensive analysis that is the text of this chapter.

Anti-Mullerian hormone

A member of the TGF-β superfamily, AMH is perhaps better known as the Sertoli cell secretion of the embryonic testes which causes regression of the Mullerian ducts during male internal genitalia differentiation [8]. However, it is detected in the granulosa cells of early primordial follicles and reaches peak concentrations in small antral follicles apparently up-regulated by growth differentiation factor-9 (GDF-9) and bone morphogenetic protein-15 (BMP-15) secreted by the maturing oocyte. AMH concentrations decrease as FSH induces further follicle development and estrogen production increases. AMH null mice display increased recruitment of primordial follicles into the growing pool, defining AMH as an inhibitor of FSH-independent follicle recruitment. AMH also indirectly inhibits FSH-dependent stages of follicle growth by suppressing growth of lesser follicles in the recruited cohort thereby preserving the major impact of dwindling FSH for stimulation of the emerging dominant follicle. As AMH levels are not affected by gonadotropins or gonadal steroid concentrations, measurement of AMH is a reliable reflection of the number of growing follicles at any point in the menstrual cycle. As such, AMH has emerged as a clinically useful marker of follicle status during ovulation induction regimens, the prognosis for current fertility, possibly an indicator of oocyte "quality" and of ovarian aging [9].

Inhibin/activin system

This system provides three critically important intrinsic as well as extrinsic endocrine functions in human reproduction [10]. As endocrine signals inhibin B secretion from the selected follicle inhibits FSH secretion. Inhibin A, produced in the luteinized granulosa of the corpus luteum, joins estradiol and progesterone in the negative feedback suppression of both LH and FSH in the luteal phase. On the other hand, the inhibin/activin system adds critical local intracrine activities in the control of H-P-O function

- The anterior pituitary gonadotrope cell release of FSH and LH: inhibin B inhibits FSH secretion not

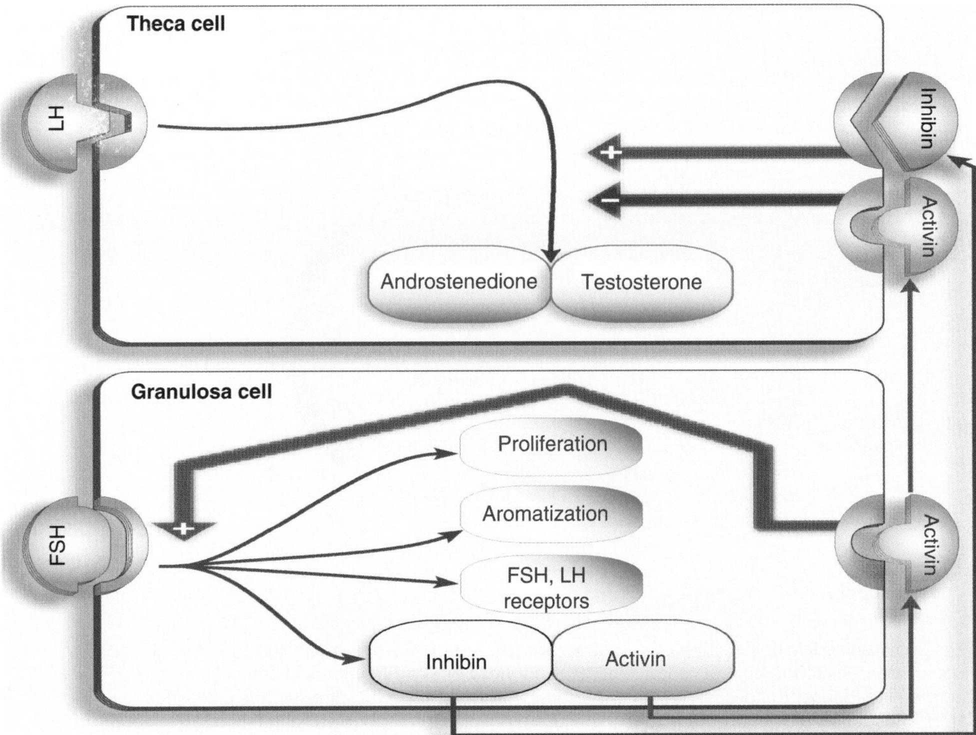

Fig. 1.4. The intrinsic function of the inhibin/activin system in early phase follicle development. Note both factors are generated in the granulosa in response to FSH but are transferred to the theca to balance LH-induced androgen synthesis. In addition, granulosa activin augments FSH action those cells to induce further proliferation, enhance aromatase function and add FSH receptors to the membrane (as well as LHR later in the cycle).

only by endocrine feedback but by local inhibition of GnRH synthesis and secretion of FSH at the gonadotrope cell. On the other hand, inhibin B increases LH by increasing GnRH receptor numbers. Local activin augments secretion of FSH by a similar process but is limited by binding to its inhibitor follistatin.

- The ovarian follicle granulosa cell: activins increase FSH receptor number and function of granulosa cells (aromatase, cell growth, and proliferation), limit thecal cell androgen production, advance oocyte maturation and growth, and possibly increase the number of surviving primordial follicles [11].
- The ovarian follicle granulosa cell inhibins: in preantral and antral follicles, inhibins increase LH-stimulated thecal cell androgen synthesis and possibly enhance AMH suppression of primary follicle generation [12]
- Both inhibins and activins enhance oocyte maturation and fertilizability [13].

Integration of the activin/inhibin system in follicle development (Fig. 1.4)

FSH stimulates inhibin and activin production by granulosa cells [1 (pp. 210–12)]. In autocrine mode, activin increases the functional impact of FSH by accelerating granulosa cell proliferation and aromatase capacity by up-regulation of FSH receptors in these cells. Granulosa cell inhibin, in paracrine mode, augments theca cell androgen synthesis, whereas activin modifies that stimulation. As follicle maturation progresses, granulosa cell inhibin B continues to stimulate androgen synthesis in the theca cell insuring adequate substrate for the granulosa cell aromatase system to support two essential endocrine functions of E2: (1) sufficient E2 coupled with secreted inhibin B join as negative feedback signals to inhibit pituitary FSH secretion, and (2) later in the cycle, E2 signals the LH mid-cycle surge. Activin, while continuing to exert its important modulating control of androgen synthesis in the theca, prepares the granulosa cell for luteal phase function by assisting FSH in the induction of LH receptors on these cells. At the same time, as the putative luteinizing inhibiting factor (LI), activin limits the synthesis of progesterone in the pre-ovulatory ovary by inhibiting premature luteinization (Fig. 1.5). Finally, and in a crucial step in selection of the dominant follicle, activin stimulates further induction of FSH receptors in granulosa cells, thereby maximizing the dominant follicle's capacity to survive and continue to flourish, despite the dwindling supply of FSH (endocrine inhibin induced). Inhibin A levels rise in the late follicular phase (as LH receptors appear), reaching peak levels in the mid-luteal phase. The addition of inhibin A to progesterone and estrogen contributes to the marked sustained reduction in gonadotropin during this phase of the cycle.

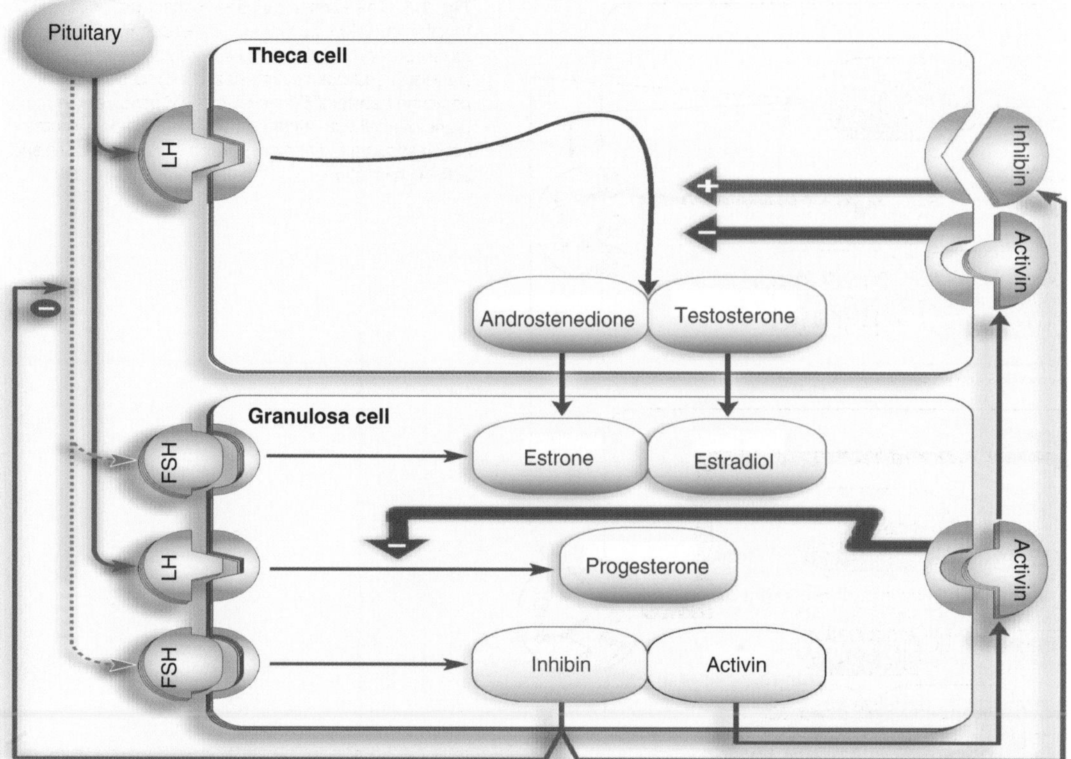

Fig. 1.5. In the late follicle pre-ovulatory phase, LH receptors appear on the granulosa (induced by intra-follicle progesterone). However, activin restrains progesterone synthesis, avoiding premature luteinization. Inhibin, now produced in increased amounts becomes an endocrine negative feedback influence on FSH, thereby avoiding supernumerary ovulation. The increased FSH receptor concentration on granulosa and the increase estradiol production leads to positive feedback on LH release.

Growth factors

Growth factors involved in follicle function include epidermal growth factor (EGF), fibroblast growth factor (FGF), various angiogenic factors such as vascular endothelial growth factor (VEGF), all of which participate in follicle and corpus luteum function. Similarly cytokines, including the interleukin-1 system, tumor necrosis factor-α (TNFα), and endothelin 1 (ET-1) are also involved. Each particular contribution of all these factors will be noted in specific portions of the text. However, certain growth factor contributions are so critical to the overall process that emphasis will be made here as well as in their specific contextual involvement.

Insulin-like growth factors (IGF-1 and IGF-2)

Formerly called somatomedins, IGF-1 and IGF-2 are peptides that have structural and functional similarity to insulin and in the case of IGF-1 mediate growth hormone (GH) action [14,15]. The majority of circulating IGF-1 is synthesized and secreted by the liver in response to GH. However, IGF-1 can be made in many tissues in response to factors other than GH and has important autocrine/paracrine activities. IGF-2 is the major IGF in the ovary and has little GH dependence. Like IGF-1, it works locally to modulate cell proliferation and differentiation.

The intrinsic IGF system in follicle development and function

Studies in human ovarian tissue demonstrate that, while both IGF-1 and IGF-2 are active, IGF-2 becomes disproportionally increased as follicle maturation proceeds (Fig. 1.6) [1 (pp. 216–19)]. Nevertheless, both stimulate DNA synthesis, steroidogenesis, aromatase activity, LH receptor synthesis, and inhibin secretion. Arising in the theca, these actions are seen in both theca cells (autocrine) and granulosa cells by paracrine signaling.

IGF-2 stimulates granulosa cell proliferation, aromatase activity, and progesterone synthesis in the human follicle and corpus luteum. In the early proliferative phase, IGF-2 is produced in the theca in response to LH. IGF-2 acts in an autocrine mode through its receptor and augments the LH-induced steroidogenesis of testosterone and androstenedione in theca cells. Furthermore, now acting in paracrine mode on granulosa cells, IGF-2 in synergy with estradiol augments FSH-directed cell proliferation, aromatase availability, and synthesis of inhibin and activin. In the pre-ovulatory follicle, when LH receptors are now present and active on the granulosa cell, thecal IGF-2 accelerates granulosa cell proliferation and assists LH in the initiation of progesterone synthesis, a property that continues into the corpus luteum phase. IGF-2 therefore is active in both stimulation of synthesis and

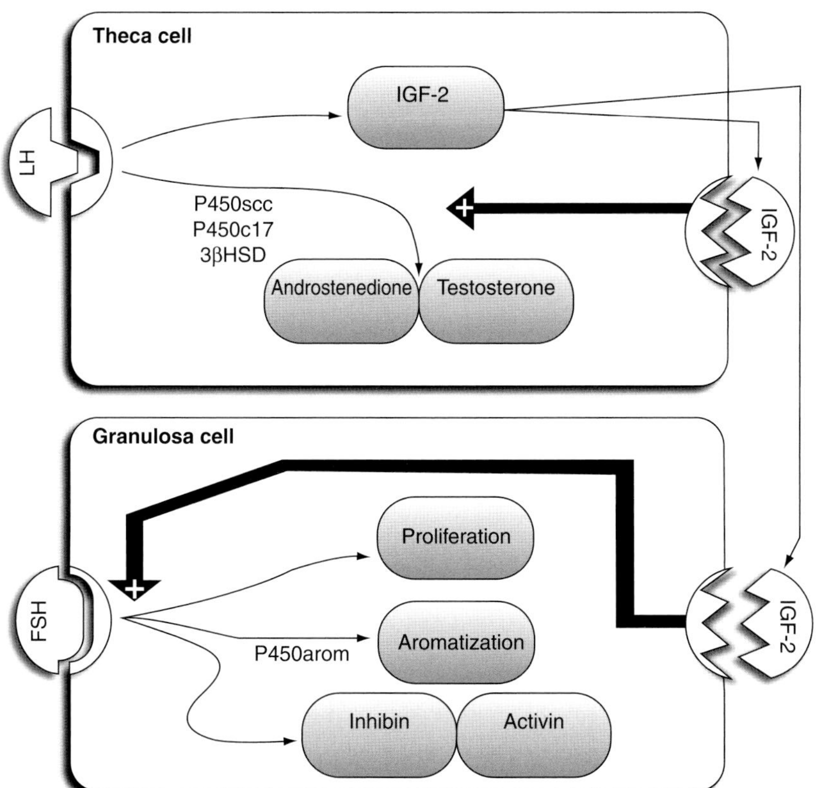

Fig. 1.6. The intrinsic function of the IGF-2 in follicle function and development. In response to LH by means of its receptor on the theca cell IGF-2 by autocrine action stimulates androgen synthesis and production. By paracrine transfer IGF-2 enhances FSH action at the granulosa cell with increased cell proliferation, aromatase action and in a bidirectional dialog, increases inhibin and activin production.

secretion of both estradiol in the follicle and progesterone in the corpus luteum.

Although IGF-2 is the primary ligand, both IGF-1 and IGF-2 receptors exist and IGF-2 activates both receptors. Of clinical interest, human theca cells encode receptors for insulin, opening the possibility that systemic metabolic syndrome-associated insulin resistance and reactive hyperinsulinemia could induce excess thecal androgen with adverse local ovarian inhibition and systemic hyperandrogenicity.

IGF, like E2, serves a major facilitatory but not sufficient function in follicle dynamics. That successful induction of ovulation in IGF-1–deficient women can be accomplished with exogenous human menopausal gonadotropin HMG/HCG therapy confirms the IGF system acts in a facilitatory supportive role in follicle maturation and emphasizes, as in enzymatic impaired hypoestrogenism, the genetic survival pressure to equip the follicle with multiple enhancing but not uniquely essential systems to achieve ovulation [16].

Steroids

Estradiol

Although the pivotal stimulatory role of estradiol in granulosa cell growth and differentiation in the rodent depicted prominently in the "two-cell" theory of follicle function is unquestioned, some observations in the primate have cast doubt on whether estradiol is a participant, let alone required, for *human intra-ovarian processes* involved in folliculogenesis, oocyte maturation, and ovulation [17,18]. While its *endocrine* role in the HPO axis is undisputed, lessons learned from successful exogenous gonadotropin induction of follicle enlargement (antral expansion), retrievable and fertilizable oocytes, as well as with cleavable and apparently transferable embryos in women with markedly reduced to non-existent intra-follicular and circulating concentrations of estradiol are the basis for this uncertainty. These clinical demonstrations include profoundly hypogonadotropic women or those treated with GnRH agonist gonadotropin suppression as well as women with steroid synthesis abnormalities, such as 3β-hydroxysteroid dehydrogenase deficiency, aromatase deficiency, and in particular 17α hydroxylase/17,20-lyase deficiency [19–21].

On the other hand, studies on the human fetal ovary by Fowler et al. [18] have materially strengthened the critical importance of intrafollicular estradiol in humans:

- The capacity of granulosa cells to synthesize E2 is well known, but it is now evident that the oocyte also produces estradiol.
- The human oocyte possesses demonstrable ER-β subtype expression and immuno-histochemical presence establishing intracrine E2-ER-β activity.
- Direct estrogen impact by means of granulosa–oocyte gap junction interchange exists. Similarly non-genomic membrane-mediated estrogen may also play an important role in oocyte biology.

- Human granulosa cells possess E receptors. Both reception and activity are induced by estrogen in the human ovary and represent the net impact generated by the relative contributions of these receptors at both the nuclear and "non-classical" non-genomic level (Tables 1.1 and 1.2).
- As shown in several primate studies, an estrogen free/poor follicle is associated with decrements in the rates of meiotic maturation and fertilization efficiency.

Taken together, the human fetal ovary expresses the machinery to produce, detect, and respond to estrogenic, progestogenic, and androgenic signaling. Furthermore, E2 is required for human follicle generation with the oocyte not only expressing ERβ but the ability to generate E2 acting as a key component of the process.

In summary, while intra-follicular estradiol alone may not be absolutely sufficient, it plays a significant contributory role in ovarian development, selection of the dominant follicle, and an essential role in oocyte maturation. In this regard, the importance of non-classical modes of hormone action should be emphasized. In addition to nongenomic mechanisms, ligand-independent steroid receptor activation by signaling pathways stimulated by growth factors such as EGF and IGF-2 should be considered in the rare clinical demonstrations of ovulatory capacity in follicles equipped with estrogen receptors but without significant presence of the provocative ligand estradiol.

Finally, the crucial importance of estradiol as an endocrine signal expressing dominant follicle readiness and instructing synthesis and release of the LH surge remains an uncontroversial and axiomatic element of the human H-P-O system.

Progesterone

Although not active in human follicle genesis, differentiation, or development, and is best known for its function in the luteal phase as will be seen later in this chapter, progesterone has important endocrine and intraovarian functions at ovulation. These include oocyte maturation (meiosis I completion), and the mechanisms leading to follicle rupture and oocyte release [22].

Table 1.1. The genes and signaling pathways which are involved in the formation of germ cells, follicle assembly, and follicle activation

Gene product/role	Role	Function
PGC formation		
BMP-2 (bone morphogenetic protein-2)	TGF-β member; extra-cellular growth factor	PGC formation
BMP-4 (bone morphogenetic protein-4)	TGF-β member; extra-cellular growth factor	PGC formation
BMP-8B (bone morphogenetic protein-8b)	TGF-β member, extra-cellular growth factor	PGC formation
Fragilis	An interferon-inducible system	Germ cell competence
Stella	A protein with a SAP-like domain and a splicing factor motif-like structure	Retention of germ cell fate and pluripotency
Smad-l	Signaling molecule of TGF-β ligands	PGC formation
Smad-5	Signaling molecule of TGF-β ligands	PGC formation
Nanos3	RNA-binding zinc-finger protein	Maintenance of germ cell lineage during migration
Blimp l (Prdm l)	A transcriptional repressor	PGC formation
Prdm l 4	A transcriptional regulator	PGC formation
TIAR	A RNA recognition motif/ ribonucleoprotein-type RNA-binding protein	PGC formation
Pog	Unknown	PGC proliferation
Stra8	Cytoplasmic factor	Premeiotic DNA synthesis and meiotic progression
W (c-Kit receptor) and steel (KL)	Tyrosine kinase receptor growth factor	PGC migration and proliferation
LIF	A cytokine with pleiotropic actions	PGC proliferation

PGC, primordial germ cells.

Conclusion: intrinsic factors at work

Whereas the catalog of the genes and signaling pathways involved in the formation of germ cells, specification of ovarian development, follicle assembly, and follicle activation (Tables 1.1, 1.2) [2] is a comprehensive listing of the "cast of characters" involved, it does little justice to the "plot," the essential interplay, multidirectional dialogue by which these elements modulate gonadal development and function leading to nothing less than reproduction and preservation of the species. The complex cross-talk linking the several intra-ovarian signaling systems and control (check and balance) mechanisms, although not exclusive, is best demonstrated in Figure 1.3, which displays the particular actions of the TGF-β superfamily of ligands and receptors in these processes. These intra-follicular factors working in concert with systemic signals (LH and FSH), the timely availability of which is directed in large measure by steroid and peptide feedback signals, coordinates follicle recruitment and progression. Obvious overlap and redundancy in these systems exists in that several locally produced ligands share responsibility for eliciting similar target responses. Receptor "promiscuity" further ensures functional competence. This redundancy of effects creates a system of checks and balances: limitation of the number of dominant follicles that ovulate (corresponding to the reproductive "limitations" in the capacity of the human female uterus and breasts), preservation of ovarian follicle reserves (prevention of premature ovarian failure), modulating the crucial balance of androgen substrate and aromatase capacity, and follicle readiness for ovulation. Finally, not shown in these graphics (but detailed later in the text) are mechanisms to protect and nurture oocytes during their long period of dormancy.

Table 1.2. The genes and signaling pathways involved in primordial follicle formation and activation

Gene product/role	Transcription factor	Primordial follicle formation pellucid genes
Notch	Signaling pathway	Primordial follicle formation
Daz la	Cytoplasmic protein	Primordial follicle formation
Nerve growth factor	Growth factor	Primordial follicle formation
SPO I I (sporulation protein homology)	Meiotic proteins	Primordial follicle formation
DMCI [disrupted meiotic cDNA I homolog (human)]	Meiotic proteins	Primordial follicle formation
MSH5 [mutS homolog 5 (*Escherichia coli*)]	Meiotic proteins	Primordial follicle formation
Zfx	Zinc-finger protein	Primordial follicle formation; oocyte survival and proliferation
ATM	A member of the phosphatidylinositol 3-kinase-like kinases	Meiotic recombination; mitotic cell cycle regulator kinase DNA damage-induced mitotic cell-cycle checkpoints
Nobox	An oocyte-specific homeobox gene	Follicles are replaced by fibrous tissue in female mice lacking nobox; survival factor for primordial follicles; also transition of primordial follicles to primary stage is abolished
Foxo3	Forkhead transcription factor	Primordial follicle activation Foxo3a$^{-/-}$ female mice exhibit global follicular activation leading to oocyte death, early depletion of functional ovarian follicles, and secondary infertility
AMH	TGF-β member	There is an increased recruitment of primordial follicles into growing pool in AMH null mice suggesting a negative effect of AMH on primordial–to–primary follicle transition; a hormonal marker of ovarian reserve used at clinical settings
PTEN-PI3K	PTEN, tumor suppressor, a major negative regulator of phosphatidylinositol 3-kinase	In mice lacking PTEN the entire primordial follicle pool becomes activated and all primordial follicles become depleted in early adulthood, causing POF Germline mutations in *PTEN* cause Cowden disease, a rare autosomal dominant syndrome characterized by multiple hamartomas of the skin, intestine, breast, and thyroid and with increased risk of breast, uterus, thyroid, or brain tumors
Tsc/mTORCI signaling	Tumor suppressor Tscl	Negatively regulates mammalian target of rapamycin complex I (mTORCI), and keeps primordial follicles quiescent; in mutant mice lacking Tscl in oocytes, the entire pool of primordial follicles is activated prematurely due to elevated MTORCI activity in the oocytes, ending up with follicular depletion in early adulthood and causing POF
p27	Cyclin-dependent kinase inhibitor IB [commonly known as p267(kipl)]	Premature activation of the primordial follicle pool initiated by oocyte growth and proliferation and differentiation of pregranulosa cells; early follicular growth depletion and POF.
Fox12	Winged-helix transcription factor	Premature growth of oocytes: arrested proliferation and differentiation of pregranulosa cells; lack of primary follicles

Extrinsic factors (Fig. 1.7)

In its simplest formulation, the classic view of ovarian follicle development is dependent on a tightly controlled interactive endocrine reciprocal servomechanism called the hypothalamic–pituitary–ovarian "axis" (H-P-O): Gonadotropin-releasing hormone (GnRH) controls the release of the gonadotropic hormones follicle-stimulating hormone (FSH) and luteinizing hormone (LH), and in response to that stimulation, secreted ovarian steroids exert both negative and positive regulatory effects on GnRH and gonadotropin secretion. It now appears that the H-P-O cascade and the systems which regulate it are more complicated: it involves additional internal and higher central nervous system (CNS) center controlling input imagined but undefined in the original concept. New modulating systems, such as the Kisspeptin-GPR54 system modulation of GnRH neurons and GnRH pulse generation have expanded the understanding of how environmental factors, internal and external, can influence basic reproductive physiology.

The Kisspeptin/GPR54 (KISS1 receptor) system

Kisspeptins are a family of peptides encoded by the *KISS1* gene that bind to the G protein coupled membrane receptor GPR54 (now named KISS1 receptor) on the cell membranes of hypothalamic GnRH neurons [23]. They have emerged as essential neuropeptide regulators of reproductive maturation and function, including puberty onset, neuroendocrine control of ovulation, and metabolic regulation of fertility [23,24]. Mapping of Kisspeptin neurons in rodents has identified two populations located in the arcuate (ARC) and anteroventral periventricular (AVPV) nuclei of the hypothalamus. Efferent projections from these nuclei connect both directly to GnRH neurons as

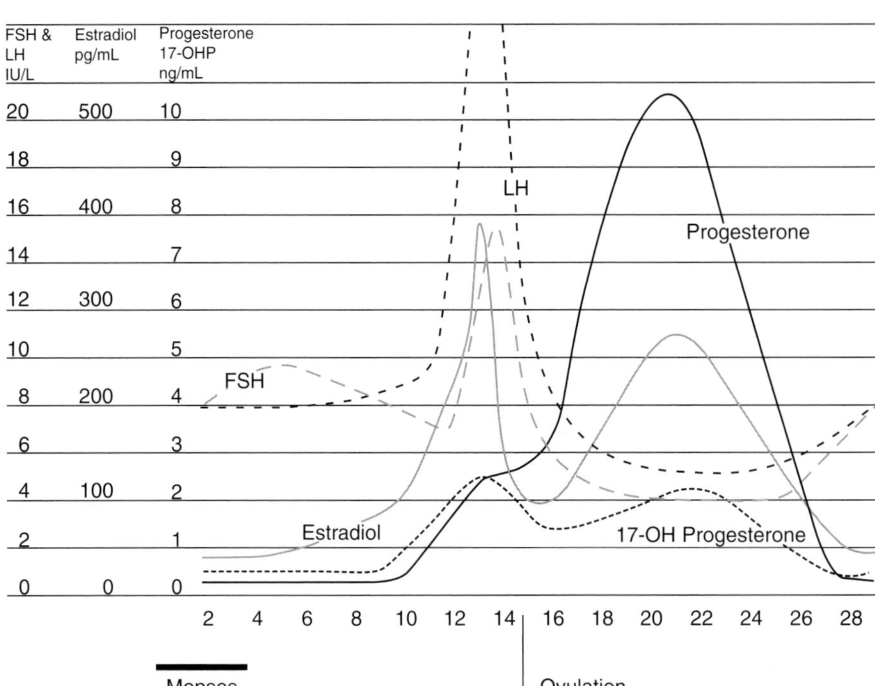

Fig. 1.7. Depiction of the integration of peptide-steroid hormone endocrine signaling interactions during an ovulatory human menstrual cycle.

well as indirectly by means of trans-synaptic connections. The GnRH releasing effect of Kisspeptin-KISS-1R involves activation of phospholipase-C (PLC), mobilization of intracellular Ca^{2+}, and recruitment of ERK 1–2 and P38 kinases. Membrane depolarization occurs by activation of cation and inhibition of potassium channels. Unlike gonadotropin activity, it is independent of adenylcyclase/cAMP pathways. The combined effect is synthesis of GnRH peptide as well as GnRH release [25].

The rodent AVPV neurons are responsive to positive feedback effects of estradiol in the generation of the preovulatory LH surge, whereas ARC conveys the tonic suppressive effects of sex steroids on gonadotropin release [26]. Thus far in primates (including humans), only inhibitory responses have been documented in ARC neurons; how Kisspeptin is involved in positive feedback has not been determined. In addition to the KISS1 system's putative role in ovulatory cyclicity and in the initiation of puberty (in itself an intriguing story of pubescent accumulation of fat stores, i.e., adequate energy sufficient to sustain pregnancy as signaled by the adipokine leptin to induce Kisspeptin-GPCR-GnRH activation and puberty) – information on higher center CNS regulation of hypothalamic Kisspeptin neurons has emerged. These include photoperiod adjustments (melatonin), stress reactivity (the opiate system, corticotrophin releasing hormone [CRH], vasopressin), and nutritional status (neuropeptide Y and IGF-1). In sum, although still fragmentary, the kisspeptin/KISS-1R system emerges as more than the putative initiator of puberty. Rather, it appears to have the potential to be the central regulator of reproductive function by integrating the internal and external signals relevant to reproduction. As such, it represents a "final common pathway" by which normal adult gonadal physiology is sustained but may be modified by stress and adverse energy balance.

Gonadotropin-releasing hormone (GnRH)

The sine qua non-factor in the maintenance and function of the HPO system is GnRH [27]. This peptide is synthesized by hypothalamic neurons located in the medio-basal hypothalamic pre-optic area and arcuate nucleus. Throughout the entire ovarian cycle, "appropriate" stimulation of gonadotropin release from anterior pituitary gonadotrope cells is achieved by pulsatile release of GnRH from these neurons [28]. How these pulses are organized and controlled is complex, multifactorial, but not totally resolved. While the Kisspeptin-GPR54 (KISS1R) system in rodents provides a basis for the positive and negative feedback controls of cyclic gonadotropin availability, it cannot explain the cycle-sensitive discrete bursts of GnRH release underlying the functional concept of the presence of a "GnRH pulse generator."

By the same token, the modification of pulse generation by positive and/or negative input from catecholamines, opiates, neuropeptide Y, CRH, or prolactin, although often dramatically suppressive, cannot account for the exquisite cycle related pulse and amplitude patterning of GnRH release. Congenital GnRH deficiency (idiopathic hypothalamic hypogonadism) caused by mutations in the GPR54 gene suggests two potential mechanisms for GnRH pulse profiles. First, as the GTPα subunit activates other messengers, adenylate cyclase or ion channels, intrinsic GTPase activity quickly hydrolyzes the GTPα to GDPα with reassociation of G protein subunits and return to inactivity. In addition to the stimulatory GPα, the presence of a GPiα inhibitory protein may be another albeit imperfect explanation for intermittent stimulating/inhibiting signals [1 (pp. 100–3)].

The control of GnRH pulses on gonadotropin release has been documented by frequent blood sampling in many experimental models and by GnRH pump induction of ovulation and recovery of gonadal function in GnRH-deficient anosmic individuals. Using long-acting GnRH derivative agonists an initial transient agonist rise in gonadotropin is followed by a dramatic and prolonged hypogonadal state, GnRH receptor desensitization, and elimination of gonadotropin release. Primate experiments using a calibrated pump to administer GnRH pulses determined that 1 μg GnRH per minute X6 pulses each hour yields a 2 ng GnRH portal vein concentration. For induction of ovulation in hypogonadotropic hypogonadal women, GnRH pump pulses administered at 2–5 μg every 60–90 minutes induces ovulation [29] [1 (pp. 166–9)].

Estradiol and the combination of estradiol and progesterone appear to alter GnRH pulse frequencies as the ovarian cycle evolves [30,31]. Using LH pulse as a surrogate marker of GnRH secretion, while pulse amplitude varies little over the follicular phase, pulse frequency rate increases to a maximum of an hourly peak during the ovulatory phase. In the luteal phase, however, LH pulses occur at intervals as long as 200 minutes apart. Of interest, the excess frequency of GnRH pulses induced by the combined feedback of elevated testosterone and insulin seen in anovulatory polycystic ovary syndrome (PCOS) women, results in sustained, non-oscillating elevated LH and lower FSH release [29,32].

Finally, complicating theories of extracellular input, immortalized GnRH neurons continue to release GnRH in a pulsatile manner in vitro, suggesting the presence of an independent intrinsic pulse generating mechanism [33].

In summary, GnRH neurons demonstrate neuronal and endocrine response functions. Excitatory neuronal input by means of GPR54 leads to stimulation of synthesis and release of GnRH. Responsiveness to neurotransmitters from higher CNS centers also modulates GnRH function. Finally, responses to ovarian hormonal feedback alter gonadotropin pulse frequency leading to cycle-specific release of GnRH. GnRH is transferred to the anterior pituitary gonadotrope cells by means of contact of its axonal extensions with the primary capillary plexus of the hypothalamic–anterior pituitary (H-P) portal vascular system.

Anterior pituitary gonadotropin secretion

Pulsatile GnRH reaches the gonadotrope cells of the anterior pituitary by means of the secondary capillary plexus of the H-P portal vessel system [1 (pp. 170–2)]. The GnRH G protein coupled membrane receptor function is calcium dependent. Activation leads to cyclic release of calcium ions from intracellular stores, opening cell membrane channels to allow entry of extra cellular Ca^{2+} ions, and by using inositol triphosphate (PIP3) and 1,2 diacylglycerol [1,2 DG] as second messengers stimulating protein kinase and cyclic AMP activity. GnRH gonadotrope cell receptors are regulated by many factors including GnRH itself, inhibin, activin, and gonadal steroids. GnRH has a self-priming effect on its own receptor number; as GnRH pulses increase (before ovulation), the number of receptors increase yielding even greater signal response capability. This self-priming amplification is enhanced by the combination of high mid-cycle E2 concentrations and initial pre-ovulatory progesterone secretion. The rate-limiting step in gonadotropin synthesis is the availability of the beta subunits of each glycoprotein. Thereafter, the gonadotropin is packaged, stored at the membrane, and secreted; each step induced by GnRH.

Multiple CNS peptides not only influence GnRH hypothalamic secretion but also interact with GnRH at the pituitary. A direct effect of these peptides may influence gonadotropin dynamics (e.g., CRH, neuropeptide Y) at the gonadotrope cell. However, the primary mechanism for gonadotropin function relies on GnRH input, and much like the ovarian follicle, by means of the local autocrine and paracrine activities of the activin/inhibin/follistatin system within the gonadotrope cells of the anterior pituitary.

The intracrine role of activin/inhibin system gonadotropin release patterns

This system presents possible answers to the question: if FSH and LH are made and secreted in the same cell and both depend on GnRH stimulation, what explains the disparate release of gonadotropins during the cycle [34]?

Inhibin action on the gonadotrope cell *inhibits* FSH both by endocrine input from the ovary and intracellular actions. On the other hand, *inhibin increases* LH by increasing GnRH receptor numbers. Since local *activin augments secretion of FSH by a similar process* (increasing GnRH receptors), the inverse release of gonadotropins may reflect competition between inhibin and activin for the GnRH receptor. In addition, follistatin is produced and active in gonadotrope cells. It suppresses synthesis and secretion of FSH by competitive inhibition (binding) of activin. The disparate FSH responses to GnRH signaling during the menstrual cycle can be explained best by a combination of GnRH input and steroid feedback modifying the balance between FSH inhibiting factors (inhibin, follistatin) and the stimulatory action of activin. Currently, there is no indication that LH secretion is regulated by any of these systems and is exclusively positively regulated by GnRH pulse frequency.

Regulatory mechanisms of gonadotropins controlling follicle growth, differentiation, and readiness for ovulation [35]

- FSH: Although the early stages of follicle formation and growth occur independent of FSH, FSH is required for *antral* granulosa cell differentiation, proliferation, and function. FSH activates adenyl cyclase by means of its cell membrane receptor FSHR, leading to cAMP activation of protein kinase A and stimulation of the targets, i.e., activin and inhibin, aromatase, up-regulation of its own receptor FSHR and ERβ (estradiol receptor β) [36]. In addition, FSH activates other signaling cascades; pathways stimulating cell cycle progression, avoidance of apoptosis, and cell nurture (RAS, glycogen synthase 3β kinase [GSK3β], and PI3K) [37]. As will be seen, many of these FSH stimulatory pathways are modulated by local follicular activin, inhibin, and follistatin. However, in addition to these TGFβ family members, growth factors, nitric oxide, prostaglandins, angiotensin II, TNFα, vasoactive intestinal peptide-(VIP), VEGF, even locally generated GnRH participate in FSH pathway regulation and function.

  In summary, FSH is the survival factor that prevents follicle atresia and induces enhancement of surviving follicles. As such, FSH is both necessary and sufficient as the endocrine agent for survival, selection, and generation of the dominant pre-ovulatory follicle.

- LH: Binding of luteinizing hormone (LH) to its receptor on the evolving thecal cell component of the follicle activates the adenyl cyclase-cyclic AMP pathway by means of the G protein mechanism. Generation of the crucial levels of estradiol needed for both intrinsic and eventual endocrine function depend on both FSH stimulation of aromatase in granulosa but also LH-stimulated theca androgen production as the essential substrate for estradiol biosynthesis. Therefore, LH in the folliculogenesis stage plays an important but relatively limited facilitatory role in the sustained survival of growing and selected follicles. As will be seen, LH performs its primary expanded and essential role at ovulation and during the corpus luteum phase [35].

Gonadal formation and folliculogenesis

The development of the ovary

At approximately 5 weeks of gestation, the mammalian gonad is first seen developing adjacent to the urogenital ridges overlying the mesonephric ducts [2–4,38]. It is termed a "bipotential" or indifferent gonad, because from all appearances it develops identically at this time in both male and female embryos. Differentiation into a testis or ovary occurs later after the primordial germ cells (PGCs) have migrated from the yolk sac and colonized the indifferent gonad. Thus, the earliest recognizable gonad is a mound of somatic cells derived from coelomic epithelium and mesonephric duct tissue consolidated in a mesenchymal matrix. As noted, the differential pattern of gonadal development does not begin until the arrival of the PGCs on the gonadal ridge at approximately 7 weeks.

Thereafter, several factors determine whether the indifferent gonad will become a testis or an ovary (Tables 1.1 and 1.2). The traditional view assigned an active, uniquely male genetic role in determination of a testis and, absent these factors, a passive "default" mode for development for the ovary. This view was founded on the earlier formation of the testis and delay in ovarian differentiation during embryogenesis. This concept is no longer tenable.

Gonadogenesis in the female requires the concerted action of genes such as WNT4 (wingless), RSP01, DAX1 (dosage-sensitive sex reversal adrenal hyperplasia critical region on chromosome X gene 1), and FOXL2 (forkhead box L2) to both *repress* testis defining genes in the SRY–S0X9 pathway and also *positively promote* ovarian development [2,39]. Mice lacking both WNT4 and FOXL2 exhibit complete and functional sex reversal of the ovary into a testis despite retaining an XX chromosomal genotype [40].

Primordial germ cells

Primordial germ cells (PGCs) first appear as a cluster of approximately of 100 cells in the endoderm on the dorsal wall of the yolk sac near the allantois [2]. They are differentiated from the proximal epiblast adjacent to the extraembryonic endoderm by ectoderm derived BMP-4 and BMP-8b and extra-embryonic-derived BMP-2 [41]. Epiblast takes on germ cell features through the influence of BMP-4. Germ cell "competence" is marked by the expression of an interferon-inducible transmembrane protein (fragilis), which induces the expression of Stella, a gene expressed exclusively on lineage-restricted germ cells. Together, these actions retain PGC pluripotency and escape from somatic cell differentiation and specification [42].

PGCs begin migration to the hindgut and dorsal mesentery during the 4th and 5th weeks of gestation, and by a combination of embryonic growth and chemotaxis reach the gonadal ridge by the 7th week and colonize the indifferent gonad. Germinal cell proliferation and migration involve stem cell factor kit ligand (KL) and expression of its receptor C-kit [5,43,44]. The presence of germ cells is essential for the differentiation of the gonad; in their absence, the gonad degenerates into fibrous cord-like structures. On the other hand, PGCs survive only in the gonadal ridge; they can be found nowhere else in the embryo.

Once the PGCs have arrived in the gonad, they undergo extensive proliferation; their numbers rapidly increasing from 10,000 (6 weeks) to 600,000 (8 weeks), and by the 20th week of gestation, reaching a peak of 6,000,000 oogonia and oocytes [45]. In humans, somatic cell activin appears to drive female germ cell proliferation before their entrance into the meiotic division phase. After reaching the peak number, oogonal mitosis declines and ends at 28 weeks. From this point on, gonadal germ cell (oocyte) content will irretrievably decrease until some 50+ years later at formal menopause less than 1,000 remain in the ovary. The vast majority of oocytes will undergo atresia; less than 400,000 are present at puberty. The rate of loss is not linear; it declines most rapidly in utero, with 1,000,000 remaining in the neonate and as noted 400,000 at puberty.

Several factors are responsible for the massive loss of oocytes in the second half of pregnancy; substantial numbers do not survive meiosis, others degenerate because they fail to be encased in the somatic cell (granulosa) envelope as primordial follicles, others are shed into the peritoneal cavity. Once encased in follicles, loss of oocytes proceeds only through reactivation, variable follicle growth followed by apoptosis (atresia) [46].

In summary, three sequential partially overlapping processes – the degree of oogonal proliferation and survival, successful initiation of meiosis 1 with conversion of ognia to oocytes, and encapsulation of the oocyte by pregranulosa cells into the primordial follicle – establish the "fixed endowment," the reserve pool of ovarian primordial follicles available for function throughout the remainder of the woman's life.

Transition of oogonia to oocytes and formation of primordial follicles

In the last several rounds of mitosis, oogonia assemble in a syncytial-like cluster [2,47,48]. Entry into meiosis begins between 8 and 13 weeks of gestation, well before follicle formation. DNA replication, meiotic chromosomal condensation, cohesion, synapsis, and recombination (i.e., initiation of meiosis) occur simultaneously in these clusters of oogonia [49]. A product of the gene Stra 8 appears to be the signal that triggers meiotic entry and is carried to each oogonium through connecting cytoplasmic bridges. Transformation of individual oogonia continues over the remainder of fetal life [50].

Formation of primordial follicles

The first primordial follicles appear in the human fetus as early as the 15th week of gestation and full conversion is completed shortly after birth [51]. The cellular cortex is gradually perforated by vascular channels originating in the deeper medullary areas, marking the beginning of follicle formation. As blood vessels invade and penetrate, they divide the previously solid cortical cell mass into smaller and smaller segments. Drawn in with the blood vessels are cells that originate in either the mesonephros or the coelomic epithelium or both. These cells give rise to the pregranulosa cells that surround the oocytes, which have initiated the first stage of meiosis. The resulting unit is the primordial follicle: an oocyte arrested in prophase of meiosis-1, enveloped by a single layer of squamous-shaped pregranulosa cells, surrounded by a basement membrane. Eventually, all surviving oocytes are covered in this manner. Residual mesenchyme not used in primordial follicle formation is found in the interstices between follicles, forming the primitive ovarian stroma. Envelopment by pregranulosa cells to form the primordial follicle provides the oocyte protection (at least temporarily) from atresia. Further meiotic progression is prevented by a granulosa cell oocyte meiosis inhibitor (OMI). At this point, the primordial follicle enters a "dormant' or "arrested" phase [52].

Dormancy and survival of mammalian primordial follicles

Each primordial follicle has three possible developmental fates: (1) remain quiescent and survive in dormancy for various lengths of time (in humans potentially many decades); (2) be activated into the growing follicle pool followed by atresia (or for very few, postpubertal dominant follicle status); or (3) undergo death directly from the dormant state [3,53,54]. Insights into molecular mechanisms underlying this "triage" control of dormancy such that the majority of primordial follicles are maintained in a dormant state have emerged. These factors are functionally divided between *suppressors of follicle activation* (Figs. 1.8, 1.9) (PTEN, Tsc, FOXO3a, P27, and AMH) and *maintenance of primordial follicle survival* (PDK1 and rps 6). Acting in a paracrine and autocrine manner, these controls arise from granulosa cells or are produced and act on the oocyte itself. Deletions in genes encoding molecules that maintain dormancy in primordial follicles in mouse models (*P10, Tsc-1, Tsc-2, FOXSO3a,* and *P27*) lead to premature and irreversible activation and depletion of the primordial follicle pool. The survival of the primordial follicle is maintained by molecules such as PI3K, PDK1, mTOR, and rpS6. Loss of genes encoding these molecules leads to follicular loss directly from their dormant state [55,56].

There is ample evidence for the importance of the phosphatidylinositol-3 pathway in general biology, including cell survival, growth, migration, and also in pathologic processes such as cancer and diabetes [57,58]. The main function of PI3K is to phosphorylate inositol-4, 5-bisphosphate (PIP2) to phosphoinositol-3, 4, 5-triphosphate (PIP3) at the cellular membrane where it acts as a second messenger docking with PDK1 (3 phosphoinositide-dependent kinase 1) and activating Akt/PKB (protein kinase B). Activated Akt promotes cell survival, cell proliferation, and growth by *inactivating* an array of downstream apoptosis promoting and inducing targets (FOXO1 family) and inhibiting BCL-2 family members (BAD), a combined action which turns off the intrinsic cell death machinery. PTEN modulates the PI3K pathway by reversing the initial PIP2 to PIP3 phosphorylation step, achieving a balanced action preserving dormancy [58,59].

Follicle development from arrest to early antral formation

The precise mechanisms of initiation and control of timing of activation of human arrested follicles, whether in milliseconds or decades, remains a mystery [60,61]. However, once begun, multidirectional communication systems linking all elements of the follicle (oocyte, granulosa, theca, and stroma cells) kick in. Growth of the follicle is first seen as conversion of the single layer of squamous-like pregranulosa envelope into a layer of cuboidal distinct cells and oocyte expansion. At this point in the primary follicle stage the zona pellucida is formed.

Activation of arrested primordial follicles and transition to primary follicles

The reactivation and recruitment of dormant primordial follicles into the growing follicle cohort starts in fetal life (immediately after oocyte "encapsulation") and continues until depletion at menopause [62]. The mechanisms that reactivate arrested follicles are multi-factorial (and probably incomplete), but it is certainly an intra-gonadal, primarily intra-follicular-driven event. The rate at which primordial follicles join the growing pool is positively related to the size of the remaining ovarian reserves, i.e., among many clinical examples, the age of menopause is about the same in women using prolonged steroidal contraception, after unilateral oophorectomy, voluntarily prolonged lactational amenorrhea, even grand multipara [3,62]. It is not a gonadotropin-related event as anencephalics [63], hypophysectomized women, individuals with absent FSH, or others with congenital absence of FSH receptors still undergo this relentless conversion and proceed to atresia [64]. Several elements are involved in the multi-directional interaction among oocyte, granulosa, theca and extracellular matrix, and growth factors in the reactivation and initial follicle growth stage [2,5].

"Reactivation" from arrest: reversal of inhibition

Loss of the inhibiting mechanisms that maintain follicle dormancy leads to follicle activation (Fig 1.9) [53]. These

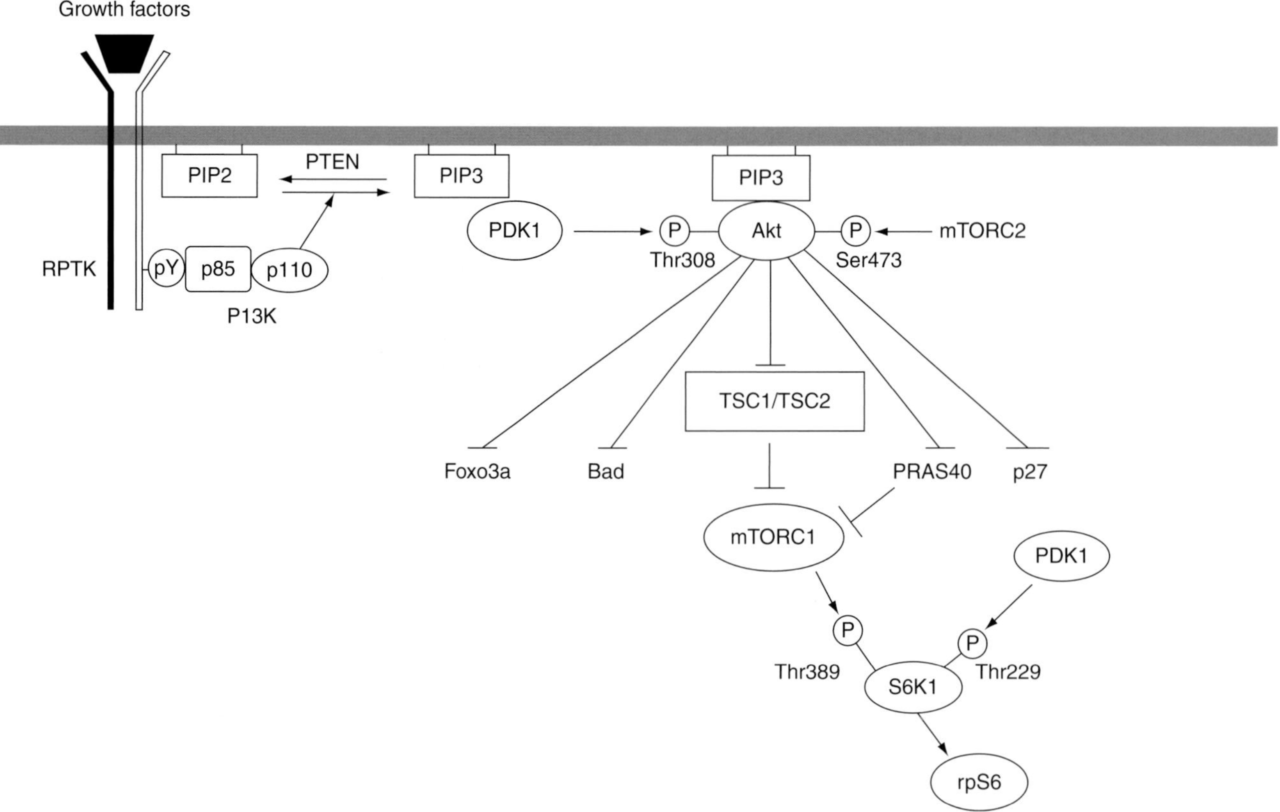

Fig. 1.8. Illustration of the PI3K pathway as well as molecules that maintain dormancy of primordial follicles Foxo3a, p27 and the TSC1/TSC2 complexes; complexes that maintain survival of primordial follicles including P13K, PDK1 mTORC1, S6K1, and rpS6. Reproduced from reference [53], with permission.

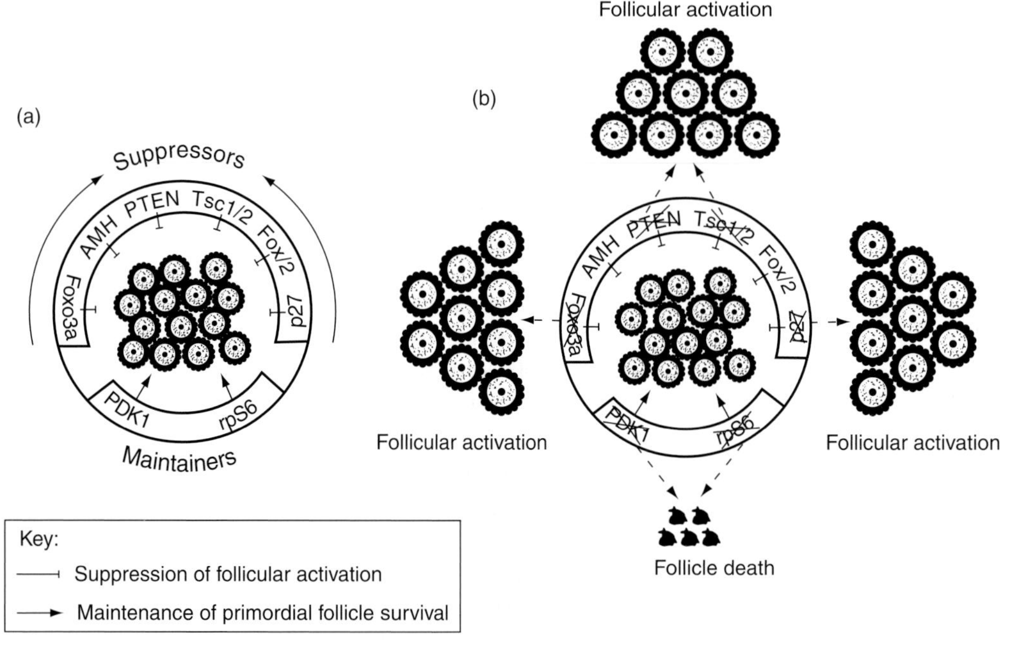

Fig. 1.9. Molecules that maintain quiescence and survival of primordial follicles include suppressors of activation and maintenance of survival during arrest. Whereas loss of suppressor molecules leads to follicle activation (primordial to primary follicle), loss of maintainers leads to primordial follicle death. Reproduced from reference [53], with permission.

inhibitors include tumor suppressor tuberous sclerosis complex (Tsc-1), phosphatase and tensin homolog deleted on chromosome 10 (PTEN), FOX3a, p27, and FOXL2. Experimentally, loss of any of these factors leads to accelerated activation and early exhaustion of the follicle pool. However, only the FOXL2 mutation has been linked to premature ovarian failure (POF) in humans. A rare syndrome composed of POF and blepharophimosis ptosis epicanthus inversus has been

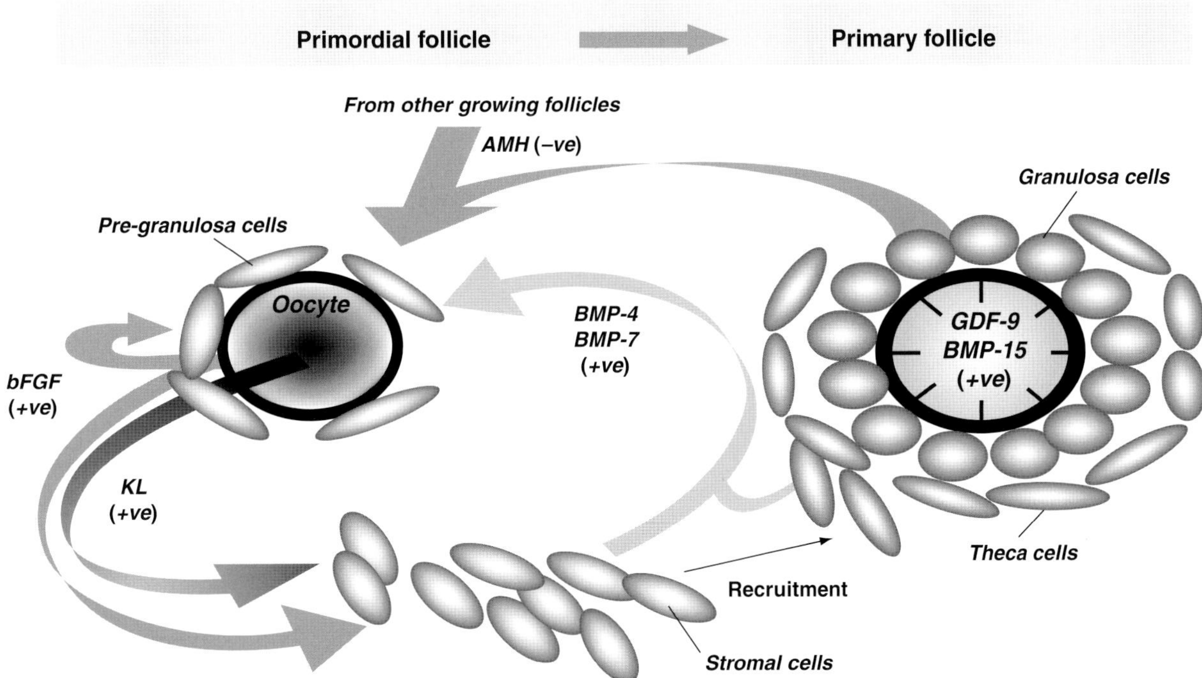

Fig. 1.10. Intercellular communication in the mammalian follicle. The conversion of a primordial follicle to primary follicle involves interactions among activated oocyte and pregranulosa production of FGF and KL which stimulate stromal cells to at once stimulate further primordial follicle activity as well as convert stroma into theca cells. As the primary follicle evolves, the oocyte stimulates further granulosa and theca cell proliferation. Finally AMH, produced by the granulosa of the evolving primary and secondary follicles inhibits primordial follicle activation. FGF = fibroblast growth factor; KL = kit ligand; (+ ive) = positive input; (-ive) = negative input. Reproduced from reference [5], with permission.

identified. On the other hand PTEN loss or mutation frequently cited as a factor in many human cancers does not appear associated with POF. Finally, mutations or common single nucleotide polymorphisms (SNPs) of the FOXO3a gene in mice are not associated with POF in humans.

TGF-β superfamily promotion of primordial to primary follicle transition (Fig. 1.10)

Theca/stroma-derived BMPs

Studies in rodents and ruminants demonstrate positive roles for BMP-4 and BMP-7 of pre-thecal and/or stromal origin in promoting the transition to primary follicle status as well as enhancing follicle survival [5,65,66]. In model systems, addition of recombinant BMP-7 or BMP-4 caused depletion of primordial follicles and increased conversion to primary, pre-antral, and antral follicle forms (Fig. 1.10). On the other hand, neutralizing or inhibiting antibodies of BMP-4 led to progressive loss of oocytes and somatic cells through apoptosis.

Oocyte-derived TGF-β ligands [67,68]

Although species differences exist, three members of the TGF-β superfamily GDF-9, BMP-15, and BMP-6, are selectively expressed by oocytes in rodents and primordial follicles in ruminants [67,68]. Furthermore, the various type I and type II receptors for each of these ligands are expressed by pregranulosa cells and granulosa cells. Mice with null mutations of the GDF-9 gene are infertile and show arrested follicle development at the primary stage. Treatment with GDF-9 in vivo and in vitro enhances progression of early to late stage primary follicles in the rat. The arrested follicles in GDF-9KO mice fail to acquire a theca layer of cells. Interestingly oocyte growth and zona pellucida acquisition proceeds in these mice. Unlike the GDF-9KO, mice with null mutations in BMP-15 or BMP-6 have minimal effects on follicle development or fertility. However, ewes with point mutations in these genes show profound infertility. Ewes immunized against BMP-15 or GDF-9 fail to develop follicles beyond the primary stage.

In summary, some evidence points to oocyte-derived GDF-9 (rodents) or both GDF-9 and BMP-15 (sheep) as having critically important effects on somatic cells of primordial and primary follicles that are essential for transition and further follicle progression.

Pregranulosa cell inhibition by anti-Mullerian hormone

As opposed to other members of the TGF-β superfamily, anti-Mullerian hormone (AMH) exerts a negative, suppressive effect on follicle development [69]. Mice with targeted deletion of AMH gene show an increased rate of follicle recruitment of primordial follicles resulting in premature depletion of follicle reserve. In vitro exposure of mouse neonatal ovaries to AMH halves the number of growing follicles. AMH expression is absent in primordial follicles, but is present in granulosa cells at the primary stage and in later follicle development as well. Expression of AMH type II receptors on pregranulosa cells indicates that AMH inhibition is exerted at the pregranulosa/granulosa stage of development.

AMH attenuates FSH function at later stages of follicle development. However, that function does not apply to AMH inhibition of primordial follicle activation because the FSH receptor is not present at this stage of FSH-independent follicle development.

Growth factors and cytokines (Fig. 1.10)

Pregranulosa growth factors and cytokines stimulate formation of primary follicles [2]. These include kit ligand (KL) and leukemia inhibitory factor (LIF) [70]. The receptor for KL is expressed by oocyte and theca/interstitial cells and presumably receptors for LIF. Both have been shown in vitro to promote the transition of primordial follicles into primary follicles, stimulate oocyte growth, and recruitment and proliferation of theca cells from surrounding stroma cells [72]. Other growth factors stimulate formation of primary follicles; these include keratinocyte growth factor (KGF) from stroma and basic fibroblast growth factor (FGF-2). KGF is a paracrine delivered, positive regulator of KL expression in granulosa cells, thereby amplifying KL-positive effects on pre-theca/theca cell proliferation and oocyte growth. FGF-2 is expressed by oocytes in the primordial stage and has at least two functions: it regulates KL expression in pregranulosa cells thereby promoting KL-positive effects on theca cell recruitment, proliferation, and by an autocrine process promotes oocyte expansion [71].

A "fixed oocyte endowment" versus oogonia stem cell "reserve"

A central dogma in reproductive medicine and widely accepted by women in general states that the number of ovarian follicles available for reproduction is fixed at mid-gestation and relentlessly diminishes over time without the possibility (as in the testis) of replacement or replenishment [73].

The concept of a fixed oocyte endowment which can only be depleted, is reinforced by the documented reduction in fertility and fecundability as residual follicles "age" in women beyond 35 years of age. In developed societies, principally as limitation in family size is chosen and women have increasingly joined the work force, these axioms have led to revision of family planning strategies by women and the clinical management of the physicians who serve them.

But the lack of oogonial stem cells (female germ stem cells, FGSCs) thesis has been challenged. Mice FGSCs have been identified in bone marrow and peripheral blood [74]. Under laboratory conditions FGSCs have undergone oogenesis and even fetuses have been unequivocally produced from fertilized oocytes derived from FGSCs. These results provide compelling evidence of the existence of FGSCs in some species of mammalian ovaries. The predictable debate these findings provoke revolves around whether these results can be confirmed not only in mice under stringent experimental conditions but with the human ovary and with a viable normal offspring as a result.

Replenishment of the human ovarian follicle reserve is a major challenge for reproductive endocrinologists, maternal fetal medicine specialists, as well as ethicists. It requires, indeed demands thorough investigation. How this process proceeds, and at what pace will be influenced by the recent ART successes in improved blastomere genetic assessment, vitrification and storage of selected 6–8 cell embryos, determination of the timing of implantation of single embryos – all associated with the prospects of doubling "take home" baby rates in IVF [75].

Progression of primary follicles to early antral stage (Fig. 1.11) [2,3]

The development of primary follicles to the late preantral/early antral stages involves oocyte enlargement, zona pellucida formation, multi-layered, granulosa cell proliferation, formation of a prominent basal membrane separating the avascular granulosa from the distinct outer envelope of initially, and progressively vascularized theca cells (Fig. 1.11). Pockets of fluid-filled spaces appear in the granulosa cell mass which gradually coalesce to form a single antral cavity. Progression from primordial follicle activation and recruitment into the irreversible stage of further follicle development is a protracted process, far longer than previously imagined. It is now estimated to take more than 120 days to pass from primary to secondary follicle stages and perhaps more than an additional 70 days are needed for the secondary group to reach the early antral stages.

The forces driving this progression continue to be the same intra-follicle and interstitial factors involved in the conversion from arrest and transition from primordial to primary follicle stages but in different proportions. These include growth and angiogenic factors but even more importantly members of the TGF-β superfamily [5,75]. In addition, particularly during the later stages of development, some degree of FSH "sensitivity" but not yet total dependence appears.

TGF-β superfamily regulators [76]

The same factors implicated in the primary to secondary follicle transition continue to be positive regulators of subsequent follicle growth to the late preantral and early antral stage. These include GDF-9 and BMP-15 of oocyte origin, granulosa cell activins, BMP-4 and BMP-7 of theca origin, and TGF-β from theca and granulosa cells. Finally, AMH performs its continued negative role in inhibiting preantral follicle development [77].

Oocyte-derived GDF-9 and BMP-15

In vitro exposure of human ovarian tissue to GDF-9 promotes primary follicle progression by stimulating granulosa proliferation and function. GDF-9 null mice, naturally occurring inactivating mutations in the GDF-9 gene, or immunization against

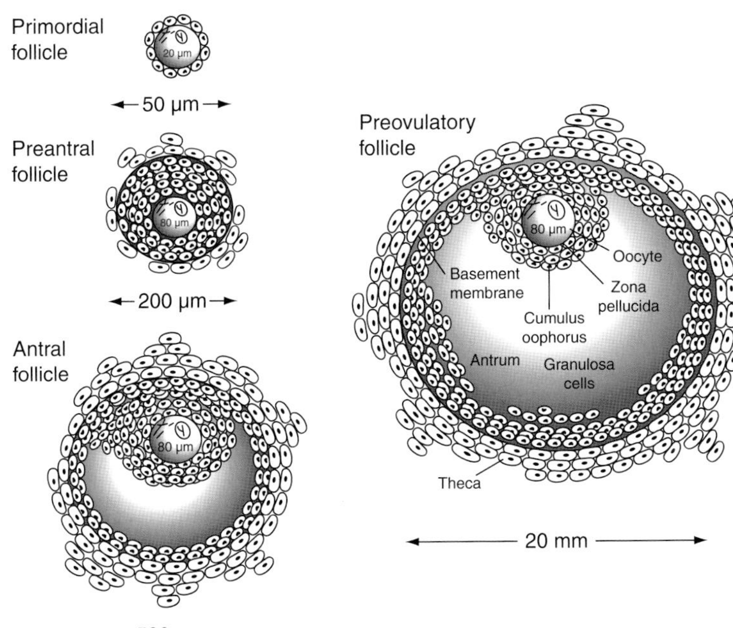

Fig. 1.11. The various stages of follicle development. Note the evolution from the primordial follicle (arrested in meiosis 1 and surrounded by a single layer of pregranulosa cells) through activation (proliferation of granulosa cells, a distinct increasingly vascularized and luteinized thecal mantle) to the preantral stage. The antral follicle and pre-ovulatory follicle display increased accumulation and distension of the antral cavity and the formation of distinct cumulus oophorus.

GDF-9 all inhibit growth beyond the primary follicle stage. The obligatory role of GDF-9 appears early in the oocyte during this transition. Oocyte-derived BMP-15 continues to induce granulosa cells in some species.

Theca cell participation

Thecal production of BMP-4 and BMP-7 stimulation continues from primary follicle stage through antral formation. Injection of BMP-7 into ovaries of rats increases the number of preantral follicles by paracrine stimulation of granulosa cells. BMP-4 exerts similar positive actions in cultured neonatal rat ovaries.

Granulosa cell activin/inhibin

Expressions of activin/inhibin and their receptors are detectable in folliculogenesis from the early primary–secondary transition stage forward. Rodent preantral follicles secrete activin-promoting, autocrine-induced growth of granulosa cells and paracrine growth instructions to oocyte and theca. Each effect is inhibited by the binding effects of follistatin. At this stage of follicle development (preantral/early antral), more activin and less inhibin is available.

TGF-β from oocyte and theca cells

TGF-β bioactivity by means of cognate receptors is seen in all compartments: granulosa, theca, and oocyte. TGF-β isoform function varies in species and in timing, however; TGF-β is active in human antral follicles but is less functional in earlier follicle development.

AMH

This member of the TGF-β superfamily is first detected in granulosa cells of primary follicles, but its production continues in increasing amounts to the mid-antral stages of follicle development in humans. The highest level of expression is observed in granulosa cells of secondary, preantral, and small antral follicles (≤ 4 mm diam). It imposes negative effects on pre-antral follicle development even beyond the primordial–primary oocyte follicle transition.

Growth factors

As noted earlier, thecal cells produce hepatocyte keratinocyte factor (KGF) and fibroblast growth factor, which by paracrine effect, induce granulosa production of KL. In response, KL promotes FGF and KGF production in theca cells; the KL↔KGF, FGF bidirectional "loop" synergistically stimulates both somatic elements that govern granulosa and theca growth and function [70,71].

FSH

Three observations suggest some FSH input in progression to the multi-layered granulosa preantral and early antral follicle stages exists. Exogenous gonadotropin therapy swiftly induces ovulation in ovaries of women with (1) profound hypogonadotropism due to anosmia (women who rarely display multi-layer follicle development) [78]. (2) Women with profound hypogonadotropic, hypogonadal, hypoestrogenism, and no observable follicle activity on ultrasound also can be brought to ovulation and fertility with impressively short courses of exogenous gonadotropin stimulation. (3) Pre-antral follicle granulosa may have some FSH receptors present [79].

Taken together, although spontaneous progression to this stage is not FSH dependent, some gonadotropin sensitivity may exist, performing a permissive role in this process. As we shall see, *total* FSH dependency emerges and is mandatory in the later full antral stages of development.

Follicle development from antral stage to ovulation

The emergence of FSH dependence: the feedback system and puberty

The feedback system

Studies in a variety of rodent models have established the presence of feedback centers in the hypothalamus responsive to steroids [1 (pp. 184–91)] with release of GnRH and variable secretion of FSH and LH [80]. Release of GnRH results from coordinated interactions among neurohormones, GnRH, the pituitary gonadotropins, estrogen, and progesterone in a mechanism known as positive and negative feedback.

The hypothalamus and anterior pituitary

The increased biologic impact of the mid-cycle surge of both gonadotropins enhances follicle ovulation mechanisms, maximizes FSH induction of LHR on granulosa cells, and assists in the repair and proliferation of the granulosa post-ovulation in preparation for its function as the corpus luteum [82]. Finally, FSH biologic activity is essential during the inter-menstrual transition phase in the rescue and selection of the next cycle's dominant follicle.

In physiologic experiments in mice, FSH levels are inversely regulated by estrogen negative inhibitory feedback signals. In the case of LH, negative feedback inhibition occurs at low levels of estrogen but a positive stimulatory feedback signal is generated by high levels of estrogen. The control centers for these E-FSH and E-LH responses were thought to be exclusively located in what were called hypothalamic "tonic" (negative feedback) and "cyclic" (positive feedback) centers [4,81]. In this thesis, the hypothalamus, specifically the GnRH neurons concentrated in the medial ventral hypothalamus, were the master controllers of the H-P-O axis.

Studies in primates necessitated modifications in this doctrine by documenting the essential participation of the anterior pituitary gonadotrope cells in the feedback loop [83,84]. Evidence defining this pituitary involvement is compelling:

- Radiofrequency destruction of the medial basal hypothalamus or complete division of both elements of the pituitary stalk (primarily disconnection of the portal vessels) led to loss of gonadotropin release [85]. Replacement of pulsatile GnRH by intra-venous pump restored gonadotropin secretion.

However,

- Further studies in primates support a positive partnership rather than a simple permissive role of GnRH in the feedback system control of LH release. When GnRH is administered in an IV bolus in the absent hypothalamus model, LH and FSH blood levels increase almost immediately, reaching peak concentrations for LH 20 to 25 minutes later and 45 minutes later for FSH. After several hours of gradual decline, the gonadotropins return to basal levels. On the other hand, if GnRH is administered in low concentrations by constant infusion, the rapid rise in gonadotropin recurs, then falls to a plateau but not to basal levels. After 200–240 minutes of sustained low level GnRH infusion, gonadotropins rise again to a second increased release of gonadotropin which persists as long as GnRH is available. These findings demonstrate the positive actions of GnRH on gonadotropin synthesis, storage and secretion; synthesis of a storage (reserve) pool of glycoproteins, a shift to a readily releasable pool (first response) and a second delayed release drawn from the stored reserve. Clearly, estradiol affects all phases of GnRH input [83–86].

Ovarian steroids

- Feedback concentrations of estradiol influence pituitary gonadotropin secretion in three ways [87–89]:
  - As estradiol levels increase at mid-cycle, FSH and LH are secreted in molecular forms possessing greater biologic activity as indicated by the disparity of gonadotropin concentrations measured by immunoassay versus bioassay [90]
  - Estradiol enhances the self-priming by GnRH on its own GnRH receptor number and sensitivity on gonadotrope cell membranes
  - Negative feedback of estrogen on FSH is achieved by estrogen-induced decrease of pituitary expression of activin and by direct inhibition of FSH beta subunit gene expression [91].
- Estradiol has a direct effect on GnRH hypothalamic neurons by means of its ER beta receptor subtype and is involved in altering the basal autorhythmicity of GnRH pulses. At ovulation, E2 by frequency perhaps more than amplitude of GnRH pulses, influences pituitary gonadotropin release responses. Peak E2 induces physiologic GnRH pulses (every 60 min), which maximize LH and FSH release. More rapid pulse frequency dissociates gonadotropin release as in PCOS, where increased LH and diminished FSH secretion prevails. Less rapid GnRH pulses during the luteal phase (every 200 min) reduces both LH and FSH concentrations typical of this phase of the cycle [92].
- Still low but rising progesterone concentrations at mid-cycle [93,94] facilitate the primarily estrogen-induced gonadotropin release at the pituitary gonadotrope cell level. On the other hand, the high luteal phase levels of progesterone abetted by sustained levels of E2 inhibit LH and FSH release at both the hypothalamic and pituitary levels by inducing slower frequencies of GnRH pulses.

While the combination of E and P in pregnancy and the therapeutic levels achieved by combined oral contraceptives replicate this luteal phase gonadotropin suppression, the anti-ovulatory contraceptive efficacy of Depo-Provera alone confirms the unique negative feedback effects of increased sustained progesterone availability.

The ontogeny of the hypothalamic–pituitary–ovarian axis (Fig. 1.12)

Fritz and Speroff have [1 (pp. 193–7, 391–7)] reviewed the topic in detail. For the purposes of this chapter, only the essential elements of the entrainment of this fundamental reproductive endocrine circuitry will be described.

The basic elements of the reproduction axis, that is, the hypothalamic GnRH pulse generator [96,97], the anterior pituitary gonadotrope cells and ovaries, are all in place early in fetal life and by mid-pregnancy are fully functional and capable of generating ovarian follicle maturation, estrogen synthesis and secretion, and waves of follicle activation, growth, and atresia (Fig. 1.12) [95]. Ovarian histology and identification of the molecular mechanisms for estrogen production are persuasive evidence of this activity which is diluted to non-recognition in the ocean of non-gonadal feto-placental production of estrogen and progesterone.

By mid-gestation, gonadotropins are present in quantities surpassing adult levels but sharply decline in response to the negative feedback imposed by the combined E and P of pregnancy. The expression within the fetal H-P-O system of sensitivity to negative feedback is confirmed by events after birth. As a result of the acute loss of placental and maternal hormones, the neonate's H-P-O system is released from negative suppression and responds with resumption of GnRH stimulation and FSH and LH release [98]. The gonadotropins rise promptly, the FSH and LH levels exceed those seen in normal adult menstrual cycles, peak at 6 months, and then decline [99]. During this interval, ovarian follicle development is stimulated and estrogen secretion equivalent to the mid-proliferative phase is achieved. This H-P-O activity is transient; well before 2 years of age gonadotropin and estrogen concentrations fall and remain at extremely low levels for the remainder of infancy and childhood until resumption of function at puberty, an interval as long as 8 to 10 years.

Although some evidence suggests an ultra-sensitive negative feedback function early in infancy, it was unlikely that the extremely low estradiol concentrations (less than 10 pg per milliliter) usually associated with high castrate levels of gonadotropin could be functioning over the decade of infancy and childhood. A more plausible biologic explanation was that a powerful suppressive force, not feedback but central in origin, was depressing GnRH function. The clinical demonstration of H-P-O readiness to function is displayed in instances of constitutional precocious puberty (premature but normal H-P-O function) and primate experiments in which pre-pubertal female monkeys can be induced to ovulate with as few as three cycles of exogenous GnRH pump infusions [100].

These experiments not only demonstrate readiness for full function at any age but that neither the anterior pituitary nor gonad was the limiting factor in the infancy and childhood inactivity. The issue was clarified when cross-sectional and longitudinal studies of women with gonadal dysgenesis (Turner's syndrome) revealed a similar "diphasic" pattern of gonadotropin secretions. Gonadotropin levels in these girls are markedly elevated in infancy, decline to very low levels during childhood, only to rise again to castrate levels at puberty [101]. These agonadal women, incapable of negative feedback, confirmed the presence of central inhibition of GnRH pulsatile secretion as the major factor in the juvenile H-P-O quiescence.

The accepted paradigm explaining these observations is the existence of a "neuroendocrine switch" for the GnRH pulse generator. It is "on" during late fetal and early neonatal life, turns off during childhood, and returns to an "on" position at initiation of puberty. Several central factors have been suggested as the putative inhibitors of GnRH; gamma-amino butyric acid (GABA) [102,103], neuropeptide Y [104–106], and inhibition of glutamate [103].

Epidemiologic correlations and clinical observations on the timing of initiation and the rate of progression of human female puberty has coupled peripheral (largely metabolic)

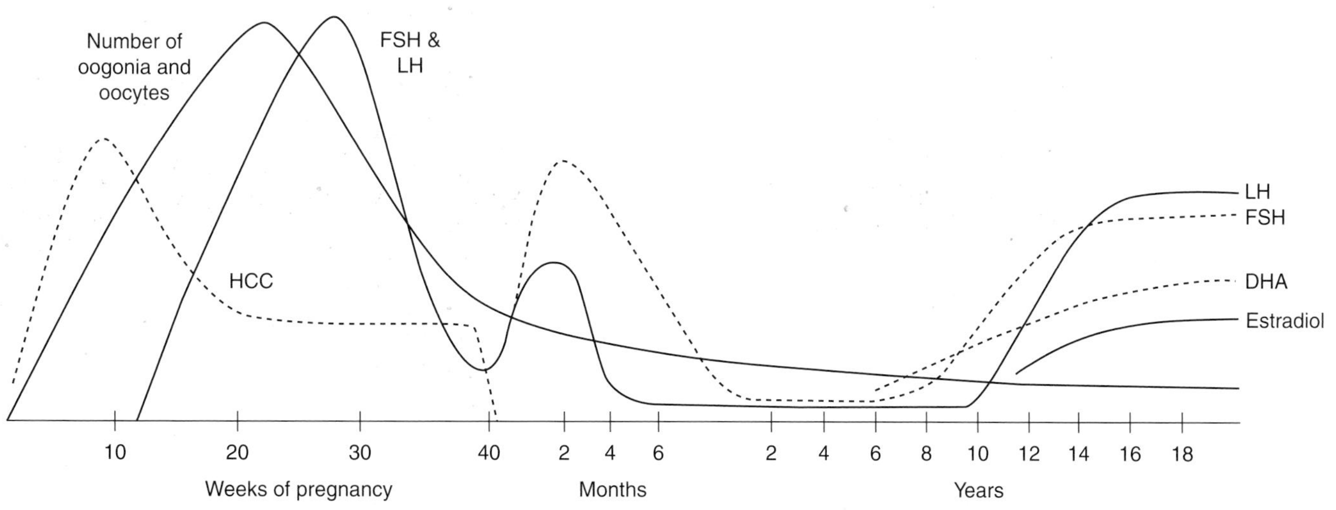

Fig. 1.12. Peptide and steroid hormone production in the fetus, neonate, infant, and child. Note evidence of H-P-O function in the fetus, the presence of feedback in utero, central gonadotropin inhibition throughout childhood, and recrudescence of gonadotropin and steroid function at puberty. Note also relentless loss of follicle numbers after peak "endowment" of oogonia/primordial follicles in mid-gestation.

feedback signaling and the activation of a central processor that turns "on" the neuroendocrine GnRH switch [107].

In addition to genetic/genomic factors in the family history of timing pubertal initiation, geographic location, population density, psychologic stress, and energy balance all influence the timing of puberty. Residence at low altitude, closeness to the equator, and urban living all promote earlier development. While mildly obese girls reach puberty earlier (earlier age of puberty is common in developed and developing societies), negative energy balance, as seen in low weight intense dieting, malnutrition, famine, excess exercise [108], and anorexia, display delayed even absent puberty changes. This suggests a critical body weight threshold or more likely critical body composition [109] as the important factor in pubertal timing. Among the many metabolic signals, the adipokine leptin has emerged as the major metabolic feedback signal of female readiness to reproduce, sustain pregnancy, and nourish the newborn.

Leptin

Leptin is produced by adipocytes, and serum concentrations are closely correlated with body fat and changes in body fat content. Accordingly, leptin has been implicated as the feedback metabolic signal to the central elements controlling the hypothalamic pulse generator and the onset of puberty.

In human females, leptin concentrations rise throughout puberty [110] with an increase in mean serum leptin concentration to 12.2 μg/L (corresponding to 29.7% body fat and a body mass index of 22.3) at menarche. Each increase in serum leptin lowers the age of the menarche by 1 month.

Evidence from studies in children with congenital leptin deficiency has provided insights into the potential importance of leptin as a somatic stimulus for the onset of puberty. In affected pubertal age children, treatment with recombinant leptin induces endocrine changes consistent with the onset of puberty [111]. Adults with congenital leptin receptor deficiency have severe hypogonadotropic hypogonadism. Recombinant human leptin administered to severe anorectic hypogonadotropic women retrieves function of the H-P-O axis, including ovulation within three cycles of therapy [112]. Of note, this stimulation is achieved despite absent change in eating habits, lifestyle, or BMI of the recipients who remained profoundly anorexic. Importantly, similar treatment in young children has not induced premature puberty.

These clinical observations suggest that leptin plays an important but only permissive role in the onset of puberty. Nonetheless, they are consistent with the notion that a circulating signal reflecting energy status might have the ability to activate the hypothalamic GnRH pulse generator. Some central response mechanism sensitive to energy balance and the metabolic status of women must be present and activated to initiate puberty [113].

Puberty

About 1 year before thelarche (breast budding) or about age 10, nocturnal pulses of gonadotropin secretion emerge with LH levels exceeding those of FSH [114,115]. These nocturnal gonadotropin pulses become strong enough to generate detectable increases in serum estradiol (which accounts for initiation of breast development). E2 increments also increase LH secretion substantially more than increments in FSH [116]. The combination of E2 and the self-priming effect of GnRH on its own receptors (upregulation) increase gonadotrope capacity for response to GnRH by synthesis and later full secretion of gonadotropins [117].

Further into pubescence, gonadotropin pulses become diurnal, which in turn increases and prolongs E2 secretion still further. As the pace of puberty quickens, the amplitude of LH pulses continues to increase, reflecting the enhancing influence of rising E2 levels at both the hypothalamus and pituitary. The progressive, accelerating, self-priming, steroid feedback sensitization of the H-P-O circuitry of the evolving pubescent child into young adulthood is thereby entrained.

Accordingly, in response to increasing gonadotropin secretion estrogen levels rise. Furthermore, endocrine levels of inhibin B (which were undetectable in pre-pubertal girls) increase significantly by mid-puberty. This combination of granulosa cell maturation and capacity to generate signals both of restraint (inhibin) and positive feedback (E2) initiate cyclic gonadotropin oscillations [118].

Menarche, cycle length, and menstrual "control" characteristics vary until feedback fully matures and repetitive ovulations become established.

In summary, after a decade of quiescence, pulsatile GnRH secretion resumes, inducing reactivation of the H-P-O axis. The "reignition" of the signal appears to be the level of leptin, reflecting the positive presence of sufficient metabolic energy stores (fat) to sustain the energy requirements of a successful month pregnancy. FSH and LH levels rise around the time of thelarche first at night but gradually expand to day time, but still with chaotic spikes of secretion. Nevertheless, estradiol concentrations increase initiating evolution of secondary sexual characteristics but also engaging a "snowballing" amplification of the H-P-O interactive circuitry. Finally, positive feedback is achieved and with increased synchrony among the endocrine and intracrine events that link successful function of the H-P-O (accurate feedback representation of follicle status and central maturity to react in a timely sequence of gonadotropin concentrations) gradually and then permanently repetitive adult ovulatory cycles emerge.

At this stage, full FSH dependence and a mature antral follicle prepared to maximize FSH instructions must be in place. The "SELECTION" process begins.

The menstrual cycle: from arrest to ovulation

Follicle development: selection of the dominant follicle

The mature antral follicle is a large entity easily visible by ultrasound (Fig. 1.13) [2,3]. The increased size is due to the expanding antral cavity filled with fluid rich in hormones, growth factors, and cytokines. This rich intracrine "nutrient

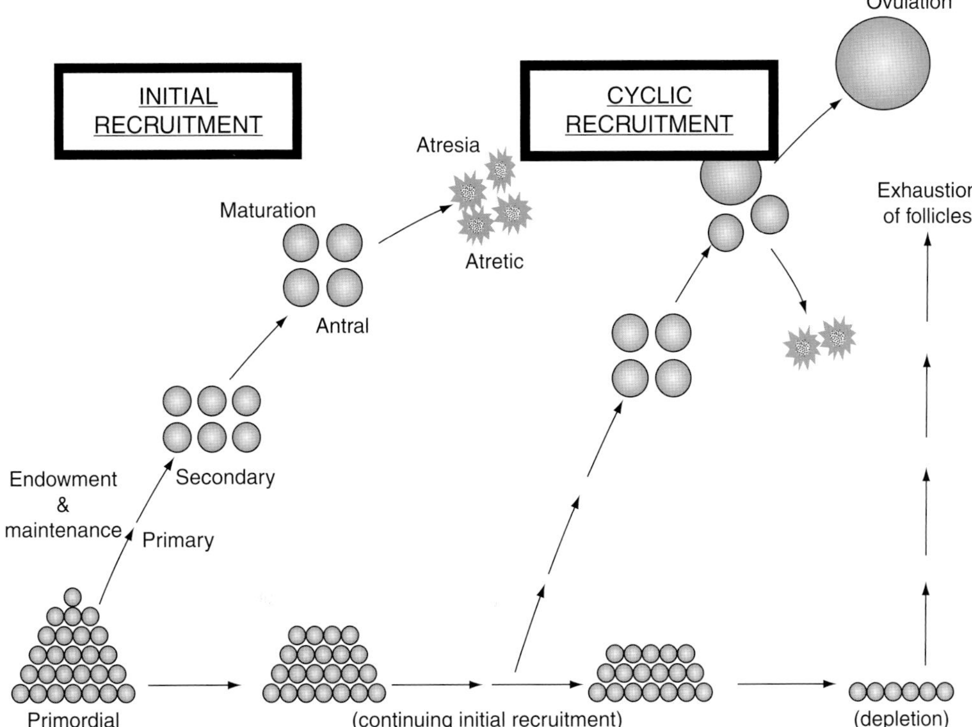

Fig. 1.13. Initial versus cyclic follicle recruitment. With puberty and the production of FSH a small group of early antral follicles are "rescued" from total loss and from this small group of "survivors" the dominant follicle is selected and matured to Graafian follicle (pre-ovulatory) status. Note relentless loss of follicle reserve independent of cyclic recruitment.

soup" compensates in part for the geometric separation of the follicle components induced by antral expansion and consequent loss of intimate paracrine contact. For example, the steroid concentrations found in antral fluid exceed levels [118] found concurrently in peripheral plasma [119].

The mural granulosa layer retains its paracrine contact with the expanding size and function of the thecal cell mantle but must rely on direct access to the antral fluid for additional support and functional directives. The thecal compartment is now richly vascularized and displays early luteinization [120]. Finally, in a remarkable response to antral expansion, the oocyte preserves its essential bidirectional interactions with granulosa through the preservation of the specialized mantle of granulosa called the cumulus oophorus (COC) [121].

As noted in the later stages of puberty, the H-P-O feedback interaction circuitry has matured. In addition to diurnal circadian fluctuations, more purposeful frequency and amplitude of gonadotropin negative and positive feedback signaling produces the increasing oscillatory shifts of gonadotropins. The combination of total follicle dependence on FSH for survival and the inter-menstrual transitional cyclic rise in FSH are the sine qua non elements of dominant follicle selection and progression [122].

The single functional composite word "selection" denotes at least three factors determining follicle destiny: (1) selection describes the rescue of the follicle from inevitable apoptosis (atresia), (2) promotion of further growth of the selected follicle to pre-ovulatory and ovulatory competence, and (3) elaboration of inhibiting factors which induce atresia in other members of the recruited cohort. This unique status of "selection" is the follicle's possession of maximum FSH receptor number, FSH receptor sensitivity, and the highest level of intracrine estradiol, activin, and other growth factors [123].

The FSH-dependent stage (3)

Reproductive endocrinologists are well aware of the fundamental importance of FSH as the necessary and sufficient driving force in ovarian follicle progression to ovulatory capacity [122]. The effectiveness of early cycle administration of Clomid in normogonadotropic anovulation, the dramatic and swift reversal of ovarian status induced by recombinant human FSH (rhFSH) or human menopausal gonadotropin (HMG) in profoundly hypogonadotropic hypo-estrogenic women attests to the unique importance of FSH in gonadal physiology. In laboratory experiments, in the absence of the beta subunit of FSH, antral follicles are formed but growth beyond that stage to ovulation does not occur.

After a minimum of 10 to 12 or a maximum of 40+ years in the arrested primordial follicle state, reactivation and progressive growth and differentiation (about 120 days), and the development of some degree of FSH "sensitivity," a small number, perhaps 3 to 15, of early antral follicles (2 to 5 mm in diameter), precariously ambivalent in their prospects, reach the state whereby they become entirely FSH dependent and resolution of their destiny defined [3]. This decisive failsafe point is reached in a 7 to 10 day endocrine window beginning late in the previous luteal phase (menses −3 or 4 days) to menses +7 days into the next follicle phase, i.e., an interval bridging the inter-cycle transition [122,124].

At this time, GnRH pulses increase from the luteal low of every 200 minutes to perhaps every 90 minutes having been released from the negative feedback of combined progesterone, estradiol, and inhibin A. This increase in GnRH pulses stimulates an FSH secretion increase (from 4 IU/L to 10 IU/L units) during the first stimulatory portion (see Fig. 1.14) of the transition [125]. The dominant follicle destined to ovulate is identified ["selected"] between menses −1 to +3 of this stimulatory rise in FSH secretions. Thereafter FSH concentrations decline (see Fig. 1.15, Part B) in response to the initial negative feedback endocrine secretions of the selected follicle (rising estradiol and inhibin B) [126], and intracrine follicle suppression by AMH [127].

This combination of endocrine and intracrine actions exposes the weakness of the less prepared follicles, condemning them to atresia. The widening gap between the accelerating growth of the emerging dominant pre-ovulatory follicle and decline of its cohort siblings is increasingly evident in the remaining days of this portion of the cycle.

The stimulatory phase: rising FSH

The stimulatory phase of follicle maturation (Fig. 1.14, stage A) is defined by two factors: the inter-menstrual rise in FSH concentrations, and the concurrent increase in number and sensitivity of FSH receptors on the granulosa cells of the selected follicle [2–4]. The intra-follicle elements responsible for FSH effectiveness are as important as the rising levels of the gonadotropin in producing maximum FSH responses.

- Granulosa cell and *oocyte*: in response to all members of the TGF-β family, TGF-β, BMPs, GDF-9, but at this stage particularly activin, arising in concert from the oocyte and granulosa (both mural and cumulus) contribute to an intracrine environment that induces increased granulosa cell numbers of FSH receptors (1500/cell), increased aromatase capacity and activity, further proliferation of granulosa cells, further oocyte development/progression, and enhanced thecal cell responses to LH [5,128]
- Thecal cell: BMP-4 and-7, enhanced by granulosa cell activin (and to a lesser extent inhibin), increase LH stimulation of androgen synthesis by increased P450scc, P450c17, among others, to provide substrate availability for granulosa aromatase estradiol production [129]
- IGF increases both LH receptor numbers (many thousands of LHR on theca cells) and by paracrine transfer from the theca, IGF-2, increases granulosa cell activin and inhibin [1,130,131]

Collectively, the intracrine environment of IGF, activin, inhibin, EGF, VEGF, and nitric oxide (NO)-increased ERβ enhances follicle growth, antral expansion, vascularization, and balanced steroidogenesis in the antral follicle destined for selection and ovulation. However, all these elements play important supportive roles for the prime drivers to dominance, the interplay between follicle estradiol and FSH [3] [1 (pp. 207–9)].

FSH and estradiol participate in an amplifying, positive feed-forward and positive feedback interactive sequence that maximizes follicle dominance [132]. FSH acting by means of its FSH receptor on granulosa induces cell proliferation, increases granulosa activin and inhibin elaboration, and most important induces increased aromatase capacity and efficiency. In response, granulosa aromatase synthesizes increasing quantities of estradiol. Rising local estradiol concentrations (not yet an important secretory product in this phase) in a positive

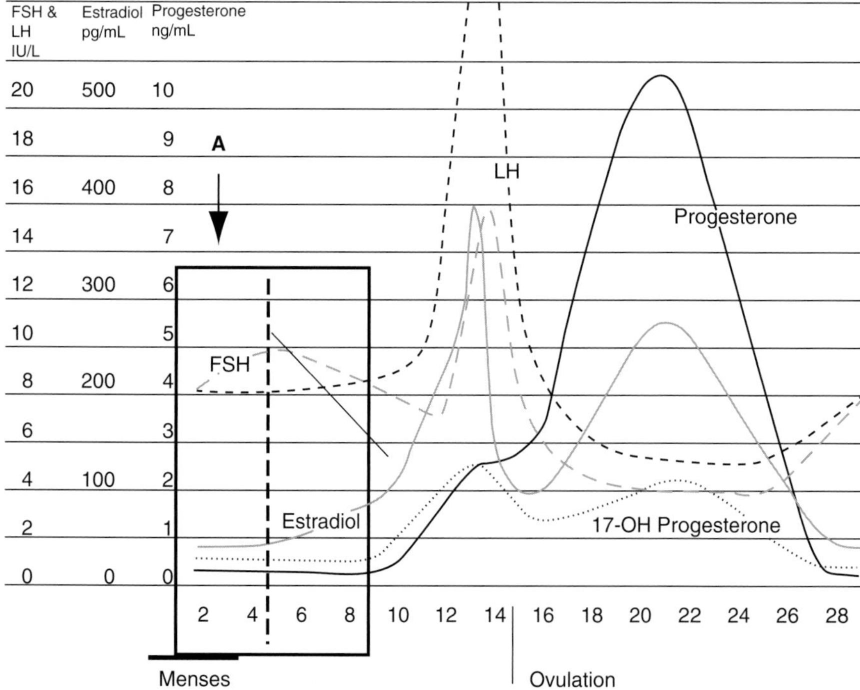

Fig. 1.14. The FSH-dependent stages: the FSH stimulatory phase (A) of rising FSH. With the demise of the prior cycle corpus luteum and withdrawal of negative feedback on gonadotropin secretion (E2, progesterone, inhibin A) the luteal–follicle intercycle menstrual-related rise in FSH leads to cyclic recruitment and selection of available preantral follicles.

intracrine loop increases FSH receptor numbers and sensitivity on granulosa cell membranes. Estradiol is a local FSH accelerant (catalyst) in this phase.

Balanced control of thecal androgen production is also critical: too little androgen leads to inadequate estrogen and follicle failure; too much androgen production of non-aromatizable, 5α-reduced androgens reduces E2 concentrations and also acts as an anti-estrogen and causes follicle failure [129,130].

In summary, this phase of antral follicle selection and further progression to dominance is dependent on the rise and maximization of FSH concentrations arriving at the follicle and the ability of local estradiol to increase FSH receptors on follicle granulosa cells.

Phase of FSH decline (Fig. 1.15)

In phase B (Fig. 1.15), endocrine factors originating in both the pituitary and ovary lead to the decline in FSH concentrations and accelerate the disparate evolution of the antral follicle cohort; one survives and prospers, while the remainder enters irreversible apoptosis and dissolution.

As noted, the selected follicle will resist dwindling FSH because of maximization of its FSH receptor content by estradiol. But the selected follicle, by dint of its success, also engineers further negative feedback on FSH at this stage by secreting increased levels of estradiol and inhibin B (combined negative feedback), thus accelerating and ensuring the demise of less competent members of the cohort [123,126].

Despite the decline in FSH concentrations during menses +3 to +8 days, the dominant follicle continues to develop. By day 5, it is functionally capable of estradiol secretion, which emerges slowly at first but then progressively increases in a trajectory that will lead to pre-ovulatory peak concentrations. At the same time, inhibin B concentrations increase to maximum on day 5, plateau through days 9 and 10, thereafter declining to pre-ovulatory basal levels.

Although a change has occurred in the intra-follicular balance between mutually opposing granulose-derived activins and inhibins such that inhibins become dominant locally and are secreted as an endocrine factor (hence the decline in FSH), local inhibin activity enhances thecal androgen synthesis necessary to accommodate the substrate requirements for the accelerated estradiol synthesis and secretion in the pre-ovulatory and anticipated ovulatory surge [132]. In addition, the enhanced thecal LH stimulation increases thecal cell number and LHR activity [128,133]. By day 9, VEGF promotes increased vascularity and delivery of cholesterol for thecal steroid synthesis [134].

Despite the inhibin/activin shift, sufficient activin action persists, particularly in the anatomic and functional intimacy of the cumulus enveloped oocyte as well as the rich antral fluid resources available to sustain and enhance further progression of the pre-ovulatory follicle [131]. The shift from activin to inhibin dominance may be the result of the emerging FSH-induced LHR presence on the granulosa cell of the dominant pre-ovulatory follicle. These receptors will have an important function as LH begins to rise toward the mid-cycle LH surge. Local progesterone synthesis and modest accumulation of that steroid in antral fluid imposes local intracrine functions but not yet in sufficient quantities to achieve endocrine secretion [135]. Local oocyte production of GDF-9, BPM-6, and BPM-15 modulates progesterone synthesis on the cumulus and mural granulosa to avoid premature luteinization [2,5].

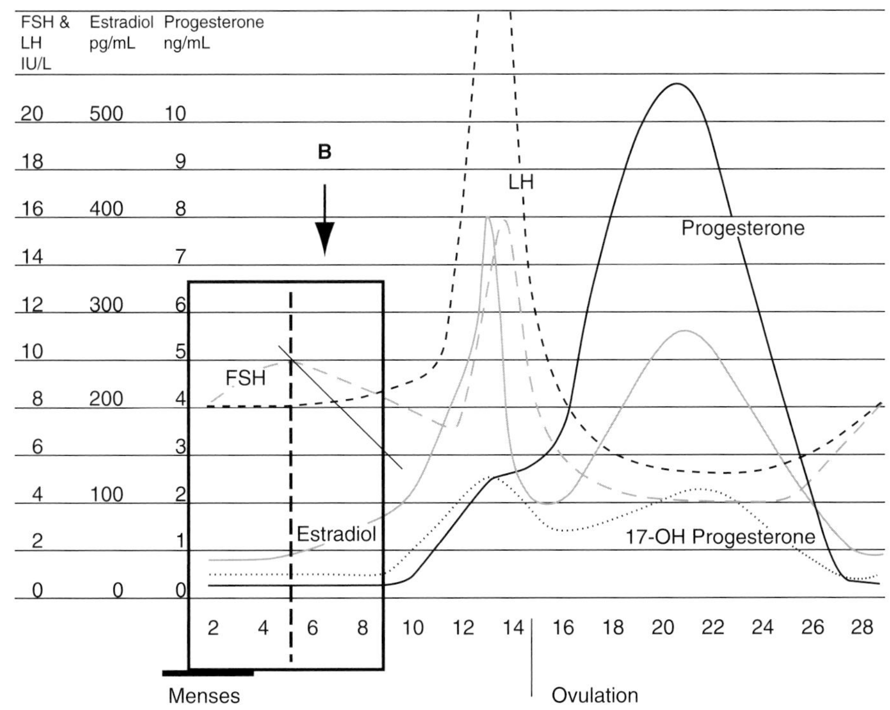

Fig. 1.15. The FSH-dependent stages: the stage of declining FSH(B). With selection of the lead follicle destined to dominance, the granulosa of that follicle produces rising E2 and inhibin B which induce negative feedback on FSH. The dwindling levels of FSH and intra-gonadal AMH induce atresia in the remaining follicle cohort.

Ovulation

As a result of the positive feedback effects of rising estradiol, stimulation of massive LH release and the dominant follicle's abundant thecal (and increasingly granulosal) LH receptor number and function, a cascade of endocrine and intrinsic factor events occurs as the dominant (now traditionally named Graafian follicle) achieves ultimate maturity (Fig. 1.16) [1 (pp. 228–33), 4,136]. Estradiol concentrations become sufficient to achieve and sustain the required threshold requirements for positive feedback on LH (200–400 pg/mL for 50 hours) and induction of the dramatic LH surge (rising from 6–8 IU/L to 35–40 IU/L).

Acting through its receptors, LH initiates major changes in the ovulating follicle: "loosening" of the matrix and expansion of the cumulus-oocyte-complex ("COC"), loss of anchoring of the complex to the basal lamina, completion of meiosis 1, progressive luteinization of the granulosa, shifting granulosa steroid synthesis to yield both estradiol but also increasing progesterone synthesis now of sufficient quantity to achieve endocrine secretion, full antral expansion, distensibility, protease- and collagenase-induced weakening, and finally rupture of the follicle wall and extrusion of the oocyte. LH achieves all these biologic effects by activating its own post-receptor cascade of molecular mechanisms, by stimulating the further production of progesterone as well as the induction of the diverse local biologic functions of prostaglandins [4].

Mechanisms of ovulation

Classically, the effects of the LH surge were described in simple terms; luteinization (the accumulation of cholesterol in "luteinized" granulosa cells), progressive synthesis of progesterone with concentrations first seen as accumulation in the antral fluid followed by initial appearance of secreted progesterone and 17αOH progesterone in peripheral blood [137]. Prostaglandin production was inferred from the gradual dissolution of the cumulus and formation of the surface "stigma" – the site of follicle wall dissolution ("rupture") followed by extrusion of the antral fluid and the oocyte with attached fragments of cumulus granulosa cells.

The general term "the effects of LH on ovulation" has now been dissected into specific, distinct molecular events and programs. These may act separately, concurrently, or in sequence to induce the various elements involved in the general term "ovulation induction." The major participants in these concurrent processes are primarily LH itself, progesterone, the prostaglandins, and FSH.

LH

LH interaction with its granulosa cell receptors activates the cAMP/PKA, PI3K/AkT, and RAS signaling pathway (see Fig. 1.17) [4]. These steps include expression of EGF-like factors (amphiregulin-AREG and epiregulin-EREG), which together bind to their receptors and induce expression of ERK1–2. ERK1–2 (extracellular signal regulated kinase 1 and 2) are elements of the MAPK program and act as the "master switch" which controls the global reprogramming of granulosa cells. The targets of ERK 1–2 include [138]:

- Nuclear receptor activating proteins 1 (NRIP-1) which enhances the expression of growth factors AREG and EREG

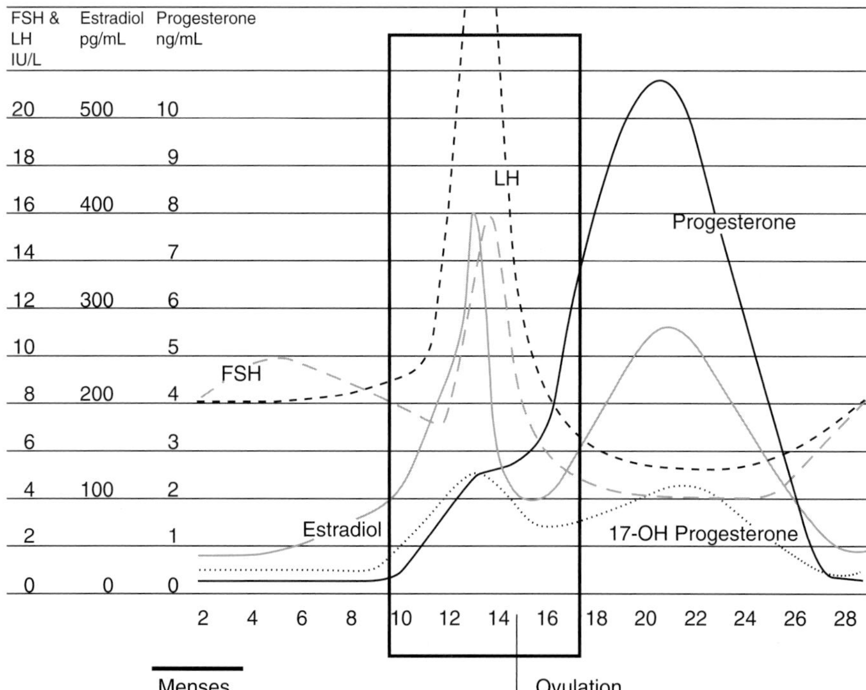

Fig. 1.16. Ovulation. The LH surge in response to stimulatory concentration and duration of E2. Note also a minor but still significant rise in FSH in response to initial rise in progesterone.

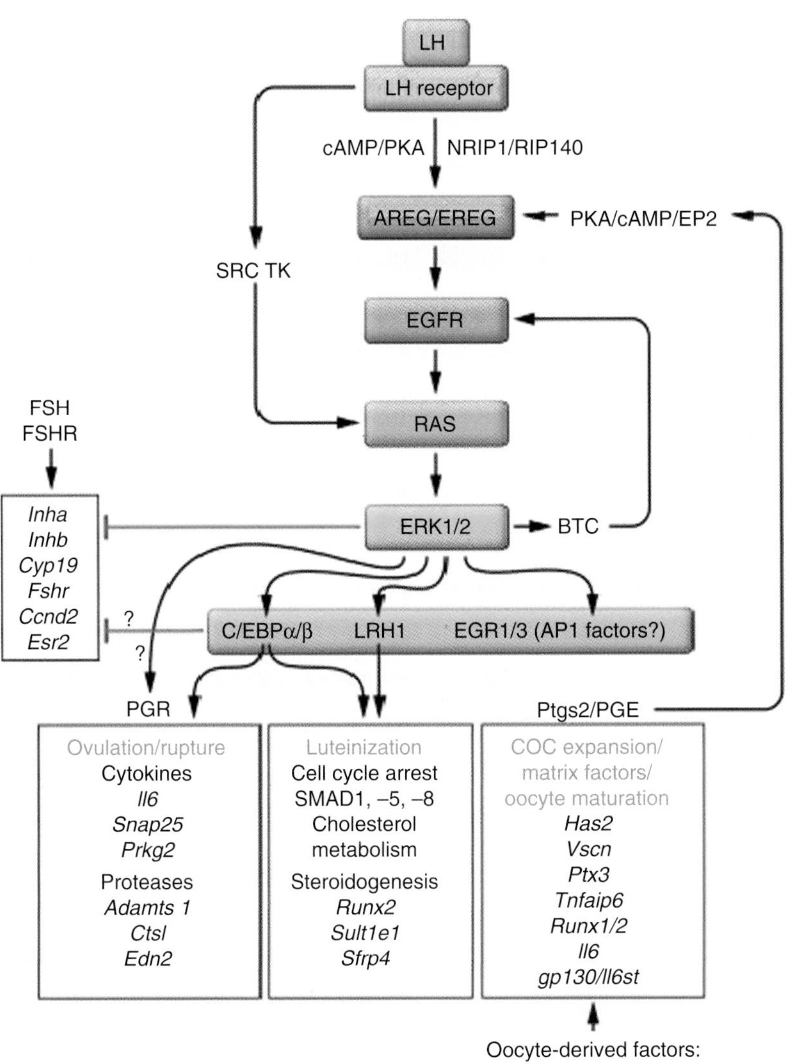

Fig. 1.17. LH mediated pathways to ovulation and luteinization. Note the presence of the "master switch" ERK1/2 which programs follicle rupture, granulosa luteinization and steroidogenesis, and cumulus-oocyte detachment and extrusion. Reproduced from reference [4], with permission.

- NR5A2 or LRH-1 (liver receptor homolog 1) and NR5A1 or SF-1 (steroidogenic factor 1). Both are essential to reorganizing, reprogramming, and stimulating steroid synthesis and granulosa luteinization
- C/EBP alpha/beta (enhancer binding proteins) are active in both luteinization, cholesterol metabolism, steroidogenesis, and particularly in the activation of progesterone receptor functions, i.e., promoting cytokine and protease activity in the mechanics of "ovulation," such as stigma formation and fracture of the follicle membrane
- EGR 1/3 (early growth response proteins 1/3) which activate prostaglandin synthase (prostaglandin F2 alpha and prostaglandin E) as well as Endothelin-1, each of which are involved in cumulus expansion and disruption and oocyte maturation (meiosis inhibition/dis-inhibition).

Taken together, LH directly influences the transformation of the ovulating follicle into a vascularized, luteinized granulosa cell structure with enhanced steroid synthetic capabilities. Through its direct effect on the COC by means of hyaluronidase action, it dissolves cell and cell–cell matrix integrity, weakens the cumulus anchoring to the basement membrane – all in preparation for ovulatory extrusion.

LH achieves these actions by inducing the ERK1–2 "master switch" which catalyzes the ovulatory follicle's synthesis of estradiol and progesterone, prostaglandins, nitric oxide synthesis and release, and targets innate immune response elements such as IL-6 and hyaluran synthesis. LH therefore expands and activates cumulus separation, luteinization, and progesterone and prostaglandin production and function.

Progesterone

As a result of the LH surge, local intra-follicular progesterone synthesis is stimulated by several factors [137]. These include increased LH receptor concentration and sensitivity on follicle granulosa cells, increased granulosa cell luteinization, increased cholesterol availability and function, and increased activity of steroid biosynthetic enzymes for progesterone synthesis (such as Star, P450scc).

As the COC expands and cell-to-cell paracrine function declines, local GDF-9, activin, and BMP-15, each specific inhibitors of luteinization and progesterone synthesis, are withdrawn. Progesterone synthesis therefore proceeds apace as a result of positive LH input and withdrawal of the inhibition imposed when the granulosa component of the cumulus was intact and autocrine paracrine inhibition was active.

Endocrine effects of progesterone

With ever-increasing ovarian progesterone synthesis and secretion still modest but rising, mid-cycle progesterone levels now achieve endocrinologic function [139,140]. Together with estradiol, these rising levels of progesterone enhance estradiol-positive feedback on both GnRH pulse and anterior pituitary LH surge responses. Progesterone also induces mid-cycle increased FSH secretion. Eventually, as progesterone concentrations increase still further into the luteal phase, progesterone negative feedback acts to terminate the LH surge at both the pituitary and hypothalamic GnRH levels.

Intra-follicular effects of progesterone

Complexing with its receptor PR, P induces three important features of ovulation:

- In partnership with prostaglandin, progesterone induces changes in follicle wall elasticity permitting additional antral distention and expansion [141]
- Stimulates proteolytic enzyme cascades with weakening and final rupture of the distended follicle at its stigma [142]
- Accelerates and completes oocyte meiosis [143]

LH concentrations rise early in the LH surge and intra-follicular progesterone concentrations increase and active secretion begins. In addition to its central effects on the FSH surge, progesterone increases the distensibility of the follicle wall by changing its elastic properties. This flexibility is necessary to compensate for the rapid increase in the follicular fluid volume which reflects the function of VEGF. This volume expansion occurs just before ovulation but is unaccompanied by a significant change in intra-follicular pressure. FSH and LH indirectly and progesterone directly stimulate the activity of proteolytic enzymes resulting in digestion of collagen in the follicular wall and increased distensibility. The proteolytic enzymes are activated in an orderly sequence. The granulosa cells produce plasminogen activators in response to the gonadotropin surge. Plasminogen activators produced by granulosa cells activate plasminogen in the follicle fluid to produce plasmin. Plasmin in turn generates active collagenase to disrupt the follicle wall.

"Ovulation" is the result of proteolytic digestion at the follicular apex, a site called the stigma. The matrix metalloproteinase enzymes and their endogenous inhibitors TIMPs increase in response to LH and progesterone and are also participants in modulating this event.

Acceleration and completion of meiosis 1

The role of progesterone in the progression and completion of meiosis 1 is well documented in amphibians [144,145]. In association with MAPK activity, progesterone stimulates chromosomal condensation, germinal vesicle breakdown, and spindle formation by means of CdC2/cyclin B promotion. A similar process exists in mammalia. In this instance, the MAPK induction of meiosis 1 is inhibited until ovulation by an oocyte meiosis inhibitor (OMI) produced in granulosa which maintains arrest by its action on Gs-linked receptor (GPR3) on the oocyte membrane.

Activation of GPR3 leads to cyclic AMP/PKA inhibition of the MAPK meiosis 1 program. Intra-follicular progesterone accumulation at the LH surge *reactivates* this MAPK meiosis 1 system by inhibiting the oocyte GPR3 receptor, eliminating possible activation of cyclic AMP. In addition, P induces cyclic nucleotide phosphodiesterase 3A, further diminishing cyclic AMP availability. Finally, granulosa OMI, the ligand for GPR3 (probably activin), is lost as paracrine contact between the oocyte and cumulus disintegrates during COC expansion and disruption.

Similarly, the factors inhibiting premature luteinization of the pre-ovulatory granulosa (oocyte GDF-9 and BMP-15), previously termed "LI-luteinization inhibiting factor," are also lost as paracrine gap junction transfer between oocyte and cumulus is withdrawn. Taken together, both the identity of the heretofore elusive but biologically critical OMI and LI, and the mechanisms by which LH and progesterone mitigate their function, are now more clearly understood.

Prostaglandins

Separately but also in overlapping synergism with other factors, prostaglandin activity promotes proteolysis, induces hyperemia, accentuates antral fluid accumulation and follicle distention, and induces peri-follicular smooth muscle contractions [146,147]. In addition, prostaglandins enhance the growth factor elements of the ERK1–ERK2 master switch pathway.

In response to the LH surge, prostaglandins E2 and F2α concentrations increase markedly in the pre-ovulatory follicle antral fluid reaching peak concentrations at ovulation. Inhibition of cyclooxygenase 2 (COX-2) synthesis of these products blocks follicle rupture without affecting the other LH-induced processes of luteinization or oocyte maturation. Prostaglandins act to free proteolytic enzymes within the follicle wall, and promote angiogenesis and hyperemia in an inflammatory-like response. LH and PGE2 both activate the epidermal growth factor-like signaling pathway that leads to cumulus expansion and resumption of oocyte meiosis.

Prostaglandins also contract smooth muscle cells identified in the peri-follicular wall thereby aiding the extrusion of the oocyte–cumulus cell mass. The ovulatory role of prostaglandins is so well documented that infertility patients should be advised to avoid the use of drugs that inhibit prostaglandin synthesis during diagnostic evaluation and ovulation induction therapy.

The role FSH

The mid-cycle FSH peak that responds to and is dependent on the pre-ovulatory rise of progesterone induces important ovulatory phase functions [4,148,149]. In a process called "expansion" (more appropriately the disruption and dissolution of the previously tight metabolic and mechanical linkage between oocyte and the cumulus granulosa cells – the COC), these cells respond to the FSH surge with secretion of hyaluronic acid, which disperses the cumulus cells and detaches the fragmenting COC complex from its anchor to the basal lamina. These changes allow the COC cell mass to become free-floating in the antral fluid immediately before follicle rupture and extrusion of the COC at ovulation.

On the other hand, the mural granulosa cells still attached to the basement membrane enclosing the follicle remain after ovulation and become the luteal cells of the corpus luteum. The mid-cycle surge of FSH repairs mechanical damage to these mural cells, stimulates further cellular proliferation (cell numbers) and induces the appropriate complement of LH receptors (functional capacity) necessary to support their physiologic responsibilities during the luteal phase.

Summary: the importance of H-P-O synchrony in ovulation

Simply an adequate gonadotropin surge does not ensure ovulation. The follicle must be at the appropriate stage of maturity in order for it to respond to the ovulating stimulus. In the normal cycle, gonadotropin release and final maturation of the follicle coincide because the timing of the gonadotropin surge is controlled by the level of estradiol which in turn reflects the degree of follicle growth, function, and maturation. Ovulatory gonadotropin release and Graafian maturity are exquisitely coordinated in time. In the majority of human cycles, this system of requisite feedback relationships, both in the early follicle selection phase (FSH) and at ovulation (LH) permit only one follicle to reach the point of ovulation. These "natural" physiologic feedback restraints are abrogated in exogenous recombinant FSH or Human Menopausal Gonadotropin induction of multiple ovulations.

The corpus luteum

The transformation of the dominant follicle to a corpus luteum

Before rupture of the follicle and release of the oocyte, the mural granulosa cells have begun to enlarge, become vacuolated and fill with lutein as part of the luteinization process and transformation into the new functional unit, the corpus luteum. In the first few days after ovulation, granulosa cell enlargement begins to compress the now vacant antral cavity and will eventually form a solid cell mass of brightly luteinized yellow granulosa. With dissolution of the basal lamina, capillaries penetrate the granulosa cell mass [150]. Often the central cavity will transiently fill with blood, which swiftly re-absorbs as granulosa enlargement and vascularization progresses. This rapid and intense angiogenesis is essential as the afferent route for cholesterol substrate delivery to support the massive demands for steroid (progesterone) synthesis and the efferent channels for maximal secretion [151].

LH-induced VEGF and angiopoietins promote and stabilize this vascular network. Within 8 days of ovulation, the former avascular granulosa cells of the follicle are now fully vascularized and luteinized. The thecal mantle, so prominent in the dominant follicle, with dissolution of the basal lamina becomes an almost indistinguishable element in the granulosa-dominated corpus luteum structure. Such robust vascularization does carry some clinical risks. Possessing among the highest blood flows per unit mass, formation of the corpus luteum in women with bleeding disorders or on anticoagulant therapy carries the risk of hemorrhage occasionally severe enough to require surgical intervention.

The cells of the corpus luteum

The corpus luteum should not be viewed solely as a luteinized granulosa cell organ [152]. In addition to the luteal cells, the total cell population is made up of endothelial cells, leukocytes, and fibroblasts, and all are critical to corpus luteum maintenance and stability. Together the non-steroidogenic cells produce prostaglandins, growth factors, angiogenic factors, cytokines, and blood flow regulators. Cross-talk among the various cell groups is essential to normal function. Endothelia contribute vasoactive controls, while steroids influence angiogenesis.

TGF-beta promotes growth, whereas TNF-alpha constrains and limits growth. Nitric oxide synthesis and production is balanced by the vasoconstrictor endothelin-1. Finally, cell growth and maintenance are also balanced by pro- and anti-apoptotic programs. Not even the luteal cells are homogeneous; large and small cells exist. The large cells, presumably former granulosa cells, possess the steroid synthetic enzymatic machinery to produce estradiol and progesterone: particularly, limited P450 C-17 permitting excess progesterone secretion but adequate aromatase substrate for ample estradiol synthesis and secretion.

Large cells also produce a variety of peptides, including oxytocin, relaxin, inhibin A, growth factors, and prostaglandins. Gap junctions regulated by oxytocin connect large cells to small cells presumably originally theca which possess LH and hCG receptors [153]. This LH/HCG reaction system is essential to sustain the endocrine function of the corpus luteum and is maintained by local action of endogenous progesterone which increases LH receptor number and sensitivity to the low gonadotropin LH levels of the luteal phase.

The luteal phase

The importance of luteal phase progesterone

LH stimulation of LHR regulates the LDL/cholesterol transport and availability of cholesterol substrate for steroidogenesis, principally progesterone production. LDL binding to its receptor, internalization of the LDL-cholesterol complex, and post-receptor processing is entirely LH dependent [151]. Cholesterol is then transported to the mitochondria in the first steps of progesterone synthesis. Progesterone secretion increases by day 3 of the corpus luteum phase and rises swiftly to peak as high as 30 ng/mL at day 8 of the luteal phase.

Progesterone must (1) induce secretion of nutrients from the endometrial glands in sufficient quantity and quality to meet the needs of the morula/blastocyst as it enters the uterine cavity but remains unattached; (2) stimulate endometrial superficial capillary and arteriolar complexity; (3) prepare and support the endometrium for trophoblast attachment, implantation, and development of the rudimentary hemo-chorial placenta; (4) induce mechanical stability by decidualization of superficial stromal cells; (5) with estrogen, suppress gonadotropin to avoid supernumerary ovulation, and (6) with estrogen, stabilize the endometrium to avoid premature tissue dissolution and disruption. All this must be accomplished within the luteal phase programmed life span of 14 days and/or until the corpus luteum is rescued by rising levels of hCG. Without this salvage mechanism luteolysis occurs, P, E2, and inhibin A are withdrawn, and menses begin.

The importance of gonadotropins

Although negative feedback of serum estradiol and progesterone leads to suppression of FSH and LH during the luteal phase, continued availability of gonadotropins even at low levels is essential [154]. For LH, this dependence is graphically demonstrated in ovulation induction practices in hypophysectomized women. Either longer acting hCG or daily administration of LH is necessary to sustain corpus luteum function. GnRH agonist suppression of LH promptly induces luteolysis substantiating the importance of GnRH pulses, despite the prolonged frequency interval (roughly every 200 min) [155].

As noted, LH plays a critical role in progesterone biosynthesis and secretion by its classic induction of cholesterol side chain cleavage and up-regulation of the variety of steroidogenic enzymes, which ensures continued high-level progesterone secretion. Finally, LH ensures delivery of these steroids by inducing extensive corpus luteum angiogenesis and vascularization.

Like LH, FSH also provides important support for the corpus luteum. In addition to the mid-cycle surge of FSH which is crucial to enhance granulosa cell repair, capacity, and function, the low level of FSH throughout the luteal phase continues to support granulosa cell integrity and sustains adequate numbers of LH receptors on these cells.

Luteolysis

In the normal cycle, the lifespan of the corpus luteum is tightly controlled [156]. The interval between the mid-cycle LH surge and menses is consistently close to 14 days with a "normal" range of 11–17 days. Cycle length varies as follicle phase duration varies; the luteal phase remains constant in all non-pregnancy ovulatory cycles [157]. Luteolysis (programmed death) of the corpus luteum is an active process. The corpus luteum can be preserved for no more than 6–8 weeks into gestation and only as a result of the availability and rapidly increasing rescuing levels of hCG secreted from an expanding mass of healthy growing trophoblast of an implanted pregnancy. Uterine bleeding in ectopic gestation occurs due to corpus luteum demise despite elevated but insufficient, plateauing levels of hCG.

The luteolytic program is initiated approximately 9–11 days post-ovulation. Whereas how the corpus luteum is formed and the details of how it functions are reasonably understood and appear straightforward, the luteolytic mechanisms in humans remain a mystery. It is unclear why the corpus luteum dies, why its functional duration is so tightly controlled, what prompts its activation and why it is so resistant to reversal except by means of semi-log increments of hCG. Some fundamental elements of the mystery have been clarified.

- Maintenance of LH secretion by GnRH pump does not alter the onset or pace of luteolysis. It is not LH receptor or GnRH dependent [158]
- Contrary to the process of luteolysis in ruminants, removal of the human uterus does not change the ovarian cycle; women with Mullerian agenesis display cyclic repetitive ovulations. The uterus is not the source of luteolytic PGF 2α as in ruminants [156]
- Corpus luteum cell death is a local phenomenon. Current theories of luteolytic mechanism (among others):
  - Increased matrix metalloproteinases (MMPs). Fibroblasts release MMPs and do not possess LHRs but do react to activin with synthesis and release of MMPs [159]
  - Leukocytes produce interleukins which induce cytolytic enzymes. This reaction is induced by a buildup of peroxynitrites by the relative hypoxia secondary to endothelin-1 vasoconstriction [160,161]

In summary, the hypothetical mechanisms of luteolysis are numerous – PGF2α and endothelin 1 (vasoconstriction), local GnRH (downregulation of LH receptors), estrogen-induced apoptosis, and so on are all biologically plausible but remain unproven.

The luteal–follicular transition

The events which occur following luteolysis, during an interval called the luteal–follicular transition phase (Fig. 1.18) have crucial bearing on the success of the next follicle phase [162]. Specifically, the decline of the corpus luteum sets in motion the cyclic recruitment of available antral follicles for possible ovulation in the next cycle [162]. The demise of the corpus luteum results in decline of serum estradiol, progesterone and inhibin A [163]. The withdrawal of these inhibitory influences eliminates the negative feedback on FSH and LH that prevails throughout the luteal phase. In the absence of negative feedback, GnRH pulses gradually return to early follicle phase frequency and amplitude, leading to increased synthesis and secretion of FSH [124,164].

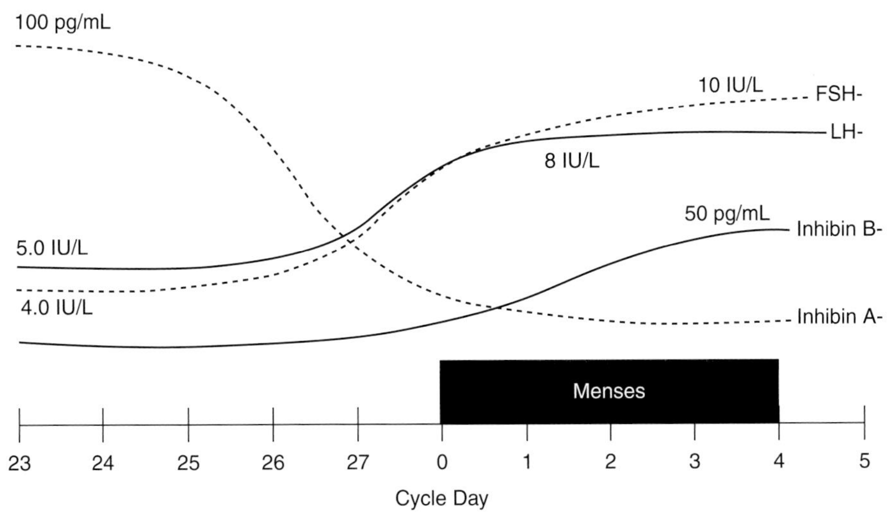

Fig. 1.18. The luteal–follicular phase transition, with the demise of the corpus luteum, withdrawal of the combined negative feedback of inhibin A, estradiol and progesterone, FSH and to a lesser extent LH resume secretion from the anterior pituitary. The impact of this renewed FSH stimulus on the "rescued" recruited follicles can be seen in the increased concentrations of inhibin B.

The combination of withdrawal of inhibin A and the low levels of estradiol typical of menses and the early follicle phase magnify the increased FSH secretory response to rising GnRH pulses and frequency [122]. The rise in FSH (from luteal phase levels of 4 IU/L to early follicular phase 10 IU/L) meet the dual physiologic requirements of concentration threshold and appropriate duration of availability to rescue a cohort of small antral follicles from atresia and propel some of this cyclically recruited group to further selection and generation of the next dominant follicle.

Conclusion: the regulation of the ovarian cycle

This chapter has focused on the chronicle of hypothalamic–anterior pituitary–ovarian follicle events which involve intrinsic and where appropriate endocrine events in gonadogenesis, primordial follicle formation, follicle arrest, reactivation, recruitment, selection, dominance, ovulation, and corpus luteum function. In this depiction, the crucial importance of the timely appearance, concentrations, and sequence of gonadotropins FSH and LH was emphasized. As seen in normal ovulatory cycles, this sequence involves timely interactions between steroid and peptide hormones. The feedback signals of the ovary (0) to the hypothalamus (H) and to the gonadotropins of the anterior pituitary (P) involve both negative and positive feedback instructions, a circumstance unique to the female H-P-O.

The efferent portion of the link involves FSH and LH. The sustaining importance of GnRH pulses in the synthesis, packaging, transport to the cell membrane, and timely secretion of gonadotropin is an absolute requirement for the normal function of this system. The influence of the Kisspeptin/GPR54 system, corticotropin-releasing hormone (CRH), opioids, TSH/thyroid hormone, ACTH, prolactin, and insulin among others, affects the integrity of this basic system and underscores how perturbations in each might cause dysfunction and disease are recognized.

It is instructive to view the H-P-O cyclic process as a sequence of three mandatory recycling events by which the ovary asserts its readiness to proceed successfully through each phase of the cycle.

Recycling event 1: rescue, recruitment, and selection of the dominant follicle

This crucial transitional luteal–follicular phase step provides the necessary FSH to rescue and recruit an emerging, available group of small antral follicles. As corpus luteum function declines, GnRH and FSH are freed from intense negative feedback induced by luteal progesterone, estradiol, and inhibin A. These factors must fall to levels low enough and over a sufficient period of time to allow FSH to meet the concentration and duration requirements for follicle rescue recruitment and selection. A rise in potential FSH inhibiting levels of estradiol and inhibin B is *delayed* to later in the cycle but not so long as to permit superovulation.

Recycling event 2: ovulation and corpus luteum formation

This step involves the positive feedback of estradiol and the initiation of the ovulatory LH surge. The dominant follicle signifies its readiness to ovulate by this endocrine message because it reflects directly the number and function of the granulosa cells of the pre-ovulatory follicle but also indirectly the entire array of support factors involved in dominant follicle generation and oocyte maturation. The physiologic parameters of estradiol feedback and the threshold for LH stimulation leading to an LH surge are achieved within a very narrow and highly specific window. Experience with exogenous gonadotropin stimulation of ovulation has underlined the detrimental effects of too early or excessive delay in LH or hCG administration.

If these elements (follicle readiness and an LH surge) are in correct alignment, then mandatory recycling event number 2 (ovulation and the formation of the corpus luteum) is successfully completed. The earlier decline in inhibin B and the delay in the rise of inhibin A well into the luteal phase permits an ancillary FSH secretory surge with benefit to granulosa cell repair and appropriate LH receptor endowment of the new corpus luteum.

Recycling event 3: corpus luteum rescue or luteolysis

The corpus luteum has a programmed life span of roughly 2 weeks. Luteolysis will take place unless rescue levels hCG becomes available. Recycling event number 3 depends upon whether the life of the corpus luteum is extended and the suppressive feedback of estradiol, progesterone and inhibin A is sustained. In the absence of pregnancy and absence of HCG, luteolysis proceeds unimpeded, and the events associated with mandatory recycling event number 1 are reopened.

Summary

In this chapter, the advances in ovarian endocrinology, molecular biology, molecular genetics, and the powerful transgene and knockout technologies have provided a new and exciting insight into the life history of the human ovarian follicle, corpus luteum formation, and function. Both the intrinsic, intra-follicle, and extrinsic endocrine factors controlling these events have been described and emphasized. Accordingly, the emphasis has been less on morphology and more on the exquisitely timed, interactive, interdependent synchronized molecular events which drive the crucial elements which promote and sustain the self-perpetuating, repetitive recycling events leading to successful reproduction.

References

1. Fritz MA, Speroff L. Clinical Gynecologic Endocrinology and Infertility. 8th edition. Philadelphia: Lippincott, Williams and Wilkins; 2011.
2. Oktem O, Urman B. Understanding follicle growth in vivo. Hum Reprod. 2010;**25**(12): 2944–54.
3. McGee EA, Hsueh AJ. Initial and cyclic recruitment of ovarian follicles. Endocr Rev. 2000;**21**(2): 200–14.
4. Richards JS, Pangas SA. The ovary: basic biology and clinical implications. J Clin Invest. 2010;**120**(4):963–72.
5. Knight PG, Glister C. TGF-beta superfamily members and ovarian follicle development. Reproduction. 2006;**132**(2):191–206.
6. Mais V, Kazer RR, Cetel NS, et al. The dependency of folliculogenesis and corpus luteum function on pulsatile gonadotropin secretion in cycling women using a gonadotropin-releasing hormone antagonist as a probe. J Clin Endocrinol Metab. 1986;**62**(6):1250–5.
7. Trombly DJ, Woodruff TK, Mayo KE. Roles for transforming growth factor beta superfamily proteins in early folliculogenesis. Semin Reprod Med. 2009;**27**(1):14–23.
8. Visser JA, Themmen AP. Anti-Müllerian hormone and folliculogenesis. Mol Cell Endocrinol. 2005;**234**(1–2):81–6.
9. van Rooij IA, Broekmans FJ, Scheffer GJ, et al. Serum antimullerian hormone levels best reflect the reproductive decline with age in normal women with proven fertility: a longitudinal study. Fertil Steril. 2005;**83**(4):979–87.
10. Pangas SA, Jorgez CJ, Tran M, et al. Intraovarian activins are required for female fertility. Mol Endocrinol. 2007;**21**(10):2458–71.
11. Zhao J, Taverne MA, van der Weijden GC, et al. Effect of activin A on in vitro development of rat preantral follicles and localization of activin A and activin receptor II. Biol Reprod. 2001;**65** (3):967–77.
12. Smitz J, Cortvrindt R. Inhibin A and B secretion in mouse preantral follicle culture. Hum Reprod. 1998;**13** (4):927–35.
13. Alak BM, Coskun S, Friedman CI, et al. Activin A stimulates meiotic maturation of human oocytes and modulates granulosa cell steroidogenesis in vitro. Fertil Steril. 1998;**70**(6):1126–30.
14. Giudice LC. Insulin-like growth factors and ovarian follicular development. Endo Rev. 1992;**13**:641–69.
15. el-Roely A, Chen X, Roberts VJ, et al. Expression of insulin-like growth factor-I (IGF-I) and IGF-II and the IGF-I, IGF-II, and insulin receptor genes and localization of the gene products in the human ovary. J Clin Endocrinol Metab. 1993;77(5):1411–18.
16. Dor J, Ben-Shlomo I, Lunenfeld B, et al. Insulin-like growth factor-I (IGF-I) may not be essential for ovarian follicular development: evidence from IGF-I deficiency. J Clin Endocrinol Metab. 1992;**74**(3):539–42.
17. Palter SF, Tavares AB, Hourvitz A, Veldhuis JD, Adashi AY. Are estrogens of import to primate/human ovarian folliculogenesis? Endocr Rev. 2001;**22**:389–424.
18. Fowler PA, Anderson RA, Saunders PT, et al. Development of steroid signaling pathways during primordial follicle formation in the human fetal ovary. J Clin Endocrinol Metab. 2011;**96**:1754–62.
19. Ben-Chetrit A, Gotlieb L, Wong PY, et al. Ovarian response to recombinant human follicle-stimulating hormone in luteinizing hormone-depleted women: examination of the two cell, two gonadotropin theory. Fertil Steril. 1996;**65**(4):711–17.
20. Karnitis VJ, Townson DH, Friedman CI, et al. Recombinant human follicle-stimulating hormone stimulates multiple follicular growth, but minimal estrogen production in gonadotropin-releasing hormone antagonist-treated monkeys: examining the role of luteinizing hormone in follicular development and steroidogenesis. J Clin Endocrinol Metab. 1994;**79**(1):91–7.
21. Rabinovici J, Blankstein J, Goldman B, et al. In vitro fertilization and primary

embryonic cleavage are possible in 17 alpha-hydroxylase deficiency despite extremely low intrafollicular 17 beta-estradiol. J Clin Endocrinol Metab. 1989;**68**(3):693–7.

22. Robker RL, Akison LK, Russell DL. Control of oocyte release by progesterone receptor-regulated gene expression. Nucl Recept Signal. 2009;**7**:e012.

23. Tena-Sempere M. Kisspeptin signaling in the brain: recent developments and future challenges. Mol Cell Endocrinol. 2010;**314**(2):164–9.

24. Roa J, Aguilar E, Dieguez C, et al. New frontiers in kisspeptin/GPR54 physiology as fundamental gatekeepers of reproductive function. Front Neuroendocrinol. 2008;**29**(1):48–69.

25. Oakley AE, Clifton DK, Steiner RA. Kisspeptin signaling in the brain. Endocr Rev. 2009;**30**(6):713–43.

26. Roa J, Castellano JM, Navarro VM, et al. Kisspeptins and the control of gonadotropin secretion in male and female rodents. Peptides. 2009;**30**(1):57–66.

27. Whitlock KE. Origin and development of GnRH neurons. Trends Endocrinol Metab. 2005;**16**(4):145–51.

28. Marshall JC, Dalkin AC, Haisenleder DJ, et al. Gonadotropin-releasing hormone pulses: regulators of gonadotropin synthesis and ovulatory cycles. Recent Prog Horm Res. 1991;**47**:155–87.

29. Filicori M, Santoro N, Merriam GR, et al. Characterization of the physiological pattern of episodic gonadotropin secretion throughout the human menstrual cycle. J Clin Endocrinol Metab. 1986;**62**(6):1136–44.

30. Ottowitz WE, Dougherty DD, Fischman AJ, et al. [18F]2-fluoro-2-deoxy-D-glucose positron emission tomography demonstration of estrogen negative and positive feedback on luteinizing hormone secretion in women. J Clin Endocrinol Metab. 2008;**93**(8):3208–14.

31. Chappel SC, Resko JA, Norman RL, et al. Studies in rhesus monkeys on the site where estrogen inhibits gonadotropins: delivery of 17 beta-estradiol to the hypothalamus and pituitary gland. J Clin Endocrinol Metab. 1981;**52**(1):1–8.

32. Wildt L, Hutchison JS, Marshall G, et al. On the site of action of progesterone in the blockade of the estradiol-induced gonadotropin discharge in the rhesus monkey. Endocrinology. 1981;**109**(4):1293–4.

33. Wetsel WC, Valença MM, Merchenthaler I, et al. Intrinsic pulsatile secretory activity of immortalized luteinizing hormone-releasing hormone-secreting neurons. Proc Natl Acad Sci U S A. 1992;**89**(9):4149–53.

34. Winters SJ, Moore JP. Paracrine control of gonadotrophs. Semin Reprod Med. 2007;**25**(5):379–87.

35. Richards JS, Fitzpatrick SL, Clemens JW, et al. Ovarian cell differentiation: a cascade of multiple hormones, cellular signals, and regulated genes. Recent Prog Horm Res. 1995;**50**:223–54.

36. Deroo BJ, Rodriguez KF, Couse JF, et al. Estrogen receptor beta is required for optimal cAMP production in mouse granulosa cells. Mol Endocrinol. 2009;**23**(7):955–65.

37. Parakh TN, Hernandez JA, Grammer JC, et al. Follicle-stimulating hormone/cAMP regulation of aromatase gene expression requires beta-catenin. Proc Natl Acad Sci USA. 2006;**103**(33):12435–40.

38. Van Wagenen G, Simpson ME. Embryology of the Ovary and Testes in "*Homo sapiens* and *Macaca mulatta*." New Haven, CN: Yale University Press; 1965.

39. Tomizuka K, Horikoshi K, Kitada R, et al. R-spondin1 plays an essential role in ovarian development through positively regulating Wnt-4 signaling. Hum Mol Genet. 2008;**17**(9):1278–91.

40. Ottolenghi C, Pelosi E, Tran J, et al. Loss of Wnt4 and Foxl2 leads to female-to-male sex reversal extending to germ cells. Hum Mol Genet. 2007;**16**(23):2795–804.

41. Ying Y, Qi X, Zhao GQ. Induction of primordial germ cells from murine epiblasts by synergistic action of BMP4 and BMP8B signaling pathways. Proc Natl Acad Sci USA. 2001;**98**(14):7858–62.

42. Ohinata Y, Ohta H, Shigeta M, et al. A signaling principle for the specification of the germ cell lineage in mice. Cell. 2009;**137**(3):571–84.

43. Saitou M, Barton SC, Surani MA. A molecular programme for the specification of germ cell fate in mice. Nature. 2002;**418**(6895):293–300.

44. Thomas FH, Vanderhyden BC. Oocyte-granulosa cell interactions during mouse follicular development: regulation of kit ligand expression and its role in oocyte growth. Reprod Biol Endocrinol. 2006;**4**:19.

45. Baker TG. A quantitative and cytological study of germ cells in human ovaries. Proc R Soc Lond B Biol Sci. 1963;**158**:417–33.

46. De Pol A, Vaccina F, Forabosco A, et al. Apoptosis of germ cells during human prenatal oogenesis. Hum Reprod. 1997;**12**(10):2235–41.

47. Pangas SA, Rajkovic A. Transcriptional regulation of early oogenesis: in search of masters. Hum Reprod Update. 2006;**12**(1):65–76.

48. Maheshwari A, Fowler PA. Primordial follicular assembly in humans – revisited. Zygote. 2008;**16**(4):285–96.

49. Baltus AE, Menke DB, Hu YC, et al. In germ cells of mouse embryonic ovaries, the decision to enter meiosis precedes premeiotic DNA replication. Nat Genet. 2006;**38**(12):1430–4.

50. Kezele P, Nilsson E, Skinner MK. Cell–cell interactions in primordial follicle assembly and development. Front Biosci. 2002;**7**:d1990–6.

51. Fortune JE, Cushman RA, Wahl CM, et al. The primordial to primary follicle transition. Mol Cell Endocrinol. 2000;**163**(1–2):53–60.

52. Skinner MK. Regulation of primordial follicle assembly and development. Hum Reprod Update. 2005;**11**(5):461–71.

53. Reddy P, Zheng W, Liu K. Mechanisms maintaining the dormancy and survival of mammalian primordial follicles. Trends Endocrinol Metab. 2010;**21**(2):96–103.

54. Hansen KR, Knowlton NS, Thyer AC, et al. A new model of reproductive aging: the decline in ovarian non-growing follicle number from birth to menopause. Hum Reprod. 2008;**23**(3):699–708.

55. John GB, Gallardo TD, Shirley LJ, et al. Foxo3 is a PI3K-dependent molecular switch controlling the initiation of oocyte growth. Dev Biol. 2008;**321**(1):197–204.

56. Reddy P, Adhikari D, Zheng W, et al. PDK1 signaling in oocytes controls reproductive aging and lifespan by manipulating the survival of primordial follicles. Hum Mol Genet. 2009;**18**(15):2813–24.

57. Cantley LC. The phosphoinositide 3-kinase pathway. Science. 2002;**296**(5573):1655–7.

58. Engelman JA, Luo J, Cantley LC. The evolution of phosphatidylinositol 3-kinases as regulators of growth and metabolism. Nat Rev Genet. 2006;7(8):606–19.

59. Vanhaesebroeck B, Ali K, Bilancio A, et al. Signalling by PI3K isoforms: insights from gene-targeted mice. Trends Biochem Sci. 2005;**30**(4):194–204.

60. Oktem O, Oktay K. The ovary: anatomy and function throughout human life. Ann N Y Acad Sci. 2008;**1127**:1–9.

61. Skinner MK. Regulation of primordial follicle assembly and development. Hum Reprod Update. 2005;**11**(5):461–71.

62. Gougeon A, Ecochard R, Thalabard JC. Age-related changes of the population of human ovarian follicles: increase in the disappearance rate of non-growing and early-growing follicles in aging women. Biol Reprod. 1994;**50**(3):653–63.

63. Baker TG, Scrimgeour JB. Development of the gonad in normal and anencephalic human fetuses. J Reprod Fertil. 1980;**60**(1):193–9.

64. Halpin DM, Jones A, Fink G, Charlton HM. Postnatal ovarian follicle development in hypogonadal (hpg) and normal mice and associated changes in the hypothalamic-pituitary axis. J Reprod Fertil. 1986;**77**:287–96.

65. Shimasaki S, Moore RK, Otsuka F, et al. The bone morphogenetic protein system in mammalian reproduction. Endocr Rev. 2004;**25**(1):72–101.

66. Nilsson EE, Skinner MK. Bone morphogenetic protein-4 acts as an ovarian follicle survival factor and promotes primordial follicle development. Biol Reprod. 2003;**69**(4):1265–72.

67. Hreinsson JG, Scott JE, Rasmussen C, et al. Growth differentiation factor-9 promotes the growth, development, and survival of human ovarian follicles in organ culture. J Clin Endocrinol Metab. 2002;**87**(1):316–21.

68. Hanrahan JP, Gregan SM, Mulsant P, et al. Mutations in the genes for oocyte-derived growth factors GDF9 and BMP15 are associated with both increased ovulation rate and sterility in Cambridge and Belclare sheep (*Ovis aries*). Biol Reprod. 2004;**70**(4):900–9.

69. Salmon NA, Handyside AH, Joyce IM. Oocyte regulation of anti-Müllerian hormone expression in granulosa cells during ovarian follicle development in mice. Dev Biol. 2004;**266**(1):201–8.

70. Parrott JA, Skinner MK. Thecal cell–granulosa cell interactions involve a positive feedback loop among keratinocyte growth factor, hepatocyte growth factor, and Kit ligand during ovarian follicular development. Endocrinology. 1998;**139**(5):2240–5.

71. Nilsson EE, Skinner MK. Growth and differentiation factor-9 stimulates progression of early primary but not primordial rat ovarian follicle development. Biol Reprod. 2002;**67**(3):1018–24.

72. Nilsson EE, Skinner MK. Kit ligand and basic fibroblast growth factor interactions in the induction of ovarian primordial to primary follicle transition. Mol Cell Endocrinol. 2004;**214**(1–2):19–25.

73. Zou K, Yuan Z, Yang Z, et al. Production of offspring from a germline stem cell line derived from neonatal ovaries. Nat Cell Biol. 2009;**11**(5):631–6.

74. Woods DC, Tilly JL. The next (re)generation of ovarian biology and fertility in women: is current science tomorrow's practice? Fertil Steril. 2012;**98**(1):3–10.

75. Findlay JK, Drummond AE, Dyson ML, et al. Recruitment and development of the follicle; the roles of the transforming growth factor-beta superfamily. Mol Cell Endocrinol. 2002;**191**(1):35–43.

76. Juengel JL, McNatty KP. The role of proteins of the transforming growth factor-beta superfamily in the intraovarian regulation of follicular development. Hum Reprod Update. 2005;**11**(2):143–60.

77. Visser JA, Themmen AP. Anti-Müllerian hormone and folliculogenesis. Mol Cell Endocrinol. 2005;**234**(1–2):81–6.

78. Goldenberg RL, Powell RD, Rosen SW, et al. Ovarian morphology in women with anosmia and hypogonadotropic hypogonadism. Am J Obstet Gynecol. 1976;**126**(1):91–4.

79. Oktay K, Briggs D, Gosden RG. Ontogeny of follicle-stimulating hormone receptor gene expression in isolated human ovarian follicles. J Clin Endocrinol Metab. 1997;**82**(11):3748–51.

80. Nakai Y, Plant TM, Hess DL, et al. On the sites of the negative and positive feedback actions of estradiol in the control of gonadotropin secretion in the rhesus monkey. Endocrinology. 1978;**102**(4):1008–14.

81. Marshall JC, Dalkin AC, Haisenleder DJ, et al. Gonadotropin-releasing hormone pulses: regulators of gonadotropin synthesis and ovulatory cycles. Recent Prog Horm Res. 1991;**47**:155–87.

82. Mais V, Kazer RR, Cetel NS, et al. The dependency of folliculogenesis and corpus luteum function on pulsatile gonadotropin secretion in cycling women using a gonadotropin-releasing hormone antagonist as a probe. J Clin Endocrinol Metab. 1986;**62**(6):1250–5.

83. Yen SS, Lein A. The apparent paradox of the negative and positive feedback control system on gonadotropin secretion. Am J Obstet Gynecol. 1976;**126**(7):942–54.

84. Hoff JD, Quigley ME, Yen SS. Hormonal dynamics at midcycle: a reevaluation. J Clin Endocrinol Metab. 1983;**57**(4):792–6.

85. Ferin M, Rosenblatt H, Carmel PW, et al. Estrogen-induced gonadotropin surges in female rhesus monkeys after pituitary stalk section. Endocrinology. 1979;**104**(1):50–2.

86. Herbison, AE. Multimodel influence of estrogen upon gonadotropin-re;easing neurons. Endocr Rev. 1998;**19**:302–38.

87. Hrabovszky E, Shughrue PJ, Merchenthaler I, et al. Detection of estrogen receptor-β messenger ribonucleic acid and 125I-estrogen binding sites in luteinizing hormone-releasing hormone neurons of the rat brain. Endocrinology. 2000;**141**:3506–9.

88. Abraham IM, Han S-K, Todman MG, Kroach KS, Herbison AE. Estrogen receptor β mediates rapid estrogen actions on gonadotropin-releasing hormone neurons in vivo. J Neurosci. 2003;**23**(13):5771–7.

89. Radovick S, Ticknor CM, Nakayama Y, et al. Evidence for direct estrogen regulation of the human gonadotropin-releasing hormone gene. Clin Invest. 1991;**88**:1649–55.

90. Urban RJ, Veldhuis JD, Dufau ML. Estrogen regulates the gonadotropin-releasing hormone-stimulated secretion

of biologically active luteinizing hormone. J Clin Endocrinol Metab. 1991;**72**(3):660–8.

91. Evans NP, Dahl GE, Mauger D, Karsch FJ. Estradiol induces both qualitative and quantitative changes in the pattern of gonadotropin-releasing hormone secretion during the presurge period in the ewe. Endocrinology. 1995;**136**:1603–9.
92. Liu JH, Yen SS. Induction of midcycle gonadotropin surge by ovarian steroids in women: a critical evaluation. J Clin Endocrinol Metab. 1983;**57**(4):797–802.
93. Waring DW, Turgeon JL. A pathway for luteinizing hormone releasing-hormone self-potentiation: cross-talk with the progesterone receptor. Endocrinology. 1992;**130**:3275–82.
94. Wildt L, Hutchison JS, Marshall G, et al. On the site of action of progesterone in the blockade of the estradiol-induced gonadotropin discharge in the rhesus monkey. Endocrinology. 1981;**109**(4):1293–4.
95. Plant TM. Hypothalamic control of the pituitary-gonadal axis in higher primates: key advances over the last two decades. J Neuroendocrinol. 2008;**20**:719–26.
96. Kaplan SL, Grumbach MM, Aubert ML. The ontogenesis of pituitary hormones and hypothalamic factors in the human fetus: maturation of central nervous system regulation of anterior pituitary function. Recent Prog Horm Res. 1976;**32**:161–243.
97. Kaplan SL, Grumbach MM. Pituitary and placental gonadotrophins and sex steroids in the human and sub-human primate fetus. Clin Endocrinol Metab. 1978;7(3): 487–511.
98. Winter JS, Hughes IA, Reyes FI, et al. Pituitary-gonadal relations in infancy: 2. Patterns of serum gonadal steroid concentrations in man from birth to two years of age. J Clin Endocrinol Metab. 1976;**42**(4):679–86.
99. Burger HG, Yamada Y, Bangah ML, McCloud PI, Warne GL. Serum gonadotropin, sex steroid, and immunoreactive inhibin levels in the first two years of life. J Clin Endocrinol Metab. 1991;**72**(3):682–6.
100. Wildt L, Marshall G, Knobil E. Experimental induction of puberty in the infantile female rhesus monkey. Science. 1980;**207**(4437):1373–5.
101. Conte FA, Grumbach MM, Kaplan SL. A diphasic pattern of gonadotropin secretion in patients with the syndrome of gonadal dysgenesis. J Clin Endocrinol Metab. 1975;**40**(4):670–4.
102. Mitsushima D, Hei DL, Terasawa E. Gamma-aminobutyric acid is an inhibitory neurotransmitter restricting the release of luteinizing hormone-releasing hormone before the onset of puberty. Proc Natl Acad Sci USA. 1994;**91**(1):395–9.
103. Mitsushima D, Marzban F, Luchansky LL, et al. Role of glutamic acid decarboxylase in the prepubertal inhibition of the luteinizing hormone-releasing hormone release in female rhesus monkeys. J Neurosci. 1996;**16** (8):2563–73.
104. Pau KY, Berria M, Hess DL, et al. Hypothalamic site-dependent effects of neuropeptide Y on gonadotropin-releasing hormone secretion in rhesus macaques. J Neuroendocrinol. 1995;7(1):63–7.
105. El Majdoubi M, Sahu A, Ramaswamy S, et al. Neuropeptide Y: a hypothalamic brake restraining the onset of puberty in primates. Proc Natl Acad Sci U S A. 2000;**97**(11):6179–84.
106. Gore AC, Mitsushima D, Terasawa E. A possible role of neuropeptide Y in the control of the onset of puberty in female rhesus monkeys. Neuroendocrinology. 1993;**58**(1):23–34.
107. Braun DW. Excitatory amino acids: evidence for a role in the control of reproduction and anterior pituitary hormone secretion. Endocr Rev. 1997;**18**:678–700.
108. Frisch R, Revelle R. Variation in body weights and the age of the adolescent growth spurt among Latin American and Asian populations, in relation to calorie supplies. Hum Biol. 1969;**41**(2):185–212.
109. Frisch RE, Revelle R, Cook S. Components of weight at menarche and the initiation of the adolescent growth spurt in girls: estimated total water, lean body weight and fat. Hum Biol. 1973;**45**(3):469–83.
110. Roemmich JN, Rogol AD. Role of leptin during childhood growth and development. Endocrinol Metab Clin North Am. 1999;**28**(4): 749–64.
111. Farooqi IS, Jebb SA, Langmack G, et al. Effects of recombinant leptin therapy in a child with congenital leptin deficiency. N Engl J Med. 1999;**341** (12):879–84.
112. Ahima RS. Body fat, leptin and hypothalamic amenorrhea. N Eng J Med. 2004;**351**:959–62.
113. Farooqi IS. Leptin and the onset of puberty: insights from rodent and human genetics. Semin Reprod Med. 2002;**20**(2):139–44.
114. Apter D, Bützow TL, Laughlin GA, et al. Gonadotropin-releasing hormone pulse generator activity during pubertal transition in girls: pulsatile and diurnal patterns of circulating gonadotropins. J Clin Endocrinol Metab. 1993;**76** (4):940–9.
115. Mitamura R, Yano K, Suzuki N, et al. Diurnal rhythms of luteinizing hormone, follicle-stimulating hormone, testosterone, and estradiol secretion before the onset of female puberty in short children. J Clin Endocrinol Metab. 2000;**85**(3):1074–80.
116. Oerter KE, Uriarte MM, Rose SR, et al. Gonadotropin secretory dynamics during puberty in normal girls and boys. J Clin Endocrinol Metab. 1990;**71**(5):1251–8.
117. Legro RS, Lin HM, Demers LM, et al. Rapid maturation of the reproductive axis during perimenarche independent of body composition. J Clin Endocrinol Metab. 2000;**85**(3):1021–5.
118. Sehested A, Juul AA, Andersson AM, et al. Serum inhibin A and inhibin B in healthy prepubertal, pubertal, and adolescent girls and adult women: relation to age, stage of puberty, menstrual cycle, follicle-stimulating hormone, luteinizing hormone, and estradiol levels. J Clin Endocrinol Metab. 2000;**85**(4):1634–40.
119. Andersen CY. Characteristics of human follicular fluid associated with successful conception after in vitro fertilization. J Clin Endocrinol Metab. 1993;**77** (5):1227–34.
120. Erickson GF, Magoffin DA, Dyer CA, et al. The ovarian androgen producing cells: a review of structure/function relationships. Endocr Rev. 1985;**6**(3):371–99.
121. Eppig JJ, Chesnel F, Hirao Y, et al. Oocyte control of granulosa cell development: how and why. Hum Reprod. 1997;**12**(11 Suppl):127–32.

122. Schipper I, Hop WC, Fauser BC. The follicle-stimulating hormone (FSH) threshold/window concept examined by different interventions with exogenous FSH during the follicular phase of the normal menstrual cycle: duration, rather than magnitude, of FSH increase affects follicle development. J Clin Endocrinol Metab. 1998;**83**(4):1292–8.

123. Gore MA, Nayudu PL, Vlaisavljevic V. Attaining dominance in vivo: distinguishing dominant from challenger follicles in humans. Hum Reprod. 1997;**12**(12):2741–7.

124. Welt CK, Pagan YL, Smith PC, et al. Control of follicle-stimulating hormone by estradiol and the inhibins: critical role of estradiol at the hypothalamus during the luteal-follicular transition. J Clin Endocrinol Metab. 2003;**88**(4):1766–71.

125. Chikazawa K, Araki S, Tamada T. Morphological and endocrinological studies on follicular development during the human menstrual cycle. J Clin Endocrinol Metab. 1986;**62**(2):305–13.

126. Rivier C, Rivier J, Vale W. Inhibin-mediated feedback control of follicle-stimulating hormone secretion in the female rat. Science. 1986;**234**(4773):205–8.

127. Durlinger AL, Visser JA, Themmen AP. Regulation of ovarian function: the role of anti-Müllerian hormone. Reproduction. 2002;**124**(5):601–9.

128. Filicori M, Cognigni GE, Tabarelli C, et al. Stimulation and growth of antral ovarian follicles by selective LH activity administration in women. J Clin Endocrinol Metab. 2002;**87**(3):1156–61.

129. Sawetawan C, Carr BR, McGee E, et al. Inhibin and activin differentially regulate androgen production and 17 alpha-hydroxylase expression in human ovarian thecal-like tumor cells. J Endocrinol. 1996;**148**(2):213–21.

130. Magoffin DA. Regulation of differentiated functions in ovarian theca cells. Semin Reprod Endocrinol. 1991;**9**:321.

131. Lockwood GM, Muttukrishna S, Ledger WL. Inhibins and activins in human ovulation, conception and pregnancy. Hum Reprod Update. 1998;**4**(3):284–95.

132. Andersen CY, Byskov AG, Estradiol and regulation of anti-Müllerian hormone, inhibin-A, and inhibin-B secretion: analysis of small antral and preovulatory human follicles' fluid. J Clin Endocrinol Metab. 2006;**91**:4064–9.

133. Filicori M, Cognigni GE, Ciampaglia W. Effects of LH on oocyte yield and developmental competence. Hum Reprod. 2003;**18**(6):1357–8; author reply 1358–60.

134. Suzuki T, Sasano H, Takaya R, et al. Cyclic changes of vasculature and vascular phenotypes in normal human ovaries. Hum Reprod. 1998;**13**(4):953–9.

135. Chaffkin LM, Luciano AA, Peluso JJ. Progesterone as an autocrine/paracrine regulator of human granulosa cell proliferation. J Clin Endocrinol Metab. 1992;**75**:1404–8.

136. Temporal relationships between ovulation and defined changes in the concentration of plasma estradiol-17 beta, luteinizing hormone, follicle-stimulating hormone, and progesterone. I. Probit analysis. World Health Organization, Task Force on Methods for the Determination of the Fertile Period, Special Programme of Research, Development and Research Training in Human Reproduction. Am J Obstet Gynecol. 1980;**138**(4):383–90.

137. Fritz MA, McLachlan RI, Cohen NL, et al. Onset and characteristics of the midcycle surge in bioactive and immunoactive luteinizing hormone secretion in normal women: influence of physiological variations in periovulatory ovarian steroid hormone secretion. J Clin Endocrinol Metab. 1992;**75**(2):489–93.

138. Fan HY, Liu Z, Shimada M, et al. MAPK3/1 (ERK1/2) in ovarian granulosa cells are essential for female fertility. Science. 2009;**324**(5929):938–41.

139. Liu JH, Yen SS. Induction of midcycle gonadotropin surge by ovarian steroids in women: a critical evaluation. J Clin Endocrinol Metab. 1983;**57**(4):797–802.

140. Collins RL, Hodgen GD. Blockade of the spontaneous midcycle gonadotropin surge in monkeys by RU 486: a progesterone antagonist or agonist? J Clin Endocrinol Metab. 1986;**63**(6):1270–6.

141. Peng X-R. Regulation of the fibrinolytic system during gonadotropin induction of ovulation in mice with inactivation of the genes encoding tPA, uPA or PAI-1. Fibrinolysis. 1994;**8**:101.

142. Jones PB, Vernon MW, Muse KN, et al. Plasminogen activator and plasminogen activator inhibitor in human preovulatory follicular fluid. J Clin Endocrinol Metab. 1989;**68**(6):1039–45.

143. Lösel R, Wehling M. Nongenomic actions of steroid hormones. Nat Rev Mol Cell Biol. 2003;**4**(1):46–56.

144. Zhu Y, Bond J, Thomas P. Identification, classification, and partial characterization of genes in humans and other vertebrates homologous to a fish membrane progestin receptor. Proc Natl Acad Sci U S A. 2003;**100**(5):2237–42.

145. Mehlmann LM, Saeki Y, Tanaka S, et al. The Gs-linked receptor GPR3 maintains meiotic arrest in mammalian oocytes. Science. 2004;**306**(5703):1947–50.

146. Markosyan N, Duffy DM. Prostaglandin E2 acts via multiple receptors to regulate plasminogen-dependent proteolysis in the primate periovulatory follicle. Endocrinology. 2009;**150**(1):435–44.

147. Lumsden MA, Kelly RW, Templeton AA, et al. Changes in the concentration of prostaglandins in preovulatory human follicles after administration of hCG. J Reprod Fertil. 1986;**77**(1):119–24.

148. Wayne CM, Fan HY, Cheng X, et al. Follicle-stimulating hormone induces multiple signaling cascades: evidence that activation of Rous sarcoma oncogene, RAS, and the epidermal growth factor receptor are critical for granulosa cell differentiation. Mol Endocrinol. 2007;**21**(8):1940–57.

149. Gonzalez-Robayna IJ, Falender AE, Ochsner S, et al. Follicle-stimulating hormone (FSH) stimulates phosphorylation and activation of protein kinase B (PKB/Akt) and serum and glucocorticoid-induced kinase (Sgk): evidence for A kinase-independent signaling by FSH in granulosa cells. Mol Endocrinol. 2000;**14**(8):1283–300.

150. Wulff C, Dickson SE, Duncan WC, et al. Angiogenesis in the human corpus luteum: simulated early pregnancy by HCG treatment is associated with both angiogenesis and vessel stabilization. Hum Reprod. 2001;**16**(12):2515–24.

151. Brannian JD, Shiigi SM, Stouffer RL. Gonadotropin surge increases fluorescent-tagged low-density lipoprotein uptake by macaque granulosa cells from preovulatory follicles. Biol Reprod. 1992;**47**(3):355–60.

152. Lei ZM, Chegini N, Rao CV. Quantitative cell composition of human and bovine corpora lutea from various reproductive states. Biol Reprod. 1991;**44**(6):1148–56.

153. Maas S, Jarry H, Teichmann A, et al. Paracrine actions of oxytocin, prostaglandin F2 alpha, and estradiol within the human corpus luteum. J Clin Endocrinol Metab. 1992;**74**(2):306–12.

154. Hutchison JS, Zeleznik AJ. The rhesus monkey corpus luteum is dependent on pituitary gonadotropin secretion throughout the luteal phase of the menstrual cycle. Endocrinology. 1984;**115**(5):1780–6.

155. Fraser HM, Lunn SF, Morris KD, et al. Initiation of high dose gonadotrophin-releasing hormone antagonist treatment during the late follicular phase in the macaque abolishes luteal function irrespective of effects upon the luteinizing hormone surge. Hum Reprod. 1997;**12**(3):430–5.

156. Auletta FJ, Flint AP. Mechanisms controlling corpus luteum function in sheep, cows, nonhuman primates, and women especially in relation to the time of luteolysis. Endocr Rev. 1988;**9** (1):88–105.

157. Lenton EA, Landgren BM, Sexton L, et al. Normal variation in the length of the follicular phase of the menstrual cycle: effect of chronological age. Br J Obstet Gynaecol. 1984;**91**(7):681–4.

158. McCracken JA, Custer EE, Lamsa JC. Luteolysis: a neuroendocrine-mediated event. Physiol Rev. 1999;**79**(2):263–323.

159. Duncan WC, McNeilly AS, Illingworth PJ. The effect of luteal "rescue" on the expression and localization of matrix metalloproteinases and their tissue inhibitors in the human corpus luteum. J Clin Endocrinol Metab. 1998;**83**(7):2470–8.

160. Vega M, Urrutia L, Iñiguez G, et al. Nitric oxide induces apoptosis in the human corpus luteum in vitro. Mol Hum Reprod. 2000;**6**(8):681–7.

161. Miceli F, Minici F, Garcia Pardo M, et al. Endothelins enhance prostaglandin (PGE(2) and PGF(2alpha)) biosynthesis and release by human luteal cells: evidence of a new paracrine/autocrine regulation of luteal function. J Clin Endocrinol Metab. 2001;**86**(2): 811–17.

162. Vermesh M, Kletzky OA. Longitudinal evaluation of the luteal phase and its transition into the follicular phase. J Clin Endocrinol Metab. 1987;**65**(4):653–8.

163. Wunder DM, Bersinger NA, Yared M, et al. Statistically significant changes of antimüllerian hormone and inhibin levels during the physiologic menstrual cycle in reproductive age women. Fertil Steril. 2008;**89**(4):927–33.

164. Welt CK, Martin KA, Taylor AE, et al. Frequency modulation of follicle-stimulating hormone (FSH) during the luteal-follicular transition: evidence for FSH control of inhibin B in normal women. J Clin Endocrinol Metab. 1997;**82**(8):2645–52.

Chapter 2

The normal human ovary part II: how steroid hormones work

Nathan G. Kase, MD

Introduction

Estrogen (E) and progesterone (P) play central roles in both the endocrine and intracrine regulation of all aspects of female reproduction [1–3]. In the reproductive system they act at the level of the hypothalamus, anterior pituitary, ovary, and uterus to coordinate neuroendocrine-directed pulsatile secretion of gonadotropin releasing hormone, cyclic release of gonadotropins FSH and LH, ovulation, and endometrial development in preparation for implantation and maintenance of the fertilized embryo. In addition, both hormones are essential for pubescent and pregnancy mammary gland development (a complex set of multiple instructions condensed in simplest terms as ductal morphogenesis in the case of E and further ductal branching with lobulo-alveolar differentiation in the case of P).

However, the physiologic activities of these steroids are not limited to reproductive system functions; their roles, particularly those of estradiol (E2), the primary estrogen, also include regulation of lipid and carbohydrate metabolism, the integrity of the cardiovascular system, the central nervous system, and skeletal homeostasis. It is in this broad spectrum of effects that the *general* understanding of the biology of these hormones has been expanded, distilled, and crystallized in cell- and tissue-specific receptor and post-receptor functional contexts. It is in the unraveling of the complexities of how these steroids work that the most revealing biologic and pharmacologic information has emerged. Among these new insights are: (1) ligand availability, variability, and tissue specificity; (2) new signaling pathways responsive to variable ligand/receptor aggregates localized in various cellular sites; (3) new modes of genomic and non-genomic action; (4) fuller understanding of the formation of receptor complexes with assemblies of either activators or repressors (transcriptomes and signalsomes); and (5) the translational and post-translational epigenetic accommodations which achieve signal-specific functional impact. Exploiting these mechanistic insights has disclosed unique opportunities for diagnostic and therapeutic interventions with the potential of identifying, modifying, and possibly reversing dysfunction and disease. Accordingly, reassessment of the roles of the E receptor subtypes ERα and ERβ and the therapeutic potential of subtype selective modulators in cardiovascular disease and diabetes mellitus type II (DMII), bone homeostasis (osteoporosis), dysfunctional brain behavior in general, and depression in particular as well as neurodegenerative diseases such as Alzheimer's disease (AD) and multiple sclerosis (MS) has emerged. Even applications in cancer await clinical assessment and validation.

This chapter will focus on the mechanism of action of the principal steroid secretory products of the ovary-E2 and ovary-P. Before undertaking a detailed examination of these functions in reproduction as well as their involvement in non-reproductive systems, the general principles of steroid hormone action will be reviewed [4]. There is a single, pervasive message here: how a single universal agonist such as E2 is interpreted and transduced by target cells to support cell-specific unique function – the concept of functional cellular context – will be repeatedly alluded to and emphasized.

The "functional context" of steroid–target cell interactions

General principles of steroid hormone–cognate receptor–DNA transcription activation

To understand how hormones produce different effects in different tissues at different times, it is necessary to consider the numerous variables which might dramatically change the final biological result of the basic steroid hormone receptor–DNA transcription activation cascade [5,6]. These include:

- Steroid structure, concentration (secretion and production rate), delivery mode, and site (autocrine, paracrine, endocrine)
- Concentration, distribution, temporal expression, and "sensitivity" of cognate receptors in various tissues
- The concentration and distribution of receptor subtypes and receptor isoforms of each receptor in a specific cell
- Whether a receptor is located in the nucleus and/or on the plasma membrane or membranes of various sub-cellular, cytosolic constituents such as mitochondria and endoplasmic reticulum
- The degree to which *steroid action* may proceed *without* involvement in genomic transcriptional processes or *without* interaction with its cognate receptor
- The degree to which *receptor activity* may be initiated in the absence of its classic steroid ligand

Altchek's Diagnosis and Management of Ovarian Disorders, ed. Liane Deligdisch, Nathan G. Kase, and Carmel J. Cohen. Published by Cambridge University Press.

- The existence of interactive "cross-talk" between diverse receptors and signaling pathways within a cell
- Cellular and hormone-specific variations in the conformational shape of the ligand–receptor dimer complex affecting DNA binding and recruitment of co-regulatory proteins
- Differential nuclear assemblies ("transcriptomes" or "signalsomes") of steroid receptor co-regulators, both co-activators and co-repressors
- Cell-specific induction of epigenomic processes (genome methylation, nucleosome compaction, lysine "tail" histone modification, and post-translational protein modification), which alter target cell response
- Cell-specific ("nuclear compaction") induction of higher order chromatin organization enabling genome-wide multiple response element occupancy by a single transcription factor forming single signal–multi gene networks ("interactomes"), which engage genes on distant sites on the same chromosome as well as genes on adjacent chromosomes [7].

The multiple possibilities for signal generation contribute to the *functional diversity* of steroid hormone action – "cellular context" – of cells displayed in different organ systems. It defines the capacity of various systems to "fine tune" cell responses. The ability to achieve either positive or negative influences on the transcription mechanism inherent in the conformational shape of the receptor and the cellular context response has given impetus to the development of *selective receptor modulators* capable of generating tissue-specific effects (whether stimulatory or repressive) with documented clinical utility [8,9,14].

In summary, the complexity and diversity of cellular context elements allows ligand, tissue, and promoter-specific interactions with selected subsets of regulators capable of elaborating distinct physiological responses to a "universal" agonist signal such as E2.

The mechanisms of E2 and E receptor signaling (Fig. 2.1)

Since the cloning of the first ER cDNA more than 20 years ago, the remarkable complexity of the molecular mechanisms underlying the diverse physiologic actions of E2 and its many natural and synthetic ligands is now emerging [4].

As would be anticipated from the general principles described in the previous section, several possible molecular mechanisms for E2 signaling are now appreciated:

- Classical nuclear (genomic) ligand-dependent ("transcriptomes")
- Cell membrane (non-genomic) ligand-dependent aggregates ("signalsomes")
- Ligand-independent ER activity
- DNA binding-independent ER activity
- Cell- and tissue-specific E2 receptor subtype distribution and their functions as homo- or heterodimers
- Ligand–receptor complex-induced cell-specific aggregates incorporating recruited co-activators or co-repressors
- Cell-specific remodeling of chromatin, DNA methylation status, nucleosome and histone tail modifications, and polycomb island-directed microRNA targeting
- Cell-specific higher order chromatin organization and the elaboration of transcription factor "networks" ("interactomes") permitting engagement of response elements to a single transcription signal ("transcriptome") at multiple distant sites on a chromosome or gene on a combination of chromosomes.

Taken together collective interaction of several modifying elements such as receptor subtypes, co-regulator (stimulatory and repressive) generation, and cross talk between steroid receptor and other signaling pathways reinstruct these modular mechanisms to yield tissue/cellular specificity (i.e., "context").

Nuclear genomic: ligand-dependent E2 action

The specificity of the reaction of a cell to E2 "instructions" is due in large part to the presence of initially unoccupied, heat-shock protein inactivated target cell ligand-specific receptor protein [4,10–12]. In the absence of hormone, the receptor is sequestered in a multiprotein inhibitory complex either within the nucleus or the cytosol of target cells. The binding of E2 (the ligand) to its cognate receptor induces activation of the complex.

The pathway follows these steps:

1. Free E2, because of its small size, enters the target cell by passive diffusion through the plasma membrane and binds with high affinity to its cognate receptor.
2. The E receptor is composed of several domains (Fig 2.1a). A constitutive transcription activation function 1 (AF-1) located in the *N-terminus A/B domain* is essential for interaction with co-regulatory proteins and for autonomous, hormone-independent transcriptional activity. The A/B domain also comprises amino acid targets for post-translational modifications by kinases of growth factor pathways which stimulate AF1 activity. *The DNA binding domain* (C) is vital for sequence-specific binding of the ligand bound ERs to DNA and positioning them to enable transcriptional regulation of target genes. The "*hinge*" *domain* (D) permits conformational flexibility and by means of two zinc fingers each containing amino acid sequences that promote nuclear localization and initiation of function and others that are targets for post-translational modification affecting ER activity and degradation. The major part of the C terminal hormone binding *E/F domain* consists of ligand-binding elements, cofactor binding, receptor dimerization, and the interaction of the ER complex with co-regulatory proteins by means of the *ligand-dependent* transcription activation function 2 (AF-2).
3. Two ER subtypes exist: ERα and ERβ. The classic mechanism through which the ER modulates gene expression is by binding to E response elements on DNA as either homodimers (ERα: ERα or ERβ: ERβ) or heterodimers (ERα: ERβ). Other reported mechanisms of ER-mediated gene transcription are binding to non-E

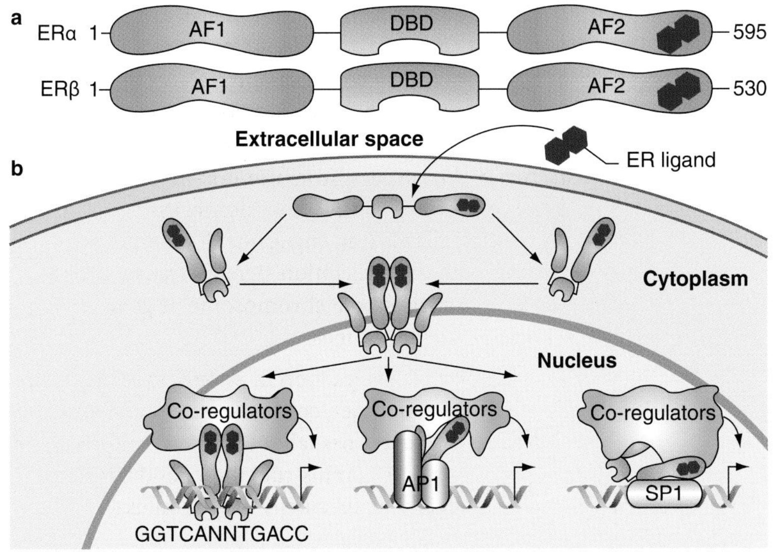

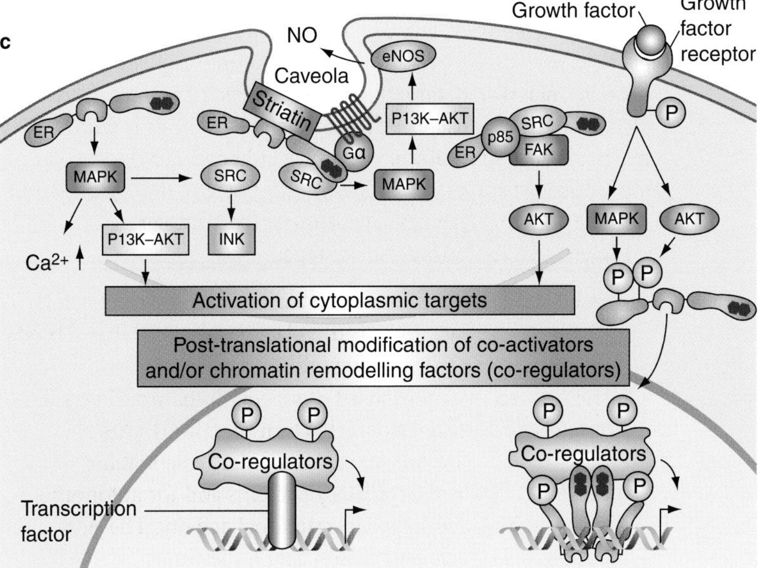

Fig. 2.1. Summary: Estrogen receptors and their mode of nuclear and cytoplasmic activity. a: Architecture of the ERα and ERβ receptors. Note amino terminal activation function 1 (AF1), the DNA-binding domain (DBD) and the carboxy terminal AF 2 containing a multifunctional ligand-binding domain (LBD). Note presence of ligand E2. b: ER ligand enters cell through diffusion and binds to ERs located in the cytoplasm; following binding the E–ER complex translocates to the nucleus, undergoes conformational changes and dimerizes. In the nucleus E–ER either binds in classic mode directly to specific estrogen receptor elements (ERE) on DNA or by tethering onto other transcription factors such as activator protein 1 (AP1) or specificity protein 1 (SP1). Note in each case coregulators and chromatin modification modulate gene expression. c: Various cytoplasmic signaling pathways are available to ligand-bound ERs in the cytoplasm or plasma membrane. Note rapid activation of non-nuclear cytoplasmic targets or additional integration with nuclear regulation of gene expression. Finally growth factors acting through their membrane receptors may also activate ERs through phosphorylation. eNOS, endothelial nitric oxide synthase; FAK, focal adhesion kinase; JNK, c-Jun N-terminal kinase; MAPK, mitogen-activated protein kinase; NO, nitric oxide PI3K, phosphoinositide 3-kinase. Reproduced from reference [3], with permission.

response elements on DNA and tethering to other transcription factors already bound to their specific sites on DNA. ER subtype polymorphisms have been identified (Fig. 2.2) and have been preliminarily linked to breast cancer susceptibility, bone mineral density and osteoporosis, hypertension, spontaneous abortion, and body height. Thus far, insufficient information as to whether these isoforms have a major clinical role remains to be determined [35].

4. With binding, E2 receptor (ER) undergoes activation, a process which involves release from heat shock protein, receptor dimerization, and tertiary and quatenary conformational changes which expose high affinity DNA binding sites (Fig. 2.1b).
5. Critical to the ligand and tissue specificity of this cascade, in addition to the conformational changes in the receptor complex following steroid binding, the activated receptor not only binds to specific enhancer DNA elements in the promoters of specific genes (Fig. 2.1b) but also recruits co-regulatory proteins which interact with the general transcriptional machinery to elaborate and/or modify hormone triggered changes. The agonist (stimulatory) properties of the ligand–receptor complex are achieved by binding of co-activator proteins, which promote transcription. On the other hand, co-repressors inhibit transcription.
6. The activated steroid–receptor (E–ER) complex binds with specific DNA sequences referred to as E response elements (EREs) which are enhancers located within the regulatory regions of target genes.
7. The activated steroid receptor complex functions as a transcription factor modulating the synthesis of specific mRNAs and proteins, which are responsible for the cellular action of the hormone.
8. The activity of the E receptor is controlled by the binding of the endogenous hormone E2 or by exogenous (synthetic, i.e., SERMS) non-steroidal compounds to the ligand-binding domain [13]. Binding triggers several events such as

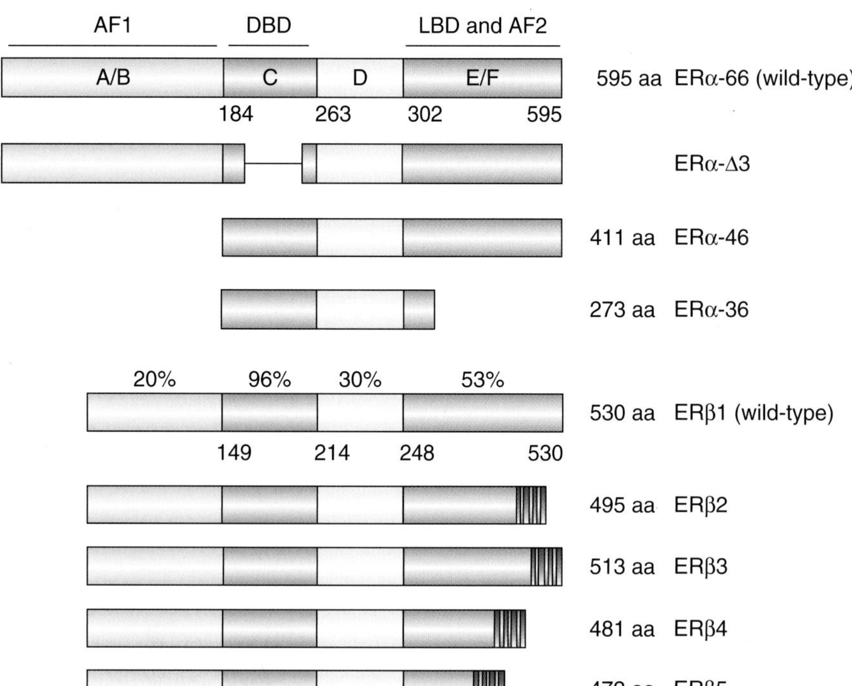

Fig. 2.2. The estrogen receptor subtypes, ERα and ERβ and their functional domains. The structural domains are labeled A–F with the amino acid numbers used to define these domains. The amino-terminal A/B regions contain a transactivation domain (AF1) with ligand-independent function and a co-regulatory domain that is responsible for recruitment of co-activators and co-repressors. The C region corresponds to the DNA-binding domain (DBD) which is required for binding to specific estrogen response elements (EREs) in the proximal promotor region or at distal regulatory elements of estrogen-responsive genes. The carboxy-terminal regions (E and F) contain the ligand-binding domain (LBD) and have a ligand-dependent transactivation function (AF2). This region is also responsible for binding to co-regulatory and chaperone proteins, as well as for receptor dimerization and nuclear translocation. Finally, the D region contains several functional domains including the hinge domain, part of the ligand-dependent activating domain and the nuclear localization signal. Human ERα and ERB variants are presented below the wild type forms. Most of these variants are expressed in malignant tissues and influence cancer biology. Reproduced from reference [35], with permission.

receptor dimerization conformational changes, binding to specific E response elements on DNA, and interaction with co-regulators (chromatin remodelers, co-activators, and co-repressors). Each class of ER ligand induces a unique ER conformation, which promotes specific co-regulatory protein interactions and association with the ER N- and C-terminal transcription activation functions, AF-1 and AF-2 [14–16] (Fig. 2.3).

9. Transcription leads to translation, mRNA-mediated protein synthesis on the ribosomes and generation of specific biologic activity. Although activated steroid hormone receptors are thought of as primarily affecting gene transcription, they also regulate posttranslational events.
10. Biologic activity is maintained only while the nuclear site is occupied with the hormone–receptor complex. The dissociation rate of the hormone from its receptor, as well as the half-life of the nuclear chromatin-bound complex are factors in the biologic response of the hormone. Thus, *duration of exposure to a hormone is as important as concentration.*
11. An important action of E is the generation of its own hormone activity by affecting ER concentrations. In a process called *replenishment*, E increases target tissue responsiveness to itself and to progestins and androgens by increasing the concentration of its own receptor and that of the intracellular progestin and androgen receptors. P and clomiphene, on the other hand, limit tissue response to E in part by blocking the replenishment mechanism, thus decreasing the concentration of E receptors over time. Replenishment, the synthesis of the sex hormone receptors, takes place in the cytoplasm, but in the case of E and progestin receptors, synthesis is quickly followed by transport ("shuttling") into the nucleus.
12. The fate of the hormone–receptor complex after gene activation is referred to as hormone-receptor *processing*. In the case of E receptors, processing involves the conversion of high-affinity E receptor sites to a rapidly dissociating form followed by loss of binding capacity and degradation by a ubiquitin-proteasome pathway.

The generation of functional diversity

Steroid receptor co-regulators

A crucial element in generation of functional diversity in the reaction to estradiol is the reality of a unique "cellular" context. This concept explains how the same hormone can produce different responses in different cells. One important contributor to unique cell responses "context" is the recruitment of available cell-specific co-regulator signal modifying proteins. For detailed reviews of this at once dauntingly complex but physiologically and clinically important element of steroid hormone action and the potential for pharmacologic manipulation and modification, please see reviews [17–19].

Co-activators and their mechanism of action (see Figs. 2.4–2.6), (Table 2.1, 2.2)

Literally hundreds of putative co-activators have been identified. As the number of potential co-activators clearly exceeds the capacity for direct interaction with a single receptor, it is likely that different protein complexes can act either sequentially, combinatorially, or in parallel. Co-activators are characterized by their interaction with the transcription machinery and activation of the functional domains of nuclear receptors. Three types of multi-protein complex are identified: (1) complexes which alter chromatin structure, (2) complexes involved primarily in histone acetylation, and (3) mediator complexes

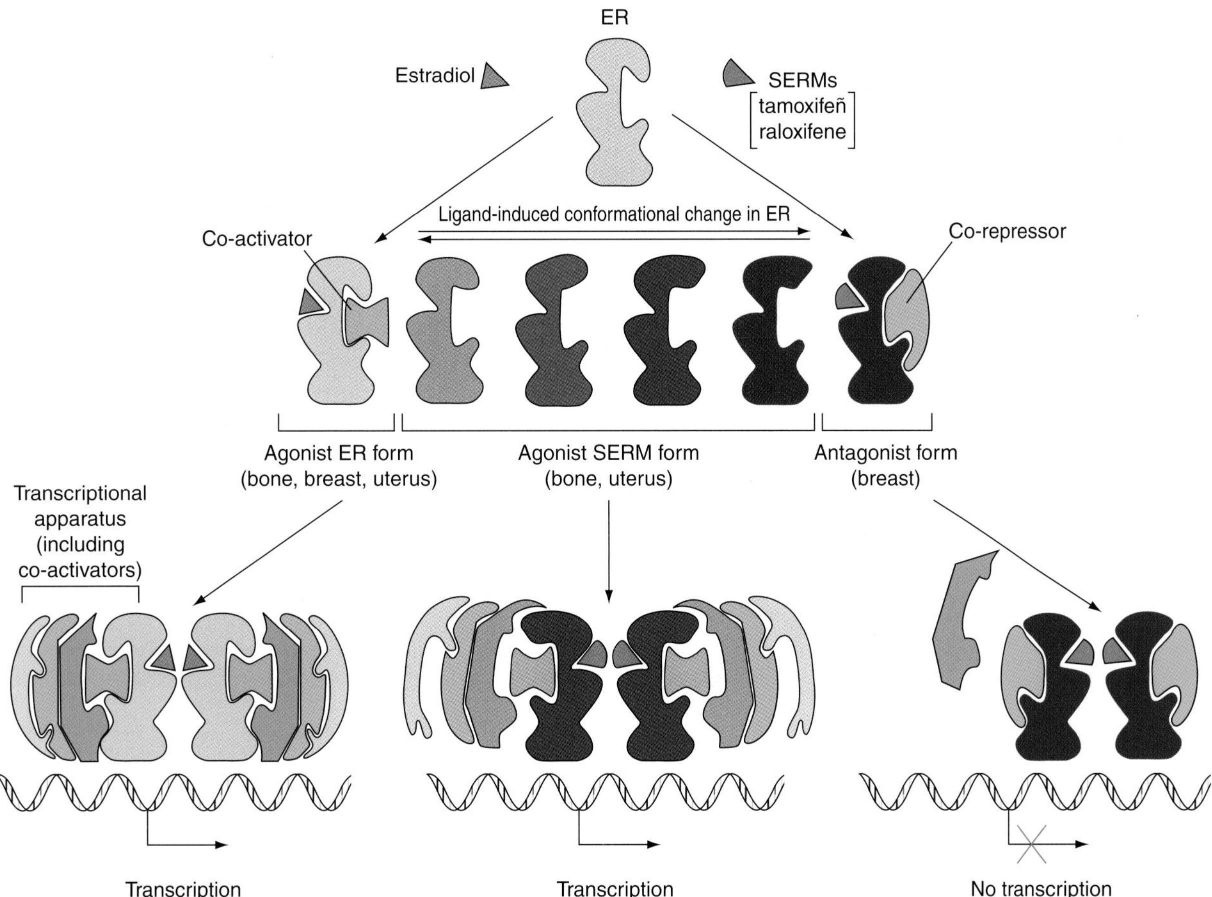

Fig. 2.3. SERM agonists/antagonists influence on ER structure and co-regulatory recruitment. After binding with E2 or SERM ligand specific conformational changes in ligand–receptor complex result in 3-dimensional "distortions" of the ligand–receptor complex. Recruitment of unique sets of co-activators/co-repressors are specific to the cellular and promotor context of differentiated tissues.

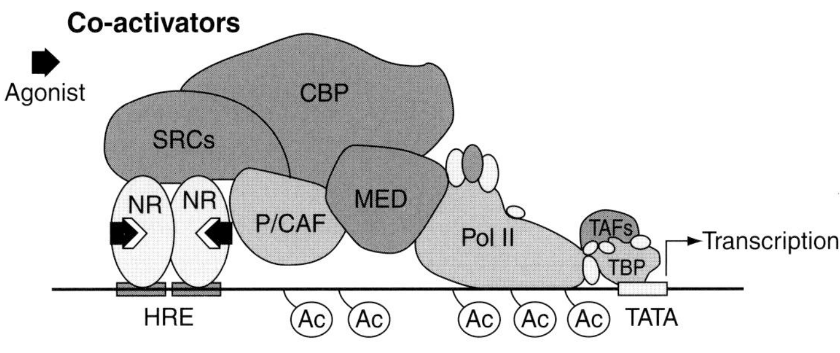

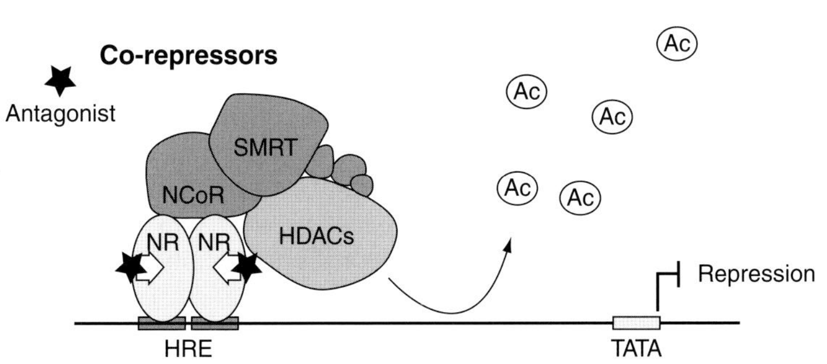

Fig. 2.4. Simplified models of co-activator and co-repressor "amalgams." Top panel shows how agonist-bound nuclear receptors associate with co-activators and other proteins to regulate gene transcription. Co-activators can increase gene transcription by means of the acetylation of histones and through the recruitment and stabilization of the transcriptional complex. Bottom panel shows how antagonist bound nuclear receptors can associate with co-repressors and additional proteins to repress gene transcription. Co-repressors can repress gene expression by causing the deacetylation of histones by means of the recruitment of HDACs to the genome. HRE, hormone response element; NR, nuclear receptor; SRCs, p160 steroid receptor co-activator family; CBP, CREB-binding protein; P/CAF, p300/CBP-associated factor; MED, mediator complex; HDACs, histone deacetylases; Ac, acetyl groups; Pol II, RNA polymerase II; TBP, TATA-binding protein; TAFs, TBP-associated factors; TATA, TATA box. Reprinted from: Tetel MJ, Auger AP, and Charlier TD. Who's in charge? Nuclear receptor co-activator and corepressor function in brain and behaviour. Front Neuroendocrinol, 2009;**30**(3):328-42. With permission from Elsevier.

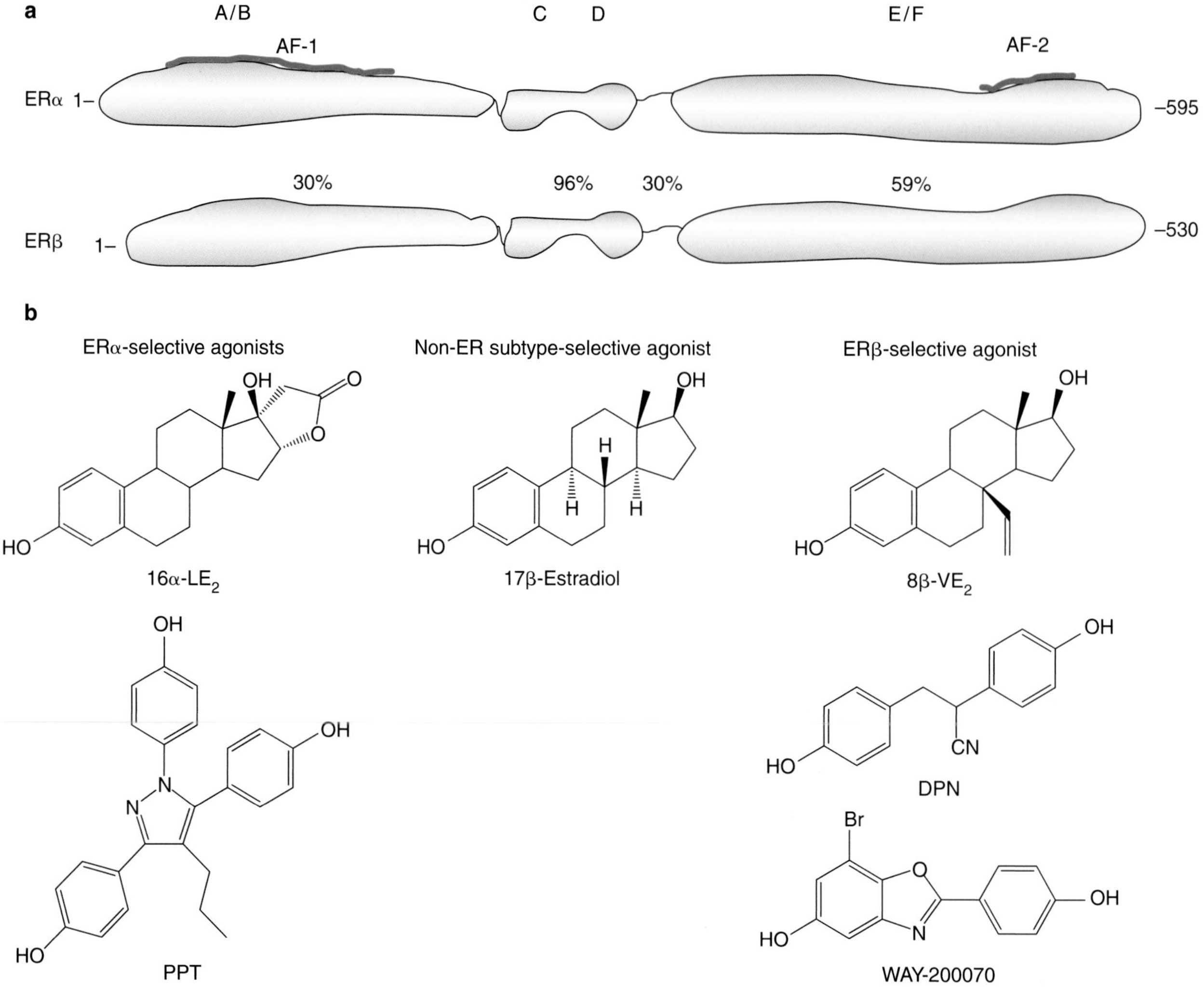

a

A/B C D E/F

AF-1 AF-2

ERα 1– –595

30% 96% 30% 59%

ERβ 1– –530

b

ERα-selective agonists

Non-ER subtype-selective agonist

ERβ-selective agonist

16α-LE_2

17β-Estradiol

8β-VE_2

PPT

DPN

WAY-200070

Fig. 2.5. Structures of ERα and ERβ affinity selective agonists compared with the nature of 17β-estradiol, which binds equally to both ER subtypes. Reproduced from reference [21], with permission.

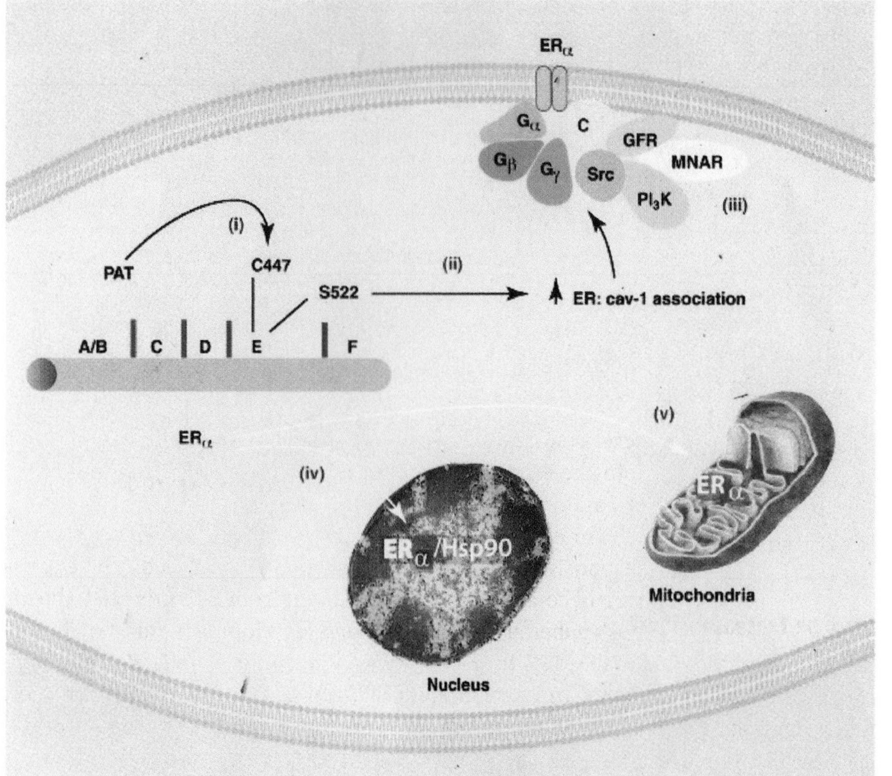

Fig. 2.6. i–iii: ERα translocation to the cell membrane. Palmitoylation of cysteine 447 on ERα. Palmitoylation is necessary for ERα association with caveolin-1. ER-caveolin raft association is transported to the cell membrane where it is joined in a signalsome complex which can be activated by E2 binding to the ERα now located in the cell membrane. iv, v: Similar chaperone functions (e.g., heat shock protein 90 transport ERα to the nucleus) may also transport ERα to the mitochondria membrane or the endoplasmic reticulum. Note: signalsome "amalgam" demonstrates how ERα physically associates with and activates G protein sub units initiating multiple early signals including proximal kinase activation (e.g., Src), growth factors (GFR), and PI3K. Reproduced from reference [27], with permission.

Table 2.1. Diverse functions of co-regulators

Function	Co-regulators
Acetyltransferases	SRC/p160, CBP/p300, and pCAF
Ubiquitin ligases	E6-AP
ATPases	BRG-1
Methylases	CARM-1 and PRMT-1
RNA transcription	SRA
Cell cycle regulators	Cdc-25B
RNA helicases	P72
Direct contact with basal transcription factors	TRAP/DRIP/mediator

involved in activation of RNA polymerase II and initiation of transcription. In the presence of agonist-bound steroid receptors, co-activators are recruited to DNA to induce both histone acetylation and unwinding of the DNA with separation of nucleosomes thereby promoting access and more efficient gene expression. Groups of co-adaptor proteins have now been identified as components of the resulting multiprotein "transcriptome." These include enzymes such as ligases, ATPases, and methylases as well as proteins that serve as cell cycle regulators, RNA helicases, and docking proteins which bridge to basal transcription factors. Specific structural domains on each co-activator recruit and assemble this amalgam of instructional transcription machinery. For example, a "division of labor" among co-activators would lead to the sequence of chromatin remodeling, followed by acetyltransferase activity, protein bridging, and finally complexes of co-activators that enhance RNA polymerase II recruitment to the promoter.

Co-repressors and their mechanism of action

Compared with co-activators, relatively less is known about co-repressors (Table 2.3). A true co-repressor contains autonomous repression domains and directly interacts with the receptor. It also interacts with components of the transcription machinery to repress transcription of a specific gene. The repression of transcription may be due to competition among molecules which bind to DNA or direct silencing of the basal transcription machinery. Several lines of investigation suggest that co-repressors associate with nuclear hormone receptors and recruit histone deacetylases (HDAC) and other isoforms that mediate histone deacetylation. Gene transcription is also repressed by nucleosomal condensation as well as failure to recruit elements of the basal transcription machinery.

Similar to co-activators, the prototype co-repressors SMRT and N-COR are molecular modular proteins containing multiple repression domains. These repress transcription by recruitment of the aforementioned HDACs which are inactive until they bind to the co-repressor [1].

The balance of co-activation/co-repression in health and disease

Modifications of expression of co-regulator proteins and steroid receptors in different mammalian tissues combined with generation of knockout mouse models or null mutations of

Table 2.2. Co-activators and their interaction with nuclear receptors

	Interaction	
Co-activators	in vitro	in vivo
SRC	PR, RAR, RXR, TR	ER, GR, PR, TR, RXR
ERAP160/$_p$160	ER, RAR, RXR	ER
GRIPI/TIF2	ER, AR, GR, TR, PR, RAR, RXR	ER, AR, GR, PR
SRC-2/NcoA-2	PPAR	VDR, RAR, RXR
ACTR/AIBI/ RAC3	ER, PR, TR, VDR, RAR, RXR, VDR, PPAR	ER. PR. TR. RAR
p/CIP	ER,RAR	ER, PR, TR, RAR
ERAP140/P140	ER	Not available
RIP140	ER, PPARα, RT, RAR, RXR	ER
RIP160/P160	ER	Not available
p/CAF	ER, AR, GR, RAR, RXR	RAR/RXR
CBP/P300	ER, GR, RT, RAR, RXR	ER,TR, RAR, RXR
ARA70	AR	AR, ER, GR, PR (weak)
Ada3	ER, TR, RXR	ER, RXR
Rap-46	ER, AR, GR, AR, PR, TR	Not available
GRIP170	GR	GR
PGC-1	ERα, PPARχ, ERα, RARα, TRβ	PPARχ/RARα,TRβ/RXRα
PGC-2	PPARχ, ERα, TRβ	PPARχ, ERα
SPT6	ER	ER
SW12/SNF2 (Brahma)	GR (SW13, ER	ER, GR, RAR
SNURF	With DBD of AR, ER, Pr	AR
TRAP220	TR, VDR, RAR, RAR, RXR, PPARα, PPARχ, ER	TR
TRAP100	ER, RXR, PPARα, PPARχ, RAR and RXR associate with a different complex	VDR
DRIP	TR, VDR, PPARχ	VDR
RAC3	AR, ER	AR, ER
NSD	ER, RXR	Bifunctional factor
	TR, RAR	Repression and activation
RSP5/RPF1	No direct interaction	GR, PR, but not ER
PGC-I	PPAR, liver X receptor	PPAR, liver X receptor
AR14	AR	AR
GZ/FHL2	ERα	ERα
Ubc9/PIAs	ERα	ERα

several co-regulatory proteins have yielded important insights into the essential role of these proteins in mediating selective steroid responses in health and disease.

For example, expression of co-regulator proteins in steroid-responsive tissues is developmentally controlled. The expression of co-activator SRC-1 is absent from E reactive cells during post-pubertal mammary gland development but can be co-localized with E-receptor-positive breast cells during pregnancy. In addition, aberrant expression of co-regulator proteins has been found in breast cancer. These reports *show increased*

Table 2.3. Co-repressors and their interaction with nuclear receptors

	Interaction	
Co-repressors	In vitro	In vivo
SMRT/TRAC-2	RAR,TR, v-ErbA, PPARχ, RXR (weak)	RAR, TR, PPARχ
N-CoR/RIP13	TR, Rev Erb, RAR, PPARχ	TR. Rev Erb, RAR
SUN-CoR	TR, Rev Erb	TR, Rev Erb
Ssn6/Tup1	Not available	ER, PR
TRUP	TR	TR, RAR
Calreticulin	GR, AR	GR, AR, RAR
REA	ER	ER
ZNF 366	ERα	ER
RIP 140	AR, ERα	AR, ERα
MTA	ERα	ERα
NM23-H2	ERβ	ERβ
AIB	ERα	ERα

co-activator levels associated with tumorigenesis while the expression of co-repressors is diminished. For example, levels of CBP, TRAP220, and several SRC family members, all co-activators, are elevated in certain breast tumors. Conversely levels of the co-repressor N-COR are decreased and even more dramatically in invasive compared with in situ disease. N-COR is also decreased in the mouse model of tamoxifen-resistant breast cancer [2].

In summary, variable abnormal co-regulatory function may contribute to a variety of hormone-related dysfunctions and diseases, including steroid resistance syndromes such as androgen insensitivity syndrome (AIS), reproductive dysfunction and steroid-responsive cell tumorigenesis.

Clinicians are all too familiar with both the virtues and disadvantages of selective estrogen receptor modulators in clinical practice. The induction of intense vasomotor reactions in some women frequently limits sustained compliance. The appearance of tamoxifen-resistant breast cancer recurrences and endometrial neoplasia after years of use are examples of too proximal insertion of SERM, leading to misdirection in the mechanism of estrogen action. At this point, the next generation of pharmaceutical approaches to tissue-specific steroid action modulation will reflect identification and perturbation of particular cell-specific co-regulatory proteins and ER subtype manipulations.

Nuclear receptor subtypes

Receptors for E are expressed as two structurally related subtypes designated as E receptor alpha (ERα) and E receptor beta (ERβ) (Fig. 2.2) [20,21]. ERα is translated from 6.8-kb mRNA derived from a gene on the long arm of chromosome 6. ERβ is encoded by a gene localized to chromosome 14,q22q24.

Both proteins show a high degree of amino acid conservation in the DNA-binding domains (96%) and lesser but still significant (55%) homology in the hormone-binding domain. However, substantial differences exist between α and β in their activation factor (AF) domains, as well as the hinge and the E domains which confer the "flexibility" necessary for differential conformational phenotypes.

Two functionally distinct AF domains exist in both receptor proteins. The first (AF-1) is located in the poorly conserved amino terminal domain and a second (AF-2) located in the ligand-binding domain. AF-1 and AF-2 may contribute either independently or synergistically to either agonist ligand-receptor transcription activity or ligand-independent phosphorylation pathways of receptor activation. Furthermore, their relative activities vary depending on the specific cellular and promoter contexts. For example, transcriptional responses of each receptor to E2 (a universal agonist ligand with which they both bind with equal affinity) varies significantly in part due to sequence divergence in their AF-1 domains and to a differential preference for specific co-regulatory proteins (a property inherent in AF-2).

Both ERα and ERβ are targets for post-translational modifications. Phosphorylation leads to enhanced ER-mediated gene transcription; acetylation is claimed to enhance ER DNA-binding activity, hormone sensitivity, and transcriptional activity; sumoylation is claimed to have effects on ER ligand-dependent transcriptional activity; nitrosylation impairs ER-mediated genomic events; myristoylation and palmitoylation have roles in targeting the ERs to the membrane, thereby influencing enzyme activities and signal transduction in a hormone-dependent manner; and ubiquitination targets the ERs for degradation.

In some organs, ERα and ERβ are expressed at similar levels, sometimes in different cell types within the same organ, and in others, one or the other subtype predominates. ERα is predominantly expressed in the uterus, prostate (stroma), ovary (theca cells), testes (Leydig cells), epididymis, bone, breast, liver, kidney, white adipose tissue, and various regions of the brain. ERβ is predominantly expressed in the colon, prostate (epithelium), testis, ovary (granulosa cells and oocyte), bone marrow, salivary gland, vascular endothelium, lung, bladder, and certain regions of the brain.

Genomic receptor subtype distribution and function in the reproductive system

Immuno-cytochemical localization of ERα and β in human reproductive organs demonstrates cell-specific localization for each of the ER subtypes [22–25]. In the ovary, ERβ immune-reactivity is found in the nuclei of somatic cells and in the oocyte in all stages of follicle growth (from primary to mature follicles). However, in the uterus and vagina, ERα is the subtype involved in the action of E: strong ERα immuno-reactivity is detected in epithelial, stromal, and myometrial cells (ERβ provides a much weaker signal). Only ERα is detected in the vagina. In the mammary gland, both ER subtypes are equally observed in epithelial cells and stromal cells.

Selective ablation of ERα (αERKO), ERβ (βERKO), and combined α and βER (αβERKO) in mice has provided definitive evidence that these receptor subtypes mediate distinct physiologic responses bearing on reproduction.

ERα is the dominant subtype expressed throughout the female mouse reproductive tract and its ablation (αERKO) results in infertility due to defects in sexual behavior, neuroendocrine gonadotropin regulation, ovulation, uterine function, and post-pubertal mammary gland development. For example, the αERKO ovary is characterized by the presence of large, hemorrhagic, and cystic follicles, a sparse number of early antral stage follicles, and a complete absence of corpora lutea. Prolonged treatment with a GnRH agonist leads to a resolution of this polycystic ovary like phenotype in αERKO mice, suggesting that it is chronic gonadotropin hyper-stimulation due to a defect in anterior pituitary ERα function that causes these polycystic changes. In contrast, βERKO results in a sub-fertile phenotype due exclusively to intrinsic germ cell and follicle somatic cell dysfunction. Fewer follicles are developed and fewer ovulate. In the gonadotropin-induced superovulation model, βERKO display diminished capacity to conclude meiosis 1 as well as a high frequency of unruptured follicles.

Compound knockout mice (αβERKO) exhibit phenotypes that resemble those of αERKO. However, in these animals, the ovaries show progressive germ cell loss and re-differentiation of the surrounding somatic cells, indicating that both ER forms are necessary in formation and maintenance of the gonad in rodents.

When hypophysectomized or gonadotropin-releasing hormone antagonist-treated female rats were treated with an ERβ-selective agonist (8β-VE2), it led to stimulation of early folliculogenesis, a decrease in follicular atresia, and stimulation of late follicular growth, followed by an increase in the number of ovulated oocytes. Treatment of wild-type, cycling female rats with E2 or with an ERα-selective agonist (16α-LE2) resulted in inhibition of the ovulation rate; treatment with the ERβ-selective agonist 8β-VE2 did not have this effect. The inhibitory effect of E2 and the ERα agonist are attributable to the effects on the hypothalamic–pituitary–gonadal axis and the observed decrease in serum LH levels.

Furthermore, treatment of ovariectomized rats with E2 or an ERα-selective agonist (16α-LE2), respectively, resulted in suppressed levels of LH and follicle-stimulating hormone; treatment with an ERβ-selective agonist (8β-VE2) did not have this effect. Taken together, these findings indicate that ERα is the primary ER subtype exerting feedback control of circulating gonadotropin levels.

ERα-selective (PPT or 16α-LE2) but not ERβ-selective (DPN or 8β-VE2) agonists stimulated uterine growth and weight in ovariectomized rats, confirming similar findings in ER knockout mice, namely, that ERα mediates uterotrophic effects in response to E2, whereas ERβ is no-nuterotrophic [21].

These models have contributed substantially to understanding the distributive functions of ERα and ERβ in mediating the tissue-specific reproductive physiologic responses to E. In addition, they have demonstrated that embryonic development of the female reproductive tract proceeds normally in the absence of E–ER interaction. In this respect, they have validated the existence of alternate signaling pathways independent of either E-ligand or E-receptor functions. Most compelling is the fact that, despite abnormal reproductive function, both the αERKO and the βERKO mice have normal life spans.

Genomic receptor subtype distribution and function in non-reproductive systems

Given the wide distribution of ER subtypes, it is understandable that the physiologic roles of E are not limited to reproductive function and include regulation of lipid and carbohydrate metabolism, the cardiovascular system (particularly the effect on endothelial physiology), the structural integrity and functions of the central nervous system, and skeletal homeostasis [3,21].

As noted the relative levels of ERα and ERβ in a given cell are important determinants of its response to E2 and synthetic, non-hormonal agonists and antagonists. For example, in mice, the level of expression of genes induced by E2 in bone were, on average, 85% higher in the absence of ERβ than in its presence, suggesting ERβ has an opposing effect on ERα-mediated gene transcription. In cells that express both ERα and ERβ, a unique set of genes (to a large extent distinct from those regulated by homodimers of ERα and ERβ) are regulated by ERα/β heterodimers. Moreover, when cells expressing both ER subtypes are treated with the ER subtype-selective agonists, such as PPT (4,4′,4″-(4-propyl-(1*H*)-pyrozole-1,3,5-triyl) trisphenol), an ERα selective agonist, and DPN (2,3-bis(4-hydroxyphenyl)-propionitrile), an ERβ-selective agonist, the cellular responses are distinct for the two treatments, and each distinct from the response induced by non-selective agonist E2. In a subsequent portion of this chapter, the receptor subtype distribution in each organ system and their clinical importance will be explored. For instance, while βERKO mice display normal body fat distribution and insulin secretion, αERKO mice developed visceral adiposity and insulin resistance.

Cell-surface, non-genomic steroid signaling (Table 2.4, Fig. 2.1c)

The rapid biologic effects of E2 in bone, breast, vasculature, and nervous system suggest that E may work through non-genomic processes [26,27]. A large body of data supports the existence of steroid effects which cannot be explained by the classic model of steroid–target cell nuclear interaction. These non-genomic processes possess the following characteristics: (1) the activity is too rapid for involvement of changes in mRNA and protein synthesis, (2) are seen in cells unable to accomplish mRNA and protein synthesis (spermatozoa) or in cells lacking steroid

Table 2.4. Non-genomic actions of sex steroids

Non-receptor-mediated actions at the plasma membrane	Membrane fluidity: ligand at millimolar concentrations
Steroid activation on non-nuclear receptors at the plasma membrane	Ion channels and G protein coupled receptors: insensitivity to antagonists
Rapid signaling through membrane-bound steroid receptors	2% of pool, estrogen receptor ERα and ERβ or progesterone receptor

nuclear receptors, (3) activity can be induced even by steroids coupled with high molecular weight substances that prevent passage through the nuclear membrane, (4) are not blocked by antagonists of the classic, genomic steroid receptor, and (5) are highly specific because steroids with similar but not identical structure may show various degrees of inductive potencies. In sum, these rapid effects are compatible with activation of signal transduction mechanisms similar to those activated by peptide hormones after interaction with their membrane receptors.

E receptors exist in discrete cellular pools outside the nucleus. Furthermore, at least with respect to plasma cell membrane-associated ERs, these are the same ERα and ERβ subtypes functioning in the classic mechanism of nuclear ER action. ERs have also been found in discrete cytoplasmic organelles including mitochondria. Each ER pool contributes to the overall integrated effects of E-associated biologic outcomes. In this section, the contributions to the overall impact of cell function by membrane ERs, their separate and combined interactions with nuclear receptor and other cytoplasmic membrane signaling molecules such as adapter proteins, G protein coupled receptors, ion channels, growth factors, and protein kinases, will be described.

Rapid signaling by ERs at the plasma membrane (Table 2.4, Fig. 2.1c)

As in the classic cascade, membrane-localized ERs exist as monomers but rapidly form homodimers in response to E or compounds with estrogenic activities [28–30]. As dimers, the membrane-localized ERs induce cell-specific assemblies of proteins – the "signalsome" – comprising G protein-coupled receptor subunits and receptor tyrosine kinases (Src), lipid kinases (PI3K), linker/scaffold proteins, and threonine/serine kinases. These signalsome assemblies followed by subsequent phosphorylations of other proteins modulate cell differentiation, cell migration, survival, and proliferation. Finally, signaling from the membrane enhances transcriptional effects of nuclear ER gene transcription (as seen in endothelium nitric oxide synthesis and activity).

Thus, the same steroid ligand can simultaneously or consecutively activate a membrane-associated receptor *and* the classic nuclear receptor. The resultant steroid effect on the cell represents a superimposition of distinct receptor-mediated events in which one may condition, synergize with, or modify the other. For example, non-genomic and genomic synergism may cause biphasic effects that have both rapid onset and long-lasting persistence.

Ligand-independent activation of ER: interaction with peptide growth factors (Fig. 2.7)

ER function can be modulated by extracellular signals in the absence of E2. The polypeptide growth factors such as epidermal growth factor (EGF), and insulin-like growth factor-1 (IGF-1) can activate ER and increase the expression of ER target genes by inducing activating phosphorylation of AF-1 [31–35]. Steroid membrane receptors are located in close proximity to binding sites for peptide hormones. This finding raises the

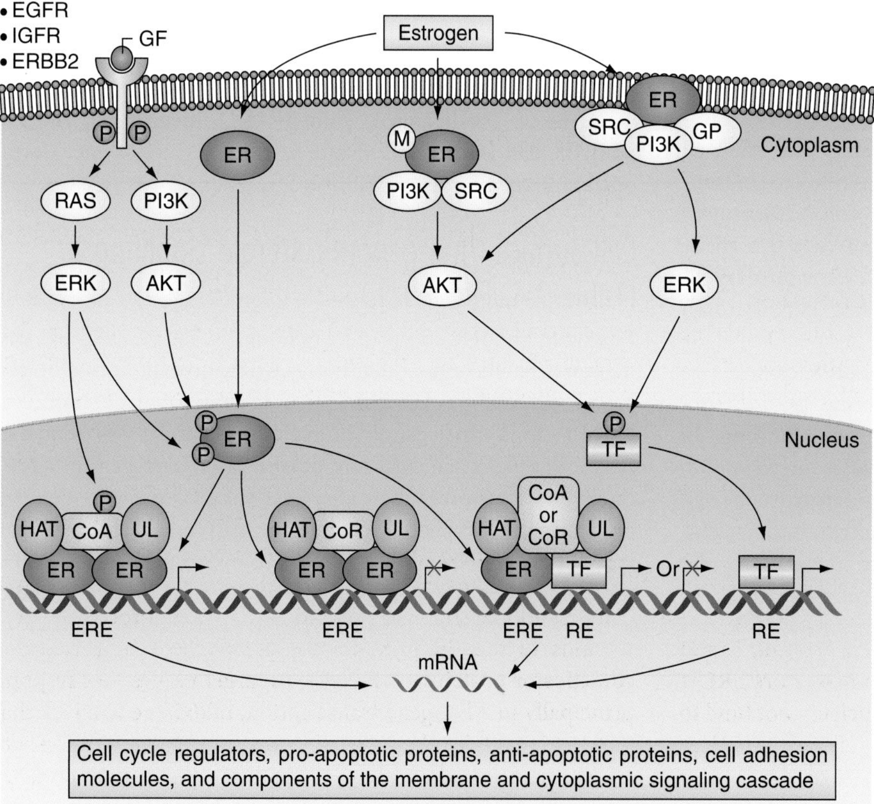

Fig. 2.7. Multiple molecular mechanisms of ER action. The classical mechanisms of ER action (E–ER binding, dimerization, binding to ERE) and recruitment of multiprotein coregulatory complexes (to activate or repress transcription). Alternatively ERs regulate gene expression by interacting with other direct DNA binding transcription factors. In this model, ERs bind directly to ERE motifs near the response element of the interacting transcription factor or indirectly through tethering to the partner transcription factor. Estrogen-bound ERs located in the membrane or in the cytoplasm can interact with Src, PI3K, and G proteins to initiate non-genomic ERE signaling – activation of protein kinase cascades leading to phosphorylation and activation of target transcription factors (TFs) which then regulate transcription at their own reactive elements (RE). Finally growth factor receptors (EGFR, IGFR, HER2/neu) in response to growth factors can activate ERK and AKT serine/threonine kinases which can phosphorylate and activate ERs in a ligand-independent manner. Reproduced from reference [35], with permission.

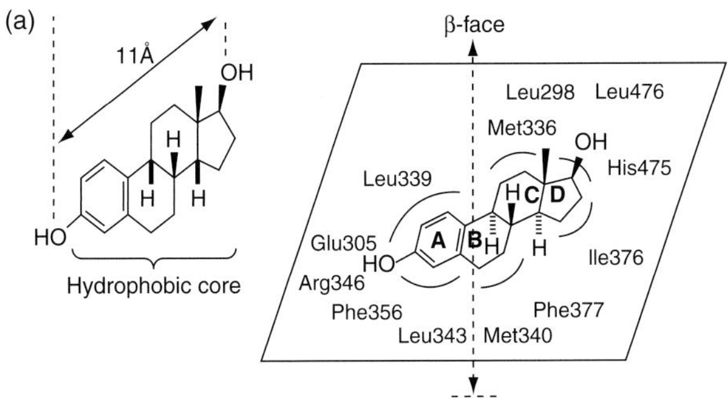

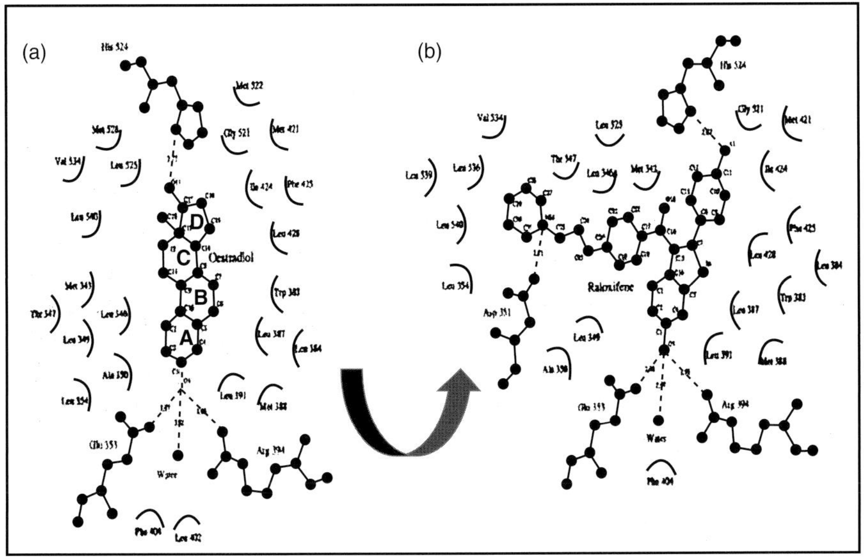

Fig. 2.8. ER agonist and antagonist binding modes. Electron density mapping for ER LBD-E2 complex (a) and ER-LBD raloxifene (RAL) complex (b). Note that as a result of rotation, reorientation, structural differences, and hydrogen bonding, residues that interact with ligand, and/or line the cavity are different. The differences are responsible for unique ligand and specific co-activators and/or co-repressors recruitment. Top panel reproduced from reference [3], with permission. Bottom panel reproduced from reference [14], with permission.

probability that a complex system of cell regulation involves not only steroid and peptide hormone action on the same target cells but also using the same intracellular messengers, and modulating the same signaling pathways. Biologically, these hormone-independent growth factor pathways may enhance function of ER positive tissues or sustain ER activation in the presence of low E2 levels. Accordingly, each pathway may be dependent on the other for full manifestation of either response. For example, an EGF response will be diminished or obliterated by administration of a full E antagonist or in an αERKO mouse model.

DNA-independent genomic actions of ER

E2–ER can lead to gene activation and regulation in the absence of direct DNA binding as in the absence of an ERE site [26]. This is seen in E2–ERα activation of IGF-1 and collagenase expression mediated through interaction with Fos and Jun at AP-I binding sites by means of the p160 co-activators SRC-1 and GRIP-1. In mice, mutant forms of ER which cannot bind to ERE still demonstrate feedback inhibition of LH secretion, indicating E–ER binding receptor can lead to cell responses independent of classical pathways.

SERMs as "proof of principle" (Figs. 2.3, 2.8, Table 2.5)

SERMs are a class of synthetic compounds that stimulate a spectrum of tissue-specific E action which exploits the availability of multiple cellular pathways of ER action in different target tissues [14]. The classical receptor theory that agonists function to turn on inherently inactive ERs, whereas antagonists competitively inhibit agonist binding and "lock" the ER in a latent state, does not explain the mixed agonist/antagonist properties of SERMs. The activity of these synthetic ER ligands is the affirmation of the classic E–ER complex physiology: The conformational shape produced after binding "instructs" modification of actions depending on recruitment of cell context-specific co-regulatory proteins. For example, the unique conformational shape of the SERM raloxifene produced when it binds to the ER prevents the involvement of a required co-activator protein at AF-2 site. In target tissues that respond principally to AF-2 gene transcription, raloxifene will lack that estrogenic activity. However, in tissues with the appropriate cellular context of proteins, E action will be preserved by means of AF-1 activation. On the other hand, in tissues that

Table 2.5. SERMs as proof of principle

Feature	Binding site residues involved		Subtype-selective ligands	
	ERα	ERβ	ERα	ERβ
Cavity height	Leu384, Met421	Met336, Ile373	None known	Genistein and other "flat ligands
B-face	Leu384	Met 3336	None known	8β-VE2
α-face	Met421	Ile373	PPT-16α-LE2	Fluorenone
B-ring cavity	Val392	Met344	None known	4-benzyl Chromanol

16α-LE2: 16α-lactone estradiol; 8β-VE2: 8β-vinylestradiol; ER: estrogen receptor; PPT: propyl pyrazole triol.

respond primarily to ERβ which lacks AF-1 activity or when target tissues lack co-activators that interact with AF-1 these agents will have antagonist activities. Thus by virtue of variations in conformational shape in the SERM–receptor complex and the specific cellular co-regulatory context, drugs have been developed to produce beneficial effects in certain target systems while avoiding deleterious action in other tissues: beneficial effects on bone, brain, and cardiovascular tissues without the mitogenic and possibly carcinogenic actions on breast and endometrium. These synthetic ligands differ from pure E antagonists in that the latter oppose E activity in all tissues both in vitro and in vivo by inhibition of dimerization of the ligand-bound receptor, prevention of DNA binding and disproportionate cytoplasmic metabolism of receptor without compensatory replenishment.

Functional diversity of E action in health and disease

As noted in previous sections, our appreciation of the mechanism of action of E has significantly increased over the past several decades. We know that E acts in a variety of tissues by activating and coordinating diverse cellular mechanisms which lead to cell, tissue, organ, and organ system biologic outcomes [21].

Efforts to dissect, analyze, and understand these complicated examples of systems biology function and dysfunction are under way using innovative genetic and pharmacologic manipulations of hormone activity. These include singly or in combination use of selective agonists for ERα and ERβ, universal E antagonists, models of general and organ-specific receptor subtype knock outs (KO), biosynthetic modifications such as aromatase inhibitors and aromatase knockouts (AromKO) as well as membrane only (MOER) knock out of α and β receptors [36] and membrane receptor only ligands such as the E dendrimer conjugate (EDC) [37]. In the following section, selected specific organ and organ system effects elucidated by these measures will be described.

The role of E in skeletal maturation and homeostasis

Abundant clinical evidence, derived from examples of prolonged hypoestrogenism (e.g., in loss of ER, FSHR, aromatase deficiency, premature ovarian failure, untreated oophorectomized women, anorexia nervosa, and, particularly, in postmenopausal women) shows the association with marked increase in the rate of bone resorption leading to osteoporosis. All these entities define the importance of physiologic E2 in maintenance of bone homeostasis (balanced serial sequential resorption and bone formation) [38–40]. Furthermore, sustained replacement E therapy (even micro amounts) attenuates the pace of bone resorption restoring homeostatic balance, and even permits modest incremental bone growth [41].

Studies of growth plate (epiphyseal) fusion and bone homeostasis dynamics in rodent models confirm the association of E deficiency and E sensitivity (therapy) in the maintenance of bone integrity seen in humans. An approximation of the "critical" thresholds for bone maturation and bone homeostatic stability is E2 greater than 20–40 pg/mL and bone loss increase at less than 10–20 pg/mL [42]. Comparing wild-type mice with both female and male αERKO, βERKO, and gonadectomy, in each instance treatment with selective ERα and ERβ agonists indicates the dominant role of *ERα* in maintenance of bone mass density (BMD), trabecular bone architecture, and cortical bone integrity. ERβ selective stimulation had no such protective homeostatic properties [43]. Therapy with E, CEE (conjugated equine E), raloxifene, and tamoxifen all appear to operate through similar ERα agonist function [21].

On the other hand, rapid signaling by means of membrane-based ER in bone operates in a ligand-independent manner. Mechano-transduction (from micro-fracture) stimulates both membrane ERα and ERβ to activate ERK, leading to osteocyte and osteoblast survival and repair function at the injured site probably by bone morphogenic protein-2 (BMP-2), signaling enhanced osteoblast differentiation [44].

The role of E in regulation of fuel homeostasis and metabolism (Fig. 2.9)

Maintenance of fuel homeostasis represents a concerted interaction between the hormones of reproduction and energy metabolism [45]. Extreme conditions of disrupted energy balance such as obesity and particularly anorexia negatively affect reproduction. Fundamental aspects of energy metabolism are regulated differently in males and females. To cite one evolutionary example of genetic pressure, the female responsible for successful gestation and lactation has been genomically engineered to resist loss of body energy stores during prolonged periods of famine by deposition of

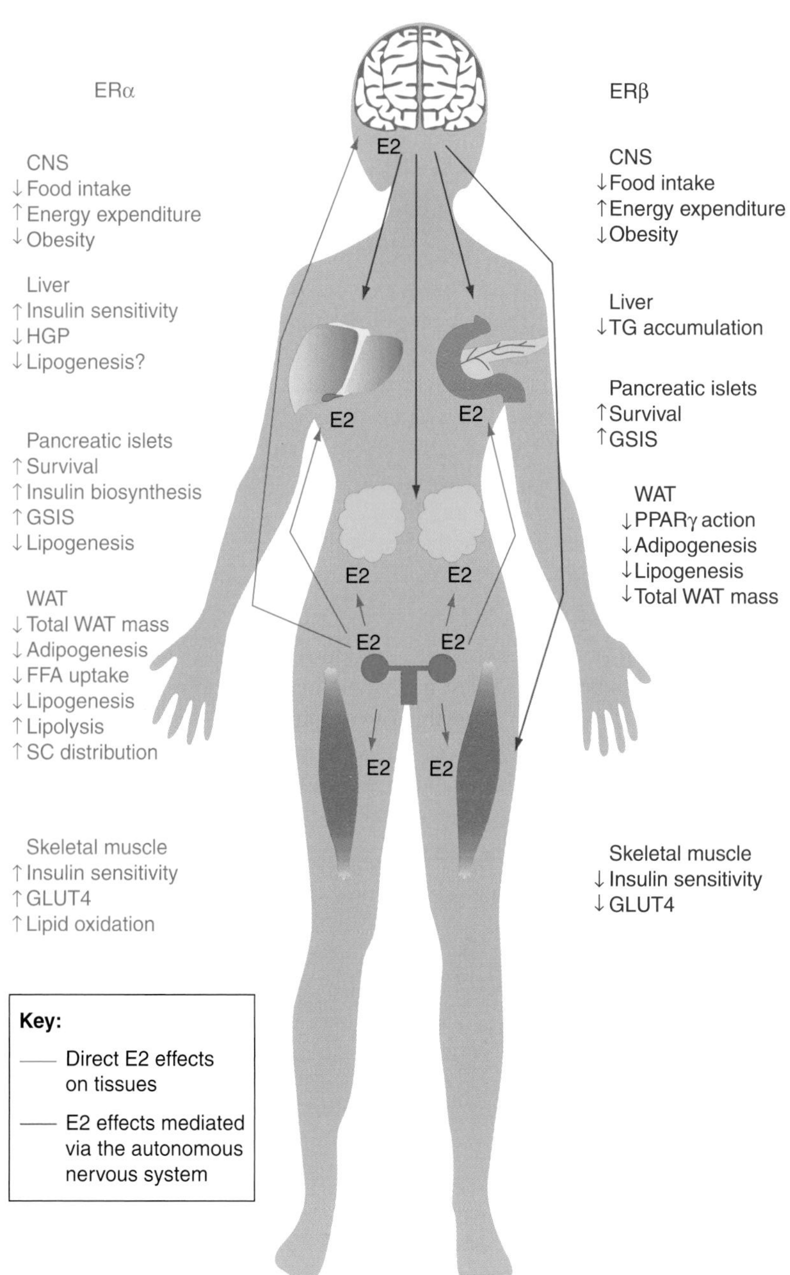

Fig. 2.9. Metabolic effects of ERα and ERβ activation in females. Both ERα and ERβ activation in CNS suppress food intake, increase energy expenditure, and decrease body weight. *Activation of ERα* improves peripheral energy and glucose homeostasis by (1) preventing *liver* steatosis and gluconeogenesis, improving insulin sensitivity; (2) increasing *skeletal muscle* lipid oxidation, GLUT4 expression, and insulin sensitivity; (3) increasing subcutaneous white adipose tissue (WAT) distribution, decreasing WAT fatty acid uptake and lipid synthesis, and increasing lipolysis; (4) *Enhancing pancreatic* β cell survival and function, increasing insulin synthesis and glucose-stimulated insulin release (GSIS). *Activation of ERβ* affects peripheral energy and glucose homeostasis by (1) enhancing β cell survival, increasing GSIS; (2) preventing obesity and decreasing WAT mass; but (3) promoting insulin resistance in the absence of ERα activation. Reproduced from reference [45], with permission.

fat in hip and thigh, areas with low lipolytic activity. Conversely, males deposit fat in visceral central areas with greater lipolytic activity enabling them to mobilize energy stores acutely for swift and effective maximum muscle activity. It is believed that circulating gonadal hormones, specifically androgen and E, control these sexually dimorphic differences particularly sustaining gender-specific energy balance between the onset of puberty and menopause. In modern cultures, women live well beyond reproductive capacity (or necessity); women spend one-third of their lives in post-menopausal E deficiency, a condition which correlates with the emergence of the metabolic syndrome, type II diabetes, and increased CVD events [46,47].

Mechanisms of ER action in regulation of fuel homeostasis

E2 activates rapid signaling by means of extra-nuclear and membrane associated forms of ERs and G protein-coupled ERs, activation of ion channels, and protein kinases [45]. Although reproductive functions are mostly mediated by means of the classic nuclear ERs acting as ligand-activated transcription factors, a large component of ER action related to energy metabolism involves extra-nuclear ERs indirectly modulating gene expression or acting independent of nuclear events. Acting through the ER α and β subtypes, E controls energy intake and expenditure, suppresses lipogenesis in white adipose tissue and liver, enhances insulin sensitivity, and has beneficial effects on β cell function and survival. Activation of ERα in the central nervous system suppresses food intake, increases energy expenditure, and decreases body weight. In addition, activation of ERα improves peripheral energy and glucose homeostasis in several ways: (1) preventing liver steatosis and suppressing hepatic gluconeogenesis thereby reducing insulin resistance; (2) enhancing skeletal muscle lipid oxidation, Glut 4 expression, and insulin sensitivity; (3) enhancing subcutaneous white adipose tissue (WAT) distribution while decreasing overall WAT mass by decreasing WAT FFA uptake and lipid synthesis, at the same time increasing lipolysis; (4) favoring pancreatic β cell survival and function by preventing pro-apoptotic injury, increasing insulin biosynthesis and glucose-stimulated insulin release. Similarly, activation of ERβ in brain also suppresses food intake, increases energy expenditure and prevents high fat diet (HFD)-induced obesity. Activation of ERβ also affects peripheral energy and glucose homeostasis in favoring pancreatic β cell survival and function and also by preventing pro-apoptotic injury. However, ERβ in the absence of ERα activation promotes insulin resistance.

In summary: The metabolic actions of ERα and ERβ both on peripheral tissues and central action on autonomic nervous systems, yield positive effects on fuel homeostasis, energy expenditure, insulin dynamics, and adipogenesis.

The role of E in metabolism (Fig. 2.9)

E deficiency in women resulting from a variety of genetic and biosynthetic disorders, but particularly in untreated post-menopausal women, leads to increased risk of cardiovascular and metabolic dysfunctions. These include body fat accumulation (weight gain) and redistribution of adiposity to visceral sites, increased free fatty acid (FFA), higher triglyceride concentrations, higher LDL-C, lower HDL-C, insulin resistance, impaired glucose tolerance, impaired glucose clearance, increased hepatic gluconeogenesis, decreased fibrinolytic potential but increased thrombogenicity, increased inflammatory markers (hsCRP), internal carotid wall thickening, and elevated coronary artery calcium scores. In short, the full expression of the metabolic syndrome is associated with increased atherosclerotic vascular changes and risk of cardiovascular disease events [46,47].

Studies in αERKO, βERKO, αβERKO, AromKO, and application of ER subtype selective ligands (+ and −) confirm the relationship among E ligand levels, E receptor activation, and the regulation of metabolic homeostasis in females, with ligand signaling by means of ERα the controlling factor of metabolic status and function [21]. Furthermore, in studies using MOER (models of membrane only ER), signal transduction through ERK and PI3K was equivalent in wild-type and MOER liver models, but completely absent in αERKO liver animals, suggesting that membrane-localized ERα is crucial, perhaps even sufficient to account for the importance of ERα in fuel and metabolic homeostasis [48].

Vascular biology

Unlike the primary role of ERα in metabolic homeostasis, both ERα and ERβ demonstrate positive roles in the endothelium (by distinct as well as overlapping mechanisms) in prevention of atherosclerotic plaque formation and progression, stimulation of vasodilatation of coronary arteries, and induction of endothelial repair (by recruitment of circulating endothelial stem cells to site of local endothelial injury) [49,50]. Whereas ERα agonists increase cyclo-oxygenase and PGI_2 (vasodilatation), both ERα and ERβ antagonists reduce endothelial NO function. The mechanisms by which selective engagement of membrane-localized ER and ER subtypes protect the endothelium have been examined. Using an E dendrimer conjugate (EDC) as the E receptor, when E2 binds to the EDC, because of the large size of EDC, the complex cannot be transferred to the nucleus and, thus, acts solely at the membrane. There it activates membrane Gα-dependent NO release. In addition, agonist stimulation of ERβ membrane function decreases atherogenic plaque development and reduces foam cell formation. Finally, a specific ERβ agonist (8B-VE2) lowers blood pressure and prevents myocardial hypertrophy and fibrosis [49,51].

Taken together, the beneficial effects of E on endothelial integrity and function appear to result from a combination of distinct as well as overlapping E–ER mechanisms which are cell, membrane/nuclear, as well as receptor subtype specific [39,45–52].

E and E receptor subtype and brain function (Table 2.6)

The general role of E

In mice, E appears to be essential for normal brain development and maintenance of function. E modulates learning and memory, mood, and behavior, "executive," and cognitive function. The primary mechanisms by which E exerts these influences are through general effects on neurogenesis, neuronal protection, synaptic plasticity, as well as specific actions in specialized brain centers. As in other organ systems, most hormone effects are achieved by means of ERα and ERβ. Again, similar to other systems but more dramatically true of the brain, is the diverse regional distribution of the receptor subtypes. Previously E receptors were *not* thought to exist in the brain in great abundance, but newer techniques have shown wide distribution; some areas possessing only ERα and ERβ, whereas in others overlapping content exists.

Table 2.6. ER subtype influences on select brain functions

	ERα	ERβ
Anxiety	Activation: anxiogenic	Anxiolytic Anti-depressant
Aggressive behavior	Increases aggressive behavior	Reduces aggression
Cognitive performance	No effect	Enhanced cognitive performance
Spatial learning	Alpha suppressive	Enhanced
E_2 acts at both receptors and can induce unpredictable results		

Brain functions can be broadly divided into three categories: affect (mood or emotion), behavior, cognition (learning and memory). Estrogen, as an unrestricted agonist, has a strong influence on all three, but these are inconsistent and paradoxical: E_2 can reduce, increase or have no effect on these activities.

Similar to other organ systems, E action in the central nervous system (CNS) may combine actions as transcription factors operating at cell nucleus, by rapid effects and cross-talk by means of the cell membrane, and less well-defined cytosolic pathways [21].

On the other hand, two substantial differences are apparent: (1) gender differences in brain function [53], and (2) dimorphic vulnerability to dysfunction in the neuro-protective effects of local E production [54]. The gender effects of E undoubtedly reflect basic gender differences in brain morphology, neurochemistry, and neuronal wiring established in development and differentiation in the embryonic and early postnatal life, as well as modified epigenetically throughout the remainder of the life cycle. In humans, hormone-based sexual dimorphism is a contributing factor in female–male differences in the prevalence, progression, and severity of brain-associated disorders such as Alzheimer's disease (AZD) (two-fold higher in women), multiple sclerosis (MS, young women predominate), Parkinson's disease (greater in men), and finally depression (women dramatically predominate).

Brain aromatase and local E neuro-protection

Disparate concentrations of E2 secretions from the ovary compared with circulating levels of E in blood and particularly hormone production locally in organs (skin, muscle, fat, brain, liver) underline the important clinical concept that circulating levels of E do not necessarily reflect concentrations existing within target cells [55]. This is particularly true in postmenopausal women where local target synthesis from androgen precursors produce most E activities. Crucial to this local synthesis is the aromatase enzyme system which converts androgen substrates to E. Numerous sites in the brain express the cytochrome P450 aromatase enzyme. Its effectiveness is seen in the fact that, while constitutively active in the local production of E2 from aromatizable substrates, this action is markedly increased in response to brain injury which results in increased local production of E2 at the site of injury. Furthermore, in an example of homeostatic positive feedback, both ERα and ERβ are up-regulated in response to injury thus maximizing the impact of local injury-generated E2.

Accordingly, aromatase activity has been studied in several brain challenging experimental settings, such as reaction to cellular toxins, experimental ischemia, and aging, and using various conditions, i.e., alterations in aromatase substrates, gonadectomy, aromatase deficiency (AromKO), and administration of aromatase inhibitors each followed by replacement with end product E2. In each instance, the necessity of a fully functional aromatase enzyme, adequate (aromatizable) substrate availability, and sufficient E2 production protect against neuronal damage from cellular toxins, effects of ischemia, and the inroads of aging. The effects of deficiencies in any element of the system, but particularly the aromatase system, were more dramatic in female test animals. Furthermore, the effects of replacement E as well as ERα and ERβ agonist applications in AromKO animals were more protective against vulnerability to these toxic and traumatic challenges in females. Importantly, the salutary effects were protective only before damage or apoptosis was entrained; thereafter, reversibility of damage was not achieved by any of these manipulations.

Estrogen and depression

The prevalence of affective disorders and symptoms of depression are more common in women than in men; the relationship between fluctuations in E levels and the manifestations of these symptoms during the menstrual cycle and intensifying during the pre-menopause to post-menopause transition implicate E levels in the modulation of mood and induction of depressive behavior [21,56]. During this transition period, there is an overall increase in symptoms of depression in previously asymptomatic individuals as well as recurrence in individuals who have experienced depression earlier in their lives. Dysfunction of the serotonergic/noradrenergic neurotransmitter systems has been implicated in the development of depression because these systems are located in brain areas involved in mood, cognition, and anxiety. Clinical studies have demonstrated a beneficial effect of E therapy alone and particularly when added to standard anti-depressive therapy where greater anti-depressive efficacy is seen with combined E and SSRI therapy as opposed to SSRI alone.

The relationship of E and mood disorders and depression, and the relationship to specific brain area distribution and function of ER subtypes in the different substructures and neuronal distributions involved in the monoamine systems is informative.

Thus far, all evidence indicates that the salutary effects of E2 in the serotoninergic/noradrenergic neurotransmitter systems are carried out by means of the ERβ subtype: this positive effect is reflected in increased serotonin release and decreased monoamine oxidase resulting in increased extracellular serotonin. βERKO animals display decreased serotonin, decreased dopamine, and increased anxiety in various tests. Similarly, in the dopaminergic system (where inhibition of re-uptake also has anti-depressive efficacy), ERβ is also instrumental in the anxiolytic and anti-depressive effects as shown by an ERβ agonist. In both monoamine systems, ERα has no effect [56].

In addition to the monoamine neurotransmitter systems, additional aspects of depressive systems are displayed in selected brain areas associated with mood and affective disorders. Hippocampal and dentate gyrus neurogenesis is required for the anti-depressive efficacy of therapies. Both E2 and ER selective agonists (PPT-ERα, DPN-ERβ agonists) increase cell proliferation and differentiation in neurones. With regard to neuroplasticity, ERβ subtype agonists, but not ERα agonists, mediate hippocampal synaptic activities increasing cognition and enhanced memory-dependent test completion.

Finally, a dramatic difference in the subtype function is displayed in the activity of the hypothalamic pituitary adrenal (H-P-A) system and its relation to traumatic stress and depressive behavior. Whereas ERα agonists increase H-P-A reactivity to stress and impair dexamethasone negative feedback, ERβ agonists reduce stress-induced activation of the H-P-A, reduce ACTH secretion, and reduce corticosterone concentration – all conducive to stress modification and anti-depressive effects [56].

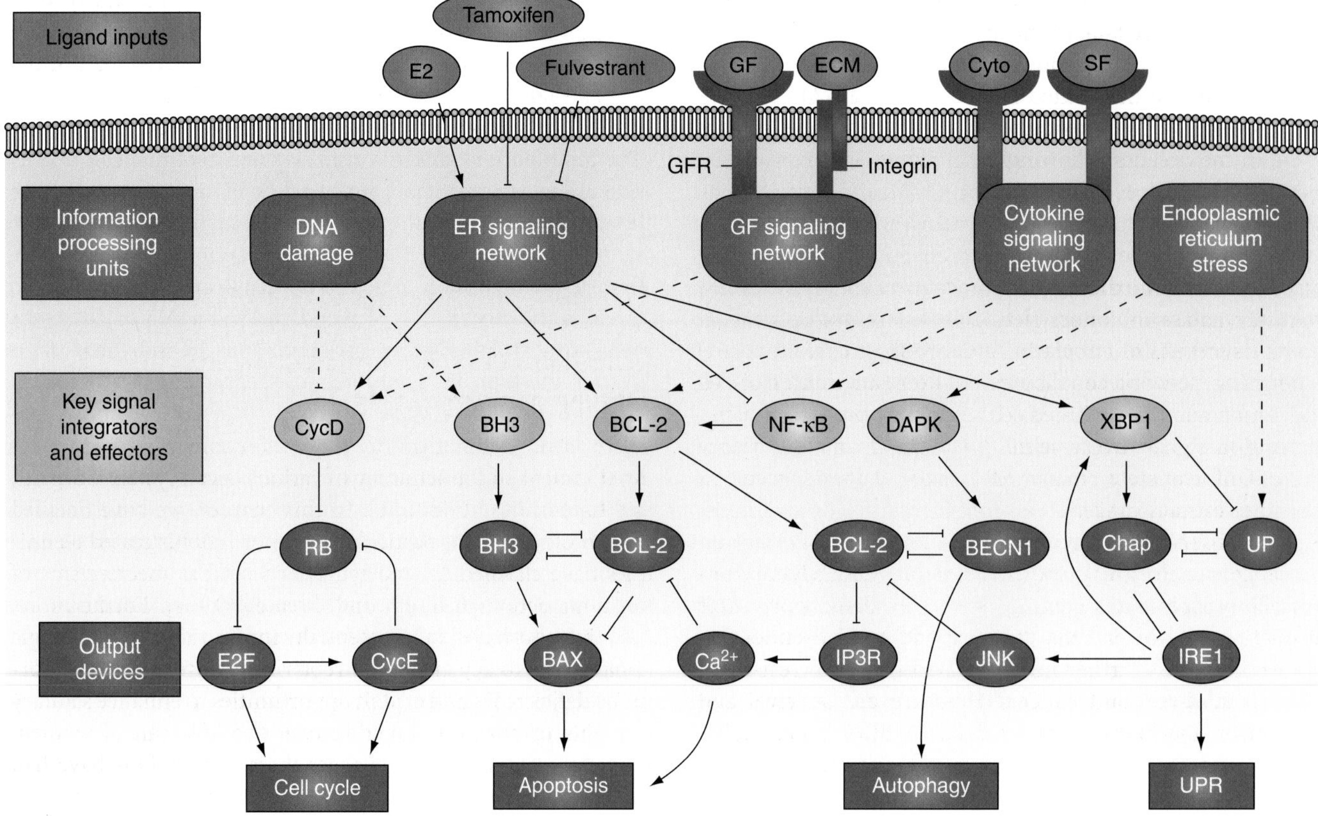

Fig. 2.10. The estrogen signaling "cross-talk" network in breast epithelial cells. Extracellular agonist signals such as estrogen (and antagonists), growth factors (GF), survival factors (SF), cytokines (Cyto), and extracellular matrix molecules (ECM) such as integrins bind to their receptor proteins and collectively initiate a complex series of reactions beginning with their specific information processing units (signaling networks) and leading to a set of key signal integrators and effectors which in turn drive output devices governing the cell cycle, apoptosis, autophagy and stress response mechanisms. Positive and negative signals promoted by these activities govern normal (and in pathology abnormal) cell growth, cell nutrition, cell replenishment, cell repair, and exclusion of damaged, "worn out," or unneeded cells. Reproduced from reference [60], with permission.

Taken together, the differential effects of E2 in wild-type, αERKO, and α βERKO, and the application of subtype agonists α and β, all unequivocally establish ERβ subtype as a major modulator of the anxiolytic anti-depressant cognitive and memory enhancement effects of E [21,56].

Breast tissue responses to E, ERs, SERMS, and subtype-selective ER agonists (Fig. 2.8)

The role of E in breast development and function

E is required for full elongation and branching of the mammary ducts as well as subsequent development of lobular-alveolar end buds [3]. Not surprising therefore is the absence of breast development pre-pubertally, and in all congenital E-deficient states. However, exogenous E supplementation in these instances leads to normal pre- and post-pubertal ductal development.

Both ER subtypes are expressed in mammary tissue. Female αERKO mice show impaired mammary development, despite elevated circulating E2 and/or replacement with E. However, female βERKO mice exhibit normal breast development under the same conditions. ERα expression in the stroma is essential for E2 stimulation of ductal epithelial growth. Studies in aromatase KO and αERKO confirm the defining role of ERα in the development of the mammary gland, whereas βERKO treatment of ovariectomized rats (deficient E) or with an ERβ-selective agonist results in no observable effects on mammary tissue. In sum, as opposed to ERα, ERβ and ERβ-selective agonists are non-mammotropic [21,57–59].

The role of ERα and ERβ in breast cancer (Figs. 2.10, 2.11)

For a thorough review of this topic, see Tyson [60]. Breast cancer, similar to other cancers, is characterized by misregulation of the bio-molecular pathways that control cellular metabolism and growth, DNA replication and repair, mitosis and cell division, autophagy and apoptosis, dedifferentiation, motility, and angiogenesis (Fig. 2.10). Like all cells, the breast ductal epithelial cell can be viewed as an information processing system that receives signals from its environment and its own internal state; it interprets these signals and makes appropriate cell fate decisions such as growth and division, movement, differentiation, self-replication, or cell death. In normal cells, this processing leads to "appropriate" development, function, survival, and cell replication. Cancer cells on the other hand make faulty decisions: proliferate when they should be quiescent, survive when they should die, or move around when they should remain immobile. In sum, normal cells make decisions that promote the functional survival of the organ/organism as a whole, whereas cancer cells make decisions that promote their own survival and are fatal to the organism.

Of the 180,000 cases of invasive breast cancer newly diagnosed each year in the United States, more than 70% express ERα (ER⊕ cells). Paradoxically, over 80% of these tumors emerge in the decades following menopause; an environment notably E deficient. However, tumor growth is stimulated by exogenous E therapy and E combined with progestins. Many tumors are responsive (at least initially) to endocrine inhibiting therapy such as tamoxifen, which binds to and neutralizes ER, and/or aromatase inhibitors (letrozole or exemestane) which block the synthesis of circulating and locally produced E. The ER signaling network contributes to the relative rates of cell proliferation and programmed cell death with pro-survival and proliferation signals overwhelming pro-death and quiescence signals. Unfortunately, many ER-positive tumors recur as endocrine-resistant cancers.

These observations invite a series of questions: Why do ER⊕ cancers evolve and grow in a low endogenous E environment? How does ER signaling drive this disproportionate malfunction in cancer cells that respond to anti-endocrine therapy? How is it further mis-regulated in anti-E resistance and aromatase-resistant cancer? How are cell survival and proliferation mechanisms maintained in ER⊖ cancer cells? Figure 2.10 demonstrates the E receptor signaling network in breast epithelial cells and the cross-talk among various signaling network modules (receptors, integrators, and effectors) which regulate cell growth and division, cell death (apoptosis), and autophagy. The importance of this cross-talk is demonstrated in the variable function of some of the key regulatory components and their interactions. For example, nuclear factor-κB (NFκB) is a pro-survival transcription factor over-expressed in hormone-resistant versus hormone sensitive cells; interferon regulatory factor 1 (IRF1), a pro-death transcription factor, is down-regulated in endocrine-resistant cells; x-box-binding protein 1(XBP1) is involved in the unfolded protein response (UPR) to reactive oxygen species (ROS) excess. Although analysis of these interactions has only begun, some evidence of the relation of ER subtype function and adverse cross-talk promotion has been uncovered. In these studies, ERβ has emerged as a potential prognostic marker predictive of endocrine therapy responsivity. The presence of ERβ is associated with significantly improved survival in post-menopausal breast cancer [21,58,59]. As would be predicted, knockdown of ERβ expression in both normal breast and breast cancer cell lines results in a significant increase in cell growth, elevated levels of cyclin A_2 expression and decreased expression of cyclin-dependent growth inhibitors. The ability of ERβ to induce breast cancer cell type apoptosis was also displayed when a selective ERα agonist PPT caused proliferation while the ERβ agonist DPN led to decreased cell numbers due to apoptosis. Expression of ERβ in breast cancer cell lines inhibits E stimulated cell growth and appears to potentiate the anti-proliferative and apoptotic effects of tamoxifen. In summary in all studies reported, ERβ activity does not stimulate tumor formation or progression, whereas ERα stimulation led to equivocal tumor growth responses. Clearly, there is a strong basis for pursuit of ERβ selection therapies in ER⊕ breast cancer.

E is of fundamental importance in the development of the normal mammary gland and ERα is the primary ER subtype mediating the proliferative effects of E. ERβ however apparently plays an important role in controlling the mammotropic effects of ERα and as noted above may be a novel target for endocrine therapy in breast cancer.

The next frontiers of estrogen function

Molecular endocrine targeted therapy using ERβ subtype agonists (Table 2.5)

There is no doubt that E2 plays a fundamental role in the development and functioning of various organ systems, organs, and tissue in the body [21]. In this chapter, we have detailed these biologic effects particularly as more sophisticated techniques have clarified the molecular and cellular mechanisms of hormone action in health and disease [61–64]. Furthermore, these insights have led to potentially innovative pharmacologic applications to replenish and repair the consequences of hormone deficiencies and exploit opportunities to enhance salutary elements of hormone function over the life span of women. Unfortunately, in some instances these applications have had adverse consequences: initiation and progression of gynecologic tumors (endometrium and breast) and in some vulnerable populations, coronary heart disease, pulmonary embolism, and stroke [61]. Although circumvention of these inherent liabilities of E2 as a universal agonist in all target tissues by deployment of selective E receptor modulators (SERMs) has improved the benefit/burden profile somewhat, even here disappointing effects have emerged, including vasomotor reactions, thrombogenesis, and VTE, uncertain cardiovascular protection, stimulation of endometrial tumors and the emergence of SERM-resistant breast cancer.

Existing and newer ER subtype-selective agonists will not only continue to be vital experimental tools in deciphering the specific roles of E action in health and disease, evidence is now in hand to consider their clinical applications. Both ER subtype agonists have been reported to alleviate vasomotor symptoms. However, whereas ERα targeting has adverse mammatropic and uterotrophic effects, ERβ agonist applications provide a safer profile and induce significant biologic benefits. Although ERα seems more important in lipid and cholesterol metabolism and pancreatic β cell function, both ERα and ERβ reduce food intake, increase energy expenditure, and decrease obesity, WAT mass, and lipogenesis. Both seem to protect against development of atherosclerosis. Most important, ERβ activation leads to diverse, multi-system positive effects: ERβ does not activate breast epithelial proliferation, has a beneficial impact on brain status (neurogenesis, neuroplasticity, neuro-protection), possesses antidepressant, anxiolytic properties, has a positive effect on feeding behavior and energy expenditure, dampens pain perception as well as possesses anti-atherosclerosis properties. In sum, ERβ agonist molecular targeted therapy presents an exciting clinical prospect.

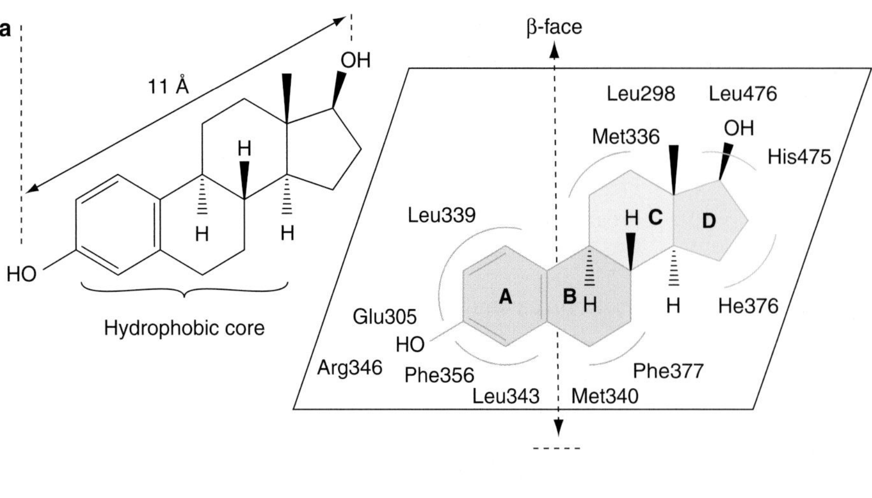

Fig. 2.11. Comparison of the classic universal agonist estradiol (a), its placement in the ligand-binding domain of ERα and the structural similarities (planar structure) and hydroxyl group electron density similarities of 27-hydroxycholesterol, an *endogenous* selective estrogen receptor modulator. Top panel reproduced from reference [3], with permission.

OH

HO

27-OH Cholesterol

27-Hydroxycholesterol: an endogenous SERM as a contributor to the morbidity and mortality of the metabolic syndrome in aging women (Fig. 2.11)

Detailed in Chapter 20 (menopause), arguably the most quality of life-disrupting, disabling, and life-threatening syndrome complex facing women is at once the paradoxical juxtaposition of the post-menopausal emergence of coronary heart disease, breast cancer, and osteoporosis. Paradoxical in that, while the absence of E might account for the progression of the detrimental imbalance on bone homeostasis leading to excess bone resorption over replacement, and the absence of an E "protective" effect on endothelium, what explains the concurrent dramatic emergence of ER+ and PR+ breast cancer in the decades defined by profound loss of endogenous E?

A clue to understanding this phenomenon has emerged from the appreciation that all three disorders share a single metabolic relationship: obesity and particularly the hypercholesterolemic element of the metabolic syndrome [65–67]. Specifically, evidence derived from a variety of in vivo and in vitro studies has identified a metabolically active metabolite of cholesterol – 27-OHC – as an *endogenously* produced selective E receptor modulator which interacts with and modulates the transcriptional activity of both ER subtypes and induces agonist and antagonist activity similar to non-steroid pharmacologic administration of SERMs (Fig. 2.11).

27-OHC is the most prevalent circulating oxysterol derivative of cholesterol; its serum levels and selected tissue concentrations increase in direct proportion to elevations in circulating total cholesterol. 27-OHC is converted from cholesterol and deposited locally by resident macrophages, epithelial cells, and endothelial cells.

It functions (as an ER ligand) at physiologic concentrations but with lower efficacy than E2. However, 27-OHC sustains its SERM activity in concentrations that accumulate over time but still remain within the Km of the catabolic enzyme governing its further metabolism and clearance, thereby maintaining local concentrations that saturate available E2 receptor. It appears that 27-OHC can perform much like an E because of its three-dimensional characteristics: it is a planar, all transverse oxysterol compound with high polarities of electron density at both ends of its structure. As such it can fit, albeit imperfectly and at a rotational shift, in the relatively large LBD groove of the ER. This is particularly true when competing E2 is low as in the post-menopausal woman. Evidence accumulated from animal and cellular models supports the role of 27-OHC as an agonist/antagonist endogenous SERM affecting coronary artery endothelial cells [65], normal and human breast carcinoma cells [66], and bone [67]. It must be remembered that interactive dynamics of the competition between E2 and 27-OHC normally favors E2. However, as 27-OHC climbs and E2 concentrations fall (post-menopause), the 27-OHC–ER complex prevails.

27-Hydroxycholesterol and coronary artery endothelium

27-OHC is found in high concentrations in developing atherosclerotic lesions where its levels rise sufficient to saturate the ER (in the absence of E2) thereby inhibiting E2 "normal" protective vasoactive effects of E2–ER–dependent actions [65]. 27-OHC for example inhibits E2-dependent association of ERβ with the transcriptional activator SRC-1. As a result, it inhibits (or eliminates) the usual E2-dependent increases in inducible NOS (iNOS) and endothelial NOS (eNOS). As such 27-OHC is an ER ligand that inhibits both the genomic and non-genomic activities of E2 in coronary artery endothelium. Also, by an ill-defined mechanism, 27-OHC inhibits the E2-dependent re-endothelialization endothelial injury repair process achieved by bone marrow-derived, circulating endothelial stem cells (ESCs) to the injury site. Therefore, 27-OHC in coronary artery endothelium is a competitive vascular ER antagonist. These findings suggest that, as endogenous E decreases in post-menopause, the anti-E effects of 27-OHC accumulate in the atherosclerotic coronary vasculature and accentuate the loss of circulating E2 cardio-protective effects seen in pre-menopausal women. Furthermore, the activity of 27-OHC as an endogenous ER antagonist confirms the large body of evidence supporting the ability of endogenous as well as exogenous E2 to protect castrate primates on high fat diets (HFD) from developing significant atherosclerotic plaques [66]. Once established, however, interventions do not reverse established plaque formation. Furthermore, the ability of E2 to compete effectively for ERα and ERβ, thereby inhibiting 27-OHC–ER activity, perhaps explains the "window of opportunity" observed in a variety of studies (including WHI ERT only study) that ERT begun within 4 years of menopause reduces coronary artery calcium scores (CAC) and reduces CHD events compared with untreated controls [63–65].

27-Hydroxycholesterol and breast cancer

As noted, breast cancer incidence increases with age and obesity [66]. The incidence accelerates unabated after menopause; up to 85% of human breast cancer occurs in the post-menopausal decades. Despite the decline of circulating E2 in these women, ER⊕ and PR⊕ breast cancer is the prevalent form of this cancer in this age group. Studies show 27-OHC is an endogenous SERM which displays *partial agonist* activity in cellular models of normal human breast and breast cancer cell lines, where it functions at physiologic concentrations (but with lower efficacy than E2) and at concentrations well below the Km of the catabolic enzyme governing its further metabolism and clearance. 27-OHC displays only partial agonist behavior by antagonizing E2 activation of ERα, in competitive assays. Both E2 and 27-OHC activate the transcriptional activity of ERα (the dominant ER subtype in breast epithelium) in exogenous reporter assays, in target gene expression, and in recruitment of ERα to the DNA ERE, as well as triggering ligand-mediated receptor degradation. 27-OHC, like E2, induces biologic activity by increasing concentrations of progesterone receptor (PR) protein and proliferation of ERα-positive breast CA cells (with associated increase in cyclin D1 expression). In conclusion, 27-OHC is a physiologically relevant ERα ligand by inducing ERα activation in the absence of E2. In addition, unlike its antagonist properties in coronary artery endothelium, 27-OHC is a tissue-specific endogenous SERM in breast where it is an agonist. These observations carry important implications in obese/hypercholesterolemic women and their increased risk of breast cancer, breast cancer progression, worse breast cancer prognosis, and because of its agonist properties, resistance to anti-E as well as aromatase inhibitor therapies.

27-Hydroxycholesterol and skeletal homeostasis

As noted elsewhere in this chapter as well as in Chapter 20, osteoporosis is a major clinical and public health problem affecting to some degree 50% (mostly women but also men) over 50 years of age [67]. E signaling is critical for maintaining proper bone density by balancing bone resorption and bone formation. However, nutritional and metabolic status can also influence bone biology thereby suggesting a possible role of 27-OHC in bone homeostasis. Using two genetically altered mouse models, Dusell et al. [62] assessed the effect of either absent 27-OHC (models incapable of synthesizing 27-OHC) or pathologically raised levels of the oxysterol (absence of the enzyme that eliminates 27-OHC). In addition, a group of mice lacking the biosynthetic enzyme were injected with exogenous 27-OHC to replenish the missing endogenous 27-OHC. Increasing 27-OHC concentrations led to decreased BMD (by decreased bone formation and increased bone resorption), evidence that the oxysterol had an E antagonist effect. To prove this point, in the animals with excess 27-OHC, when E2 was administered exogenously, normal BMD was restored. 27-OHC competitively reduces E signaling at the ER and its co-regulatory constituents. This inhibition of bone homeostasis becomes more prominent when E2 levels fall with menopause and aging and as women become obese and hypercholesterolemic. However, the dual findings of 27-OHC and its implications in breast cancer and osteoporosis combined with the epidemiologic observation that breast cancer women are also likely to be osteoporotic are intriguing.

Progesterone: functions and mechanism of actions

The major physiologic roles of progesterone in the female mammal include [1,68–70]:

- release of mature oocytes, facilitation of implantation, and maintenance of pregnancy
- breast lobulo-alveolar development, differentiation, and function in preparation for milk secretion and suppression of milk protein synthesis before parturition
- mediating signals in the brain required for sexually responsive behavior
- diverse non-reproductive systems such as bone (regulation of bone mass and protection against bone loss).

Similar to the previous description of the mechanism of action of E, the effects of P are primarily mediated through the nuclear P receptor (PR), which interacts with transcriptional co-regulators, moves into nuclear aggregates, i.e., "transcriptomes"

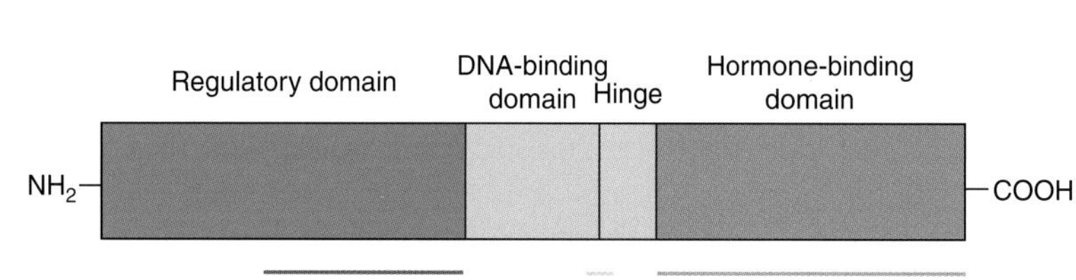

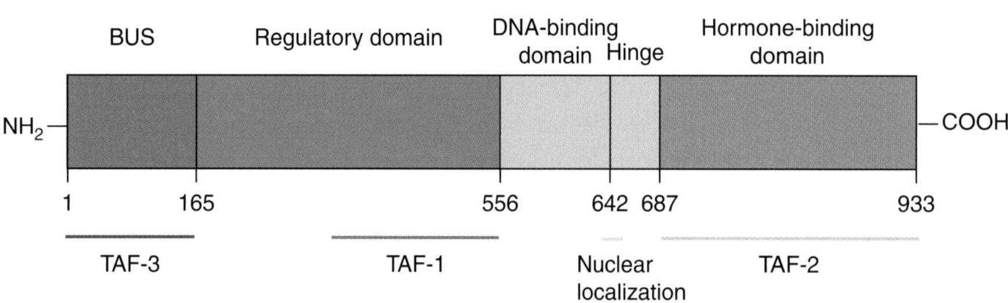

Fig. 2.12. The two isoforms of the progesterone receptor (PR). PRA and PRB and their functional domains. Note that PRB has three transcription activation factor components.

or membrane "signalsomes" to direct target cell gene expression and function [68]. Although P plays a pivotal role in normal physiology, reproductive exposure to its analogs in exogenous hormone formulations is sometimes associated with deleterious effects, most notably an explicit progestin-driven increase in breast cancer risk [61,64,71].

The following paragraphs describe the role of nuclear localization of PR and its cell-specific recruitment and association with select assemblies of co-regulators. Unlike the E–ER subtype dependence, it will be seen that the co-regulator complement in target tissues, not receptor subtype, is the more important contributor to the biologic identity of P function in normal and malignant target tissues. The non-nuclear membrane action of P will be mentioned, but far less is known about this area.

The progesterone receptor (Fig. 2.13)

P effects are mediated by binding to the nuclear P receptor (PR) or its membrane forms. The P receptor is induced by estrogens at transcription and decreased by progestins at both the transcriptional level and by post-translational modifications [72–74]. Similar to the ER, as a member of the large family of ligand-activated nuclear transcription regulators, the PR is organized into specific functional domains (Fig. 2.12). PR is made up of a central DNA-binding domain (DBD) and a carboxyl-terminal ligand-binding domain (LDB). In addition, the receptor contains multiple activation (AF) and inhibitory (IF) functional elements, which enhance or repress transcriptional activation of PR by association of these regions with transcriptional co-regulators. Newly transcribed cytoplasmic PR is assembled in an inactive multi-protein chaperone complex. Progestin binding to PR causes conformational changes leading to dissociation of chaperones, dimerization, nuclear transport, binding to progestin response elements in the promoters of target genes, and recruitment of specific co-regulators and general transcription factors [75–78] (Fig. 2.13).

PR nuclear receptors have also been demonstrated at the plasma membranes (mPR) particularly in breast cancer cells where they rapidly signal cell proliferation and survival [79,80]. When ligand activated, mPR associates with specific domains of SRC kinase, activating SRC signaling to ERK, MAPK and transactivation of EGF or IGF-1 receptors. This transactivation of kinase cascades is typical of the membrane G protein-coupled receptor-initiated functions of angiotensin, adrenergic and dopaminergic receptors as well as the steroid membrane receptor group. Thus, the PR reactive signalsome at the membrane of specific target cells either associates with or initiates cross-talk with multiple proteins including GPCRs and growth factor (GF) receptors to activate second messenger cascades. Scaffolding of these unique assemblies results in the generation of cell-specific rapid PR signaling [81–86]. These effects may include P negative feedback on GnRH (by means of reduced cAMP) and the anti-apoptotic effect of P on ovarian cancer models undergoing cisplatin exposure. But mPR signaling also includes regulation of nuclear (genomic) PR function, such as in the case of histone/chromatin genomic remodeling of mouse mammary tumor cells leading to co-activator and RNA polymerase recruitment. Progesterone also has the ability to induce activity at the cell membrane independent of complexing with a progesterone receptor.

In summary, P-dependent action of PR occurs in a cell type- and promoter-specific manner and proceeds by means of nuclear as well as cytoplasmic- and membrane-generated signals.

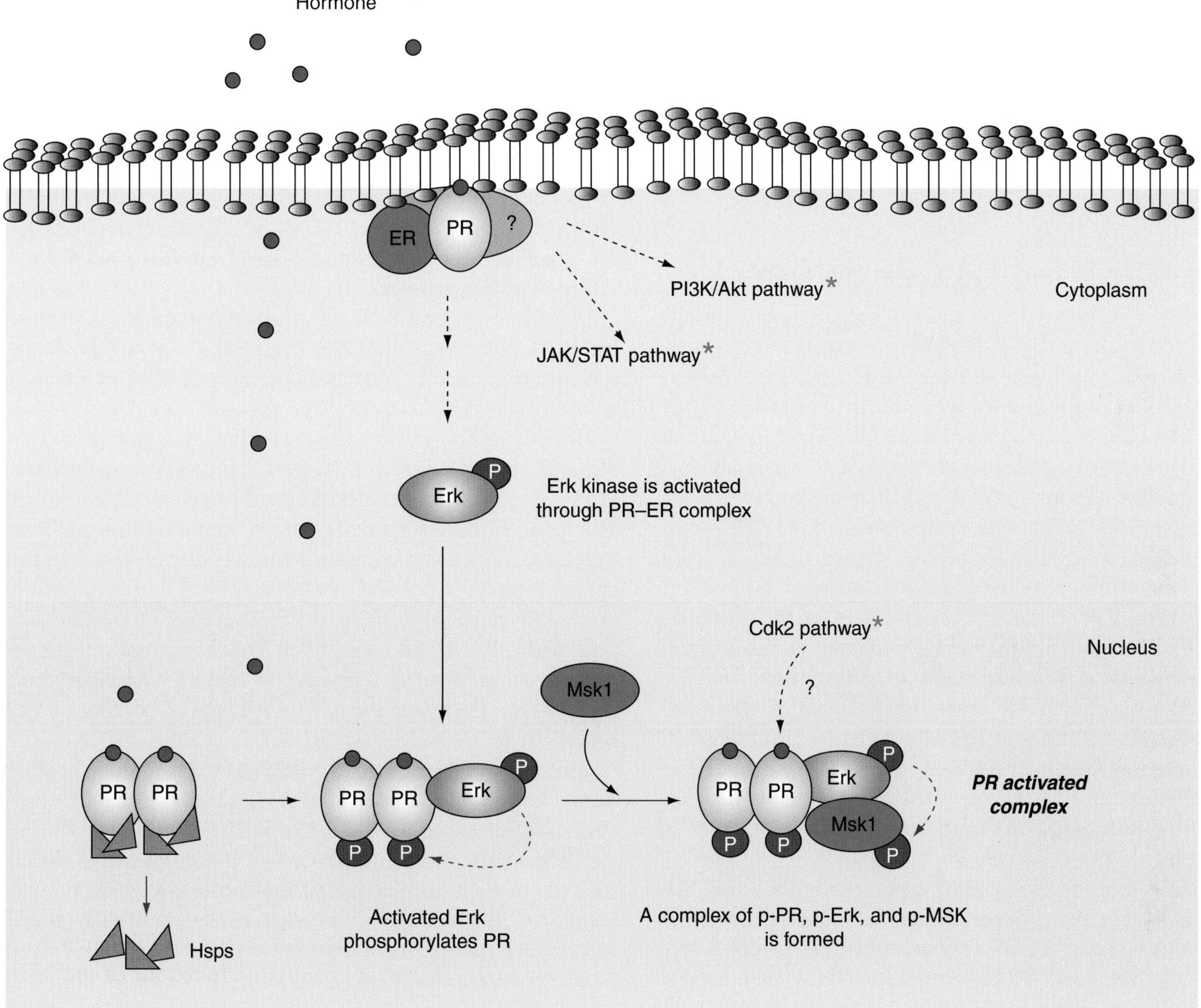

Fig. 2.13. Combined nuclear and membrane actions of P-PR. Progestins bind to PR/ER complex anchored in the cell membrane and activate the Src/Ras/Erk pathway. In this manner signal cascades through PI3K/Akt or JAK/STAT pathways are activated. Activated ERK kinase (phosphorylated) accumulates in nucleus. The majority of PR is located in the nucleus (silenced by chaperone heat shock proteins (Hsps)). Hormones (progestins) enter the cell, pass into the nucleus and bind with PR. On ligand binding Hsps are shed, homo or hetero dimers are formed and attach to PRE DNA. In this instance a fraction of the PR membrane dimer is phosphorylated by pERK with the eventual formation of PR activated complex including Erk and Mskl (mitogen- and stress-activated protein kinase 1) leading to cell proliferation. JAK/Stat, Janus kinase; P13K, phosphatidylinositol kinase; Akt, serine-threonine kinase. Reproduced from reference [83], with permission.

Progesterone action is mediated by two PR isoforms [68,74,75]

In the human, the effects of P are mediated by two distinct forms of the PR transcribed from a single gene (on chromosome 11 at q22–23) by alternate initiation of transcription from two distinct promoters giving rise to transcripts encoding two protein isoforms, PRA and PRB. PRA and PRB are identical in sequence, except that PRA lacks 164 amino acids at the N-terminus, making it the shorter of the two proteins (see Fig. 2.12) [68,74,75]. Structure–function studies suggest that the AF3 domain located within the PRB upstream sequence region, which is absent in PRA, contributes to PRB transcriptional activity by suppressing the activity of an inhibitory domain (ID) contained within the sequences common to PRA and PRB. Evidence suggests that the two receptors adopt distinct conformation within the cell allowing PRA to interact with a set of co-regulators that are different from those that regulate PRB.

Relative expression of the PR isoforms contributes to selectivity of PR action

In mice, because either PRA or PRB is expressed in different cells within the reproductive system, the homodimer is the critical contributor to P action, consistent with the divergent and tissue-specific roles identified for these proteins in knockout studies [68,87,88]. In human physiology, however, the majority of PR-positive cells express both PRA and PRB at equivalent levels, and cells that express only one PR isoform are uncommon. In the human therefore, P exerts its effects in cells that co-express both PR isoforms, making the PRA–PRB heterodimer the dominant molecular formulation.

It was once thought that PRA exerted a dominant negative effect on PRB as well as other members of the nuclear receptor family. However, it now appears that PRA can only exert this dominant effect in experimental conditions where PRA expression is in very significant excess, a circumstance unlikely to exist under physiologic conditions in humans but that may exist in aggressive breast cancer.

PR expression in target tissues in the human

PR proteins are expressed in a variety of human tissues, including the uterus, mammary gland, brain, pancreas, bone, ovary, testes, and tissues of the lower urinary tract [68,69].

As noted, in contrast to the predominant expression of one PR isoform frequently observed in animal tissues, in normal human tissues in vivo, including the breast and uterus, all PR⊕ epithelial cells co-express PRA and PRB at similar levels. This suggests that co-location and heterodimerization of PRA and PRB mediates PR action in the human. However, there is some evidence that differential hormonal regulation of the two PR isoforms occurs in special circumstances as in the glandular epithelial cells of the endometrium. During the secretory phase of the menstrual cycle, when high circulating levels of P are associated with altered PR expression (as well as decreased ER expression), PRA is preferentially decreased, resulting in a distinct predominance of PRB in these cells at this time. Potential effects of this change in the secretory endometrium in ovulation-induced PCOS women will be discussed later in this chapter.

Also in contrast to the balanced expression of PRA and PRB in normal human tissues, progression of breast and endometrial tissues to malignancy is frequently accompanied by progressive unbalancing changes in PR isoform expression. Unlike normal breast or in benign conditions, as breast cancer evolves, PRA predominance emerges in a significant proportion of ductal carcinomas in situ (DCIS) and invasive cancers [82]. In endometrial cancers, one PR isoform is frequently lost [89], and PR isoform loss is often associated with higher histological grade.

In summary, PRA and PRB to work together to modulate the complex and divergent pathways of P action in normal physiology. However in malignancy, the abnormal unbalancing of PR isoform expression and its effect on the ligand–dimer complex configuration and conformational state adversely alters transcriptional responses in large part by recruitment of unphysiologic inappropriate co-regulators which contribute to cell dysfunction.

The role of PR co-regulators in P action in human tissue

Binding of ligand to PR leads to receptor dimerization, conformational change, association with specific response element sequences in proximal and distal regions of target genes and regulation of transcription. This transcriptional regulation is a complex multistep process, which involves the sequential recruitment of several primary and secondary co-regulators (see Table 2.6) [68,89,90]. The complex combinatorial process of chromatin remodeling, co-regulator recruitment and initiation of transcription by nuclear receptors has been described in detail elsewhere in this chapter.

The ligand-dependent change in PR conformation promotes recruitment of a group of p160 co-activators, histone acetylases, DNA helicases, ubiquitin ligases (such as E6-AP), methylases, and the steroid receptor-specific RNA activator SRA. The resulting histone modifications and remodeling of the local chromatin allows recruitment and activation of the RNA polymerase II holocomplex, and increased RNA transcription of target genes [83].

Because PRA and PRB are equivalently expressed in most human target tissues, but the effects of P are highly tissue-specific, variations in the level and type of PR co-regulators with distinct affinities for the two PR isoform heterodimers is the mechanism by which a tissue-specific functional reaction is achieved [91–93]. As seen in Table 2.7, the level of co-regulator expression is critical in determining the overall transcriptional activity of PR in target tissues, as well as aberrant co-regulator expression or activity in disease including cancer. For example, although the co-repressors N-CoR and SMRT play no role in normal PR physiology, these proteins have been found to associate with PR and ER when bound to the mixed antagonists such as tamoxifen, to suppress the agonist effects of these compounds. Decreased expression of these co-repressors may contribute to the tamoxifen-resistance phenotype.

In summary, in the case of P action perhaps more than other steroid hormones, variations in the recruitment of co-activators and co-repressors to the P–PR heterodimer complex represents the determining mechanism by which P induces tissue-specific function in both normal and malignant tissues in the human. Identifying the tissue distribution and regulation of co-regulator expression is an important key to understanding the diversity of P effects in disease progression and cancer (see Table 2.7).

Summary and conclusion

When bound to P, PR activates target gene transcription in a diverse range of target tissues such as the breast, uterus, brain, and central nervous and cardiovascular systems. The effects of P on these target tissues are diverse, with co-regulators playing a critical role in regulating the magnitude and nature of these biological responses. PR heterodimers recruit tissue-specific regulators that activate unique sets of P-regulated genes and in target tissues. This differs from the importance of the variations in the presence of either ERα and ERβ subtypes and their contributions to E-specific activity in tissues and cells.

The next frontier in progesterone function

"Progesterone resistance"

Polycystic ovary syndrome (PCOS) is characterized by oligo-anovulation and hyperandrogenism. Standard methods of ovulation induction in these patients yield relatively poor reproductive outcomes (lower pregnancy rates and higher rates of early pregnancy loss). PCOS women are also at risk

Table 2.7. Reported patterns of PR co-regulator expression in human tissues

Co-regulator	Pattern of detection in human	RNA/ protein
SRC1	• Predominant p160 isoform in normal mammary gland. Detected in normal endometrium, myometrium and ovary • Predominant p160 isoform in normal endometrium and stroma. Highest during proliferative phase (Shiozawa) or menstruation (Weiser) • Detected in normal brain. Rodent studies suggest colocalization with PR	RNA Protein Protein
SRC-2	• Present in epithelial cells of mammary gland and prostate, endometrial epithelium, and stroma. Expression pattern suggestive of PR colocalization • Expressed in normal endometrium and uterine stroma • Normal mammary gland, ovary, endometrium, and myometrium • Detected in normal brain. Over-expressed in meningioma	Protein Protein RNA Protein
SRC-3	• Expressed in normal mammary gland, ovary, endometrium, myometrium, testis, pituitary gland, and muscle. Weak detection in bone marrow and heart • Detected in normal endometrium. Highest in secretory phase Elevated with polycystic ovarian syndrome and endometrial cancer. Over-expression in endometrial cancer correlated with ER/PR • Amplified and over-expressed in breast cancer • Transcripts correlated with elevated protein in breast cancer • Amplification correlated with ER/PR • Elevated transcript expression in endometrial cancer	RNA Protein DNA/RNA RNA/Protein DNA/Protein RNA
SRA	• High in pituitary, adrenal gland, and liver Low in breast, ovary, uterus, and prostate Elevated specifically in hormone-dependent cancers	RNA
E6-AP	• High in lymph gland, pineal gland, and bladder Moderate in placenta, uterus, brain, bone, and liver Low in mammary gland, ovary, adrenal gland, and blood • Decreased expression in invasive breast cancer. Inversely correlated with ER in breast cancer and AR in prostate cancer	RNA Protein
N-CoR/ SMRT	• Present in normal mammary gland. N-CoR markedly higher than SMRT in mammary gland. Present in endometrium and myometrium Elevated expression in breast and endometrial cancers • N-CoR protein, but not SMRT, detected in proliferative phase endometrium, absent in secretory phase tissue	RNA Protein
CBP/P300	• Present in normal breast, endometrium, and myometrium • Abundant protein expression in endometrium, highest in proliferation	RNA Protein
pCAF	• Present in endometrium and myometrium	RNA
PPMID	• Amplified and over-expressed in breast cancers and cell lines	DNA/RNA

Note: The findings of studies reporting expression of known PR co-regulators at the transcript or protein level in human tissues are summarized.

for higher rates of endometrial hyperplasia and cancer. Comparison of gene expression by microarray analysis of endometrial samples obtained from normal fertile controls and women with PCOS demonstrate *lower* expression of P-regulated genes such as leukemic inhibitory factor (LIF) which is critical to endometrial support of implantation and placentation, up-regulation of cell proliferative genes such as those for cyclin B1 and cyclin E2, and down-egulation of the growth suppressor mitogen-inducible gene 6. Concurrently, the E–ERα signaling pathway is aberrantly up-regulated by recruitment of decreased co-repressors and increased co-adaptors while PR activity is down regulated. This combination leads to less inhibited and overall increased E function. These findings of reduced P function despite availability of normal mid-secretory P circulating concentrations support the thesis that local "P resistance" may be responsible in part for the reproductive dysfunction and increased endometrial cancer risks in PCOS women [94].

The paradoxical effects of progesterone/progestin on breast cancer and osteoporosis (Fig. 2.14)

Mammary stem cells (MaSCs) give rise to all the cells of the mammary gland including P receptor expressing PR⊕ cells. In adult post-pubertal women, progesterone induces proliferation directly on mature mammary epithelial cells. During pregnancy however, in preparation for increased demands of impending lactation and breast feeding, in addition to the proliferation induced by the massive elevations in circulating maternal

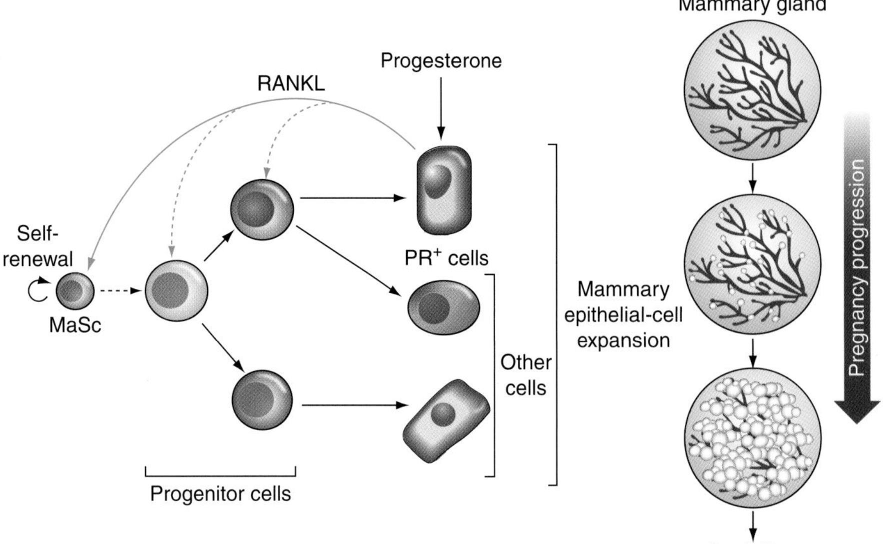

Fig. 2.14. Mammary stem cells (MaSCs) give rise to all cells of the mammary gland including PR⁺ (progesterone receptor expressing) cells. P-PR activation leads to cell proliferation. During pregnancy, in response to rising P levels, PR⁺ cells secrete RANKL which activates MaSCs (and other progenitor cells – dotted line) proliferation programs with mammary epithelial proliferation necessary for adequate lactation capacity. As noted in the text, continuous exposure to high levels or pharmacologic progestin may result in adverse growth responses, and in the presence of a malignant clone evolution of breast cancer. Reprinted from Lydon J. Stem cells: cues from steroid hormones. Nature, 2010;**465**:695–6.

progesterone and E2, progesterone activation of PR⊕ cells also induces secretion of the bone cytokine RANKL (ligand for receptor activator for NFκB). Although primarily thought of as essential for bone osteoblast development and initiator of the bone resorption-replacement sequence, RANKL also signals MaSC proliferation resulting in expansion of the mammary epithelial compartment and significant functional augmentation of the breast. Several studies, in particular the WHI report of increased breast cancer in the HRT (conjugated equine estrogen plus progestin) women compared with controls and ERT-only recipients have documented the unique stimulatory effect of progestins on breast cancer incidence [95–98]. This finding opens the question, could endogenous or exogenous P stimulate PR⊕ cancer cells to proliferate not only by direct action but also by RANKL induction of MaSC stem cell expansion of a malignant epithelial clone? This thesis is reinforced by the epidemiologic observation of an inverse association between bone loss (osteoporosis) and increased breast cancer. Furthermore, an experimental mouse model of P-dependent breast cancer demonstrated a marked decrease in incidence and delayed onset of breast cancer in RANKL *inactivated* mammary epithelium. Similarly, transgenic mice with RANKL *gain of function expression* exhibited accelerated mammary tumor formation. Pharmacologic inhibition of RANKL reduced P-inducible breast cancer in wild type mice. Denosumab, a monoclonal antibody inhibitor of RANKL, now FDA approved for treatment for osteoporosis, is also approved as a therapeutic agent for control of metastatic disease in bone from breast and prostate cancer. Accumulating evidence emphasizes the involvement of RANKL in the development of carcinogen-induced mammary tumorigenesis in mice in the setting of P treatment and provides proof of concept that RANKL inhibition may attenuate this process not only in bone metastatic disease but in PR⊕ primary breast cancer [98].

Progesterone is a powerful hormone; physiologically it can be essential, benevolent, and benign, but like Janus especially as a therapeutic agent (progestin), it may at once curtail malignant transition (endometrium) or stimulate cancer (breast).

How ovarian steroid hormones work: overall conclusion

As has been suggested throughout this chapter, substantial direct and circumstantial evidence links "how steroid hormones work" with almost all aspects of human physiology and clinical medicine. These insights, however complex, uncertain, or even barely defined, provide a basis for optimism that some of the mechanisms underlying the worst aspects of human dysfunction and disease such as cardiovascular disease and cancer can be addressed more successfully. Not only does a detailed understanding of these processes carry implications for diagnosis and possible prevention, it may also provide opportunities for development of new targeted therapies directed to correct aberrant pathophysiologic mechanisms.

References

1. Wierman ME. Sex steroid effects at target tissues: mechanisms of action. Adv Physiol Educ. 2007;**31**(1):26–33.
2. Kase NG. The human ovary part II. How steroid hormones work. In: Altcheck A, Deligdisch L, Kase NG (Eds.). Diagnosis and Management of Ovarian Disorders, Chapter 2B. San Diego, CA: Academic Press; Elsevier Science; 2003, pp. 33–50.
3. Nilsson S, Koehler KF, Gustafsson JA. Development of subtype-selective oestrogen receptor-based therapeutics. Nat Rev Drug Discov. 2011;**10** (10):778–92.

4. Speroff L, Fritz MA. Mechanism of action for steroid hormones. In: Clinical Gynecologic Endocrinology and Infertility, 6th edition. Philadelphia: Lippincott Williams & Wilkins; 2005, pp. 60–4.
5. Conneely OM. Perspective: female steroid hormone action. Endocrinology. 2001;**142**(6):2194–9.
6. Hall JM, Couse JF, Korach KS. The multifaceted mechanisms of estradiol and estrogen receptor signaling. J Biol Chem. 2001;**276**(40):36869–72.
7. Biddie SC, John S, Hager GL. Genome-wide mechanisms of nuclear receptor action. Trends Endocrinol Metab. 2010;**21**(1):3–9.
8. Tanenbaum DM, Wang Y, Williams SP, et al. Crystallographic comparison of the estrogen and progesterone receptor's ligand binding domains. Proc Natl Acad Sci U S A. 1998;**95**(11):5998–6003.
9. Lonard DM, O'Malley BW. The expanding cosmos of nuclear receptor coactivators. Cell. 2006;**125**(3):411–14.
10. Ascenzi P, Bocedi A, Marino M. Structure-function relationship of estrogen receptor alpha and beta: impact on human health. Mol Aspects Med. 2006;**27**(4):299–402.
11. Mangelsdorf DJ, Thummel C, Beato M, et al. The nuclear receptor superfamily: the second decade. Cell. 1995;**83**(6):835–9.
12. Parker MG. Structure and function of estrogen receptors. Vitam Horm. 1995;**51**:267–87.
13. Beato M, Sánchez-Pacheco A. Interaction of steroid hormone receptors with the transcription initiation complex. Endocr Rev. 1996;**17**(6):587–609.
14. Brzozowski AM, Pike AC, Dauter Z, et al. Molecular basis of agonism and antagonism in the oestrogen receptor. Nature. 1997;**389**(6652):753–8.
15. McKenna NJ, Lanz RB, O'Malley BW. Nuclear receptor coregulators: cellular and molecular biology. Endocr Rev. 1999;**20**(3):321–4.
16. Robyr D, Wolffe AP, Wahli W. Nuclear hormone receptor coregulators in action: diversity for shared tasks. Mol Endocrinol. 2000;**14**(3):329–47.
17. Smith CL, O'Malley BW. Coregulator function: a key to understanding tissue specificity of selective receptor modulators. Endocr Rev. 2004;**25**(1):45–71.
18. Lonard DM, Lanz RB, O'Malley BW. Nuclear receptor coregulators and human disease. Endocr Rev. 2007;**28**(5):575–87.
19. Thakur MK, Paramanik V. Role of steroid hormone coregulators in health and disease. Horm Res. 2009;**71**(4):194–200.
20. McKenna NJ, O'Malley BW. Combinatorial control of gene expression by nuclear receptors and coregulators. Cell. 2002;**108**(4):465–74.
21. Nilsson S, Gustafsson JA. Estrogen receptors: therapies targeted to receptor subtypes. Clin Pharmacol Ther. 2011;**89**:44–55.
22. Speroff L, Fritz MA. Mechanism of action for steroid hormones. In: Clinical Gynecologic Endocrinology and Infertility, 6th edition. Philadelphia: Lippincott Williams & Wilkins; 2005, pp. 53–69.
23. Couse JF, Korach KS. Estrogen receptor null mice: what have we learned and where will they lead us? Endocr Rev. 1999;**20**(3):358–417.
24. Couse JF, Hewitt SC, Bunch DO, et al. Postnatal sex reversal of the ovaries in mice lacking estrogen receptors alpha and beta. Science. 1999;**286**(5448):2328–31.
25. Dupont S, Krust A, Gansmuller A, et al. Effect of single and compound knockouts of estrogen receptors alpha (ERalpha) and beta (ERbeta) on mouse reproductive phenotypes. Development. 2000;**127**(19):4277–91.
26. Hammes SR, Levin ER. Extranuclear steroid receptors: nature and actions. Endocr Rev. 2007;**28**(7):726–41.
27. Levin ER. Plasma membrane estrogen receptors. Trends Endocrinol Metab. 2009;**20**(10):477–82.
28. Levin ER. Minireview: extranuclear steroid receptors: roles in modulation of cell functions. Mol Endocrinol. 2011;**25**(3):377–84.
29. Revankar CM, Cimino DF, Sklar LA, et al. A transmembrane intracellular estrogen receptor mediates rapid cell signaling. Science. 2005;**307**(5715):1625–30.
30. Filardo EJ, Quinn JA, Bland KI, et al. Estrogen-induced activation of Erk-1 and Erk-2 requires the G protein-coupled receptor homolog, GPR30, and occurs via trans-activation of the epidermal growth factor receptor through release of HB-EGF. Mol Endocrinol. 2000;**14**(10):1649–60.
31. Björnström L, Sjöberg M. Mechanisms of estrogen receptor signaling: convergence of genomic and nongenomic actions on target genes. Mol Endocrinol. 2005;**19**(4):833–42.
32. Britton DJ, Hutcheson IR, Knowlden JM, et al. Bidirectional cross talk between ERalpha and EGFR signalling pathways regulates tamoxifen-resistant growth. Breast Cancer Res Treat. 2006;**96**(2):131–46.
33. Kousteni S, Bellido T, Plotkin LI, et al. Nongenotropic, sex-nonspecific signaling through the estrogen or androgen receptors: dissociation from transcriptional activity. Cell. 2001;**104**(5):719–30.
34. Shupnik MA. Crosstalk between steroid receptors and the c-Src-receptor tyrosine kinase pathways: implications for cell proliferation. Oncogene. 2004;**23**(48):7979–89.
35. Thomas C, Gustafsson J-A. The different roles of ER subtypes in cancer biology and therapy. Nat Rev Cancer. 2011;**11**:597–608.
36. Pedram A, Razandi M, Kim JK, et al. Developmental phenotype of a membrane only estrogen receptor alpha (MOER) mouse. J Biol Chem. 2009;**284**(6):3488–95.
37. Harrington WR, Kim SH, Funk CC, et al. Estrogen dendrimer conjugates that preferentially activate extranuclear, nongenomic versus genomic pathways of estrogen action. Mol Endocrinol. 2006;**20**(3):491–502.
38. Smith EP, Specker B, Bachrach BE, et al. Impact on bone of an estrogen receptor-alpha gene loss of function mutation. J Clin Endocrinol Metab. 2008;**93**(8):3088–96.
39. Zirilli L, Rochira V, Diazzi C, et al. Human models of aromatase deficiency. J Steroid Biochem Mol Biol. 2008;**109**(3–5):212–18.
40. Hillisch A, Peters O, Kosemund D, et al. Dissecting physiological roles of estrogen receptor alpha and beta with potent selective ligands from structure-based design. Mol Endocrinol. 2004;**18**(7):1599–609.
41. Anderson GL, Limacher M, Assaf AR, et al. Effects of conjugated equine estrogen in postmenopausal women with hysterectomy: the Women's Health Initiative randomized controlled trial. JAMA. 2004;**291**(14):1701–12.

42. Vandenput L, Ohlsson C. Estrogens as regulators of bone health in men. Nat Rev Endocrinol. 2009;**5**(8):437–43.
43. Hertrampf T, Seibel J, Laudenbach U, et al. Analysis of the effects of oestrogen receptor alpha (ERalpha)- and ERbeta-selective ligands given in combination to ovariectomized rats. Br J Pharmacol. 2008;**153**(7):1432–7.
44. Aguirre JI, Plotkin LI, Gortazar AR, et al. A novel ligand-independent function of the estrogen receptor is essential for osteocyte and osteoblast mechanotransduction. J Biol Chem. 2007;**282**(35):25501–8.
45. Mauvais-Jarvis F. Estrogen and androgen receptors: regulators of fuel homeostasis and emerging targets for diabetes and obesity. Trends Endocrinol Metab. 2011;**22**(1):24–33.
46. Carr MC. The emergence of the metabolic syndrome with menopause. J Clin Endocrinol Metab. 2003;**88**(6):2404–11.
47. Janssen I, Powell LH, Crawford S, et al. Menopause and the metabolic syndrome: The Study of Women's Health Across the Nation (SWAN). Arch Intern Med. 2008;**168**(14):1568–75.
48. Roepke TA, Bosch MA, Rick EA, et al. Contribution of a membrane estrogen receptor to the estrogenic regulation of body temperature and energy homeostasis. Endocrinology. 2010;**151**(10):4926–37.
49. Chow RW, Handelsman DJ, Ng MK. Minireview: rapid actions of sex steroids in the endothelium. Endocrinology. 2010;**151**(6):2411–22.
50. Mendelsohn ME, Karas RH. HRT and the young at heart. N Engl J Med. 2007;**356**(25):2639–41.
51. Mendelsohn ME, Karas RH. Molecular and cellular basis of cardiovascular gender differences. Science. 2005;**308**(5728):1583–7.
52. Hodgin JB, Maeda N. Minireview: estrogen and mouse models of atherosclerosis. Endocrinology. 2002;**143**(12):4495–501.
53. Gillies GE, McArthur S. Estrogen actions in the brain and the basis for differential action in men and women: a case for sex-specific medicines. Pharmacol Rev. 2010;**62**(2):155–98.
54. Brann DW, Dhandapani K, Wakade C, et al. Neurotrophic and neuroprotective actions of estrogen: basic mechanisms and clinical implications. Steroids. 2007;**72**(5):381–405.
55. Azcoitia I, Sierra A, Veiga S, et al. Brain aromatase is neuroprotective. J Neurobiol. 2001;**47**(4):318–29.
56. Osterlund MK. Underlying mechanisms mediating the antidepressant effects of estrogens. Biochim Biophys Acta. 2010;**1800**(10):1136–44.
57. Helguero LA, Faulds MH, Gustafsson JA, et al. Estrogen receptors alfa (ERalpha) and beta (ERbeta) differentially regulate proliferation and apoptosis of the normal murine mammary epithelial cell line HC11. Oncogene. 2005;**24**(44):6605–16.
58. Nilsson S, Gustafsson JA. Biological role of estrogen and estrogen receptors. Crit Rev Biochem Mol Biol. 2002;**37**(1):1–28.
59. Hartman J, Ström A, Gustafsson JA. Estrogen receptor beta in breast cancer – diagnostic and therapeutic implications. Steroids. 2009;**74**(8):635–41.
60. Tyson JJ, Baumann WT, Chen C, et al. Dynamic modelling of oestrogen signalling and cell fate in breast cancer cells. Nat Rev Cancer. 2011;**11**(7):523–32.
61. Rossouw JE, Anderson GL, Prentice RL, et al. Risks and benefits of estrogen plus progestin in healthy postmenopausal women: principal results from the Women's Health Initiative randomized controlled trial. JAMA. 2002;**288**(3):321–33.
62. Manson JE, Allison MA, Rossouw JE, et al. Estrogen therapy and coronary-artery calcification. N Engl J Med. 2007;**356**(25):2591–602.
63. Hodis HN. Assessing benefits and risks of hormone therapy in 2008: new evidence, especially with regard to the heart. Cleve Clin J Med. 2008;**75**(Suppl 4):S3–12.
64. LaCroix AZ, Chlebowski RT, Manson JE, et al. Health outcomes after stopping conjugated equine estrogens among postmenopausal women with prior hysterectomy: a randomized controlled trial. JAMA. 2011;**305**(13):1305–14.
65. Umetani M, Domoto H, Gormley AK, et al. 27-Hydroxycholesterol is an endogenous SERM that inhibits the cardiovascular effects of estrogen. Nat Med. 2007;**13**(10):1185–92.
66. DuSell CD, Umetani M, Shaul PW, et al. 27-hydroxycholesterol is an endogenous selective estrogen receptor modulator. Mol Endocrinol. 2008;**22**(1):65–77.
67. DuSell CD, Nelson ER, Wang X, et al. The endogenous selective estrogen receptor modulator 27-hydroxycholesterol is a negative regulator of bone homeostasis. Endocrinology. 2010;**151**(8):3675–85.
68. Scarpin KM, Graham JD, Mote PA, et al. Progesterone action in human tissues: regulation by progesterone receptor (PR) isoform expression, nuclear positioning and coregulator expression. Nucl Recept Signal. 2009;**7**:e009.
69. Graham JD, Clarke CL. Physiological action of progesterone in target tissues. Endocr Rev. 1997;**18**(4):502–19.
70. Conneely OM, Lydon JP. Progesterone receptors in reproduction: functional impact of the A and B isoforms. Steroids. 2000;**65**(10–11):571–7.
71. Santen RJ, Pinkerton J, McCartney C, et al. Risk of breast cancer with progestins in combination with estrogen as hormone replacement therapy. J Clin Endocrinol Metab. 2001;**86**(1):16–23.
72. Giangrande PH, Kimbrel EA, Edwards DP, et al. The opposing transcriptional activities of the two isoforms of the human progesterone receptor are due to differential cofactor binding. Mol Cell Biol. 2000;**20**(9):3102–15.
73. Kastner P, Krust A, Turcotte B, et al. Two distinct estrogen-regulated promoters generate transcripts encoding the two functionally different human progesterone receptor forms A and B. EMBO J. 1990;**9**(5):1603–14.
74. Kraus WL, Montano MM, Katzenellenbogen BS. Cloning of the rat progesterone receptor gene 5'-region and identification of two functionally distinct promoters. Mol Endocrinol. 1993;**7**(12):1603–16.
75. Allan GF, Tsai SY, Tsai MJ, et al. Ligand-dependent conformational changes in the progesterone receptor are necessary for events that follow DNA binding. Proc Natl Acad Sci U S A. 1992;**89**(24):11750–4.
76. Weigel NL. Receptor phosphorylation. In: Tsai MJ, O'Malley BW (Eds.). Mechanism of Steroid Hormone Regulation of Gene Transcription. Austin, TX: R.G. Landes; 1994, pp. 93–110.
77. Gronemeyer H. Transcription activation by estrogen and progesterone

receptors. Annu Rev Genet. 1991;**25**:89–123.

78. Tata JR. Signalling through nuclear receptors. Nat Rev Mol Cell Biol. 2002;**3**(9):702–10.
79. Levin ER. Minireview: extranuclear steroid receptors: roles in modulation of cell functions. Mol Endocrinol. 2011;**25**(3):377–84.
80. Thomas P. Characteristics of membrane progestin receptor alpha (mPRalpha) and progesterone membrane receptor component 1 (PGMRC1) and their roles in mediating rapid progestin actions. Front Neuroendocrinol. 2008;**29**(2):292–312.
81. Sleiter N, Pang Y, Park C, et al. Progesterone receptor A (PRA) and PRB-independent effects of progesterone on gonadotropin-releasing hormone release. Endocrinology. 2009;**150**(8):3833–44.
82. Faivre EJ, Lange CA. Progesterone receptors upregulate Wnt-1 to induce epidermal growth factor receptor transactivation and c-Src-dependent sustained activation of Erk1/2 mitogen-activated protein kinase in breast cancer cells. Mol Cell Biol. 2007;**27**(2):466–80.
83. Vicent GP, Nacht AS, Zaurín R, et al. Minireview: role of kinases and chromatin remodeling in progesterone signaling to chromatin. Mol Endocrinol. 2010;**24**(11):2088–98.
84. Lonard DM, Lanz RB, O'Malley BW. Nuclear receptor coregulators and human disease. Endocr Rev. 2007;**28**(5):575–87.
85. Lange CA, Richer JK, Shen T, et al. Convergence of progesterone and epidermal growth factor signaling in breast cancer. Potentiation of mitogen-activated protein kinase pathways. J Biol Chem. 1998;**273**(47):31308–16.
86. Lange CA. Integration of progesterone receptor action with rapid signaling events in breast cancer models. J Steroid Biochem Mol Biol. 2008;**108**(3–5):203–12.
87. Mote PA, Balleine RL, McGowan EM, et al. Colocalization of progesterone receptors A and B by dual immunofluorescent histochemistry in human endometrium during the menstrual cycle. J Clin Endocrinol Metab. 1999;**84**(8):2963–71.
88. Arnett-Mansfield RL, Graham JD, Hanson AR, et al. Focal subnuclear distribution of progesterone receptor is ligand dependent and associated with transcriptional activity. Mol Endocrinol. 2007;**21**(1):14–29.
89. Mote PA, Bartow S, Tran N, et al. Loss of co-ordinate expression of progesterone receptors A and B is an early event in breast carcinogenesis. Breast Cancer Res Treat. 2002;**72**(2):163–72.
90. Wolf IM, Heitzer MD, Grubisha M, et al. Coactivators and nuclear receptor transactivation. J Cell Biochem. 2008;**104**(5):1580–6.
91. Lanz RB, Chua SS, Barron N, et al. Steroid receptor RNA activator stimulates proliferation as well as apoptosis in vivo. Mol Cell Biol. 2003;**23**(20):7163–76.
92. Jackson TA, Richer JK, Bain DL, et al. The partial agonist activity of antagonist-occupied steroid receptors is controlled by a novel hinge domain-binding coactivator L7/SPA and the corepressors N-CoR or SMRT. Mol Endocrinol. 1997;**11**(6):693–705.
93. Lavinsky RM, Jepsen K, Heinzel T, et al. Diverse signaling pathways modulate nuclear receptor recruitment of N-CoR and SMRT complexes. Proc Natl Acad Sci U S A. 1998;**95**(6):2920–5.
94. Savaris RF, Groll JM, Young SL, et al. Progesterone resistance in PCOS endometrium: a microarray analysis in clomiphene citrate-treated and artificial menstrual cycles. J Clin Endocrinol Metab. 2011;**96**(6):1737–46.
95. Gonzalez-Suarez E, Jacob AP, Jones J, et al. RANK ligand mediates progestin-induced mammary epithelial proliferation and carcinogenesis. Nature. 2010;**468**(7320):103–7.
96. Schramek D, Leibbrandt A, Sigl V, et al. Osteoclast differentiation factor RANKL controls development of progestin-driven mammary cancer. Nature. 2010;**468**(7320):98–102.
97. Asselin-Labat ML, Vaillant F, Sheridan JM, et al. Control of mammary stem cell function by steroid hormone signalling. Nature. 2010;**465**(7299):798–802.
98. Hofbauer LC, Rachner TD, Hamann C. From bone to breast and back – the bone cytokine RANKL and breast cancer. Breast Cancer Res. 2011;**13**(3):107.

Chapter 3

Gonadal dysgenesis: ovarian function and reproductive health in Turner syndrome

Paul Saenger, MD, and David Rodriguez-Buritica, MD

Turner syndrome (TS) affects approximately one in 2500 liveborn females [1]. This disorder presents the clinician with a challenging array of genetic, developmental, endocrine, cardiovascular, psychosocial, and reproductive issues. For the purpose of this chapter, Turner syndrome will be used to describe the patient with an abnormality of the chromosomal karyotype involving loss of part or all of the X chromosome associated with phenotypic abnormalities that include short stature and the potential for or the presence of ovarian failure.

Definition

The diagnosis of TS requires the presence of characteristic physical features in phenotypic females coupled with complete or partial absence of the second sex chromosome, with or without cell line mosaicism [2–4]. Individuals with a 45,X cell population but without clinical features are not considered to have TS. Phenotypic males are also excluded from the diagnosis of TS, regardless of karyotype. Whether to diagnose individuals with sex chromosome structural abnormalities as having TS requires clinical judgment. Abnormalities such as ring X and Xq isochromosomes are common in patients with classic TS features, and many of these patients have phenotypes indistinguishable from that of patients with apparently non-mosaic monosomy X (45,X) [4]. Patients with small distal short arm deletions (Xp-) including the SHOX gene frequently have short stature and other TS-associated skeletal anomalies, but most are at low risk of ovarian failure and should generally not be diagnosed with TS if band Xp22.3 is not deleted [5]. Individuals with deletions of the long arm distal to Xq24 frequently have primary or secondary amenorrhea without short stature or other TS features [6]; the diagnosis of premature ovarian failure is more appropriate for them. Table 3.1 summarizes the cytogenetic findings in TS patients.

Prenatal diagnosis

Sex chromosome abnormalities are increasingly detected prenatally by chorionic villous sampling or amniocentesis, and genetic counseling before any prenatal diagnostic procedure should always include discussion of the possibility of detecting them. Certain ultrasound findings indicate an increased likelihood of TS. Increased nuchal translucency on ultrasound is frequently seen in TS but may also be observed in autosomal trisomy syndromes. The presence of cystic hygromas makes the diagnosis of TS more likely [7]. Other ultrasound findings suggestive of TS are coarctation of the aorta and/or left-sided cardiac defects, brachycephaly, renal anomalies, polyhydramnios, oligohydramnios, and growth retardation [8]. Abnormal triple or quadruple maternal serum screening (α-fetoprotein, human chorionic gonadotropin, inhibin A, and unconjugated estriol) may also suggest the diagnosis of TS [9]. Ultrasound and maternal serum screening are not diagnostic, and to make a prenatal diagnosis of TS, karyotype confirmation is obligatory.

The postnatal outcome and constitutional karyotype of individuals with prenatally diagnosed sex chromosome monosomy are uncertain, especially in mosaic cases. Therefore, chromosomes should be reevaluated postnatally in all cases. The degree of mosaicism detected prenatally is not generally predictive of the severity of the TS phenotype [10,11]. In general, any of the features of TS may be seen with virtually any of the common chromosome constitutions [4]. Non-mosaic 45,X fetuses with pleural effusion or cystic hygroma often spontaneously abort [12]. Nevertheless, a 45,X karyotype, even with ultrasound evidence of cystic hygroma, lymphedema, and effusions, is compatible with delivery of a viable newborn.

Many pregnancies diagnosed prenatally with TS are currently terminated [13,14]. Decisions regarding pregnancy termination are difficult; thus, it is critical that the best available information be provided to parents. Although upholding personal choice about reproduction is a widely embraced ethical principle, decisions to terminate a fetus with TS should never be based upon misunderstood or unbalanced information [15]. Many studies providing genotype–phenotype correlations are subject to considerable ascertainment bias. Individuals with 45, X mosaicism detected because of an abnormal antecedent ultrasound study are more likely to have clinical TS than those with 45,X mosaicism detected incidentally by screening on the basis of advanced maternal age [10,11], which itself is not associated with an increased incidence of TS [16]. Outcomes of incidentally detected 45X/46,XX mosacism are difficult to predict prenatally, but high-resolution ultrasound often provides useful prognostic information. Not unexpectedly, prenatally diagnosed children tend to be less affected than those diagnosed postnatally on clinical grounds [10,11].

Physicians and genetic counselors involved in pre- and postdiagnostic counseling need to be fully informed about the

Altchek's Diagnosis and Management of Ovarian Disorders, ed. Liane Deligdisch, Nathan G. Kase, and Carmel J. Cohen. Published by Cambridge University Press.

Table 3.1. Summary of the cytogenetic findings in 207 patients with Turner syndrome

No.	%	Karyotype	
112	54.6	45,X	
34	16.6	46,X,i(Xq)	22: 45,X/46,X,i(Xq) 11: 46,X,i(Xq) 1: 45,X/46,X,i(Xq)/46,XXp2
26	12.6	45,X/46,XX	24: 45,X/46,XX 1: 45,X/46,XX1mar* 1: 45,X/45,X1mar†
11	5.3	46,X,r(X)	All: 45,X/46,X,r(X)
10	4.9	45,X/46,XY‡	
5	2.4	46,XXq2	2: 45,X/46,XXq2 3: 46,XXq2
4	1.9	46,XXp2	2: 46,XXp2 1: 45,X/46,XXp2 1: 45,X/46,XXp2/46,X1mar
4	1.4	45,X/47,XXX	
1	0.5	46,X,t(X;15)	(q22.1;q24)

* DNA was examined with Y chromosome–specific probes and found to contain Y sequences. Gonadal streaks were removed, and an in situ gonadoblastoma was found.
† Leukocytes examined by fluorescent in situ hybridization with X- and Y-specific pericentromeric probes showed presence of one cell line positive only for X probe and one cell line positive for both probes. Gonadal streaks were removed and were tumor free.
‡ Eight patients had removal of gonadal streaks. One macroscopic calcified gonadoblastoma and three in situ gonadoblastomas were found. Two patients who did not have surgery were lost to follow-up.

prognosis, complications, and quality of life of individuals affected with TS as well as of recent advances in management. The clinical spectrum of TS is much broader and often less severe than that described in many textbooks. Prenatal counseling should always involve discussion of the variability of features, the likelihood of short stature and ovarian failure, and their management. It should be emphasized that most individuals with TS have intelligence scores in the normal range, although they may have specific types of learning disabilities. Most adults with TS function well and independently. Girls and women in one study indicated that struggling with their infertility was the greatest challenge they faced in adapting to a life with TS [17]. Speaking with children and adults with TS and their families is important for prospective parents faced with a decision about pregnancy and can be facilitated by support organizations, e.g., Turner syndrome societies.

Postnatal diagnosis

All individuals with suspected TS (see below) should have a karyotype performed. A standard 30-cell karyotype is recommended by the American College of Medical Genetics and identifies at least 10% mosaicism with 95% confidence [18], although additional metaphases may be counted or fluorescence in situ hybridization (FISH) studies performed if there is a strong suspicion of undetected mosaicism [19]. The cytogeneticist should be consulted in this case. Although a peripheral blood karyotype is usually adequate, if there is a strong clinical suspicion of TS, despite a normal blood karyotype, a second tissue, such as skin, may be examined.

Numerous studies have examined the relationship between the chromosomal karyotype and the phenotypic characteristics that appear in Turner syndrome. In a classic article by Ferguson-Smith the karyotypes of 307 patients with various forms of gonadal dysgenesis were correlated with their clinical findings [4]. He noted that short stature was the only clinical finding invariably associated with the 45,X karyotype. Complete gonadal insufficiency was not always present because seven patients with a 45,X karyotype demonstrated evidence of spontaneous puberty. He also noted that as a whole patients with mosaic karyotypes, including one normal XX line (i.e., 45,X/46,XX), tended to have fewer phenotypic abnormalities.

Save for a very few mosaic patients who were not short, however, on physical examination individual patients with mosaicism could not be readily distinguished from patients with the monosomic karyotype. Finally, he proposed that the area of the X chromosome responsible for the disturbance in growth was localized to the short arm of the X chromosome. Although banding studies were not yet available at the time of this study, the majority of these observations are still valid. A subsequent study of a large group of patients, which included banding, confirmed that short stature is the only characteristic present in virtually 100% of patients [20]. Table 3.2 shows the clinical findings commonly described in patients with Turner syndrome.

Testing for Y chromosome material should be performed in any TS patient (or fetus) with a marker chromosome (a sex chromosomal fragment of unknown origin, i.e., X vs. Y). This can be achieved by DNA studies or FISH using a Y centromeric probe, supplemented as necessary by short- and long-arm probes. The presence of virilization in a TS patient should prompt a search for a gonadal, adrenal, or midline tumor as well as investigation of the karyotype for Y material. The prevalence and clinical significance of cryptic Y material detected only by FISH or DNA analysis in patients without virilization or a marker chromosome needs additional investigation. False positives may be a problem with highly sensitive PCR-based Y detection methods [21].

The patient and/or her parents should be informed of the finding of Y chromosome material with the utmost sensitivity regarding gender identity issues to minimize psychological harm. The presence of Y chromosome material is associated with an approximately 12% risk of a gonadoblastoma, according to a recent analysis of pooled data [22]. Gonadoblastomas may transform into malignant germ cell neoplasms; hence, the current recommendation is for laparoscopic, prophylactic gonadectomy [23]. It is often assumed that gonads in patients with TS and Y chromosome mosaicism have no reproductive potential, but spontaneous pregnancies in such women have been reported [24]. Thus, preservation of follicles or oocytes may be a future option for some patients undergoing gonadectomy. The gene responsible for gonadoblastoma has not been identified, but mapping data indicate that it is distinct

Table 3.2. Clinical findings commonly described in patients with Turner syndrome

Primary defects	Secondary features	Incidence (%)
Physical features		
Skeletal growth disturbances	Short stature	100
	Short neck	40
	Abnormal upper-to -lower segment ratio	97
	Cubitus valgus	47
	Short metacarpals	37
	Madelung deformity	7.5
	Scoliosis	12.5
	Genu valgum	35
	Characteristic facies with micrognathia	60
Lymphatic obstruction	Webbed neck	25
	Low posterior hairline	42
	Rotated ears	Common
	Edema of hands/feet	22
	Severe nail dysplasia	13
	Characteristic dermatoglyphics	35
Unknown factors	Strabismus	17.5
	Ptosis	11
	Multiple pigmented nevi	26
Physiologic features		
Skeletal growth disturbances	Growth failure	100
	Otitis media	73
Germ cell chromosomal defects	Gonadal failure	90
	Infertility	95
Unknown factors – embryogenic	Cardiovascular anomalies	55
	Hypertension	7
Unknown factors	Strabismus	17.5
	Renal and renovascular anomalies	39
Unknown factors – metabolic	Hashimoto thyroiditis	34
	Hyperthyroidism	10
	Alopecia	2
	Vitiligo	2
	Gastrointestinal disorders	2.5
	Carbohydrate intolerance	40

from SRY, the male sex-determining gene [25,26]. Routine testing for SRY or the presence of Y chromosome material in 45,X individuals without masculinization is not clinically warranted at present.

Indications for karyotype

The diagnosis of TS should be considered in any female with unexplained growth failure or pubertal delay or any constellation of the following clinical findings: edema of the hands or feet, nuchal folds, left-sided cardiac anomalies, especially coarctation of the aorta or hypoplastic left heart, low hairline, low-set ears, small mandible, short stature with growth velocity less than the 10th percentile for age, markedly elevated levels of FSH, cubitus valgus, nail hypoplasia, hyperconvex uplifted nails, multiple pigmented nevi, characteristic facies, short fourth metacarpal, high arched palate, or chronic otitis media (OM).

Newborn screening

Under-diagnosis and delayed diagnosis of TS remains a problem [27]. Importantly, early detection permits identification of cardiovascular system malformations such as bicuspid aortic valve that require treatment to prevent complications. Moreover, early diagnosis facilitates prevention or remediation of growth failure, hearing problems, and learning difficulties. Finally, it may be possible in future years to prevent infertility in some individuals with TS by harvesting eggs or ovarian tissue for cryopreservation from girls while they still have viable follicles [28]. PCR-based screening methods to detect sex chromosome aneuploidy are feasible [29] but have not yet been validated on a newborn population sample, and have failed to detect 40% of the patients with Turner syndrome that have mosaicisms or partial X-chromosome deletions [30]. Another promising technique for large-scale screening is the pyrosequencing-based method for genotyping of single-nucleotide polymorphism (SNP) [31]. However, the standardization of the technique for large populations as a screening method is still in process. When molecular screening for TS is offered, positive findings will need karyotype confirmation, an infrastructure for follow-up and treatment of the patients with sex chromosome abnormalities, and support services to help parents and caregivers deal with the uncertainties inherent in this type of diagnosis. By extrapolation from experience with prenatal diagnosis, it is highly likely that newborn screening will also identify sex chromosome abnormalities of no clinical consequence in some phenotypically normal individuals; this risk must be weighed against the benefit of early detection of TS and other X-chromosome disorders.

Cardiovascular anomalies

The most serious, life-threatening consequences of X-chromosome haploinsufficiency involve the cardiovascular system. Several recent imaging studies have investigated the prevalence of aortic coarctation and bicuspid aortic valve (BAV) in large groups of girls and women with TS [32–36]. These studies suggest that on average, approximately 11% have coarctation and approximately 16% have BAV. Aortic coarctation and BAV are each almost four-fold more frequent in patients with webbed necks, e.g., 37% of patients with neck webbing have a BAV compared with 12% in those without webbing [34]. It is important to note that coarctation may not be detected in infancy and may be first diagnosed in older children or adults, and magnetic resonance imaging (MRI) studies frequently identify cases missed by echocardiography [37–43]. The presence of an abnormal aortic valve is usually clinically silent in young patients and detected only as a result of screening. Recent studies suggest a broader spectrum of cardiovascular system abnormalities in TS than previously recognized. Magnetic resonance angiographic screening studies of asymptomatic individuals with TS have identified a high prevalence of vascular anomalies of uncertain clinical significance [37,38,40,41].

Almost 50% have an unusual angulation and elongation of the aortic arch termed elongated transverse arch by Ho et al. [40]. By itself the elongated transverse arch does not appear to be clinically significant, but there is concern that it may reflect an abnormal aortic wall prone to dilation and perhaps dissection. Additional vascular anomalies found in magnetic resonance angiographic studies include partial anomalous pulmonary connection (PAPVC) and persistent left superior vena cava, each affecting approximately 13% versus less than 1% in the general population [40]. PAPVC in TS frequently involves the left upper pulmonary vein, which is less common than the typical right-sided presentation in the general population, and makes echocardiographic detection more challenging. Whether this defect is clinically significant depends upon the degree of the left-to-right shunt [45–47].

Adults with TS have a high prevalence of electrocardiographic conduction and repolarization abnormalities. Right axis deviation, T wave abnormalities, accelerated AV conduction, and QTc prolongation are significantly more common in women with TS than normal, age-matched controls [50,51].

A major concern in TS remains the rare but often fatal occurrence of aortic dilation, dissection, or rupture in relatively young individuals. Dissecting aortic aneurysm in TS is usually associated with additional risk factors including BAV or other abnormalities of the aortic valve, coarctation or dilatation of the aorta, and systemic hypertension [43,53]. Systemic hypertension is common in TS and therefore may be the most important treatable risk factor for aortic enlargement and dissection [44,48,49].

Normal ascending aortic diameter is related to body size and age. Because most individuals with TS are small, one would expect their aortic diameter to be smaller than the average for age-matched control females, but in general it is larger [41,44]. All measurements of the aorta should be done at the end of systole. The ascending aorta should be measured at the level of the annulus at the hinge points of the valve, at the level of the sinuses of Valsalva perpendicular to the ascending aorta long axis, and at the ascending aorta 10 mm above the sino-tubular junction. Normative data for aortic diameters as a function of body surface area are available [60]. Additional measurements that are not as well standardized include measurement of the transverse aortic arch and the descending aorta.

Data on aortic diameters normalized to body surface area for adults with TS are available [44], and a range of absolute diameters from both echo and MRI for women with TS and age-matched controls are also available [41]. Review of these data (including echocardiographic ascending aorta diameters measured at the annulus and MRI diameters measured at the level of the bifurcation of the pulmonary arteries) suggests that unadjusted values greater than 28–32 mm will identify patients with diameters greater than 95% of controls, which would clearly be abnormal for women with TS who are generally smaller. When aortic root enlargement is found, medical therapy [56–59] and serial imaging are recommended. Aggressive control of blood pressure should aim for low-normal values. Because many individuals with TS demonstrate nocturnal hypertension, 24-hr monitoring may be helpful in obtaining optimal control [52,54,55,61]. In hypertensive patients with aortic root enlargement who also have resting tachycardia, β-adrenergic receptor blockade is an excellent therapeutic option. β-blockers have been shown to reduce the rate of aortic dilation and dissection in Marfan syndrome, although efficacy in treating aortic dilatation in TS has not yet been investigated [62].

Pregnancy

Spontaneous or assisted pregnancy in TS should be undertaken only after thorough cardiac evaluation. Alarming reports of fatal aortic dissection during pregnancy and the postpartum period have raised concern about the safety of pregnancy in TS [63]. If pregnancy is being considered, preconception assessment must include cardiology evaluation with MRI of the aorta. A history of surgically repaired cardiovascular defect, the presence of BAV, or current evidence of aortic dilatation or systemic hypertension should probably be viewed as relative contraindications to pregnancy. For those who become pregnant, close cardiology involvement throughout pregnancy and the post-partum period is essential.

Growth-promoting therapy

The goals of growth-promoting therapies are to attain a normal height for age as early as possible, progress through puberty at a normal age, and attain a normal adult height[70]. The centerpiece of growth-promoting therapy is GH, which increases growth velocity and final adult stature. Girls with TS generally have a normal GH secretory pattern [71]. Provocative GH testing should be performed only in those whose growth is clearly abnormal relative to that expected for TS, determined by plotting lengths and heights on TS-specific growth curves [64–67,72,73].

It is well established that GH therapy is effective in increasing final adult height. However, the magnitude of the benefit has varied greatly depending upon study design and treatment parameters. In the first randomized controlled trial to follow GH-treated TS subjects to final height the Canadian GH Advisory Committee corroborated the increases in adult stature reported by studies with historical controls [74–78]. In the Canadian study, girls with TS (aged 7–13 years) who were randomized to receive GH (0.3 mg/kg per week; maximum weekly dose, 15 mg) achieved a final adult stature 7.2 cm taller than the control group after an average of 5.7 years. Factors predictive of taller adult stature include a relatively tall height at initiation of therapy, tall parental heights, young age at initiation of therapy, a long duration of therapy, and a high GH dose [79–84].

The optimal age for initiation of GH treatment has not been established. Preliminary data from the Toddler Turner Study, in which 88 girls between the ages of 9 months and 4 years (mean age, 2.0 years) were randomized to GH or no GH therapy, indicate that GH therapy is effective beginning as early as 9 months of age [85]. In addition, the safety profile appears to be similar to that observed in older TS children. Treatment with GH should be considered as soon as growth failure (decreasing height percentiles on the normal curve) is demonstrated and its potential risks and benefits have been discussed with the family.

GH therapy in the United States is generally initiated at the FDA-approved dose of 0.375 mg/kg per week. This is most effective when given daily and customarily administered in the evening. The dose can be adapted according to the patient's growth response and IGF-1 levels. Daily doses substantially higher than those approved by the FDA (0.054 mg/kg = 0.162 IU/kg = ~4.8IU/m^2) produce a relatively small gain in final height, although there is no apparent increase in short-term adverse events [86]. For example, in a study by the Dutch Working Group, the mean gain in final height in groups treated daily with 4 IU/m^2 (0.045 mg/kg), 6 IU/m^2 and 8 IU/m^2 averaged 11.9 ± 3.6, 15.7 ± 3.5, and 16.9 ± 5.2 cm, respectively [75]. However, when GH was given at the higher doses, IGF-1 levels were often above the normal range, and ideally, prolonged exposure to elevated IGF-1 levels should be avoided because of theoretical concern about potential long-term adverse effects [87].

For girls below approximately 9 years of age, therapy is usually started with GH alone. In older girls, or those with extreme short stature, consideration can be given to using higher doses of GH and adding a nonaromatizable anabolic steroid, such as oxandrolone [71,77]. The daily dose of oxandrolone should be 0.05 mg/kg or less, and liver enzymes should be monitored. Higher doses are likely to result in virilization (clitoral enlargement, acne, lowering of the voice, etc.) and more rapid skeletal maturation. Therapy may be continued until a satisfactory height has been attained or until little growth potential remains (bone age ≥ 14 years and growth velocity < 2 cm/year). GH therapy should be directed by a pediatric endocrinologist and the child monitored at intervals of 3–6 months. Evaluation for orthopedic problems as well as growth velocity should be part of the regular physical examination. Development of scoliosis or kyphosis does not necessarily preclude GH therapy; however, close collaboration with an orthopedic surgeon is required [68,69].

Puberty induction

Absent pubertal development is one of the most common clinical features of TS, although up to 30% or more of girls with TS will undergo some spontaneous pubertal development, and 2–5% may achieve spontaneous pregnancy [88–90]. Ultimately, over 90% of individuals with TS will have gonadal failure. Before initiation of estrogen therapy, serum gonadotropin levels should be determined to exclude the possibility of delayed spontaneous pubertal development.

When estrogen therapy is required to induce pubertal development, the form, dosing, and timing should reflect the process of normal puberty. Delaying estrogen therapy until 15 years of age to optimize height potential, as previously recommended, seems unwarranted. This emphasis on stature tends to undervalue the psychosocial importance of age-appropriate pubertal maturation and may be deleterious to bone and other aspects of the child's health [91–93,95]. Furthermore, recent evidence suggests that some treatment regimens using estradiol that begin replacement at the age of 12 years permit a normal pace of puberty without interfering with the positive effect that GH has on final adult height [92,96–98].

Many forms of estrogen are available, and oral estrogens have been most often used. However, both transdermal and injectable depot forms of estradiol may be more physiological alternatives [92,96,97,99]. Low-dose estradiol therapy can be initiated as early as 12 years of age. Replacement is usually begun at one tenth to one eighth of the adult replacement dose and then increased gradually over a period of 2–4 years. The following are equivalent doses that achieve estradiol levels in the normal range for young adult women: oral estradiol, 2 mg/d; transdermal estradiol, 0.1 mg/d; and injectable estradiol cypionate, 2.5 mg/month. To allow for normal breast and uterine development, it seems advisable to delay the addition of progestin at least 2 years after starting estrogen or until breakthrough bleeding occurs. The use of oral contraceptive pills to achieve pubertal development is best avoided, because the synthetic estrogen doses in most formulations are too high and the typical synthetic progestin may interfere with optimal breast and uterine development. It is important to educate the patient that estrogen replacement is usually required until the time of normal menopause to maintain feminization and prevent osteoporosis [94].

During the process of pubertal development, it is important to engage the patient in a gradual discussion about how TS and its treatment may impact her sexual development and function and reproductive potential. In addition, when appropriate, counseling for the prevention of sexually transmitted diseases (and unwanted pregnancy for those with endogenous ovarian function) should also be provided.

Transition management

The transition from pediatric to adult health care should occur at the completion of growth and puberty during late-stage adolescence (usually by age 18 years). However, the transition should be initiated as a staged process. Beginning at approximately age 12, the center of care should be shifted incrementally from the parent to the adolescent with TS. The health care focus also shifts from maximizing height to inducing feminization, counseling the adolescent with TS about the evolving impact of her condition into adulthood and promoting the development of independent self-care behaviors.

Transition is an appropriate time to assess individual risks for potential adult morbidities and promote healthy lifestyles. To help ensure adequate bone mineral accrual, girls with TS are encouraged to have calcium intake of more than 1,000 mg of elemental calcium daily in the preteen years and 1,200–1,500 mg daily after 11 years of age. This will generally require oral supplementation. Counseling as to healthy eating and exercise habits and maintaining a healthy weight are essential. During late-stage transition, the pediatric endocrinologist should engage the transition patient in developing an adult care plan in close collaboration with her new health care provider to help assure that they will continue to receive the careful monitoring that they need to optimize adult health and longevity [150].

Medical care for adults with TS

Medical follow-up and estrogen replacement therapy

Adult women with TS require careful medical follow-up. Early medical intervention may decrease the substantially increased morbidity and mortality and improve the quality of life of women with TS [99–102]. Ideally, the process of transition should take place over a period of 2–3 years during the late pubertal period as described above and should involve an adult endocrinologist and a gynecologist with expertise in premature ovarian failure. A multidisciplinary team including specialists in endocrinology, cardiology, hearing and ear-nose-throat, infertility/gynecology, and psychology may be developed at a tertiary care center. The agenda for such a specialist service should be developed in partnership between medical professionals and Turner support groups. Regrettably, late diagnosis of TS, even in adults, is still a problem. No matter what the age of the patient, a full work-up with assessment of congenital malformations should be performed, including all screening tests recommended for younger patients.

Upon transfer to an adult care clinic, the young woman with TS should undergo a comprehensive medical evaluation, addressing not only the specific problems associated with TS but also screening for osteoporosis, hypertension, diabetes, and dyslipidemia, which are increased in TS [100]. All medical problems present during childhood should be followed in adults, especially congenital cardiovascular issues, thyroid and celiac disease [121], and hearing loss. Annual medical history and general physical evaluation should be performed, including blood pressure, heart auscultation, clinical evaluation of thyroid size and function, breast examination, and Pap smear. As in children, regular otological examination is important, because about 60% of adults with TS experience sensorineural hearing loss. The hearing loss is progressive but tends to occur more rapidly after about 35 years of age, leading to early presbyacusis [103]. Hearing aids are frequently necessary. Otological screening should be conducted at least every 2–3 years in patients who are asymptomatic and have previous documented normal hearing and more frequently as indicated for those with established hearing loss or new symptoms of hearing loss.

Many of the problems of adult life in patients with TS are compounded by obesity partly because of low physical fitness and a sedentary lifestyle [104–107]. Lifestyle education with advice on diet and exercise must be included in a program of prevention of diabetes, osteoporosis, and hypertension. Women with TS should aim to have a body mass index less than 25 kg/m^2 and a waist/hip ratio less than 0.80. Any exercise program should be developed with consideration of individual skeletal or cardiovascular problems, and a physical rehabilitation specialist or trainer may be of great value in designing individualized programs for patients with physical limitations.

Laboratory tests

Laboratory testing of women with TS should be carried out at 1- to 2-year intervals and include measurements of usual screening tests, such as hemoglobin, white blood cell count, renal function (creatinine and blood urea nitrogen), but should especially include fasting blood glucose lipid profile, liver enzymes, TSH, and total or free T_4.

Recommendations for breast evaluation, self-examination, and mammography are the same as for the general population.

Hepatic disease

Liver enzymes, especially γ-glutamyl transferase, alanine amino transferase, aspartate amino transferase, and alkaline phosphatase, are commonly raised in women with TS, but their relationship to chronic liver disease is unknown [105,106]. Hepatitis serology can be checked if indicated, although the prevalence of viral hepatitis is not raised in TS. Usually, elevated liver enzymes do not progress to overt hepatic disease, but regenerative nodular hyperplasia and other architectural abnormalities or biliary lesions are seen on biopsy, as is portal hypertension, which should be treated according to hepatology guidelines [109]. Estrogen treatment is not associated with adverse effects on the liver and usually lowers liver enzymes in TS and thus is not contraindicated in patients that have elevated liver enzymes [108]. If elevated liver enzymes persist for more than 6–12 months, an ultrasound should be performed to rule out hepatic steatosis. If steatosis is not present and liver enzymes remain elevated or increase, a hepatology consult may be obtained with consideration of biopsy guided by the use of hepatic ultrasound with assessment of blood flow by Doppler. Potentially hepatoxic drugs such as statins and glitazones have to be prescribed with caution in affected patients.

Renal function

Although congenital structural anomalies of the kidney are found in about 30% of TS patients, renal function is usually normal, with the only common complication being urinary infections related to obstruction. Thus, individuals with known renal collecting-system anomalies may require more frequent screening for urinary tract infections.

Bone metabolism

Fractures are increased in older patients with TS, but these patients may not have received optimal estrogen treatment in the past. Most studies using dual-energy x-ray absorptiometry find decreased bone mineral density (BMD), but small size may lead to underestimation of BMD by dual-energy X-ray absorptiometry [106,110,111]. When adjusted for size, women that have received appropriate estrogen treatment usually have normal BMD in trabecular bone, e.g., the spine [106,111]. However, there seems to be an intrinsic, estrogen-independent deficit in cortical bone in TS [106,112,113]. A baseline BMD should be obtained at the initial visit in the adult clinic, with follow-up depending on the initial result. If the BMD is normal (adjusting for size), additional evaluation need not take place until age 40–50 years or when the patient plans to discontinue estrogen treatment. If BMD is low in a young woman with TS, one needs to investigate and treat possible contributory factors such as estrogen replacement non-compliance, tobacco use, excessive alcohol use, possible celiac disease, or vitamin D deficiency. Proper estrogen treatment improves BMD and is the mainstay of bone protection. Adequate calcium and vitamin D intake is essential because many women have low levels of vitamin D. Weight-bearing exercise is very important in achieving and maintaining BMD and should be encouraged.

Bisphosphonates or other anti-osteoporotic pharmaceuticals are not recommended for treating osteopenia in young women with TS, because reduced cortical BMD in TS is not proven to lead to increased fractures and bisphosphonates have not been shown to be effective in enhancing cortical BMD in TS. Furthermore, these agents may blunt treatment with newer modalities in the future and are contraindicated in women who might attempt pregnancy. For women with confirmed osteoporosis, especially those at risk for fracture, or who have already sustained a low-impact fracture, the usual medical treatment for osteoporosis is indicated.

Risk factors for coronary artery disease

In addition to their burden of congenital cardiovascular disease, women with TS are at increased risk for atherosclerosis. Hypertension affects as many as 50% of young adult patients. Blood pressure should therefore be closely monitored and hypertension treated vigorously [107,118–120]. Increased heart rate and altered autonomic innervation of the heart are common in TS [121]. Type 2 diabetes is common in TS. An oral glucose tolerance test uncovers impaired glucose tolerance or diabetes in more than 50% of cases, usually associated with an insulin secretory defect in TS [114,118]. Insulin sensitivity may be normal in many patients but reduced in those with obesity or a strong family history of type 2 diabetes. Often, the diabetes is relatively mild and responsive to weight loss or monotherapy.

Low-density lipoprotein cholesterol and triglycerides are elevated, and lipid particle size is reduced in women with TS compared with age and body-mass-index-matched women with karyotypically normal ovarian failure, suggesting that the X chromosome deletion per se, apart from the effects of premature ovarian failure, is associated with dyslipidemia [115,116].

Thyroid and celiac disease

Screening for thyroid and celiac diseases may continue throughout adult life because of an increased risk of developing overt disease [119].

Ovarian hormone replacement

It is recommended that women with TS receive cyclical estrogen and progestin. Sufficient estrogen should be prescribed to prevent the symptoms, signs, and sequelae of estrogen deficiency. An estrogen dose equivalent to 2 mg estradiol daily suffices for most adult women with TS, but individual requirements may vary from 1 to 4 mg/d. Ideally, natural estradiol and progesterone, rather than analogs, should be delivered by transdermal or transmembranous routes so as to mimic age-appropriate physiological patterns as closely as possible. However, regimens that meet each individual woman's tolerance and preference vary widely, and the most important consideration is that women actually take ovarian hormone replacement. This is critical because the risk of clinically significant osteoporosis with spontaneous fractures is very high in young women with TS not taking estrogen [122]. As with other women receiving estrogen replacement therapy, pelvic ultrasonography and endometrial biopsy should be considered when abnormal vaginal bleeding occurs. Androgen concentrations are reduced in many women with TS and androgen substitution therapy may be of value in some instances [117]. This is an area that needs additional investigation. The duration of estrogen therapy should be individualized, and readjustment of dosage or discontinuation should occur at the age of normal menopause (Table 3.3).

Ovarian function and reproductive health in Turner syndrome patients

As mentioned above, spontaneous puberty has been described in up to 37% of patients with TS, and in up to 50% of those with a mosaic karyotype; 5–10% might experience menarche, but this number could be higher due to the mosaic TS that are undiagnosed. Even though spontaneous pregnancies have been described in up to 2–5%, and pregnancies have also been described in TS women without prior menarche, most of them are infertile, and up to 90% will develop premature ovarian failure at some point in their lives [150]. The critical period when the oocyte number decreases is not well characterized, but TS girls have a normal number of oocytes during fetal life, and up to the 18th week of pregnancy [123–125]. During early life, the follicles experience an accelerated process of atresia; however, recent data suggest that this process is not as absolute as it was thought before. Histologic evidence suggests that the ovary of the fetus with a 45,X karyotype (and presumably the ovary of the fetus with karyotypes with X chromosome deletions, rings, or mosaicism) undergoes an initial phase of differentiation that is the same as that in the 46,XX fetus. The triggering mechanism for this premature follicular atresia is postulated to be in part secondary to meiotic pairing anomalies in prophase [126]. The molecular mechanisms presumably involve the acceleration of an oocyte-intrinsic apoptosis defect regulated by members of the Bcl-2 gene family and the caspase family of proteases [127]. The processes of oocyte loss and fibrosis are, however, neither absolute nor inevitable.

The presence of viable oocytes in tissue samples from ovaries removed from TS girls with Y-chromosome material, and subsequent studies of ovarian biopsies demonstrated that despite a high reduction of the follicular number, Turner syndrome girls still have a reserve of viable follicles. Follicles containing oocytes were found in a group of 10 girls that had ovarian biopsies by Hreinsson and Hovatta, between the ages

Table 3.3. Ovarian hormone replacement treatment in Turner syndrome

Age (yr)	Age-specific suggestions	Comments
10–11	Monitor for spontaneous puberty by Tanner staging and FSH level	Low-dose estrogen treatment may not inhibit GH-enhanced growth in stature
12–13	If no spontaneous development and FSH elevated, begin low dose E2	Equivalent initial E2 doses: depot (im) E2, 0.2–0.4 mg/month; transdermal E2, 6.25 μg daily;[a] micronized E2, 0.25 mg daily by mouth
12.5–15	Gradually increase E2 dose over about 2 yr (e.g., 14, 25, 37, 50, 75, 100, 200 μg daily by means of patch) to adult dose	Usual adult daily dose is 100–200 μg transdermal E2, 2–4 mg micronized E2, 20 μg EE2, 1.25–2.5 mg CEE
14–16	Begin cyclic progesterone treatment after 2 yr of estrogen or when breakthrough bleeding occurs	Oral micronized progesterone best option at present; usual adult dose is 200 mg/d on d 20–30 of monthly cycle or d 100–120 of 3-month cycle
14–30	Continue full doses at least until age 30 because normally estrogen levels are highest between age 15 and 30 yr	Some women may prefer using oral or transdermal contraceptive for HRT; monitor endometrial thickness
30–50	The lowest estrogen dose providing full protection vs. osteoporosis is 0.625 CEE or equivalent	Monitor osteoporosis risk factors, diet, exercise; obtain BMD and begin regular screening mammography by age 45 yr
>50	Decision on estrogen use based on same considerations as for other post-menopausal women	New HRT options are appearing, and these recommendations may need updating in near future

CEE, conjugated equine estrogens; E2, estradiol; EE2, ethinylestradiol; HRT, hormone replacement treatment.
[a] The lowest-dose commercially available E2 transdermal patches deliver 14 and 25 μg daily; it is not established whether various means of dose fractionation (e.g., administering a quarter patch overnight or daily or administering whole patches for 7–10 days per month) are equivalent.

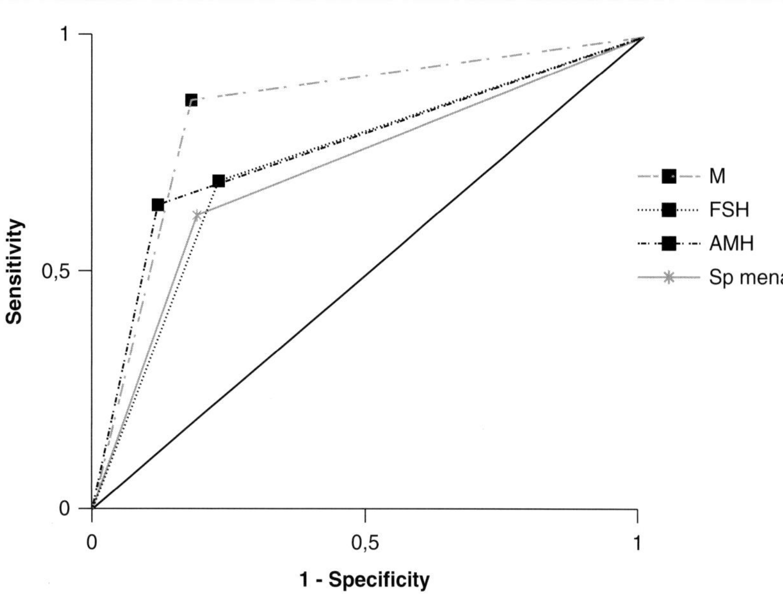

Fig. 3.1. Receiver operating characteristic curves showing the relationship between sensitivity and specificity regarding the four investigated variables with the highest sensitivity.

of 12–19; only two (aged 17 and 19 years) did not have any oocytes. The density of follicles correlated inversely with the FSH level [128]. Additionally, they demonstrated that most of the follicles are present in the cortex of the ovary, and a larger subsequent study of 57 Swedish Turner syndrome girls gathered information that helped identify factors related to the density of ovarian follicles. Prognostic factors like the onset of puberty, mosaic karyotype, normal serum concentration of FSH, normal serum concentration of AMH, and age 12–14 years are associated with the presence of viable follicles in girls and adolescents (Fig. 3.1) [128].

Anti-Mullerian hormone (AMH) has been shown to be particularly useful to predict the ovarian reserve of follicles. In 2010, Hagen et al. demonstrated that the levels of AMH correlate with the karyotype and the presence of ongoing ovarian function, being very low for those TS patients with absent spontaneous puberty and higher for those with present ovarian function [130]. Serum concentrations of AMH levels in 926 healthy female subjects in infancy, childhood, and adolescence were compared with AMH levels in 172 TS patients. In healthy individuals, AMH levels rise during infancy, and remain stable from childhood to early adulthood; an AMH level of 8 pmol/L or higher was associated with functional ovaries in TS girls (Fig. 3.2). AMH is produced by primary and pre-antral follicles, and in adults it has been used as a marker of viable follicle reserve associated with fertility. Recently, serum levels of AMH

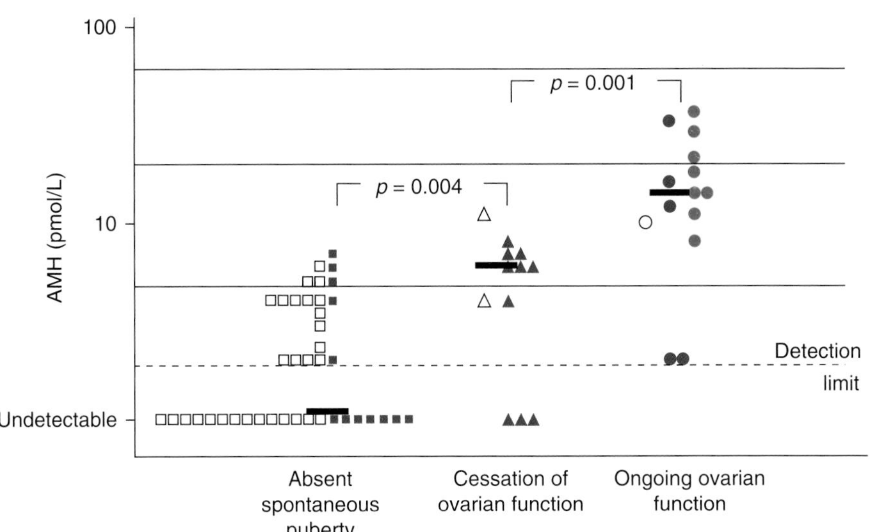

Fig. 3.2. AMH levels and ovarian function at time of AMH measurement in patients with TS, aged 12–25 years. Dotted line represents the detection limit of the assay. Squares, patients with absent puberty; triangles, patients with cessation of ovarian function; circles, patients with ongoing ovarian function. Thick black bars, median of AMH. Black, patients with 45,X; blue, miscellaneous karyotypes; red, 45,X/46,XX.

levels have been a useful adjunct as a marker of the remaining ovarian function in Turner syndrome. The fact that changes in AMH levels are seen in the early phases of ovarian failure and the absence of fluctuations during the menstrual cycle, give AMH advantages compared with other markers of ovarian failure during childhood. The FSH elevation and the inhibin B decrease are not seen until the time of expected puberty. It is during midchildhood when AMH might be useful to predict the future outcome of ovarian failure. Additionally, AMH escapes the regulation by other hormones compared with FSH levels that are affected by hormone replacement therapy; and undetectable inhibin B is a normal finding in 18% of healthy females and this affects its positive predictive value. As happens with adult females, AMH seems to be a promising marker of the reserved follicular function in TS girls, and might be helpful with regard to fertility potential [130].

Cryopreservation of recovered oocytes has been an alternative for fertility preservation in patients before they undergo cancer chemotherapy [129,130], however the results for this technique in TS patients have only been proven efficacious in case reports of patients with mosaic karyotypes, and large series are still expected. Different approaches have been used for these purposes, and include techniques like extraction of ovarian tissue by laparoscopy or transvaginal oocyte retrieval [131,132]. Huang et al. reported a case of fertility preservation in a 16-year-old female with TS who underwent laparoscopic ovarian wedge resection followed by in vitro maturation (IVM) of the recovered oocytes [133]. In another case report, Kavoussi et al. described a 28-year-old female with TS mosaic karyotype that had successful transvaginal oocyte retrieval [134]. More recently, Oktay et al. reported a case of a 14-year-old TS patient with mosaic karyotype (45X/46XX), spontaneous puberty at 11 years, and deteriorating ovarian function that had successful oocyte cryo-preservation after controlled ovarian stimulation [135].

Oocyte or embryo donation are more feasible alternatives with pregnancy rates as high as 53%, very similar to those reported for women with other types of ovarian failure [136,137]. Initially, the miscarriage rates for these techniques were as high as 50–60%, and it was thought that they were associated to the size of the uterus, and with intrinsic characteristics of the endometrium that were not beneficial for the embryo implantation [138]. Nowadays, rates of miscarriage have dropped as low as 25–40%; very close to those seen in receptors of oocyte donation or embryo transfer due to other etiologies of ovarian failure [139].

The improvement in the hormonal treatment explains in part the success in the pregnancy rates. A hormonal treatment with adequate dosages of estrogen and progesterone supports an endometrium with optimal thickness to accept the embryo. A thickness of 5–7 mm, very close to those of normal adult women, is the objective of the hormonal replacement before the implantation [130]. Uterine size is another important factor that explains the miscarriage rates in Turner syndrome women [140]. McDonell et al. showed a cohort of 18 Turner syndrome girls that received adequate estrogen supplementation, during induction of puberty, and had normal uterine length of 5.8–8.6 cm (mean 7.04) within the normal adult range (5–8 cm) [141]. Follow-up of the uterine size during the puberty induction treatment seems to be a critical aspect for the prospective fertility of Turner syndrome patients; however the exact method of treatment, in regards to the uterine size, is still controversial. Features like the route (oral vs. transdermal) as well as the timing and duration have to be investigated further [142,143].

Pregnancy increases the inherent risk of cardiovascular complications in Turner syndrome patients, particularly high blood pressure and aortic dissection. Up to 30% of the pregnancies are complicated with high blood pressure, 57% of these have pre-eclampsia, and aortic dissection has been described in 2% of the cases. Women in the general population that are oocyte recipients have an increased risk of pregnancy-associated high blood pressure that could be as high as 23–38% [144]. In pregnant Turner syndrome women the risk seems to be very similar, despite the fact that Turner syndrome patients are younger at the time of the fertility treatment. In the French cohort of Chevalier et al. 31 out of 82 (37%) developed pregnancy-induced hypertension; 17 out of these developed preeclampsia (20.7%) and 5 had severe preeclampsia (6%) [145].

Eight cases of aortic dissection in pregnant women with Turner syndrome have been documented in the literature: three women had a history of aortic coarctation; one of these with bicuspid aortic valve; one had bicuspid aortic valve only; one had aortic insufficiency with mild aortic root dilation; one had bicuspid aortic valve with mild aortic root dilation; and two had no recordable congenital heart disease. Six of the women had the aortic dissection during the last trimester: two immediately after the pregnancy, and only two survived. In non-pregnant Turner syndrome women, dissection occurred at a young age, 30.7 (range, 4–64) years, compared with the general population. A total of 15% of those cases had associated high blood pressure only, 30% had associated congenital heart disease only, and 34% had both, however, 11% of the cases of aortic dissection did not have high blood pressure or congenital heart disease associated [146]. The risk of aortic dissection is well established in adult Turner syndrome women, and the finding of an aortic size index >2.0 cm/m^2 requires close cardiovascular monitoring [147]; unfortunately, there is not enough information to establish specific guidelines for pregnant women with Turner syndrome, and until new information emerges, following the guidelines for adult Turner syndrome is advised. This includes calculation of the aortic size index, which is not routinely measured in adults, using MRI interpreted by an experienced cardiologist. A fatal case report raised concerns about the importance of the MRI after Boissonnas et al. described a 33-year-old French woman with Turner syndrome and normal cardiac evaluation (including echocardiogram), before she received a single embryo transfer. At 16 weeks of gestation, an echocardiogram performed at a specialized center, revealed a bicuspid aortic valve with aortic root dilation of 39 mm. The patient died of a total aortic rupture after having an emergency cesarean section and aortic dissection repair at 38 weeks of gestation [148]. In a subsequent study, Boissonnas showed that 7 out 18 women with Turner syndrome seeking oocyte donation had cardiac abnormalities when examined by an experienced cardiologist compared with no abnormalities described by a cardiologist without experience with Turner syndrome [149].

Special interest should be placed in the assessment of the cardiovascular risk before pregnancy induction, or in those patients with functional ovaries who want to become pregnant. Magnetic resonance imaging before, and continuous blood pressure monitoring and close follow-up with echocardiogram by experienced personnel during the pregnancy are the recommendations. Despite these recommendations, only 50% of the patients that became pregnant had a cardiac work-up before the fertility treatment [150].

Most of the pregnant women with Turner syndrome deliver by means of cesarean section due to their small size, and their newborns are born at a younger gestational age but are appropriate for gestational age. In a series by Hagman et al., birth defects did not differ between TS and controls [151]. In the American cohort of Bondy et al. only one child had cerebral palsy out of 14 live births; the others were chromosomally normal, but some other case reports have suggested that pregnancies of TS patients have an increased risk of fetal malformations, and chromosomal defects, especially trisomy 21 [152].

References

1. Nielsen J, Wohlert M. Chromosome abnormalities found among 34,910 newborn children: results from a 13-year incidence study in Arhus, Denmark. Hum Genet. 1991;**87**:81–3.
2. Turner HH. A syndrome of infantilism, congenital webbed neck, and cubitus valgus. Endocrinology. 1938;**23**:566–74.
3. Ullrich O. Über typische Kombinationsbilder multipler Abartungen. Z Kinderheilk. 1930;**49**:271–6.
4. Ferguson-Smith MA. Karyotype-phenotype correlations in gonadal dysgenesis and their bearing on the pathogenesis of malformations. J Med Genet. 1965;**2**:142–55.
5. Ross JL, Scott C Jr, Marttila P, et al. Phenotypes associated with SHOX deficiency. J Clin Endocrinol Metab. 2001;**86**:5674–80.
6. Maraschio P, Tupler R, Barbierato L, et al. An analysis of Xq deletions. Hum Genet. 1996;**97**:375–81.
7. Nicolaides KH, Azar G, Snijders RJ, et al. Fetal nuchal oedema: associated malformations and chromosomal defects. Fetal Diagn Ther. 1992;**7**:123–31.
8. Bronshtein M, Zimmer EZ, Blazer S. A characteristic cluster of fetal sonographic markers that are predictive of fetal Turner syndrome in early pregnancy. Am J Obstet Gynecol. 2003;**188**:1016–20.
9. Ruiz C, Lamm F, Hart PS. Turner syndrome and multiple-marker screening. Clin Chem. 1999;**45**:2259–61.
10. Gunther DF, Eugster E, Zagar AJ, et al. Ascertainment bias in Turner syndrome: new insights from girls who were diagnosed incidentally in prenatal life. Pediatrics. 2004;**114**:640–4.
11. Koeberl DD, McGillivray B, Sybert VP. Prenatal diagnosis of 45, X/46, XX mosaicism and 45, X: implications for postnatal outcome. Am J Hum Genet. 1995;**57**:661–6.
12. Hook EB, Warburton D. The distribution of chromosomal genotypes associated with Turner's syndrome: livebirth prevalence rates and evidence for diminished fetal mortality and severity in genotypes associated with structural X abnormalities or mosaicism. Hum Genet. 1983;**64**:24–7.
13. Baena N, De Vigan C, Cariati E, et al. Turner syndrome: evaluation of prenatal diagnosis in 19 European registries. Am J Med Genet A. 2004;**129**:16–20.
14. Hamamy HA, Dahoun S. Parental decisions following the prenatal diagnosis of sex chromosome

abnormalities. Eur J Obstet Gynecol Reprod Biol. 2004;**116**:58–62.

15. Hall S, Abramsky L, Marteau TM. Health professionals' reports of information given to parents following the prenatal diagnosis of sex chromosome anomalies and outcomes of pregnancies: a pilot study. Prenat Diagn. 2003;**23**:535–8.
16. Warburton D, Kline J, Stein Z, et al. Monosomy X: a chromosomal anomaly associated with young maternal age. Lancet. 1980;**1**:167–9.
17. Sutton EJ, McInerney-Leo A, Bondy CA, et al. Turner syndrome: four challenges across the lifespan. Am J Med Genet A. 2005;**139**:57–66.
18. Hook EB. Exclusion of chromosomal mosaicism: tables of 90%, 95% and 99% confidence limits and comments on use. Am J Hum Genet. 1977;**29**:94–7.
19. Wiktor AE, Van Dyke DL. Detection of low level sex chromosome mosaicism in Ullrich-Turner syndrome patients. Am J Med Genet A. 2005;**138**:259–61.
20. Palmer CG, Reichman A. Chromosomal and clinical findings in 110 females with Turner syndrome. Hum Genet. 1976;**35**:35.
21. Nishi MY, Domenice S, Medeiros MA, et al. Detection of Y-specific sequences in 122 patients with Turner syndrome: nested PCR is not a reliable method. Am J Med Genet. 2002;**107**:299–305.
22. Cools M, Drop SL, Wolffenbuttel KP, et al. Germ cell tumors in the intersex gonad: old paths, new directions, moving frontiers. Endocr Rev. 2006;**27**:468–84.
23. Brant WO, Rajimwale A, Lovell MA, et al. Gonadoblastoma and Turner syndrome. J Urol. 2006;**175**(5):1858–60.
24. Landin-Wilhelmsen K, Bryman I, Hanson C, et al. Spontaneous pregnancies in a Turner syndrome woman with Y-chromosome mosaicism. J Assist Reprod Genet. 2004;**21**:229–30.
25. Salo P, Kaariainen H, Petrovic V, et al. Molecular mapping of the putative gonadoblastoma locus on the Y chromosome. Genes Chromosomes Cancer. 1995;**14**:210–14.
26. Tsuchiya K, Reijo R, Page DC, et al. Gonadoblastoma: molecular definition of the susceptibility region on the Y chromosome. Am J Hum Genet. 1995;**57**:1400–7.
27. Gravholt CH, Juul S, Naeraa RW, et al. Prenatal and postnatal prevalence of Turner's syndrome: a registry study. BMJ. 1996;**312**:16–21.
28. Hreinsson JG, Otala M, Fridstrom M, et al. Follicles are found in the ovaries of adolescent girls with Turner's syndrome. J Clin Endocrinol Metab. 2002;**87**:3618–23.
29. Meng H, Hager K, Rivkees SA, et al. Detection of Turner syndrome using high-throughput quantitative genotyping. J Clin Endocrinol Metab. 2005;**90**:3419–22.
30. Wolff DJ, Van Dyke DL, Powell CM. Laboratory guideline for Turner syndrome. Gene Med. 2010;**12**:52–5.
31. Rivkees S, Hager K, Hosono S, et al. A highly sensitive, high-throughput assay for the detection of Turner syndrome. J Clin Endocrinol Metb. 2011;**96**(3):699–705.
32. Loscalzo ML, Van PL, Ho VB, et al. Association between fetal lymphedema and congenital cardiovascular defects in Turner syndrome. Pediatrics. 2005;**115**:732–5.
33. Berdahl LD, Wenstrom KD, Hanson JW. Web neck anomaly and its association with congenital heart disease. Am J Med Genet. 1985;**56**:304–7.
34. Gotzsche C, Krag-Olsen B. Prevalence of cardiovascular malformations and association with karyotypes in Turner's syndrome. Arch Dis Child. 1994;**71**:433–6.
35. Mazzanti L, Prandstraller D, Tassinari D, et al. Heart disease in Turner's syndrome. Helv Paediatr Acta. 1998;**43**:25–31.
36. Volkl TM, Degenhardt K, Koch A, et al. Cardiovascular anomalies in children and young adults with Ullrich-Turner syndrome: the Erlangen experience. Clin Cardiol. 2005;**28**:88–92.
37. Chalard F, Ferey S, Teinturier C, et al. Aortic dilatation in Turner syndrome: the role of MRI in early recognition. Pediatr Radiol. 2005;**35**:323–6.
38. Castro AV, Okoshi K, Ribeiro SM, et al. Cardiovascular assessment of patients with Ullrich-Turner's syndrome on Doppler echocardiography and magnetic resonance imaging. Arq Bras Cardiol. 2002;**78**:51–8.
39. Dawson-Falk KL, Wright AM, Bakker B, et al. Cardiovascular evaluation in Turner syndrome: utility of MR imaging. Australas Radiol. 1992;**36**:204–9.
40. Ho VB, Bakalov VK, Cooley M, et al. Major vascular anomalies in Turner syndrome: prevalence and magnetic resonance angiographic features. Circulation. 2004;**110**:1694–700.
41. Ostberg JE, Brookes JAS, McCarthy C, et al. A comparison of echocardiography and magnetic resonance imaging in cardiovascular screening of adults with Turner syndrome. J Clin Endocrinol Metab. 2004;**89**:5966–71.
42. Sybert VP. Cardiovascular malformations and complications in Turner syndrome. Pediatrics. 1998;**101**:E11.
43. Lin AE, Lippe B, Rosenfeld RG. Further delineation of aortic dilation, dissection, and rupture in patients with Turner syndrome. Pediatrics. 1998;**102**:E12.
44. Elsheikh M, Casadei B, Conway GS, et al. Hypertension is a major risk factor for aortic root dilatation in women with Turner's syndrome. Clin Endocrinol (Oxf). 2001;**54**:69–73.
45. Bechtold SM, Dalla Pozza R, Becker A, et al. Partial anomalous pulmonary vein connection: an underestimated cardiovascular defect in Ullrich-Turner syndrome. Eur J Pediatr. 2004;**163**:158–62.
46. Shiroma K, Ebine K, Tamura S, et al. A case of Turner's syndrome associated with partial anomalous pulmonary venous return complicated by dissecting aortic aneurysm and aortic regurgitation. J Cardiovasc Surg (Torino). 1997;**38**:257–9.
47. van Wassenaer AG, Lubbers LJ, Losekoot G. Partial abnormal pulmonary venous return in Turner syndrome. Eur J Pediatr. 1988;**148**:101–3.
48. Ostberg JE, Donald AE, Halcox JPJ, et al. Vasculopathy in Turner syndrome: arterial dilatation and intimal thickening without endothelial dysfunction. J Clin Endocrinol Metab. 2005;**90**:5161–6.
49. Baguet JP, Douchin S, Pierre H, et al. Structural and functional abnormalities of large arteries in Turner syndrome. Heart. 2005;**91**:1442–6.
50. Bondy CA, Van PL, Bakalov VK, et al. Prolongation of the cardiac QTc interval in Turner syndrome. Medicine (Baltimore). 2006;**85**:75–81.

51. Liao AW, Snijders R, Geerts L, et al. Fetal heart rate in chromosomally abnormal fetuses. Ultrasound Obstet Gynecol. 2000;**16**:610–3.

52. Gravholt CH, Hansen KW, Erlandsen M, et al. Nocturnal hypertension and impaired sympathovagal tone in Turner syndrome. J Hypertens. 2006;**24**:353–60.

53. Mazzanti L, Cacciari E. Congenital heart disease in patients with Turner's syndrome. Italian Study Group for Turner syndrome (ISGTS). J Pediatr. 1998;**133**:688–92.

54. Nathwani NC, Unwin R, Brook CG, et al. The influence of renal and cardiovascular abnormalities on blood pressure in Turner syndrome. Clin Endocrinol (Oxf). 2000;**52**:371–7.

55. Gravholt CH, Naeraa RW, Nyholm B, et al. Glucose metabolism, lipid metabolism, and cardiovascular risk factors in adult Turner's syndrome. The impact of sex hormone replacement. Diabetes Care. 1998;**21**:1062–70.

56. Radetti G, Crepaz R, Milanesi O, et al. Cardiac performance in Turner's syndrome patients on growth hormone therapy. Horm Res. 2001;**55**:240–4.

57. Sas TC, Cromme-Dijkhuis AH, de Muinck Keizer-Schrama SM, et al. The effects of long-term growth hormone treatment on cardiac left ventricular dimensions and blood pressure in girls with Turner's syndrome. Dutch Working Group on Growth Hormone. J Pediatr. 1999;**135**:470–6.

58. Bondy CA, Van PL, Bakalov VK, et al. Growth hormone treatment and aortic dimensions in Turner syndrome. J Clin Endocrinol Metab. 2006;**91**:1785–8.

59. van den Berg J, Bannink EM, Wielopolski PA, et al. Aortic distensibility and dimensions and the effects of growth hormone treatment in the Turner syndrome. Am J Cardiol. 2006;**97**:1644–9.

60. Roman MJ, Devereux RB, Kramer-Fox R, et al. Two-dimensional echocardiographic aortic root dimensions in normal children and adults. Am J Cardiol. 1989;**64**:507–12.

61. Nathwani NC, Unwin R, Brook CG, et al. Blood pressure and Turner syndrome. Clin Endocrinol (Oxf). 2000;**52**:363–70.

62. Shores J, Berger KR, Murphy EA, et al. Progression of aortic dilatation and the benefit of long-term β-adrenergic blockade in Marfan's syndrome. N Engl J Med. 1994;**330**:1335–41.

63. Karnis MF, Zimon AE, Lalwani SI, et al. Risk of death in pregnancy achieved through oocyte donation in patients with Turner syndrome: a national survey. Fertil Steril. 2003;**80**:498–501.

64. Ranke MB, Pfluger H, Rosendahl W, et al. Turner syndrome: spontaneous growth in 150 cases and review of the literature. Eur J Pediatr. 1983;**141**:81–8.

65. Rongen-Westerlaken C, Corel L, van de, Broeck J, et al. Reference values for height, height velocity and weight in Turner's syndrome. Swedish Study Group for GH treatment. Acta Paediatr. 1997;**86**:937–42.

66. Gravholt CH, Weis Naeraa R. Reference values for body proportions and body composition in adult women with Ullrich-Turner syndrome. Am J Med Genet. 1997;**72**:403–8.

67. Binder G, Fritsch H, Schweizer R, et al. Radiological signs of Leri-Weill dyschondrosteosis in Turner syndrome. Horm Res. 2001;**55**:71–6.

68. Elder DA, Roper MG, Henderson RC, et al. Kyphosis in a Turner syndrome population. Pediatrics. 2002;**109**:e93.

69. Kim JY, Rosenfeld SR, Keyak JH. Increased prevalence of scoliosis in Turner syndrome. J Pediatr Orthop. 2001;**21**:765–6.

70. Sas TC, Muinck Keizer-Schrama SM, Stijnen T, et al. A longitudinal study on bone mineral density until adulthood in girls with Turner's syndrome participating in a growth hormone injection frequency-response trial. Clin Endocrinol (Oxf). 2000;**52**:531–6.

71. Stahnke N, Keller E, Landy H, et al. Favorable final height outcome in girls with Ullrich-Turner syndrome treated with low-dose growth hormone together with oxandrolone despite starting treatment after 10 years of age. J Pediatr Endocrinol Metab. 2002;**15**:129–38.

72. Lyon AJ, Preece MA, Grant DB. Growth curve for girls with Turner syndrome. Arch Dis Child. 1985;**60**:932–5.

73. Davenport ML, Punyasavatsut N, Stewart PW, et al. Growth failure in early life: an important manifestation of Turner syndrome. Horm Res. 2002;**57**:157–64.

74. The Canadian Growth Hormone Advisory Committee. Impact of growth hormone supplementation on adult height in Turner syndrome: results of the Canadian Randomized Controlled Trial. J Clin Endocrinol Metab. 2005;**90**:3360–6.

75. van Pareren YK, de Muinck Keizer-Schrama SM, Stijnen T, et al. Final height in girls with Turner syndrome after long-term growth hormone treatment in three dosages and low dose estrogens. J Clin Endocrinol Metab. 2003;**88**:1119–25.

76. Rosenfeld RG, Attie KM, Frane J, et al. Growth hormone therapy of Turner's syndrome: beneficial effect on adult height. J Pediatr. 1998;**132**:319–24.

77. Rosenfeld RG, Frane J, Attie KM, et al. Six-year results of a randomized, prospective trial of human growth hormone and oxandrolone in Turner syndrome. J Pediatr. 1992;**121**:49–55.

78. Pasquino AM, Pucarelli I, Segni M, et al. Adult height in sixty girls with Turner syndrome treated with growth hormone matched with an untreated group. J Endocrinol Invest. 2005;**28**:350–6.

79. Ranke MB, Lindberg A, Chatelain P, et al. Prediction of long-term response to recombinant human growth hormone in Turner syndrome: development and validation of mathematical models. KIGS International Board. Kabi International Growth Study. J Clin Endocrinal Metab. 2000;**85**:4212–18.

80. Reiter EO, Blethen SL, Baptista J, et al. Early initiation of growth hormone treatment allows age-appropriate estrogen use in Turner's syndrome. J Clin Endocrinol Metab. 2001;**86**:1936–41.

81. Quigley CA, Crowe BJ, Anglin DG, et al. Growth hormone and low dose estrogen in Turner syndrome: results of a United States multi-center trial to near-final height. J Clin Endocrinol Metab. 2002;**87**:2033–41.

82. Carel JC, Mathivon L, Gendrel C, et al. Growth hormone therapy for Turner syndrome: evidence for benefit. Horm Res. 1997;**48**:31–4.

83. Sas TC, de Muinck K, Stijnen T, et al. Normalization of height in girls with Turner syndrome after long-term growth hormone treatment: results of a randomized dose-response trial. J Clin Endocrinol Metab. 1999;**84**:4607–12.

84. Hofman P, Cutfield WS, Robinson EM, et al. Factors predictive of response to growth hormone therapy in Turner's

syndrome. J Pediatr Endocrinol Metab. 1997;**10**:27–33.

85. Davenport ML, Quigley CA, Bryant CG, et al. A Effect of early growth hormone (GH) treatment in very young girls with Turner syndrome (TS). Seventh Joint European Society for Paediatric Endocrinology/Lawson Wilkins Pediatric Endocrine Society Meeting, Lyon, France, 2005.
86. Sas TC, Muinck Keizer-Schrama SM, Stijnen T, Aanstoot HJ, Drop SL. Carbohydrate metabolism during long-term growth hormone (GH) treatment and after discontinuation of GH treatment in girls with Turner syndrome participating in a randomized dose-response study. Dutch Advisory Group on Growth Hormone. J Clin Endocrinol Metab. 2000;**85**:769–75.
87. Park P, Cohen P. The role of insulin-like growth factor I monitoring in growth hormone-treated children. Horm Res. 2004;**62**(Suppl 1):59–65.
88. Boechat MI, Westra SJ, Lippe B. Normal US appearance of ovaries and uterus in four patients with Turner's syndrome and 45, X karyotype. Pediatr Radiol. 1996;**26**:37–9.
89. Pasquino AM, Passeri F, Pucarelli I, Segni M, Municchi G. Spontaneous pubertal development in Turner's syndrome. J Clin Endocrinol Metab. 1997;**82**:1810–13.
90. Hovatta O. Pregnancies in women with Turner's syndrome. Ann Med. 1999;**31**:106–10.
91. Chernausek SD, Attie KM, Cara JF, et al. Growth hormone therapy of Turner syndrome: the impact of age of estrogen replacement on final height. Genentech, Inc., Collaborative Study Group. J Clin Endocrinol Metab. 2000;**85**:2439–45.
92. Rosenfield RL, Devine N, Hunold JJ, et al. Salutary effects of combining early very low-dose systemic estradiol with growth hormone therapy in girls with Turner syndrome. J Clin Endocrinol Metab. 2005;**90**:6424–30.
93. Carel JC, Ecosse E, Bastie-Sigeac I, et al. Quality of life determinants in young women with Turner's syndrome after growth hormone treatment: results of the StaTur population-based cohort study. J Clin Endocrinol Metab. 2005;**90**:1992–7.
94. Hogler W, Briody J, Moore B, et al. Importance of estrogen on bone health in Turner syndrome: a cross-sectional and longitudinal study using dual-energy x-ray absorptiometry. J Clin Endocrinol Metab. 2004;**89**:193–9.
95. Ross JL, Quigley CA, Cao D, et al. Growth hormone plus childhood low-dose estrogen in Turner's syndrome. N Engl J Med. 2011;**364**:1230–42.
96. Ankarberg-Lindgren C, Elfving M, Wikland KA, et al. Nocturnal application of transdermal estradiol patches produces levels of estradiol that mimic those seen at the onset of spontaneous puberty in girls. J Clin Endocrinol Metab. 2001;**86**:3039–44.
97. Soriano-Guillen L, Coste J, Ecosse E, et al. Adult height and pubertal growth in Turner syndrome after treatment with recombinant growth hormone. J Clin Endocrinol Metab. 2005;**90**:5197–204.
98. van Pareren YK, de Muinck Keizer-Schrama SM, Stijnen T, et al. Final height in girls with Turner syndrome after long-term growth hormone treatment in three dosages and low dose estrogens. J Clin Endocrinol Metab. 2003;**88**:1119–25.
99. Elsheikh M, Conway GS, Wass JA. Medical problems in adult women with Turner's syndrome. Ann Med. 1999;**31**:99–105.
100. Gravholt CH, Juul S, Naeraa RW, et al. Morbidity in Turner syndrome. J Clin Epidemiol. 1998;**51**:147–58.
101. Price WH, Clayton JF, Collyer S, et al. Mortality ratios, life expectancy, and causes of death in patients with Turner's syndrome. J Epidemiol Community Health. 1986;**40**:97–102.
102. Swerdlow AJ, Hermon C, Jacobs PA, et al. Mortality and cancer incidence in phromosome abnormalities: a cohort study. Ann Hum Genet. 2001;**65**:177–88.
103. Hultcrantz M. Ear and hearing problems in Turner's syndrome. Acta Oto-Laryngol. 2003;**123**:253–7.
104. Elsheikh M, Conway GS. The impact of obesity on cardiovascular risk factors in Turner's syndrome. Clin Endocrinol (Oxf). 1998;**49**:447–50.
105. Gravholt CH, Naeraa RW, Fisker S, et al. Body composition and physical fitness are major determinants of the growth hormone-insulin-like growth factor axis aberrations in adult Turner's syndrome, with important modulations by treatment with 17β-estradiol. J Clin Endocrinol Metab. 1997;**82**:2570–7.
106. Gravholt CH, Lauridsen AL, Brixen K, et al. Marked disproportionality in bone size and mineral, and distinct abnormalities in bone markers and calcitropic hormones in adult Turner syndrome: a cross-sectional study. J Clin Endocrinol Metab. 2002;**87**:2798–808.
107. Landin-Wilhelmsen K, Bryman I, Wilhelmsen L. Cardiac malformations and hypertension, but not metabolic risk factors, are common in Turner syndrome. J Clin Endocrinol Metab. 2001;**86**:4166–70.
108. Elsheikh M, Hodgson HJ, Wass JA, et al. Hormone replacement therapy may improve hepatic function in women with Turner's syndrome. Clin Endocrinol (Oxf). 2001;**55**:227–31.
109. Roulot D, Degott C, Chazouilleres O, et al. Vascular involvement of the liver in Turner's syndrome. Hepatology. 2004;**39**:239–47.
110. Landin-Wilhelmsen K, Bryman I, Windh M, et al. Osteoporosis and fractures in Turner syndrome: importance of growth promoting and oestrogen therapy. Clin Endocrinol (Oxf). 1999;**51**:497–502.
111. Bakalov V, Chen M, Baron J, et al. Bone mineral density and fractures in Turner syndrome. Am J Med. 2003;**115**:257–62.
112. Bechtold S, Rauch F, Noelle V, et al. Musculoskeletal analyses of the forearm in young women with Turner syndrome: a study using peripheral quantitative computed tomography. J Clin Endocrinol Metab. 2001;**86**:5819–23.
113. Bakalov VK, Axelrod L, Baron J, et al. Selective reduction in cortical bone mineral density in Turner syndrome independent of ovarian hormone deficiency. J Clin Endocrinol Metab. 2003;**88**:5717–22.
114. Bakalov VK, Cooley MM, Quon MJ, et al. Impaired insulin secretion in the Turner metabolic syndrome. J Clin Endocrinol Metab. 2004;**89**:3516–20.
115. Cooley M, Bakalov V, Bondy CA. Lipid profiles in women with 45, X vs 46, XX primary ovarian failure. JAMA. 2003;**290**:2127–8.
116. Van PL, Bakalov VK, Bondy CA. Monosomy for the X chromosome is associated with an atherogenic lipid profile. J Clin Endocrinol Metab. 2006;**91**:2867–70.
117. Hojbjerg Gravholt C, Svenstrup B, Bennett P, et al. Reduced androgen levels in adult Turner syndrome: influence of female sex steroids and growth hormone status. Clin Endocrinol (Oxf). 1999;**50**:791–800.

118. Gravholt CH, Naeraa RW, Nyholm B, et al. Glucose metabolism, lipid metabolism, and cardiovascular risk factors in adult Turner's syndrome. The impact of sex hormone replacement. Diabetes Care. 1998;**21**:1062–70.

119. Nathwani NC, Unwin R, Brook CG, et al. Blood pressure and Turner syndrome. Clin Endocrinol (Oxf). 2000;**52**:363–70.

120. Bonamico M, Pasquino AM, Mariani P, et al. Prevalence and clinical picture of celiac disease in Turner syndrome. J Clin Endocrinol Metab. 2002;**87**:5495–8.

121. Gravholt CH, Hansen KW, Erlandsen M, et al. Nocturnal hypertension and impaired sympathovagal tone in Turner syndrome. J Hypertens. 2006;**24**:353–60.

122. Hanton L, Axelrod L, Bakalov V, et al. The importance of estrogen replacement in young women with Turner syndrome. J Womens Health (Larchmt). 2003;**12**:971–7.

123. Weiss L. Additional evidence of gradual loss of germ cells in the pathogenesis of streak ovaries in Turner's syndrome. J Med Genet. 1971;**8**(4):540–4.

124. Reynaud K, Cortvrindt R, Verlinde F, et al. Number of ovarian follicles in human fetuses with the 45, X karyotype. Fertil Steril. 2004;**81**(4):1112–19.

125. Singh RP, Carr DH. The anatomy and histology of XO human embryos and fetuses. Anat Rec. 1965;**155**:369.

126. Speed RM. The possible role of meiotic pairing anomalies in the atresia of human fetal oocytes. Hum Genet. 1988;**78**:260.

127. Bergeron L, Perez GI, Macdonald G, et al. Defects in regulation of apoptosis in caspase-2-deficient mice. Gene Dev. 1998;**12**:1304.

128. Hreinsson JG, Otala M, Fridström M, et al. Follicles are found in the ovaries of adolescent girls with Turner's syndrome. J Clin Endocrinol Metab. 2002;**87**(8):3618–23.

129. Borgström B, Hreinsson J, Rasmussen C, et al. Fertility preservation in girls with turner syndrome: prognostic signs of the presence of ovarian follicles. J Clin Endocrinol Metab. 2009;**94**(1):74–80. Erratum in: J Clin Endocrinol Metab. 2009;94(4):1478.

130. Hagen CP, Aksglaede L, Sørensen K, et al. Serum levels of anti-Müllerian hormone as a marker of ovarian function in 926 healthy females from birth to adulthood and in 172 Turner syndrome patients. J Clin Endocrinol Metab. 2010;**95**(11):5003–10.

131. Martin JR, Patrizio P. Options for fertility preservation in pediatric populations undergoing cancer chemotherapy. Pediatr Endocrinol Rev. 2009;**6**(Suppl 2):306–14.

132. Levine J, Canada A, Stern CJ. Fertility preservation in adolescents and young adults with cancer. J Clin Oncol. 2010;**28**(32):4831–41.

133. Huang JY, Tulandi T, Holzer H, et al. Cryopreservation of ovarian tissue and in vitro matured oocytes in a female with mosaic Turner syndrome: case report. Hum Reprod. 2008;**23**:336–9.

134. Kavoussi SK, Fisseha S, Smith YR, et al. Oocyte cryopreservation in a woman with mosaic Turner syndrome: a case report. J Reprod Med. 2008;**53**:223–6.

135. Oktay K, Rodriguez-Wallberg KA, Sahin G. Fertility preservation by ovarian stimulation and oocyte cryopreservation in a 14-year-old adolescent with Turner syndrome mosaicism and impending premature ovarian failure. Fertil Steril. 2010;**94**(2):753.e15–19.

136. Hovatta O. Pregnancies in women with Turner's syndrome. Ann Med. 1999;**31**(2):106–10.

137. Bryman I, Sylvén L, Berntorp K, et al. Pregnancy rate and outcome in Swedish women with Turner syndrome. Fertil Steril. 2011;**95**(8):2507–10.

138. Yaron Y, Ochshorn Y, Amit A, et al. Patients with Turner's syndrome may have an inherent endometrial abnormality affecting receptivity in oocyte donation. Fertil Steril. 1996;**65**(6):1249–52.

139. Foudila T, Soderstrom-Anttila V, Hovatta O. Turner's syndrome and pregnancies after oocyte donation. Hum Reprod. 1999;**14**:532–5.

140. Khastgir G, Abdalla H, Thomas A, et al. Oocyte donation in Turner's syndrome: an analysis of the factors affecting the outcome. Hum Reprod. 1997;**12**(2):279–85.

141. McDonnell CM, Coleman L, Zacharin MR. A 3-year prospective study to assess uterine growth in girls with Turner's syndrome by pelvic ultrasound. Clin Endocrinol (Oxf). 2003;**58**(4):446–50.

142. Bannink EM, van Sassen C, van Buuren S, et al. Puberty induction in Turner syndrome: results of oestrogen treatment on development of secondary sexual characteristics, uterine dimensions and serum hormone levels. Clin Endocrinol (Oxf). 2009;**70**(2):265–73.

143. Taboada M, Santen R, Lima J, et al. Pharmacokinetics and pharmacodynamics of oral and transdermal 17{beta} estradiol in girls with Turner syndrome. J Clin Endocrinol Metab. 2011;**96**:3502–10.

144. Sheffer-Mimouni G, Mashiach S, Dor J, et al. Factors influencing the obstetric and perinatal outcome after oocyte donation. Hum Reprod. 2002;**17**(10):2636–40.

145. Chevalier N, Letur H, Lelannou D, et al. Materno-fetal cardiovascular complications in Turner syndrome after oocyte donation: insufficient prepregnancy screening and pregnancy follow-up are associated with poor outcome. J Clin Endocrinol Metab. 2011;**96**(2):E260–7.

146. Carlson M, Silberbach M. Dissection of the aorta in Turner syndrome: two cases and review of 85 cases in the literature. J Med Genet. 2007;**44**(12):745–9.

147. Matura LA, Ho VB, Rosing DR, Bondy CA. Aortic dilatation and dissection in Turner syndrome. Circulation. 2007;**116**(15):1663–70.

148. Boissonnas CC, Davy C, Bornes M, et al. Careful cardiovascular screening and follow-up of women with Turner syndrome before and during pregnancy is necessary to prevent maternal mortality. Fertil Steril. 2009;**91**(3):929.e5–7.

149. Chalas Boissonnas C, Davy C, Marszalek A, et al. Cardiovascular findings in women suffering from Turner syndrome requesting oocyte donation. Hum Reprod. 2011;**26**(10):2754–62.

150. Bondy CA; Turner Syndrome Study Group. Care of girls and women with Turner syndrome: a guideline of the Turner Syndrome Study Group. J Clin Endocrinol Metab. 2007;**92**(1):10–25.

151. Hagman A, Källén K, Barrenäs ML, et al. Obstetric outcomes in women with Turner karyotype. J Clin Endocrinol Metab. 2011;**96**:3475–82.

152. Hadnott TN, Gould HN, Gharib AM, et al. Outcomes of spontaneous and assisted pregnancies in Turner syndrome: the U.S. National Institutes of Health experience. Fertil Steril. 2011;**95**(7):2251–6.

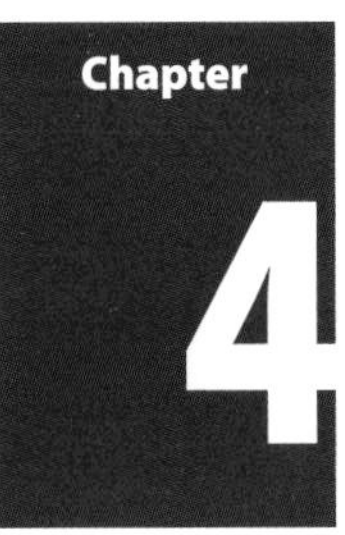

Pathology of benign and malignant ovarian epithelial tumors

Liane Deligdisch, MD

Introduction

The surface ovarian epithelium is considered to be the most common origin of ovarian neoplasms, both benign and malignant. Composed of a single layer of cuboidal cells, as an extension of the peritoneal mesothelium, the ovarian surface epithelium is closely related to the adjacent ovarian cortical stroma and some tumors arising in the area include both epithelial and stromal elements. Recent studies suggest that the fallopian tube epithelium, benign or malignant, that implants on the ovary is the source of low-grade and high-grade serous carcinoma [1].

Benign ovarian tumors of epithelial origin are fortunately far more common than malignant ovarian tumors. Borderline ovarian malignancy will be discussed in a separate chapter (Chapter 5) due to their complex and often controversial clinical–pathologic correlations. The histogenesis of ovarian epithelial tumors, their classification, grading, and interrelationship has recently been the object of extensive research and of fundamental changes, based on new molecular and genetic discoveries. This process is still unfolding, although several established facts have contributed to a revision of previously accepted histopathologic categories.

This chapter includes the gross and microscopic description of the most common pathologic entities, their diagnostic criteria and clinical significance. The classification of the described pathological entities is somehow different from the classical World Health Organization (WHO) classification and is based on histological and immuno-histochemical, molecular, and genetic data. The latter are still evolving along with new technologies. It is expected that future identification of subcellular–molecular elements will be used for targeted therapeutical purposes [2].

Pathology of ovarian benign epithelial tumors

1. *Ovarian benign serous tumors.* These account for about 40% of all ovarian tumors. The most common are serous cystadenomas, adenofibromas, and cystadenofibromas, representing about two-thirds of benign ovarian epithelial tumors and the majority of ovarian serous tumors. They occur in patients of all ages. They may be asymptomatic or elicit symptoms related to their volume, due to compression of neighboring organs. About 20% are bilateral. The histologic diagnosis of serous cystadenomas is based on the presence of an epithelial lining of the cystic cavity. Grossly a serous cyst may resemble a functional ovarian cyst, especially in pre-menopausal women: in follicle and luteal cysts the cyst lining is composed of granulosa or luteinized cells. Some functional cysts are lined by flat cells due to the pressure by the fluid content thus resembling serous cystadenomas.
   (a) *Serous cystadenomas* are unilocular or multilocular cysts containing serous, clear, occasionally mucoid fluid. Their external surface is usually smooth, with a visible vascular pattern, occasionally with papillations that may also be found on the inner surface (Fig. 4.1).
   (b) *Cystadenofibromas* include solid components, connected to cystic cavities lined by benign epithelium. Their size is variable, reaching up to 30 cm in diameter, but are usually smaller, around 5–10 cm in diameter.
   Histologically the cystic cavity(ies) lining consists of one layer, sometime pseudostratified, of tubal-type epithelium with secretory and ciliated cells. The cells are often cuboidal or flattened due to the compression by the fluid content. Epithelial proliferation with papillary structures is not uncommon (Fig. 4.2); if more than 10% of the inner surface of the cyst displays complex papillations, with multi-layered and detached clusters of epithelial cells, the lesion may be an atypical proliferating serous tumor (APST, Chapter 6).
   (c) *Adenofibromas* are benign, solid tumors of the ovary histologically composed of cortical stromal cells and variable amounts of collagen fibers, with scattered glandular structures lined by benign cuboidal cells, occasionally with papillary or endometrioid patterns.
2. *Ovarian benign mucinous tumors.* Benign mucinous cystadenomas are the most common ovarian mucinous tumors, while malignant mucinous tumors are considered now as rarely primary ovarian. They represent about 13% of

Altchek's Diagnosis and Management of Ovarian Disorders, ed. Liane Deligdisch, Nathan G. Kase, and Carmel J. Cohen. Published by Cambridge University Press.

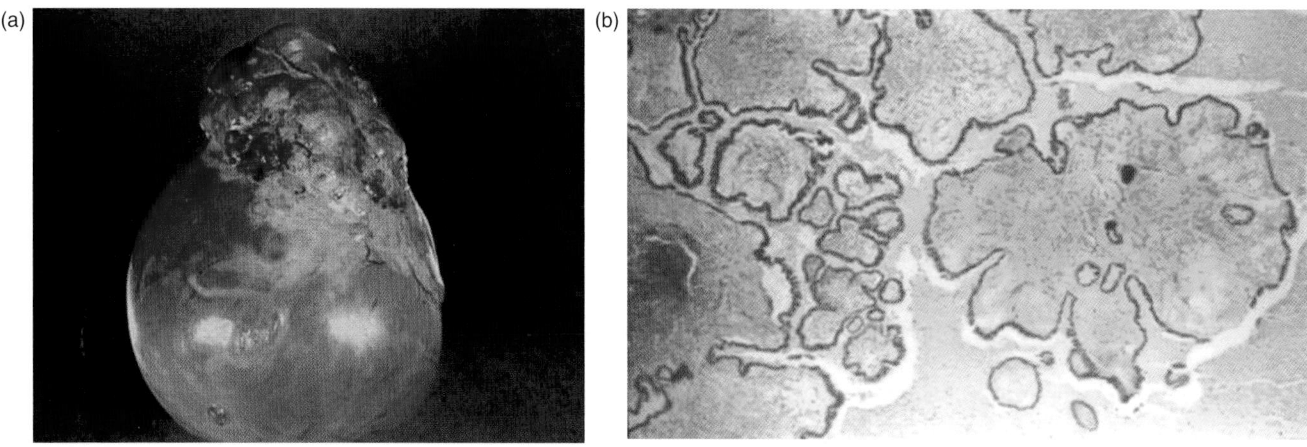

Fig. 4.1. Ovarian serous cystadenoma. (a) Appearance. (b) Internal surface displaying papillations.

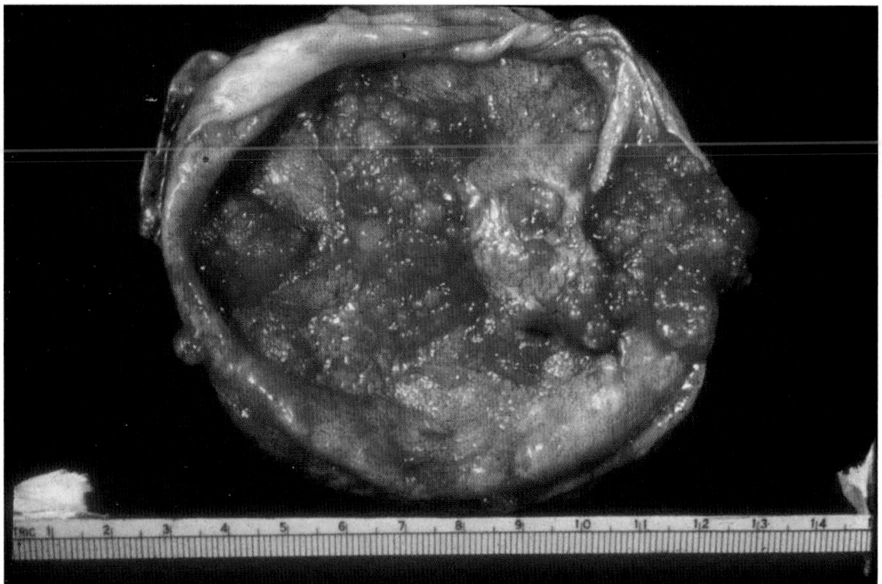

Fig. 4.2. Cystadenofibroma with papillary proliferation.

benign ovarian neoplasms and may occur at any age, with an average at 50 years. Grossly, these are more often multilocular cystic tumors of various sizes, often reaching large dimensions especially in geographic areas with difficult or no access to medical care (Fig. 4.3a). The external surface is thick and whitish and the cystic cavity(ies) contain gelatinous white-gray sticky material (Fig. 4.3b).

Histologically the glands and cysts are lined by simple layers of mucin-secreting cells resembling gastric foveolar-type, intestinal type goblet cell, type or endocervical epithelium (Fig. 4.3c).

At the periphery of the tumor, the epithelium may appear more crowded, focally with atypical proliferation involving not more than 10% of the tumor, with occasional mitotic activity and mild nuclear hyperchromasia. Leakage of mucus with reactive changes such as pseudoxanthoma or luteinized cells can be present.

Sero-mucinous cystadenomas are lined by columnar cells similar to those of endocervical glands. Tumors composed of both mucinous cystadenomas and adenofibromas are rare; they are benign but may recur if not completely excised.

3. *Brenner tumors.* These are common incidental findings about 2 cm or smaller, may rarely exceed 10 cm, firm, solid and well circumscribed, and occasionally cystic. Microscopically there are nests of epithelial cells in a dense fibrous stroma (Fig. 4.4). The epithelial cells are reminiscent of urothelial (transitional) epithelium, are uniform, with oval nuclei showing a longitudinal groove. The epithelial nests often display a central cystic cavity containing mucin, lined by metaplastic mucinous epithelium. Mucinous cystadenomas are often associated with Brenner tumors. The surrounding stroma is fibrous with various degrees of cellularity and common calcified areas. These are benign tumors in their majority; atypical ("borderline") proliferative and malignant Brenner tumors are uncommon.

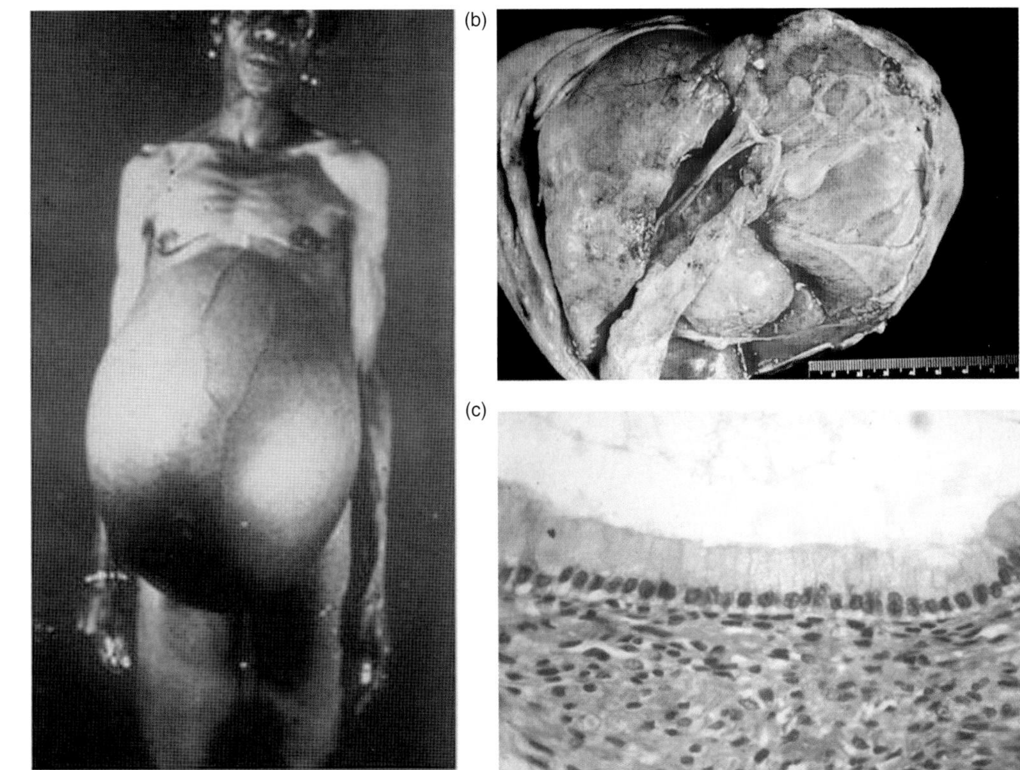

Fig. 4.3. (a) Patient with large ovarian mucinous cystadenoma. (b) Ovarian mucinous cystadenoma with multiloculated cavities with gelatinous sticky content. (c) Columnar mucus-secreting epithelial lining, similar to endocervical epithelium. Hematoxylin & eosin; original magnification, ×100.

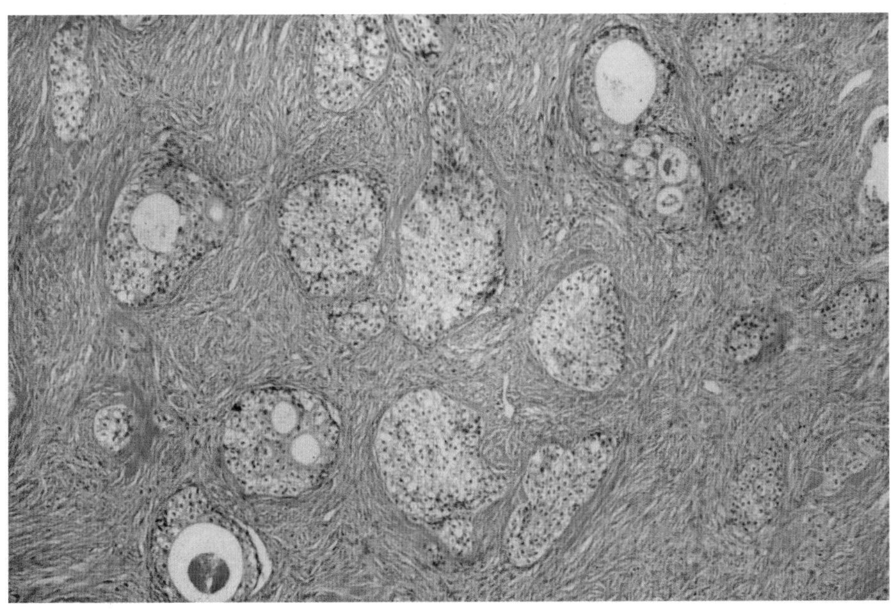

Fig. 4.4. Brenner tumor of ovary: nests of epithelial cells with occasional mucin-containing central cavities surrounded by a dense fibrous stroma. Hematoxylin & eosin; original magnification, ×40.

Pathology of ovarian malignant epithelial neoplasms

Nearly 90% of all ovarian malignant neoplasms are of epithelial origin, therefore named "carcinomas."

Based on histologic, genetic, molecular, and immunohistologic phenotype studies, correlated with clinical and statistical data, ovarian carcinomas (OC) are now classified into two broad categories: type I or low-grade and type II or high-grade carcinomas, the latter being by far the most common and most challenging [3]. Their carcinogenesis is different (Table 4.1).

A. *Type I OC, or low-grade OC (LGOC)* include tumors with different histologic patterns: low-grade serous carcinomas, mucinous, endometrioid, and clear cell carcinomas.

Despite their phenotypical and immuno-histochemical diversity, they have in common a potential origin in benign and/or borderline tumors, a slower and less invasive growth compared with the type II OC, and a better prognosis due to their more frequent earlier stage diagnosis [4].

1. *Invasive low-grade serous carcinomas* are much less common than high-grade serous OC representing about 6% of all serous carcinomas [5]. They often originate in borderline micropapillary serous tumors and are also classified as invasive well-differentiated serous papillary carcinomas. In addition to the invasion of the ovarian parenchyma beyond 5 mm depth, they are more often associated with peritoneal invasive implants.

   The patients' age is lower than that of high-grade OC, and symptoms are likely to appear in advanced stages, i.e., with peritoneal involvement by tumor. About 80% are bilateral, and often diagnosed in advanced stage [5]. Bilateral and exophytic tumors are more likely associated with advanced stage disease. The tumors are well differentiated, papillary, with little or no necrosis.

   Histologically, they resemble the non-invasive micropapillary serous carcinomas (MSPC) also described as a variant of borderline tumors (Chapter 6). Microscopically, they display micropapillae with a non-hierarchical branching pattern, nests, and gland-like structures, with clear clefts and abundant psammomatous calcifications. If the latter predominate in >75% of the papillae, the tumor is designated as psammocarcinoma and characterized by an extensive peritoneal involvement. The epithelial tumor cells tend to be rounded with scant cytoplasm, moderate atypia, and low mitotic activity (Fig. 4.1).

   Associated peritoneal implants are frequently invasive and regional lymph node involvement is not uncommon [6].

2. *Ovarian mucinous adenocarcinoma* (invasive mucinous carcinoma). These are mucinous carcinomas of intestinal type which are rarely primary ovarian and comprise about 2–3% of all ovarian carcinomas. They are usually large (18–22 cm), unilateral, multicystic, mucus-containing tumors with areas of necrosis (Fig. 4.5) and have to be distinguished from the atypical proliferative mucinous tumors which are histologically composed of seromucinous, endocervical type glands, are often bilateral and associated with endometriosis, and seem to have a benign biological behavior [7]. Microscopically, the invasive mucinous carcinomas are usually well differentiated and are often found adjacent to atypical proliferative (borderline) mucinous tumors. Destructive invasive growth into the ovarian stroma is associated with confluent glandular or expansile growth and consists of markedly crowded glandular epithelium inter-connected in a confluent pattern, with little or no

Table 4.1. Two types of ovarian carcinogenesis

Type 1 low-grade CA	Type 2 high-grade CA
• Low-grade micropapillary serous, mucinous, endometrioid, clear cell carcinomas	• High-grade serous, endometrioid (?), peritoneal, fallopian tube carcinoma, MMMT
• Slow progression	• Rapid progression
• BRAF, K-Ras, PTEN	• P53 (signature: mutation of suppressor gene, DNA damage)
• Genetic (relative) stability	• Genetic instability
• Precursors: Borderline serous and mucinous tumors, endometriotic cysts, stepwise progression	• Precursors: dysplasia (CIS, OIN) ovarian epithelium, fallopian tube fimbria

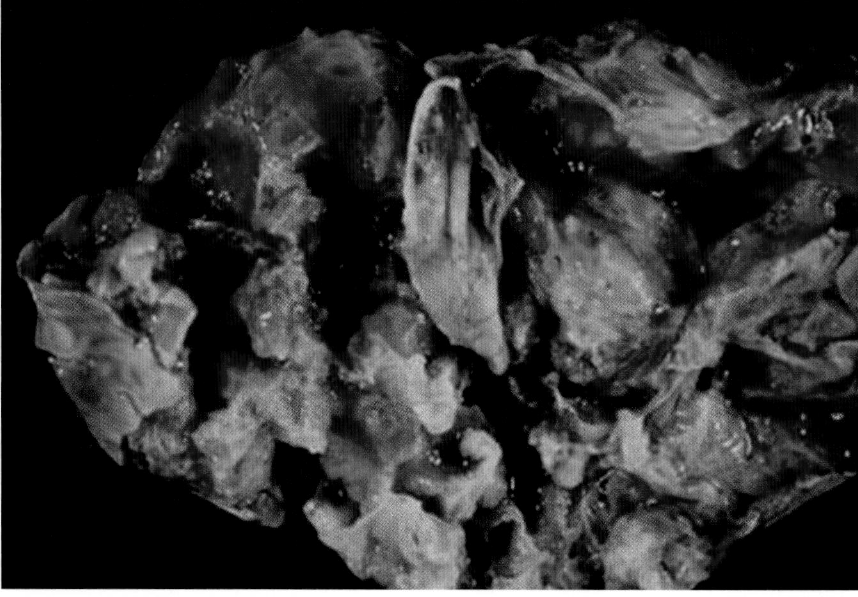

Fig. 4.5. Mucinous ovarian cystadenocarcinoma, multicystic, mucus-containing tumor with necrosis.

(a)

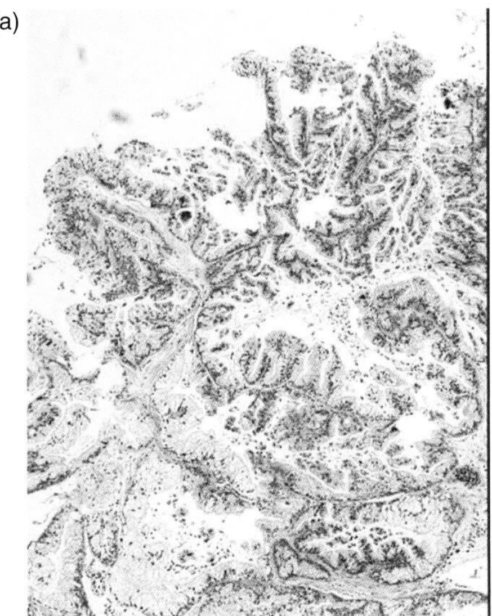

(b)

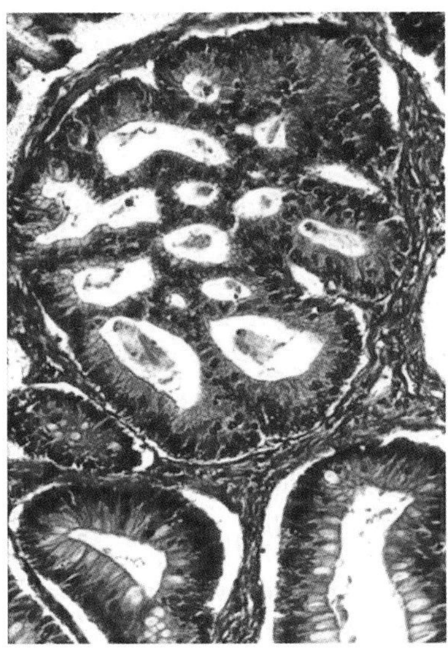

Fig. 4.6. (a) Ovarian atypical proliferating (borderline) mucinous tumor often present adjacent to malignant tumor. Hematoxylin & eosin; original magnification, ×40. (b) Ovarian well-differentiated malignant mucinous adenocarcinoma with crowded, confluent glandular pattern. Hematoxylin & eosin; original magnification, ×100.

intervening stroma (Fig. 4.6). The grading of the tumor is based on nuclear atypia rather than on tissue architecture. These tumors are immuno-reactive to cytokeratin 7, less for cytokeratin 20, and are negative for ER/PR and CA125. The most important differential diagnosis is with metastatic carcinomas which are bilateral, smaller in size (<10–12 cm), involve the ovarian surface, and present a nodular and infiltrative pattern.

Pseudomyxoma peritonei (PMP) is a syndrome including mucinous ascites and atypical epithelial structures surrounded by mucin pools. It is now considered that the origin of PMP is most often in mucinous tumors of the appendix and that the ovarian involvement is secondary. The intra-operative diagnosis of ovarian mucinous tumors at frozen section should be followed by thorough examination of the appendix, gastrointestinal, and pancreatic-biliary tract by the surgeon.

The 5-year survival rate of patients with stage I ovarian mucinous carcinomas is about 90%. These tumors are considered to evolve from benign and borderline mucinous cystadenomas: this view is supported by the finding of *KRAS* mutations in both carcinomas and adjacent cystadenomas and borderline tumors, and justifies their inclusion in the type I or low-grade epithelial carcinomas [7,8].

3. *Ovarian endometrioid adenocarcinoma (OEC)*

Endometriosis is a common condition not considered as precancerous, but suggestive of being a risk factor for ovarian carcinoma in those cases in which there is epithelial atypical proliferation, with glandular crowding and cytologic atypia, in the lining of endometriotic cysts and in endometrioid adenofibromas (Fig. 4.2). The atypical proliferation of endometrioid epithelium in the ovary resembles that seen in the uterus, both being associated with, and possibly preceding the development of endometrioid adenocarcinoma.

Endometrioid atypical proliferation in adenofibromas is not common. In these tumors, there is a glandular and papillary proliferation with complex crowding which may be confluent in the glandular component of adenofibromas. OEC arising in adenofibroma invades the surrounding stroma, often displays squamous metaplasia and necrosis. Its immuno-histologic characteristics are similar to those of uterine endometrioid adenocarcinoma.

Atypical endometrioid hyperplasia arising in endometriotic ovarian cysts and in ovarian adenofibromas is now considered as a potential precursor of OEC, that developed over a period of time during which the lesions became symptomatic and were removed surgically. Occasionally, an occult malignancy may be detected, most commonly a stage I ovarian endometrioid and rarely, a clear cell carcinoma [4]. OEC are less common than previously thought, about 10–15% or less because high-grade adenocarcinomas with endometrioid features often belong to the group of high-grade serous carcinomas [9].

Most patients are in their fifth decade, younger than those with serous carcinomas and present with painful pelvic masses due to endometriosis and often vaginal bleeding due to associated endometrial pathology [4].

The tumors measure 15 cm on average, with a higher proportion (43–50%) diagnosed in early stages, and are unilateral in most cases (13% are bilateral). Endometriosis is found in 15–20% of patients. Grossly, the tumors are solid and cystic, with brownish green mucoid content and necrosis, like endometriotic cysts with solid tumoral components.

Histologically, the tumors display a glandular confluent epithelial proliferation, with an infiltrative pattern exceeding 5 mm (the limit for microinvasion).

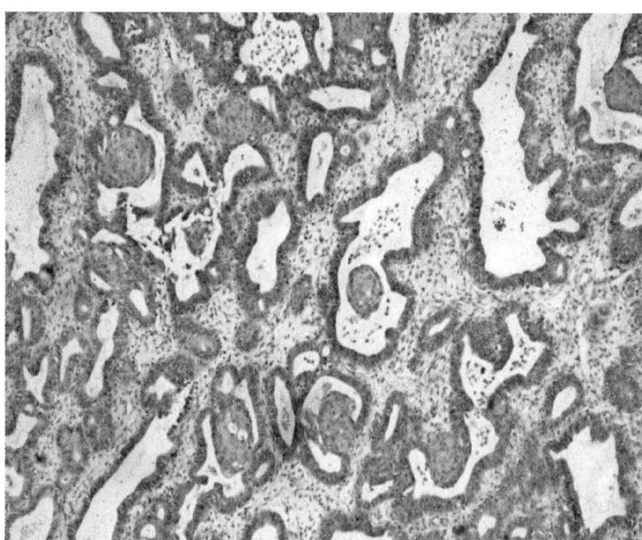

Fig. 4.7. Ovarian well-differentiated endometrioid adenocarcinoma with endometroid glandular hyperplasia and squamous metaplasia. Hematoxylin & eosin; original magnification, ×100.

There is glandular branching, budding, cribriforming, and papillary complex proliferation. The stromal invasion is mostly confluent and expansile. Squamous metaplasia is quite common and represents a criterion in the differential diagnosis from serous papillary carcinomas (Fig. 4.7). Villo glandular patterns are also common, as in endometrial adenocarcinoma. Many endometrioid adenocarcinomas of the ovary are associated with adenofibromas and endometriosis, as mentioned, and represent a progression to a type I ovarian carcinoma [10]. Moderately and poorly differentiated OEC are relatively rare: they are composed of solid sheets of tumor cells, complex glandular structures with marked nuclear pleomorphism and high mitotic activity. Many of these high-grade tumors are reclassified as serous carcinomas [10]. OEC are mostly well differentiated (75%) according to these authors while poorly differentiated tumors are likely to be variants of high-grade serous carcinomas. A small proportion (1–5%) could be mixed serous-endometrioid carcinomas.

The nuclear grade is considered as the best histologic discriminator. It should be mentioned that neither the WHO 3 grade system nor the binary system has been adequately tested for OEC [9].

There are histologic variants of OEC that are less common than the glandular pattern although often associated with it: squamous, secretory, ciliated cell variants. Unusual features are sex-cord tumor patterns, sertoliform, spindle-cell squamous, and spindle-cell stromal type components. The latter should be distinguished from carcinosarcomas diagnosed on unequivocally sarcomatous characteristics. Rare variants are neuro-endocrine tumor components. When histo-pathologic diagnosis was limited to routine stains, endometrioid ovarian carcinoma was considered as "the great imitator" and the most often misdiagnosed ovarian cancer! Immuno-histologic stains and molecular studies have improved the differential diagnosis from other ovarian tumors, especially from serous high-grade carcinomas, the natural history, management, and prognosis of which are quite different.

Immuno-histochemistry is relevant for diagnostic purposes: the most positive markers for OEC are CK7, EMA, ER/PR, followed by less positive: vimentin, CEA, CA125. Loss of staining for $hMLH_1$ and $hMSH_2$ proteins occurs in the majority of tumors with high microsatellite instability phenotype representing about 20% of OEC [11]. Well differentiated OEC share molecular features with their uterine counterpart such as mutations of tumor suppressor genes (*PTEN*), oncogenes, and genes involved in DNA repair [12]. *TP53* mutations are common in both uterine and ovarian endometrioid carcinoma, in a greater percentage in high-grade tumors [13].

Overall, OEC have a better prognosis than serous OC and are diagnosed in stage I in a higher proportion. OEC occur also in a different clinical setting, in younger women often with history of infertility, endometriosis, and uterine pathology, ranging from benign polyps to endometrial hyperplasia and neoplasia [4].

Approximately 14% of women with OEC also have endometrial carcinoma, often both are well differentiated and non-invasive, representing separate primary neoplasms [14]. Recent discovery of AT-rich interactive domain 1A gene (*ARID1A*) mutations in OEC, clear cell carcinoma (CCC), and adjacent endometriosis support the potential cancer-precursor nature of endometriosis [15]. Metastatic tumors of the ovaries from endometrial carcinoma are bilateral and nodular. Primary and metastatic OEC share the same histologic characteristics, often including associated areas of endometrial hyperplasia with squamous metaplasia.

4. Ovarian clear cell carcinoma

This is the ovarian carcinoma most often associated with endometriosis, and also with thrombo-embolic events and paraneoplastic hypercalcemia, and it is more often diagnosed in stage I [16].

Grossly, the tumors are solid and cystic, sometimes multiloculated, often arising in endometrioid cysts or adenofibromas. The histological patterns include solid, papillary, and tubulo-cystic features. The papillary pattern displays often hyalinized cores. The tumor cells have a clear granular eosinophilic cytoplasm, and contain glycogen and hyaline globules that are PAS positive. The nuclei are small and round, and often atypical in size and shape, located at the luminal border of the cell ("hobnail cells") (Fig. 4.8). Mitotic activity is usually low. Clear cell carcinoma arising in endometriosis is usually cystic and may display transition areas between the tumor and atypical endometrioid lining. The association with endometriosis is very frequent, according to some reports up to 90% [16].

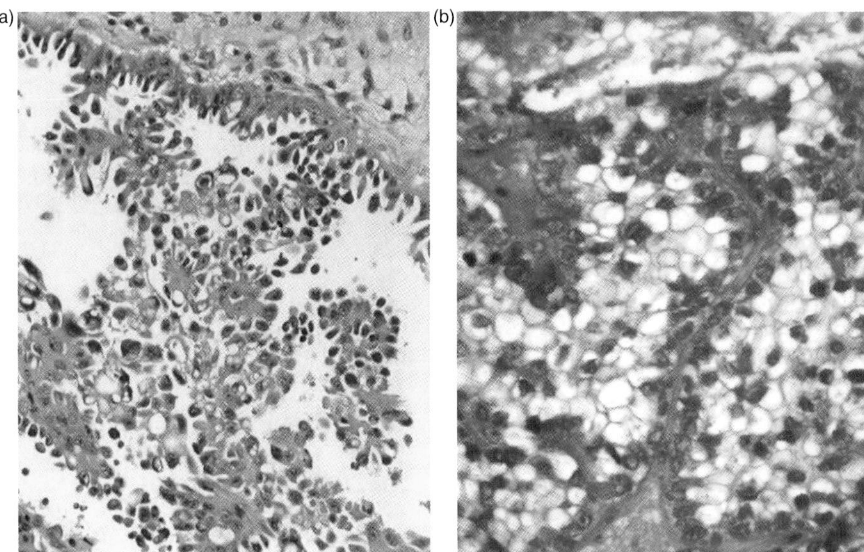

Fig. 4.8. (a) Ovarian clear cell carcinoma with "hobnail" cell pattern. Hematoxylin & eosin; × 40. (b) Ovarian clear cell carcinoma. Note small nuclei and clear cytoplasm. Hematoxylin & eosin; × 100.

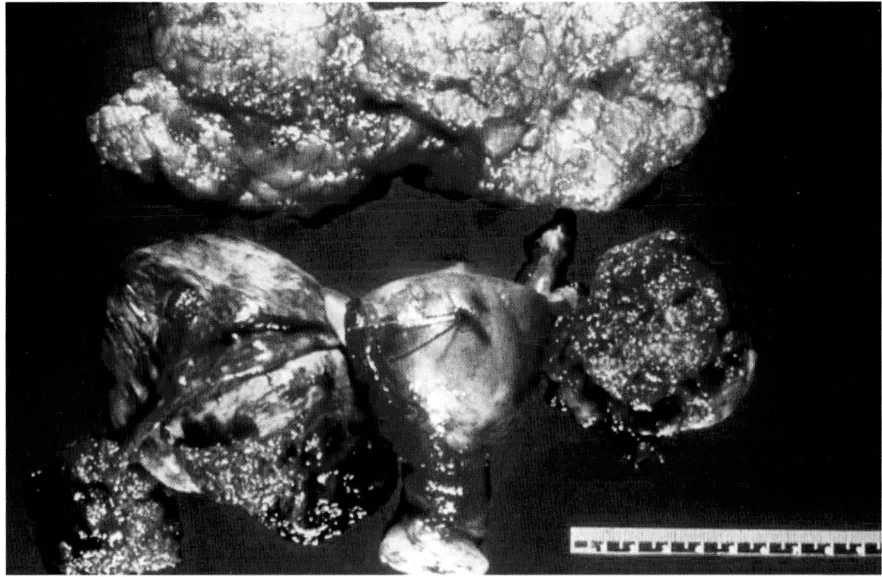

Fig. 4.9. High-grade ovarian carcinoma, bilateral, and "omental cake."

Immuno-histologic findings are positive for epithelial markers and negative for p53 and for alpha-fetoprotein. The latter is used for the differential diagnosis from the clear tumor cells seen in endodermal sinus (yolk sac) tumors. BRCA and Ca125 have been reported to be positive [17].

ER/PR are negative in the malignant tissue while adjacent endometriotic tissue is positive.

Upregulated hepatocyte nuclear factor 1β (HNF-1β) appears to play an important role in the pathogenesis of CCC [17].

High-grade serous carcinoma (HGOC)

This is the most common type of ovarian cancer. It most often occurs in the sixth and seventh decade and includes ovarian, fallopian tube, and peritoneal carcinomas. Some authors propose the term serous pelvic carcinoma [18]. Ovarian high-grade carcinoma presents in most cases in advanced stage with tumor usually disseminated in the pelvic and abdominal cavities and ascites.

Abdominal pain and distention and palpable masses are late symptoms. Gastrointestinal and urinary symptoms are nonspecific and are often ignored.

Over two-thirds of HGOC are bilateral and often extend to pelvic, peritoneal, recto-sigmoid, broad ligament structures due to contiguous growth.

Grossly, they range from microscopic to >20 cm in greatest dimension. They are often multi-cystic tumors with soft friable areas and areas of necrosis, and associated with large omental tumors forming "omental cakes" (Fig. 4.9). Grossly normal-appearing omentum contains microscopic tumor in 22% of cases [19].

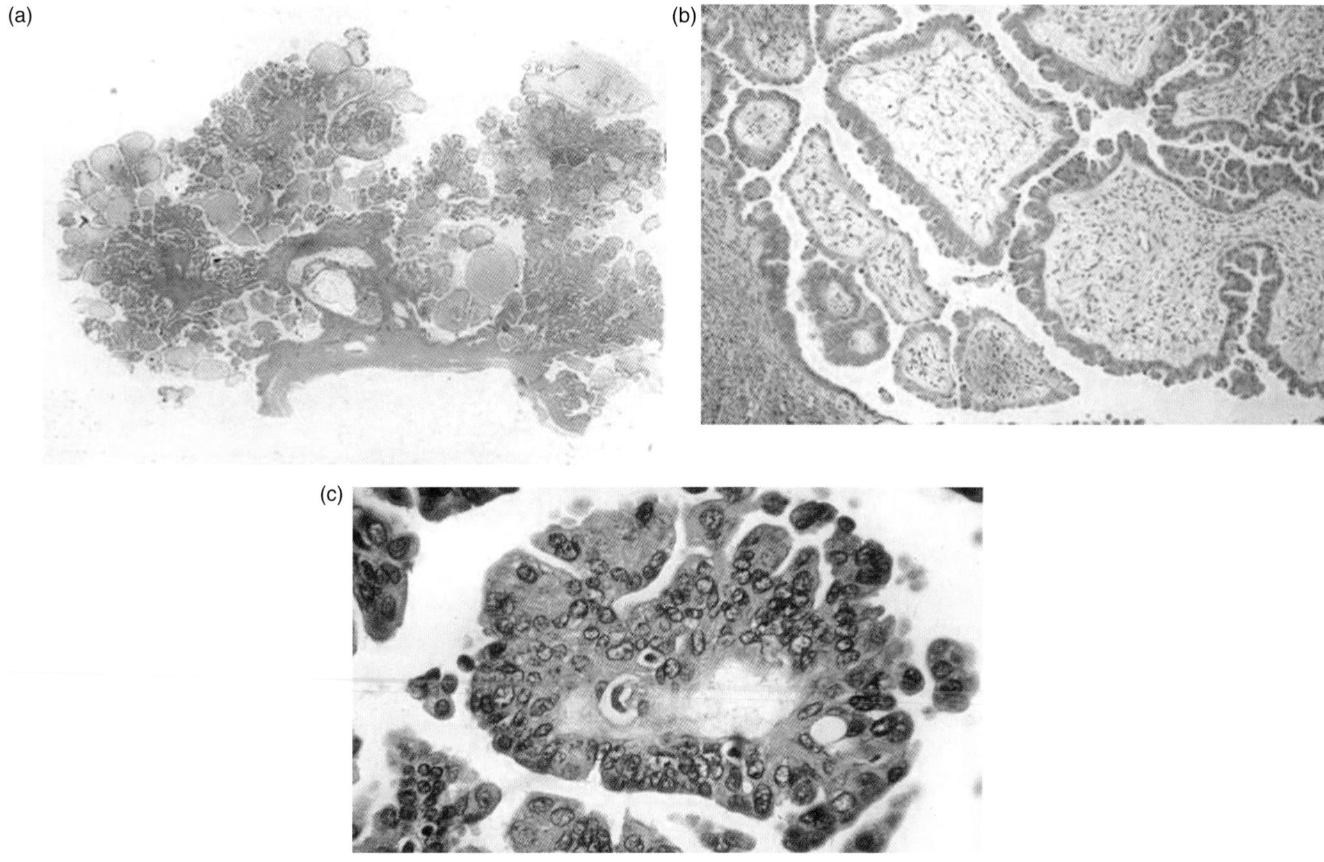

Fig. 4.10. (a) Whole-mount image of ovarian serous papillary carcinoma. (b) HGOC papillary carcinoma with "hierarchical" papillary branching. (c) HGOC with marked nuclear atypia.

Microscopic findings. The vast majority of HGOC are serous papillary epithelial tumors that display complex papillary and solid patterns with marked cytologic atypia.

The histologic basic pattern in most cases is papillary consisting of "hierarchical" branching with large papillae branching into smaller ones, different from the "non-hierarchical" branching of the low-grade, micropapillary serous tumors. Coalescing papillae form complex lace-like patterns, with slit-like spaces and areas of glandular and papillary patterns. The main characteristics of the HGOC are the high degree of nuclear atypia, bizarre-shaped large (>50 μm) often multinucleated cells, and numerous and atypical mitotic figures (Fig. 4.10). Also often seen in HGOC, as opposed to their low-grade counterparts, are large areas of necrosis and hemorrhage. Psammoma bodies are present in 25% of cases.

Traditionally, ovarian serous papillary carcinomas were divided into three grades: well, moderately and poorly differentiated tumors (Grade 1, 2, 3 respectively), based on the proportion between the epithelial tumor tissue and the connective tissue stalks of the papillary structures, and on the degree of nuclear atypia. This classification has been challenged and a two-tier (binary) system was proposed based on the fact that in the group of "moderate" or grade 2 tumors the nuclei lack BRAF and KRAS mutations (characteristic for low-grade tumors) and display p 53 mutations in >90% of cases, the hallmark of HGOC; therefore moderately and poorly differentiated serous tumors appear to belong to the same category [20]. Their prognosis supports this binary system as well [21]. In HGOC, usually there are >12 mitoses per 10 high power fields; however, mitotic counting is not included in the histologic criteria.

This new approach to grading ovarian serous carcinomas is clinically significant because it appears that the 5-year survival is 75% for the low-grade and 35% for the high-grade tumors. It should be kept in mind, however, that the high mortality in HGOC occurs in patients who are almost two decades older, on average, therefore possibly sicker (comorbidity) with a lower life expectancy [22].

HGOC, as mentioned, is mostly composed of serous tumors. A smaller and somewhat controversial group of HGOC are OEC displaying histologic characteristics such as glandular and cribriform patterns with squamoid and spindle cell differentiation, villo-glandular structures, with high-grade nuclear atypia and high mitotic activity, traditionally classified as poorly differentiated endometrioid carcinomas.

HGOC may display areas resembling clear-cell carcinoma with papillary and solid tumor tissue composed of cells with clear cytoplasm, as well as solid tumors with no differentiation displaying marked cellular atypia and high mitotic activity, large and bizarre cells with irregular nuclei and multinucleated cells, generally classified as "undifferentiated." They probably represent serous carcinomas as well. Uncommon variants of undifferentiated carcinomas are non-small cell neuroendocrine and small cell hypercalcemic carcinomas, the latter occurring in young women (<40 years) with a dismal prognosis.

The basis for including these "undifferentiated" tumors into the large group of ovarian high-grade serous carcinomas is the immuno-reactivity of the tissue. p53 positivity is the hallmark of serous carcinomas; CK7, EMA, WT1, and BRCA1 are positive in the majority of cases. By difference from endometrioid carcinomas, only a minority of serous carcinomas are ER positive. Malignant Brenner tumors are rare and display transitional cell carcinoma features; most are now considered as variants of high-grade serous carcinomas.

TP53 mutations were found in more than 50% of HGOC and may also represent an early event in their development [23,24].

Chromosomal instability is more pronounced in HGOC than in low-grade tumors; this may be causally related to invasion, metastases, and chemoresistance [25].

Malignant mixed Mullerian tumor (MMMT-carcinosarcoma) is not as rare as previously thought, representing 7.5% of ovarian carcinomas. These are large tumors (15–20 cm) histologically similar to MMMT of the endometrium which are more common. Both are seen in older patients and are high-grade neoplasms composed of epithelial (high-grade serous/endometrioid) elements and malignant stromal elements with sheets of spindle-shaped cells displaying marked nuclear atypia and brisk mitotic activity.

Heterologous components such as cartilage, rhabdomyoblasts, osteoid, or adipose tissue are not uncommon (Fig. 4.11). The stromal-appearing tumor tissue often is immuno-reactive to epithelial markers, and the tumor tissue has been shown to be monoclonal, suggesting that some of these tumors are metaplastic carcinomas [26]. They belong to the group of HGOC, and their biological behavior is probably even more aggressive.

The classification into the two-tier system was recently challenged because type 1 includes multiple distinct entities [15].

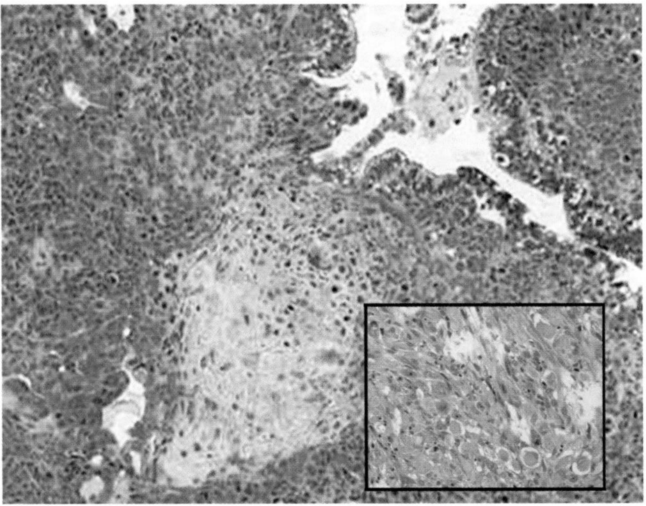

Fig. 4.11. Ovarian malignant mixed Mullerian tumor heterologous type with malignant epithelial and stromal tumor cells and area of chondroid differentiation. Inset: right lower corner: rhabdomyoblasts. Hematoxylin & eosin; original magnification, ×40.

Conclusion

Ovarian carcinomas are not the most common malignant gynecological tumors but they are the most lethal. As shown in other chapters, their high mortality rate has changed little over the past decades, despite the intense clinical and basic research of the subject. Early detection, identification of reliable tumor markers, and targeted chemotherapy are needed. The process of revealing the molecular and genetic subcellular mechanisms of ovarian carcinogenesis is still unfolding raising perhaps more questions than finding the answers! New paradigms are proposed: For example, while the role of the fallopian tube fimbriae in the inception of HGOC has been supported by numerous studies [27–29], recently it was reported that low-grade ovarian carcinoma may be initiated by fallopian tube lesions as well [30]. A significant breakthrough to change the poor outcome of the majority of HGOC is still elusive. The role of pathological descriptions and classifications is to define as accurately as possible the neoplastic entities for their optimal therapeutic management. The interpretation of histopathologic patterns described in this chapter may change in the years to come, as they have changed due to recently acquired knowledge since the prior editions of this book.

References

1. Kurman RJ, Shih IeM. Molecular pathogenesis and extraovarian origin of epithelial ovarian cancer- shifting the paradigm. Hum Pathol. 2011;**42**(7):918–31.
2. Lalwani N, Prasad SR, Vikram R, et al. Histologic, molecular, and cytogenetic features of ovarian cancers: implications for diagnosis and treatment. Radiographics. 2011;**31**(3):625–46.
3. Kurman RJ, Shih IeM. The origin and pathogenesis of epithelial ovarian cancer: a proposed unifying theory. Am J Surg Pathol. 2010;**34**(3):433–43.
4. Deligdisch L, Pénault-Llorca F, Altchek A, et al. Stage I ovarian carcinoma: different clinical pathologic patterns. Fertil Steril. 2007;**88**(4):906–10.
5. Gershenson DM, Sun CC, Lu KH, et al. Clinical behavior of stage II–IV low-grade serous carcinoma of the ovary. Obstet Gynecol. 2006;**108**(2):361–8.
6. Shroff R, Brooks RA, Zighelboim I, et al. The utility of peritoneal biopsy and omentectomy in the upstaging of apparent early ovarian cancer. Int J Gynecol Cancer. 2011;**21**: 1208–12.
7. Dubé V, Roy M, Plante M, et al. Mucinous ovarian tumors of Mullerian-type: an analysis of 17 cases including borderline tumors and intraepithelial, microinvasive, and invasive carcinomas. Int J Gynecol Pathol. 2005;**24**(2):138–46.
8. Soslow RA. Mucinous ovarian carcinoma: slippery business. Cancer. 2011;**117**(3):451–3.

9. Seidman JD, Cho KR, Ronnett BM, et al. Blaustein's pathology of the female genital tract, 6th edition. In: Kurman RJ, Hedrick Ellenson L, Ronnett BM (Eds.). Epithelial Tumors of the Ovary. New York: Springer Science & Business Media; 2011, p. 753.
10. Köbel M, Kalloger SE, Baker PM, et al. Diagnosis of ovarian carcinoma cell type is highly reproducible: a trans-Canadian study. Am J Surg Pathol. 2010;**34**(7):984–93.
11. Liu J, Albarracin CT, Chang KH, et al. Microsatellite instability and expression of hMLH1 and hMSH2 proteins in ovarian endometrioid cancer. Mod Pathol. 2004;**17**(1):75–80.
12. Di Cristofano A, Ellenson LH. Endometrial carcinoma. Annu Rev Pathol. 2007;**2**:57–85.
13. Kolasa IK, Rembiszewska A, Janiec-Jankowska A, et al. *PTEN* mutation, expression and LOH at its locus in ovarian carcinomas. Relation to TP53, K-RAS and BRCA1 mutations. Gynecol Oncol. 2006;**103**(2):692–7.
14. Seidman JD, Cho KR, Ronnett BM, et al. Blaustein's pathology of the female genital tract, 6th edition. In: Kurman RJ, Hedrick Ellenson L, Ronnett BM. (Eds.). Epithelial Tumors of the Ovary. New York: Springer Science & Business Media; 2011, p. 757.
15. J. Prat. New Insights into ovarian cancer pathology. Annals Oncol. 2012;**23** (Suppl 10):x111–17.
16. Veras E, Mao TL, Ayhan A, et al. Cystic and adenofibromatous clear cell carcinomas of the ovary: distinctive tumors that differ in their pathogenesis and behavior: a clinicopathologic analysis of 122 cases. Am J Surg Pathol. 2009;**33**(6):844–53.
17. Howell NR, Zheng W, Cheng L, et al. Carcinomas of ovary and lung with clear cell features: can immunohistochemistry help in differential diagnosis? Int J Gynecol Pathol. 2007;**26**(2):134–40.
18. Crum CP, Drapkin R, Miron A, et al. The distal fallopian tube: a new model for pelvic serous carcinogenesis. Curr Opin Obstet Gynecol. 2007;**19**(1):3–9.
19. Seidman JD, Cho KR, Ronnett BM, et al. Blaustein's pathology of the female genital tract, 6th edition. In: Kurman RJ, Hedrick Ellenson L, Ronnett BM. (Eds.). Epithelial Tumors of the Ovary. New York: Springer Science & Business Media; 2011, p. 727.
20. Malpica A, Deavers MT, Lu K, et al. Grading ovarian serous carcinoma using a two-tier system. Am J Surg Pathol. 2004;**28**(4):496–504.
21. Seidman JD, Horkayne-Szakaly I, Cosin JA, et al. Testing of two binary grading systems for FIGO stage III serous carcinoma of the ovary and peritoneum. Gynecol Oncol. 2006;**103**(2):703–8.
22. Seidman JD, Cho KR, Ronnett BM, et al. Blaustein's pathology of the female genital tract, 6th edition. In: Kurman RJ, Hedrick Ellenson L, Ronnett BM. (Eds.). Epithelial Tumors of the Ovary. New York: Springer Science & Business Media; 2011, p. 730.
23. Singer G, Stöhr R, Cope L, Dehari R, et al. Patterns of p53 mutations separate ovarian serous borderline tumors and low- and high-grade carcinomas and provide support for a new model of ovarian carcinogenesis: a mutational analysis with immunohistochemical correlation. Am J Surg Pathol. 2005;**29**(2):218–24.
24. Leitao MM, Soslow RA, Baergen RN, et al. Mutation and expression of the TP53 gene in early stage epithelial ovarian carcinoma. Gynecol Oncol. 2004;**93**(2):301–6.
25. Meng Q, Xia C, Fang J, et al. Role of PI3K and AKT specific isoforms in ovarian cancer cell migration, invasion and proliferation through the p70S6K1 pathway. Cell Signal. 2006;**18**(12):2262–71.
26. Jin Z, Ogata S, Tamura G, et al. Carcinosarcomas (malignant mullerian mixed tumors) of the uterus and ovary: a genetic study with special reference to histogenesis. Int J Gynecol Pathol. 2003;**22**(4):368–73.
27. Guo DH, Pang SJ, Shen Y, et al. [Morphological features of the fimbria of the fallopian tube in pelvic serous adenocarcinoma]. [Article in Chinese] Zhonghua Zhong Liu Za Zhi. 2011;**33**(4):287–90.
28. Auersperg N. The origin of ovarian carcinomas: a unifying hypothesis. Int J Gynecol Pathol. 2011;**30**(1):12–21.
29. Rosen DG, Yang G, Liu G, et al. Ovarian cancer: pathology, biology, and disease models. Front Biosci. 2009;**14**:2089–102.
30. Li J, Abushahin N, Pang S, et al. Tubal origin of 'ovarian' low-grade serous carcinoma. Mod Pathol. 2011;**24**:1488–99.

Chapter 5

Ovarian tumors of borderline malignancy

Peter Schlosshauer, MD

Introduction

The category of "ovarian tumors of borderline malignancy" was introduced by the World Health Organization (WHO) in 1971. By then it was recognized that there is a subset of relatively rare ovarian surface-epithelial tumors exhibiting pathomorphological features intermediate between clearly benign adenofibromas and clearly malignant adenocarcinomas, and that some of these intermediate tumors would behave in a malignant manner. The "borderline" terminology was meant to be a provisional one, until detailed studies would reveal definite criteria to classify these tumors as either benign or malignant.

Now, 40 years later, we know a lot more about these tumors, there is a plethora of literature about them (very disproportionate to their actual incidence), and several attempts have been made to eliminate the unfortunate "B" word. In fact, the latest edition of one of the major gynecologic pathology textbooks declares the "serous borderline" category as no longer needed [1]. However, no general consensus about the terminology has been achieved, and these tumors continue to cause considerable controversy among the experts. "Borderline" is still an accepted, if not the preferred term by the majority of pathologists and gynecologic oncologists.

The somewhat lengthy designation "ovarian tumor of borderline malignancy" is often substituted by the abbreviated, albeit less accurate, term "borderline tumor." Of course, these lesions are true tumors in the sense of space-occupying masses; in fact, mucinous borderline tumors are among the biggest tumors encountered in humans. What is borderline about them is our ability to predict their clinical behavior. Terms used more or less synonymously with "borderline tumor" are "tumor of low malignant potential" and "atypical proliferative tumor," see below.

Ovarian borderline tumors are surface-epithelial neoplasms, and similar to ovarian adenofibromas and adenocarcinomas, there are several subtypes depending on the phenotypic differentiation of the epithelial tumor cells. The WHO distinguishes serous, mucinous, endometrioid, clear cell, and transitional cell borderline tumors. Their definitions vary slightly, but basically they are defined as ovarian tumors of low malignant potential exhibiting an atypical epithelial proliferation greater than that seen in their benign counterparts but without destructive stromal invasion [2].

The incidence of ovarian borderline tumors in the United States is 2.5 per 100,000 women per year, including all subtypes; 3.6% of all ovarian epithelial tumors are borderline tumors.

Additional images of ovarian borderline tumors can be found on the website of the University of Illinois at Chicago (http://borderlineovariantumors.pathology.uic.edu).

Serous borderline tumors

General features

According to the Bethesda Borderline Ovarian Tumor Workshop from 2003, the "borderline" terminology is preferred for serous tumors by the majority of experts. The terms "tumor of low malignant potential" and "atypical proliferative tumor" were believed to not adequately convey the potentially aggressive nature of the lesion, discourage the clinician from performing a complete staging procedure, and interfere with cancer registry reporting and international comparison/research efforts [3].

Being the most frequent subtype, serous borderline tumors (SBT) comprise less than 2% of all ovarian surface-epithelial tumors, 10% of all ovarian serous tumors and about 50% of all ovarian borderline tumors. They occur at a mean age of 42 years; up to 55% are bilateral and 40% have extra-ovarian disease ("implants") at the time of diagnosis. Most patients have an excellent prognosis with 10-year survival rates around 95%, which includes cases with microinvasion, lymph node involvement, and advanced stage cases with noninvasive extra-ovarian implants (see below). Tumors may recur after many years; recurrent cases still carry a good prognosis as long as the tumor shows the same morphologic "borderline" features and has not become invasive. Primary SBT arising from the peritoneum outside the ovaries have been described, but are exceedingly rare.

Morphologically, SBT tend to form well circumscribed unilocular solid-cystic ovarian masses with papillary excrescences protruding into the cyst cavity or involving the ovarian surface. Tumors are soft and friable, but necrosis is not usually seen. Microscopically, the papillae tend to display a hierarchical branching pattern, with smaller papillae emanating from larger ones. The epithelial layer is stratified, i.e., several cells thick ("tufting"), as opposed to the single cell layer seen in

Altchek's Diagnosis and Management of Ovarian Disorders, ed. Liane Deligdisch, Nathan G. Kase, and Carmel J. Cohen. Published by Cambridge University Press.

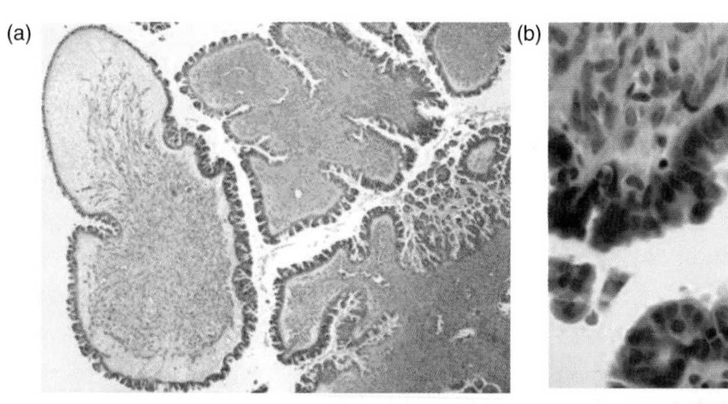

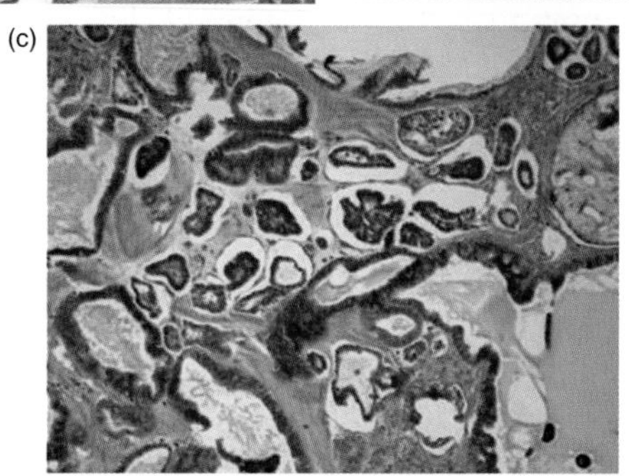

Fig. 5.1. (a) Ovarian serous borderline tumor (SBT). Note tangentially sectioned tips of papillae, appearing as "free floating" cell clusters in right half of image. Hematoxylin & eosin original magnification 40×. (b) Ovarian SBT. Note atypical epithelial proliferation, evident as multilayered epithelium. Some cells are ciliated. Hematoxylin & eosin; original magnification 400×. (c) Ovarian SBT, focus of microinvasion, microinvasive carcinoma-type. Cell clusters and micropapillary structures are separated by clefts from the surrounding stroma. Hematoxylin & eosin; original magnification, ×100.

benign serous cystadenomas and cystadenofibromas. Tangential sectioning of the tips of epithelial tufts results in characteristic "free floating" cell clusters (Fig. 5.1a). Epithelial cells resemble those of the fallopian tube or mesothelial cells. Ciliated cells may be present. Cytologic atypia is mild and mitotic activity is low, with a mitotic index of less than 4 mitotic figures per 10 high power (40× objective) microscopic fields (Fig. 5.1b). Variable amounts of psammoma bodies are seen in 50% of cases.

Some tumors show a morphologic spectrum ranging from cystadenoma to borderline features. A diagnosis of SBT is warranted if more than 10% of the epithelial-lined surfaces exhibit stratified (as opposed to single cell layer) epithelium. The designation "serous cystadenoma with focal atypical epithelial proliferation" is recommended for those lesions with less than 10% "borderline" features [3].

For histopathological examination, it is crucial that SBT be thoroughly sampled. While obviously malignant tumors can be diagnosed with relatively few sections, borderline tumors may require many more sections to rule out the presence of occult invasive disease. Surgical pathology's golden rule of one section per centimeter tumor diameter may not be sufficient and is granted an exception for ovarian borderline tumors. Especially for tumors with a solid component bigger than 10 cm in greatest dimension, two or more sections per cm are recommended (based on the fact that tumor volume increases exponentially with tumor radius, assuming a spherical shape). Not surprisingly, the more sections taken, the more likely one will find foci of invasion.

Microinvasion

Foci of microinvasion are reported in up to 25% of all SBTs, and even more frequently when extra-ovarian implants are present. Definitions vary slightly among authors, but most consider invasive foci of less than 5 mm in greatest dimension or less than 10 mm^2 as micro-invasion. There may be multiple separate foci of micro-invasion within the same tumor. Any larger confluent areas of invasion lead to a diagnosis of invasive carcinoma. Different growth patterns of micro-invasion have been described. The more frequent "eosinophilic type" is characterized by small clusters of cells and individual cells with abundant eosinophilic cytoplasm and bland cytologic features, growing into the stroma of tumor papillae. Occasional cases show cell clusters and micropapillary structures, separated by spaces from the surrounding stroma. The latter variant has been termed "micro-invasive carcinoma" by some authors (Fig. 5.1b). At this time, it is uncertain whether these morphologic variants bear a different biologic significance. Of note, microinvasion is seen more frequently in tumors from pregnant women. Microinvasion has been associated with increased risk of bilaterality and extra-ovarian disease [4]. Recent analyses suggest that – contrary to earlier beliefs – the presence of microinvasion in SBTs may be associated with an increased risk for tumor progression and adverse outcome [5–9].

Implants

Extra-ovarian lesions of similar "borderline" morphologic features are present in 40% of all SBT patients and 56% of bilateral SBT cases. These lesions, known as "implants," are most frequently found on the serosal surface of the peritoneal cavity, including the pelvis and the omentum. The term "implant" does not suggest an understanding of its pathogenesis. The debate whether "implants" are independent synchronous/metachronous lesions or secondary lesions derived from the ovarian tumor is ongoing; several lines of evidence suggest that the latter is the case at least in some instances [10–12].

For clinical purposes, the distinction between "non-invasive" and "invasive" implants is of great importance:

Non-invasive implants account for 75% of all implants and are further subdivided into "epithelial" and "desmoplastic" implants. Epithelial implants morphologically closely resemble the ovarian tumor, i.e., they are well circumscribed, show a hierarchical branching pattern and epithelial tufting. They are attached to the serosal surface of the involved intraperitoneal structure and lack a stromal reaction. In contrast, desmoplastic implants are composed of a serous epithelial component and a granulation tissue-like stromal component. The volume of the stromal component may by far outweigh the epithelial component. Other morphologic features that identify desmoplastic implants include their superficial location on the serosa and the close attachment of epithelial cells to the surrounding stromal cells ("merging" appearance; Fig. 5.2a). Like many other terms in this context, the designation "desmoplastic" is an unfortunate and confusing one: In any other tumor type, a "desmoplastic" stromal response describes a phenomenon that is associated with invasive (i.e., malignant) disease. Therefore, it needs to be emphasized that unlike anywhere else, "desmoplastic implants" of an ovarian SBT are considered benign, because they have a good prognosis.

Approximately 25% of all implants are classified as "invasive." They are distinguished from their non-invasive counterparts by deeper location within the tissue, haphazard growth pattern, a predominantly epithelial component outgrowing the stromal tissue, destructive growth pattern, and close resemblance to low-grade (well-differentiated) ovarian papillary serous carcinomas (Fig. 5.2b). In addition, the finding of epithelial cell clusters separated from the surrounding stroma by slit-like spaces and formation of micropapillae have been associated with progressive disease and poor outcome [13]. Invasive implants are considered synonymous with low-grade (well-differentiated) papillary serous carcinoma [3]. The distinction between non-invasive and invasive implants may be very difficult in individual cases. A combination of non-invasive and invasive implants may occur in the same patient.

Non-invasive or invasive implants involving the very ovary that harbors the SBT are known as "auto-implants." Because non-invasive desmoplastic autoimplants carry a good prognosis, it is important not to over diagnose them as invasive implants/carcinoma.

The finding of invasive implants significantly worsens the prognosis: One study found a survival rate of 66% after a mean follow-up of 7.4 years [14]. In fact, the presence of invasive implants is the only feature of clinical importance for further treatment short of a diagnosis of frank ovarian carcinoma. It is for this reason that thorough staging is recommended for all bilateral ovarian SBTs and SBTs with micropapillary features (see below).

Both non-invasive and invasive implants count for tumor staging. For example, a non-invasive desmoplastic implant in the omentum outside the pelvis results in a Fédération Internationale de Gynécologie et d'Obstétrique (FIGO) stage III. Likewise, in the TNM system endorsed by the American Joint Committee on Cancer (AJCC), the same case would be classified as T3 (but not M1) [15]. For complete definition of ovarian tumor stages see Chapter 28 of this book.

Endosalpingiosis

Small inclusion cysts lined by serous-type epithelium are found underneath the peritoneum or within pelvic lymph nodes in 40–65% of patients with ovarian SBTs (as opposed to 5–14% in unselected women) and are known as "endosalpingiosis." If present in lymph nodes, they tend to be located at the periphery of the lymph node, often within its capsule (Fig. 5.3a). Again, the debate is ongoing as to whether this is an independent metachronous phenomenon or secondary to the ovarian primary tumor [11,16]. Endosalpingiosis may show small papillary structures and psammoma bodies. It is considered benign and does not count toward tumor staging.

(a)

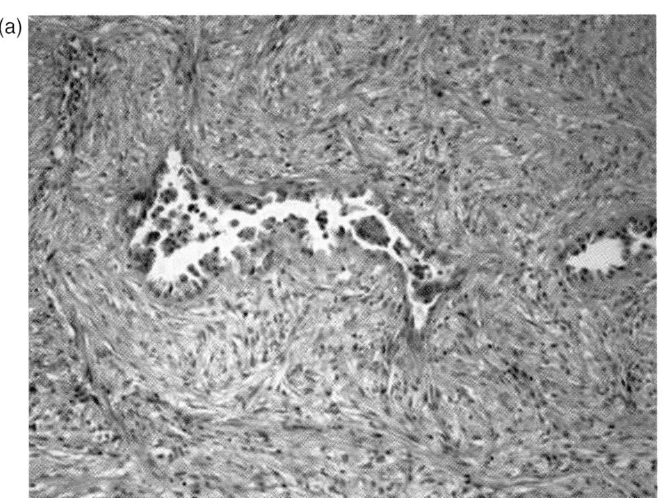

(b)

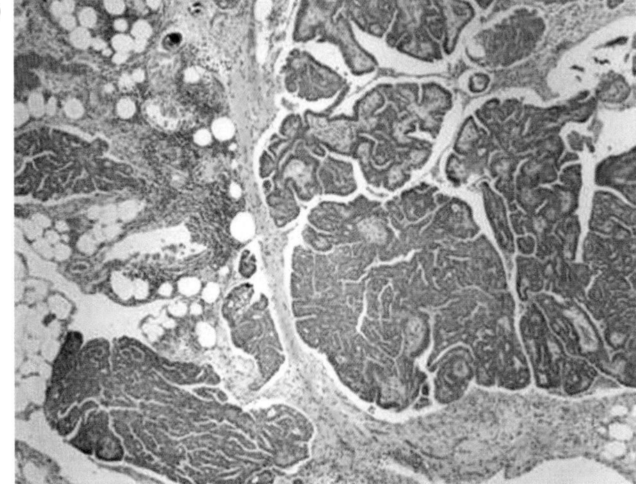

Fig. 5.2. (a) Non-invasive desmoplastic implant associated with an ovarian SBT. Epithelial cells are attached to and merge with the abundant surrounding granulation tissue-like stroma. Hematoxylin & eosin original magnification, ×100. (b) Invasive implant associated with an ovarian SBT. Abundant epithelial proliferation with micropapillary features and surrounding clefts, located deep within the omentum. Hematoxylin & eosin; original magnification, ×40.

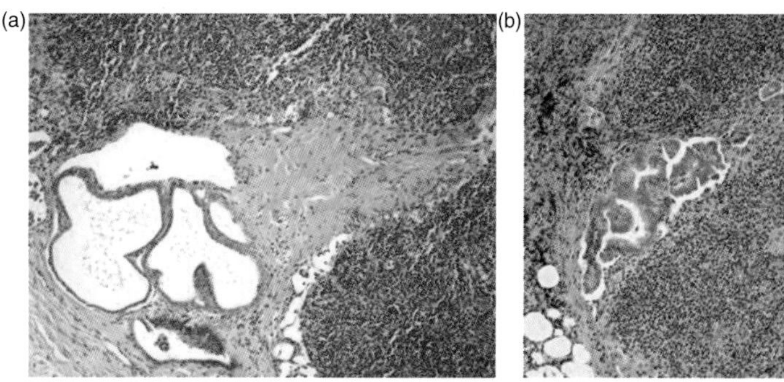

Fig. 5.3. (a) Endosalpingiosis. Simple cystic structures lined by serous-type epithelium, located within the lymph node capsule. Hematoxylin & eosin; original magnification, ×100. (b) Lymph node involvement in patient with ovarian SBT. Serous-type cells forming clusters and papillary structures, extending deep into the lymph node. Hematoxylin & eosin; original magnification, ×100.

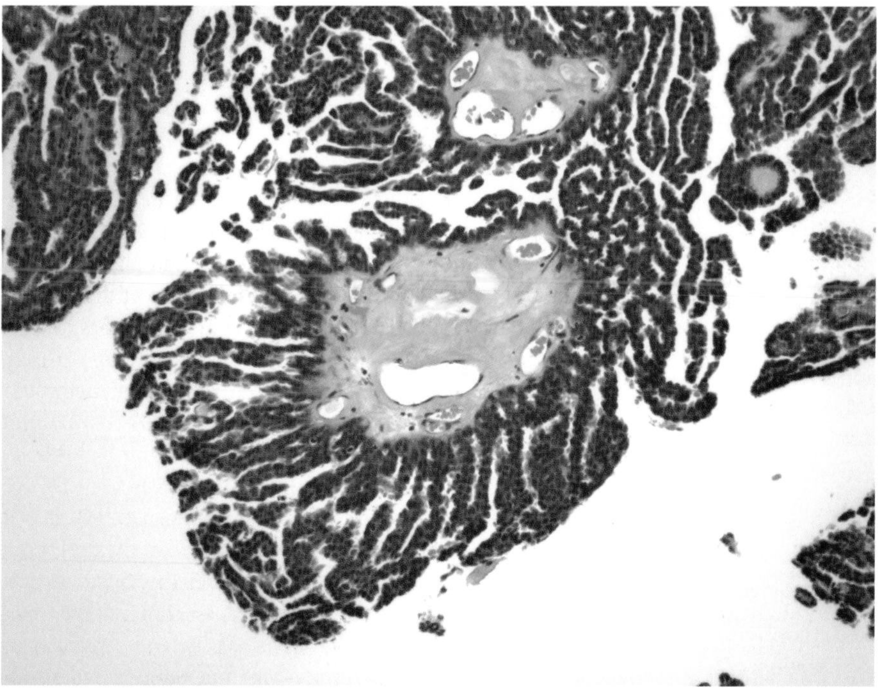

Fig. 5.4. Micropapillary tumor. Filigree epithelial papillae emanating from a relatively broad fibrovascular stalk ("caput medusae" appearance). Hematoxylin & eosin; original magnification 100×.

Lymph node involvement

The finding of serous-type epithelial cell clusters or papillary structures within the sinuses or the actual lymph node tissue is referred to as "lymph node involvement" (Fig. 5.3b). This is seen in 30% of SBT patients. Pathogenetically, these cell clusters are thought to have been "deported" – meaning that they originated from the ovarian SBT and were passively transferred to the lymph node by means of lymph drainage (as opposed to active invasion of frank cancer cells). It has been hypothesized that ovarian tumor cells shed into the peritoneal cavity may enter the lymphatic vascular network of the peritoneal surfaces [17]. Lymph node involvement by itself does not appear to have an impact on overall survival, but often coexists with other potentially adverse features, especially extra-ovarian implants. Nodular aggregates of epithelial cells exceeding 1 mm in greatest diameter have been associated with decreased disease-free interval [18].

Unlike endosalpingiosis, lymph node involvement does count for tumor staging. For example, involvement of a pelvic lymph node results in a FIGO stage IIIC and AJCC N1, respectively.

Micropapillary tumors

A subset of SBTs shows "micropapillary" features, defined as slender epithelial papillae with no or minimal fibrovascular support, which are at least five times longer than wide. For the purpose of this chapter and due to disagreement among authors about the nomenclature, tumors exhibiting continuous micropapillary areas greater than 5 mm in diameter will be discussed as micropapillary serous tumors. Smaller areas of similar appearance can be seen within "regular" SBTs, and do not warrant separating the lesion into a different diagnostic category. Micropapillary serous tumors tend to display a less hierarchical branching architecture than "regular" SBTs, resulting in microapillary fronds emanating directly from relatively broad fibrovascular stalks. This appearance, when seen in histologic cross-section, has been likened to a "caput medusae" (Fig. 5.4). Some authors consider micropapillary tumors a separate entity with significantly worse prognosis and hence prefer the term "micropapillary serous carcinoma," but most experts prefer to classify these tumors within the "borderline" category [19–23]. Some, although not all, studies on micropapillary tumors conclude that they are associated with increased risks of bilaterality, advanced stage, and invasive implants when compared with "regular" SBTs [4,7,14,20,22,24–28]. Others argue that the only feature impacting clinical outcome is the presence or absence of invasive extra-ovarian implants. Because invasive implants can be seen with both micropapillary tumors and "regular" SBTs, the separation of the ovarian tumors may be more of academic but not practical interest [29,30].

Clinical implications

Several studies published during recent years have found that recurrent SBTs can be easily resected without compromising the good prognosis, as long as there is no evidence of invasive disease. Therefore, recommendations for the surgical approach of SBTs have become more conservative, especially in patients of childbearing age [31–33]. Cystectomy or unilateral salpingo-oophorectomy is considered acceptable if there is no evidence of more widespread disease at the time of surgery. Thorough surgical exploration and full staging is recommended in all cases of extra-ovarian disease, ovarian tumors exceeding 8 cm in diameter, and tumors with micropapillary features [34].

At the upper end of the spectrum of ovarian SBTs, we encounter an interesting diagnostic dilemma: how to differentiate SBTs with invasive implants from well-differentiated (low-grade, FIGO grade 1) serous carcinomas? In fact, despite the vast amount of literature on SBTs, this issue has hardly ever been formally addressed. One study came to the apparently logical conclusion that all "invasive implants" should be named "invasive low-grade carcinoma" [13]. Subsequently, a formal consensus was obtained that the terms "invasive implant" and "invasive carcinoma" are synonymous [3]. The "invasive" feature may pertain only to the extra-ovarian disease, while it is possible that no invasive tumor was identified within the ovarian (presumed primary) tumor. Again: the only feature that clinically matters is the presence of invasive implants, which implies malignant behavior and poor prognosis. Tumor stage, lymph node involvement, and micropapillary features within the ovarian tumor do not impact treatment. Most gynecologic oncologists will treat a patient diagnosed with "invasive implants" the same way as a patient with low-grade (well-differentiated) ovarian serous carcinoma, which may include chemotherapy. Recent studies, however, suggest that low-grade serous carcinomas do not respond as well as high-grade ovarian serous carcinomas to platinum-based chemotherapy [35–39]. Conversely, adjuvant chemotherapy is not usually administered in the absence of invasive implants.

Given the rarity of these tumors, the confusing terminology, and the significant impact on patient treatment of the trigger word "invasive implant," it is prudent to obtain second and even third opinions by expert pathologists as well as gynecologic oncologists before determining a treatment plan for any patient with an ovarian SBT.

Mucinous borderline tumors

General features

Mucinous borderline tumors (MBTs) account for 30–40% of all ovarian borderline tumors, and approximately 12% of all mucinous ovarian tumors are "borderline." As mentioned before, they are among the largest tumors encountered in humans. Extreme examples have reached a weight of more than 100 kg. Two subtypes are distinguished: The intestinal type represents 85% of MBTs and exhibits intestinal-type differentiation of its epithelium, including numerous goblet cells. The vast majority (94%) of intestinal-type MBTs are unilateral. In contrast, "seromucinous" (Mullerian) borderline tumors are characterized by a Müllerian-type endocervical mucinous epithelium. They share a high frequency (40%) of bilaterality with their serous counterparts, may be seen in association with endometriosis, and may rarely exhibit extra-ovarian implants. Both subtypes have an excellent prognosis with 10-year survival rates exceeding 95%. Hence, primary ovarian MBTs are basically benign tumors. Nevertheless, the term "mucinous borderline tumor" continues to be used to ensure that both pathologists and clinicians use special caution during examination and follow-up of these cases. Given the large size of these lesions, it is conceivable that despite adequate sampling a focus of carcinoma within the tumor may be missed, which may give rise to recurrence and metastatic disease. The terms "atypical proliferative mucinous tumor" and "mucinous tumor of low malignant potential" are used synonymously, the latter term being the least favored [40].

As opposed to serous tumors, MBTs are typically multiloculated. At the low end of the spectrum, a minimum of 10% of the lining epithelium is required to be stratified to distinguish an MBT from a mucinous cystadenoma. At the high end, MBTs can display a bewildering degree of architectural complexity (Fig. 5.5a). Cytologic features are bland, i.e., the mucinous epithelial cells are well differentiated and exhibit abundant mucin-containing cytoplasm and low mitotic activity (Fig. 5.5b). Intraepithelial carcinoma can be seen within a MBT and is defined by severe (grade 3) cytologic atypia of the epithelial cells, as manifested by high nuclear/cytoplasmic ratio, nuclear pleomorphism, cytoplasmic mucus depletion and increased mitotic activity (Fig. 5.5c). Microinvasion may occur multifocally with each focus measuring less than 5 mm in greatest diameter. Both intra-epithelial carcinoma and microinvasion have no impact on the prognosis. However, rarely a "mural nodule" is found, in which the tumor may dedifferentiate into a highly aggressive malignant neoplasm (e.g., anaplastic carcinoma, sarcoma) with poor prognosis (Fig. 5.5d). Thorough sampling is crucial for accurate pathologic diagnosis and may require two or more sections per centimeter of solid tumor diameter, especially in tumors larger than 10 cm in diameter.

It is currently thought that primary ovarian MBTs practically never develop extra-ovarian disease/implants. Intestinal-type MBTs always present as stage I tumors, although rarely they are bilateral. Except in the rare case of a seromucinous (Mullerian, endocervical-type) MBT, extra-ovarian disease is to be considered metastatic disease from an ovarian or

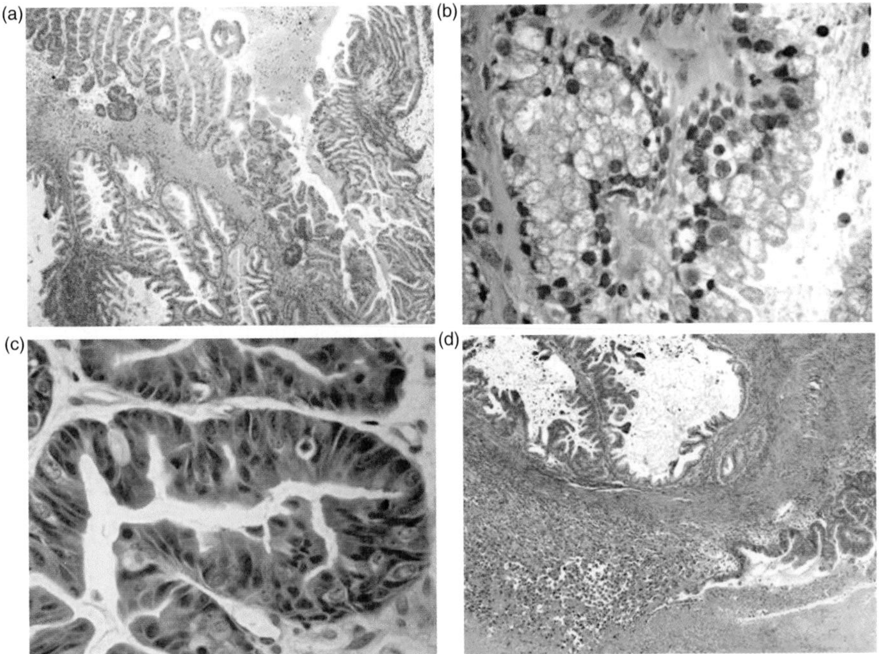

Fig. 5.5. (a) Ovarian mucinous borderline tumor (MBT). The tumor shows a complex architecture and epithelial stratification, but no stromal invasion. Hematoxylin & eosin; original magnification 40×. (b) Ovarian MBT showing bland cytologic features. Hematoxylin & eosin; original magnification, ×400. (c) Focus of intra-epithelial carcinoma within an ovarian MBT. Same patient as in (a). Note severe cytologic atypia (high nuclear/cytoplasmic ratio, mucus depletion, mitotic activity) compared with (b). Hematoxylin & eosin; original magnification, ×400. (d) Mural nodule with anaplastic carcinoma (lower left side of image) arising from an ovarian MBT with intra-epithelial carcinoma. Hematoxylin & eosin; original magnification 40×.

non-ovarian primary carcinoma. Reports of advanced stage ovarian mucinous borderline tumors tend to date from the 1990s and earlier. Based on today's understanding, those cases likely represented misclassified non-ovarian primary neoplasms with secondary ovarian involvement in the setting of pseudomyxoma peritonei (see below).

Pseudomyxoma peritonei and pseudomyxoma ovarii

The term "pseudomyxoma peritonei" describes a clinical scenario in which the patient presents with mucinous ascites. This condition is usually associated with abdominal tumors, which in females often involve one or both ovaries. Over the past two decades, it has become evident that the vast majority of such neoplasms originate not in the ovaries, but in the intestinal tract, typically in the appendix. Ovaries are secondarily involved. The histologic correlate of this condition is mucus dissecting the stroma of the involved tissue (Fig. 5.6a). In 66% of females with "pseudomyxoma peritonei," the ovarian tissue shows similar changes, known as "pseudomyxoma ovarii."

Clinically, two variants can be distinguished: a relatively indolent form exhibits abundant tissue dissecting mucin pools with few bland-appearing mucinous epithelial cells on histologic examination. Often an appendiceal mucinous adenoma is found as the primary lesion. Involvement of lymph nodes or other organs is rare. Although the mucin-producing cells show only minimal morphologic atypia, low mitotic rate, and no tendency of invasive destructive growth, the condition is complicated by notorious recurrences and the necessity of repeated surgery. This condition has been termed disseminated peritoneal adenomucinosis (DPAM) [41]; alternatively, some authors prefer the designation "low-grade mucinous adenocarcinoma" in view of the overall guarded prognosis (5-year survival rate 75%) [42].

On the other hand, a peritoneal mucinous carcinomatosis (PMCA) is diagnosed when there are abundant mucin-producing cells exhibiting severe cytologic atypia, high mitotic rate, and stromal invasion. Signet ring cells may be present. In these cases, there is usually a primary mucinous adenocarcinoma of the intestinal tract, including appendix, colon, or small intestine. Involvement of lymph nodes and other organs is frequent. This condition represents a high stage (metastatic) mucinous adenocarcinoma and has a poor prognosis with 5-year survival rates around 15% [41].

Intermediate forms between these extremes occur.

Mucinous tumors involving the ovaries with borderline-like appearance

Some primary non-ovarian mucinous carcinomas may metastasize to the ovaries and then morphologically perfectly mimic a primary ovarian MBT. Therefore, whenever an ovarian mucinous tumor with borderline features is encountered, the possibility of a secondary mucinous tumor involving the ovary needs to be ruled out. This includes but is not limited to patients with pseudomyxoma peritonei. Metastases from an intestinal, pancreatic, biliary, gastric, or endocervical adenocarcinoma may appear deceptively bland on histologic examination, lack invasive growth pattern, and thus look like a primary ovarian MBT (Fig. 5.6b,c).

The following histopathological features help distinguish primary from secondary mucinous ovarian tumors (Table 5.1): Primary ovarian mucinous tumors tend to present unilaterally as large tumors (> 15 cm in diameter), are multiloculated, and confined to the ovarian stroma. Various primary ovarian non-mucinous tumors (including Brenner tumors, mature cystic teratomas, Sertoli–Leydig cell tumors) may be seen in association with a mucinous neoplasm, in which cases

Table 5.1. Pathomorphologic features distinguishing primary from metastatic ovarian mucinous tumors

Primary ovarian	Metastatic
Unilateral	Bilateral
> 15 cm	< 10 cm
Confined to ovarian stroma	Ovarian stroma and surface involvement
Multiloculated cysts	Nodular or infiltrative growth pattern
Associated Brenner tumor, teratoma, Sertoli–Leydig cell tumor	Associated pseudomyxoma peritonei
Immuno-histochemistry of epithelial cells: CK7+; CK20–/+; CDX2–/+; MUC2–/+; PAX8+	Immuno-histochemistry if primary tumor located in the lower GI tract: CK7–/+; CK20+; CDX2+; MUC2+; PAX8–

CK, cytokeratin; –/+, negative or focally/weakly positive.

the mucinous component can be assumed to have originated in the ovary. In contrast, metastatic mucinous tumors tend to involve both ovaries, are on average smaller (< 10 cm in diameter), involve the ovarian surface and typically show a nodular or infiltrative growth pattern. The finding of lymphvascular involvement within the ovary favors a metastatic tumor. As mentioned above, the presence of pseudomyxoma peritonei strongly suggests an extra-ovarian (intestinal, appendiceal) primary tumor.

At the time of frozen section, the term "ovarian MBT" should be used with caution, especially if the full clinical history is not known to the pathologist. On the other hand, a diagnosis of MBT on frozen section should prompt the surgeon to carefully examine the abdomen, including the appendix and the pancreaticobiliary tract, and to consider an appendectomy, especially if the ovarian tumor is located on the right side (i.e., next to the appendix). It is not unusual for non-serous ovarian tumors that a frozen section "borderline" diagnosis will be

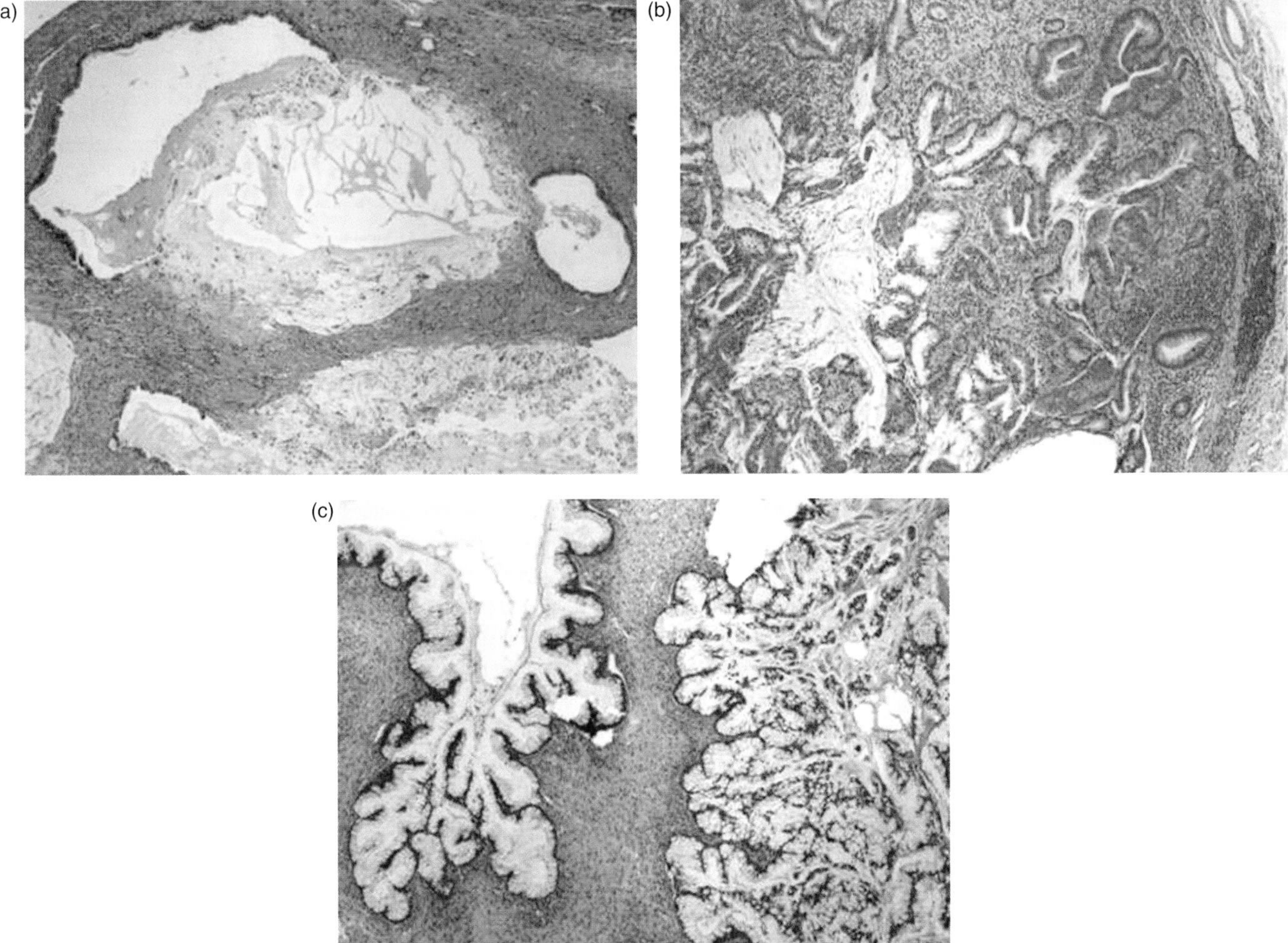

Fig. 5.6. (a) Pseudomyxoma peritonei/ovarii. Mucus dissecting the stroma. Bland appearing mucin-producing epithelium. Hematoxylin & eosin; original magnification, ×40. (b) Primary appendiceal mucinous carcinoma. Hematoxylin & eosin; original magnification 40×. (c) Metastatic appendiceal carcinoma to the right ovary. Same patient as in (b). Note juxtaposition of non-invasive "borderline" pattern (left half of image) and more complex architecture (right half of image). Hematoxylin & eosin; original magnification, ×40.

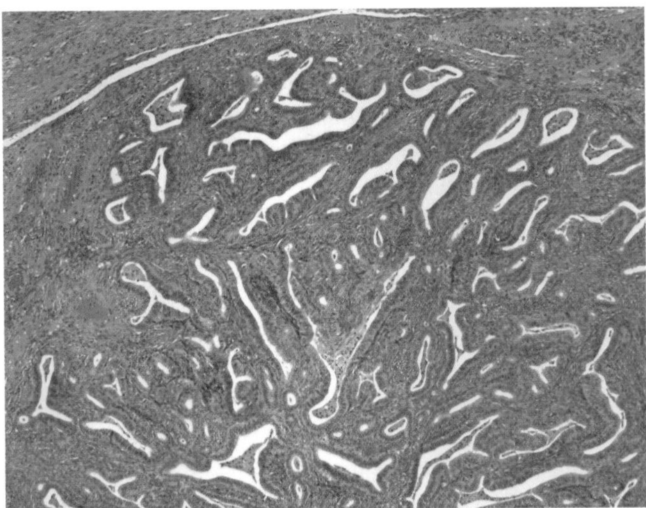

Fig. 5.7. Ovarian endometrioid borderline tumor. Complex epithelial proliferation, resembling endometrial complex hyperplasia. Hematoxylin & eosin; original magnification, ×40.

upgraded to a "carcinoma" diagnosis, once additional permanent sections become available [34,43].

In this context, immuno-histochemical stains on tissue sections may be helpful to determine the origin of a mucinous tumor encountered in the ovary. To distinguish primary ovarian from lower intestinal (including appendiceal) tumors, a panel including some or all of the following immuno-stains will be most informative: PAX-8 is positive in most tumors of Mullerian origin, but negative in gastrointestinal epithelia. Mucinous epithelium from primary ovarian tumors tends to express cytokeratin (CK) 7 and may also be positive for CK 20 in over 80% of cases. Epithelium from the lower GI tract tends to be positive for CK20 and negative for CK 7. CDX-2 and MUC-2 are positive in most tumors from the GI tract, including almost all appendiceal carcinomas, but may be positive in up to 40% of primary ovarian mucinous tumors [44]. Hence, considerable overlap in expression patterns occurs specifically among intestinal-type ovarian tumors and primary lower intestinal tumors. However, the relative staining intensity often still points in one direction or the other. To identify a metastatic endocervical adenocarcinoma, HPV analysis or a p16 stain may be of value: both are positive in most endocervical adenocarcinomas. Loss of Dpc-4 (Smad-4) expression has been reported in approximately 50% of metastatic mucinous tumors of primary pancreaticobiliary origin [45].

Endometrioid borderline tumors

These tumors constitute less than 1% of ovarian surface epithelial tumors. The distinction from an endometrioid adenofibroma is poorly defined. Lack of invasive growth pattern sets them apart from endometrioid adenocarcinomas. They are unilateral in 95% of cases and often associated with ovarian or extra-ovarian endometriosis. Concomitant endometrial hyperplasia or endometrioid adenocarcinoma is not infrequent. Endometrioid borderline tumors are composed of fibrous and epithelial elements to variable proportions. The epithelial component resembles hyperplastic endometrium and may display an equivalent morphologic spectrum ranging from simple to complex architecture, with or without cytologic atypia (Fig. 5.7). Squamoid metaplasia/morules are seen in up to 50% of cases. The prognosis is excellent with 95–100% 10-year survival rates.

Ovarian borderline tumors, other types

- Transitional cell (Brenner) borderline tumors are rare. They tend to be multiloculated cystic and exhibit a papillary transitional-type epithelium resembling low-grade non-invasive transitional cell carcinoma of the urinary tract. Like regular Brenner tumors, they may be associated with ovarian mucinous tumors or teratomas. The prognosis is good. Concomitant transitional cell carcinomas of the urinary bladder have been described.
- Clear cell borderline tumors are extremely rare – much rarer than clear cell carcinoma. Hence, this diagnosis should only be made after careful exclusion of a clear cell carcinoma. Clear cell borderline tumors tend to be unilateral. Histologically, they display an epithelium of glycogen-containing cells with translucent cytoplasm and moderate nuclear atypia, "hobnailing," and a mitotic rate of less than 3 mitotic figures per 10 high power (40× objective) microscopic fields. Absence of invasion differentiates them from their malignant counterparts.

Ovarian borderline tumors and their relation to invasive carcinoma

Improved understanding of clinical and molecular genetic features observed in ovarian tumors has led to a dualistic model of ovarian carcinogenesis, according to which ovarian carcinomas can be classified into two major groups [46,47]:

Type I carcinomas include low-grade (FIGO grade 1) serous carcinomas, mucinous carcinomas, endometrioid carcinomas, malignant Brenner tumors, and clear cell carcinomas. They have in common that putative precursor lesions have been identified, namely the respective borderline tumors and/or endometriosis in cases of ovarian endometrioid and clear cell carcinomas. On occasion, a carcinoma can be seen emerging from a background borderline tumor, supporting this concept (Fig. 5.8). Molecular analyses have shown a similar spectrum of genetic aberrations in borderline tumors and their malignant counterparts. For example, mutations of the *BRAF* and *KRAS* genes are frequent in both SBT and low-grade serous carcinoma [48,49].

In contrast, type II carcinomas include high-grade (FIGO grade 2 and 3) serous carcinomas, undifferentiated carcinomas, and malignant mixed Mullerian tumors (MMMT). The existence and recognizability of putative precursor lesions for these tumors are controversial, which has resulted in the "de novo" carcinogenesis theory. Type II carcinomas display a different spectrum of genetic aberrations, most frequently mutations in the p53 tumor suppressor gene, and a high degree of genetic instability [50]. Their clinical behavior is more aggressive than that of type I carcinomas.

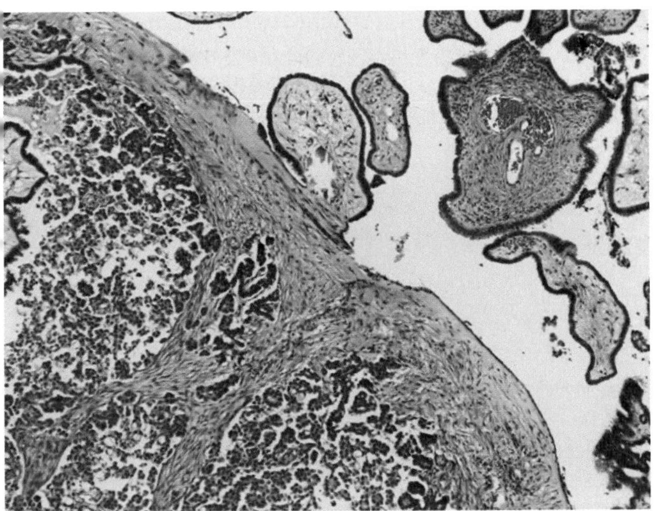

Fig. 5.8. Low-grade invasive serous carcinoma (lower left half of image) arising in a background of SBT (upper right half of image). Hematoxylin & eosin; original magnification ×40.

Based on the above, low-grade and high-grade ovarian serous carcinomas are to be considered completely different entities, despite the apparent morphologic continuum ranging from serous cystadenomas to borderline tumors to low-grade carcinomas to high-grade carcinomas. However, occasional SBTs and low-grade serous carcinomas (type I) have been reported to progress to high-grade carcinomas (type II), meaning the distinction is not absolute and exceptions do exist.

Concluding remarks

Although the "borderline" category was introduced with the intention to be abolished as soon as possible, this goal has not yet been achieved. While most borderline tumors will behave in an entirely benign manner, some may still surprise with unexpected recurrences and/or progression to frank carcinoma. Therefore reasons for maintaining the "borderline" category at this time include the following: Serous borderline tumors may be associated with extra-ovarian disease, which may have been missed at the time of primary surgery, and which in the case of invasive implants may result in malignant behavior. Mucinous borderline tumors tend to be very large, and the possibility of an occult carcinoma cannot be ruled out despite adequate sampling [23]. Hence, close follow-up and a high index of suspicion for recurrent disease are warranted.

Important progress has been made during the past decades regarding the understanding of tumor pathogenesis and establishment of prognostically important features. Specifically the identification of invasive extra-ovarian disease in serous tumors as the single most important prognostic factor, and the clarification of the origin of mucinous tumors involving the ovary have set new standards for diagnosis and treatment of these tumors. On the other hand, occasional cases still behave in an unpredictable manner, like the rare high-grade serous carcinoma that apparently emerged from a serous borderline tumor. Recent years have shown a tendency toward less aggressive treatment of borderline tumors of all subtypes, especially in women of childbearing age. The role of chemotherapy for advanced stage ovarian SBTs and low-grade serous carcinomas is currently unclear. Before embarking on a treatment plan, extensive inter-and intra-disciplinary consultation involving experts in this field, as well as comprehensive patient education will be invaluable to define expectations regarding prognosis and treatment results.

References

1. Seidman JD, Cho KR, Ronnett BM, Kurman RJ. Surface epithelial tumors of the ovary. In: Kurman RJ, Hedrick Ellenson L, Ronnett BM (Eds.). Blaustein's Pathology of the Female Genital Tract, 6th edition. New York: Springer; 2011, pp. 679–784.
2. Tavassoli FA, Devilee P. Tumours of the Breast and Female Genital Organs. Lyon, France: IARC Press; 2003.
3. Seidman JD, Soslow RA, Vang R, et al. Borderline ovarian tumors: diverse contemporary viewpoints on terminology and diagnostic criteria with illustrative images. Hum Pathol. 2004;**35**:918–33.
4. Prat J, De Nictolis M. Serous borderline tumors of the ovary: a long-term follow-up study of 137 cases, including 18 with a micropapillary pattern and 20 with microinvasion. Am J Surg Pathol. 2002;**26**:1111–28.
5. Bell DA, Scully RE. Ovarian serous borderline tumors with stromal microinvasion: a report of 21 cases. Hum Pathol. 1990;**21**:397–403.
6. McKenney JK, Balzer BL, Longacre TA. Patterns of stromal invasion in ovarian serous tumors of low malignant potential (borderline tumors): a reevaluation of the concept of stromal microinvasion. Am J Surg Pathol. 2006;**30**:1209–21.
7. Longacre TA, McKenney JK, Tazelaar HD, et al. Ovarian serous tumors of low malignant potential (borderline tumors): outcome-based study of 276 patients with long-term (> or =5-year) follow-up. Am J Surg Pathol. 2005;**29**:707–23.
8. Cusido M, Balaguero L, Hernandez G, et al. Results of the national survey of borderline ovarian tumors in Spain. Gynecol Oncol. 2007;**104**:617–22.
9. Ren J, Peng Z, Yang K. A clinicopathologic multivariate analysis affecting recurrence of borderline ovarian tumors. Gynecol Oncol. 2008;**110**:162–7.
10. Sieben NL, Kolkman-Uljee SM, Flanagan AM, et al. Molecular genetic evidence for monoclonal origin of bilateral ovarian serous borderline tumors. Am J Pathol. 2003;**162**:1095–101.
11. Diebold J, Seemuller F, Lohrs U. K-RAS mutations in ovarian and extraovarian lesions of serous tumors of borderline malignancy. Lab Invest. 2003;**83**:251–8.
12. Sieben NL, Roemen GM, Oosting J, et al. Clonal analysis favours a monoclonal

origin for serous borderline tumours with peritoneal implants. J Pathol. 2006;**210**:405–11.

13. Bell KA, Smith Sehdev AE, Kurman RJ. Refined diagnostic criteria for implants associated with ovarian atypical proliferative serous tumors (borderline) and micropapillary serous carcinomas. Am J Surg Pathol. 2001;**25**:419–32.
14. Seidman JD, Kurman RJ. Ovarian serous borderline tumors: a critical review of the literature with emphasis on prognostic indicators. Hum Pathol. 2000;**31**:539–57.
15. AJCC Cancer Staging Handbook, 7th edition. New York: Springer; 2010.
16. Alvarez AA, Moore WF, Robboy SJ, et al. K-ras mutations in Mullerian inclusion cysts associated with serous borderline tumors of the ovary. Gynecol Oncol. 2001;**80**:201–6.
17. Fadare O, Orejudos MP, Jain R, et al. A comparative analysis of lymphatic vessel density in ovarian serous tumors of low malignant potential (borderline tumors) with and without lymph node involvement. Int J Gynecol Pathol. 2008;**27**:483–90.
18. McKenney JK, Balzer BL, Longacre TA. Lymph node involvement in ovarian serous tumors of low malignant potential (borderline tumors): pathology, prognosis, and proposed classification. Am J Surg Pathol. 2006;**30**:614–24.
19. Burks RT, Sherman ME, Kurman RJ. Micropapillary serous carcinoma of the ovary. A distinctive low-grade carcinoma related to serous borderline tumors. Am J Surg Pathol. 1996;**20**:1319–30.
20. Seidman JD, Kurman RJ. Subclassification of serous borderline tumors of the ovary into benign and malignant types. A clinicopathologic study of 65 advanced stage cases. Am J Surg Pathol. 1996;**20**:1331–45.
21. Eichhorn JH, Bell DA, Young RH, et al. Ovarian serous borderline tumors with micropapillary and cribriform patterns: a study of 40 cases and comparison with 44 cases without these patterns. Am J Surg Pathol. 1999;**23**:397–409.
22. Deavers MT, Gershenson DM, Tortolero-Luna G, et al. Micropapillary and cribriform patterns in ovarian serous tumors of low malignant potential: a study of 99 advanced stage cases. Am J Surg Pathol. 2002;**26**:1129–41.
23. McCluggage WG. The pathology of and controversial aspects of ovarian borderline tumours. Curr Opin Oncol. 2010;**22**:462–72.
24. Uzan C, Kane A, Rey A, et al. Prognosis and prognostic factors of the micropapillary pattern in patients treated for stage II and III serous borderline tumors of the ovary. Oncologist. 2011;**16**:189–96.
25. Gilks CB, Alkushi A, Yue JJ, et al. Advanced-stage serous borderline tumors of the ovary: a clinicopathological study of 49 cases. Int J Gynecol Pathol. 2003;**22**:29–36.
26. Slomovitz BM, Caputo TA, Gretz HF III, et al. A comparative analysis of 57 serous borderline tumors with and without a noninvasive micropapillary component. Am J Surg Pathol. 2002;**26**:592–600.
27. Chang SJ, Ryu HS, Chang KH, et al. Prognostic significance of the micropapillary pattern in patients with serous borderline ovarian tumors. Acta Obstet Gynecol Scand. 2008;**87**:476–81.
28. Park JY, Kim DY, Kim JH, et al. Micropapillary pattern in serous borderline ovarian tumors: Does it matter? Gynecol Oncol. 2011;**123**:511–16.
29. Leitao MM Jr. Micropapillary pattern in newly diagnosed borderline tumors of the ovary: what's in a name? Oncologist. 2011;**16**:133–5.
30. Morice P, Camatte S, Rey A, et al. Prognostic factors for patients with advanced stage serous borderline tumours of the ovary. Ann Oncol. 2003;**14**:592–8.
31. Song T, Choi CH, Park HS, et al. Fertility-sparing surgery for borderline ovarian tumors: oncologic safety and reproductive outcomes. Int J Gynecol Cancer. 2011;**21**:640–6.
32. Eskander RN, Randall LM, Berman ML, et al. Fertility preserving options in patients with gynecologic malignancies. Am J Obstet Gynecol. 2011;**205**:103–10.
33. Lenhard MS, Mitterer S, Kumper C, et al. Long-term follow-up after ovarian borderline tumor: relapse and survival in a large patient cohort. Eur J Obstet Gynecol Reprod Biol. 2009;**145**:189–94.
34. Shih KK, Garg K, Soslow RA, et al. Accuracy of frozen section diagnosis of ovarian borderline tumor. Gynecol Oncol. 2011;**123**:517–21.
35. Schmeler KM, Sun CC, Bodurka DC, et al. Neoadjuvant chemotherapy for low-grade serous carcinoma of the ovary or peritoneum. Gynecol Oncol. 2008;**108**:510–4.
36. Shih KK, Zhou QC, Aghajanian C, et al. Patterns of recurrence and role of adjuvant chemotherapy in stage II-IV serous ovarian borderline tumors. Gynecol Oncol. 2010;**119**:270–3.
37. Trimble CL, Kosary C, Trimble EL. Long-term survival and patterns of care in women with ovarian tumors of low malignant potential. Gynecol Oncol. 2002;**86**:34–7.
38. Bristow RE, Gossett DR, Shook DR, et al. Recurrent micropapillary serous ovarian carcinoma. Cancer. 2002;**95**:791–800.
39. Gershenson DM, Sun CC, Lu KH, et al. Clinical behavior of stage II-IV low-grade serous carcinoma of the ovary. Obstet Gynecol. 2006;**108**:361–8.
40. Ronnett BM, Kajdacsy-Balla A, Gilks CB, et al. Mucinous borderline ovarian tumors: points of general agreement and persistent controversies regarding nomenclature, diagnostic criteria, and behavior. Hum Pathol. 2004;**35**:949–60.
41. Ronnett BM, Zahn CM, Kurman RJ, et al. Disseminated peritoneal adenomucinosis and peritoneal mucinous carcinomatosis. A clinicopathologic analysis of 109 cases with emphasis on distinguishing pathologic features, site of origin, prognosis, and relationship to "pseudomyxoma peritonei". Am J Surg Pathol. 1995;**19**:1390–408.
42. Bradley RF, Stewart JH IV, Russell GB, et al. Pseudomyxoma peritonei of appendiceal origin: a clinicopathologic analysis of 101 patients uniformly treated at a single institution, with literature review. Am J Surg Pathol. 2006;**30**:551–9.
43. Houck K, Nikrui N, Duska L, et al. Borderline tumors of the ovary: correlation of frozen and permanent histopathologic diagnosis. Obstet Gynecol. 2000;**95**:839–43.

44. Vang R, Gown AM, Wu LS, et al. Immunohistochemical expression of CDX2 in primary ovarian mucinous tumors and metastatic mucinous carcinomas involving the ovary: comparison with CK20 and correlation with coordinate expression of CK7. Mod Pathol. 2006;**19**:1421–8.

45. Meriden Z, Yemelyanova AV, Vang R, et al. Ovarian metastases of pancreaticobiliary tract adenocarcinomas: analysis of 35 cases, with emphasis on the ability of metastases to simulate primary ovarian mucinous tumors. Am J Surg Pathol. 2011;**35**:276–88.

46. Kurman RJ, Shih I. Pathogenesis of ovarian cancer: lessons from morphology and molecular biology and their clinical implications. Int J Gynecol Pathol. 2008;**27**:151–60.

47. Kurman RJ, Shih I. The origin and pathogenesis of epithelial ovarian cancer: a proposed unifying theory. Am J Surg Pathol. 2010;**34**:433–43.

48. Sieben NL, Macropoulos P, Roemen GM, et al. In ovarian neoplasms, BRAF, but not KRAS, mutations are restricted to low-grade serous tumours. J Pathol. 2004;**202**:336–40.

49. Singer G, Oldt R III, Cohen Y, et al. Mutations in BRAF and KRAS characterize the development of low-grade ovarian serous carcinoma. J Natl Cancer Inst. 2003;**95**:484–6.

50. Singer G, Stohr R, Cope L, et al. Patterns of p53 mutations separate ovarian serous borderline tumors and low- and high-grade carcinomas and provide support for a new model of ovarian carcinogenesis: a mutational analysis with immuno-histochemical correlation. Am J Surg Pathol. 2005;**29**:218–24.

Chapter 6

Precursors of ovarian epithelial tumors

Liane Deligdisch, MD

Introduction

Ovarian carcinoma (OC) arising from the surface epithelium and its invagination into the ovarian stroma is the most lethal gynecologic tumor. About 22,000 new cases with a mortality of about 14,000 are predicted for 2013. No significant statistical changes occurred over the past decades, despite a voluminous and sophisticated body of research. OC is less frequent than cervical and endometrial cancer, but it has a higher mortality than both of them combined. The continuously decreasing morbidity due to invasive cancer of both cervical and endometrial cancers, and their resulting lower mortality is due to their earlier diagnosis and to the detection of cancer precursors (dysplasia in the cervix, atypical hyperplasia in the endometrium) that made a systematic implementation of screening possible and effective, even in the absence of symptoms as is the case with cervical cancer precursors.

There is no screening for ovarian cancer at the present time, and unfortunately early diagnosis is rare and erratic (see Chapter 22). Women at known high risk due to family clusters of breast and ovarian cancer represent a minority, and even those closely followed with pelvic examinations, transvaginal ultrasound examinations and serologic markers often present in late stages of the disease, as do most of the sporadic ovarian cancer patients.

Carcinogenic factors have been documented for cervical (viral) and endometrial (hormonal) cancer. For OC, the need for early clinical detection is also compounded by the need for understanding the carcinogenic process that underlies the structural changes of the ovarian epithelial carcinogenesis. Molecular and genetic studies have unveiled several sequential events that may precede the microscopic changes [1–4].

At this point however, the diagnosis of potential cancer precursors is based on the visualization of microscopic, immunohistologic, morphometric structural changes, the dynamics of which remain to be revealed by processes that depend both on the cell biologic carcinogenic mechanism and on the host genomics and defenses. The identification of tissue changes is indispensable for elaborating a screening program, therefore the accessibility of the ovaries by laparoscopic surgery, and the availability of prophylactically removed adnexae offer possibilities for the study of lesions that may be potential cancer precursors.

The ovaries are a pair of organs situated in a secluded location in the posterior abdominal/pelvic area, with a paucity of sensorial nerves, therefore not always easy to reach by simple pelvic examination and not likely to elicit pain or other symptoms when the tumor is confined to the organ. The detection of early stage tumors of small dimensions is uncommon and the detection of precursors of cancer is mostly elusive.

Ovarian low-grade (type I) cancer precursors

Ovarian carcinoma has been re-classified relatively recently into low-grade and high-grade tumors, the latter unfortunately being by far more frequent (see Chapter 4).

The low-grade (type I) ovarian carcinomas include serous micropapillary, mucinous, endometrioid, and clear cell carcinomas. The presumptive origin of these neoplasms is in benign and/or borderline tumors which can be diagnosed in earlier stages due to their slower growth. These tumors are relatively genetically stable and have gene mutations such as *KRAS*, *BRAF*, *PTEN*, *ERBB2*, and beta-catenin. The histologic phenotype of the precursor lesions is different for each type: the serous papillary borderline tumor considered to precede the invasive low-grade serous tumor is characterized by a micropapillary pattern, relatively uniform cells with rather small nuclei, low mitotic activity, and papillary branching with non-hierarchic ramifications (Fig. 6.1).

The precursors of endometrioid and clear cell adenocarcinoma are the best documented [5]. They are considered to be the atypical epithelial endometrioid lining of endometriotic cysts involving the ovary most often, but also extra-ovarian locations, such as the pelvic and abdominal peritoneal surfaces and rarely organs such as the bladder, intestinal wall, abdominal wall, etc.

Endometriosis is a very common condition (see Chapters 12, 14) usually occurring in a hyperestrogenic clinical environment, and fortunately ovarian endometrioid and clear cell carcinomas are relatively rare. There are however cases of ovarian cancer detected incidentally in endometriotic cysts displaying endometrioid histologic patterns, similar to uterine endometrioid adenocarcinoma, often arising in a background of endometrial glandular hyperplasia, simple, cystic, complex, and atypical, as seen in the endometrioid uterine carcinoma. Separate primary coexisting carcinomas of the uterus and ovaries are not uncommon [6]. Careful histologic and immuno-histologic observation of the transition area between the benign endometriosis and the malignant tumor often reveals atypical changes of the epithelial endometrioid lining, piling up of the layers in an

Altchek's Diagnosis and Management of Ovarian Disorders, ed. Liane Deligdisch, Nathan G. Kase, and Carmel J. Cohen. Published by Cambridge University Press.

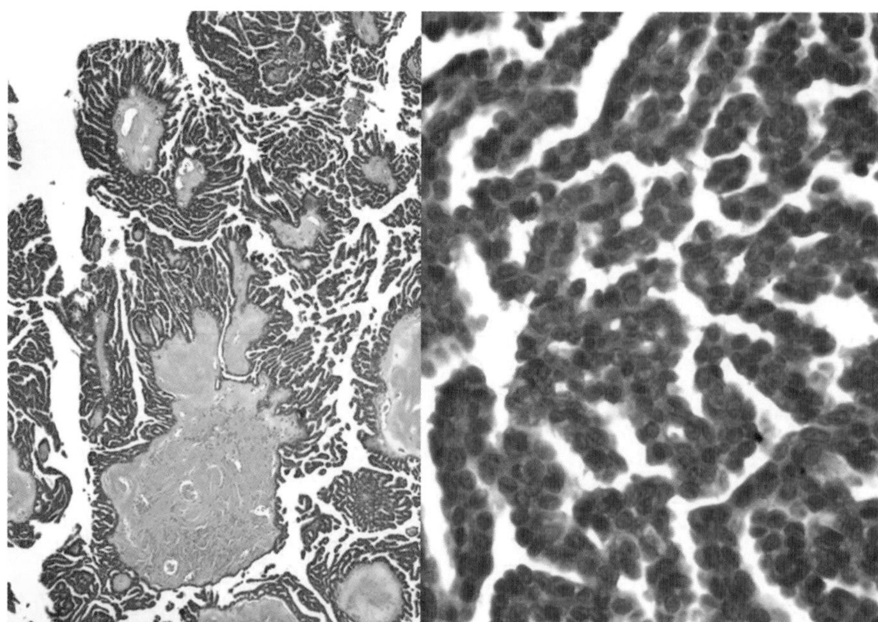

Fig. 6.1. Ovarian serous micro-papillary tumor of borderline malignancy, presumable precursor of invasive, low-grade serous carcinoma (left, hematoxylin and eosin stain; original magnification ×40). Micropapillary pattern with slender, non-hierarchic papillary branching; nuclei are rather small and uniform (right, hematoxylin and eosin stain; original magnification, ×400).

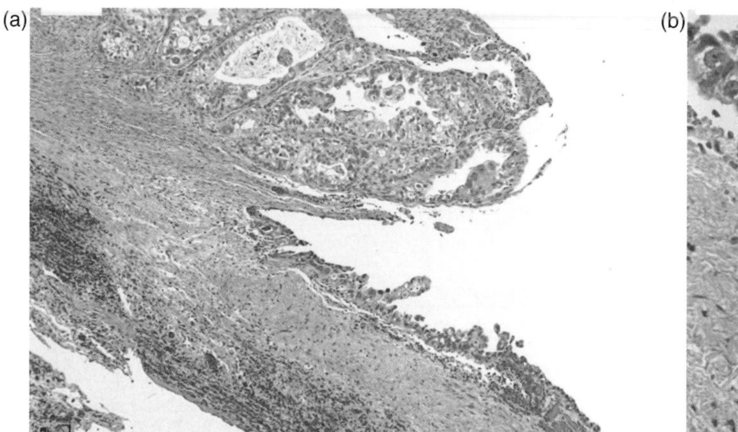

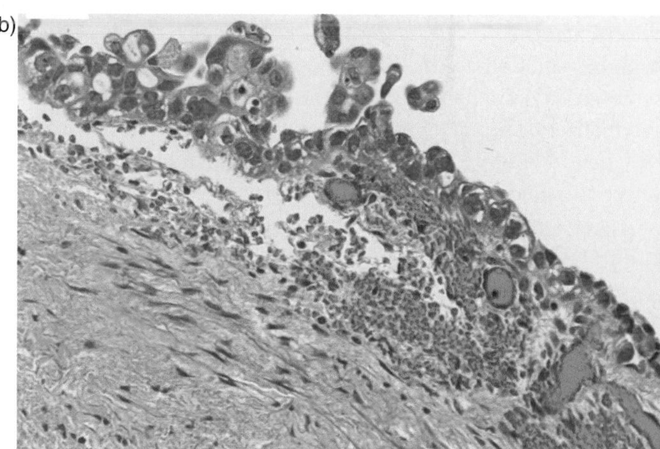

Fig. 6.2. (a) Ovarian endometrioid adenocarcinoma and adjacent atypical epithelial lining. Hematoxylin and eosin stain; original magnification, ×10. (b) Irregular piling up of cells, nuclei with coarse chromatin clumping. Hematoxylin and eosin stain; original magnification, ×40, 100.

irregular pattern, enlarged and abnormal nuclei with coarse chromatin clumping (Fig. 6.2) and mitotic activity, without invasion of the ovarian parenchyma through the basement membrane. Immuno-histologic studies of this atypical endometriotic epithelial tissue revealed positive reactivity to several tumor markers identified in the adjacent invasive tumor, such as PTEN, ARID1A, BCL-2, BAX, MMP9, and p53 altered protein [5]. Both histologic changes and immune-phenotypes seen in atypical endometriosis and adjacent adenocarcinoma may also be present in atypical endometrioid epithelium lining, in the absence of frankly malignant changes, raising the question of its potential precancerous nature. Ovarian clear cell carcinomas are the most commonly associated malignant OC tumors with endometriosis. A borderline clear cell carcinoma is also described in ovarian cystadenofibroma, a usually benign tumor which is occasionally lined by clear cells, epithelial cells with a clear vacuolated cytoplasm, irregular nuclei which are located sometimes at the luminal border of the cell representing the "hobnail" pattern characteristic of clear cell carcinoma. This unusual histologic pattern may also represent an ovarian carcinoma precursor and is seen occasionally in association with overt endometrioid and/or clear cell carcinomas, considered therefore to have arisen from an atypical cystadenofibroma (see Chapter 4). These tumors are associated in up to 20% of cases with endometriosis, and with LOH in the *PTEN* genes.

Mucinous adenocarcinomas of the ovaries are now considered to be quite rarely primary ovarian neoplasms [7]. Their vast majority, especially when bilateral, are metastatic from the gastrointestinal tract. Most primary mucinous carcinomas of the ovary are unilateral and well differentiated. They often reach large dimensions and display an array of histologic patterns ranging from benign mucin-secreting epithelium to borderline mucinous tumors to frankly malignant adenocarcinomas, with identifiable transition areas. They usually present clinically in earlier stages than their serous counterparts because of compression of neighboring organs due to their large size.

The above described histo-pathologic entities included in the group of "type I" or low-grade ovarian carcinomas represent a

Table 6.1. Ovarian dysplasia (OIN)

	Benign ovarian epithelium	Malignant ovarian epithelium	Dysplastic ovarian epithelium
Architectural changes Crowding, no. of cells per unit of basement membrane	160	400	240
Stratification, loss of polarity. Distance from nuclear center to basement membrane	33 μm	150 μm	78 μm
Nuclear profiles Nuclear area	18–23 μm^2	50–70 μm^2	33–44 μm^2
Minimal chord, perimeter circularity factor	Statistically not significant		
Nuclear texture	Quantification of dark, light and gray nuclear areas. Progressively decreasing correlation between nuclear area and textons with increasing malignancy		
Auto correlation factor β	Tridimensional surface plots showing increasingly irregular surfaces as the nuclear surface becomes less homogenous (Fig. 6.5)		

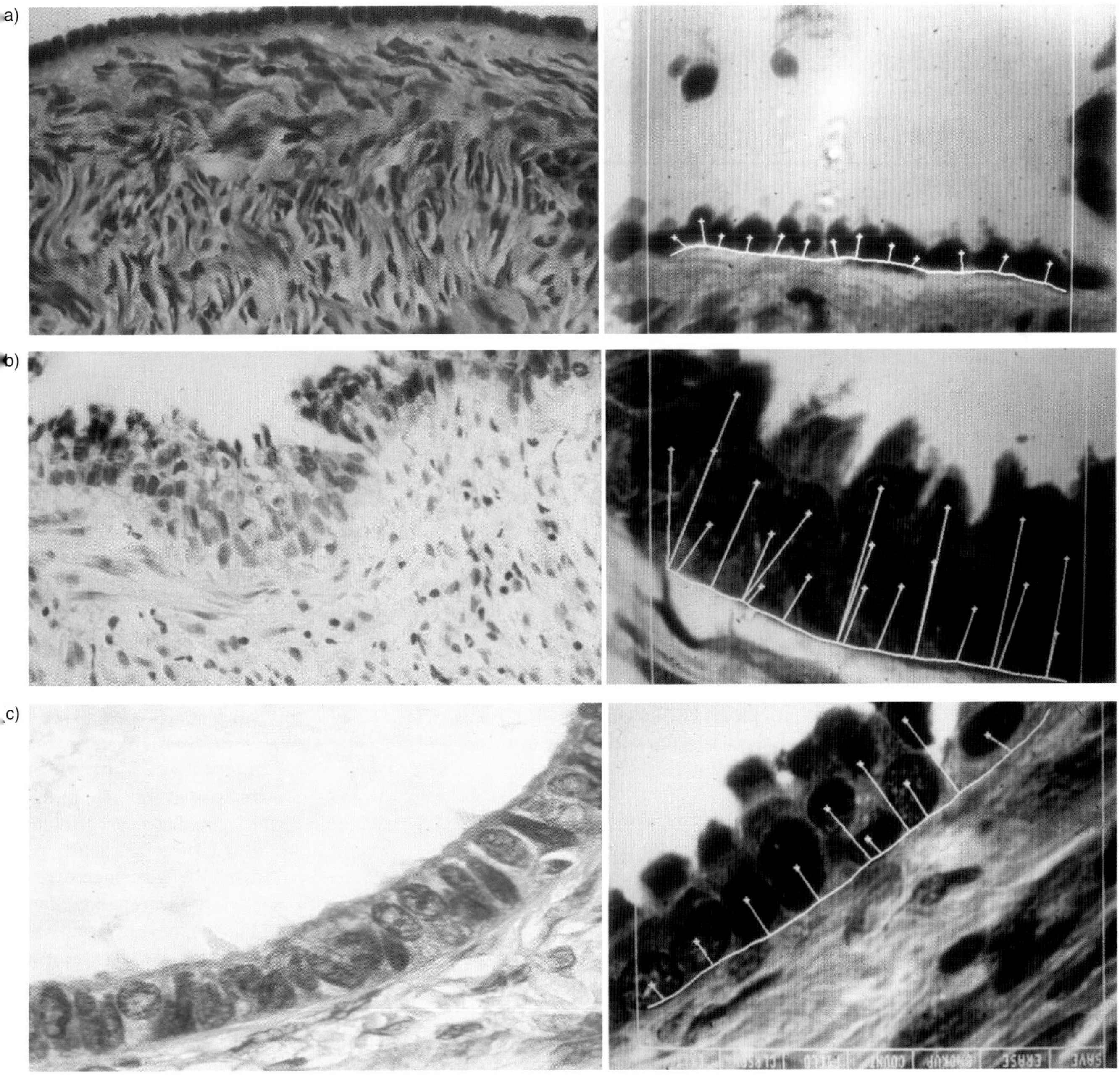

Fig. 6.3. Stratification, loss of polarity, and cellular crowding as assessed by computerized image analysis by measuring the shortest distance between the center of the nuclei and the basement membrane. (a) Normal ovarian epithelium; (b) malignant ovarian epithelium; (c) dysplastic ovarian epithelium.

(a)

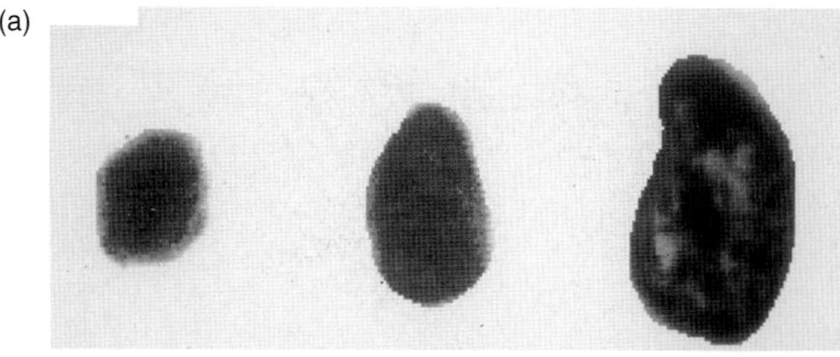

(b)

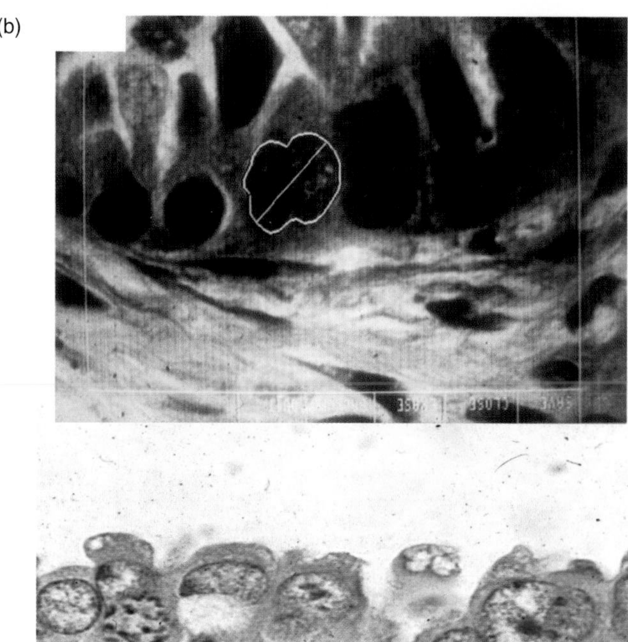

Fig. 6.4. (a) Nuclear profiles of dysplastic cells are intermediate between benign and malignant epithelial cells (from left to right normal 18 μm, dyplasic 33 μm, and cancerous 60 μm). (b) Note loss of polarity and irregular nuclear chromatin.

minority of ovarian epithelial tumors. Their more favorable prognosis is due to their detection in earlier stages being associated with symptomatic, possibly slower growing pelvic and abdominal masses (see Chapter 22).

Ovarian type II or high-grade ovarian serous carcinoma precursors

The majority (up to 87% of all OC, including malignant mixed Mullerian tumors) of OC are high-grade serous papillary carcinomas characterized by a rapid destructive growth while still asymptomatic. Detecting their precursors is obviously more difficult because the surgical specimens removed most commonly are stage III–IV ovarian cancers that overgrew the neighboring tissues at the time of their detection. This is why it was believed that they arise "de novo."

Studies performed on specimens from high-risk patients, such as identical twin sisters of patients with ovarian carcinoma, on ovaries detected fortuitously in stage I, and on ovaries removed prophylactically from BRCA1- and BRCA2-positive patients revealed changes that were diagnosed as dysplastic or ovarian intra-epithelial neoplasia (OIN), therefore potentially precursors of malignancy [8–10]. These changes were described histologically as architectural and cytological and were validated by computerized image analysis (morphometry). The immuno-reactivity of the dysplastic ovarian epithelial cells was similar to that of the invasive ovarian serous adenocarcinomas, in a manner analogous to the atypical endometriosis or clear cell tumors and endometrioid OC as well as that described in other locations in situ of dysplastic lesions (uterine cervix, larynx, colon, breast). Dysplastic changes may potentially progress to overt cancer, may not change and may regress as it was shown in HPV-induced dysplasia of the uterine cervix. However, their identification is crucial for the implementation of a screening program as well as for the insight into early epithelial carcinogenesis. In other words, you have to know what the cellular and subcellular structural changes are to identify the potential cancer precursors.

Ovarian dysplasia: ovarian intra-epithelial neoplasia (OIN)

The histologic criteria for diagnosing ovarian dysplasia or intra-epithelial neoplasia consist of changes in the tissue architecture (piling up of ovarian epithelial cells, loss of polarity, and crowding), and cytologic changes: (increased nucleocytoplasmic ratio, increased nuclear surface, nuclear hyperchromasia, abnormal nuclear texture) (Table 6.1). While these changes may be subtle and overlooked in the presence of an adjacent overt cancer, morphometric measurements have validated their objective characteristics situating ovarian dysplastic cells at the mid-distance between normal and cancer cells [11]. Computerized statistical evaluation was verified by neural network procedures, a highly discriminatory method [12,13].

Stratification, loss of polarity, and cellular crowding were established by measuring the shortest distance from the nuclear center to the basement membrane and by counting the number of cells per unit of basement membrane (Fig. 6.3).

Dysplastic ovarian cellular characteristics were assessed by measuring the longest nuclear chord, perimeter, and area (Fig. 6.4).

Because for the histopathological diagnosis of most malignancies, nuclear changes are of prime importance, further studies were undertaken to evaluate nuclear texture, which represents the distribution of chromatin and thereby reflects the proliferative activity of cells. Histogram-derived "textons" representing contiguous areas with similar levels of dark, light, or gray material from individual nuclei were quantitated in terms of their areas and numbers. A multivariate analysis of the results, based on the progressively decreasing correlation between the size of the textons and the size of the containing nucleus as the degree of malignancy increases, confirmed the existence of the three

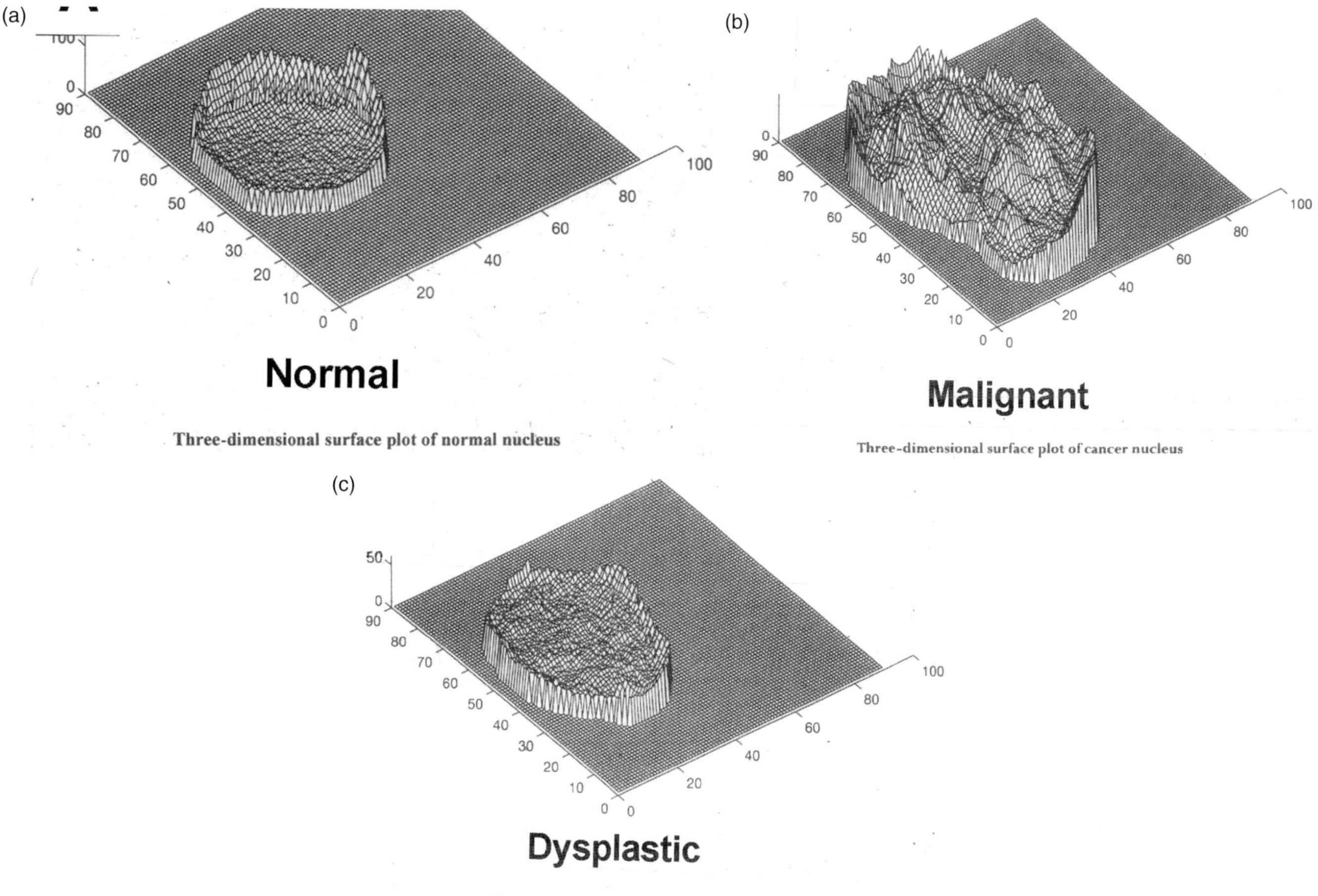

Fig. 6.5. Tridimensional images obtained by autocorrelation. (a) Flat surface for normal nuclei; (b) abrupt peaks and depressions for malignant nuclei; and (c) intermediate values for dysplastic nuclei, reflecting, respectively, homogeneous, highly irregular, and intermediate chromatin patterns.

diagnostic categories: benign, malignant, and dysplastic [12]. The accuracy of the evaluation of intra-nuclear texture was further enhanced by using the autocorrelation procedure [10]. This method yielded three-dimensional surface plots showing increasingly irregular surfaces as the nuclear structure becomes less homogeneous. Thus, for normal nuclei the surface appears flat, reflecting the homogeneity of the chromatin, for malignant nuclei the surface exhibits abrupt peaks and depressions, reflecting the marked irregularity of the nuclear chromatin, and for the dysplastic nuclei the surface was intermediate between the two. The three-dimensional images correlated with the nuclear areas, which also corresponded to the respective diagnostic category (Fig. 6.5).

The autocorrelation method is based on shifting the nuclear image by three to four pixels and comparing the similarity of regions of the nuclei with their relationship among neighboring pixels [10].

This method was used for the assessment of ovarian dysplasia in women undergoing prophylactic oophorectomies for *BRCA1* and *BRCA2* mutations and family history of ovarian cancer. Statistical analysis asserted the presence of incidental ovarian dysplasia in about two-thirds of the prophylactically removed ovaries, and of 15 cases of adjacent dysplasia in 23 patients with ovaries removed for carcinoma. No significant morphometric differences were found between the incidental and adjacent dysplastic nuclei [10].

Ovarian dysplasia has been studied in epithelial inclusion cysts. The measurements taken from dysplastic lesions in two different groups or clinical settings, incidental in grossly normal ovaries, and adjacent to overt carcinoma, were analyzed by artificial neural networks. No significant differences were found between the two groups, thus confirming the potentially precancerous nature of the "incidentally" diagnosed changes in non-cancerous ovaries as they were not different from those seen adjacent to overt cancer [13]. It should be mentioned that similar dysplastic precancerous changes were described in other tissues, such as adjacent to colon cancer, in polyps, and in dysplastic nevi adjacent to malignant melanoma.

More recently, dysplastic changes and carcinoma in situ were also described in the fallopian tubes, especially in the fimbriae, and even considered to precede ovarian and peritoneal neoplastic changes (Fig. 6.6). Their histologic characteristics are based on changes in stratification, nuclear size, and texture [14,15].

Computerized image analysis has made it possible to create a database of the measurements (see Table 6.1) of normal, malignant, and dysplastic nuclei.

Ovarian dysplasia is encountered in two clinical settings: adjacent to the overt carcinoma, most often high-grade serous papillary carcinoma which is also the most common malignant tumor of the ovary, and incidental, in ovaries removed either preventively for high risk or for other reasons, with no associated overt OC.

Ovaries "at risk"

In many specimens from prophylactic salpingo-oophorectomies, several histologic changes were described as "cancer prone phenotype." They consisted of deep invaginations of the surface epithelium, psammoma bodies, epithelial inclusion cysts, cortical stroma hyperplasia, etc. [16]. Specimens from prophylactic salpingo-oophorectomies performed on women at high risk to develop ovarian carcinoma are valuable study material and may reveal occasionally hidden ovarian cancer (Fig. 6.7). The incidence of precursor changes in a group of BRCA1- and BRCA2-positive patients, of Ashkenazi Jewish origin, was found to be significantly higher than in control cases as mentioned before (Fig. 6.8).

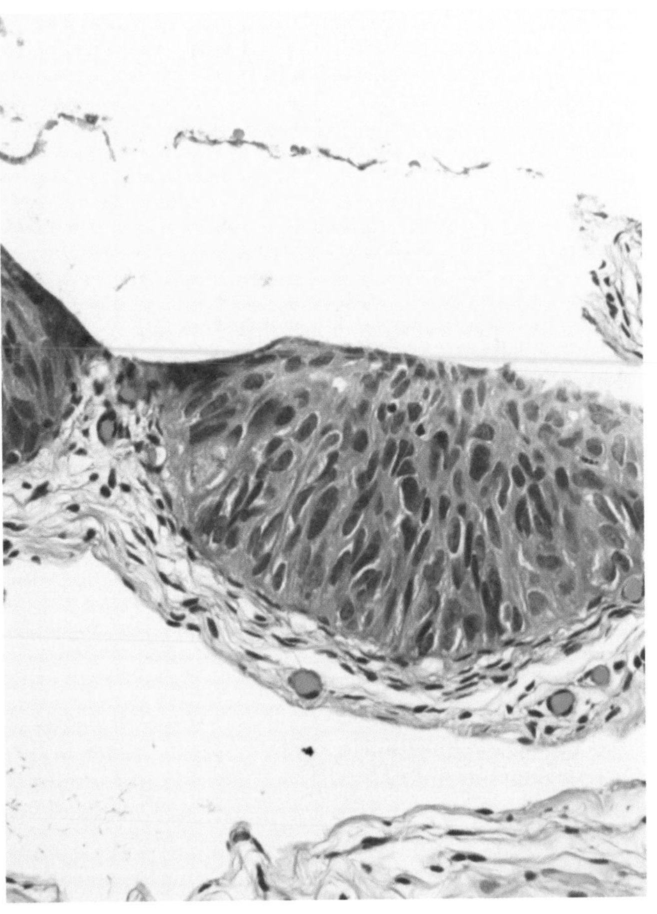

Fig. 6.6. Focal carcinoma in situ of fallopian tube fimbria. Hematoxylin and eosin stain; original magnification, ×100. A 48-year-old patient is BRCA1 positive and had previous breast carcinoma.

Occasionally, dysplastic lesions as well as "cancer-prone phenotypes" were described in contralateral ovaries from cases of unilateral ovarian carcinoma. Ovarian histo-pathological abnormalities have also been described in infertile patients undergoing ovulation induction therapy, especially those with multiple stimulating cycles, resulting in irreversible dysplastic changes after 7 years or more [17]. It should however be noted that ovarian dysplasia/neoplasia may be associated with the underlying infertility and that a causal relationship between ovulation stimulation and ovarian carcinogenesis is still a controversial issue.

Although grossly and often microscopically normal in appearance, specimens removed by prophylactic salpingo oophorectomy should be sectioned entirely with special care to identify the changes of the tubal fimbriae. The search for a "cancer prone phenotype" may reveal subtle changes in the tissue structures and subcellular molecular changes manifested by the presence of p53 mutations [15]. More than 75% of type II OC have *TP53* mutations. Increased percentage of Mib-1 nuclear staining as well as increased CA125 immuno-reactivity was also reported [18].

The histologic and morphometric study of subtle changes presumed to be cancer precursors in prophylactically removed ovaries and fallopian tubes from women "at risk" was correlated with molecular, subcellular analysis of this tissue (Fig. 6.9). Phenotypically normal cells exhibited the "p53 signature," considered the hallmark of serous pelvic carcinoma, were also identified in malignant endometrium, ovaries, fallopian tube fimbriae, and peritoneum [15].

Overexpression of Ki67 proliferation marker and of the p53 tumor suppressor gene product in the ovarian epithelium suggest a proliferation abnormality and the loss of cell cycle control, clonal expansion, and acquisition of potential invasive growth properties. Like other cancers, OC arise through a multistep process in which clonal selection acts on cells with somatic mutations and altered gene expression.

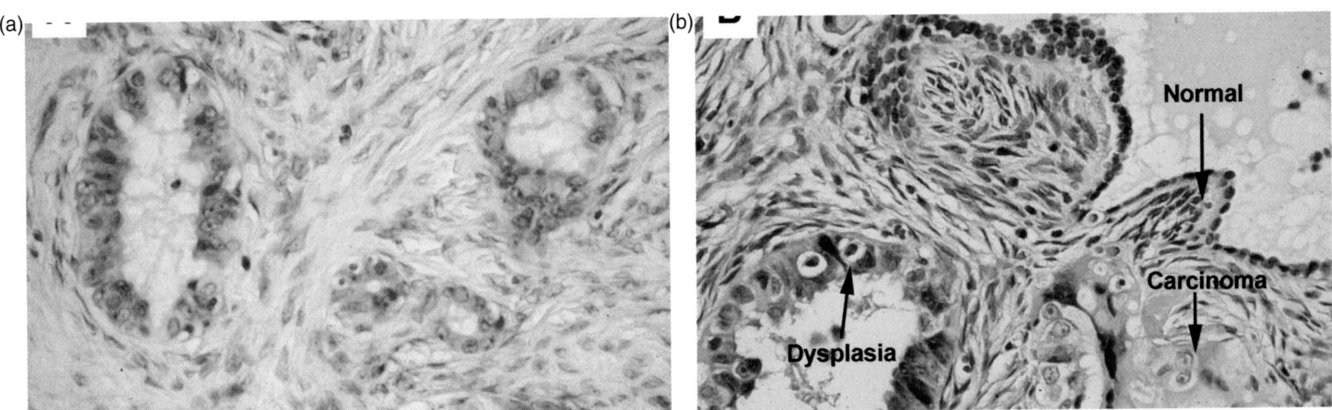

Fig. 6.7. Histologic sections from prophylactic salpingo-oophorectomy. Grossly normal ovaries reveal dysplastic changes (A) and normal, dysplastic and overtly malignant changes. B: Hematoxylin and eosin stain; original magnification, ×100. The patient is 58 years old and BRCA1 positive.

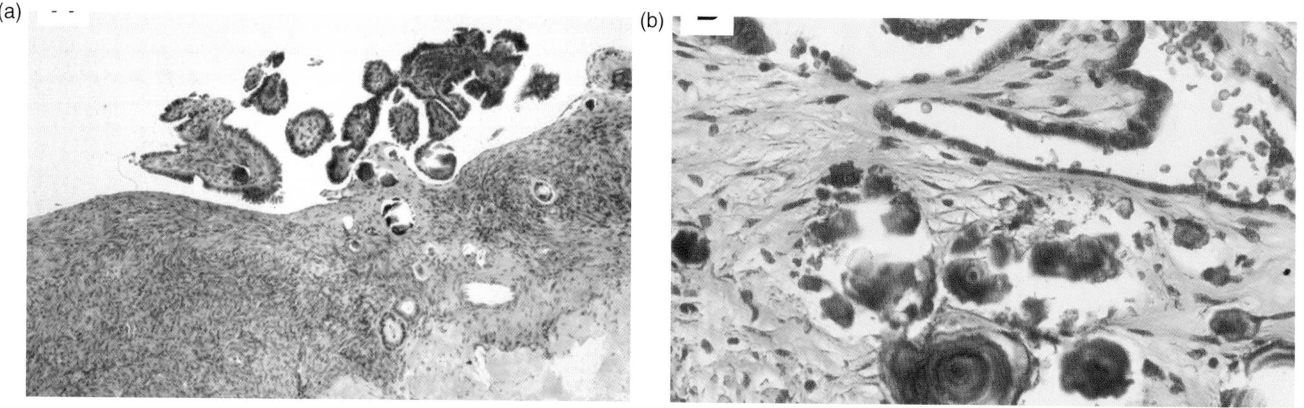

Fig. 6.8. "Ovaries at risk." Prophylactic salpingo-oophorectomy specimen, grossly normal, exhibiting surface papillations, psammoma bodies, and clusters of small epithelial inclusion cysts. (a) Hematoxylin and eosin stain; original magnification, ×40. (b) Hematoxylin and eosin stain; original magnification, ×400). The patient is 46 years old, BRCA1 positive.

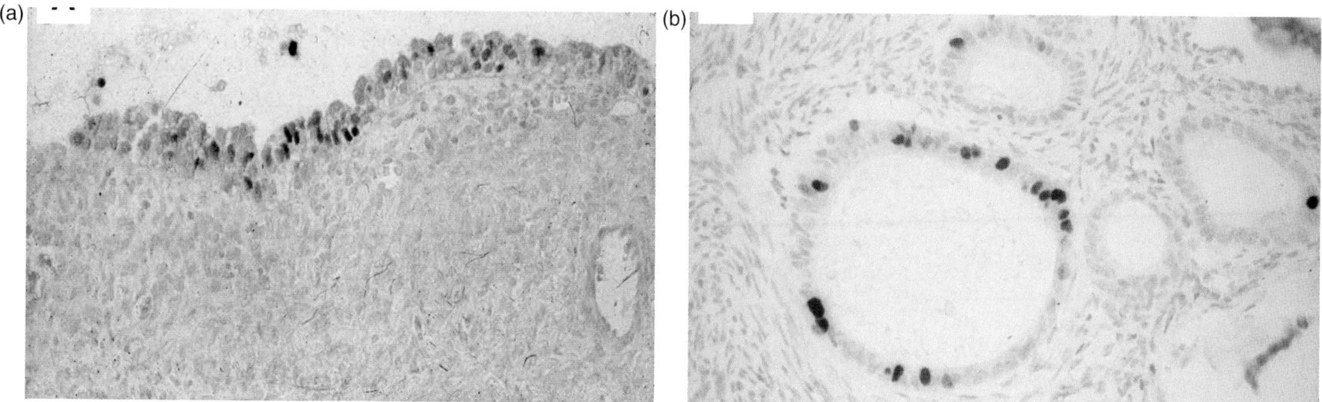

Fig. 6.9. (a) Positive immuno-histologic stain for p53 on dysplastic surface epithelium. (b) K67 (Mib-1) positive in epithelial inclusion cyst. The patient is 42 years old, BRCA1 positive, and underwent prophylactic salpingo-oophorectomy.

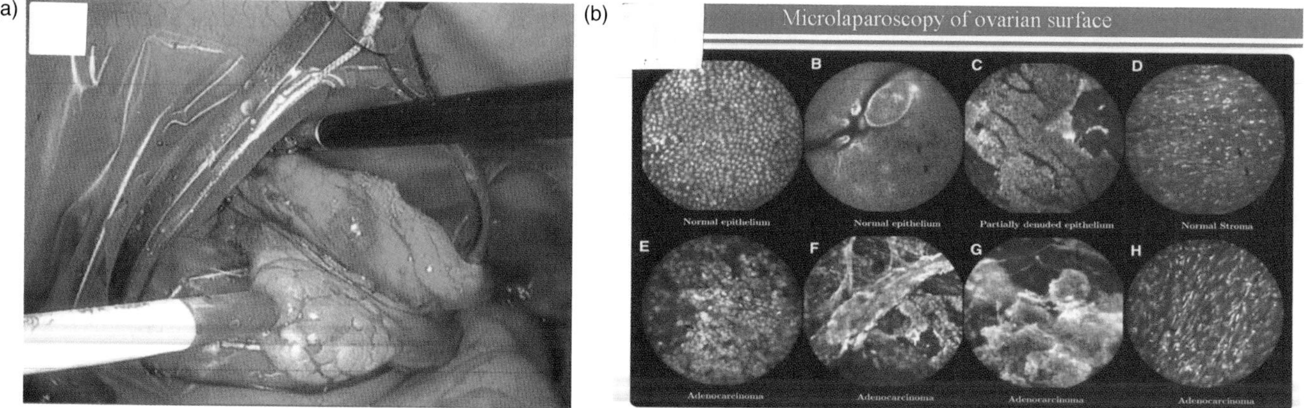

Fig. 6.10. (a) Pelvic laparoscopy with confocal microscopy. (b) Images of ovarian normal surface (above, A–D) with regular small nuclei (left) and ovarian cancer with disorganized surface structures and irregular nuclei (below E–H). Reprinted from reference [21], with permission from Elsevier.

A neoplastic process arising in these cells is a multi-step, time-related process associated with a multitude of genetic events, including hereditary mutations, suppressor-gene inhibition, apoptosis, and suppression of certain genes. The sequence and end-result of these are still poorly understood. A preneoplastic change in the ovarian tissue could be identified by histologic examination and morphometric evaluation which established it objectively, using computerized multivariate statistical discriminatory methods, as an entity intermediate between normal and neoplastic, consistent with dysplasia or OIN. Dysplasia had been described in other epithelial tissues in the body, such as the colon, larynx, skin, and uterine cervix. The progression from dysplasia to cancer, however, is unpredictable depending on several still poorly understood carcinogenic factors.

Laparoscopic confocal optic biopsy

At the present time, in the absence of reliable serum tumor markers and of early symptoms, by analogy with cervical precancer detection, it seems essential to identify the structural and tissue immuno-phenotypical characteristics of ovarian cancer precursors. Advances in surgical technology that consist of pelvic laparoscopy enhanced recently by the addition of confocal optic biopsies may offer an insight into the ovarian epithelial tissue analogous to that of the colposcope for cervical epithelial cancer precursors (Fig. 6.10). Currently in use for detection of gastrointestinal early cancer and cancer precursors, confocal laparoscopic biopsies could perform a histologic evaluation of the ovarian surface without unnecessary tissue removal. Precancerous lesions of the uterine cervix were also described using confocal optic biopsies based on the assessment of nuclear profiles and stratification patterns [19]. The diagnosis of precancerous lesions is based on the previously described architectural and nuclear cytological criteria, which are actually quite similar to those used for the gastrointestinal endoscopic confocal biopsies to detect precancerous lesions such as enlarged irregular nuclear profiles and abnormal stratification [20]. Laparoscopic confocal biopsies could also detect occult cancer, before any clinical manifestations. The fact that ovarian carcinomas, in their majority, arise on the surface of the organ makes them particularly suitable for laparoscopic optic biopsy exploration [21]. The visualization of early cancer precursors correlated with genetic and molecular analysis of early carcinogenic mechanisms may contribute to an understanding of the inception of this deadly neoplasm, and most importantly, to its detection and physical removal. Future progress in laparoscopic optic biopsy performance adding safe contrast substances for visualization of the lesions and depth beyond the presently existing 250 μm could considerably enhance the suitability of this method in detection and removal of precancerous ovarian lesions [22].

It should be kept in mind that "every invasive carcinoma is in fact a missed intra-epithelial tumor," a late stage of development from a precursor lesion [23].

The challenge remains to identify also the aberrant molecular signatures of precursor lesions in time to allow either effective screening or earlier intervention to improve clinical outcomes.

References

1. Singer G, Shih IeM, Truskinovsky A, et al. Mutational analysis of K-ras segregates ovarian serous carcinomas into two types: invasive MPSC (low-grade tumor) and conventional serous carcinoma (high-grade tumor). Int J Gynecol Pathol. 2003;**22**(1):37–41.
2. Levanon K, Crum C, Drapkin R. New insights into the pathogenesis of serous ovarian cancer and its clinical impact. J Clin Oncol. 2008;**26**(32):5284–93.
3. Kurman RJ, Shih IeM. Pathogenesis of ovarian cancer: lessons from morphology and molecular biology and their clinical implications. Int J Gynecol Pathol. 2008;**27**(2):151–60.
4. Landen CN Jr, Birrer MJ, Sood AK. Early events in the pathogenesis of epithelial ovarian cancer. J Clin Oncol. 2008;**26**(6):995–1005.
5. Ogawa S, Kaku T, Amada S, et al. Ovarian endometriosis associated with ovarian carcinoma: a clinicopathological and immunohistochemical study. Gynecol Oncol. 2000;**77**(2):298–304.
6. Irving JA, Catasús L, Gallardo A, et al. Synchronous endometrioid carcinomas of the uterine corpus and ovary: alterations in the beta-catenin (CTNNB1) pathway are associated with independent primary tumors and favorable prognosis. Hum Pathol. 2005;**36**(6):605–19.
7. Seidman JD, Cho KR, Ronnett BM, et al. In: Blaustein's pathology of the female genital tract, 6th edition. Kurman RJ, Hedrick Ellenson L, Ronnett BM. (Eds.). Mucinous Adenocarcinomas. New York: Springer; 2011. p 735.
8. Gusberg SB, Deligdisch L. Ovarian dysplasia. A study of identical twins. Cancer. 1984;**54**(1):1–4.
9. Plaxe SC, Deligdisch L, Dottino PR, et al. Ovarian intraepithelial neoplasia demonstrated in patients with stage I ovarian carcinoma. Gynecol Oncol. 1990;**38**(3):367–72.
10. Deligdisch L, Gil J, Kerner H, et al. Ovarian dysplasia in prophylactic oophorectomy specimens: cytogenetic and morphometric correlations. Cancer. 1999;**86**(8):1544–50.
11. Deligdisch L, Gil J. Characterization of ovarian dysplasia by interactive morphometry. Cancer. 1989;**63**(4):748–55.
12. Deligdisch L, Miranda C, Barba J, et al. Ovarian dysplasia: nuclear texture analysis. Cancer. 1993;**72**(11):3253–7.
13. Deligdisch L, Einstein AJ, Guera D, et al. Ovarian dysplasia in epithelial inclusion cysts. A morphometric approach using neural networks. Cancer. 1995;**76**(6):1027–34.
14. Crum CP, Drapkin R, Miron A, et al. The distal fallopian tube: a new model for pelvic serous carcinogenesis. Curr Opin Obstet Gynecol. 2007;**19**(1):3–9.
15. Folkins AK, Jarboe EA, Saleemuddin A, et al. A candidate precursor to pelvic serous cancer (p53 signature) and its prevalence in ovaries and fallopian tubes from women with *BRCA* mutations. Gynecol Oncol. 2008;**109**(2):168–73.
16. Salazar H, Godwin AK, Daly MB, et al. Microscopic benign and invasive malignant neoplasms and a cancer-prone phenotype in prophylactic oophorectomies. J Natl Cancer Inst. 1996;**88**(24):1810–20.
17. Chene G, Penault-Llorca F, Le Bouëdec G, et al. Ovarian epithelial dysplasia after ovulation induction: time and dose effects. Hum Reprod. 2009;**24**(1):132–8.
18. Schlosshauer PW, Cohen CJ, Penault-Llorca F, et al. Prophylactic oophorectomy: a morphologic and immunohistochemical study. Cancer. 2003;**98**(12):2599–606.
19. De Palma GD. Confocal laser endomicroscopy in the "in vivo" histological diagnosis of the gastrointestinal tract. World J Gastroenterol. 2009;**15**(46):5770–5.
20. Carlson K, Pavlova I, Collier T, et al. Confocal microscopy: imaging cervical precancerous lesions. Gynecol Oncol. 2005;**99**(3 Suppl 1):S84–8.

21. Tanbakuchi AA, Udovich JA, Rouse AR, et al. In vivo imaging of ovarian tissue using a novel confocal microlaparoscope. Am J Obstet Gynecol. 2010;**202**(1):90.e1–9.
22. Deligdisch L. Optic biopsy in gynecology: anatomic pathology consideration. Bull Acad Natl Med. 2011;**195**:35–41.
23. Levanon K, Crum C, Drapkin R. New insights into the pathogenesis of serous ovarian cancer and its clinical impact. J Clin Oncol. 2008;**26**(32):5284–93.

Chapter 7

Peritoneal and tubal serous carcinoma

Anna Laury, MD, Eric C. Huang, MD, PhD, Christopher P. Crum, MD, and Jonathan Hecht, MD, PhD

Introduction

In recent studies of the origin(s) of pelvic serous carcinoma, two concepts have emerged: the fallopian tube as a major source for these tumors and a carcinogenic sequence in the distal fallopian tube. The first has immediate implications for both the early detection and classification of this disease. The second impacts on the pathogenesis of tubal malignancies and has important implications for the histologic diagnosis. In particular, the discovery of benign-appearing secretory cell outgrowths (SCOUTs) in the fallopian tube that contain functional gene perturbations shared with cancer requires a reassessment of the concept of intra-epithelial neoplasia. This exercise requires the separation of innocuous clonal expansions or outgrowths of no clinical significance from those with the potential, albeit low, to metastasize.

In this chapter, we introduce the term "intra-epithelial neoplasia" to denote the latter, preferring to relegate epithelial processes of lesser degree to a descriptive category that although linked to cancer, do not belong in the diagnostic lexicon. In this spectrum may lie the genetic changes that mark the acquisition of the metastatic phenotype. We emphasize that, while this progression is most closely linked to serous carcinomas, it can occur with other phenotypes, including endometrioid and, rarely, mucinous neoplasia. Finally it is important to superimpose this new information on the existing concept of ovarian and peritoneal carcinoma. In both instances, it is useful to look at both low- and high-grade serous neoplasms and the potential contribution of the fallopian tube in their pathogenesis.

Background

Fallopian tube cancer was first described by Renaud in 1847 [1]. Subsequently, Rokitansky recorded the first microscopic description in 1861, and Orthmann followed with what is considered the first reported case in 1888 [2]. Primary fallopian tube serous carcinoma has been considered a rare, but highly aggressive carcinoma, accounting for less than 1% of all gynecological malignancies, with 5-year survival rates varying between 22% and 57%, depending on stage [3,4]. The most frequently occurring clinical symptoms are vaginal bleeding, pelvic pain, and a pelvic mass, the latter occurring in approximately 65% of patients [5]. However, a cardinal sign is unexplained profuse vaginal discharge. The majority of women with primary tubal carcinoma are diagnosed after age 50 years, with a peak incidence of between 60 and 64 years. Caucasian women (including Hispanics) have a 14% higher incidence rate than African-American women [6]. In the United States, the Surveillance, Epidemiology, and End Results program (SEER program) reported an age-adjusted incidence rate of 3.3 per million among Caucasian women during the period 1995–1999 [7]. Likewise, the incidence for the entire United Kingdom was 2.19 per million in 2000 [8].

Based on the World Health Organization (WHO) definition and criteria set forth by other authors, the following must be met to establish the diagnosis of primary tubal carcinoma: (1) the main tumor is in the fallopian tube and arises from the endosalpinx; (2) histologic features reflect a tubal differentiation pattern; (3) if the tubal wall is involved, the transition between malignant and benign tubal epithelium should be detectable; and (4) the fallopian tube contains more tumor than any other sites (i.e., ovary, endometrium or peritoneum) [9–12].

Tumors meeting all the above criteria are uncommon, making primary tubal carcinoma an extremely rare entity, which explains in part the fact that this disease is reported at a rate of less than one in 30 ovarian carcinomas. Much of this disparity is rooted in criteria 1 and 4 above, i.e., the requirement that the main portion of the tumor be centered in the tube and comprise the bulk of the tumor mass. Moreover, the term "ovarian cancer" has had an unshakeable grip on both laymen and the medical profession for the past 50 years, both eluding efforts to seriously reassess the origins of pelvic serous cancer and continuously fostered by programs that stressed serologic detection in the face of a disease that invariably presented at high stage, even in closely followed high-risk populations.

This chapter challenges these prior assumptions and puts forth the most recent evidence in support of a tubal origin for pelvic serous cancer. The areas discussed include the fallopian tube of women at risk (BRCA+), the precursor spectrum, an algorithm for defining three categories of tubal intra-epithelial neoplasia, and finally, the link between low- and high-grade pelvic serous cancers and the fallopian tube.

The fallopian tube from women at risk (BRCA+)

Historically, primary fallopian tube malignancies have been viewed as uncommon relative to conventional ovarian carcinomas, and

Altchek's Diagnosis and Management of Ovarian Disorders, ed. Liane Deligdisch, Nathan G. Kase, and Carmel J. Cohen. Published by Cambridge University Press.

some estimates have placed the oviduct as nearly 50 times less common to be the initiating site [7,8]. Part of this disparity was attributed to the stringent criteria for the diagnosis of a primary tubal malignancy. Criteria include the presence of a dominant tumor mass in the fallopian tube plus a tubal intra-epithelial carcinoma (TIC). Tumors fulfilling this requirement were uncommon, with an estimated incidence of 0.41 per 100,000. In retrospect, the reason for both the lack of frequency and this particular presentation was the need for both a tumor arising in the endosalpinx and fimbrial adhesions, which effectively barred the tumor from exiting the fallopian tube. This guaranteed that the tumor would carry out the initial stages of its natural history within the tubal lumen.

In the population carrying *BRCA1* or *BRCA2* mutations (*BRCA+*), most *symptomatic* serous carcinomas are designated as ovarian in origin according to the traditional method of primary site assignment mentioned above. However, examination of prophylactically removed fallopian tubes and ovaries has made it possible to intercept these tumors early in their course. Thus, pathology exams have shown that a large number of early serous carcinomas involve the fallopian tube, either as an invasive or intra-epithelial carcinoma. Between 57% and 85% of these patients have exhibited involvement of the fimbriated end of the fallopian tube or its immediate vicinity (Table 7.1) [13–20]. These observations have increasingly focused attention to the distal fallopian tube as an initiating point for high-grade serous malignancies (Table 7.1).

In the fallopian tube model, serous tubal intra-epithelial carcinoma (STIC) is the earliest morphologic manifestation of serous carcinoma. STICs are composed of "secretory cells," the non-ciliated population of the endosalpinx. These cells, when neoplastic, exhibit three important features; (1) variable stratification, (2) increased nuclear cytoplasmic ratio and (3) loss of nuclear polarity, often with intra-epithelial fractures or detached micro-clusters of cells in the tubal lumen. Most but not all STICs will show strong nuclear staining with antibodies to p53 as well as an increased proliferation index (MIB-1) compared with the background tubal epithelium (Fig. 7.1) [21].

The precursor spectrum in the fallopian tube

In the uterine cervix, cancer precursors are almost uniformly associated with human papillomaviruses. This leads to a powerful link between the presence of HPV and the morphologic changes that typify the precursor spectrum. Various terms, including dysplasia, CIN, and "intra-epithelial lesion" can be held synonymous in as much as they all pertain to a single definable entity. In the fallopian tube, it is virtually impossible to assign a single term to the plethora of epithelial alterations that are associated with either cancer or increased risk. Each may have a different risk associated with them, and may in many instances be incidental or inconsequential. Thus, it is most logical to separate this spectrum into two discrete subsets; those with minimal atypia and a low proliferative index, which we can term latent precursors, and those with worrisome histologic features, increased proliferative index, and an immunophenotype that befits an association with malignancy. The former are descriptive, the latter are intra-epithelial neoplasms.

Latent precursors in the fallopian tube: secretory cell outgrowths (SCOUTs)

Although the cervix is the prototype for a viral-induced carcinogenic sequence – one which is repeated in other anogenital sites and the oropharynx – the pathway to malignancy in other epithelial surfaces in other organs is one of accumulated genetic changes. This scenario is seen in the bladder, esophagus (Barrett's metaplasia), prostate, pancreas, and colon [22–26]. Each organ has a continuum of microscopic epithelial changes that reflect the gradual, age-related accumulation of genetic or epigenetic disturbances in gene function. Until recently, such a spectrum was not appreciated in the fallopian tube because the field of ovarian cancer concentrated primarily on an ovarian source. However, of late, the concept of precursors in the fallopian tube has emerged, initiated by the reports of p53 positive foci within the oviductal mucosa and subsequently, the direct link between these benign or "latent" precursors and early malignancy [27,28]. Finally, the discovery of so-called "precursor correlates" – mucosal events remote to the most

Table 7.1. Frequency of tubal intra-epithelial neoplasia (TIC) in risk-reducing salpingo-oophorectomies of women with *BRCA1* or *BRCA2* mutations

Author	No.	Tumors (%)	Tubal involvment (%)
Colgan (2001) [13]	39	5(13)	4(80)
Leeper (2002) [15]	30	5(17)	3(60)
Powell (2005) [16]	67	7(10)	4(57)
Carcangiu (2006) [17]	50	6(12)	4(67)
Finch (2006) [18]	159	7(4)	6(86)
Callahan (2007) [19]	100	7(7)	7(100)[a]
Hirst (2009) [20]	45	4(9)	4(100)
TOTAL	490	41(8)	32(78)

[a] Updated to 2010, 17/20 associated with TIC (85%).

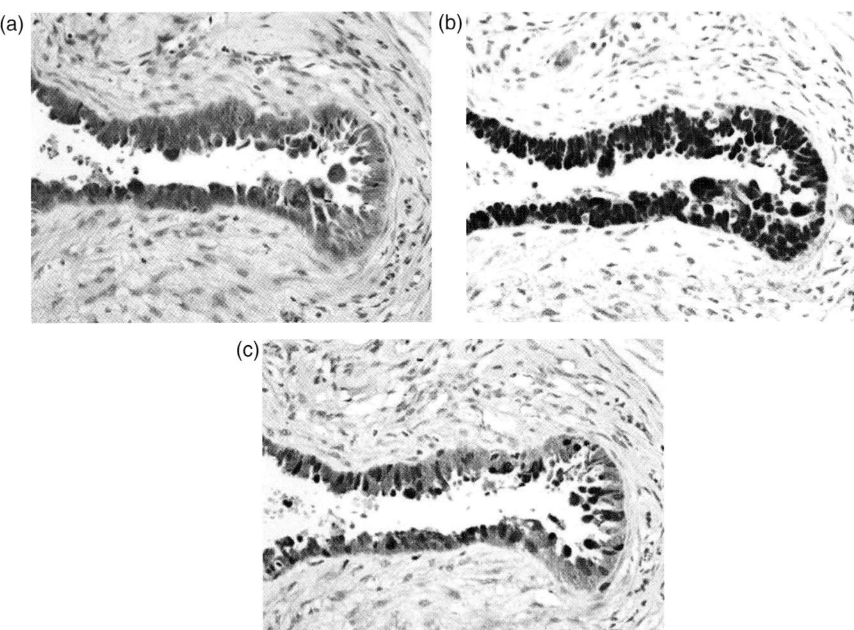

Fig. 7.1. Serous tubal intra-epithelial neoplasia (STIC) with nuclear atypia and epithelial stratification and loss of cell polarity (a). There is strong positivity for p53 (b) and a high proliferative index (c).

common site of tumor initiation but emblematic of the same functional gene perturbations – introduces the notion that the carcinogenic sequence can be separated in both space and time [29]. The underpinning of these site specific and more globally distributed changes in the oviduct is the "secretory cell outgrowth" or SCOUT [30–32].

Secretory cell outgrowths with increased p53 immuno-staining (p53 signatures)

It is widely accepted that a precursor lesion often precedes an invasive carcinoma. This can be seen in the cervix where a cervical intra-epithelial neoplasia can progress to an invasive carcinoma. However, such precursor lesion was never previously identified in serous carcinogenesis. In the fallopian tube, STICs are presumed to be an early and non-invasive carcinoma, but potentially lethal phase of malignancy that will eventually spread if not detected; hence, STICs cannot be considered as precursor lesions. While the normal fallopian tubal epithelium consists of a mixture of ciliated and secretory cells, STIC and invasive serous carcinoma are comprised of only secretory cells. Piek et al. noted that prophylactically removed fallopian tubes from BRCA-positive patients contained dysplastic changes that had an increase in *p53* expression and are secretory cell type [27]. Because *p53* mutation is considered integral to the development of both STICs and invasive carcinomas, Lee et al. analyzed a series of BRCA-positive women and controls for p53 positivity [28]. They required the presence of at least 12 consecutive secretory p53-positive nuclei, given that these cells sometimes inter-mixed with normal ciliated cells. Discrete segments of secretory cells with strong nuclear p53 immunostaining in benign-appearing tubal mucosa were identified and were designated as "p53 signature" (Fig. 7.2a) [28]. These precursor lesions of the fallopian tube epithelium share many features with high-grade serous carcinomas, including the cell type involved, evidence of DNA damage, and p53 mutations. In addition, the p53 signatures were found most commonly in the fimbria, a site similar to STICs, supporting a tubal precursor lesion. A series of studies have identified numerous links between p53 signatures and pelvic serous cancer, establishing this entity as either a direct precursor or a reflection of the early events leading to pelvic serous carcinoma [33–35].

Secretory cell outgrowths with preserved p53 function and loss of PAX2 expression

p53 signature is characterized by a linear expansion of a homogeneous population of tubal secretory cell outgrowth (SCOUTs), presumably as a result of interruption in the process of normal differentiation. This process is most conspicuous in the setting of p53 mutations and DNA damage, as demonstrated by intense p53 nuclear staining and γ-H2AX staining [28,36]. However, because carcinogenesis is classically multigenic, we surmised that the oviductal mucosa could also give rise to benign clonal expansions (SCOUTs) that reflected disturbances in genes other than p53. Recently, down-regulation of Pax2, a member of the pair box (*PAX*) gene family expressed in Müllerian duct derivatives, has been documented in both early endometrial carcinogenesis, including normal endometrial glandular epithelium, and pelvic serous carcinomas, implicating this gene in the carcinogenesis of gynecologic tract malignancy [37,38]. We have recently demonstrated that *PAX2* expression is consistently down-regulated in SCOUTs (Fig. 7.2B) [29,31]. Hence, similar to the endometrium, SCOUTs appear to signify a latent serous precancer commonly harboring loss of Pax2. The subset of p53-positive SCOUTs (e.g., "p53 signatures") seen in continuation with STICs and associated invasive serous carcinomas show concomitant loss

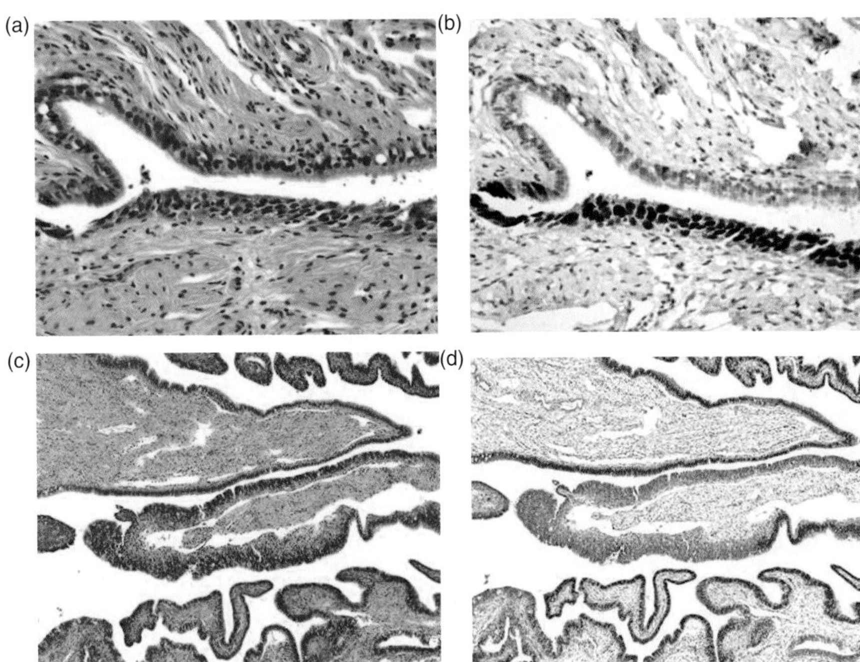

Fig. 7.2. Secretory cell outgrowths in the fallopian tube. The p53 signature (a) has strong nuclear positivity for p53 (b) and is considered a direct precursor to STIC. Most other secretory cell outgrowths (c) do not have loss of p 53 but are distinguished by loss of *PAX2* expression (d, center).

of both Pax2 and p53 function, further linking the fallopian tube precursor to pelvic serous carcinogenesis and supporting the accepted multi-hit model for this malignancy [29]. It is still not entirely clear whether Pax2 and p53 function in the same pathway leading to serous carcinogenesis. Several pieces of evidence suggest that Pax2 and p53 might function independently. First, p53 signatures (inactivation of p53 function) occur more frequently in the fimbria [28]. In contrast, SCOUTs are more widely distributed in the fallopian tube [29,31]. Thus, exposure to genotoxic injury, while sufficient in some loci to produce p53 signatures, is not required to produce dysregulation of Pax2. This supports the concept of functional gene disturbances separated in both space and time.

Tubal intra-epithelial neoplasia

Secretory cell outgrowths, including most with p53 mutations, are not accompanied by either atypia or more than a mild increase in proliferative index and are very common in the fallopian tube. Over one half of controls will exhibit an uninterrupted sequence of secretory cells with strong p53 immuno-staining. PAX2-null outgrowths with variable ciliated differentiation are seen in a high percentage of fallopian tubes, albeit more commonly in women in the older age groups or with co-existing pelvic serous cancer. In contrast, expansile or proliferative p53, positive epithelia, variously termed *proliferative p53 signatures* or *tubal intra-epithelial lesions in transition*, are uncommon and bear some resemblance to tubal intra-epithelial carcinomas. In contrast, they exhibit preserved epithelial polarity, a lower proliferative index, frequent admixtures of ciliated cells and in our experience, less consistent staining for markers associated with ovarian cancer such as p16. Because they are much larger than most p53 signatures, often spanning hundreds of nuclei, they merit consideration as intra-epithelial neoplasms (TIN).

The following descriptive criteria for TIN are not intended for routine pathologic diagnosis, where the simple distinction of STIC from a lesser atypia is all that is required for managing women with *BRCA1* or *BRCA2* mutations. Rather this classification is intended to highlight three separable forms of p53-positive (or less commonly p53 null) oviductal epithelium, each with a different implication.

Type 1 tubal intra-epithelial neoplasms (TIN1) (Fig. 7.3a): TIN1 is in essence an expansile or proliferative p53 signature. The size criteria are not fixed, but they typically encompass at least an entire plical surface or its equivalent. They are presumed benign but clearly have acquired a growth advantage and conform to the definition of "new growth" assigned to neoplasms. When discovered in prophylactic specimens, TIN1 is typically overlooked or when identified ultimately classified as epithelial atypia that does not fulfill the criteria for malignancy.

Tubal intra-epithelial carcinomas differ from proliferative p53 signatures by the presence of a higher proliferative index, high nuclear-cytoplasmic ratio and most importantly, conspicuous loss of polarity with variable stratification. The latter is often associated with small clusters of un-polarized cells on the surface, or small intra-epithelial fractures splitting off groups of cells. Immuno-stains for a Mib1 will typically reveal an index of greater than 70% in at least a portion of the lesion although the most important parameters are histologic. These can be divided into "early" and "late" tubal intra-epithelial carcinomas. Early ones are typically encountered in risk-reducing salpingo-oophorectomy specimens and may not display the striking atypia seen in intra-epithelial carcinomas accompanying stromal invasion or metastases.

These can be viewed as *type 2 tubal intra-epithelial neoplasms (TIN2)* (Fig. 7.3b). The implication is that they are intra-epithelial carcinomas, carry some risk but not an absolute risk of recurrence.

(a)
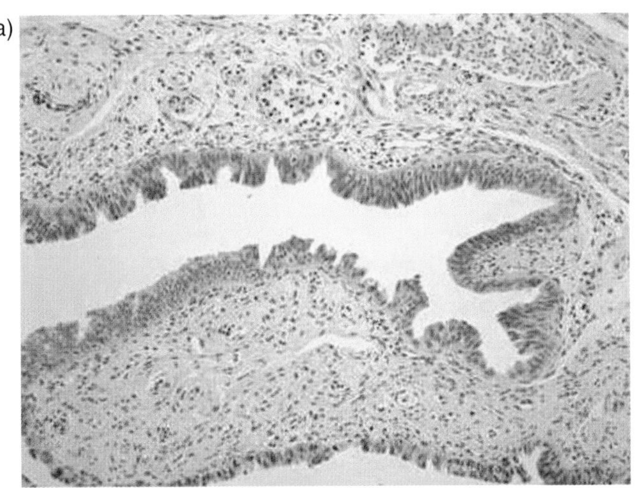
(b)
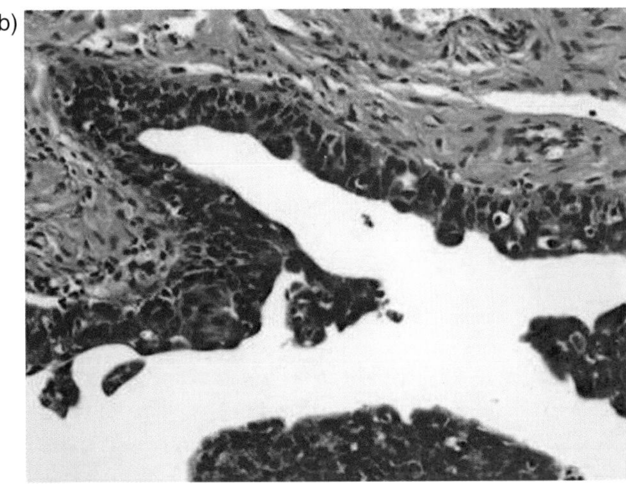
(c)
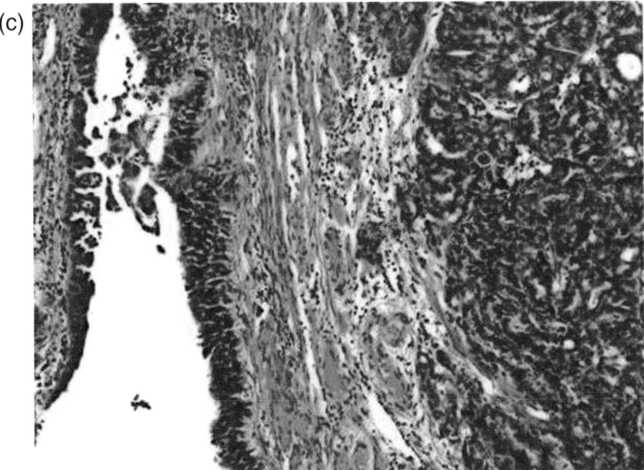

Fig. 7.3. Three biologically different types of tubal intra-epithelial neoplasia, including (a) an expansile or proliferative p53 signature sufficiently large to signify a acquisition of new growth (type 1), (b) tubal intra-epithelial carcinoma that has not yet metastasized (type 2), and (c) tubal intra-epithelial carcinoma that is associated with metastatic carcinoma (type 3).

The tubal intra-epithelial carcinomas associated with invasion and/or metastasis can be viewed as *type 3 tubal intra-epithelial neoplasms (TIN3)* (Fig. 7.3c). The clinical implications of the above classification should be clear. Any intra-epithelial lesion classified as grade 2 or 3 carries a risk of recurrence, with the definition of grade 3 TIN self-fulfilling. The importance of separating the intra-epithelial neoplasms from the latent precursors is obvious; the latter confer no risk to the patient. In the event that one should be classified as a tubal intra-epithelial neoplasm, it will be grade 1, connoting no risk to the patient.

The link between low- and high-grade serous cancer and peritoneal disease

The majority of extra-uterine pelvic carcinomas in women with Mullerian differentiation have traditionally been assumed to be ovarian in origin. This assumption has encouraged studies focusing on the ovarian surface epithelium (OSE) as the source of the pelvic carcinomas [39]. The traditional view of ovarian carcinogenesis has been that the various tumors are presumed to arise from the ovarian surface epithelium (mesothelium), or derived from ovarian cortical epithelial inclusions, which exhibit the morphologic features of reproductive tract epithelium (Müllerian), and that subsequent metaplastic changes lead to the development of the different cell types [40]. Three possible mechanisms for their development include: (1) exfoliation or tubal-ovarian adhesions from the distal fallopian tubal epithelium (endosalpingiosis), (2) invagination and incorporation of the OSE into the cortex (cortical inclusion cysts), and (3) implantation of cells from the endometrium by means of retrograde menstruation (endometriosis) [41]. No cells in normal ovaries resemble any of these epithelia, leading to the controversy of whether ovarian epithelial neoplasms arose by means of trans-differentiation and transformation of the OSE or from cells transported to the ovary from other Mullerian sites, including the fallopian tube.

Resolving the above controversy is not a simple matter. The fact that most ovarian endometrioid and mucinous carcinomas arise from ovarian endometriosis is unchallenged. The origin of borderline and low-grade serous carcinomas has been assigned to the ovaries or peritoneum, although emerging data implicate the tube, at least indirectly, in some instances. The link between high-grade serous carcinoma and the tube is gaining increased attention, but is not irrefutable. The purpose of this section is to address this association by the available evidence, which is more compelling the *earlier* in the natural history pelvic serous carcinoma is intercepted. In addressing this relationship between the tube and pelvic serous cancer, we will review five different scenarios, or levels of certainty. When placed in an

Table 7.2. Frequency of serous tubal intra-epithelial carcinoma in high-grade serous carcinomas

Author	Diagnosis	No.	(%)
Kindelberger (2007) [42]	OVCA	44	20 (45)
Carlson (2008) [43]	PPCA	19	9 (47)
Roh (2010) [47]	OVCA	78	28 (36)
Przybycin (2010) [46]	OVCA/PPCA	41	24 (59)
Seidman (2011) [44]	PPCA	51	28 (56)
Leonhardt (2011) [45]	PPCA	9	3 (33)

algorithm, it may be possible to assign a relative degree of certainty for a tubal origin based on the strength of the evidence. These levels are viewed from the strongest to the weakest likelihood that the tumor arose in the tube.

Level 1: pelvic serous carcinoma with normal fallopian tubes

In our experience, most pelvic serous cancers involve the endosalpinx. In approximately 15% of cases the endosalpinx is both evaluable and appears pristine. In these cases it can be said that there is no evidence of a tubal origin as we know it.

Level 2: pelvic serous carcinoma with involvement of the endosalpinx

This category includes both microscopic involvement of the endosalpinx without STIC or complete replacement of ovary and tube such that the mucosa cannot be evaluated. In this setting, the tube can neither be confirmed nor excluded as the source of the tumor. This comprises from 30–40% of pelvic serous cancers.

Level 3: disseminated pelvic serous carcinoma associated with serous tubal intra-epithelial carcinoma

This scenario comprises roughly half of the cases of pelvic serous cancer. Kindelberger et al. examined a consecutive series of pelvic serous carcinomas using the SEE-FIM protocol [42]. Approximately 70% of these cases involved the endosalpinx with nearly one-half of tumors classified as ovarian serous carcinomas co-existed with a STIC. In a small series of five cases, p53 mutation was identified in both the tubal and ovarian cancers. In addition, of seven tumors classified as a primary peritoneal serous carcinoma, six also involved the endosalpinx and four demonstrated clear evidence of an early cancer arising in the fallopian tube. Carlson et al. demonstrated that 47% of the patients with primary peritoneal serous carcinomas also have STIC [43]. Based on these findings and that of others, it is conceivable that many so-called peritoneal and ovarian serous carcinomas originate in the inner lining of the distal fallopian tube (Table 7.2) [42–47].

By definition, STICs contain *p53* mutations, which is integral to serous carcinogenesis. About 80% of STICs will be highlighted by immuno-chemical nuclear accumulation of mutated p53 protein. Negative p53 staining can be attributed to upstream mutation that is not targeted by the immunohistochemical analysis, mutations that result in the conformational change of p53 protein thereby preventing antigen recognition or null mutations. In our experience with early serous cancers, all cases with thorough p53 sequencing scored positive for a mutation [47].

Level 4: irrefutable primary tubal carcinoma

This scenario has two presentations. In the first there is a *dominant bulky mass in the tube associated with a STIC.* This conforms to the time-honored image of a sausage-shaped fallopian tube, expanded from within by tumor and often sealed at the fimbriated end. The latter phenomenon likely explains the fact that many of these tumors present at stage I and underscores the potential lethality when the intra-epithelial tumor is exposed to the pelvic surfaces. If this is prevented by adhesions, it is reasonable to assume that a "grace period" exists during which the tumor can grow and expand – and possibly be detected – before extra-tubal spread takes place. In the second early serous carcinoma is microscopic and limited to the distal tube. This can be seen rarely incidentally in tubes from women undergoing surgery for benign neoplasms or, more commonly, in risk reducing salpingo-oophorectomies for genetic risk (*BRCA+*). Complete histologic sampling of the fallopian tubes and ovaries is required in prophylactic salpingo-oophorectomies for BRCA-positive patients due to the extreme small size of the tumor that cannot be visualized grossly. Using a protocol for Sectioning and Extensively Examining the FIMbria (SEE-FIM), Medeiros et al. identified five tumors with STICs where four of these tumors arose from the fimbria and one was immediately proximal in the ampullary region, confirming the tubal fimbria as the most common site of origin for Müllerian carcinoma in a prophylactic adnexectomy series from BRCA-positive patients, which was also validated by others [14,18,48].

Although the number of cases reported is small, evidence suggests that many early tubal carcinomas do not metastasize, of if they do, will present months to years later as pelvic recurrences. This further underscores the certainty with which an isolated intra-epithelial carcinoma can be viewed as a primary neoplasm.

Level 5: serous borderline tumors (SBT) and the fallopian tube

There is indirect evidence implicating the fallopian tube in the genesis of borderline serous tumors. First, both adenofibromas and papillary mucosal proliferations can occur in the fallopian tubes that resemble benign or borderline tumors (Fig. 7.4) [32,49,50]. However, they are distinctly uncommon and not present in most cases of SBT. Second, loss of *PAX2*, in the form of *PAX2*-null SCOUTs, is more common in the tubes of women with SBTs and loss of *PAX2* can also be seen in the latter [32]. Third, the cell types of the fallopian tube are identical to those of SBTs [51]. What remains unclear is the mechanism by which

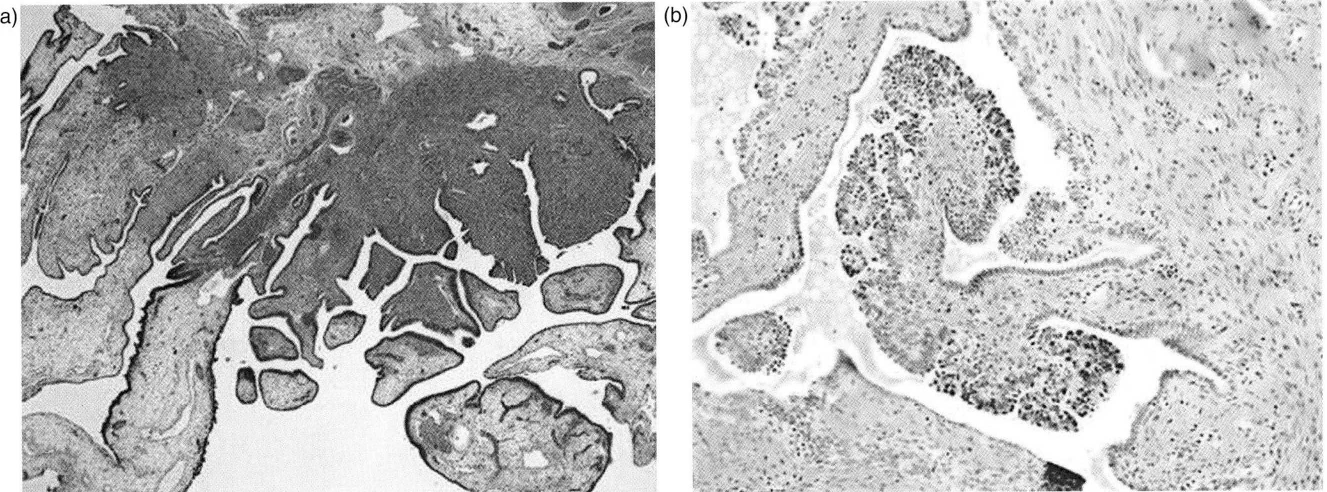

Fig. 7.4. The fallopian tube can also give rise to benign adenofibromas (a) and occasionally to papillary proliferations reminiscent of borderline serous tumors (b).

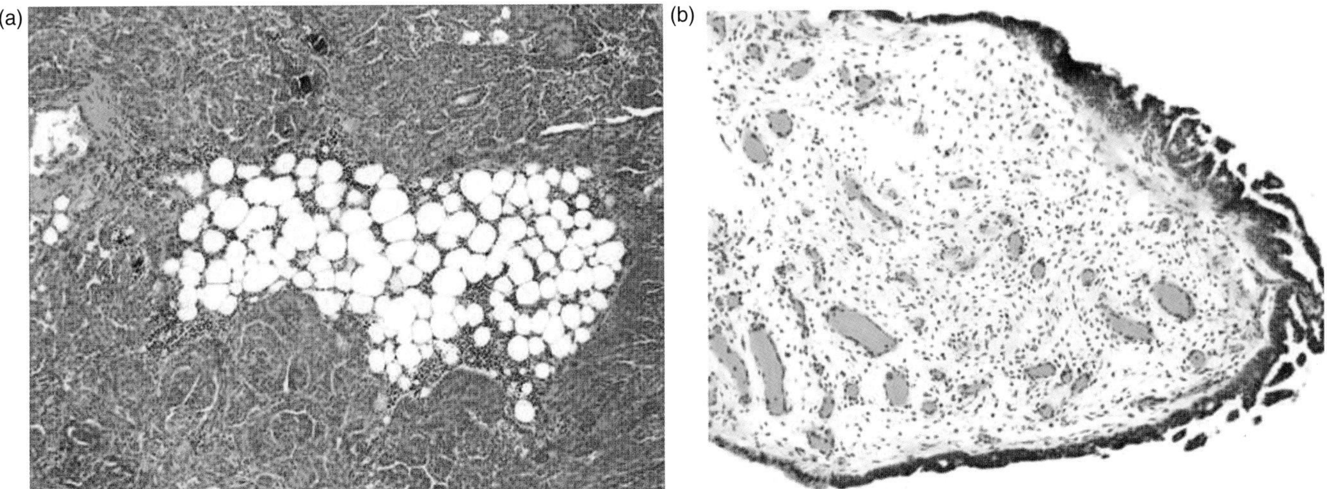

Fig. 7.5. Widespread omental involvement (a) associated with STIC. One half of cases otherwise classified as primary peritoneal carcinomas will display a microscopic tubal intra-epithelial carcinoma (b).

the cells make their way to the peritoneal or ovarian surface and whether this migration takes place in the form of benign (endosalpingiosis) rather than proliferating serous epithelium. If the former, the link between the tube and SBTs is considerably less direct than that proposed for high-grade serous cancers.

Do peritoneal carcinomas come from tubal intra-epithelial neoplasms?

So-called primary peritoneal serous cancers are so defined because there is disseminated disease without a clear source. We know that they bear a close resemblance to presumed fimbrial/ovarian carcinomas and that in approximately half of cases, a STIC can be implicated in their pathogenesis (Fig. 7.5). We also know that approximately 6% of BRCA+ women who undergo RRSO will develop a pelvic serous cancer at a later time point. We know that some of these cases are likely the consequence of a disseminated STIC, either by prospective follow-up or retrospective discovery of STIC in the RRSO specimen. What is not clear is the pathogenesis of pelvic cancers that develop despite documented normal fallopian tubes. This is difficult to establish given the fact that some STICS are sufficiently small to be overlooked. Thus, until large prospective studies are done with exhaustive examination of the oviducts, the exact percentage in which the tubes can be excluded will not be known. If occult disease in the fallopian tubes gave rise to these peritoneal tumors, there are two potential scenarios. In the first, an occult STIC would shed cells to the peritoneum that survived but did not grow immediately. The acquisition of additional mutations would result in a malignancy. In the second, normal tubal cells would become ensconced in the peritoneum and undergo malignant transformation. This is difficult to believe given the fact that the peritoneal surface is remote to the fimbrial-ovarian region, where most tumors develop and would not be exposed to the same carcinogenic stimuli. Two additional possibilities exist. The first is endometriosis, which unquestionably gives rise to high-grade Mullerian carcinomas on occasion. The last is a source in the ovary such as the ovarian surface epithelium or another cell type that has yet to be discovered.

References

1. Renaud F, Ricci JV. One Hundred Years of Gynecology. Philadelphia: Blakiston; 1945.
2. Orthmann EG. Primareskarzinom in Einertuberkulosen. Z Geburtshulfe Gynakol. 1888;**15**:211–37.
3. Baekelandt M, Jorunn Nesbakken A, Kristensen GB, et al. Carcinoma of the fallopian tube. Cancer. 2000;**89**(10):2076–84.
4. Schink JC, Lurain JR. Rare gynecologic malignancies. Curr Opin Obstet Gynecol. 1991;3(1):78–90.
5. Nordin AJ. Primary carcinoma of the fallopian tube: a 20-year literature review. Obstet Gynecol Surv. 1994;**49**(5):349–61.
6. Rosenblatt KA, Weiss NS, Schwartz SM. Incidence of malignant fallopian tube tumors. Gynecol Oncol. 1989;**35**(2):236–9.
7. Goodman MT, Shvetsov YB. Incidence of Ovarian, Peritoneal, and Fallopian tube carcinomas in the United States, 1995–2004 Cancer Epidemiol Biomarkers Prev. 2009;**18**:132–139.
8. Clayton NL, Jaaback KS, Hirschowitz L. Primary fallopian tube carcinoma – the experience of a UK cancer centre and a review of the literature. J Obstet Gynaecol. 2005;**25**(7):694–702.
9. Alvarado-Cabrero I, Cheung A, Caduff R. Tumors of the fallopian tube. In: Tavassoli FA, Devilee P (Eds.). WHO Classification of Tumors: Pathology and Genetics of Tumors of the Breast and Female Genital Organs. Lyon, France: IARC Press; 2003, pp. 206–11.
10. Hu CY, Taymor ML, Hertig AT. Primary carcinoma of the fallopian tube. Am J Obstet Gynecol. 1950;**59**(1):58–67.
11. Sedlis A. Primary carcinoma of the fallopian tube. Obstet Gynecol Surv. 1961;**16**:209–26.
12. Yoonessi M. Carcinoma of the fallopian tube. Obstet Gynecol Surv. 1979;**34**(4):257–70.
13. Colgan TJ, Murphy J, Cole DE, Narod S, Rosen B. Occult carcinoma in prophylactic oophorectomy specimens: prevalence and association with BRCA germline mutation status. Am J Surg Pathol. 2001;**25**(10):1283–9.
14. Cass I, Holschneider C, Datta N, et al. BRCA-mutation-associated fallopian tube carcinoma: a distinct clinical phenotype? Obstet Gynecol. 2005;**106**(6):1327–34.
15. Leeper K, Garcia R, Swisher E, et al. Pathologic findings in prophylactic oophorectomy specimens in high-risk women. Gynecol Oncol. 2002;**87**:52–6.
16. Powell CB, Kenley E, Chen LM, et al. Risk-reducing salpingo-oophorectomy in BRCA mutation carriers: role of serial sectioning in the detection of occult malignancy. J Clin Oncol. 2005;**23**(1):127–32.
17. Carcangiu ML, Peissel B, Pasini B, et al. Incidental carcinomas in prophylactic specimens in BRCA1 and BRCA2 germ-line mutation carriers, with emphasis on fallopian tube lesions: report of 6 cases and review of the literature. Am J Surg Pathol. 2006;**30**:1222–30.
18. Finch A, Shaw P, Rosen B, et al. Clinical and pathologic findings of prophylactic salpingo-oophorectomies in 159 BRCA1 and BRCA2 carriers. Gynecol Oncol. 2006;**100**(1):58–64.
19. Callahan MJ, Crum CP, Medeiros F, et al. Primary fallopian tube malignancies in BRCA-positive women undergoing surgery for ovarian cancer risk reduction. J Clin Oncol. 2007;**25**:3985–90.
20. Hirst JE, Gard GB, McIllroy K, et al. High rates of occult fallopian tube cancer diagnosed at prophylactic bilateral salpingo-oophorectomy. Int J Gynecol Cancer. 2009;**19**:826–9.
21. Jarboe E, Folkins A, Nucci MR, et al. Serous carcinogenesis in the fallopian tube: a descriptive classification. Int J Gynecol Pathol. 2008;**27**:1–9.
22. Cheng L, Davidson DD, Maclennan GT, et al. The origins of urothelial carcinoma. Expert Rev Anticancer Ther. 2010;**10**(6):865–80.
23. Wang X, Ouyang H, Yamamoto Y, et al. Residual embryonic cells as precursors of a Barrett's-like metaplasia. Cell. 2011;**145**:1023–35.
24. Epstein JI. Precursor lesions to prostatic adenocarcinoma. Virchows Arch. 2009;**454**:1–16.
25. Ito R, Kondo F, Yamaguchi T, et al. Pancreatic intraepithelial neoplasms in the normal appearing pancreas: on their precise relationship with age. Hepatogastroenterology. 2008;**55**(84):1103–6.
26. Zeki SS, Graham TA, Wright NA. Stem cells and their implications for colorectal cancer. Nat Rev Gastroenterol Hepatol. 2011;**8**(2):90–100.
27. Piek JM, van Diest PJ, Zweemer RP, et al. Dysplastic changes in prophylactically removed Fallopian tubes of women predisposed to developing ovarian cancer. J Pathol. 2001;**195**(4):451–6.
28. Lee Y, Miron A, Drapkin R, et al. A candidate precursor to serous carcinoma that originates in the distal fallopian tube. J Pathol. 2007;**211**(1):26–35.
29. Chen EY, Mehra K, Mehrad M, et al. Secretory cell outgrowth, PAX2 and serous carcinogenesis in the Fallopian tube. J Pathol. 2010;**222**:110–6.
30. Mehra K, Mehrad M, Ning G, et al. STICS, SCOUTs and p53 signatures; a new language for pelvic serous carcinogenesis. Front Biosci (Elite Ed). 2011;**3**:625–34.
31. Quick CM, Ning G, Bijron J, et al. *PAX2*-null secretory cell outgrowths in the oviduct and their relationship to pelvic serous cancer. Mod Pathol. 2011;**25**:449–55.
32. Laury AR, Ning G, Quick CM, et al. Fallopian tube correlates of ovarian serous borderline tumors. Am J Surg Pathol. 2011;**35**(12):1759–65.
33. Norquist BM, Garcia RL, Allison KH, et al. The molecular pathogenesis of hereditary ovarian carcinoma: alterations in the tubal epithelium of women with *BRCA1* and *BRCA2* mutations. Cancer. 2010;**116**:5261–71.
34. Shaw PA, Rouzbahman M, Pizer ES, et al. Candidate serous cancer precursors in fallopian tube epithelium of *BRCA1/2* mutation carriers. Mod Pathol. 2009;**22**:1133–8.
35. Saleemuddin A, Folkins AK, Garrett L, et al. Risk factors for a serous cancer precursor ("p53 signature") in women with inherited *BRCA* mutations. Gynecol Oncol. 2008;**111**:226–32.
36. Levanon K, Ng V, Piao HY, et al. Primary ex vivo cultures of human fallopian tube epithelium as a model for serous ovarian carcinogenesis. Oncogene. 2010;**29**(8):1103–13.
37. Monte NM, Webster KA, Neuberg D, et al. Joint loss of *PAX2* and *PTEN*

expression in endometrial precancers and cancer. Cancer Res. 2010;**70**:6225–32.

38. Tung CS, Mok SC, Tsang YT, et al. *PAX2* expression in low malignant potential ovarian tumors and low-grade ovarian serous carcinomas. Mod Pathol. 2009;**22**(9):1243–50.
39. He QY, Zhou Y, Wong E, et al. Proteomic analysis of a preneoplastic phenotype in ovarian surface epithelial cells derived from prophylactic oophorectomies. Gynecol Oncol. 2005;**98**(1):68–76.
40. Katabuchi H, Okamura H. Cell biology of human ovarian surface epithelial cells and ovarian carcinogenesis. Med Electron Microsc. 2003;**36**(2):74–86.
41. Drapkin RL, Hecht JL. Pathogenesis of ovarian cancer. In: Crum CP, Lee KR (Eds.). Diagnostic Gynecologic and Obstetric Pathology. Philadelphia: WB Saunders; 2006, pp. 793–810.
42. Kindelberger DW, Lee Y, Miron A, et al. Intraepithelial carcinoma of the fimbria and pelvic serous carcinoma: evidence for a causal relationship. Am J Surg Pathol. 2007;**31**(2):161–9.
43. Carlson JW, Miron A, Jarboe EA, et al. Serous tubal intraepithelial carcinoma: its potential role in primary peritoneal serous carcinoma and serous cancer prevention. J Clin Oncol. 2008;**26**(25):4160–5.
44. Seidman JD, Zhao P, Yemelyanova A. Primary peritoneal high-grade serous carcinoma is very likely metastatic from serous tubal intraepithelial carcinoma: assessing the new paradigm of ovarian and pelvic serous carcinogenesis and its implications for screening for ovarian cancer. Gynecol Oncol. 2011;**120**:470–3.
45. Leonhardt K, Einenkel J, Sohr S, et al. p53 signature and serous tubal in-situ carcinoma in cases of primary tubal and peritoneal carcinomas and serous borderline tumors of the ovary. Int J Gynecol Pathol. 2011;**30**: 417–24.
46. Przybycin CG, Kurman RJ, Ronnett BM, et al. Are all pelvic (nonuterine) serous carcinomas of tubal origin? Am J Surg Pathol. 2010;**34**:1407–16.
47. Roh MH, Yassin Y, Miron A, et al. High-grade fimbrial-ovarian carcinomas are unified by altered p53, PTEN and Pax-2 expression. Mod Pathol. 2010;**23**:1316–24.
48. Medeiros F, Muto MG, Lee Y, et al. The tubal fimbria is a preferred site for early adenocarcinoma in women with familial ovarian cancer syndrome. Am J Surg Pathol. 2006;**30**:230–6.
49. Bossuyt V, Medeiros F, Drapkin R, et al. Adenofibroma of the fimbria: a common entity that is indistinguishable from ovarian adenofibroma. Int J Gynecol Pathol. 2008;**27**:390–7.
50. Kurman RJ, Vang R, Junge J, et al. Papillary tubal hyperplasia: the putative precursor of ovarian atypical proliferative (borderline) serous tumors, noninvasive implants, and endosalpingiosis. Am J Surg Pathol. 2011;**35**:1605–14.
51. Li J, Abushahin N, Pang S, et al. Tubal origin of 'ovarian' low-grade serous carcinoma. Mod Pathol. 2011;**24**:1488–99.

Chapter 8

Pathology of ovarian germ cell tumors

Liane Deligdisch, MD

Introduction

Germ cell tumors (GCT) are a fascinating group of tumors exhibiting a large variety of pathological patterns and occurring in clinical settings that often include developmental, genetic, and hormonal disorders. These tumors are unique because they involve gonads of both sexes, ovaries and testes, and are seen mostly in young patients. Actually, they represent about 60% of all ovarian tumors diagnosed in patients under the age of 30. With the exception of dermoid cysts (benign, mature cystic teratomas), they are uncommon neoplasms; fortunately, the most common are benign and conversely, the malignant tumors are the least common. Their clinical outlook has changed dramatically for the better, over the past decades, due to their responsiveness to chemotherapy.

The pathologic characteristics of ovarian germ cell tumors are also unique: they are composed of multiple tissues, occurring in various degrees of maturation from their cells of origin (the germ cells) as well as in various histologic tissue combinations.

Some germ cell tumors are associated with sex-cord tissue derivatives.

Germ cell tumors represent one-third of all malignant tumors seen in young females and about 20% of all ovarian tumors in Europe and North America. In Asia and Africa, they represent a much larger proportion of ovarian tumors because the prevalence of epithelial–stromal-derived tumors is much lower.

Classification

Germ cell tumors (GCT) are classified according to the degree of differentiation of their cells of origin (see Table 8.1). Tumors composed only of primitive germ cells, which is the case for the most common malignant GCT, are dysgerminomas of ovaries and seminomas of testes. GCT composed of multiple embryonal tissues, originating in somatic primitive tissues, are embryonal carcinomas. Tumors composed of endo-, meso-, and ectodermal tissues arising in differentiated embryonic layers, especially ectodermal, are teratomas, of which the most common are benign, the mature cystic teratomas or dermoids.

Tumors arising in the most primitive embryonal tissues, preceding in their development the somatic fetal tissues, such as the yolk sac and the trophoblast, are rare and potentially highly malignant. These are the endodermal sinus tumors arising in the primitive yolk sac and the non-gestational choriocarcinoma arising in the trophoblast (Table 8.1). As mentioned before, fortunately, the most common GCT, the mature teratomas, are also the most benign. The least common tumors arising in primitive embryonal tissues are the most malignant. Their natural history however has been profoundly changed by the advent of an effective chemotherapy (Chapter 30).

Dysgerminoma

This is a tumor composed of primordial germ cells considered to be at an early stage of development before any sexual differentiation of the gonad.

Their early embryogenesis is in the yolk sac from where they migrate to the primitive gonad by means of midline structures such as the parapineal, the mediastinum, the retroperitoneum, and the sacrococcygeal regions which may (rarely) be the sites of GCT.

While many GCT represent a mixed association of tumor tissues, dysgerminomas most often occur in pure form. They are uncommon tumors, representing about 1–2% of all primary ovarian neoplasms and 3–5% of ovarian malignancies [1].

Most cases are diagnosed in the second to third decades of life; 80% of patients are under 30 years. Rare cases are seen in post-menopausal women. Some cases were reported in the same family. The presenting symptom is usually a pelvic mass, sometimes with torsion and pain. Dysgerminoma is the most common malignant ovarian tumor associated with pregnancy due to its high incidence in the child-bearing age group. About 5–10% of patients with dysgerminoma also have dysgenetic gonads and sexual abnormalities (Fig. 8.1) [2,3]. An unusual association is that with gonadoblastomas, a sex cord-GCT. Hormonal abnormalities are seen in cases with associated choriocarcinoma when human chorionic gonadotropins are found in the serum and urine. In cases with associated gonadoblastoma, the patients may present with primary amenorrhea [4].

Dysgerminomas are rapidly growing, mostly unilateral solid tumors, with a smooth capsule and a soft to rubbery consistency measuring a few centimeters up to 50 cm. The cut section displays a lobulated grayish surface.

Microscopically dysgerminomas are composed of sheets and nests of uniform large cells with large nuclei containing a double amount of DNA, as in primitive germ cells before the first meiosis. Mitotic activity is variable. The tumor cells are

Altchek's Diagnosis and Management of Ovarian Disorders, ed. Liane Deligdisch, Nathan G. Kase, and Carmel J. Cohen. Published by Cambridge University Press.

Table 8.1. Ovarian germ cell tumors

Dysgerminoma	Embryonal	Extra-embryonal
• Composed of primitive germ cells	• Ectoderm, mesoderm, endoderm A. Mature cystic (dermoid) or solid teratoma B. Monodermal teratoma Struma ovarii Carcinoid Other C. Immature teratoma	• Yolk sac: endodermal sinus tumor • Trophoblast, choriocarcinoma, non-gestational • Mixed with embryonal carcinoma

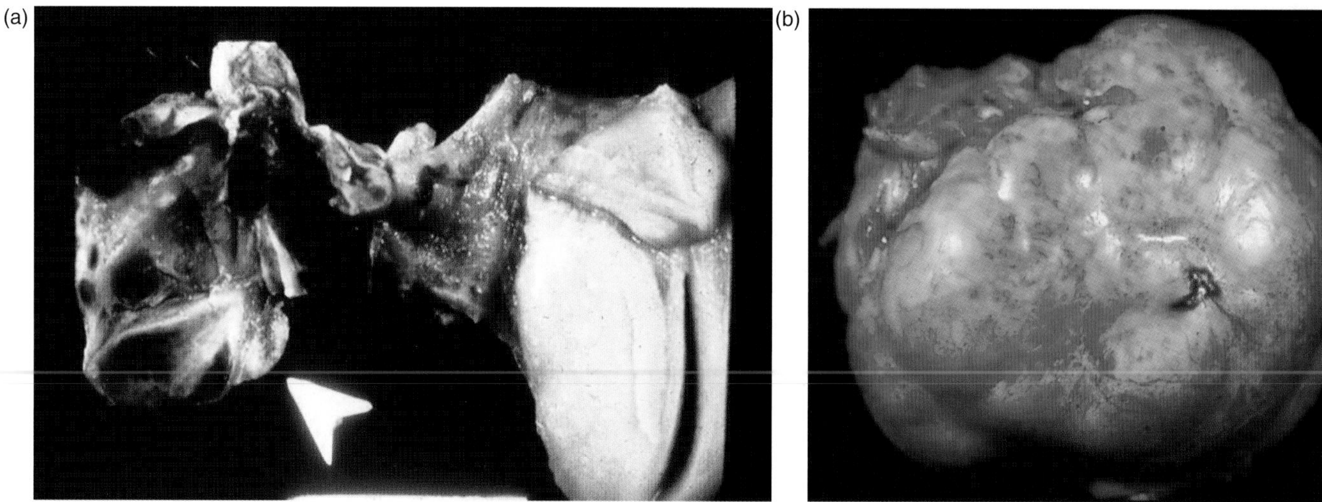

Fig. 8.1. (a) A 27-year-old patient with right side ovotestis (true hermaphrodite). (b) Same patient, with left side dysgerminoma.

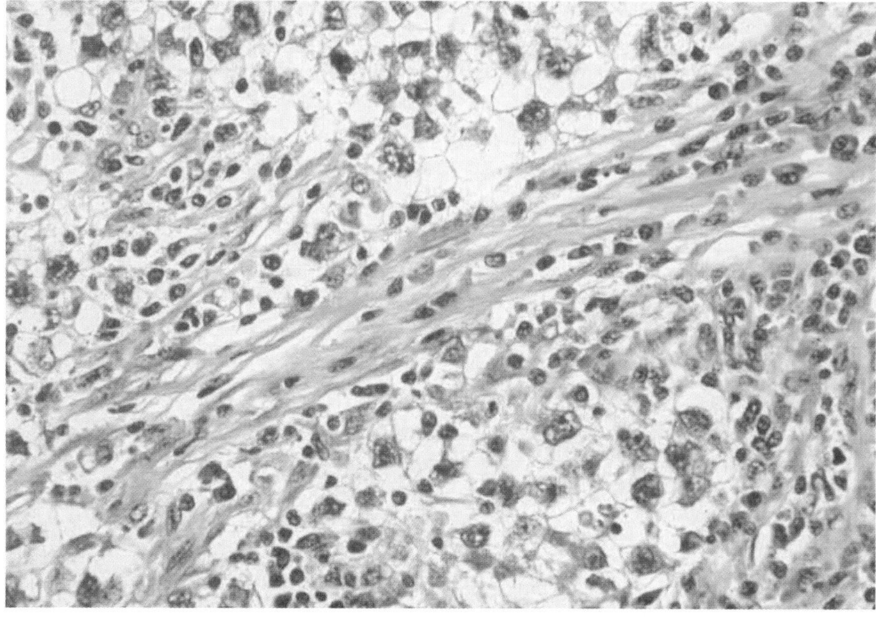

Fig. 8.2. Histologic section of dysgerminoma. Large tumor cells with large nuclei, separated by bands of connective tissue with lympho-plasma cel infiltrates. Hematoxylin and eosin stain; original magnification, ×100.

separated by bands of connective tissue infiltrated by lymphocytes (mostly T cells) (Fig. 8.2), plasma cells, polymorphonuclear leukocytes, and often multinucleated giant cells, with occasional granuloma formation. The histological appearance of an ovarian dysgerminoma is quite similar to that of the testicular seminoma.

The tumor cells stain positive with placenta-specific alkaline phosphatase (PLAP) and glycogen (PAS). Also reported is expression of the c-Kit proto-oncogene product (CD 117) [5,6] and OCT-4 nuclear staining [7]. Occasionally, there are syncytiotrophoblastic large multinucleated cells among the tumor germ cells which stain positive for HCG. The

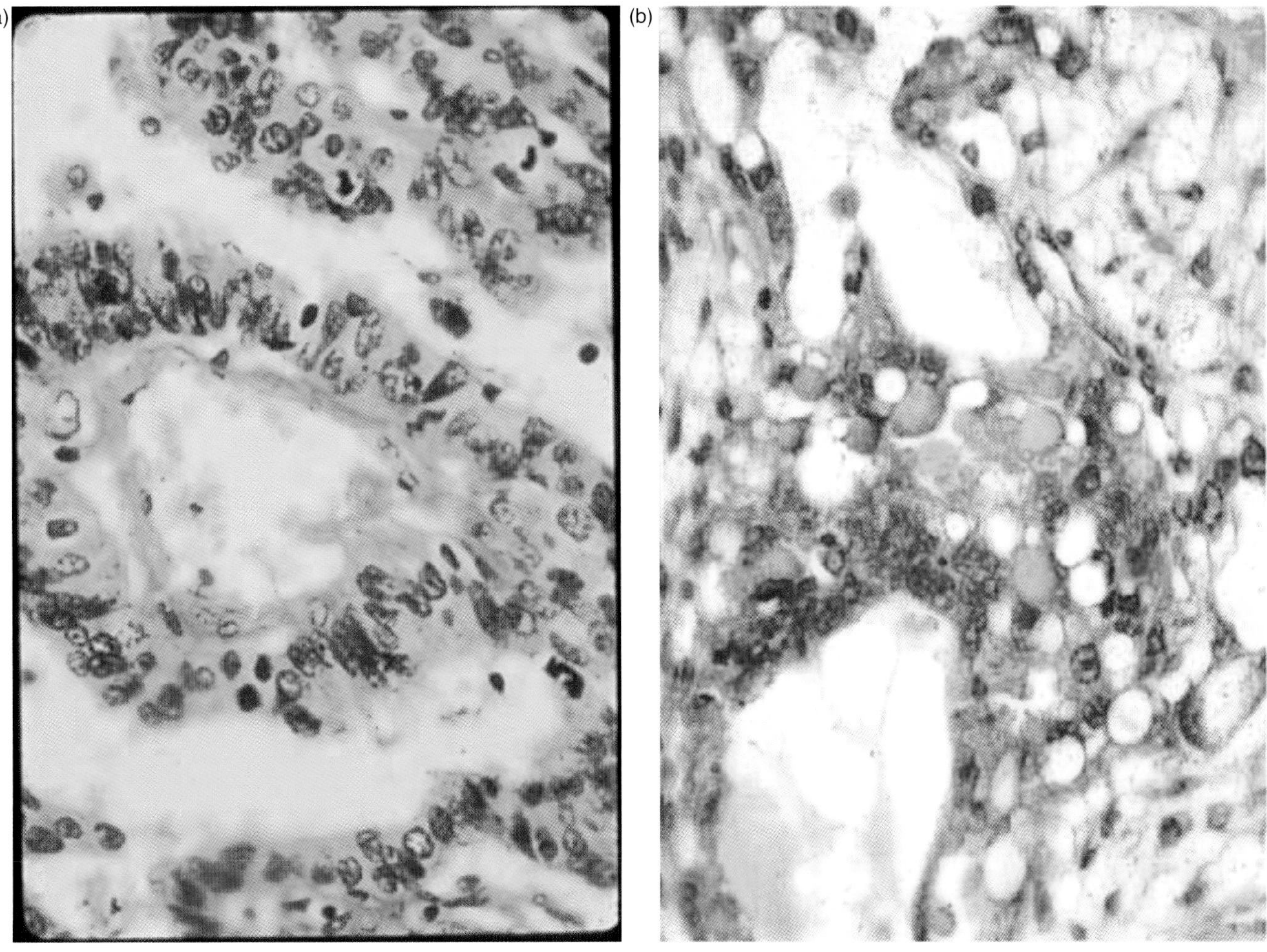

Fig. 8.3. (a) Yolk sac tumor with Schiller-Duval body composed of a central blood vessel surrounded by highly atypical epithelial cells. (b) Yolk sac tumor with eosinophilic bodies that stain positive for alpha-fetoprotein (AFP). Hematoxylin and eosin stain; original magnification, ×100.

diagnosis of choriocarcinoma, however, also requires the presence of cytotrophoblastic cells and a marked serum elevation of Beta HCG.

Dysgerminoma is an aggressively proliferating tumor invading the ovarian parenchyma, the neighboring pelvic and abdominal structures, and metastasizing later to lungs, bones, and other sites by means of hematogenous spread. The metastatic tumors may include other germ cell neoplastic elements. Elevated levels of serum lactic dehydrogenase (LDH) and their isoenzymes 1 and 2 serve as tumor markers for diagnosis and follow-ups [8]. Sa114 is highly sensitive and specific for primitive GCT including dysgerminoma [9]. Most recurrences occur in the first 2 years after diagnosis.

Yolk sac tumor (endodermal sinus tumor)

This is the second most common malignant germ cell tumor, often mixed with other GCT types. It is more often diagnosed in recent years because of better defined diagnostic criteria.

This tumor, like the dysgerminoma, is more often encountered during the second and third decade, and rarely in later life. The tumors grow rapidly, invading the ovary and surrounding tissues, and resulting in increased abdominal girth and pain. They are usually unilateral but may be associated with a contralateral dermoid cyst. Grossly, they present as soft grayish masses with necrotic and hemorrhagic areas and a moist, mucoid cut surface. Bilateral tumors are metastatic.

Their microscopic appearance includes a large variety of histologic patterns, which, therefore, may create diagnostic problems, especially when only one type of tumor tissue is present. The tumor structures repeat somehow the appearance of the primitive yolk sac as demonstrated by Teilum [10]. The polyvesicular vitelline pattern displays small cysts with a central constriction resembling a figure of eight lined by columnar to flat epithelium surrounded by connective tissue that can be loose and edematous. Other primitive embryonal structures are the hepatoid and the intestinal patterns resembling glandular elements. A fairly common histologic feature, although not always present, is the Schiller–Duval body consisting of a central blood vessel surrounded by highly atypical epithelial cells (Fig. 8.3A). Microcystic, macrocystic, and solid histologic patterns are usually seen in various combinations with other (papillary, myxomatous) features often posing diagnostic difficulties. The hallmark is the Schiller–Duval body, which, however is not always present, and the diagnosis as well as the

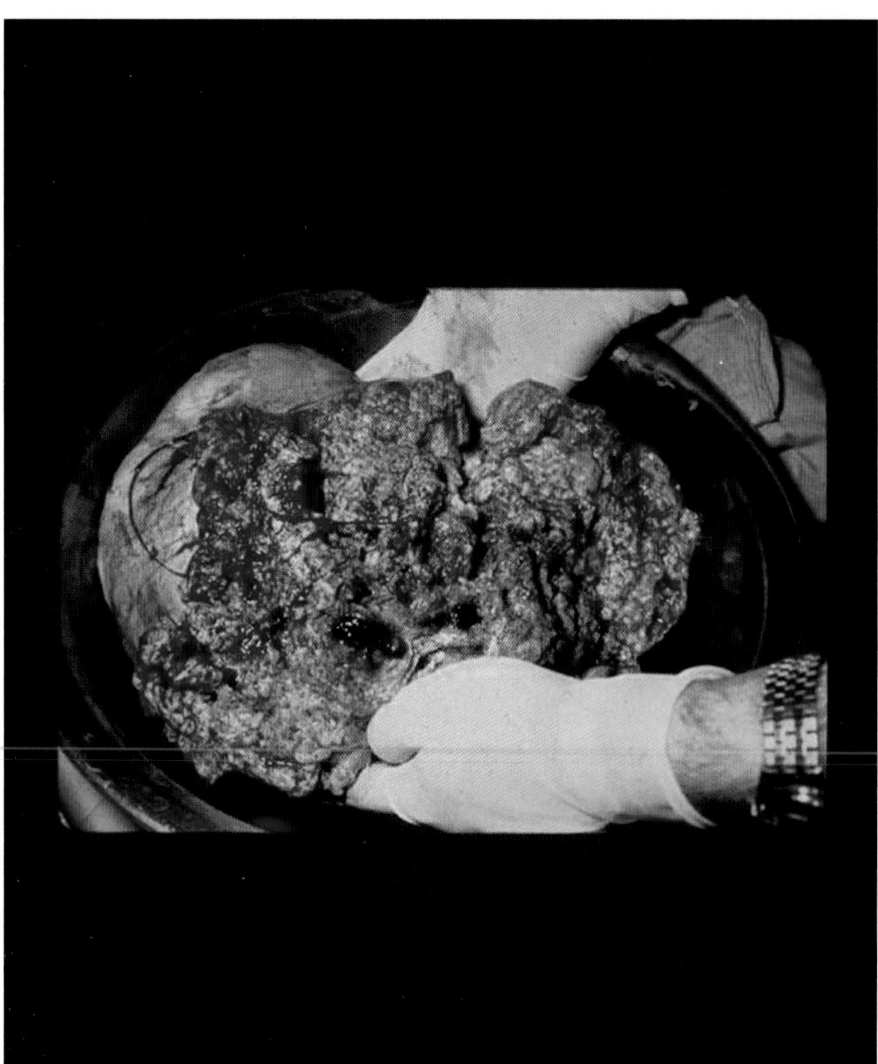

Fig. 8.4. Large embryonal tumor with hemorrhage and necrosis.

follow-up of the patient is based on alpha-fetoprotein (AFP) levels in the serum. AFP is also positive in the tumor tissue as well as low molecular keratin stains [11].

The histologic differential diagnosis is with clear cell and endometrioid carcinomas which are seen in older women and present a different immuno-reactivity [12].

In most yolk sac tumors, there are hyaline intra- and extra-cellular eosinophilic bodies (Fig. 8.3B) that stain positive with DPAS and AFP. The latter is a tumor marker that should be monitored in the patients' serum for diagnosis and follow-up during chemotherapy.

This tumor is highly malignant and diffusely invasive. Chemotherapy however is successful in most cases, especially when started early.

Clinically, the large pelvic masses may produce severe acute symptoms due to torsion of the tumor. Yolk sac tumor like dysgerminoma may be diagnosed during pregnancy because of the child-bearing age of the patients.

As mentioned, chemotherapy has considerably changed the outlook of this aggressively growing malignant tumor, especially the highly effective combination chemotherapy with complete cure in about 80% of cases (see Chapter 30).

Other rare ovarian germ cell tumors, characterized by their occurrence in young patients and aggressive growth, often presenting in combination with yolk sac tumors, are:

(1) *Embryonal carcinoma* occurs in gonads of both sexes, more often in the testes. It is rarely pure being associated with other germ cell neoplasms, like yolk sac tumors and choriocarcinoma. It is composed of primitive embryonal tissues and considered to be the least differentiated form of GCT. It occurs almost always in children and young adults and may manifest clinically with precocious puberty and positive pregnancy test (if choriocarcinoma is part of it). The tumor is large, partly hemorrhagic and necrotic (Fig. 8.4). Microscopically, there are solid aggregates of undifferentiated pleomorphic cells and occasionally non-gestational syncytial trophoblastic cells, histologically similar to those seen in gestational trophoblastic tumor.

(2) *Non-gestational choriocarcinoma* occurs rarely in pure form, usually being a component of mixed GCT. It is a large, solid, unilateral tumor with an occasional contralateral dermoid cyst. The tumor is highly malignant and invasive, hemorrhagic, and necrotic and metastasizes

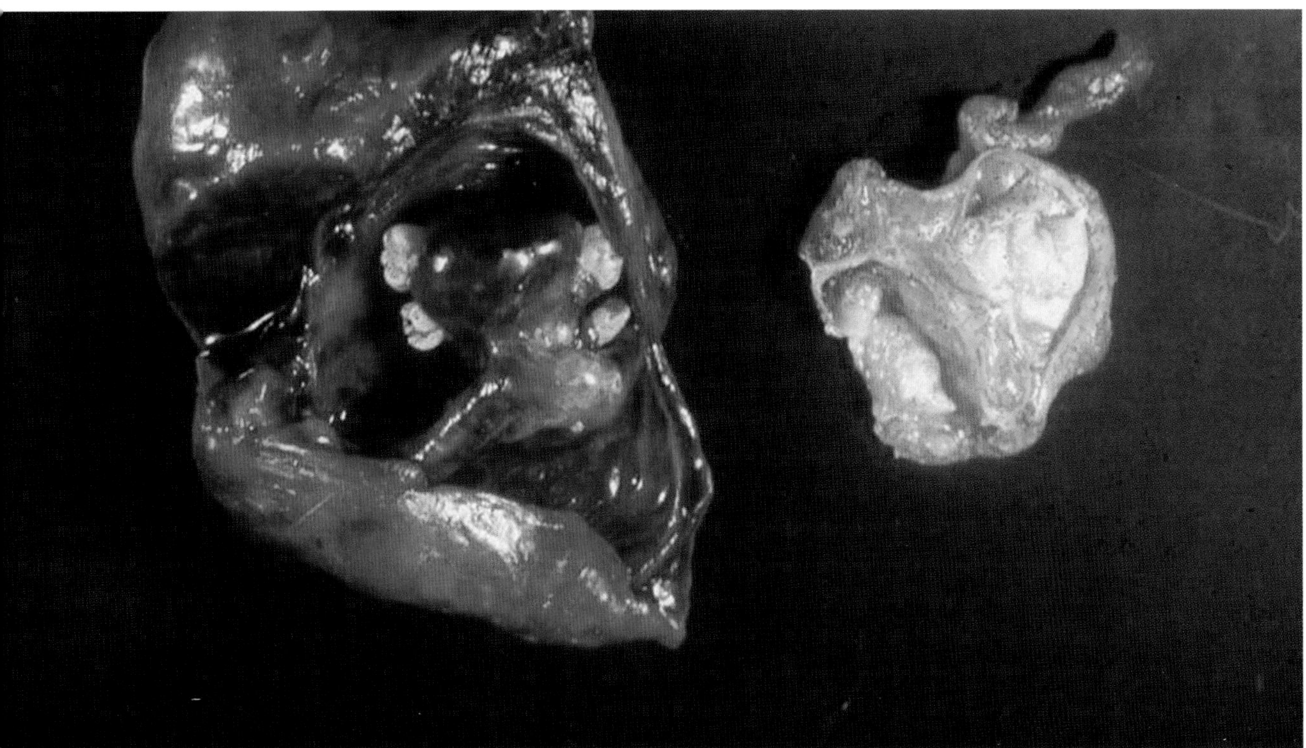

Fig. 8.5. Bilateral dermoid tumor in a 12-year-old girl. Left dermoid tumor with hemorrhagic infarction due to torsion (right).

widely as does its gestational counterpart. Histologically the pattern is biphasic being composed of cyto-and syncytiotrophoblastic cells, displaying large multinucleated cells and bizarre, irregular nuclei with a high mitotic activity. The hallmark of this tumor is the presence of elevated levels of human chorionic gonadotropins (HCG), especially of the β subunit which does not cross-react with the luteinizing hormone (LH), in the serum and urine, as well as in the tumor tissue, representing a reliable tumor marker for the diagnosis and follow-up of this neoplasm. Clinically, the patients may present with hemorrhagic masses, thyreotoxicosis, vaginal bleeding, and sometimes with signs of precocious puberty. Grossly, choriocarcinoma is a large unilateral grayish and hemorrhagic mass, and microscopically, cytotrophoblastic and syncytiotrophoblastic cells are seen in various proportions, surrounded by blood and necrotic tissue. The tumor spreads by means of both lymphatic and blood stream.

3) *Polyembryoma* is an extremely rare tumor component characterized by the presence of embryoid bodies that include a central disc and yolk sac as well as an amniotic cavity.

Ovarian teratomas

These GCT are composed of embryonal tissues differentiated along the lines of somatic embryonal development including endodermal, mesodermal and especially ectodermal tissues. Ninety-nine percent of all teratomas are benign, being composed of mature tissues (dermoid tumors). Basically, ovarian germ cell tumors that are mature are benign. In malignant teratomas the degree of malignancy is related to the extent of immature tissue present in the tumor. The histogenesis of teratomas is now considered to be through parthenogenesis because they develop during the reproductive years and their karyotype is female 46,XX. Teratomas are classified into mature (benign dermoid cysts), monodermal and immature.

A. *Mature cystic teratoma (dermoid cyst).* This is a quite common ovarian tumor representing 20% of all ovarian tumors. It is found in women of all ages, unlike the other germ cell tumors, although seen predominately during the reproductive years and sometime even in fetuses and newborns. Dermoid tumors are often incidental findings on physical examination. In younger patients, they may present with acute symptoms due to torsion and hemorrhagic infarction (Fig. 8.5). In 10% of cases, the tumor is diagnosed during pregnancy, when it may present with torsion and rare rupture of the cyst. A rare complication is hemolytic anemia. Most teratomas are cystic, uniloculated; they are bilateral in about 15% of cases. Occasionally, multiple tumors are present in the same ovary. The tissues composing a mature teratoma originate in all three embryonal layers, endoderm, mesoderm, and ectoderm, the latter being mostly represented by skin and skin appendages, and by neural tissue. In addition, the most frequent tissues observed on routine microscopic examination are adipose tissue, bone, cartilage, intestinal, bronchial, and thyroid tissue (Fig. 8.6). Arising from the cyst wall is a nipple-like protuberance covered by skin with hair, often containing bone and teeth. There is no axial arrangement of these tissues; however, there is a degree of vicinity-induced tissue organization such as skin next to subcutaneous fat and hair follicles, thyroid tissue next to cartilage, choroid plexus next to central nervous tissue, and to retinal anlage, etc. Teeth are often seen adjacent to mandibular bone. The cystic cavity contains a yellowish liquid (at temperature >34°C) material resulting from sebum secretion of the skin

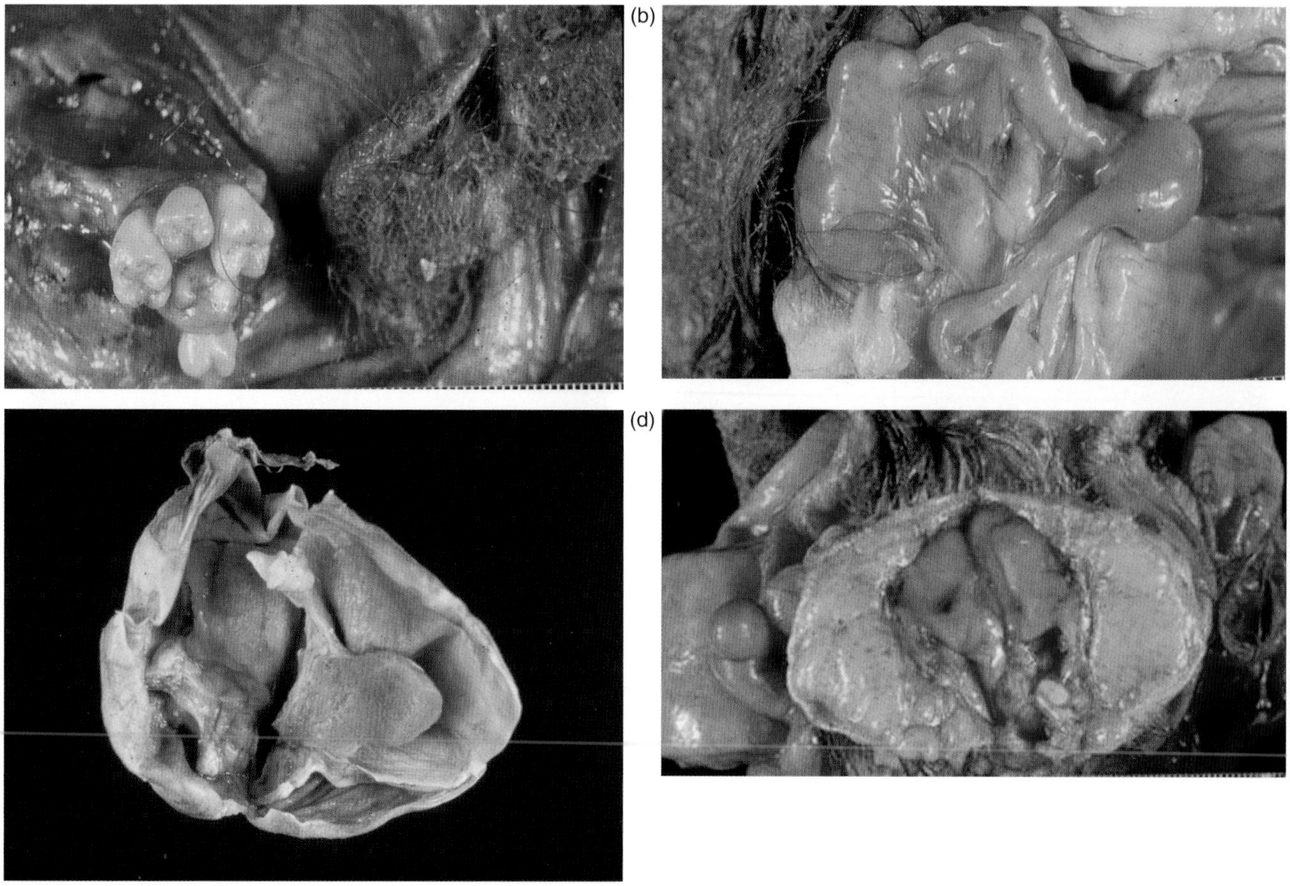

Fig. 8.6. (a) Benign cystic teratoma in a 22-year-old female with teeth and hair. (b) Benign cystic teratoma in a 17-year-old female with portion of intestine and Meckel's diverticulum. (c) Benign cystic teratoma with thyroid tissue (center). D: Dermoid cyst with hair, skin, and subcutaneous fat.

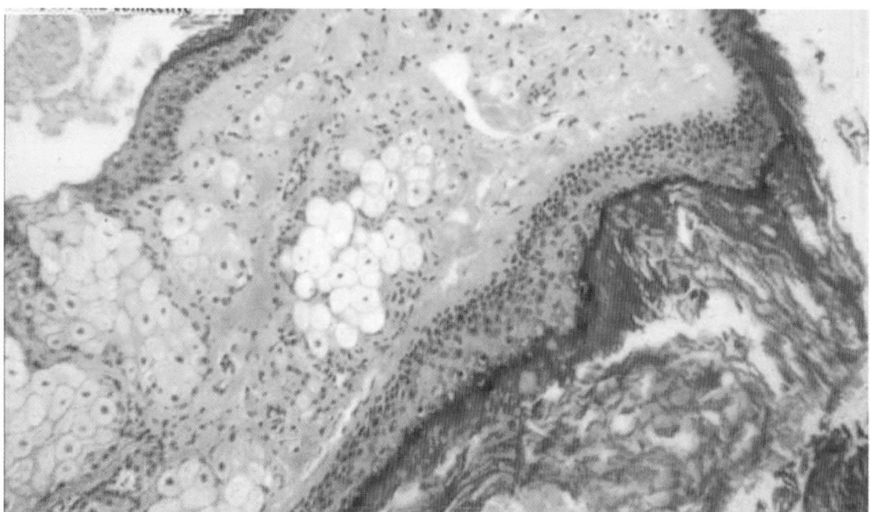

Fig. 8.7. Nipple-like structure in a dermoid tumor covered by epidermal squamous epithelium, with underlying sebaceous glands. Hematoxylin and eosin stain; original magnification, ×40.

adnexa, and hair produced by numerous hair follicles located in the dermis (Fig. 8.7). Solid mature teratomas are rare and should be sampled extensively to rule out the presence of immature tissue components.

Sebum and hair shafts often elicit a foreign body microscopic reaction with giant cells and histiocytic proliferation.

All tissues are mature. It is recommended to perform a thorough histologic examination of benign-appearing teratomas in older patients because of occasional (2% of cases) malignant transformation arising in mature tissues, such as squamous cell carcinoma of the skin (Fig. 8.8), thyroid carcinoma, chondrosarcoma, carcinoid, malignant melanoma, and mucinous adenocarcinoma arising in glandular structures. Their prognosis is unfavorable [13–15].

Mature neural tissue is found occasionally in the peritoneal cavity (gliomatosis peritonealis). Most often the neural tissue is benign; however, immature neural tissue can be identified especially in immature teratomas (Fig. 8.9).

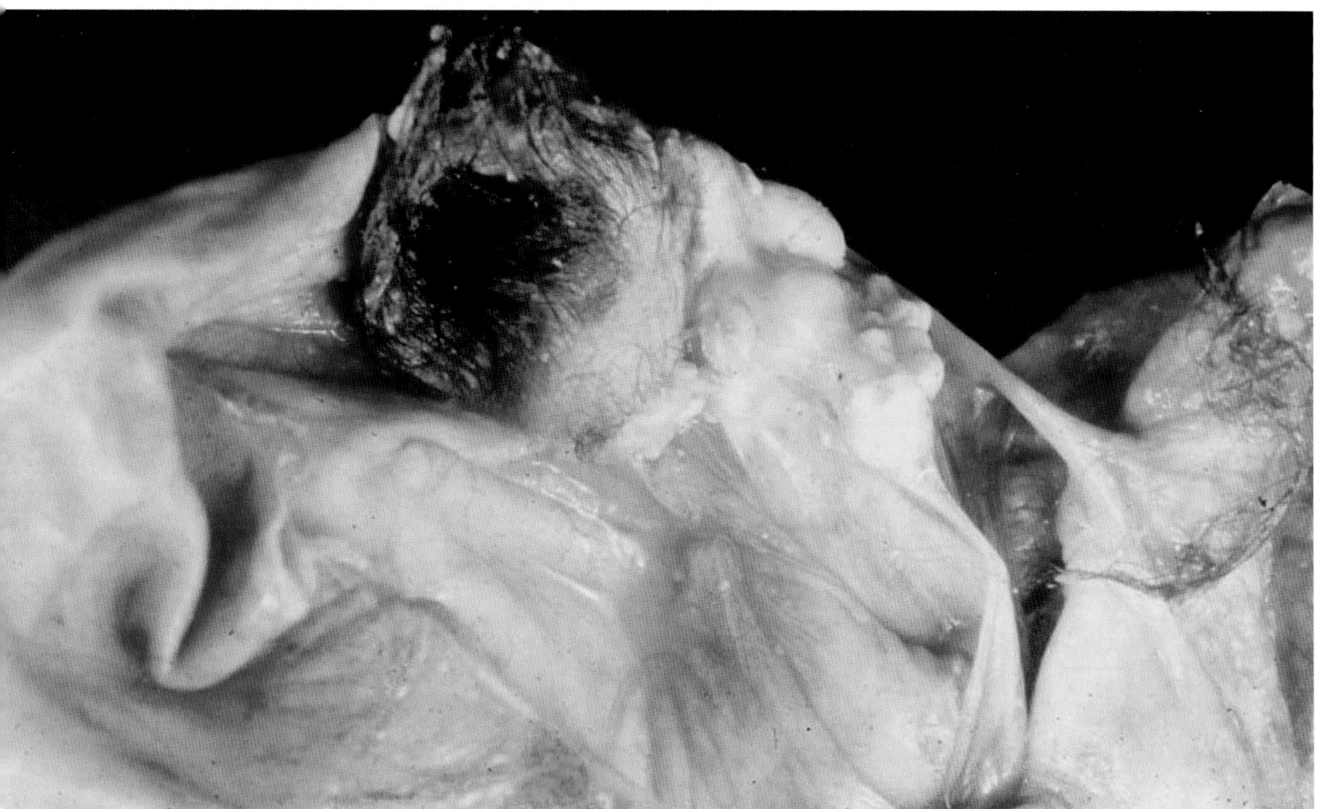

Fig. 8.8. Squamous cell carcinoma (arrow) arising in the skin of a mature teratoma with hair and teeth (dermoid tumor) removed from a 67-year-old patient.

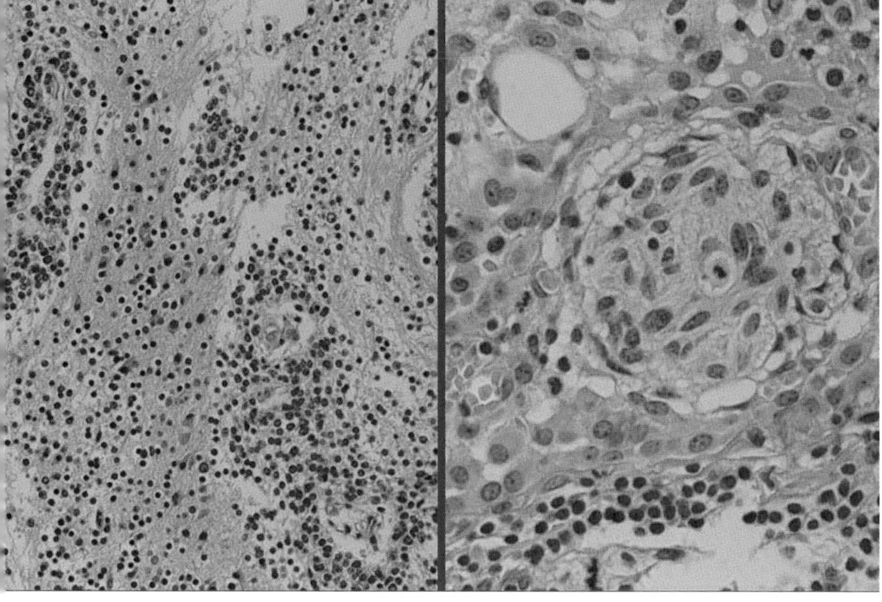

Fig. 8.9. Mature and immature neural tissue found in the peritoneum (gliomatosis peritonealis). Hematoxylin and eosin stain; original magnifications, ×100 and 400.

B. *Monodermal teratomas.* These are composed of one predominant type of tissue, the most frequent being thyroid tissue (struma ovarii) [16,17].

Struma ovarii consists of an overgrowth of thyroid tissue replacing or predominating over the other components [10] seen in patients of all ages, more often in younger individuals, grossly resembling thyroid tissue, solid or cystic, sometimes with necrosis and hemorrhage. Microscopically there are thyroid acini of various sizes, containing colloid (Fig. 8.10a) and papillary projections, with areas of nodular adenomatous-like follicles and rare atypical proliferation and/or thyroiditis. Most cases are benign, and are sometime associated with hyperthyroidism which usually disappears after the surgical removal of the lesion. Thyroid carcinomas arising in struma ovarii are rare [18]. These are papillary and follicular carcinomas, and strumal carcinoids, and their biological behavior is unpredictable; they may metastasize and/or recur in extra-ovarian locations [19,20].

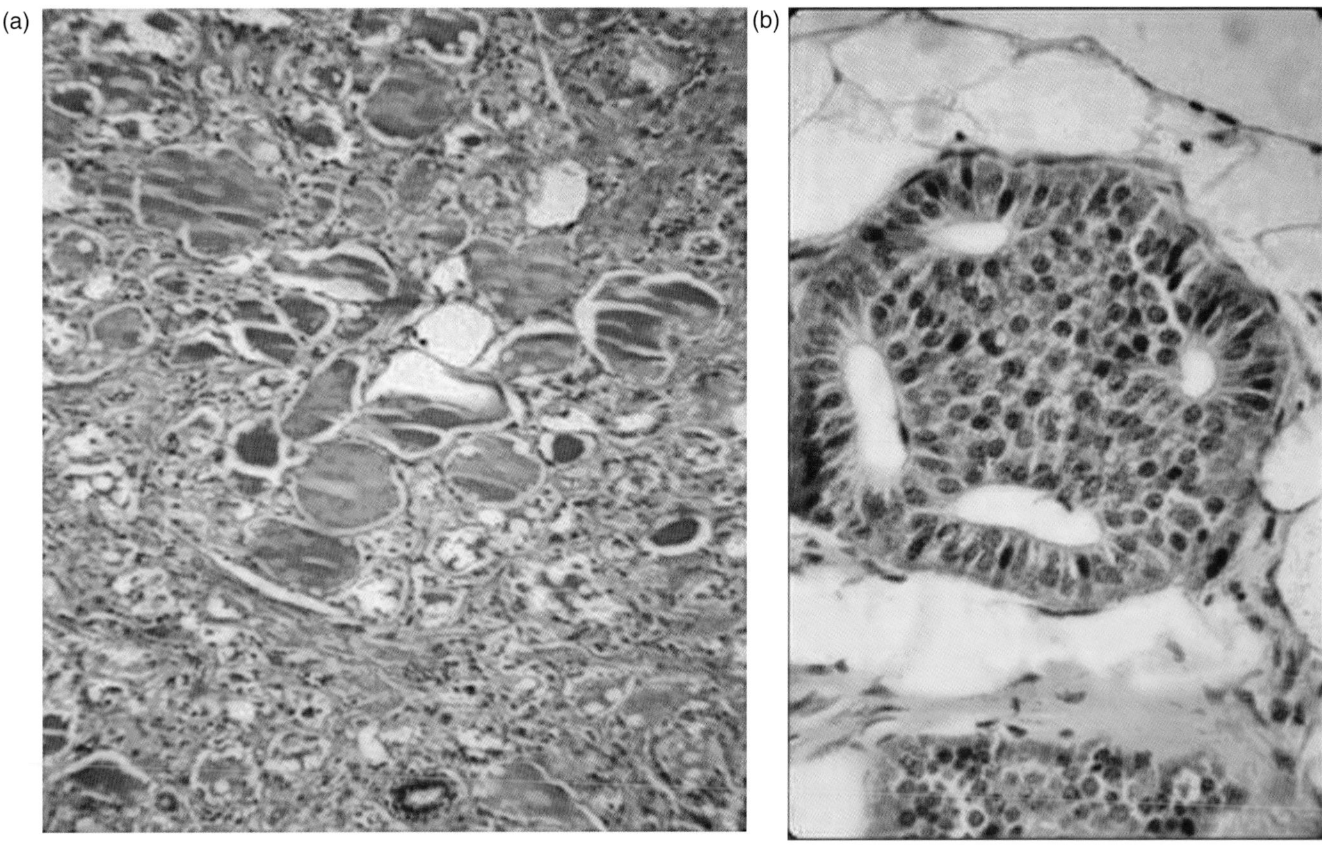

Fig. 8.10. Monodermal teratoma. (a) Struma ovarii composed of thyroid follicles with colloid content. Hematoxylin and eosin stain; original magnification, ×40. (b) Ovarian carcinoid tumor, insular type. Hematoxylin and eosin stain; original magnification, ×100.

Carcinoid tumors can be primary ovarian neoplasms arising in germ cell tumors. They are uncommon and have to be distinguished from metastatic ovarian carcinoid tumors. Histologically they are insular, trabecular, strumal, and mucinous. The most common is the insular, arising from endodermal components of the teratomas (Fig. 8.10b). Histologically the tumor cells are characteristically composed of nests of cells with neurosecretory granules staining positive for chromogranin and synaptophysin. Carcinoid syndrome is found in larger tumors and disappears after the surgical removal of the tumor [21,22].

Mucinous carcinoid is rare and has to be distinguished from metastatic appendiceal carcinoma and from Krukenberg tumor. This is a unilateral tumor that can be large, solid or cystic, composed of small glands lined by cuboidal cells, some with goblet cells distended with mucin and some with neuroendocrine cells; some tumors exhibit a mixed pattern. Immuno-histologic stains are positive for neuro-secretory granules. The tumor is more malignant than other carcinoids and is often diagnosed with metastatic spread.

Strumal carcinoid is an uncommon ovarian tumor composed of thyroid and carcinoid tissue, the latter displaying trabecular patterns merging with thyroid epithelium. It may be part of a teratoma, with other tissues present.

Mucinous tumors arising in mature cystic teratomas are not very rare (up to 11%) [23]. As the mucinous ovarian tumors arising from the surface epithelium, they may be benign cystadenomas, borderline, and adenocarcinomas, sometimes associated with pseudomyxoma ovarii. Pseudomyxoma peritonei more often originates in mucinous tumors of the appendix [24]. The microscopic lining of the glands and cysts that compose these tumors is columnar or goblet cells. These tumors are primary ovarian if other teratomatous elements can be identified [25]. Otherwise, as mentioned in Chapter 4, most malignant mucinous tumors of the ovary are metastatic from the GIT.

Other monodermal teratomas with one type of tissue over growing the other components are rare. They are neuroectodermal, vascular, sebaceous tumors, all composed of mature tissue.

Peritoneal implants are seen infrequently. Despite their extensive involvement of the peritoneal cavity their presence does not affect the prognosis.

C. *Immature teratomas*. These tumors are also composed of derivatives from the three embryonic layers containing immature and embryonal tissues admixed with mature tissues. Immature teratomas are rare compared with mature teratomas (dermoids) (1% vs. 99%) [26,27].

Immature teratomas occur more often in younger individuals, in childhood and early adolescence and grow rapidly, producing symptoms due to compression of pelvic and abdominal organs, and often torsion with acute abdominal pain.

The tumors are usually unilateral, sometime with a contralateral dermoid (10–15% of cases). They are larger than dermoid tumors and are solid and cystic with a variegated cut surface displaying cartilage, cysts, lobules, and fat (Fig. 8.11a).

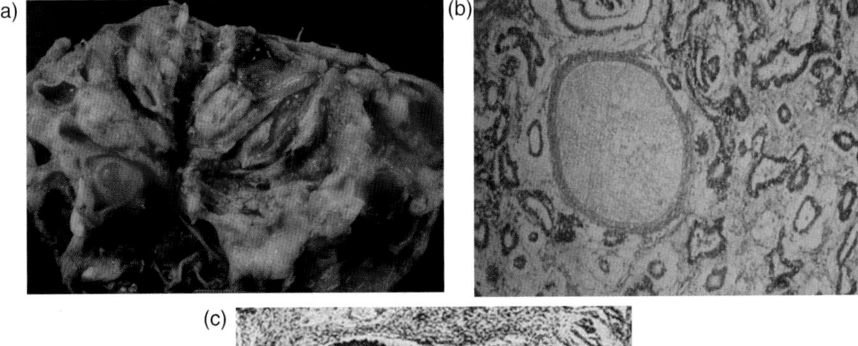

Fig. 8.11. (a) Immature teratoma in an 11-year-old female. Solid tumor with a variegated cut section. (b) Immature teratoma displaying a mixture of mature and immature tissues Hematoxylin and eosin stain; original magnification, ×40. (c) Immature teratoma: rosette-like immature neural tubules. Hematoxylin and eosin stain; original magnification, ×100.

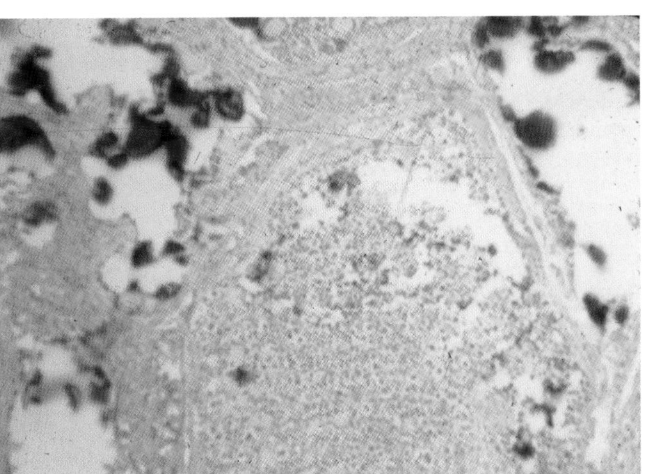

Fig. 8.12. Sex cord elements, primitive germ cells, and calcifications in gonadoblastoma. Hematoxylin and eosin stain; original magnification, ×40.

Histologically, there are derivatives of all three germ layers present, with neural tissue most often predominating. Mature tissue is seen admixed with immature elements (Fig. 8.11b). The grading of immature teratomas is based on the aggregate amount of immature neuro-epithelium on any single slide [10]. Initially, three grades were proposed but more recently two grades are considered to establish a good correlation with the clinical behavior of the tumor [28]. One block of tissue per centimeter should be sampled for histologic examination.

Any tissue component, such as mesenchymal and endodermal-originating glandular tissue may show undifferentiated areas (primitive embryonal tumor tissue) in immature teratomas. However, the grading and the subsequent management of the patient are based on the extent of immature neuro-ectodermal tissue (neuro-ectodermal rosette-like structures, immature glia) (Fig. 8.11c). The presence of yolk sac tumor components in teratomas is considered as predictive of recurrence [28]. Immature teratomas are seen more frequently in male gonads than in the ovaries. Chemotherapy is successful and curative in most cases, especially when the tumor is confined to the gonads.

The presence of peritoneal implants, both mature and immature neural tissue, is not uncommon. "Gliomatosis peritonei" consists of widespread whitish nodules on the peritoneal serosa composed of mature glial tissue. Its presence does not change the grade of the tumor. The management is based on the grading of the primary tumor.

D. *Mixed GCT.* These include multiple neoplastic germ cell tissues admixed with each other or separate. They are classified according to the predominant elements and should be sampled extensively. For example, in immature teratomas of children, the presence and extent of yolk sac tumor elements should be mentioned as it is important for the management.

Ovarian mixed GCT and sex-cord tumors

Gonadoblastoma is a rare tumor associated with abnormalities of sexual development [29,30]. Microscopically it is composed of primitive sex cord elements, sertoliform cords, and luteinized steroid-secreting cells, hyaline nodules, and dysgerminoma, often with calcified nodules (Fig. 8.12). Dysgerminoma and/or other malignant GCT may overgrow the sex-cord tumor elements resulting in a worse prognosis than that of the combined dysgerminoma – sex cord tumor.

References

1. Seidman JD, Cho KR, Ronnett BM, et al. Blaustein's pathology of the female genital tract, 6th edition. In: Kurman RJ, Hedrick Ellenson L, Ronnett BM. (Eds.). Germ Cell Tumors. Chapter 16. New York: Springer Science & Business Media; 2011, p. 850.
2. Schwartz IS, Cohen CJ, Deligdisch L. Dysgerminoma of the ovary associated with true hermaphroditism. Obstet Gynecol. 1980;**56**(1):102–6.
3. Letterie GS, Page DC. Dysgerminoma and gonadal dysgenesis in a 46,XX female with no evidence of Y chromosomal DNA. Gynecol Oncol. 1995;**57**(3):423–5.
4. Obata NH, Nakashima N, Kawai M, et al. Gonadoblastoma with dysgerminoma in one ovary and gonadoblastoma with dysgerminoma and yolk sac tumor in the contralateral ovary in a girl with 46XX karyotype. Gynecol Oncol. 1995;**58**(1):124–8.
5. Sever M, Jones TD, Roth LM, et al. Expression of CD117 (c-kit) receptor in dysgerminoma of the ovary: diagnostic and therapeutic implications. Mod Pathol. 2005;**18**(11):1411–16.
6. Hoei-Hansen CE, Kraggerud SM, Abeler VM, et al. Ovarian dysgerminomas are characterised by frequent KIT mutations and abundant expression of pluripotency markers. Mol Cancer. 2007;**6**:12.
7. Cheng L, Thomas A, Roth LM, et al. OCT4: a novel biomarker for dysgerminoma of the ovary. Am J Surg Pathol. 2004;**28**(10):1341–6.
8. Schwartz PE, Morris JM. Serum lactic dehydrogenase: a tumor marker for dysgerminoma. Obstet Gynecol. 1988;**72**(3 Pt 2):511–15.
9. Cao D, Li J, Guo CC, et al. SALL4 is a novel diagnostic marker for testicular germ cell tumors. Am J Surg Pathol. 2009;**33**(7):1065–77.
10. Teilum G. Endodermal sinus tumors of the ovary and testis. Comparative morphogenesis of the so-called mesoephroma ovarii (Schiller) and extraembryonic (yolk sac-allantoic) structures of the rat's placenta. Cancer. 1959;**12**:1092–105.
11. Ramalingam P, Malpica A, Silva EG, et al. The use of cytokeratin 7 and EMA in differentiating ovarian yolk sac tumors from endometrioid and clear cell carcinomas. Am J Surg Pathol. 2004;**28**(11):1499–505.
12. Esheba GE, Pate LL, Longacre TA. Oncofetal protein glypican-3 distinguishes yolk sac tumor from clear cell carcinoma of the ovary. Am J Surg Pathol. 2008;**32**(4):600–7.
13. Krumerman MS, Chung A. Squamous carcinoma arising in benign cystic teratoma of the ovary: a report of four cases and review of the literature. Cancer. 1977;**39**(3):1237–42.
14. Chumas JC, Scully RE. Sebaceous tumors arising in ovarian dermoid cysts. Int J Gynecol Pathol. 1991;**10** (4):356–63.
15. Gupta D, Deavers MT, Silva EG, et al. Malignant melanoma involving the ovary: a clinicopathologic and immunohistochemical study of 23 cases. Am J Surg Pathol. 2004;**28**(6):771–80.
16. Roth LM, Talerman A. The enigma of struma ovarii. Pathology. 2007;**39** (1):139–46.
17. Devaney K, Synder R, Norris HJ, et al. Proliferative and histologically malignant struma ovarii: a clinicopathologic study of 54 cases. Int J Gynecol Pathol. 1993;**12**:333–43.
18. Robboy SJ, Shaco-Levy R, Peng RY, et al. Malignant struma ovarii: an analysis of 88 cases, including 27 with extraovarian spread. Int J Gynecol Pathol. 2009;**28** (5):405–22.
19. Roth LM, Miller AWII, Talerman A. Typical thyroid type carcinoma arising in struma ovarii: a report of 4 cases and review of the literature. Int J Gynecol Pathol. 2008;**27**:496–506.
20. Garg K, Soslow RA, Rivera M, et al. Histologically bland "extremely well-differentiated" thyroid carcinomas arising in struma ovarii can recur and metastasize. Int J Gynecol Pathol. 2009;**28**(3):222–30.
21. Davis KP, Hartmann LK, Keeney GL, et al. Primary ovarian carcinoid tumors. Gynecol Oncol. 1996;**61**(2):259–65.
22. Rabban JT, Lerwill MF, McCluggage WG, et al. Primary ovarian carcinoid tumors may express CDX-2: a potential pitfall in distinction from metastatic intestinal carcinoid tumors involving the ovary. Int J Gynecol Pathol. 2009;**28**(1):41–8.
23. Vang R, Gown AM, Zhao C, et al. Ovarian mucinous tumors associated with mature cystic teratomas: morphologic and immunohistochemical analysis identifies a subset of potential teratomatous origin that shares features of lower gastrointestinal tract mucinous tumors more commonly encountered as secondary tumors in the ovary. Am J Surg Pathol. 2007;**31**(6):854–69.
24. McKenney JK, Soslow RA, Longacre TA. Ovarian mature teratomas with mucinous epithelial neoplasms: morphologic heterogeneity and association with pseudomyxoma peritonei. Am J Surg Pathol. 2008;**32** (5):645–55.
25. Hristov AC, Young RH, Vang R, et al. Ovarian metastases of appendiceal tumors with goblet cell carcinoidlike and signet ring cell patterns: a report of 30 cases. Am J Surg Pathol. 2007;**31**(10):1502–11.
26. Norris HJ, Zirkin HJ, Benson WL. Immature (malignant) teratomas of the ovary: a clinical and pathologic study of 58 cases. Cancer. 1976;**37** (5):2359–72.
27. Heifetz SA, Cushing B, Giller R, et al. Immature teratomas in children: pathologic considerations: a report from the combined Pediatric Oncology Group/Children's Cancer Group. Am J Surg Pathol. 1998;**22**(9):1115–24.
28. Talerman A, Roth LM. Recent advances in the pathology and classification of gonadal neoplasms composed of germ cells and sex cord derivatives. Int J Gynecol Pathol. 2007;**26**(3):313–21.
29. Scully RE. Gonadoblastoma. A review of 74 cases. Cancer. 1970;**25**(6):1340–56.
30. Park IJ, Pyeatte JC, Jones HW, Woodruff JD Jr. Gonadoblastoma in a true hermaphrodite with 46, XY genotype. Obstet Gynecol. 1972;**40**(4):466–72.

Chapter 9

Metastatic ovarian tumors

Angelica Mareş, MD, and Liane Deligdisch, MD

Introduction

Aside from primary ovarian malignancies, ovaries are a frequent site of metastases from other primary tumors, mostly from the gastrointestinal tract, breast, and other gynecological organs. Metastatic tumors to the ovaries are an important group of ovarian neoplasms, and their correct pathological interpretation is paramount for the right treatment of the patient.

It can be very difficult for a pathologist to diagnose metastatic disease of the ovary because it often mimics a primary ovarian malignancy. Evaluating the metastatic nature of an ovarian tumor depends on the clinician's and pathologist's knowledge about the frequency of metastases of different primary tumors, a complete clinical history, a careful evaluation and re-evaluation of the gross pathology of the specimen and also, use of special stains and immuno-histochemistry.

The diagnosis of metastatic ovarian tumor should be considered when the anatomical distribution of the disease is atypical for primary ovarian cancer, when the patient has another tumor outside the ovaries and when both ovaries are involved by the tumor, although unilaterality of the tumor is not a definite argument against one's metastatic nature (different studies show bilaterality of ovarian metastatic tumors in approximately 70% of cases) [1,2]. Other tumoral findings suggestive of metastasis are: size less than 10 cm, tumor grossly visible on the surface of the ovary, presence of multiple tumor nodules often growing in a desmoplastic stroma, and lymphatic and/or blood vessels invasion (more pronounced in the ovarian hilum).

The frequency of metastases to the ovaries varies with the different incidence of the primary tumors in different geographical areas (for instance, in Japan and in Hawaii there is a higher prevalence of gastric cancer and hence there will be a higher incidence of Krukenberg tumors, as opposed to Africa or Australia, where this type of cancer is relatively rare). Also, the age distribution of patients with ovarian metastases depends on that of the primary tumors but it was noticed that the average age of patients with ovarian metastatic involvement is significantly lower than in cases of cancer patients without ovarian spread (fact possibly explained by the higher receptivity for metastases of the richly vascularized ovaries of younger women).

For multiple reasons, it is not possible to calculate exactly the frequency of metastatic ovarian tumors. There were numerous studies done on the subject, which showed different results; these could be explained by a meta-analysis showing different inclusion criteria for different studies, such as autopsy findings versus surgical specimens, or clinically silent tumors found in prophylactic oophorectomy specimens versus incidentally detected metastatic ovarian tumors during surgery for other abdominal pathology. In practice though, the important figure for the clinician, as well as for the pathologist, is the overall probability that an ovarian neoplasm is metastatic, and this figure is about 5–10% [3,4].

Tumors spread to the ovaries from extra-genital sites or from other sites in the genital tract by several routes: hematogenous dissemination (by means of blood vessels and lymphatics), dissemination through the peritoneal fluid (from intra-abdominal cancers), direct extension (especially from other genital cancers, from mesotheliomas or from colon carcinomas), and transtubal spread (most often from endometrial or cervical carcinomas).

A concise classification of metastatic ovarian tumors is presented in Table 9.1.

Gastric cancer: metastatic tumors with signet-ring cells

The most frequent tumors to metastasize to the ovary are tumors of the gastrointestinal tract, and of these, most frequently encountered are Krukenberg tumors, defined as "metastatic tumors histologically characterized by at least 10% mucin-filled neoplastic signet-ring cells." Krukenberg tumors were originally described by Sir James Paget in 1854 but the eponym is credited to Dr. Friedrich Krukenberg who in 1896 published five case reports of these tumors which he thought to be a new type of ovarian tumor, "Ueber das Fibrosarcoma ovarii mucocellulare (carcinomates) von Dr. Friedrich Krukenberg" [5].

The main sources of these tumors are gastric carcinomas (approximately 70% of cases), followed by carcinomas of the breast, large intestine, and appendix; other rare primary tumors generating Krukenberg tumors are carcinomas of the gallbladder, pancreas, cervix, and urinary bladder. The prevalence of Krukenberg tumors varies mainly with that of gastric carcinoma in different populations; for instance, in Japan their prevalence is almost 20%, but it is much lower in other parts of the world.

Altchek's Diagnosis and Management of Ovarian Disorders, ed. Liane Deligdisch, Nathan G. Kase, and Carmel J. Cohen. Published by Cambridge University Press.

Patients are typically diagnosed with Krukenberg tumors at the average age of 45 years old. It is believed that the young age at diagnosis is related to better vascularization of these patients' ovaries, a fact that facilitates vascular metastasis [5]. Presenting symptoms usually include abdominal pain, distention, ascites, and sometimes abnormal vaginal bleeding and signs of virilization and hirsutism. Krukenberg tumors are bilateral in approximately 80% of cases. The mortality rate for Krukenberg tumors is relatively high and the majority of patients will die within 1 year of diagnosis [3].

Table 9.1. Origins of ovarian metastatic tumors

Extra-genital tumors metastatic to the ovaries
Tumors of the GI tract: carcinoma of the stomach (Krukenberg tumors), intestinal-type adenocarcinoma of the stomach, intestinal carcinoma, appendix tumors, carcinoid and neuroendocrine tumors, pancreatic tumors (UDA, mucinous cystadenocarcinoma and acinar cell carcinoma), tumors of the gallbladder and extra-hepatic bile ducts, tumors of the liver (HCC, intra-hepatic cholangiocarcinoma)
Breast carcinoma
Renal tumors
Tumors of the urinary bladder, ureter, and urethra
Adrenal gland tumors
Malignant melanoma
Pulmonary and mediastinal tumors
Extra-genital sarcomas
Female genital tract tumors metastatic to the ovaries
Fallopian tube carcinoma
Endometrial carcinoma
Cervical carcinoma
Vulvar and vaginal tumors
Peritoneal tumors metastatic to the ovaries
Peritoneal mesotheliomas
Intra-abdominal desmoplastic small round cell tumor

Gross findings: Krukenberg tumors appear as firm, white, round masses that may reach considerable sizes. In general, the outer surface of the tumor is smooth and does not present adhesions. The cut surface is tan-white, with areas of brown-red discoloration, usually uniform or sometimes with ill-defined or discrete nodules. The consistency of Krukenberg tumors is usually firm, but can also be fleshy or gelatinous (Fig. 9.1).

The microscopic findings in Krukenberg tumors can be quite variable. On low-power, distinct tumor nodules are observed, with intervening edematous stroma. The nodules are composed of signet-ring cells and ovarian stromal cells. Other epithelial elements, such as glands and cysts, may be present. The diagnosis requires the presence of signet ring cells but they vary in amount from sheets of cells to very few, barely noticeable even on high power. The architectural disposition of these cells is equally variable, from pseudotubular formations, to clusters of cells or totally random location between the stromal cell, glands, and cysts. Cytologically, signet ring cells have basophilic cytoplasm which compresses the nucleus to the periphery of the cell. Occasionally, the cytoplasm may have a large vacuole with a central eosinophilic body, giving the cell the "bull's eye" appearance (Figs. 9.2, 9.3). The stroma is more often edematous than cellular, sometimes containing pools of mucin.

Krukenberg tumors resemble many other tumors and can be misdiagnosed as Sertoli–Leydig tumors, clear cell carcinomas, mucinous carcinoids, and others. The common presence of blood vessels and lymphatics' invasion is important in the differential diagnosis because, except for other metastatic tumors, other entities in the differential do not have this feature. Also, special diagnostic stains can be used to highlight the presence of signet ring cells and immuno-histochemistry (IHC) can be used to distinguish metastatic carcinoma from primary ovarian neoplasms [6]. The ovarian tumors that are CEA positive, CK20 positive, and CK7 negative are more likely to be of colorectal origin and, hence, Krukenberg (primary ovarian tumors usually test positive for CK7 and negative for

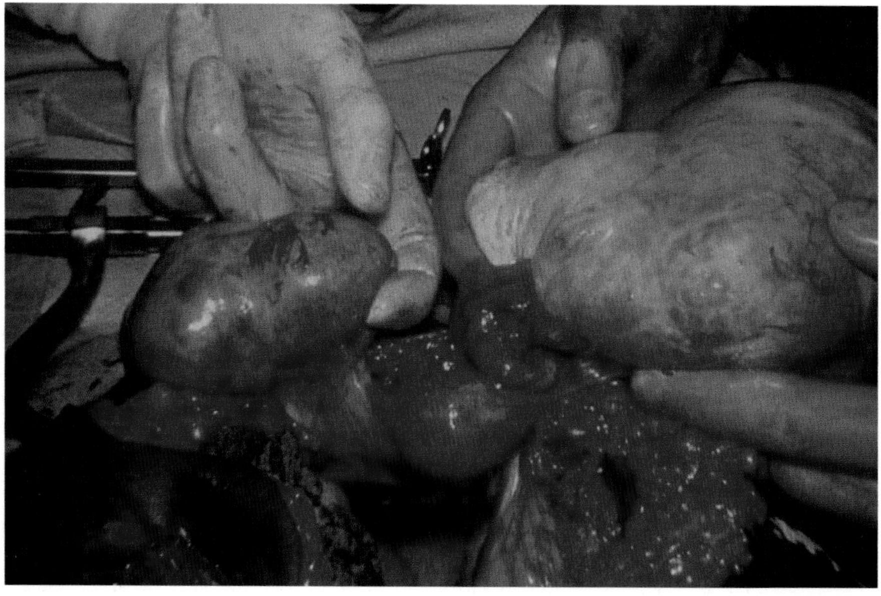

Fig. 9.1. Bilateral metastatic gastric carcinoma; gross picture.

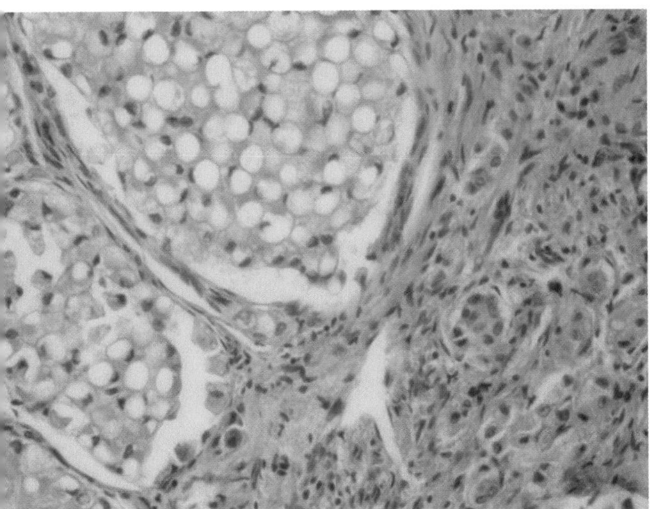

Fig. 9.2. Krukenberg tumor: signet ring cells with intra-cytoplasmic mucinous vacuoles. Hematoxylin and eosin stain.

CK20) [7]. Other immuno-histochemical stains currently under investigation include CD44v6, vascular endothelial growth factor, and matrix metalloproteinases MMP-2 and MMP-9. Tumor marker CA125 is usually elevated in patients with Krukenberg tumors and is found to decrease after tumor resection; therefore CA125 can be used for post-operative follow-up [8]. To distinguish between different primary sites of Krukenberg tumors, few panels of immuno-histochemistry stains were proposed: Muc 1, CK7, and estrogen receptor positive favor breast primary; CDX2, Hep Par 1 positive and estrogen receptor negative favor stomach primary; Muc 2, CDX2, Muc 5AC positive and Muc 1, Hep Par 1, and estrogen receptor negative favor colon primary [9].

Gastric cancer: metastatic intestinal-type adenocarcinoma of the stomach

To date, only a small number of cases of this type were documented. Lerwill and Young, in their 2006 study, showed that these patients are older than patients with Krukenberg tumors and they lack the endocrine manifestations of these mentioned tumors [10]. Grossly, the tumors are unilateral or bilateral, large, and solid (sometimes cystic), resembling metastatic colon cancer rather than gastric cancer. Microscopically, they show tubular glands arranged in a pseudoendometrioid pattern, edematous stroma, and sometime, 'dirty necrosis'. If signet ring cells are present, they will be less than 10% of total cells. Differential diagnosis of metastatic intestinal-type gastric adenocarcinoma is with metastatic colorectal carcinoma and primary ovarian endometrioid and mucinous carcinoma.

Intestinal carcinoma

The majority of metastatic ovarian tumors of intestinal origin arise from primary large intestine malignancies, with about 80% of the primaries originating in rectum or sigmoid colon and the rest of them almost equally divided among descending colon, ascending colon, and rectum; very few cases originate in

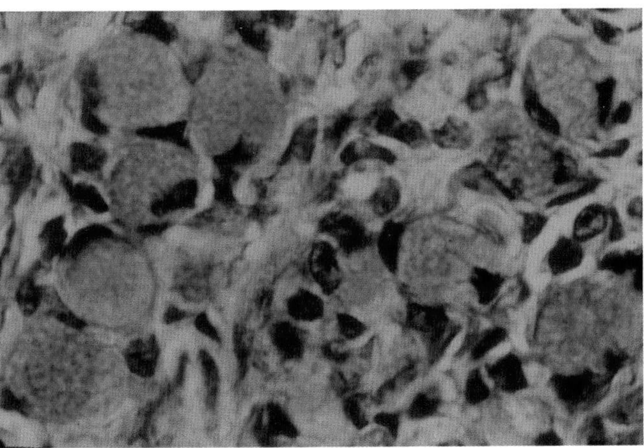

Fig. 9.3. Krukenberg tumor. Mucin stain.

primary small intestine carcinomas, especially intestinal clear cell adenocarcinoma [11].

Up to 45% of colon cancer metastases to the ovaries are clinically diagnosed as primary ovarian neoplasia and many are even misinterpreted on pathologic evaluation [12]. Approximately 4% of women with intestinal cancer will present with ovarian metastases during the evolution of the disease [13,14], and this figure increases to 18–27% if the patients are under 40 years of age [15].

These neoplasms are usually bilateral (more than half of the cases), and grossly appear as large solid masses or cystic masses (Fig. 9.4). Histologically, they are very similar to primary colonic tumors and also with primary ovarian mucinous carcinomas. Neoplastic cells form glands, usually with a cribriform architecture. Characteristic for an intestinal primary origin is intra-luminal "dirty necrosis" (formed by eosinophilic necrotic masses, nuclear debris, and inflammatory cells), glandular disposition as a garland at the periphery of necrotic areas, and focal segmental necrosis of the glandular epithelium (Fig. 9.5). Mucin-containing cells (e.g., goblet cells) are usually interspersed among epithelial cells; the latter ones can show a high degree of atypia. Tumor stroma varies from sparse to abundant and can be desmoplastic or edematous.

The main entities to be considered in the differential diagnosis are endometrioid carcinoma and mucinous adenocarcinoma. One clue to distinguish between these entities is tumor bilaterality, dominant in cases of metastatic tumors as opposed to less than 15% frequency of bilateral involvement in cases of primary endometrioid and mucinous adenocarcinomas. Other gross features helpful in the differential diagnosis are a more solid looking cut-section, with less necrosis and with cysts filled with hemorrhagic material ("chocolate cysts") in a clinical background of endometriosis, all of these traits being more specific for endometrioid adenocarcinomas. Microscopically, in cases of metastatic intestinal adenocarcinoma, epithelial glandular cells are more poorly differentiated than those in endometrioid adenocarcinomas, which more often also display squamous differentiation.

Immuno-histochemistry can be helpful in differentiating these tumors, known being the fact that colorectal carcinomas are usually CK7 negative, CA125 negative, CK20 positive, and CEA

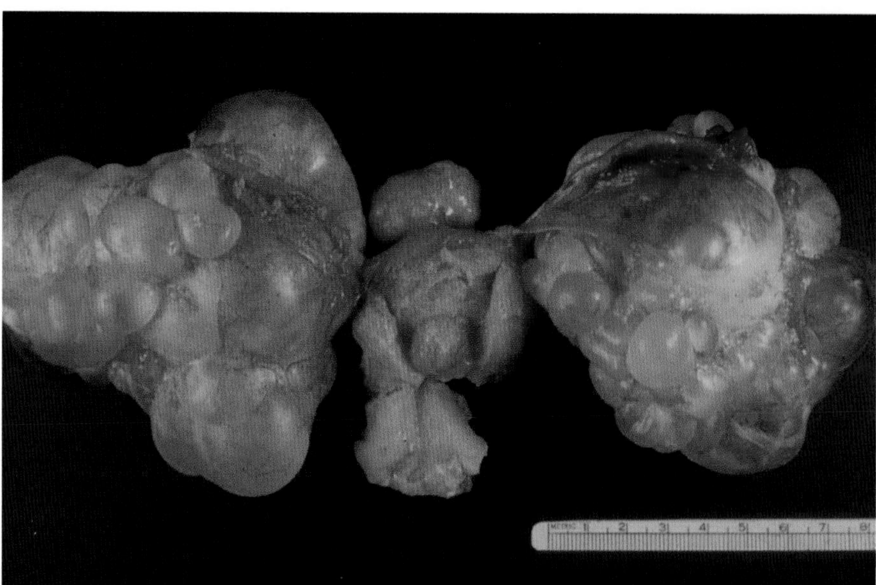

Fig. 9.4. Cystic bilateral metastatic mucinous adenocarcinoma, from recto-sigmoid primary; gross picture.

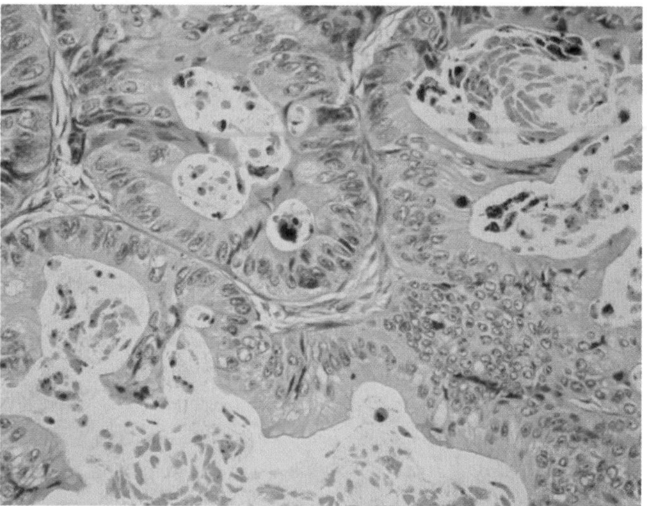

Fig. 9.5. Metastatic colon carcinoma. Intra-luminal "dirty necrosis." Hematoxylin & eosin stain.

positive, while the majority of endometrioid carcinomas have the opposite IHC profile. Also, colon carcinomas are MUC2 positive and MUC5AC usually negative, while mucinous ovarian carcinomas are MUC2 sparsely positive (limited to goblet cells) and MUC5AC positive [16]. It is important to remember that no IHC panel is 100% "typical" and for an accurate diagnosis nothing can replace the overall consideration of clinical data, gross aspect, morphological features, and special stains.

Apendiceal cancer

Ovarian metastases from the appendix are most common in cases of low-grade mucinous appendix tumors but other types of appendiceal neoplasms can involve the ovaries, e.g., intestinal type and mucinous type adenocarcinomas, colloid, and signet ring cell adenocarcinomas. Typical carcinoids of the appendix rarely metastasize to the ovaries [11].

In cases of ovarian metastases from low-grade mucinous appendiceal carcinomas, the relationship between these tumors was somehow controversial until recent years, but now a consensus was reached that ovarian tumors are recognized as metastatic from an appendiceal neoplasm despite its low grade and the fact that rupture of this primary tumor is almost always impossible to prove. Middle-aged to elderly patients usually present with symptoms related to an adnexal mass. If not removed previously, the appendix is dilated and most of the time covered with mucus; in cases of pseudomyxoma peritonei, the mucoid substance can cover the surface of all pelvic organs. Ovarian metastases are usually bilateral and can reach about 15–20 cm in diameter; on cut section, a multicystic appearance with mucoid material is common. Microscopically, these tumors present glands and cysts without a particular architecture, lined by columnar epithelial cells containing mucin toward the apex. In many cases, mucin dissects into ovarian stroma (pseudomyxoma ovarii).

Clinical association of these ovarian tumors with appendiceal pathology as well as similar histologic appearance and frequent bilateral ovarian involvement help in defining them as metastatic spread.

Carcinoid tumors

Carcinoids of any origin rarely metastasize to the ovaries. Metastatic carcinoid tumors to the ovaries represent 0.1% of all ovarian malignancies [17] and 2% of metastatic ovarian tumors. Most metastatic carcinoid tumors originate in the small intestine, with only a small percentage originating in the appendix, colon, stomach, pancreas, or lung [3,18,19].

Age at presentation is variable, but the majority of patients are in the fifth decade of life. Clinically, most of the patients have signs and symptoms of the carcinoid syndrome (flushing and diarrhea) accompanied by elevated levels of serum serotonin and urinary 5-HIAA. Also, tumoral cells express somatostatin receptors, as indicated by increased uptake of indium-111-pentetreotide on scintigraphy.

While primary carcinoid tumors of the ovary are unilateral, typically localized, and arise in the setting of a teratoma,

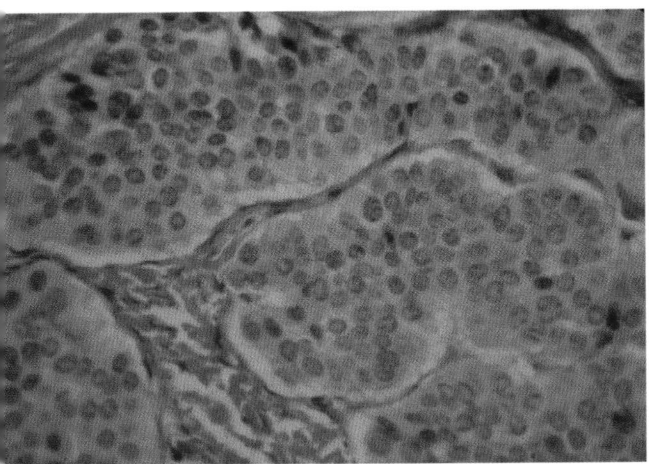

Fig. 9.6. Clusters of metastatic breast carcinoma to the ovary. Hematoxylin and eosin stain.

metastatic carcinoid ovarian tumors are bilateral and commonly associated with disseminated abdominal disease. Grossly, the ovaries are variably enlarged, with smooth or bosselated surfaces; cut sections reveal firm, whitish-yellow nodules, with possible cystic areas or areas of necrosis and hemorrhage. Microscopically, the tumor architecture displays a trabecular pattern, specific to pancreatic tumors, or a mucinous pattern, specific to appendiceal carcinoids [20]; the tumoral stroma often is extensively fibrous and hypocellular.

Different studies of carcinoid tumors metastatic to the ovaries show different survival data, between 94% [21] and 25% [22] 5-year survival, but all authors agree that the prognosis depends on the extent of the disease and the presence or absence of the carcinoid syndrome. A cure of the disease may be tried with surgery and chemotherapy, and patients should be followed-up with serial measurements of serum serotonin and urinary 5-HIAA.

Breast cancer

About 10% autopsies of breast cancer cases reveal ovarian involvement and of these, 80% are bilateral. Among the patients with breast cancer, less than 10% have signs and symptoms of distant metastases at the time of diagnosis, but about 30% of them will have metastatic disease [23]. Clinically, it is unusual that the metastatic ovarian carcinoma would come to medical attention before the primary breast carcinoma. Another important fact to be noted is that patients with breast carcinoma also have an increased incidence of ovarian carcinomas; hence, if a known patient with breast carcinoma presents with a new ovarian mass, statistically this new tumor is more likely to be ovarian primary and not breast metastasis [24].

Lobular carcinomas spread to the ovaries more frequently than ductal carcinomas, but because the incidence of the ductal type breast carcinoma is much higher, ovarian metastases of the ductal type are more common in daily practice.

Grossly, involved ovaries have irregular, bosselated surfaces and the cut surface shows firm, yellow-white nodules of different sizes. Microscopically, ovarian metastases resemble the primary tumors in terms of architecture and cytological features. In cases of lobular carcinoma, metastatic ovarian tumors show neoplastic cells arranged in small clusters (Fig. 9.6) or trabecule, the so-called characteristic 'Indian file' pattern (Figs. 9.7 and 9.8), while the ductal type show neoplastic cells forming acini or glands with a cribriform pattern.

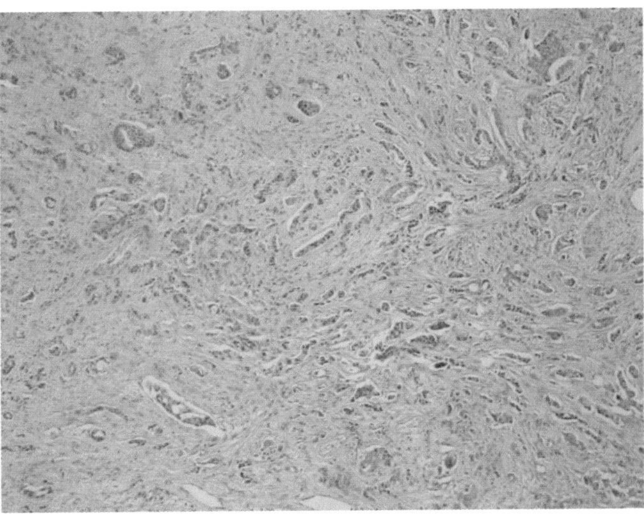

Fig. 9.7. Metastatic breast carcinoma, "Indian file." Hematoxylin and eosin, low magnification.

Differential diagnosis of ovarian metastases from breast carcinoma reflects the similarities between tumoral patterns; hence, a glandular pattern has to be distinguished from an ovarian primary carcinoma, endometrioid type; an insular pattern is similar to carcinoid tumors while diffuse patterns may be confused with granulosa cell tumors, lymphomas or undifferentiated sarcomas. In these cases, immuno-histochemistry studies may be helpful (Figs. 9.9 and 9.10). Among the most useful markers are GCDFP-15, mammoglobin, WT-1, and CA125. Gross cystic disease fluid protein-15 (GCDFP-15) is positive in the majority of ovarian metastases from breast while almost always negative in ovarian primary malignancy and strongly but focally positive in the breast carcinoma. Mammoglobin is more sensitive but less specific in showing breast origin than GCDFL-15; also, this staining is positive in the endometrioid carcinoma of the uterus. WT-1 is frequently positive in serous and transitional cell ovarian carcinomas and usually negative in breast carcinomas while CA125 is more often positive in ovarian carcinomas.

Female genital tract tumors

Endometrial carcinoma

Statistically, about 40% of autopsies of patients diagnosed with endometrial carcinoma also reveal ovarian involvement and the figure drops to 5–15% in surgical excisions (TH-BSO) [25].

When both uterus and ovaries are involved by carcinomas, pathologist and surgeon are confronted with the question of tumor origin: which one of the tumors is the primary or is that a case of synchronism of two primary tumors? For the past few decades, several criteria have been used to conclude if an ovarian tumor is primary or metastatic from a uterine primary carcinoma. Hence, if endometrial carcinoma has deep myometrial invasion, if lymphatics or blood vessels invasion is present,

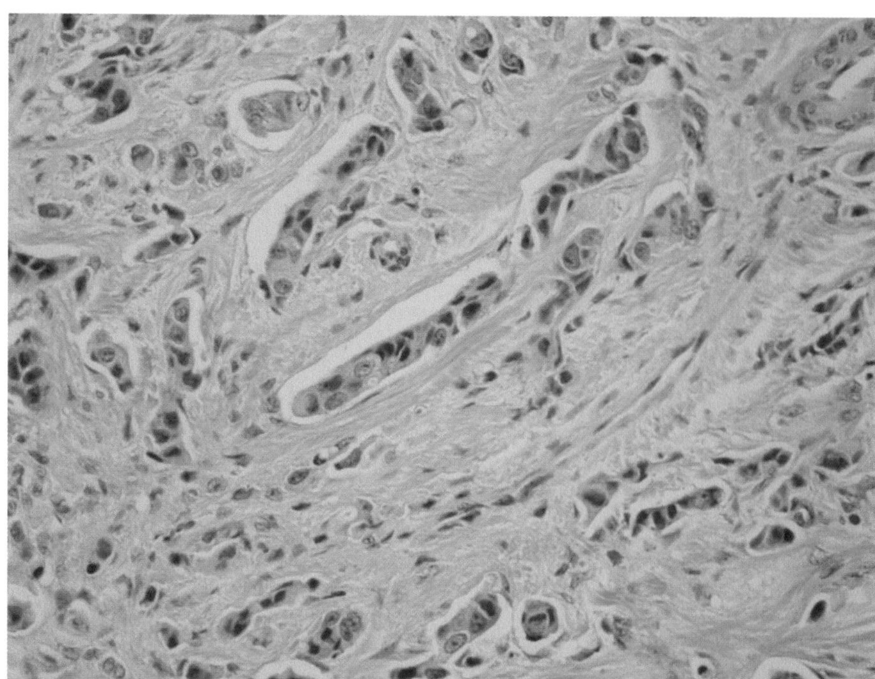

Fig. 9.8. Metastatic breast carcinoma, "Indian file." Hematoxylin and eosin, high magnification.

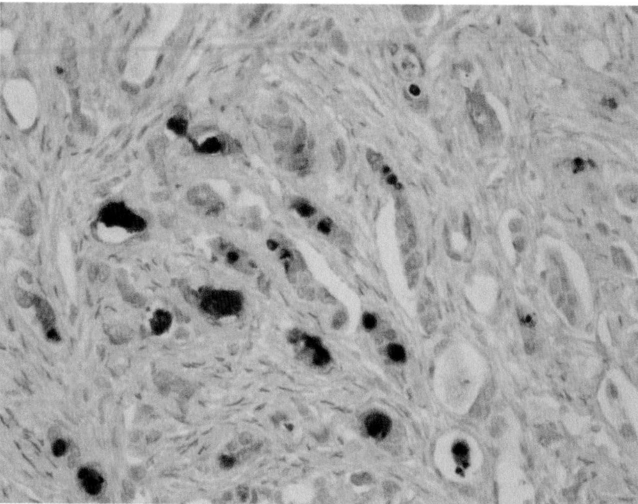

Fig. 9.9. Metastatic breast carcinoma. Positive mammoglobin stain.

if the tumor extends into the fallopian tube and if the tumor is present on the surface of the ovary or in its lymphatics or blood vessels, there is a high probability that ovarian involvement was secondary [26]. The most common mechanism of spreading of endometrial carcinoma to the ovaries appears to be lymphatic channels or direct extension of the tumor into the fallopian tubes and from here, to the ovaries.

Similarly, when endometrial carcinoma is small, does not extend to the myometrium, does not invade vessels and appears in a background of atypical hyperplasia while concomitant ovarian carcinoma arises on a background of endometriosis, then both tumors are probably synchronous primaries.

In cases of synchronous endometrial and ovarian carcinomas, most of the time both tumors are of endometrioid type and only rarely are they similar but of different type than endometrioid or of different histological types.

Tubal carcinoma

Involvement of the ovaries in fallopian tube carcinomas is seen in 10–15% of cases. Usually, the spread mechanism is direct extension of the tubal tumor, either by means of inflammatory adhesion between the tubes and ovaries or by means of direct ovarian surface implantation.

In most cases of concomitant ovarian and fallopian tube carcinomas, gross findings can usually establish which tumor is the primary. However, in practice there are cases with extensive involvement of both organs where it is impossible to ascertain the original tumor; in these situations, given the higher incidence of ovarian tumors, it used to be thought that ovarian carcinoma was the primary tumor, with secondary extension to the tubes. The problem is further compounded by the fact that most tubal carcinomas resemble serous, endometrioid, or undifferentiated carcinomas of the ovary; hence, microscopic examination does not help in establishing which carcinoma represented the primary tumor. It should be mentioned here that, due to the great rarity of primary mucinous and clear cell carcinomas of the fallopian tubes, a tumor of these histological types found in both organs should be considered an ovarian primary.

In an attempt to solve this diagnostic problem, the term 'tuboovarian carcinoma' or 'serous pelvic carcinoma' was recently considered to be more appropriate for cases of advanced high-grade disease, where the primary site of the tumor cannot be determined with confidence (see Chapter 7). A primary origin of ovarian serous carcinoma in the fallopian tube fimbriae is suggested for about 50% of cases by some authors (see Chapter 7).

Cervical carcinoma

Any histological type of cervical carcinoma (e.g., small cell carcinoma, adenosquamous carcinoma, transitional cell, carcinoid, and undifferentiated carcinoma) may spread to the

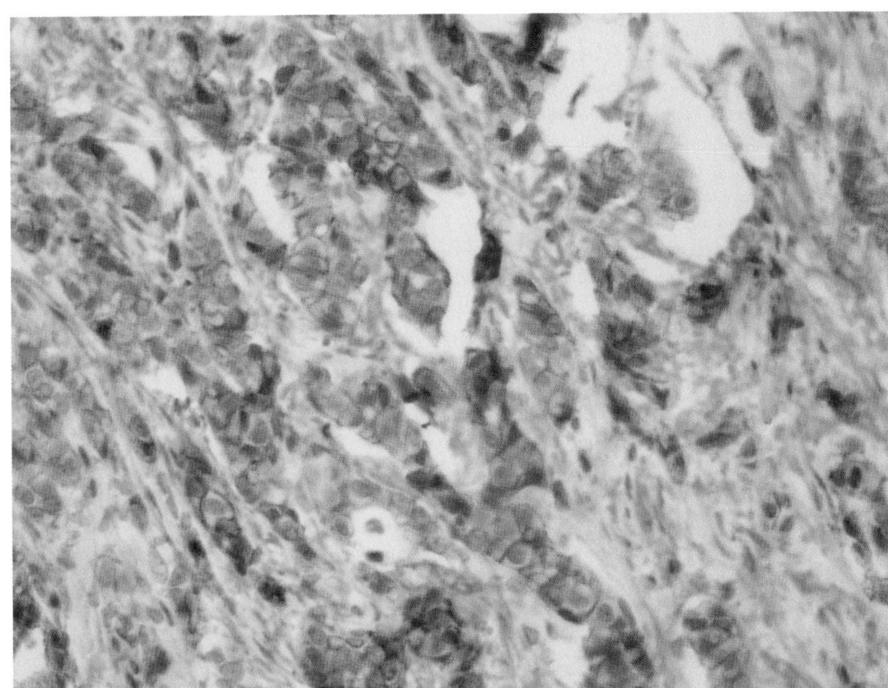

Fig. 9.10. Metastatic breast carcinoma. Positive Her-2 neu stain.

ovaries. In most of these cases, a cervical primary tumor is evident and differential diagnosis does not pose a problem as it could in cases of primary cervical adenocarcinomas or, less often, squamous cell carcinomas.

The fact that cervical adenocarcinoma spreads to the ovaries more frequently than cervical squamous cell carcinoma raises a very practical question: is ovarian conservation justified in cases of cervical adenocarcinomas? In one extensive study, the autopsies series showed that ovarian involvement in cervical squamous cell carcinomas was 17% (as opposed to 3% reported in prior studies), whereas in cervical adenocarcinoma, it was 28% [27].

In cases of ovarian metastases from cervical squamous cell carcinomas, the clinical picture is usually very evident and if needed, the diagnosis may be clarified by history and extensive sampling of the specimen. In cases of cervical adenocarcinoma metastatic to the ovaries, there are more diagnostic problems due to the fact that cervical adenocarcinomas are more often occult and also because metastatic tumors may simulate mucinous or endometrioid adenocarcinomas. Conventional traits of metastatic tumors, mentioned in the beginning of this chapter, may help in the differential diagnosis, but they may not always be present. In such cases, immuno-histochemistry may help, because HPV and P16 staining proved to be positive in cases of cervical metastases to the ovaries [28].

Other uterine, vulvar, and vaginal tumors

Other uterine tumors to metastasize to the ovaries are endometrial stromal sarcoma and leiomyosarcoma, with the former being more frequent. Vulvar and vaginal carcinomas rarely spread to the ovary; literature reports rare cases of vaginal clear cell adenocarcinoma metastases to the ovaries.

Miscellaneous other ovarian metastases

Pulmonary neoplasms can metastasize to the ovaries, but autopsies of women with lung cancer showed only ovarian involvement in 5%. The average age of presentation is 47 years, with more than half of cases having a history of lung cancer and the rest of the cases presenting synchronous tumors of ovarian tumors antedating the lung neoplasm [29]. Among the histological types, small cell carcinomas, as expected, spread more often then other types (approximately 44% of cases), with the rest of the cases being divided between adenocarcinomas and large cell carcinomas, while squamous cell carcinomas rarely spread to the ovaries. It has to be mentioned that, in cases of doubt, immuno-staining for TTF-1 usually provides strong support for pulmonary origin when positive.

Malignant melanoma can involve the ovaries in about 20% of cases. The average age at presentation is 38 years, and common symptoms are abdominal swelling or pain. In the majority of cases, there is a history of cutaneous or, rarely, choroidal melanoma. Metastatic melanomas must be distinguished from primary ovarian melanomas, which can arise in the wall of a dermoid cyst; in these cases, microscopic recognition of teratoma elements is important in determining the primary nature of an ovarian melanoma.

Other tumors that can spread to the ovaries are tumors of the pancreas, biliary tract, gallbladder, and liver. Among the pancreatic tumors, usual ductal adenocarcinomas and mucinous cystadenocarcinomas are the most frequent, although rare, followed in incidence by acinar cell carcinomas and islet cell carcinomas. Hepatocellular carcinoma spread to the ovaries is even less frequent than pancreatic tumors, while intra-hepatic cholangiocarcinoma spreads to the ovaries more frequently especially in the Far East, probably due to the higher incidence of Opisthorchis viverrini infestation in that part of the world [30,31].

Renal cell carcinomas and renal transitional cell tumors rarely spread to the ovaries, whereas among childhood tumors, Wilms' tumor and adrenal neuroblastomas are more frequent than pheochromocytomas and adrenal cortical carcinomas, although rare altogether.

Tumors from the urinary bladder, ureter, and urethra metastasize rarely to the ovaries. Differentiating between a transitional cell carcinoma of the urinary tract and a primary ovarian transitional cell carcinoma can be challenging and almost impossible if based only on morphologic aspects. In these cases, immuno-histochemical staining proves helpful because tumors of the bladder are frequently positive for CK20, uroplakin III and thrombomodulin and negative for WT-1, unlike the primary ovarian tumors which show the opposite immunohistochemistry panel.

Other tumors that may metastasize to the ovaries and are worth mentioning here are malignant mesotheliomas, desmoplastic small round cell tumors and peritoneal mesotheliomas, GIST (gastrointestinal stromal tumors), rhabdomyosarcomas, carcinomas of the thyroid and parathyroid, and lymphomas. Indeed, few are the tumors that do not metastasize to the ovaries and as Dr. Robert Young said, one "opens a Pandora box when one enters the world of secondary ovarian neoplasia" [11].

References

1. de Waal Y, Thomas C, Oei A, Sweep F, Massuger L. Secondary ovarian malignancies: frequency, origin, and characteristics. Int J Gynecol Cancer. 2009;**19**(7):1160–5.
2. Petru E, Pickel H, Heydarfadai M, et al. Nongenital cancers metastatic to the ovary. Gynecol Oncol. 1992;**44**:83–6.
3. Kurman RJ, Ellerson LH, Ronnett BM. Metastatic tumors of the ovary. Blaustein's Pathology of the Female Genital Tract, 6th edition. New York: Springer; 2011, pp. 929–97.
4. Demopoulos RI, Touger L, Dubin N. Secondary ovarian carcinoma: a clinical and pathological evaluation. Int J Gynecol Pathol. 1987;**6**(2):166–75.
5. Young RH. From Krukenberg to today: the ever present problems posed by metastatic tumors in the ovary. Part 1: historical perspective, general principles, mucinous tumors including the Krukenberg tumor. Adv Anat Pathol. 2006;**13**(5):205–27.
6. Onuigbo WIB. Early descriptions of Krukenberg tumors. J Am Coll Surg. 2005;**1**:111–12.
7. Kiyokawa T, Young R, Scully R. Krukenberg tumors of the ovary: a clinicopathologic analysis of 120 cases with emphasis on their variable pathologic manifestations. Am J Surg Pathol. 2006;**30**(3):277–99.
8. Lou G, Gao Y, Ning XM, Zhang QF. Expression and correlation of CD44v6, vascular endothelial growth factor, matrix-metalloproteinase-2, and matrix-metalloproteinase-9 in Krukenberg tumor. World J Gastroenterol. 2005;**11** (32):5032–6.
9. Chu P, Weiss L. Immunohistochemical characterization of signet-ring cell carcinomas of the stomach, breast and colon. Am J Clin Pathol. 2004;**121**:884–92.
10. Lerwill MF, Young R. Ovarian metastases of intestinal-type gastric carcinoma. A clinico-pathologic study of 4 cases with contrasting features to those of the Krukenberg tumor. Am J Surg Pathol. 2006;**31**:1382–8.
11. Young RH. From Krukenberg to today: the ever present problems posed by metastatic tumors in the ovary. Part II. Adv Anat Pathol. 2007;**14**(3):149–77.
12. Lash R, Hart W. Intestinal adenocarcinomas metastatic to the ovaries. A clinicopathological evaluation of 22 cases. Am J Surg. 1987;**11**:114–21.
13. Burt C. Prophylactic oophorectomy with resection of the large bowel for cancer. Am J Surg. 1951;**82**:572–7.
14. Birnkrant A, Sampson J, Sugarbaker P. Ovarian metastasis from colorectal cancer. Dis Colon Rectum. 1986;**29**:767–71.
15. Pitluk H, Poticha S. Carcinoma of the colon and rectum in patients less than 40 years of age. Surg Gynecol Obstet. 1983;**157**:335–7.
16. Baker P, Oliva E. Immunohistochemistry as a tool in the differential diagnosis of ovarian tumors: an update. Int J Gynecol Pathol. 2004;**24**:39–55.
17. Modlin I, Lye K, Kidd M. A 5-decade analysis of 13,715 carcinoid tumors. Cancer. 2003;**97**:934–59.
18. Ulbright T, Roth L, Stehman F. Secondary ovarian neoplasia. A clinicopathologic study of 35 cases. Cancer. 1984;**53**:1164–74.
19. Young R, Scully R. Ovarian metastases from cancer of the lung: problems in interpretation – a report of seven cases. Gynecol Oncol. 1985;**21**:337–50.
20. Talerman A. Carcinoid tumors of the ovary. J Cancer Res Clin Oncol. 1984;**107**:125–35.
21. Strosberg J, Nasir A, Cragun J, Gardner N, Kvols L. Metastatic carcinoid tumor to the ovary: A clinicopathologic analysis of seventeen cases. Gynecol Oncol. 2007;**106**:65–8.
22. Robboy S, Scully R, Norris H. Carcinoid metastatic to the ovary. A clinicopathologic analysis of 35 cases. Cancer. 1974;**33**(3):798–811.
23. Bigorie V, Morice P, Duvillard P, et al. Ovarian metastases from breast cancer. Report of 29 cases. Cancer. 2010;**116**:799–804.
24. Curtin J, Barakat R, Hoskins W. Ovarian disease in women with breast cancer. Obstet Gynecol. 1994;**84**:449–52.
25. Beck R, Latour J. Necropsy reports on 36 cases of endometrial adenocarcinoma. Am J Obstet Gynecol. 1963;**85**:307–11.
26. Ulbright T, Roth L. Metastatic and independent cancers of the endometrium and ovary. A clinicopathologic study of 34 cases. Hum Pathol. 1985;**16**:28–34.
27. Tabata M, Ichinoe K, Sakuragi N, et al. Incidence of ovarian metastasis in patients with cancer of the uterine cervix. Gynecol Oncol. 1987;**28**:255–61.
28. Elishaev E, Gilks C, Miller D, et al. Synchronous and metachronous endocervical and ovarian neoplasms. Evidence supporting interpretation of the ovarian neoplasms as metastatic endocervical adenocarcinomas

simulating primary ovarian surface epithelial neoplasms. Am J Surg Pathol. 2005;**29**:281–94.

29. Irving J, Young R. Lung carcinoma metastatic of the ovary. A clinicopathologic study of 32 cases emphasizing their morphologic spectrum and problems in differential diagnosis. Am J Surg Pathol. 2005;**29**:997–1006.

30. Low J, Chew S, Chew SP, et al. A rare case of metastatic ovarian carcinoma originating from primary intrahepatic cholangiocarcinoma. Case report. Eur J Gynaecol Oncol. 2003;**24**:85–8.

31. Khunamornpong S, Siriaunkgul S, Suprasert P, et al. Intrahepatic cholangiocarcinoma metastatic to the ovary: a report of 16 cases of an underemphasized form of secondary tumor of the ovary that may mimic primary neoplasia. Am J Surg Pathol. 2007;**31**:1788–99.

Chapter 10

Genetic etiology of sporadic ovarian cancer

Ellen L. Goode, PhD, MPH, Mine S. Cicek, PhD, Catherine M. Phelan, PhD, MD, MMS, and Brooke L. Fridley, PhD

Introduction

Ovarian cancer presents as familial clusters and as sporadic cases without strong family history. As summarized elsewhere in this book, rare mutations conferring substantially increased ovarian cancer risk (up to 50%) occur in several genes including *BRCA1* and *BRCA2* [9,10], mismatch repair genes such as *MLH1* and *MSH2* [11], and other DNA repair genes, such as *RAD51C* [12]. Yet, these high-risk variants are very rare (less than 1% in most populations), and they are estimated to account for less than 40% of the excess familial risk of ovarian cancer [13]. Here, we describe the genetic etiology of sporadic ovarian cancer (i.e., ovarian cancers that do not arise from within high-risk familial clusters). We review evidence that ovarian cancer is genetic, data on particular genes which have been studied as candidates, results from searches throughout the genome for ovarian cancer risk factors, strategies for follow-up of genomic regions harboring risk loci, and approaches for the identification and characterization of additional genetic factors.

Evidence for low-penetrance loci

The role of inherited factors in ovarian cancer susceptibility is suggested by numerous epidemiologic studies reporting increased risks from 2- to 10-fold for women with family history of ovarian cancer [14]. In fact, compared with confirmed demographic, reproductive, and lifestyle factors, positive family history is the strongest risk factor for ovarian cancer. Increased familial risk can be explained, in part, by shared environmental factors; however, studies of twins and migrants provide additional support for genetic heritability of the disease. For example, identical twins are more likely to have the same ovarian cancer disease state than fraternal twins [15]. In addition, genetic epidemiologic models suggest that a large number of additional rare high-risk variants, such as *BRCA1* or *BRCA2* is unlikely to exist [16]. Rather, combinations of common genetic variants (with minor allele frequencies, MAF, greater than 5%), which confer modest effects on disease risk are most likely to account for the residual heritability of ovarian cancer [16]. While the risk of disease for a given common allele may be small, because of their high frequency, these alleles can lead to large population attributable risks. Figure 10.1 illustrates a spectrum of types of ovarian cancer risk-associated variants by effect size and MAF. *BRCA1* belongs in the upper left of the plot, and the common variants which are discussed below are represented in the lower right of the plot.

Although linkage analysis is a powerful method for mapping Mendelian traits and even multigenic traits with highly penetrant Mendelian genes, association testing is generally more powerful to detect effects of genes in common, complex diseases. Genetic association studies involve the comparison of cases and controls (i.e., women with and without ovarian cancer). Ideally, the cases are incident, as opposed to prevalent, the cases represent the clinical spectrum of disease, and the controls are matched to cases on key characteristics such as region, race, and age. Germline DNA is readily obtained through peripheral blood, and questionnaires solicit data on lifestyle, diet, and other known or suspected ovarian cancer risk factors. Single nucleotide polymorphisms (SNPs) represent the most common and easily studied genetic variants. There are thought to be 11 million SNPs in the human genome, and much is known about them due to large-scale public studies such as the HapMap Project [17] and the 1000 Genomes Project [18], which characterized correlations among SNPs, or linkage disequilibrium (LD). Knowledge of the structure of LD throughout the genome has enabled wise selection of variants to study. Because of LD, a disease-susceptibility SNP need not be genotyped, as long as it is tagged by a SNP or set of SNPs that are genotyped. Advances in genotyping technology since 2000 have enabled efficient SNP studies in large sample sizes.

Candidate gene studies

The majority of studies seeking to discover ovarian cancer susceptibility variants have taken candidate gene approaches which assess genes with suspected roles in ovarian cancer and hypothesize that variation within these genes relate to susceptibility. These initially focused on non-synonymous SNPs in coding regions with suspected function and expanded into non-coding SNPs that may be in LD with the true causal variant. A 2011 review summarized 147 candidate gene studies in ovarian cancer published from 1990 to 2010, including more than 1,000 genetic variants in more than 200 candidate genes [19]. Only a small number of findings have been successfully replicated in other independent studies, in fact, it has been reported that two-thirds of genetic association studies do not hold up on meta-analysis [20]. The inconsistent results among genetic association studies

Altchek's Diagnosis and Management of Ovarian Disorders, ed. Liane Deligdisch, Nathan G. Kase, and Carmel J. Cohen. Published by Cambridge University Press.

Table 10.1. Ovarian cancer susceptibility loci from candidate gene studies

Gene	Locus	SNP	Histology	OR (95% CI)	*P* value	Ref.
TERT	5p15.33	rs7726159	Serous	1.30 (1.16–1.45)	5.7×10^{-6}	(1)
SYNE1	6q25.1	rs2295190	All invasive	1.11 (1.04–1.19)	0.001	(3)
PGR	11q22-q23	PROGINS*	Endometrioid	1.17 (1.01–1.36)	0.036	(4)
RB1	13q14.2	rs2854344	All invasive	0.88 (0.79–1.00)	0.041	(5)
TP53	17p13.1	rs12951053	Serous	1.65 (1.20–2.26)	–	(7)

* *PROGINS* is an intron 7 Alu insertion, which is completely correlated with rs1042838 and rs1042839; OR, odds ratio; CI, confidence interval, TERT, telomerase reverse transcriptase.

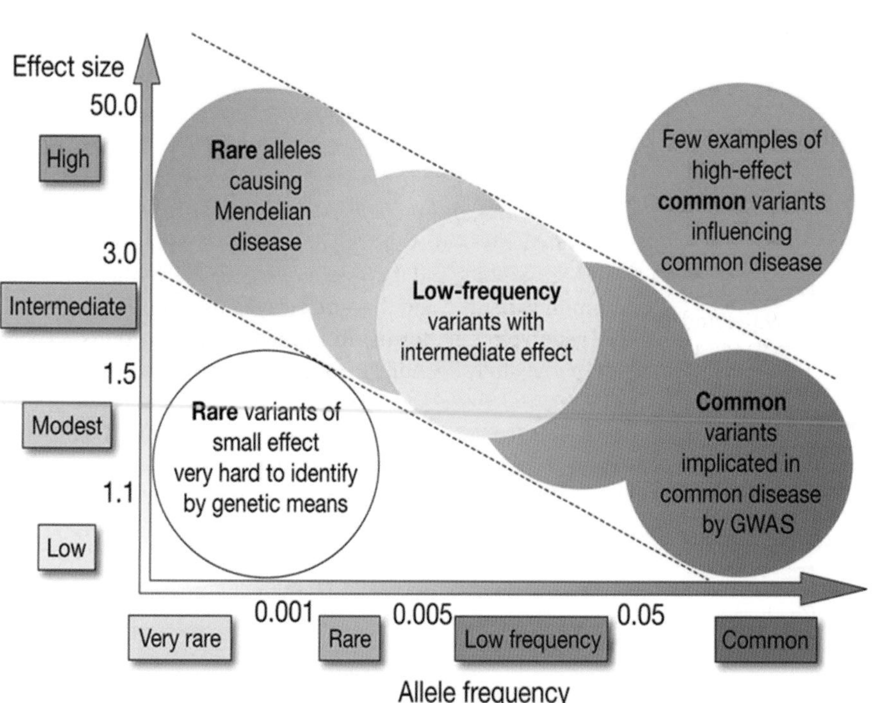

Fig. 10.1. Spectrum of genetic variants associated with ovarian cancer risk. GWAS, genomewide association study. Modified from TA Manolio et al. Nature 2009;**461**:747–53.

most often can be explained by heterogeneity across study populations as well as false-positive and false-negative results. The variants tested are expected to have low penetrance; therefore, large sample sizes and pooling of data are critical in such studies. Some of the consistently observed associations with risk of ovarian cancer include variants in *TERT*, *SYNE1*, *PGR*, *RB1*, and *TP53* genes on chromosomes 5p15.33, 6q25.1, 11q22–23, 13q14.2, and 17p13.1, respectively (Table 10.1).

Telomase reverse transcriptase: *TERT*

TERT encodes the catalytic subunit of telomerase which is essential for the replication of chromosomes. Telomerase expression plays a role in cellular senescence and deregulation of telomerase expression is involved in genomic instability. Overexpression of telomerase is key component of the transformation process in many malignant cancer cells. Combined analysis of multiple ovarian cancer case–control studies found evidence of an association between *TERT* SNP rs7726159 and risk of invasive serous tumors (odds ratio [OR], 1.30; 95% confidence interval [CI], 1.16–1.45; $P = 5.7 \times 10^{-6}$) [1]. The rs7726159 variant resides in intron 3 and has no known functional significance, but it is thought to be correlated with another causal SNP. Inherited variation in *TERT* has also been highlighted in recent studies in other cancers, and association has been reported between the *TERT* locus and multiple cancers including lung, basal cell carcinoma, and pancreatic cancer [21]. Thus, there is growing evidence that the TERT locus is a general cancer susceptibility locus.

Spectrin repeat-containing, nuclear envelope 1: *SYNE1*

SYNE1 is a large gene on chromosome 6q25.1–25.2 which encodes several isoforms and neighbors the estrogen receptor ESR1. One of many transcripts of *SYNE1*, *DROP1*, is encoded in the 5′ end of *SYNE1* and has been reported to be down-regulated in epithelial ovarian tumors, particularly stage I. Loss of DROP1 is a common feature for many types of carcinomas, including breast, uterus, cervix, lung, and pancreas. A missense SNP, rs2295190 (G>T), in the COOH terminus region of SYNE1 results in an amino acid substitution from Leu to Met. The T allele of rs2295190 (MAF 15%) was associated with increased invasive ovarian cancer risk (OR, 1.11; 95% CI, 1.04–1.19; $P = 0.001$). Among invasive ovarian cancers, this association was strongest for the mucinous subtype (OR, 1.32; 95% CI, 1.11–1.58; $P = 0.002$) [3]. The T allele is predicted to be damaging to SYNE1 protein function because the amino change is within a highly conserved region.

Progesterone receptor: *PGR*

The progesterone receptor is a member of the steroid-receptor superfamily of nuclear receptors and its gene, *PGR*, is located on 11q22-q23. The encoded protein mediates the physiological effects of progesterone. There is evidence for a protective role of progestins in ovarian cancer, and patients expressing the progesterone receptor may have a better prognosis. Epidemiologic data show an inverse association of progestin levels with risk of ovarian cancer. PGR exists in two isoforms, PGR-A and PGR-B, and the latter is the full-length receptor while the A-isoform misses the first 165 amino acid residues. They function distinctly differently; PGR-A represses estrogen receptor and PGR-B activates progesterone target genes. Several polymorphisms in *PGR* have been reported to be associated with risk of ovarian cancer [22]. A complex of three correlated polymorphisms known as *PROGINS* includes an Alu insertion, V660L in exon 4, and His770His in exon 5. In addition, two coding SNPs (S344T and G393G) and another two in the promoter region (+44C/T and +331G/A) between the two transcriptional start sites have been identified. *PROGINS* has been studied extensively and its association with ovarian cancer risk thus far has been predominantly negative. However, combined analysis of data from two studies observed decreased risk of endometrioid/clear cell ovarian cancer cases with the presence of the rs10895068 +331A allele (OR, 0.46; 95% CI, 0.23–0.92) [23]. A pooled analysis of 4,788 ovarian cancer cases and 7,641 controls from 12 case–control studies found a statistically significant association between endometrioid ovarian cancer risk and the *PROGINS* allele (OR, 1.17; 95% CI, 1.01–1.36; $P = 0.036$) [4]. These data suggest that there is evidence of histology-specific effects of the variants in ovarian cancer.

Retinoblastoma: *RB1*

RB1 is a tumor suppressor gene (13q14.2), and germline mutations in *RB1* predispose to retinoblastoma. A variety of cancers show somatic alterations in *RB1*, and *RB1* is one of the significantly mutated genes in high-grade serous ovarian cancer cases [24]. It has been suggested that the overall survival rate for epithelial ovarian cancer patients with normal *RB1* function may be better. The rare allele of a SNP in intron 17, rs2854344, was found to be protective for ovarian cancer (OR, 0.88; 95% CI, 0.79–1.00; $P = 0.041$) [5,25]. This is a non-coding SNP and not in a highly conserved region. However, it is contained in an ORF encoding a G protein coupled receptor P2RY5 in reverse orientation to the transcription of *RB1*. The involvement of this receptor has been described in other cancers. It is unlikely that this variant has a functional effect, thus it may be correlated with true causal SNP.

Tumor protein p53: *TP53*

TP53 encodes the tumor suppressor protein p53 and is located at 17p13.1. There is a very high prevalence of somatic *TP53* mutations in ovarian cases. It is involved in genomic integrity, and it has been hypothesized that polymorphisms may cause instability and therefore increased disease risk. There is evidence to suggest that alterations in *TP53* may have a significant effect on its biological function. Epidemiologic studies have evaluated association of several *TP53* variants with ovarian cancer risk [26], and two correlated SNPs have been confirmed to be associated with invasive serous ovarian cancer in a large follow-up study [7]. Risk is increased with rs2078486 (OR, 1.65; 95% CI, 1.21–2.25) and rs12951053 (OR, 1.65; 95% CI, 1.20–2.26) [7]. Several variants with putative functional significance have been identified to be in LD with these risk SNPs.

Genome-wide association studies

An alternate approach to the identification of common variants associated with ovarian cancer risk is the genome-wide association study (GWAS). GWAS also generally use the case–control study design, but unlike the candidate gene approach, no particular gene is targeted for interrogation. Rather, from 100,000 to 2.5 million SNPs throughout the genome are studied. These SNPs are within and beyond genes, they are chosen to tag common variation, and they are arrayed on commercially available genotyping platforms. In numerous human traits, GWAS have successfully identified novel loci through the use of very large sample sizes and multiple levels of replication, most often through collaborations of international consortia. Due to the large number of SNPs tested, a stringent criterion for statistical significance of $P < 10^{-8}$ is used for interpretation of results.

In ovarian cancer, the Ovarian Cancer Association Consortium (OCAC) [27,28] has published three GWAS reports to date which provide strong evidence for novel ovarian cancer susceptibility loci [2,6,8]. These describe a three-stage approach initiated in the United Kingdom with a smaller number of participants initially studied (approximately 1,800 cases, 2,300 controls, and 500,000 SNPs) and replication of subsets of the most promising SNPs in larger numbers of participants from multiple studies (e.g., 4,200 cases, 4,800 controls, 35 SNPs) [2,6,8]. Confirmed loci reside on chromosomes 2q31, 3q25, 8q24, 9p22, 17q21, and 19p13; they confer modest changes in risk and are common in populations of European descent (Table 10.2). Additional GWAS are now under way, as are combined ovarian cancer GWAS analyses through a National Cancer Institute-supported post-GWAS initiative entitled Follow-up of Ovarian Cancer Genetic Association and Interaction Studies (FOCI) (http://epi.grants.cancer.gov/pgwas/).

Only some of the six GWAS-identified ovarian cancer susceptibility SNPs reside within a gene or in a gene region, including *BNC2, TIPARP, HOXD1/3, MERIT40*, and *SKAP1* (Fig. 10.2). Interestingly, at 8q24, there are multiple independent regions (i.e., not in LD) with variants associated with ovarian cancer, prostate cancer, breast cancer, colorectal cancer, and other others. This region contains *MYC*, suggesting that this proto-oncogene may be implicated in susceptibility to each of these cancers; however, the relationships with *MYC* and between these loci appears much more complicated than initially thought and much remains unknown [29]. The 19p13 region includes *MERIT40* (or C19orf62), which interacts

Table 10.2. Ovarian cancer susceptibility loci from GWAS

					All cases	Serous cases only	
Locus	SNP	MAF	Location	Gene(s)	OR (95% CI)	OR (95% CI)	Ref
2q31	rs2072590	0.32	inter-genic	*HOXD3, HOXD1*	1.16 (1.12–1.21)	1.20 (1.14–1.25)	(2)
3q25	rs2665390	0.08	intronic	*TIPARP*	1.19 (1.11–1.27)	1.24 (1.15–1.34)	(2)
8q24	rs10088218	0.12	inter-genic	*MYC*	0.84 (0.80–0.89)	0.76 (0.70–0.81)	(2)
9p22	rs3814113	0.28	inter-genic	*BNC2*	0.82 (0.79–0.86)	0.77 (0.73–0.81)	(6)
17q21	rs9303542	0.27	intronic	*SKAP1*	1.11 (1.06–1.16)	1.14 (1.09–1.20)	(2)
19p13	rs8170	0.45	synonymous	*MERIT40*	1.12 (1.07–1.17)	1.18 (1.12–1.25)	(8)

OR, odds ratio; 95% CI, 95% confidence interval.

with *BRCA1*, and, in 3q25, TIPARP is part of an alternative DNA repair pathway and small molecule target for BRCA1- or BRCA2-deficient cells. An important feature to note about these loci is that most of these SNPs show the strongest associations with the most common serous histological subtype of ovarian cancer. This may be due to the use of primarily serous cases in initial GWAS phases. In addition, there appear to be differences in risk by histologic subtype, for example at 2q31, suggesting that GWAS focused on endometrioid, clear cell, or mucinous ovarian cancer may uncover further loci.

Characterization of confirmed loci

An important factor in the assessment of GWAS-identified SNP associations is the study design and context of the GWAS. The GWAS platform and methodologies can bias results, so must be taken into consideration. In most GWAS of complex traits, the associations are with SNPs with higher MAFs, because there is greater power to detect such associations. In addition, the majority of associations have been identified in regions of high LD where SNP coverage on commercial panels is most dense. For the majority of GWAS-identified associations in the major diseases, the identified variants are located not in coding regions but in gene deserts [29]. The associations may be due to an unknown mechanism involving transcriptional regulation by non-coding RNAs or other elements. The same is true for the GWAS-identified SNPs in loci associated with ovarian cancer. The characterization of these loci involves in silico, in vitro, and in vivo studies. The following are the main considerations involved in the characterization of GWAS-identified SNPs or genes:

1) Interrogation of known databases/publications to annotate the SNP/gene
2) Fine mapping of the locus to identify potential causal variants
3) Identification of variable regulatory elements such as enhancers
4) Investigation of tissue-specific expression in gynecologic and other human tissues and epigenetic regulation
5) Investigation of allele-specific function using expression quantitative trait loci (eQTLs), and
6) Knock-out/knock-in cell line models, murine, and other animal models.

In silico annotation

With funding agencies such as the National Institute of Health implementing data sharing requirements and the National Human Genome Research Institute project to develop and make publicly available, high quality comprehensive annotations of functional elements of the human genome, there is a wealth of genomic and genetic data from de-identified cancer patients and other individuals. The characterization of the GWAS-identified loci first involves in silico analysis and review of databases for information on known functional associations. The University of California Santa Cruz (UCSC) Human Genome Browser provides potential functional elements of a genomic region as well as gene mapping, mRNA mapping, miRNA regulatory sites, transcription factor binding sites, gene prediction, expression, regulation, and evolutionary conservation. Chromatin state profiling can pinpoint regions involved in transcription regulation. The Broad Histone data track incorporates maps of chromatin state generated by the Encyclopedia of DNA Elements (ENCODE) [30] project in the UCSC browser, and can be used to provide information on different histone modifications and chromatin states. Candidate variants are categorized by gene location (intergenic, intronic, or exonic) and by predicted effect (frameshift, in-frame insertion or deletion, synonymous substitution, nonsynonymous substitution, splice site alteration, or nonsense). Variants identified are classified using the recommended guidelines from the Human Genome Variant Study (HGVS) and structural-based computation tools are used to obtain functional predictions.

Fine mapping using additional SNPs or targeted re-sequencing

The SNPs included on GWAS platforms take advantage of the LD structure of the genome as fewer SNPs represent greater genomic area than non-tagged SNPs. LD can be further exploited by the introduction of methods to impute genotypes at untyped markers, based on genotypes at

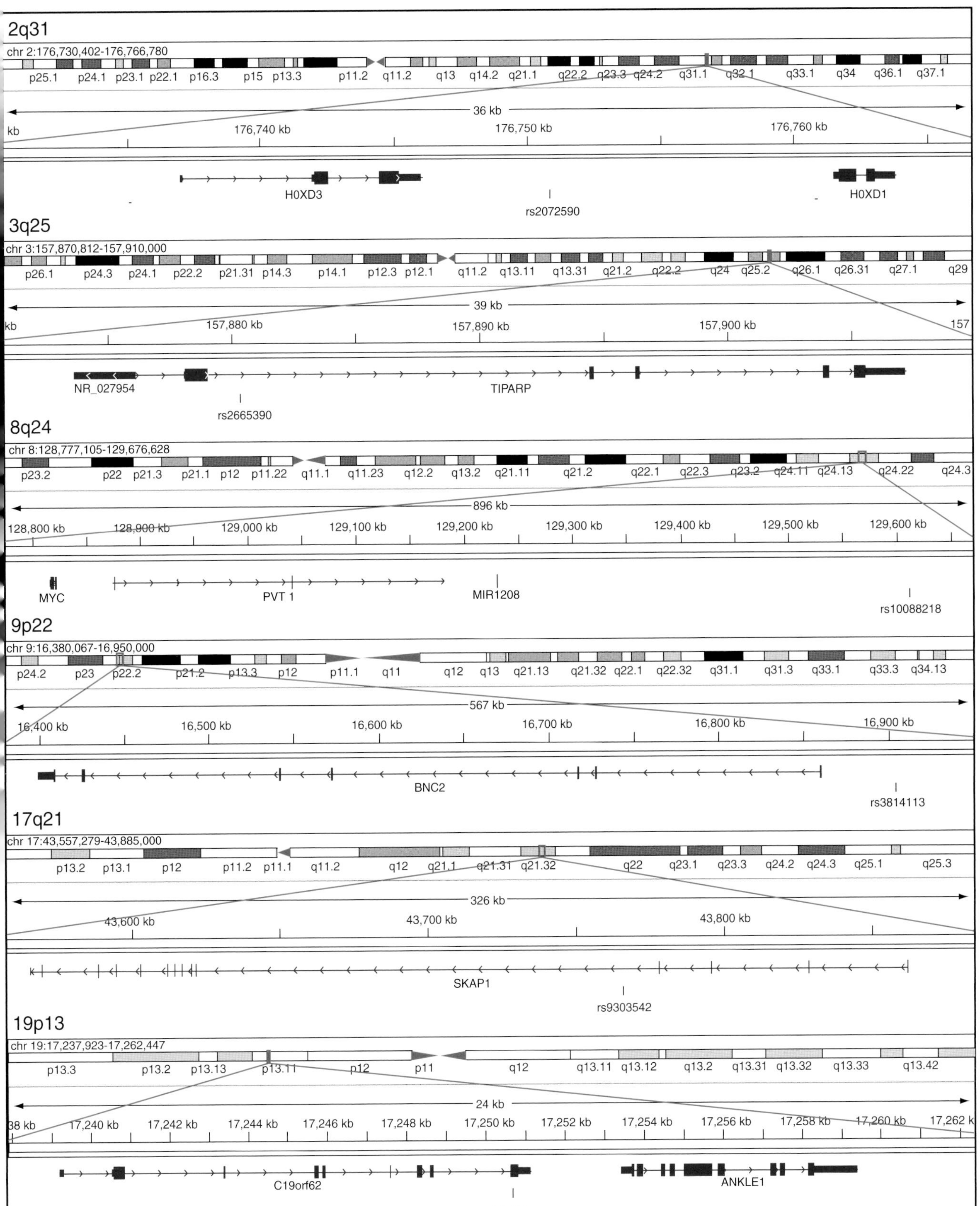

Fig. 10.2. Ovarian cancer susceptibility loci identified from GWAS. The chromosomal location of each locus is indicated (red) in the top portion of each plot and expanded in the bottom portion of each plot; SNPs associated with ovarian cancer risk are shown in green and genes are shown in blue.

typed markers and information about LD within the region based on a reference group. To better refine regions of association, one can use methods for imputation of untyped genotypes using the reference haplotypes from the 1000 Genomes Project [18] or HapMap [17]. Fine mapping of a locus for unimputable variants can involve either the genotyping of a greater number of SNPs in that locus in cases and controls or re-sequencing. The ovarian cancer GWAS were performed in mainly Caucasians of European descent, thus ideally, the fine mapping population should include individuals from different ethnic groups with less LD, such as Asians, African Americans, and Latin Americans, as has been useful in breast cancer [31]. However, there are currently very few ovarian cancer case–control studies in these populations. In both approaches, the numbers of cases and controls is an important consideration dependent of the MAF of the variant of interest.

Identification of variable regulatory elements

The study of the regulatory infrastructure of a genomic region including promoters, enhancers, insulators, and silencers for GWAS-identified loci is likely to yield information on allele-specific function and tissue-specificity of disease-associated SNPs. DNase sensitivity assays and the investigation of histone modifications using chromatin immunoprecipitation sequencing methods (ChIP-seq) are two approaches which may yield relevant information. Additional in vivo and in vitro reporter assays may provide information on enhancer elements.

Epigenetics and tissue-specific expression and regulation of the gene of interest

The expression of a particular gene in specific tissues may be due to different promoters. For example, *BNC2* in the chromosome 9p22 ovarian cancer susceptibility region has six different promoters and shows tissue-specificity for particular transcripts [6]. Investigation of protein levels in normal and tumor tissue can provide clues to the oncogenic or suppressor function of the gene of interest, as well as those in the surrounding region. In addition, while the cell of origin in ovarian cancer has been the subject of debate, it is thought that high-grade serous ovarian cancer is derived from cells in the fallopian tube, whereas low-grade serous ovarian cancer may be derived from ovarian surface epithelium [32]. Therefore, a comprehensive analysis of a spectrum of gynecologic tissues including endometrial and fallopian tubes as well as different related disease states such as endometriosis may provide valuable clues as to the etiology of the different ovarian cancer histologic subtypes. Levels of proteins of interest are also investigated in similar histologic subtypes in different cancers; for example, there is emerging evidence that clear cell carcinoma of the ovary may show similar genetic etiology to clear cell carcinoma of the kidney [33]. Epigenetic silencing through hyper- or hypomethylation is a predominant method of gene expression regulation. Therefore individual gene methylation assays as well as genome-wide methylation assays may provide mechanistic information. Although at present the top GWAS loci in ovarian cancer are not associated with methylation genes, SNPs in the methylation gene MSMB reached genome-wide significance in prostate cancer [34,35]. SNPs can also alter miRNA binding sites which may impact gene expression.

Investigation of allele-specific function using expression quantitative trait loci (eQTLs)

Most SNPs which have been reproducibly associated with complex traits are thought to have a role in expression; thus, eQTL examination for a given SNP may help to understand complex traits in terms of the biological function. The identification of novel SNPs in unexpected genes and pathways may be accurately characterized with respect to particular genes and mechanisms of effect. The main challenge in conducting eQTL experiments is to comprehensively investigate all human tissues. There are potential issues as an eQTL is tumor-specific and tissue-specific. In one study, only 30% of eQTLs were shared among the three tissue types studied including lymphoblastoid cell lines, skin, and fat, while another 29% appear exclusively tissue-specific. However, even among the shared eQTLs, a substantial proportion (10–20%) has significant differences in the magnitude of change between genotypic classes across tissues, underlining the need to account for the complexity of eQTL tissue-specificity. With the disagreement as to the cell of origin for the serous histologic subtype of ovarian cancer [32], a comprehensive eQTL assessment must include both ovarian surface epithelial cell lines and fallopian tube cancer cell lines. A database has been developed to capture eQTL data called the SNP and Copy number ANnotation (SCAN).

Cell line, murine, and other animal models

The functional consequences of SNPs in a particular gene can also be investigated using cancer cell line models. Cell lines are crucial models for a variety of biological studies, including drug screening and transporter studies. The selected cell line must carry the allele of interest to characterize the functional effect of a SNP. Thus, many investigators are now including cell lines in their GWAS study. In ovarian cancer, some investigators have genotyped normal ovarian surface epithelial cell lines and drug (cisplatin) -sensitive and -resistant parent-daughter pairs. The gene of interest must also be expressed, and the cell line model should mimic the in vivo situation as closely as possible. SNPs might affect gene expression or alter the biological function of a protein and therefore result in important phenotypic consequences for the cell, such as gene regulation, gene splicing, miRNA regulation, and transcription factor binding. Three-dimensional cell culture models of human ovarian cancers enable biological and morphological testing against two-dimensional models of the same cell lines and the primary tumors.

Animal models may also help to take the GWAS-identified loci to the next level. Animal models have been established for GWAS-identified genes in some diseases such as type 2 diabetes. Ragvin et al. [36] took the sequence within LD blocks for three loci (*HHEX, SOX4*, and *IRX3*) from the type 2 diabetes

GWAS and searched across species for highly conserved non-coding elements that potentially marked regulatory blocks. They then tested these blocks using a transgenic reporter in zebrafish embryos and correlated expression patterns with other genes in the synteny region (where the gene order is conserved between species). They then came up with the more likely candidate for involvement in type 2 diabetes in each region. However, zebrafish may show a restricted pattern of expression of particular genes and the causal gene may be rejected. Mouse models may have greater potential to characterize susceptibility loci by investigating the function of associated genes in vivo. The mouse is a good mammalian model organism for several reasons: the availability of its complete genomic sequence, genetically defined strains and extensive genetic manipulation tools; the ease and control of breeding; and the availability of a wide array of standardized phenotyping tests. Mouse models that functionally test disease-associated genes illustrate how the model can provide functional evidence to identify causative genes among GWAS data. Such models are in development for the ovarian cancer GWAS-identified genes.

Methods for identification of novel loci

From a statistical perspective, it is challenging to efficiently identify relevant genetic variation important in the etiology of ovarian cancer. To date, the genetic variants discovered by GWAS, based primarily on univariate analyses of individual SNPs, account for only a small proportion of the heritability of complex traits, including ovarian cancer [37]. Research strategies to uncover this "missing heritability" include studying rare variants, epistatic and epigenetic effects, and gene sets.

Gene–gene and gene–environment interactions

The etiology of complex diseases and phenotypes is likely controlled by networks of interacting biochemical pathways influenced by the products of many genes. Therefore, methods that detect gene–gene or gene–environment interaction may detect novel loci not detected by assessment of the marginal effects of each marker alone. However, the study of interactions poses some common and some unique challenges. Due to the low statistical power to detect interactions (compared with marginal SNP effects) and the computation required to evaluate all possible combinations, interactions are not typically reported for large-scale genetic studies. Often, a screening step is performed to reduce the number of genetic variants for consideration; however, screening steps used in genetic studies usually fail to account for potential gene–gene interactions. Gene–environment interaction analyses are additionally complicated by existence of intermediate environmental risk factors that are themselves under genetic influence.

Several methods intended to identify the complex interacting effects of genetic and environmental disease risk factors have been proposed, including both parametric and non-parametric methods. In non-parametric statistical methods, several data-mining approaches have been used to detect higher order gene–gene interactions, such as combinatorial partitioning, neural networks, and multifactor dimensionality reduction. These methods detect interactions between SNPs by reducing the dimension of the vast amount of genetic data and recognizing hidden patterns.

Other standard logistic and penalized regression models are also typically used, such as the use of the joint test for interaction. Alternatively, an empirical Bayes-style shrinkage estimation framework for studying gene–environment interactions may be used; this remains valid when the assumption of independence between the gene and environment is not met. Finally, case-only designs have been advocated as an alternative to case–control designs to study interaction.

Gene set analysis

Gene set analysis (GSA) assesses the overall evidence for association of variation among an entire set of SNPs within a gene set (or pathway) with a phenotype, such as ovarian cancer risk. A gene set is a pre-defined set of genes, such as genes within a specific biological pathway as defined in the Kyoto Encyclopedia of Genes and Genomes (KEGG) database (http://www.genome.jp/kegg/pathway.html) or genes with a gene set as defined by the Gene Ontology (GO) (http://www.geneontology.org/). GSA has the potential to detect subtle effects of multiple SNPs in the same gene set that might be missed when assessed individually. Because numerous genes can be combined into a limited number of gene sets for analysis, the multiple-testing burden may be greatly reduced using GSA. Moreover, the incorporation of biological knowledge in statistical analysis may aid in the interpretation of results.

GSA methods can be classified into two types: competitive and self-contained. Many competitive methods are based on initial identification of SNPs (or genes) that are significantly associated with a trait followed by evaluation of whether the significantly associated SNPs tend to cluster in predefined gene sets. These methods are competitive because they compare the frequency of significantly associated SNPs in a particular set of genes with the frequency of significant associations among all genes not in the set. The null hypothesis for competitive methods is thus Ho: SNPs/genes in the gene set of interest are associated with the phenotype as much as SNPs/genes outside the gene set. The commonly used gene set enrichment analysis (GSEA), extended to GWAS by Wang et al. [38], is a competitive method that assesses the enrichment of significant associations for genes in the gene set (as compared to those outside the gene set). In contrast, a self-contained GSA method considers results only within a gene set of interest and tests the null hypothesis Ho: SNPs/genes in the gene set of interest are NOT associated with the phenotype versus the alternative hypothesis Ha: SNPs/genes in the gene set are associated with the phenotype. For reviews of GSA methods, the reader is referred to Fridley and Biernacka [39]. No GSA of ovarian cancer risk has been reported; however, GSA in ovarian cancer survival show promise [40].

Genomic copy number association

Copy number variants (CNVs) occur commonly in the human genome and are largely heritable. Relative to single nucleotide polymorphism (SNPs), CNVs are a priori more likely to have larger phenotypic effects. Using current genotype SNP arrays, researchers are not only able to investigate the impact of SNP variation on phenotypes, but also CNVs (primarily CNVs > 5 kb). However, analysis of CNVs from SNP arrays poses some challenges. First, the intensity data must be normalized and adjusted for differences in the allele intensities. Following the normalization, one can complete CNV association analysis using two complementary approaches. In the first approach, which we refer to as "CNV-level testing," stage I involves estimating the number of copies present in all segments of the genome for each individual, using software such as PennCNV [41] or circular-binary segmentation [42]; this is often referred to as "CNV calling." Stage II is then carrying out a genetic association test at every segment for which copy-number variability exists.

In contrast, a second approach, referred to as "single-locus testing," consists of genetic association testing at every marker using the normalized intensity data. Stage II then pools these test results across neighboring genetic loci to determine CNV regions associated with a phenotype. In addition to applying "CNV-level" and "single-locus" and testing approaches, CNV burden analysis can also be completed. No CNV analyses of ovarian cancer etiology have been published to date.

Analysis of rare and uncommon variants

The overall hope for rare variant analyses (e.g., MAF < 0.01) is that larger effect sizes and the analytical aggregation of variants within a gene will provide ample statistical power to detect associations (Fig. 10.1). The growing need for analysis of rare variants from next generation sequencing studies has led to the development of methods to increase the power for association testing, as the power to assess each rare variant individually requires a large sample size to detect an effect with reasonable power. Many methods seek to improve power by aggregating information across a set of rare variants, for example, in a gene. Li and Leal [43] presented the combined multivariate and collapsing method, where an indicator variable is defined as 1 if the individual carries at least one variant in a particular region and 0 otherwise. A multivariate method such as Hotelling's T2 test is then used to test for association between the phenotype and the indicator variable. The inclusion of variants with effects in the opposite direction is likely to decrease power in this method, unless variants are grouped by direction of effect (e.g., number of risk variants, number of protective variants), perhaps by using univariate effect estimates in choosing groups.

Madsen and Browning [44] presented the weighted sum statistic method, which weights variants by their frequency, allowing the combined analysis of rare and common variants. This was subsequently modified by Price et al. [45] to allow variable MAF thresholds for defining rare alleles. However, when one has a choice of methods to collapse rare variants in a region for an individual, greater power is obtained when regressing on the proportion of a set of rare alleles carried by each individual rather than simple presence or absence of alleles. However, a limitation of all of these approaches is that they assume all rare variants to be deleterious. Recently, many methods have been proposed that allow for both deleterious and protective rare variants. For more details and methods on rare variants, the reader is referred to review papers by Bansal et al. [46].

Integrative genomic methods

With the wealth of data produced by current genomic technologies, collection of multiple types of genomic data on a set of samples is becoming commonplace. New methods explore a multifactor approach that combines different kinds of genomic data, sometimes referred to as "integrative genomics" or "genomic convergence," in which a multistep procedure is used to identify potential key drivers of complex traits that integrate DNA variation and gene expression data. For example, one can first determine SNPs found to be statistically associated with the phenotype. Because SNPs might control mRNA expression in a *cis* manner (within or near a gene) or *trans* manner (far from a gene), one next determines the set of genes for which the SNP is associated with levels of mRNA expression. Finally, this set of genes, in which mRNA expression was identified to be related to the phenotype-associated SNP, are then assessed for association with the phenotype. This analysis procedure produces a set of genes that can be explored for possible biological relevance with the phenotype, such as ovarian cancer susceptibility.

Another approach for integrative genomic analysis is a single, comprehensive approach, as opposed to the multistep analysis procedure outlined above. Current comprehensive modeling approaches are limited in their scope to the analysis of a small number of variables, and therefore have only been applied to candidate gene and pathway studies. However, recently, sparse canonical correlation and partial least squares have been proposed for assessing the relationship between two high-dimensional sets of data (e.g., mRNA expression and SNPs). By incorporating a "shrinkage" penalty, these new methods allow for the analysis and integration of two sets of genome-wide genomic data and have been recently extended to more than two data sets.

Finally, mRNA expression data have been used to map SNPs to genes, in addition to the standard mapping of SNPs to genes based on base-pair location. For example, gene sets usually consist of SNPs in, or near, genes thought to contribute to a particular biological process. However, the definition of a gene set could be extended to use other knowledge related to gene function. For example, mRNA expression data have been used to define gene sets that include eQTL SNPs, i.e., SNPs that have been shown to regulate the expression of a particular gene in either a *cis*- or *trans*-acting manner. Recent advances in molecular genetics are providing novel insight into the relationships between genetic variation and variation in mRNA expression, leading to identification of eQTLs at an unprecedented level.

imilar approaches could be used to understand the relationips between other types of genomic data, such as methylation ata, and their impact on the development of ovarian cancer.

ummary

dvances in genetics now make it clear that, even among cases hich do not arise from multi-case ovarian cancer families, herited factors play a role in risk of this disease. These include ariants in chromosomes 2q31, 3q25, 8q24, 9p22, 17q21, and 9p13, and, to a lesser extent, variants in a small set of genes ith known biology. Each of these variants is common (freuency more than 8%) and leads to only a modest change in risk p to 20%). Additional variants are likely to be identified with e use of larger sample sizes, examination of histologyecific risks, analysis of sets of genes in combination, considration of larger scale structural genomic variation, and intration of multiple data types. Generally, the specific function f these risk-associated variants is unknown; in fact, other orrelated variants may be driving the result, and it may not e the studied variants which are causal. Thus, a great amount f work is needed to understand how these variants affect varian cancer disease risk; such work, including in silico, in vivo, and in vitro studies is under way with the best approach depending on what is currently known about each risk region. Additional work is also needed to properly characterize the role of each variant as it relates to non-genetic risk factors, such as use of hormones. Such gene–environment interactions will be critical to translation of these findings into clinical preventive efforts.

The ultimate goals of characterizing the genetic etiology of sporadic ovarian cancer are two-fold: first, to uncover novel biological targets for prevention or treatment measures (e.g., PARP-inhibitors) and, second, to assist in counseling-based genetic risk prediction. Whether and when these hopes come to light remains to be seen. Before the clinical application of genetic tests for the identification of women at highest risk based on common susceptibility SNPs beyond high-penetrance mutations, many more loci for sporadic ovarian cancer must be elucidated, and more effective screening or prevention mechanisms must be in place. Continued cooperation between clinicians, epidemiologists, biostatisticians, and functional biologists will increase our knowledge of the biology of ovarian cancer and may lead to tailored treatments or improved management of this lethal disease.

eferences

- Johnatty SE, Beesley J, Chen X, et al. Evaluation of candidate stromal epithelial cross-talk genes identifies association between risk of serous ovarian cancer and TERT, a cancer susceptibility "hot-spot". PLoS Genet. 2010;**6**:e1001016.
- Goode EL, Chenevix-Trench G, Song H, et al. A genome-wide association study identifies susceptibility loci for ovarian cancer at 2q31 and 8q24. Nat Genet. 2010;**42**:874–9.
- Doherty JA, Rossing MA, Cushing-Haugen KL, et al. ESR1/SYNE1 polymorphism and invasive epithelial ovarian cancer risk: an Ovarian Cancer Association Consortium study. Cancer Epidemiol Biomarkers Prev. 2010;**19**:245–50.
- Pearce CL, Wu AH, Gayther SA, et al. Progesterone receptor variation and risk of ovarian cancer is limited to the invasive endometrioid subtype: results from the ovarian cancer association consortium pooled analysis. Br J Cancer. 2008;**98**:282–8.
- Ramus SJ, Vierkant RA, Johnatty SE, et al. Consortium analysis of 7 candidate SNPs for ovarian cancer. Int J Cancer. 2008;**123**:380–8.
- Song H, Ramus SJ, Tyrer J, et al. A genome-wide association study identifies a new ovarian cancer susceptibility locus on 9p22.2. Nat Genet. 2009;**41**:996–1000.

7. Schildkraut JM, Iversen ES, Wilson MA, et al. Association between DNA damage response and repair genes and risk of invasive serous ovarian cancer. PLoS One. 2010;**5**:e10061.
8. Bolton KL, Tyrer J, Song H, et al. Common variants at 19p13 are associated with susceptibility to ovarian cancer. Nat Genet. 2010;**42**:880–4.
9. Antoniou A, Pharoah PD, Narod S, et al. Average risks of breast and ovarian cancer associated with BRCA1 or BRCA2 mutations detected in case series unselected for family history: a combined analysis of 22 studies. Am J Hum Genet. 2003;**72**:1117–30.
10. Boyd J, Rubin SC. Hereditary ovarian cancer: molecular genetics and clinical implications. Gynecol Oncol. 1997;**64**:196–206.
11. Lu HK, Broaddus RR. Gynecologic cancers in Lynch syndrome/HNPCC. Fam Cancer. 2005;**4**:249–54.
12. Shulman L, Dungan J. Cancer genetics: risks and mechanisms of cancer in women with inherited susceptibility to epithelial ovarian cancer. Cancer Treat Res. 2010;**156**:69–85.
13. Holschneider CH, Berek JS. Ovarian cancer: epidemiology, biology, and prognostic factors. Semin Surg Oncol. 2000;**19**:3–10.
14. Tung KH, Goodman MT, Wu AH, et al. Aggregation of ovarian cancer with breast, ovarian, colorectal, and prostate cancer in first-degree relatives. Am J Epidemiol. 2004;**159**:750–8.
15. Lichtenstein P, Holm NV, Verkasalo PK, et al. Environmental and heritable factors in the causation of cancer – analyses of cohorts of twins from Sweden, Denmark, and Finland. N Engl J Med. 2000;**343**:78–85.
16. Pharoah PD, Antoniou A, Bobrow M, et al. Polygenic susceptibility to breast cancer and implications for prevention. Nat Genet. 2002;**31**:33–6.
17. Frazer KA, Ballinger DG, Cox DR, et al. A second generation human haplotype map of over 3.1 million SNPs. Nature. 2007;**449**:851–61.
18. The 1000 Genomes Project Consortium. A map of human genome variation from population-scale sequencing. Nature. 2010;**467**:1061–73.
19. Braem MGM, Schouten LJ, Peeters PHM, et al. Genetic susceptibility to sporadic ovarian cancer: a systematic review. Biochim Biophys Acta. 2011;**1816**:132–46.

20. Lohmueller KE, Pearce CL, Pike M, et al. Meta-analysis of genetic association studies supports a contribution of common variants to susceptibility to common disease. Nat Genet. 2003;**33**:177–82.
21. Rafnar T, Sulem P, Stacey SN, et al. Sequence variants at the TERT-CLPTM1L locus associate with many cancer types. Nat Genet. 2009;**41**:221–7.
22. Modugno F. Ovarian cancer and polymorphisms in the androgen and progesterone receptor genes: a HuGE review. Am J Epidemiol. 2004;**159**:319–35.
23. Berchuck A, Schildkraut JM, Wenham RM, et al. Progesterone receptor promoter +331A polymorphism is associated with a reduced risk of endometrioid and clear cell ovarian cancers. Cancer Epidemiol Biomarkers Prev. 2004;**13**:2141–7.
24. Cancer Genome Atlas Research Network. Integrated genomic analyses of ovarian carcinoma. Nature. 2011;**474**:609–15.
25. Song H, Ramus SJ, Shadforth D, et al. Common variants in RB1 gene and risk of invasive ovarian cancer. Cancer Res. 2006;**66**:10220–6.
26. Schildkraut JM, Goode EL, Clyde MA, et al. Single nucleotide polymorphisms in the TP53 region and susceptibility to invasive epithelial ovarian cancer. Cancer Res. 2009;**69**:2349–57.
27. Fasching PA, Gayther S, Pearce L, et al. Role of genetic polymorphisms and ovarian cancer susceptibility. Mol Oncol. 2009;**3**:171–81.
28. Bolton KL, Ganda C, Berchuck A, et al. Role of common genetic variants in ovarian cancer susceptibility and outcome: progress to date from the ovarian cancer association consortium (OCAC). J Intern Med. 2012;**271**:366–78.
29. Grisanzio C, Freedman ML. Chromosome 8q24–associated cancers and MYC. Genes Cancer. 2010;**1**:555–9.
30. Raney BJ, Cline MS, Rosenbloom KR, et al. ENCODE whole-genome data in the UCSC genome browser (2011 update). Nucleic Acids Res. 2011;**39**:D871–5.
31. Pasaniuc B, Zaitlen N, Lettre G, et al. Enhanced statistical tests for GWAS in admixed populations: assessment using African Americans from CARe and a Breast Cancer Consortium. PLoS Genet. 2011;**7**:e1001371.
32. Kurman RJ, Shih IeM. Molecular pathogenesis and extraovarian origin of epithelial ovarian cancer – shifting the paradigm. Hum Pathol. 2011;**42**:918–31.
33. McCluggage WG, Young RH. Immunohistochemistry as a diagnostic aid in the evaluation of ovarian tumors. Semin Diagn Pathol. 2005;**22**:3–32.
34. Eeles RA, Kote-Jarai Z, Giles GG, et al. Multiple newly identified loci associated with prostate cancer susceptibility. Nat Genet. 2008;**40**:316–21.
35. Waters KM, Stram DO, Le Marchand L, et al. A common prostate cancer risk variant 5’ of microseminoprotein-beta (MSMB) is a strong predictor of circulating beta-microseminoprotein (MSP) levels in multiple populations. Cancer Epidemiol Biomarkers Prev. 2010;**19**:2639–46.
36. Ragvin A, Moro E, Fredman D, et al. Long-range gene regulation links genomic type 2 diabetes and obesity risk regions to HHEX, SOX4, and IRX3. Proc Natl Acad Sci U S A. 2010;**107**:775–80.
37. Manolio TA, Collins FS, Cox NJ, et al. Finding the missing heritability of complex diseases. Nature. 2009;**461**:747–53.
38. Wang K, Li M, Bucan M. Pathway-based approaches for analysis of genomewide association studies. Am J Hum Genet. 2007;**81**:1278–83.
39. Fridley BL, Biernacka JM. Gene set analysis of SNP data: benefits, challenges, and future directions. Eur J Hum Genet. 2011;**19**:837–43.
40. Fridley BL, Jenkins GD, Tsai YY, et al. Gene set analysis of survival following ovarian cancer implicates macrolide binding and intracellular signaling genes. Cancer Epidemiol Biomarkers Prev. 2012;**21**:529–36.
41. Wang K, Li M, Hadley D, et al. PennCNV: an integrated hidden Markov model designed for high-resolution copy number variation detection in whole-genome SNP genotyping data. Genome Res. 2007;**17**:1665–74.
42. Olshen AB, Venkatraman ES, Lucito R, et al. Circular binary segmentation for the analysis of array-based DNA copy number data. Biostatistics. 2004;**5**:557–72.
43. Li B, Leal SM. Methods for detecting associations with rare variants for common diseases: application to analysis of sequence data. Am J Hum Genet. 2008;**83**:311–21.
44. Madsen BE, Browning SR. A groupwise association test for rare mutations using a weighted sum statistic. PLoS Genet. 2009;**5**:e1000384.
45. Price AL, Kryukov GV, de Bakker PI, et al. Pooled association tests for rare variants in exon-resequencing studies. Am J Hum Genet. 2010;**86**:832–8.
46. Bansal V, Libiger O, Torkamani A, et al. Statistical analysis strategies for association studies involving rare variants. Nat Rev Genet. 2010;**11**:773–85.

Chapter 11

Chronic anovulation and the polycystic ovary syndrome

Nathan G. Kase, MD

Introduction

Chapter 1 of this volume chronicled the integration of the hypothalamic–anterior pituitary–ovarian follicle events involving intrinsic and endocrine factors driving gonadogenesis, primordial follicle formation, follicle arrest, reactivation, recruitment, selection, dominance, ovulation, and corpus luteum function [1]. The crucial importance of the timely appearance, concentrations, and sequence of gonadotropins FSH and LH was emphasized. However, simply adequate gonadotropin availability does not insure ovulatory or reproductive success. The follicle must also be at the appropriate stage of functional maturity to respond to any of the selection steps leading to pre-ovulatory dominance let alone respond to the ovulation stimulus.

In the normal cycle, gonadotropin release and final maturation of the follicle coincide because the timing of the gonadotropin surge is controlled by the level of gonadal feedback signals which reflect the degree of dominant follicle growth and functional maturity. The requisite feedback relationships in both the inter-cycle early follicle selection phase and at ovulation are tightly controlled, generally permitting only one follicle to reach the point of ovulation (Fig. 11.1) [2]. This is the salient feature of the evolutionary pressure to survive as a species – the human uterus cannot sustain a litter of embryos successfully, nor has the human mother the mammary capacity to feed more than two suckling dependent neonates. Superimposed on these structural constraints is the capacity to transiently postpone reproduction when negative internal or environmental factors challenge the system – illness, starvation, chronic danger, and stress – by inducing acute or chronic anovulation.

Crucial to this extraordinary degree of coordination and timing is the Graafian follicle which signals readiness to ovulate by positive feedback levels of estradiol and progesterone, a capability only this unique entity can generate. Reviewed in Chapter 1, these cyclic processes are driven by a sequential series of three

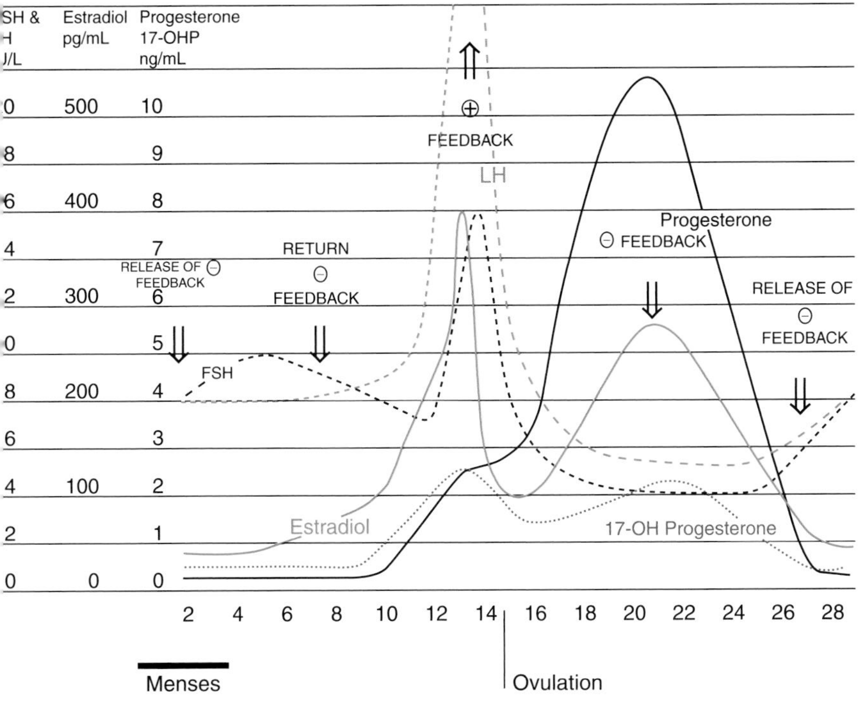

Fig. 11.1. Interactive endocrine signals driving repetitive ovulatory cycles. The hypothalamic–anterior pituitary–ovarian interactive circuitry in ovulatory menstrual cycles. Note the physiologically unique presence of sequential negative and positive signaling mechanisms generating follicle maturation, ovulation and menstruation.

Altchek's Diagnosis and Management of Ovarian Disorders, ed. Liane Deligdisch, Nathan G. Kase, and Carmel J. Cohen. Published by Cambridge University Press.

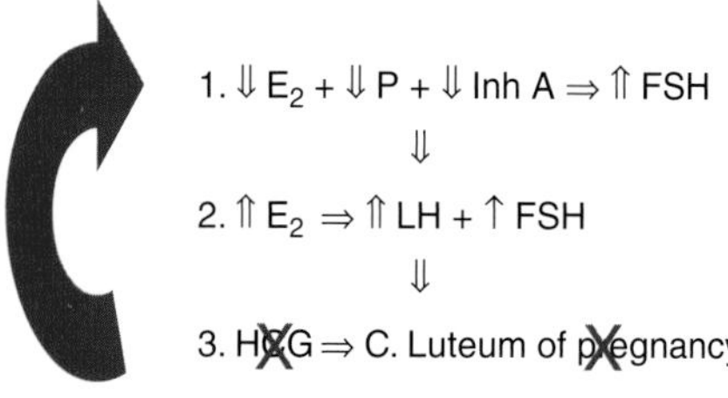

Fig. 11.2. The sequential mandatory recycling events in successful repetitive ovulation. The mandatory recycling events leading to successful, repetitive ovulatory cycles. Failure in either event 1 or 2 leads to anovulation. The presence of human chorionic gonadotropin from the implanted trophoblast of pregnancy salvages the corpus luteum by preventing luteolysis and delaying recycling.

mandatory recycling events by which the ovary achieves follicle readiness, and proceeds through each successive phase of repetitive ovulatory menstrual cycles. Failure in mandatory events 1 or 2 leads to acute and/or chronic anovulation (Fig. 11.2).

The ovulatory menstrual cycle as a vital sign of health status

Repetitive H-P-O ovulatory cycles depend on practically every regulatory mechanism in human biology. These include secretion and production rates of classic endocrine signals, intracrine, autocrine, paracrine regulation and interactions at organs of origin, at target tissues, as well as sites of signaling molecule metabolism and catabolic clearance.

The "success" of this highly synchronized interactive system depends on the specificity of signals, the sensitivity of target reception, and minimization of disruptive extraneous "noise." Because the organ systems involved are not exclusively classic "reproductive" organs *failure* of the system – anovulation – may not only indicate impending reproductive failure but also as a *sentinel signal* of the evolving often silent presence of subclinical non-reproductive system dysfunction and disease. As such anovulation represents a warning of the potential for later appearance of disease in sufficiently timely manner to permit intervention, stabilization, or even reversal of disruptive processes. Analysis of the etiologic mechanisms, consequences, and management of anovulation is the subject of this chapter.

Causes of ovulatory failure (anovulation)

Acute anovulation

Depending on the timing, intensity, and duration of the initiating stress [3], both recycling events 1 and 2 may be unfavorably altered in acute anovulation. For recycling event 2, limited quantity, perhaps biologic quality, certainly untimely release of LH, in short a deficiency of the inducer of ovulation leads to acute anovulation. The FSH response essential to recycling event 1 success may also be limited resulting in failure of adequate stimulation of follicle recruitment and selection.

The pathogenesis of either or both defects resides in suprasellar factors modifying/suppressing GnRH pulses not as a result of negative feedback but central inhibition of the GnR pulse generator. Because the specific mechanisms are unclea the catch-all phrases "environmental stress" or "hypothalam amenorrhea" are used. Sometimes a physical illness can b identified, but more commonly the disruptive factor emotional, behavioral, or "psychologic" in origin. It occurs i young women in whom by simple history possible incitin causes can be identified: academic pressures, occupation stress, positive/negative social and sexual experiences, fisc difficulties, death, or illness in the family. These are representa tive of the spectrum of stimuli for the most primitive physic logic defense mechanism, to avoid or postpone reproductio when unfavorable stressful conditions intervene. If LH o FSH dysfunction persists and spontaneous cycles do no resume, the condition converts from physiologic "reproductiv avoidance" to potentially pathophysiologic chronic anovula tory failure [4,5].

Chronic anovulation

Anovulation becomes chronic as dysfunction in mandatory recy cling event 1 (insufficient FSH to "rescue and select" the domi nant follicle) emerges as the main etiologic factor [2]. In th absence of adequate follicle development, the LH surge will als be impaired. Persistent blunting of FSH and loss of the essentia mandatory initiating step in H-P-O recycling peptide–steroi endocrine interactions results in a non-oscillating, dampene homeostatic state presenting as chronic anovulation, infertility and oligo/amenorrhea. If the disruptive process is rapidly pro gressive then hypogonadotropic, hypogonadal, hypoestrogeni amenorrhea will be the immediate clinical response. A subclinica "silent" period, if any, will be brief. On the other hand, static o slowly evolving dysfunction may not terminate in full hypgonad ism but stabilize at a prolonged "steady state" of non-oscillatin eugonadal, normo-gonadotropic, normo-estrogenic, chroni anovulation (Fig. 11.3).

In this circumstance, estradiol settles at mid follicle phas concentrations, FSH is marginally suppressed within lo normal non-oscillating basal levels. LH concentrations ar frequently slightly elevated but remain within the normal pre ovulatory range. Whatever progesterone can be detecte reflects the short luteal phase of defective ovulation.

The morphologic result of H-P-O non-oscillation is pre dictable – polycystic ovary morphology.

Etiology of chronic anovulation: a spectrum of vulnerabilities

Chronic anovulation can be described as dysfunction or diseas at any point in the cascade of events that make up the H-P-O axis (Table 11.1) [2 (pp. 495–500)]. Many can be categorized i identifiable *anatomic "compartments"*:

- *The central nervous system*: adverse hypothalamic, higher neural center reactions to environmental (internal or external) stimuli

Table 11.1. Etiology of "dampened" endocrine oscillations leading to chronic anovulation

Loss or blunting of mandatory recycling events with disruption of "normal" H-P-O ovulatory circuitry by dysfunction or disease
By anatomic compartment defects
CNS/anterior pituitary hypothalamic, higher neural centers, or environment
Gonadal (local)
By pathophysiologic signal dysregulation
Misdirecting endocrine or metabolic signals without specific anatomic origin

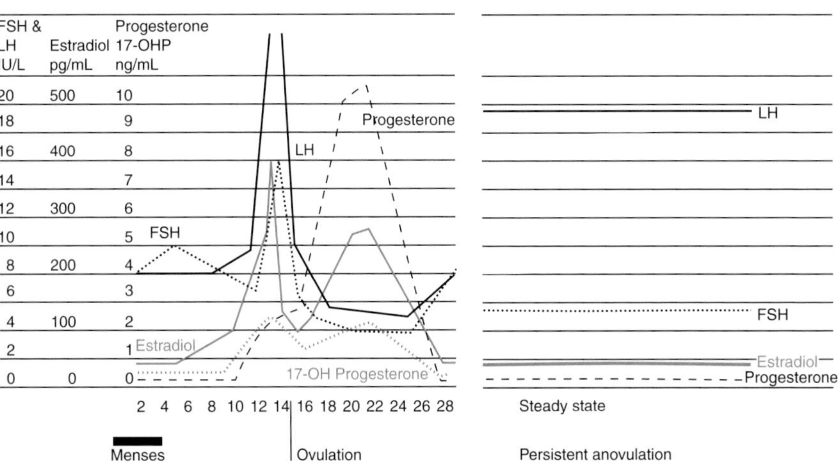

Fig. 11.3. Conversion of endocrine cyclicity to the non-oscillation state of anovulation. Conversion of cyclicity to non-oscillatory H-P-O interactions in chronic anovulation. Although basal concentrations of gonadotropins and estradiol are present, the absence of recycling event 1 and/or 2 leads to "dampening" of H-P-O circuitry resulting in normo-gonadotropic, normo-estrogenic anovulatory amenorrhea.

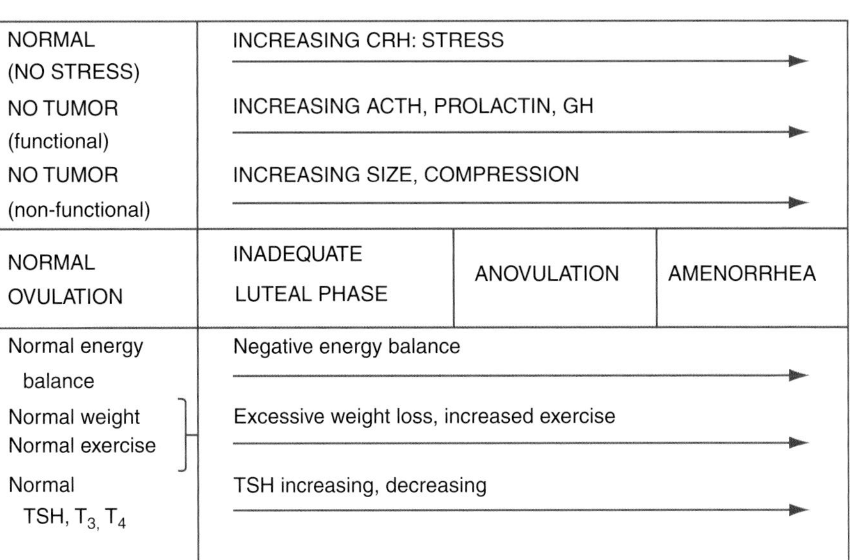

Fig. 11.4. The evolving spectrum of ovarian dysfunction with progression of disease: CNS/anterior pituitary. For example, as prolactin increases in concentration partial loss of appropriate corpus luteum formation and function leads to a "short" inadequate luteal phase. At higher prolactin levels further loss of ovulation function (blunting of recycling levels 1 and 2) occurs. Finally prolactin excess may inhibit gonadotropin completely, leading to hypogonadotropic, hypogonadal amenorrhea. Similar evolving dysfunction occurs in stress, other functional and non-functional tumors, as well as disturbances in energy balance. GH, growth hormone; TSH, thyroid-stimulating hormone; T_3, triiodothyronine; T_4, thyroxine.

- *Anterior pituitary*: induced or intrinsic abnormality or loss of gonadotrope cell function
- *Gonadal*: induced or intrinsic follicle abnormalities, dysfunction OR
- *System biology failure*: in the absence of an identifiable anatomic (organ system) etiology, dysregulation and dysfunction resulting from inappropriate or untimely misdirection of the interactive ovulation signal networks can lead to chronic anovulation.

"Central defects": CNS – anterior pituitary dysfunction/disease (Fig. 11.4)

Ovulatory gonadotropic responses (either the menstrual rise in FSH or the LH surge) require accurate reception, integration, transduction, and target responses linking GnRH and the anterior pituitary gonadotrope cells.

Two arterial blood supplies support the hypothalamus and anterior pituitary gonadotropes in the performance of these non-axonal functions. The superior hypothalamic artery delivers internal feedback to the ventral medial hypothalamic centers; long portal vessels then transfer adjusted hypothalamic signals to the anterior pituitary. This "long" system integrates higher central nervous system center secretions such as kisspeptin, norepinephrine, dopamine, endorphins, and neurokinins among others in addition to internal endocrine signal feedback to the anterior pituitary.

An inferior hypothalamic artery also exists which arrives first at the posterior pituitary, but also sends out major branches which connect to a short hypothalamic pituitary portal system. This vascular connection arises in the basal hypothalamic area and at the base of the stalk. This "short" system specifically transmits internal feedback signals directly to the anterior pituitary gonadotrope cells.

Cycle-appropriate frequency and amplitude of GnRH must be released into the primary capillary plexus of the hypothalamic anterior pituitary portal system. Similarly, the integrating function of anterior pituitary gonadotrope cells requires the capacity to react to GnRH and feedback steroid signals as well as adjustments of intracrine factors which organize cycle-specific, timely quantities of gonadotropin secretion. Adequate perfusion of the intra-sellar anterior pituitary gonadotrope cells by means of the secondary capillary plexi of the two portal systems is required for GnRH arrival at target cell receptors which drive synthesis, storage, and release of FSH and LH in both positive and negative modes.

Supra-sellar dysfunction, disease (Fig 11.4)

A wide range of central nervous system inhibiting mechanisms may lead to chronic anovulation. Although organic hypothalamic disease can disrupt these circuits these are uncommon compared with the incidence of dysfunction variously described as functional and/or psychogenic "hypothalamic" amenorrhea. The criteria dividing functional from psychogenic (or behavioral) are blurred and reflect the overlapping degrees of emotional stress and/or negative energy balance present [6,7].

The diagnosis proceeds by excluding organic disease (imaging is essential in differentiating intra-sellar vs. supra-sellar etiologies) and determining energy deficiency (low TSH, low T_3, T_4) versus psychogenic stress (increased CRH, cortisol) [4,8]. Although initiating organic disease is rarely found, nevertheless hazardous consequences do result. Most worrisome is progression across the spectrum of chronic hypothalamic "anovulation/amenorrhea" to the more serious forms of true hypogonadotropic, hypogonadal amenorrhea most often seen in adolescents or young adult white women. Either by dietary restriction [6] or intense participation in dance or sports [7], eventually severe underweight, wasting, and reduced fat and lean body mass ensues. Aside from preoccupation with and distorted attitudes about food, obsessive interest in exercise, athletic or scholastic goals, a negative or distorted body image, cycles of binging and purging – significant non-psychologic co-morbidities emerge: osteoporosis, anemia, leukopenia, thrombocytopenia, electrolyte disturbances, bradycardia, hypotension, cardiac arrhythmias, and even asystole [8].

Anorexia is an example of a potentially deadly end point of hypothalamic dysfunction that begins with normogonadotropic normo-estrogen "functional" anovulation. It serves to emphasize the point that chronic anovulation is a sentinel signal of potentially progressive disease that requires interception and stabilization well before the emergence of disabling, life-threatening disease.

Intra-sellar disease

Anterior pituitary tumors (Fig. 11.4)

Pituitary tumors [9,10] (even the rare empty sella syndromes, and even rarer auto-immune hypophysitis) of any type may cause anovulation by affecting GnRH secretion, transmission, or action at gonadotrope cells. These masses may act as expanding space-occupying lesions within the relatively unyielding boney sella turcica girdle and compress gonadotrope cells directly or interrupt delivery of vital GnRH by compressing portal vessel flow. Additionally, rather than by compression, functioning pituitary tumors may produce inhibiting secretions which modify or inhibit either GnRH or gonadotropin cell function directly.

Prolactinoma and hyperprolactinemia

The prolactin-producing prolactinoma is the prototypical example of CNS-anterior compartment disease evolving, slowly interrupting normal ovulatory dynamics by its functional secretion and less commonly as an expanding macroadenoma (>10 mm), which can escape the sella and invade the supra-sellar space, compromise visual fields, and invade sinus cavities [11]. The microadenoma (<10 mm) is a common tumor found at all ages from infancy to late age. Because its growth is slow, occurring over decades and often stabilizing at endocrinologically disruptive but non-hypogonadal levels, it is an important target in the differential diagnosis of chronic anovulation. This tumor secretes non-physiologic, non-pregnancy, and non-breast feeding-related levels of prolactin which inhibit GnRH-gonadotropin function. As prolactin levels rise well before galactorrhea is present or even provocable, FSH and LH oscillations and concentrations are suppressed, inducing a gradually evolving spectrum of ovulatory dysfunction ranging from a short luteal phase [12] to anovulatory cycles and eventually hypogonadotropic, hypogonadal, hyperprolactinemic, amenorrhea (Fig. 11.4).

The diagnosis of prolactinoma is more commonly made in women the appearance of anovulatory amenorrhea by (perhaps 80%). Men on the other hand present decades later with larger tumors causing hypogonadism, hypothyroidism, and compromise of visual fields.

The same evolving spectrum of ovulatory dysfunction (through short luteal phase and thereafter anovulation with polycystic-like ovaries) appears in Cushing's syndrome [13] as either ACTH and/or CRH increase to levels that interrupt GnRH–FSH, GnRH–LH synchrony. Similarly acromegaly [14], by function as well as compression can disrupt ovulatory function by excess growth hormone and insulin-like growth

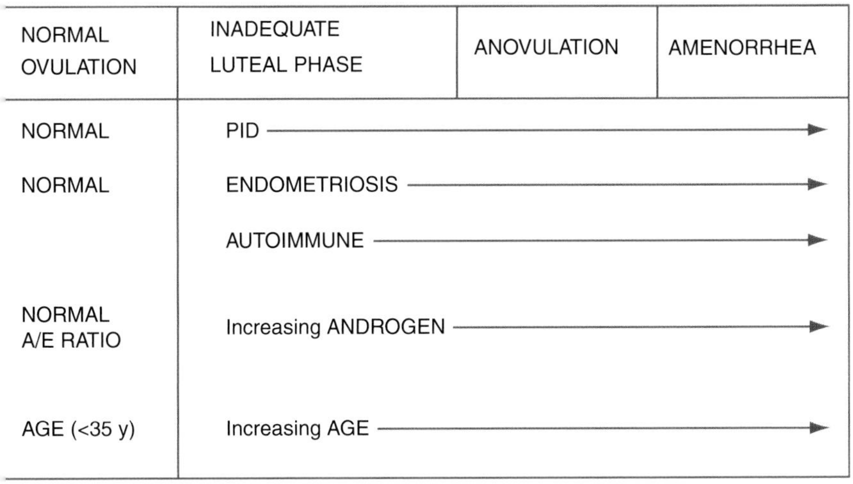

NORMAL OVULATION	INADEQUATE LUTEAL PHASE	ANOVULATION	AMENORRHEA
NORMAL	PID →		
NORMAL	ENDOMETRIOSIS →		
	AUTOIMMUNE →		
NORMAL A/E RATIO	Increasing ANDROGEN →		
AGE (<35 y)	Increasing AGE →		

Fig. 11.5. The evolving spectrum of ovarian dysfunction with progression of disease. Progressive disruption of follicle maturation resulting from a variety of local disorders (infection, endometriosis, autoimmune disease) as well as intra-gonadal, intra-follicle excess androgen. Defective oocyte maturation and follicle function occurs as women age (>35 years). PID, pelvic inflammatory disease.

factor (IGF) stimulation, producing ovaries with PCOS morphology (PCOM). Pituitary gonadotropin dysfunction is the presenting sign of autoimmune *hypophysitis* [15] which over time compromises other tropic activity (TSH, ACTH). Non-functioning space-occupying benign neoplasms or compression from non-neoplastic empty sella syndrome produce the same sustained compromise of gonadotropin functions. [16].

Not all pituitary dysfunction is primary to the gland. In the differential assessment of hyperprolactinemia, primary hypothyroidism with elevated TSH may induce lactotroph hyperplasia and secondary hyperprolactinemia. Prolactin excess may be generated from a variety of ectopic sites – dermoids, bronchogenic carcinoma by failure of renal clearance.

Loss of dopamine inhibiting restraint of prolactin occurs in a variety of forms of hypothalamic–pituitary stalk damage: trauma, tumor-related vascular compression (meningioma, craniopharyngioma, germinoma), granulomas, and even a Rathke's cyst. Neural feedback resembling suckling induced by chest wall trauma, surgery, or herpes zoster infection can induce hyperprolactinemic responses whereas cirrhosis or chronic renal disease sustains prolactin excess by disordered clearance. Finally a wide variety of drugs including anti-depressants, anti-hypertensive, neuroleptics/anti-psychotics, opiates, and opiate antagonists (altered synthesis, inhibition, and metabolism) all stimulate lactotroph release of prolactin [11]. For example, valproate treatment of epilepsy alters these signals and induces polycystic ovary morphology [17].

Although these alternate diagnostic possibilities require exclusion, the primary approach to differential diagnosis of CNS-anterior pituitary causes of chronic anovulation proceeds with initial imaging of the area to distinguish intra- from supra-sellar disease (tumor vs. functional disorders).

Gonadal factors (Fig. 11.5)

Follicle, oocyte "aging"

A disturbance in any of the intra-follicle regulatory mechanisms involved in selection and progression to dominant follicle status leads to local gonadal inhibition of ovulation and menstrual disturbance, even with increased availability of endogenous or administered FSH stimulation. The most common example of this type of dysfunction is seen in women beyond the age of 35 who experience progressively diminished fertility, fecundability, and decreased ovulatory frequency presumably reflecting age-related impairment of normal follicle development and oocyte maturation [18].

Effects of gonadal infection or disease

The assembly of intra-follicle factors is required for "successful" follicle responses to FSH and the LH surge [19]. Clinicians are aware of the adverse effects of chronic pelvic inflammatory disease, tubo-ovarian abscess formation and ovarian endometriosis/endometrioma on the diminished frequency of ovulation (and in the last instance resistance to even pharmacologic gonadotropin stimulation). Not explicitly understood or described, the effects of various pro-inflammatory cytokines, chemokines, macrophages, interleukins, and the range of interferon system responses are plausibly involved in these clinical conditions.

Adverse androgen/estrogen ratios

A delicate balance among thecal androgen production, granulosa cell aromatase function and E2 secretion is essential for normal follicle function; too little androgen, too little E2, too few FSH receptors, too little E2 secretion, no LH surge – that dysfunctional sequence is obvious [20]. However, too much androgen production will inhibit follicle development and maturity. At high local concentrations excess testosterone is converted to the androgenically powerful but non-aromatizable 5α-reduced androgens such as 5α-dihydrotestosterone (5αHT). This androgen acts as an anti-estrogen (decreased FSH receptors) and as an aromatase inhibitor (reduced E2 production) (Fig. 11.6). This is the mechanism by which an androgen-producing ovarian tumor inhibits local gonadal function by inducing PCOS morphology in the ovary bearing the tumor as well as the contra lateral ovary.

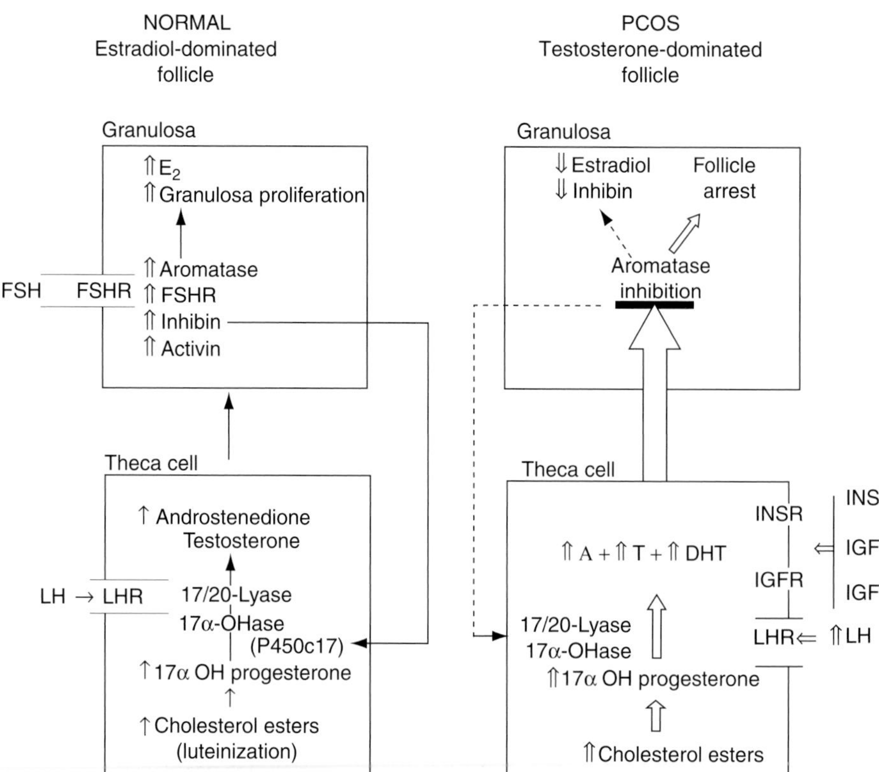

Fig. 11.6. Altered ovarian steroidogenesis in the PCOS and the inhibition of the follicle maturation and function.

Increased testosterone and DHT (non aromatizable active androgen) theca cell synthesis and delivery to granulosa inhibits granulosa cell proliferation and differentiation by reducing aromatase activity, estrogen synthesis, inhibins and activin synthesis and FSHR number and/or activity. Compounding these changes, hyperinsulinemia, increased IGF-1, and increased LH drive excess androgen availability and effects.

Local disruptive excess androgen may in rare instances reflect genetic variations in local androgen production or biologic effect. One defect is a deficiency in the aromatase enzyme system by which genetic variations in CYP19 may contribute to prenatal androgenization. A genomic variant (an intronic single nucleotide polymorphism (SNP50) of the CYP19 produces a hyperandrogenic state by both increased secretion of unused androgen substrate and reduced metabolic clearance of testosterone (as well as deficient estradiol production). It is associated with early adrenarche, pubertal hyperandrogenism, anovulation, and polycystic ovary morphology [21].

Autoimmune oophoritis

Rarely as a single organ expression, autoimmune oophoritis is most often associated with other autoimmune endocrinopathies such as adrenal cortical autoimmune insufficiency which precede ovarian involvement [22]. In 20% of adrenal autoimmune disease, ovarian autoimmune dysfunction can be identified.

Obesity

Obesity may alter menstrual cyclicity, oocyte quality, maturation and fertilizability by direct gonadal effects [23]. In application of Assisted Reproductive Technologies (ART) implantation and pregnancy rates are lower in overweight, obese subjects. In oocyte donation however no relationship between *recipient* BMI and implantation rates is seen. The oocyte or embryo of obese women, not receptivity of their endometrium, appears to be the cause of decreased pregnancy rates in obese women. Overall, as will be emphasized in the discussion of the pathophysiology of the PCOS, insulin resistance and obesity have a direct negative effect on follicle function in general and oocyte quality in particular. Nevertheless, a *direct* deleterious effect on follicle and oocyte function may exist *independent* of a generalized endocrinopathy.

Pathophysiologic system biology dysregulation (non-anatomic)

The polycystic ovary syndrome

The cause of chronic anovulation may be relatively easily demonstrated and mechanistically understood when the initiating disruptive process exists in any one of the anatomic compartments just discussed (i.e., the anovulation and PCOS ovarian morphology seen in an evolving prolactinoma, acromegaly, late onset adreno-cortical hyperplasia, excess androgen production, or valproate therapy) [2]. However H-P-O dysfunction resulting in dampened gonadotropin-gonadal steroid anovulation and distinct ovarian morphology may be an expression of physiologic

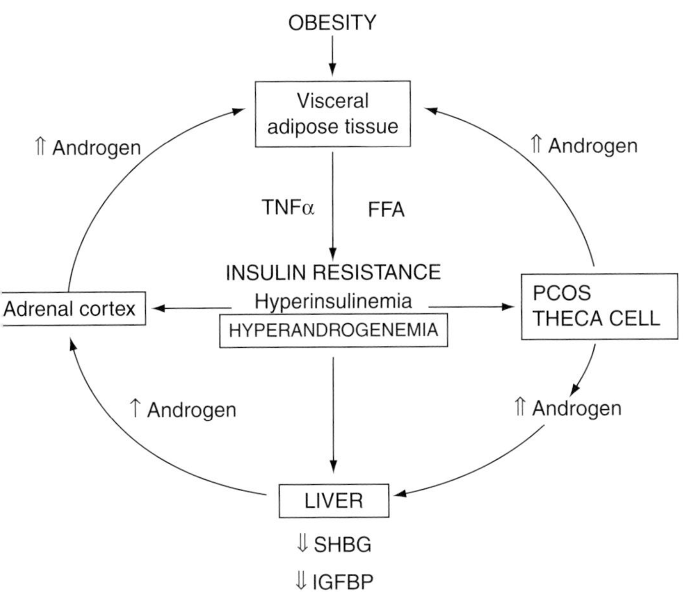

Fig. 11.7. Insulin resistance and hyperandrogenicity in the pathogenesis of PCOS. Hyperandrogenemia and hyperinsulinemia combine to promote a synergistic, positive feedforward cycle in which further increments in insulin and androgen are the result.

signal misdirection not assignable to pathology in a particular organ. In this circumstance, an assembly of several disparate mechanisms contributes to the accelerating, reinforcing "steady state" expressed as chronic anovulation. This is PCOS.

Although PCOS is conventionally described as the most common "cause" of anovulation, it does not cause anovulation. Rather it is the consequence of misdirecting HPO interactions which impose anovulatory dysfunction on the ovary. At least initially, the ovary is the victim; the unwilling participant – not the provocative agent. In that context the disorder is more accurately described as chronic anovulation displaying characteristic polycystic ovary *morphology and function*. This morphologic reaction is the entirely predictable reactive expression to chronic low FSH and relatively high LH signal input (Fig. 11.3).

Initially the ovary is a target, not a protagonist. Once established the PCO becomes not only a participant but a catalyst in its increased secretion of androgen. In the "mature" form of PCOS the ovary is a partner in a "vicious cycle" of incremental dysfunctions, the initiating origin of which cannot be absolutely identified (Fig. 11.7). Yet modification of any dysfunctional element (Clomid for FSH enhancement or Metformin for reduction of hyperinsulinemia) reestablishes the mandatory oscillating HPO recycling progression, the PCO morphology is reversed, and ovulatory cycles resume.

What is meant by "system biology dysregulation" in PCOS?

In all previous iterations of the pathophysiology of chronic anovulation, a special category entitled *"Abnormal Feedback"* was used to explain the loss of the essential interactions of the H-P-O in anovulation [24].

An example of this special category of dysfunction is the static, sustained, somewhat elevated levels of estrogen that is a feature of PCOS. A significant portion of this estrogen is not secreted by the ovaries but is produced *extra-gonadally* (hence not under gonadotropin control) by conversion of excess androgen secreted by the adrenal cortex and the theca cells of the ovary at sites which possess the aromatase enzyme system. The result is production of estrogen feedback signals from the metabolic "periphery" which *misrepresent* ovarian follicle status. This "abnormal feedback," the essence of chronic anovulation, occurs in two sequential steps:

- chronically elevated estrogen levels do not permit the essential inter-cycle increase in FSH secretion required to stimulate or sustain progressive follicle development (impairment of mandatory recycling event 1)
- as a result of deficient follicle development, the ovary is incapable of generating the increased levels of estradiol required to induce the ovulatory LH surge (impairment of mandatory recycling event 2).

Inhibiting levels of estrogen could be caused by increased production or decreased clearance and catabolism. As noted, increased production of estrogen results from secreted androgens which are irreversibly cleared from the circulation by a variety of processes (e.g., formation of the historically useful 17-ketosteroid assays in urine) but in this instance by the aromatase system which "detoxifies" one biologically active group (androgens) to another with entirely different biology – the estrogens. Adipose tissue possesses significant aromatase activity; the more adiposity the greater the facility for estrogen production.

Alternatively the clearance of estrogen can be impaired in a variety of conditions such as thyroid or hepatic disease. Both hypo- and hyperthyroidism can alter the metabolic clearance and peripheral inter-conversions of both androgens and estrogens. Similarly, hepatic disease perturbs normal clearance and metabolism of these steroids.

But abnormal feedback and misdirection of gonadotropin, while still an important element in the pathogenesis of chronic anovulation, is not the only component of the complex array of system-wide dysregulation underlying PCOS.

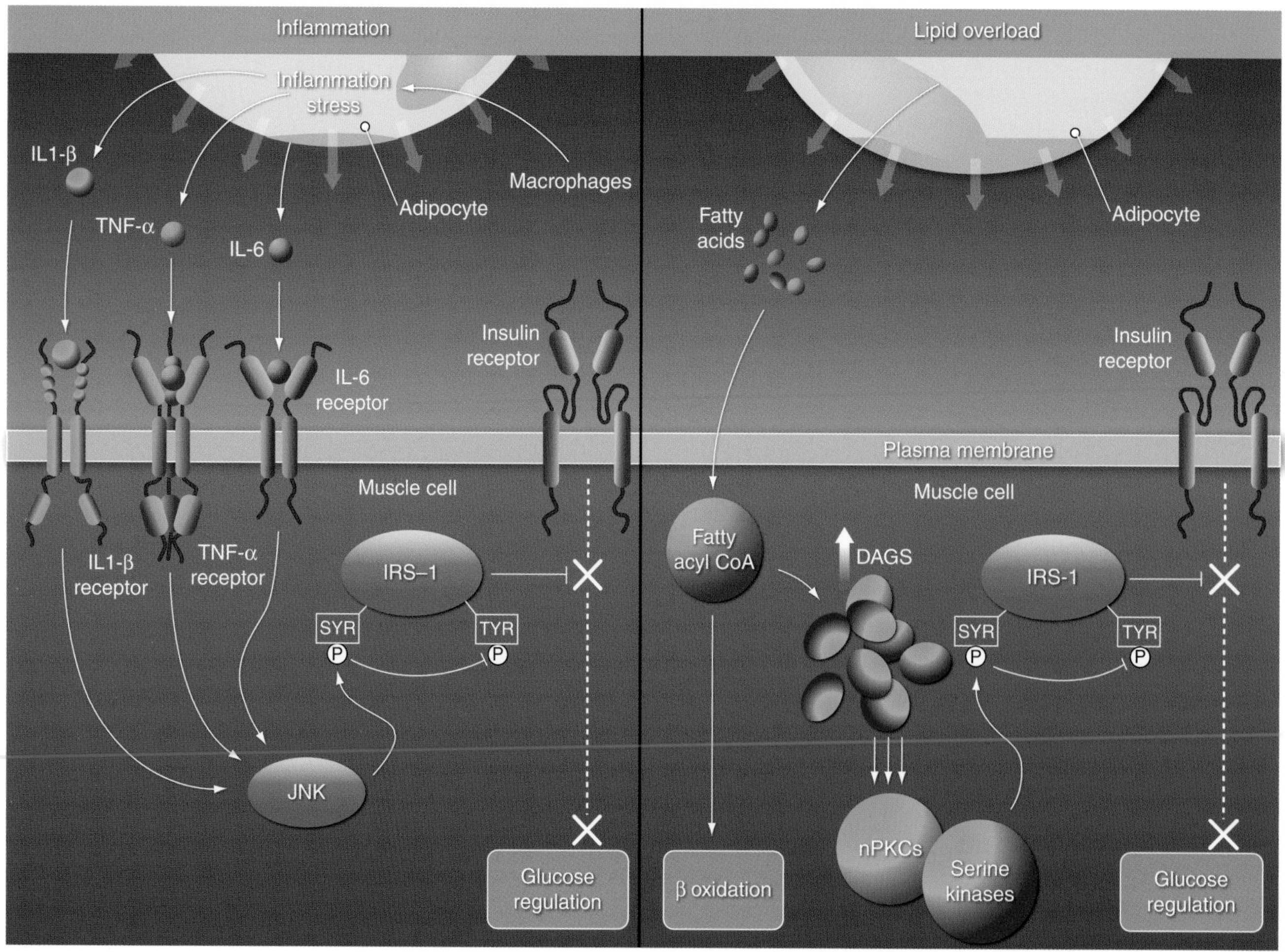

Fig. 11.8. Visceral adipose cell secretions and the induction of insulin resistance at target organs. The combination of pro-inflammatory cytokines and excess free fatt acids emanating from inflamed metabolically activated visceral adipocytes disrupts insulin receptor function. In the former, after interaction with their respective receptors, IRS-1 function is impaired by serine phosphorylation. Similarly, intracellular accumulation of diacylglycerols (DAGs) derived from FFAs also inhibits IRS-1 by the same process. In both instances the insulin receptor function is diminished leading to altered glucose intake and regulation, excess fat storage, and reactive hyperinsulinemia. Reprinted from: Taubes G. Insulin resistance: prosperity's plague. Science, 2009;**325**(5938):256–60. With permission from American Association for the Advancement of Science.

Both hyperinsulinemia (secondary to insulin resistance) and elevated testosterone concentrations are basic elements of the pathophysiology of PCOS and chronic anovulation. Their interaction is an example of how two signaling networks each of which are essential for the normal biologic function of a specific physiologic system can, by cross-talk between systems, modulate responses to stimuli with either positive or negative results.

Insulin resistance is a condition in which normal concentrations of insulin produce a tissue specific (i.e., muscle) subnormal biologic response. It occurs in acute physiological (pregnancy) and chronic pathological states (metabolic syndrome). One mechanism causing insulin receptor malfunction is altered kinase phosphorylation of insulin receptor substrate proteins (IRSs) – the large protein scaffold which serves as the docking platform for signaling protein–receptor complexes – occurring in response to pro-inflammatory cytokines, fetuin-A, interleukins, and free fatty acids (FFAs) with activation of NFκB-mediated pathways negatively regulate IRS signaling by serine phosphorylation replacing tyrosine kinase phosphorylation (Fig. 11.8) [25].

Hyperandrogenism is responsible for several clinical and biological problems in the chronically anovulatory PCOS woman. In addition to hirsutism and related cosmetic changes excess androgen inhibits follicle maturation and with insulin alters GnRH pulse frequency, increases pre-adipocyte proliferation, independently worsens the metabolic syndrome, is the substrate for extra-gonadal aromatase estrogen synthesis, and reduces hepatic production of SHBG. Accordingly it has important interactions with skin, hypothalamus, adipose tissue, and the liver, not simply organs of reproduction.

In PCOS insulin and testosterone combine to initiate and accelerate the glucotoxicity, lipotoxicity, and systemic inflammatory state underlying the endocrine, metabolic, vascular, and oncogenic burdens of PCOS. But they are also linked at the most fundamental level – the effect of high circulating FFAs on serine phosphorylation [25]:

- FFAs increase serine phosphorylation of IRS leading to insulin resistance
- FFAs increase adrenal cortical and ovarian theca cell serine phosphorylation of the biosynthetic enzyme p450c17 and 17,20-lyase which increases androgen synthesis and secretion.

Table 11.2. Definitions of the metabolic syndrome

Source	National Cholesterol Education Program/Adult Treatment Panel III	International Diabetes Federation
Measure	Presence of any three of the five clinical criteria	Presence of central obesity plus any two of the four clinical criteria
Clinical criteria	Elevated waist circumference (central obesity)> 35 in	Elevated triglycerides
	Elevated triglycerides > 150 mg/dL	Reduced HDL cholesterol
	Reduced HDL cholesterol <50 mg/dL	Elevated blood pressure
	Elevated blood pressure 130/85 mmHg or higher	Elevated fasting glucose

Table 11.3. Differential diagnosis of the polycystic ovary syndrome

Androgen-secreting tumor
Exogenous androgens
Cushing syndrome
Non-classical congenital adrenal hyperplasia
Acromegaly
Genetic defects in insulin action
Primary hypothalamic amenorrhea
Primary ovarian failure
Thyroid disease
Prolactin disorders

System biology is focused on how diverse components of natural biologic systems interact to form functional "nodes" at various scales of organization and complexity which support the survival of the organism. On the other hand as seen in this example, dysregulation by excess FFAs beginning in one of several interconnected nodes spreads throughout the multi-factorial biologic matrix promoting and sustaining progressive dysfunction and disease. For example, the liver secretory protein fetuin-A is an adaptor protein linking FFAs, pro-inflammatory cytokines, Toll-like receptor 4, and the systemic inflammatory state which impairs insulin signaling [26].

A detailed discussion of the pathogenesis, pathophysiology, genomics, differential diagnosis, and management of short- and long-term burdens and morbidity of the PCOS is the subject of the remainder of this chapter.

The polycystic ovarian syndrome

General overview

The polycystic ovary syndrome (PCOS) is a common endocrine disorder affecting from 4 to 12% of reproductive aged women (depending on criteria used – see below) [2].

For decades it was known as a cause of anovulatory oligo-amenorrhea and infertility, complicated by dysfunctional bleeding, acne, hirsutism, and the remote risk of endometrial cancer. Furthermore, when pregnant the PCOS woman and her fetus face increased intra- and post-pregnancy morbidities. PCOS is now understood as a factor in promoting progressive lifetime disease risks of type 2 diabetes mellitus (T2DM), cardiovascular disease, and cancer in the majority of affected women. This is a consequence of the confluence of hyperandrogenemia, central visceral fat accumulation, and induced insulin resistance (Ins Res) participating in a cluster of metabolic risk factors known as the metabolic syndrome (MetS) (Table 11.2).

Accordingly, PCOS is no longer entirely within the clinical purview of the gynecologist/infertility specialist; it is now a concern for all physicians caring for women.

Challenges and opportunities of PCOS

Challenges

PCOS imposes variable risks for progressive disabilities requiring sustained long-term follow-up. In addition, anovulatory oligo-amenorrhea can be secondary to any one of a broad range of etiologic possibilities, each of which requires identification and specific treatment. Meticulous initial differential diagnosis must exclude specific disorders and (Table 11.3) diseases which interrupt cyclic ovarian function and impose the PCOS phenotype.

Beyond differential diagnosis, PCOS challenges the physician caring for these women to identify, evaluate and treat disease and dysfunction *early*. PCOS affects the young – with symptoms and signs emerging in childhood well before puberty-implicating a *developmental basis* for the syndrome. PCOS also runs in families, hence a *genomic basis* must exist. More than 50% of PCOS women in the U.S. are overweight or obese – a morbidity emphasizing the presence of an *environmental/acquired* factor.

In addition there is that particular pain, not just reproductive impairment or disease risk, but the immediate cosmetic stigma of acne and hirsutism which compounds the ungainly physical dimensions of obesity. Women with PCOS have an increased prevalence of *psychiatric burdens* (mood disorders including depression (20–40%) and anxiety syndromes).

Opportunities

Challenges exist, but opportunities are also available for interception, modification, and even reversal of many of the burdens of PCOS. Differential diagnostic algorithms are in place to exclude treatable conditions to which PCOS is secondary. Widely available, reliable methods can identify and stratify the risk levels of various metabolic and vascular consequences imposed by PCOS. In many instances, effective management strategies can be applied to control and reverse the gynecologic, dermatologic, and

Table 11.4. Criteria for defining PCOS

Source	NIH (1990)	Rotterdam (2003)	Androgen-Excess and PCOS Society (2009)
Measure	Two of two criteria	Two of three criteria	Three of three criteria
Criteria	Chronic anovulation Clinical and/or biochemical signs of hyperandrogenism and exclusion of other etiologies	Oligovulation or anovation Clinical and or biochemical signs of hyperandrogenism Polycystic ovaries and exclusion of other etiologies	Hyperandrogenism (hirsutism and/or hyperandrogenemia) Ovarian dysfunction (oligovulation or anovulation and/or polycystic ovaries) Exclusion of other androgen excess or related disorders

metabolic manifestations of the syndrome. Finally, the PCOS mother and her fetus face incremental risks *during* pregnancy, at birth, as adults and even transgenerational consequences have been recognized. Preventive, intercepting strategies are implementable even in these multi-generational circumstances.

Clinical definition

PCOS is a cluster of symptoms, signs, and biochemical features resulting from variable degrees of confluence of multifactorial genomic and acquired (environmental) factors which emerge over time in various combinations and in variable degrees of intensity. But, as important issues of differential diagnosis and management confront the physician, unfortunately no single initiating clinical, biochemical, or genetic marker has been identified that unequivocally defines the syndrome.

Three consensus conferences have been convened to formulate a uniform definition of PCOS and perhaps predictably, three different definitions emerged and now are variably used. The first set was from the US National Institutes of Health (NIH) in 1990 [27]; the second set of revised criteria was formulated by the combined European Society for Human Reproduction and Embryology and the American Society of Reproductive Medicine (ESHRE-ASRM) in 2003 and now known as the Rotterdam Criteria [28]. Finally, the Androgen-Excess–PCOS Society produced their own recommendations [29]. Details of each are shown in Table 11.4.

The new criteria add two new categories of PCOS women – (a) those with hyperandrogenism, PCO morphology but *regular* cycles (possibly ovulatory), and (b) women with anovulatory oligoamenorrhea and polycystic ovaries by ultrasound but who are not hyperandrogenic. Problems applying the expanded criteria are obvious: 70% of the female population of Amsterdam can be shown to meet Rotterdam criteria at some time in their lives [30].

These definitions are not meaningful to the clinical management of PCOS either for the individual woman or in the approach of her health care provider. Periodic anovulation/amenorrhea is common and if examined by ultrasound, evidence of "multi-cystic" ovarian morphology may be found in healthy fertile women.

Accordingly, this chapter will use a more specific clinical definition of the syndrome: PCOS and the subpopulation at risk for evolving metabolic, cardiovascular disease, and cancer consist of the following:

- emergence and persistence of hyperandrogenism, anovulatory oligo/amenorrhea and insulin resistance
- a positive family history of PCOS or presence of elements of the metabolic syndrome and its consequences in first degree relatives
- increased markers of metabolic dysfunction (elevated blood pressure, impaired glucose tolerance, dysplipidemia, increased waist circumference) at initial evaluation of the patient or evolving in follow-up assessments.

In summary, to identify patients with PCOS or with impending evolving risk of developing PCOS, not only the presenting symptoms and signs, but evidence of the presence of precursors and/or emerging metabolic consequences of PCOS is required.

Pathogenesis and pathophysiology of PCOS

Introduction

PCOS presenting as hyperandrogenism, chronic oligo-anovulation, and polycystic ovarian morphology is associated with metabolic derangements, chiefly insulin resistance and compensatory hyperinsulinemia [31]. PCOS women often have psychological impairments including depression and mood disorders. Most women with PCOS are also overweight or obese, further accelerating androgen secretion and exaggerating androgen action, while impairing metabolism and reproductive functions. By definition, PCOS is not a specific disorder having a unique cause. Rather, as a complex syndrome, numerous elements interact, combine, and contribute to its pathogenesis and pathophysiology [2,32]. In the following sections, these elements will be described in detail and in particular how together they integrate into a self-sustaining self-perpetuating pathophysiologic state.

Endocrinology of PCOS

Steroids in PCOS

The average daily production of both androgens and estrogens is increased in women with PCOS, as reflected in the elevated serum concentrations of testosterone, androstenedione, dehydroepiandrosterone (DHEA), dehydroepiandrosterone sulfate (DHEA-S), 17α-hydroxprogesterone (17-OHP), and estrone.

Estrogens

Serum estrone concentrations are modestly elevated due to peripheral conversion of increased amounts of androstenedione [33]. In contrast, serum estradiol levels in PCOS fluctuate but generally remain within the range typically observed in the early follicular phase [34], reflecting continued low-level production from limited follicular development as well as non-gonadal interconversion from estrone.

Androgen excess

While androgen excess is considered an essential feature of PCOS, only 80–85% of women with clinical hyperandrogenism exhibit the "full spectrum" PCOS phenotype [35]. Acne and diffuse alopecia are even less specific. Nevertheless, visual scoring systems for the degree of hirsutism are valuable in most white or black women with PCOS [36] although not in East Asian women. Serum androgen measurements are helpful, but accurate detection of chemical hyperandrogenemia depends on the quality and type of androgen assays used and the normative values of the control population that are applied [37].

A cautionary clinical note: women with "classic" PCOS, with blatant cutaneous evidence of androgen excess often display "normal" testosterone concentrations. Circulating total and free testosterone and dehydroepiandrosterone sulfate (DHEAS) levels are elevated in 50–75% of women with PCOS if quality assays are used. The gold standard remains the FREE testosterone assay.

Given this situation any evidence of excess androgen (whether chemical or cutaneous) is sufficient for diagnosis.

Defining alterations of androgen synthesis in PCOS

In normal, non-PCOS women 25% of androstenedione and testosterone production is of ovarian origin, 25% adrenal origin and 50% is produced in peripheral tissues [2,25,38]. The adrenal cortex accounts almost entirely for the synthesis of DHEA and dehydroepiandrosterone sulfate (DHEAS) as well as that of androstenediol and 11β-hydroxy androstenedione.

Studies have documented higher PRs (due to increased secretion) for both androstenedione and testosterone in women with PCOS associated with a less pronounced increase in their MCRs [39], suggesting that factors such as peripheral conversion, reduced binding to sex hormone binding globulin as well as body size influence androgen dynamics in PCOS women. Women with excess abdominal fat accumulation have higher testosterone PR compared with those with only the subcutaneous fat phenotype [40].

Adrenal androgen production

In normal women, basal serum levels of ovarian androgens decrease only slightly with age and remain relatively stable until menopause, while a significant decrease in adrenal androgens is observed beginning at age 30 [41]. On the other hand the adrenals contribute significantly to hyperandrogenism in PCOS (40% of the overall increase), and unlike non-PCOS, women with PCOS continue enhanced adrenal androgen production until their late reproductive years [42].

In summary, the adrenal cortex, like the ovary in PCOS, synthesizes and secretes more androgen and for a longer period than in non-PCOS women.

Steroidogenesis and hyperandrogenism in PCOS [25]

In both human ovary and adrenal cortex, the 27-carbon sterol cholesterol is the precursor substrate for steroid synthesized by a series of enzymatic steps in both organs [25,43] (Fig. 11.9).

In the ovary, formation of androgen from pregnenolone or progesterone (both 21 carbon precursors) is performed in LH-stimulated thecal cells by cytochrome P450c17 (see below), leading to the synthesis of testosterone and androstenedione, both 19-carbon steroids [44]. Thereafter a portion of these androgens is converted to estrogens (18 carbon phenolic steroids) by granulosa cells which express the enzyme P450 aromatase [45]. Ovaries also directly secrete unused non-aromatized androgens into the circulation, mainly as androstenedione and testosterone. Ovarian androgens do not negatively feedback on LH production (quite the opposite!), so that even a significant excess of testosterone or androstenedione will not inhibit LH stimulation of further ovarian production of these androgens in theca cells.

The adrenal gland also contributes to androgen production. In the adrenal cholesterol may be converted to corticoids (cortisol), mineralocorticoids (aldosterone) or androgens by the presence of specific enzymes governing carbon number reduction and sequential hydroxylations in various adrenal cortex "zones" [46]. These "zones" are located in three distinct cellular layers of the cortex and each possesses distinct enzymatic cascades resulting in three different types of steroid synthesis. The outer part of the adrenal gland

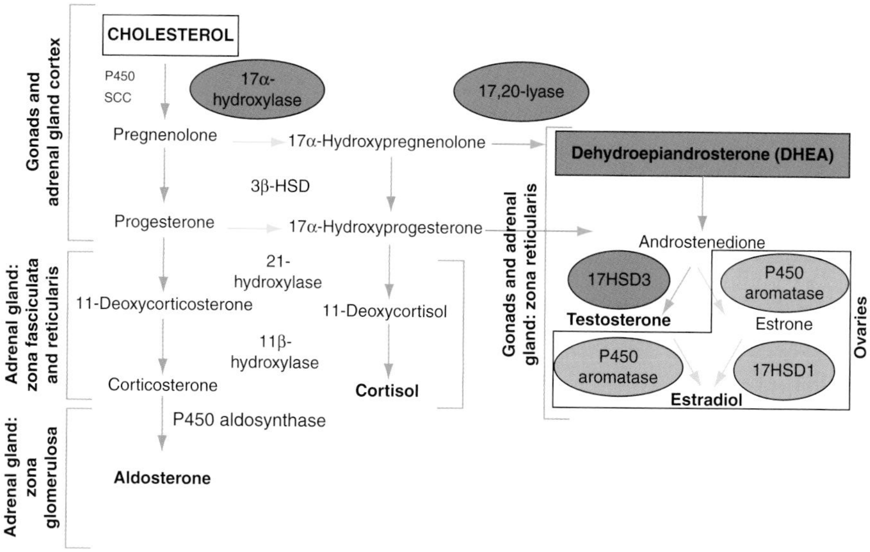

Fig. 11.9. Steroidogenesis occurring in both human gonad and adrenal gland. Reprinted from reference [25], with permission.

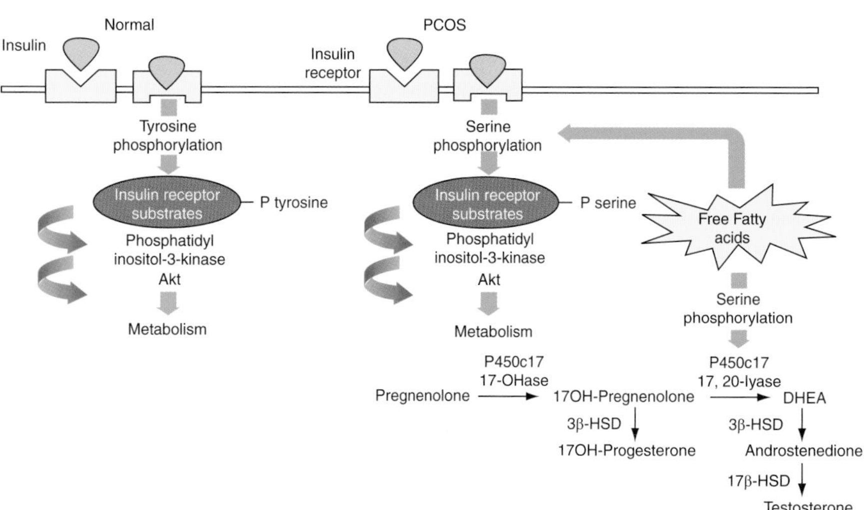

Fig. 11.10. The effect of excess free fatty acids on insulin resistance and androgen secretion in PCOS. Note the dual effects of serum phosphorylation on steroid synthesis in the adrenal cortex and ovarian theca cell. Reprinted from reference [25], with permission.

(zona glomerulosa) has the capacity to secrete mineralocorticoids such as aldosterone. In humans, the inner parts of the adrenal cortex (zona fasciculata and zona reticularis) produce cortisol and androgens such as DHEA and androstenedione. The zona fasciculata uses its abundant 17, 21, and 11 hydroxylase biosynthetic enzyme capacity and is the prime generator of cortisol synthesis. The zona reticularis on the other hand is the primary site of androgen synthesis [47]. In the absence of an aromatase system, estrogen is not a secretory product of the adrenal cortex.

The stimulus for adrenocortical steroid synthesis is adrenocorticotropin hormone (ACTH), which induces a substantial increase in secretion in all classes of adrenal steroids. Adrenal androgens do not feedback on ACTH production, which is under the control of cortisol. Neither adrenal nor ovarian androgen exert negative feedback on the tropic hormones ACTH or LH.

Are there congenital androgen biosynthetic enzyme gene defects in PCOS?

Both constitutive hyper-secretion of androgen by ovarian theca cells [48] and abnormalities of adrenal androgen production in the PCOS are well established and beg the questions: are heritable, congenital biosynthetic enzyme defects in steroidogenesis important contributors to the pathogenesis of PCOS? Is PCOS some subtle form of late onset congenital adrenal hyperplasia? On the basis of currently available evidence, the answer to these questions is NO [49].

To date, case–control and family-based studies have shown no clear evidence that variants in any of the genes involved in cortisol or androgen synthesis are the basis for the etiology of PCOS. Even suggestive genomewide studies (GWAS) findings implicate only a minor genetic involvement in this multifactorial syndrome [50,51]. *Nevertheless, interest in the function if not structure of synthetic enzymes has been pursued.*

The key enzyme for androgen biosynthesis in both ovary and adrenal cortex: P450c17 (Fig. 11.10) [25]

P450c17 is the essential biosynthetic enzyme for androgen biosynthesis. It has been described as the "qualitative regulator of steroidogenesis" because it determines which class of steroid (corticoid or androgen) will be produced. It is at once the gateway to the progressive hydroxylations that form cortisol, conversion to androgens, and indirectly by providing available substrate, for ovarian estrogen synthesis. Although P450c17 is coded by a single gene, it is directs two separate usually sequential synthetic functions – 17α-hydroxylase and 17,20-lyase activities [52]. The human adrenal gland zona fasciculata primarily expresses the 17α-hydroxylase activity, thus favoring cortisol production [53]. The 17,20-lyase-specific activity of P450c17 is weak in zona fasciculata, but strong in zona reticularis and therefore this zone produces DHEA and androstenedione [53]. In the ovary, thecal cells express both the 17α-hydroxylase and 17,20-lyase activities of the P450c17 enzyme [54].

Taken together androgen formation in any steroid producing gland is dependent upon the 17,20-lyase/17α-hydroxylase activity ratio. An increase in this ratio (more lyase) produces more androgen and is favored by the serine/threonine phosphorylation status of P450c17. The effects of excess FFAs on the serine/threonine phosphorylation property governing this ratio has crucial implications to both the hyperandrogenicity and insulin resistance that defines PCOS [25].

Origins of hyperandrogenemia in PCOS

Androgen secretion is increased in both the ovary and adrenal gland in PCOS. Unlike normal ovaries, in PCOS, the ovaries produce up to 60% of the overall increased circulating androgens, while the adrenals contribute the remaining 40% [2]. When ovarian androgen synthesis is suppressed with GnRH agonists, PCOS women continue to have higher androgen levels in comparison with normal women ascribable to adrenal overproduction of androgens. Similarly, when adrenal androgen synthesis is suppressed with dexamethasone, PCOS women again display higher androgen levels in comparison to normal women, indicating exaggerated ovarian production [55,56].

Reduced levels of sex-hormone binding globulin (SHBG) also contribute to high free testosterone levels in women with PCOS. SHBG levels are negatively correlated with the circulating levels of insulin and with the degree of insulin resistance even in non-PCOS women [57].

Chronic suppression of LH or ACTH [58] does not alter the characteristic PCOS exaggerated 17α-hydroxyprogesterone response to exogenous hCG stimulation or ACTH stimulation. On the other hand, treatments which improve insulin sensitivity in PCOS women (e.g., weight loss, metformin, D-chiro-inositol) *reduce basal androgen levels* [59]. However, the exaggerated androgenic response to LH [60] or ACTH [61] persists. *Hyperinsulinemia contributes to androgen excess, but when that stimulus is excluded, the incremental effects of tropic hormones persist.*

Gonadotropin dysfunction

Compared with normally cycling women, those with PCOS generally exhibit increased serum LH concentrations and low-normal FSH levels [62]. The increased LH results from a sustained increase in basal GnRH pulse frequency of approximately one pulse per hour and to a lesser extent in pulse amplitude [2,63]. The decrease in FSH levels reflects the impact of three factors: (1) the increased GnRH pulse frequency, (2) the negative feedback effects of chronically elevated estrone concentrations (derived from extra-gonadal aromatization of elevated androgens–androstenedione and testosterone), and (3) increased levels of inhibin B (derived from the mass of small follicles typical of PCO morphology) [64].

In addition to GnRH and LH pulse frequency, several other factors are responsible for the elevated LH in PCOS.

- Serum LH concentrations in PCOS are increased in immunoassays and, reflecting a difference in gonadotropin glycosylation, increased bioactivity in bioassay systems [65].
- Elevated LH pulses in PCOS reflect the loss of a modulating effect of progesterone feedback due to chronic anovulation [66]. During the luteal phase of the normal ovulatory cycle, progesterone reduces LH to very low levels in part by reducing GnRH pulses by means of activation of an opioid-dependent suppression of the GnRH generator. In PCOS exogenous progestin also lowers LH presumably through the same mechanism [67].
- On the other hand, treatment with exogenous estrone does not increase basal or GnRH-stimulated LH concentrations in women with PCOS [68]. Its effect is exclusively on FSH.
- Treatment with an estrogen-progestin contraceptive or with physiologic doses of exogenous estrogen and progesterone slows LH pulse frequency in women with PCOS but to a lesser extent than in normal women [69].
- Neither exogenous insulin nor therapy (Metformin) which reduces hyperinsulinemia have a significant effect on LH concentrations in PCOS. However the *combination* of increased testosterone from any source and hyperinsulinemia induces precisely the altered (increased) GnRH pulse frequencies that underlie the LH increase and FSH decrease of PCOS [70]. In this regard, flutamide (an androgen receptor antagonist) returns LH pulses to non-PCOS levels [71].

However, normally cycling women with polycystic ovary morphology may exhibit higher androgen and insulin levels and lower SHBG concentrations than women with normal-appearing ovaries despite normal LH levels [72].

Taken together, these observations suggest that while elevated LH secretion is an important contributor to the disordered follicular development and anovulation of PCOS, and adds to the androgen burden in the syndrome, it is not the sole or initiating cause of polycystic ovary morphology or of the increased ovarian androgen production in PCOS women.

Metabolic aspects of PCOS

Obesity and adipose tissue dysfunction in PCOS

The risk for developing PCOS rises with increasing obesity [73], particularly visceral obesity, as do the complicating elements of the metabolic syndrome and sleep apnea [25,74].

Insulin resistance is highly correlated with intra-abdominal obesity. Visceral fat is more active metabolically than subcutaneous fat, more sensitive to lipolysis, releases more free fatty acids and produces several cytokines involved in insulin resistance, such as tumor necrosis factor-α (TNF-α), interleukin-6, fetuin-A, leptin, and resistin [26,75]. The accumulation of free fatty acids and fetuins in muscle, liver, and adipose tissue causes insulin resistance, which reflects increased serine phosphorylation and inhibited insulin signaling [25, 76]. Even lean (by BMI) women with PCOS possess an increased percentage of body fat, a higher waist-hip ratio, and greater intra-abdominal, peritoneal, and visceral fat, compared with non-PCOS women matched for body mass index [77,78].

The overall prevalence of obesity in women with PCOS varies among different patient populations [79]. In the U.S., approximately 35% of all adult women and 60% of women with PCOS are obese. However, the overall prevalence of PCOS in the general population is approximately 7% [80]. The prevalence of PCOS among unselected women varies minimally with increasing BMI: 8.2% in underweight women (BMI <18.5), 9.8% in normal-weight women, 9.9% in overweight women (BMI 25.0–30.0), and 9.0% in obese women (BMI ≥ 30.0), 12.4% in those with a BMI between 35.0 and 40.0, and 11.5% in morbidly obese women (BMI >40.0) [81].

In summary, these observations indicate that obesity is a common, but not essential, feature of PCOS. Obesity contributes to the risk for developing PCOS and adds to the pathophysiology in already affected women.

These data also emphasize the point – the BMI metric alone does not accurately assess the metabolic burden that visceral and hepatic adiposity imposes on women.

Insulin secretion and action in PCOS: insulin resistance

Insulin resistance is recognized as a feature of a wide variety of disorders and conditions, ranging from extreme insulin resistance syndromes (auto antibodies to the insulin receptor, insulin receptor mutations, lipodystrophic states) [82] to common problems such as type II diabetes, obesity, stress, infection, starvation, puberty, pregnancy – and PCOS [25].

Insulin resistance is a common feature in obese and, to a lesser extent, lean women with PCOS; the overall prevalence ranges between 50% and 75% [83]. Insulin sensitivity is decreased by an average of 35–40% in women with PCOS, compared with normal women, similar to what is observed among women with non-insulin-dependent diabetes mellitus [84]. A total of 35% of women with PCOS exhibit impaired glucose tolerance and 7–10% meet criteria for type 2 diabetes mellitus [85]. Conversely, women with type 2 diabetes are six-fold more likely than non-diabetic women of similar age and weight to have PCOS [83].

How insulin resistance affects PCOS pathophysiology

Insulin resistance is a condition in which endogenous or exogenously administered insulin has altered effects on fat, muscle, and the liver [86]. In adipose tissue, as opposed to normal circumstances, insulin resistance results in increased hydrolysis of stored triglycerides and elevated circulating free fatty acid levels. Decreased glucose usage (primarily in muscle) and increased hepatic gluconeogenesis (which insulin normally inhibits) result in increased blood glucose concentrations and compensatory hyperinsulinemia (in those with adequate pancreatic reserve) [87].

In vitro studies demonstrate that insulin stimulates androgen production in ovarian theca cells [88]. Theca cells from women with PCOS exhibit increased sensitivity to insulin compared with cells derived from normal women. Even physiologic levels of insulin can stimulate androgen synthesis in theca cells of women with PCOS, whereas higher insulin concentrations are required in normal theca cells [89]. Insulin and LH act synergistically to stimulate ovarian androgen production [90]. The cumulative insulin response during an oral glucose tolerance test correlates positively with a rise in serum androstenedione and testosterone above baseline concentrations [91]. Moreover, suppression of serum insulin levels by treatment with diazoxide or insulin-sensitizing agent metformin decreases serum androstenedione and testosterone levels in women with PCOS [92].

Insulin stimulates ovarian androgen production acting by means of insulin receptors on theca/interstitial cells in the ovarian stroma [93]. At high concentrations, insulin also binds to IGF-11 receptors in the ovary (Fig. 11.6).

High insulin concentrations also inhibit hepatic SHBG production [57], as do elevated androgen concentrations. The combined actions of insulin and androgens lower SHGB concentrations, yielding increased free androgen levels which in turn aggravate the underlying insulin resistance. Ultimately, these conditions foster a self-propagating positive feedforward loop which increases in severity over time.

In summary, increased circulating insulin levels cause or contribute to hyperandrogenism in women with PCOS; (1) by stimulating increased ovarian androgen production, (2) by inhibiting hepatic SHBG production, 3) combined with testosterone stimulating increased LH secretion by altering GnRH pulse frequency (Fig. 11.7).

What causes insulin resistance in PCOS?

Given the complexity of PCOS more than one mechanism driving insulin resistance may be involved. The excellent study by Baptiste et al. [25] has reviewed this issue in detail.

The actions of insulin are mediated by means of its receptor and two distinct intracellular pathways. The phosphatidyl-inositol 3-kinase (PI-3K) pathway mediates the *metabolic* effects of insulin, and the mitogen-activated protein kinase (MAPK) pathway mediates the growth *stimulating actions* of insulin. Insulin binding to its receptor induces tyrosine phosphorylation of one or several insulin receptor protein substrates (IRSs) which bind and serially activate PI-3K and Akt, which is an effector molecule that plays a major role in signal transduction for glucose regulation and metabolism [25]. Akt activation potentiates the translocation of glucose transporter 4 (GLUT4) from intracellular compartments to the plasma membrane, increasing glucose uptake. Other effector molecules mediate insulin inhibition of gluconeogenesis and glycogenolysis, stimulation of lipid synthesis, and inhibition of lipid catabolism [94].

Studies in cultured skin fibroblasts, muscle, and adipocytes from women with PCOS indicate that insulin resistance results from defects early in the In-R post receptor signaling pathway [95]. The number and affinity of insulin receptors in both obese and lean women with PCOS are not decreased, but insulin receptors exhibit a constitutive increase in phosphorylation of serine residues and a decrease in insulin-stimulated phosphorylation of tyrosine residues [96,97].

Serine phosphorylation of insulin receptor substrates prevents their binding with PI-3K and thereby inhibits insulin signaling. A variety of pro-inflammatory cytokines, TNF-α, and IL6 among others can increase serine phosphorylation in insulin target tissues. Increased serine phosphorylation can also be induced by intracellular metabolites of free fatty acids, which are increased in most women with PCOS and have been demonstrated to cause insulin resistance in vivo [25] (Fig. 11.8).

As mentioned earlier in this chapter and reemphasized in various sections of PCOS pathophysiology, in a parallel phenomenon, high circulating free fatty acid levels also increase androgen production by inducing serine phosphorylation on P450c17, which results in increased 17,20-lyase activity and androgen synthesis [98]. These observations not only provide a mechanism for insulin resistance, but also further explain the link between insulin and hyperandrogenism in women with PCOS (Fig. 11.10).

Insulin resistance and hyperinsulinemia undoubtedly contribute to the pathophysiology of PCOS. However, 25–50% of women with PCOS have no demonstrable insulin resistance. Moreover, among all women with insulin resistance, the prevalence of PCOS is relatively low (approximately 15%) [75,81]. *Insulin resistance and hyperinsulinemia are not essential to the pathogenesis of PCOS.*

Hyperandrogenism as the catalyst in PCOS

The preceding paragraphs substantiated the contributing but non-essential presence of obesity, insulin resistance, gonadotropin dysregulation, and adipose tissue imposed dysfunction in the generation of PCOS. The inescapable conclusion is each of these elements contributes to PCOS but only to the degree it generates and maximizes hyperandrogenism.

As Marshall has noted, "elevated plasma androgens influence several physiologic systems with generally negative implications for the normal regulation of female reproduction and metabolism" [99]:

- excess androgen limits progression of follicle maturation by inhibition of aromatase activity and the production of non-aromatizable dihydrotestosterone (Fig. 11.6)

- elevated secretion of ovarian testosterone acts centrally to increase GnRH and LH pulse frequencies resulting in relative elevation of circulating LH
- LH stimulates increased theca cells synthesis and secretion of even higher testosterone concentrations. A positive feed-forward interplay between ovary and CNS/pituitary is engaged, yielding increased secretion and sustained overall excess production of testosterone
- androgen-induced reduction of sex hormone binding globulin (SHBG) aggravates this condition by increasing concentrations of unbound biologically active testosterone
- elevated androgens modify adipose cell function through androgen receptors primarily expressed on abdominal pre-adipocytes [100]. Hyperandrogenemia adversely modulates adipocyte production of cytokines such as TNF-α, IL-6, and plasminogen activator inhibitor-1, factors which induce insulin resistance at insulin target tissues [25]
- obese adolescents with PCOS not only suffer a higher incidence of insulin resistance and metabolic syndrome but hyperandrogenemia adds a further incremental risk for metabolic syndrome independent of changes already induced by obesity and insulin resistance [101]
- the SWAN studies indicate the metabolic syndrome emerges during the menopausal transition (not only in PCOS). Its incidence and intensity is increased by parallel increases in free testosterone concentrations [102]
- PCOM exists in female-to-male transsexuals treated with exogenous androgens [105].

The adverse effect of high local ovarian androgen concentrations in PCOS is demonstrated by the results of ovarian wedge resection and by the presence of PCOM secondary to non-PCOS hyperandrogen conditions. Wedge resection results in a sustained decrease in androgen levels that precedes the return of ovulatory cycles [103]. The effect correlates with the amount of androgen-producing stromal tissue removed; even a unilateral oophorectomy can restore menstrual cyclicity and ovulation in anovulatory women with polycystic ovaries [104]. Although laparoscopic procedures have replaced the classical wedge resection, the results achieved are similar.

Androgen excess is the central requirement in the genesis and pathophysiologic progression of PCOS.

Polycystic ovary morphology

Gross morphology and histology (Fig. 11.11)

The PCOM ovary is rotund and distended; its surface area may be doubled, with volume increasing 2–8 times normal [2,106]. The capsule is thickened by 50% and the stromal compartment increased substantially, perhaps by a factor of 5 over what is seen normally. On cut section, the ovary exhibits more than 10 discrete subcapsular follicles, 4–9 mm in diameter and peripherally arrayed to resemble a "pearl" necklace (Fig. 11.12). Surprisingly, a corpus luteum or corpus albicans may be present.

The histology of the polycystic ovary depicts an increased rate of activation and recruitment but otherwise normal follicle development and progression but which is arrested at the early antral stage. The cysts are typically lined with a few layers of granulosa cells. In contrast an unusually prominent luteinized and vascularized theca cell mantle surrounds each follicle (Fig. 11.13).

The PCO displays normal numbers of primordial "reserve" follicles and normal numbers of primary and secondary follicles serving to emphasize the inherent "normalcy" of these follicles other than the pace of their development and their failure to proceed to dominant follicle maturation [107].

Ultrasound appearance (Fig. 11.14)

Several ultrasound-based criteria for the "diagnosis" of PCOM have been advanced. According to an ACOG Bulletin [108], determination of PCOS in one or both ovaries requires either 12 or more antral follicles measuring 2–9 mm in diameter or increased

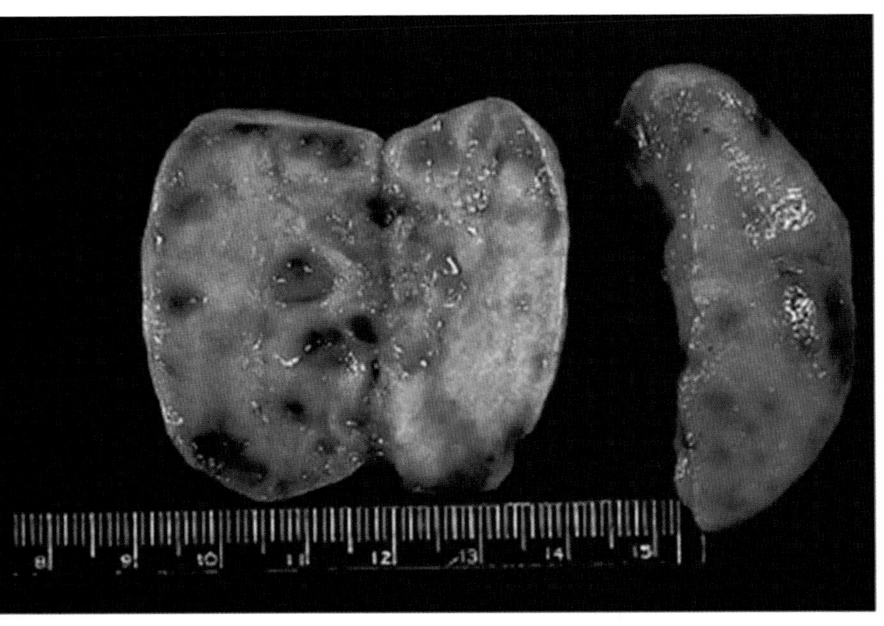

Fig. 11.11. PCOS; gross section.

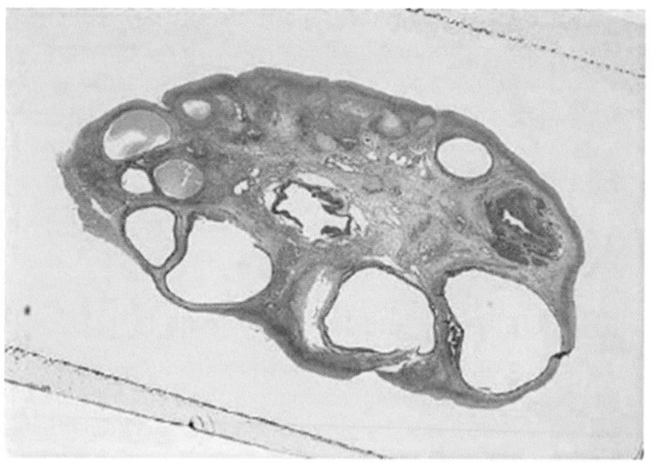

Fig. 11.12. PCOS; cut section.

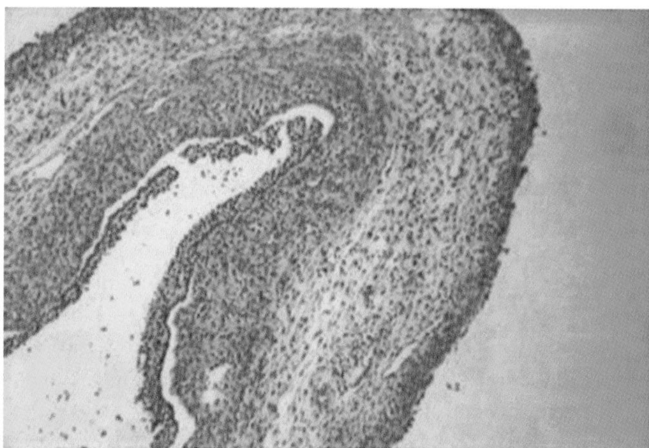

Fig. 11.13. PCOS; histology.

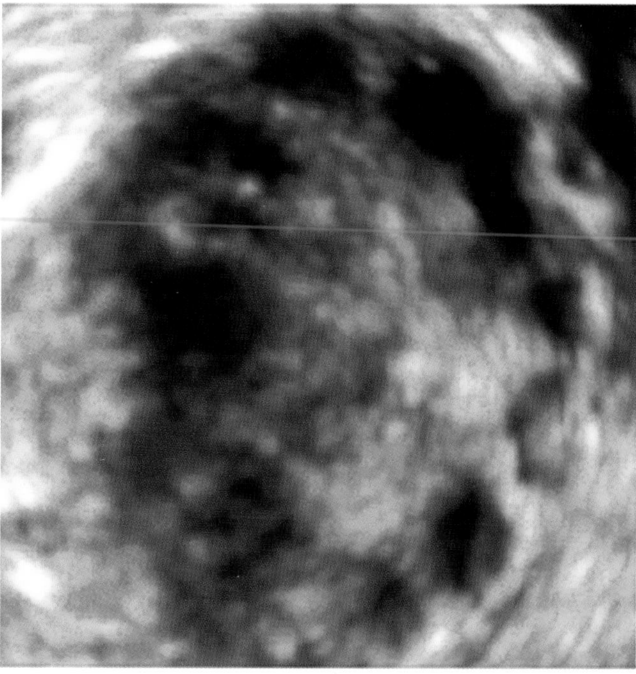

Fig. 11.14. PCOS; ultrasound.

ovarian volume (greater than 10 cm^3). Unlike other "standards" the presence of one polycystic ovary is sufficient for diagnosis. The Rotterdam ultrasound [28] criteria emphasize the total number of follicles, requiring a mean of 12 follicles measuring 2–9 mm in diameter existing in both ovaries. Still other criteria define PCO on the basis of volume alone – greater than 7.0–7.5 mL [109].

Hyperplasia of thecal stromal cells/stromal hyperthecosis [110]

The expanded stromal compartment of the PCO represents an accumulation of cells derived from the hyperplastic, hyperluteinized, hypervascularized thecal mantle surrounding the small antral follicles of PCOS. Although the follicles become atretic, the residual thecal component is retained in the subcortical stroma. These cells continue to respond to LH and continue to augment gonadal secretion of testosterone and androstenedione. When PCOS women become post-menopausal, the elevated LH stimulates further luteinization of these cells and induces persistent elevated androgen production manifested as a post-menopausal hyperthecosis syndrome of masculinization and insulin resistance. In this instance, insulin stimulation of stromal androgen synthesis adds to the combined action of androgen and insulin in the promotion of the pathologic burdens of PCOS [111].

Considering the age group affected by this entity with long-standing metabolic burdens already well established, treatment requires bilateral combined oophorectomy or GnRH agonist ovarian suppressive therapy. Although still infrequently encountered (perhaps unrecognized), its presence contributes to the understanding of the pathophysiology of PCOS; a persistent LH and insulin-driven ovarian source of excess androgen can reproduce a MetS phenotype *typical of younger PCOS women but in this instance in the absence of PCOM follicles.*

Determinants of PCOM

Clues to the pathogenesis and pathophysiology of the syndrome may be discovered by examining the mechanisms which generate the distinctive gross and microscopic appearance of PCOM. There are limited morphologic options the ovary can achieve: inactivity, various stages of development and atresia, ovulation, benign and malignant neoplasms, imposed infections, post-menopausal senescence, and atrophy. What factors lead to chronic arrest of follicle development in early antral stages when under normal circumstances this is the decisive point at which follicle fate is determined: either to proceed to selection and further development or undergo atresia? As noted normal numbers of primordial follicles exist in the PCO ovary and the rate of atresia is appropriate. What factors – local (intra-ovarian) or imposed (dysfunctional, misdirecting signals) – so dramatically blocks the next steps in follicle destiny?

Intra-ovarian regulation of ovarian morphology

Chapter 1 described the cross-talk among numerous intracrine factors linking the oocyte, granulosa, and theca participation in the activation and transition of the primordial follicle through the various stages leading to the stage of FSH dependence – the small antral follicle. All steps before this point are understood to be independent of gonadotropin presence or stimulation (defined by the absence of FSH receptors on pre-granulosa and the developing granulosa layers of pre-antral follicles) [1]. The inhibition of further progression in PCOM must be local: the "success" of ovarian wedge resection [112], the mysterious but definitive return of ovulatory cyclicity to former PCOS women age (>40 years) as their pool of remaining follicles dwindle, but most dramatic the acute steep rise in FSH and return of ovulatory cycles after "successful" laparoscopic ovarian follicle drilling – all suggest some local inhibiting elements exist, are produced by or reflective of the size of the current residual pool of 2–5 mm early antral follicles which contribute to and sustain PCOM follicle arrest. As examples:

- High local androgen concentrations contribute to the polycystic morphogenesis of the ovaries by means of local conversion to more potent 5α-reduced androgens. These androgens, unlike testosterone or androstenedione, cannot be aromatized to estrogen and inhibit both aromatase activity and FSH induction of LH receptors on granulosa cells, thereby impeding or preventing progressive follicular development (Fig. 11.6). Granulosa cells obtained from polycystic ovaries are not functionally impaired. They are sensitive to FSH and insulin-like growth factors to produce estrogen [113,114]. However, they cannot generate and maintain the estrogenic follicular milieu required to achieve more advanced stages of development because of imposed androgen inhibition of aromatase. Consequently, new follicular growth continues but arrests before full maturation, resulting in accumulation of multiple small follicular cysts (typically measuring 2–10 mm in diameter).
- *Kit ligand* (KL) [115] is an intra-ovarian cytokine that promotes multiple aspects of folliculogenesis in animal models including primordial follicle activation, follicle growth and survival, stromal cell differentiation, theca cell proliferation, and androgen biosynthesis. Perturbation of these fundamental processes occurs in anovulatory women with PCOS, in whom there is evidence for abnormal oocyte maturation, increased follicle and stromal density, thecal hypertrophy, and increased thecal cell androgen biosynthesis. Therefore, KL may play a key role in the morphogenesis of PCO, particularly in hyperandrogenic women with PCOS.

  While the specific role of KL signaling is not known, its molecular biology has interesting relevance to PCOM.

  Abnormalities of KL (Kit ligand) availability could adversely influence ovarian morphology by unbalanced development of follicle constituents; diminished granulosa and oocyte maturation, excess stromal cell differentiation and excess theca cell proliferation and function (i.e., androgen biosynthetic capacity). The disproportionate presence and function of theca versus granulosa cells resulting in adverse excess androgen substrate versus aromatase capacity could bias PCO morphology and function in response to gonadotropin.
- *AMH* [116] Anti-Mullerian hormone (AMH) is elevated in PCOS. Granulosa cell production of AMH is higher in anovulatory than ovulatory women. PCOS follicle fluid contains high concentrations of AMH. AMH's suppressive effects on folliculogenesis in normal ovaries suggest that when present in excess it may be the sought-after local inhibitor [117]. PCOS women with the lowest AMH levels respond best to induction of ovulation. Metformin inhibits AMH production in cell cultures. Perhaps best known for its inhibition of primordial to primary follicle conversion, AMH also impedes further follicle development up to the preantral follicle stage. The high concentration of local AMH issuing from the large number of small antral follicles could substantially impede new follicle recruitment as well as their further development.

In summary, it would appear that the characteristic PCO morphology is preserved and possibly initiated by high intracrine concentrations of the inhibitors of follicle development – AMH and androgen – working on a Kit-ligand-susceptible gonad.

Influence of gonadotropins on PCOM

Relative FSH insufficiency may also be an aggravating factor in follicle arrest. Basal FSH concentrations in PCOS are non-oscillating and in the low normal range. Increasing FSH (with clomiphene or exogenous hFSH) without any other manipulation *restores normal follicular growth*. This highlights the role of appropriate gonadotropin (recycling event 1) action in restoring follicular development and ovulation in PCOS women but not in the primary initiation of PCO morphology which remains governed by local inhibitors.

Despite these considerations, 8–25% of normal women and 14% of women using oral contraceptives meet the ultrasonographic criteria for polycystic ovaries [118]. Moreover, polycystic ovaries are commonly observed during normal pubertal development, and even in women with hypothalamic amenorrhea and hyperprolactinemia. Otherwise normal women with polycystic ovaries have regular menstrual cycles, exhibit normal serum gonadotropin and ovarian steroid hormone levels, and are fertile [119].

Genetics of PCOS

Powerful reasons exist to consider PCOS as a genetic, heritable syndrome [120].

Heritability of PCOS and the PCOM component [121]. Around 20–40% of first-degree relatives of PCOS women have PCOS compared with 4–12% of the general population. Nearly 50% of sisters of women with PCOS have elevated total or bio-available testosterone concentrations, and approximately 35% of mothers are also affected. A heritability factor for PCOS of 0.79 among Dutch twins suggests a genetic/genomic influence in vulnerability/development of the syndrome [122].

Heritability of the metabolic syndrome components and consequences [123]. Siblings and first-degree relatives of women with PCOS have a high prevalence of hyperinsulinemia and hypertriglyceridemia and other metabolic abnormalities such as dyslipidemia [124,125].

The search for the "culpable gene" [126]

As noted earlier, well-conducted replication studies were unable to confirm any association with genes encoding cytochrome P450 side-chain cleavage enzyme, CPY11A, insulin, aldo-keto reductase family 1, or the 17β-hydroxysteroid dehydrogenase type 5 gene [126]. An exception is deficiency in the aromatase enzyme system by which a genetic variation in CYP19 may contribute to androgenization. A common genomic variant (an intronic single nucleotide polymorphism (SNP50) of the CYP19 produces a hyperandrogenic state by both increased secretion of unused substrate androgen and reduced metabolic clearance of testosterone. This rare entity is associated with early adrenarche, pubertal hyperandrogenism and PCOS [127] (Fig. 11.15).

Genetic variation in androgen receptor (AR) sensitivity has been identified as a cause of hyperandrogenism. Clinical hyperandrogenism and androgen concentrations are increased in girls with shorter AR gene $(CAG)_n$ repeat alleles. High AR sensitivity is associated not only with greater target tissue (including visceral adipocytes) impact but through a series of positive feed-forward mechanisms with increased overall androgen production [128].

Evidence exists that reduction in SHBG in PCOS, independent of hyperinsulinism or hyperandrogenism, may also be genetically determined. Women with PCOS were more frequent carriers of less active, longer allele genotypes $(TAAAA)_n$ in the promoter region of *SHBG*, leading to lower SHBG levels than control [128] (Fig. 11.15).

Genes for which association with PCOS or its component traits have been replicated include fibrillin 3 (*FBN3*) and 17β-hydroxysteroid dehydrogenase type 6 (*HSD17B6*). An attempt to replicate the association between PCOS and variants in 26 genes found good evidence of replication with a fibrillin gene FBN3 and pro-opiomelanocortin (POMC), and nominal replication of variants in activin A receptor type 2A (*ACVR2A*), fem-1homolog B (*FEB1B*), and small glutamine-rich tetratricopeptide-containing protein alpha (*SGTA*). The contribution of these findings and recent genome wide analyses [129,130] to understanding the mechanisms underlying PCOS remains to be verified.

Conclusion

The genetic contribution to PCOS remains uncertain. There is currently no recommended genetic screening test. No specific environmental substance has been identified as a cause of PCOS. However, and an essential point to emphasize here: while the gene or genes involved may not be defective *their protein products may be altered as a result of a variety of post-translational modifications* – such as sumoylation, phosphorylation, acetylation/deacetylation, and amino acid substitutions among other possibilities. It is now recognized that "new" aggregates and assemblies, i.e., "amalgams" of multiple proteins, act as complex units as transcriptomes, signalsomes, proteosomes, interactomes, transporters (rafts), chaperones, stabilizers, co-activators, and co-repressors are the agents of signal–target cell interactions and integration (see Chapter 2). The alterations of insulin receptor activity and the P450c 17-hydroxylase/17,20-lyase enzyme dysfunction in androgen synthesis results from a shared vulnerability to excess FFAs. This is ONE example of the new prospects for analysis of PCOS pathogenesis. *The genes producing the proteins involved appear to be NORMAL.*

Maternal PCOS: pregnancy complications and the transgenerational transfer of the PCOS phenotype to female progeny

The PCO ovary in almost all instances is inherently physiologically normal and capable of ovulatory responses. Its follicular development is inhibited by imposed intra- and extra-gonadal factors. When this inhibition is eliminated or reversed normal ovulatory function can be restored. But with restoration by induction of ovulation and fertility, PCOS women and their progeny continue to encounter problems.

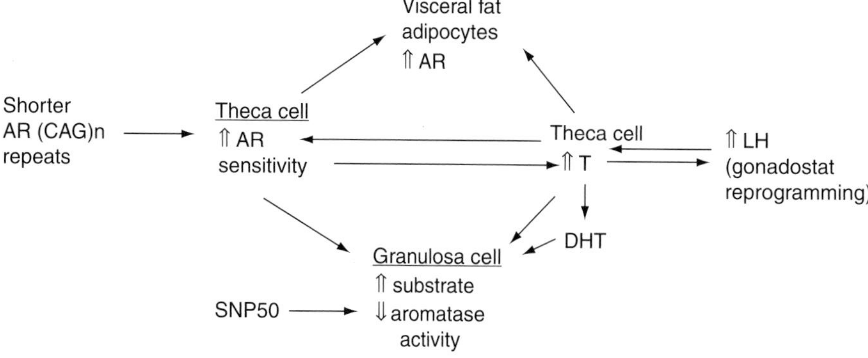

Fig. 11.15. An example of the genetic origin of PCOS. Androgen receptor "hypersensitivity" as a factor in fetal programming of PCOS by androgen excess luteinizing. As a result of ⇑ AR sensitivity, a positive feed-forward cycle is entrained in which enhanced intrauterine androgen leads to visceral fat sensitization, theca cell androgen dominance, aromatase inhibition, and "androgenization" of GNRH control of LH secretion at puberty. Each element is activated and the entire cycle synergistically accelerated by increments in LH, insulin, IGF-1, and weight gain with establishment of PCOS. AR, androgen receptor; T, testosterone; LH, luteinizing hormone; DHT, dihydrotestosterone; ⇑, increase; ⇓, decrease.

The "heritability" of PCOS in the absence of a defective gene may result from fetal *epigenetic* adjustments to maternal constraints which persist into adulthood and are even transferred to future generations [131].

One certainty exists: most PCOS women begin pregnancy already in a hyperglycemic, hyperlipidemic, insulin–resistant, incipiently hypertensive vasoconstrictive and systemic inflammatory (increased ROS) state. Two-thirds of all women in the United States are either overweight or obese at the time of conception [23].

PCOS and pregnancy complications

The PCOS woman and her fetus face significant complications [132].

1. When pregnant, PCOS mothers are at increased risk of:

   Pregnancy-associated hypertension/preeclampsia
   Gestational diabetes
   Pregnancy loss, premature delivery
   Cesarean section, birth canal trauma

2. Pregnancy in PCOS mothers adversely affects the fetus:

   Large for gestational age (LGA), macrosomia
   Small for gestational age (SGA)
   Intra-uterine growth retardation (IUGR)

3. Affects the neonate:

   Birth trauma, shoulder dystocia
   Neonatal hypoglycemia, hyperbilirubinemia
   Elevated c-peptide levels in cord blood
   Admission to NICU

4. Female progeny of PCOS mothers face life-long (infancy through late adult life) risk of PCOS as well as developing all or individual elements of the MetS and its consequences, CV disease, and DM 2 (ACOG Bulletin) [108].

Pre-pregnancy cardio/endocrine/metabolic status of the PCOS woman and the genesis of intra-pregnancy complications

Physiology of normal pregnancy

In pregnancy the feto-placental unit and maternal compartments while anatomically separate are indivisibly linked in mutual support of successful reproduction [133]:

- The feto-placental compartment provides structural insulation and a functionally selective barrier against adverse factors in the maternal internal and external environment
- Maternal molecular mechanisms protect and promote early implantation and placentation of the fetal allograft and early embryogenesis
- On the other hand the fetal placental unit signals either its "readiness" for post-natal life or its recognition of progressive and imminent exhaustion of maternal resources or placental transfer defects, and signals the need for urgent exit by initiating progressive uterine contractions, premature labor, and delivery
- Specifically related to the PCOS maternal environment during pregnancy, the fetal placental unit modulates maternal cardiovascular and metabolic status to ensure maximal placental perfusion and transfer of oxygen, glucose, and other nutrients to support fetal growth and development. This involves both specific transport systems and maintenance of favorable maternal-to-fetus nutritional gradients.

A good example of these interactions is the process by which a glucose transfer gradient from mother to fetus is maintained despite alternating maternal feed/fast nutritional intake. The feto-placental unit imposes a state of insulin resistance on the mother throughout pregnancy to ensure constant availability and transfer of glucose [134]. The fetus requires glucose for its general development and growth but primarily for the fetal brain which is almost entirely glucose dependent. This maternal endocrine and metabolic adaptation of pregnancy-induced insulin resistance is driven and maintained by placental secretions of "diabetogenic" signals including chorionic GH, CRH, cortisol, human chorionic somatomammotropin (HCS or placental lactogen) and progesterone. In addition to these hormonal signals, normal pregnancy is characterized by a state of moderate maternal systemic inflammatory reaction (MSIR) caused by increased reactive oxygen species (ROS) emanating from the placenta. In addition MSIR stimulates moderate maternal vasoconstriction to maximize placental perfusion [135].

This state of mild maternal systemic inflammatory response (MSIR) is especially beneficial to the fetus. As a result of maternal insulin resistance, the role of insulin as a "metabolic switch," directing maternal fuel distribution between storage and usage and fat versus glucose usage is modified to reinforce a steady flow of glucose to the fetus while providing compensating storage/usage of fat by the mother [136].

PCOS maternal "constraints"

As crucially important as maternal insulin resistance is to normal pregnancy, it poses *adverse* implications for the PCOS mother who even before pregnancy may be significantly insulin-resistant, hyperinsulinemic, moderately hypertensive, and if not already overtly diabetic, prone to impaired glucose tolerance (Fig. 11.16). How will the combination of the increased tendency to vasoconstriction, hyperglycemia, and thrombogenicity inherent in normal pregnancy, compounded by the already insulin-resistant, obese (hyperglycemic and hyperlipidemic) marginally hypertensive PCOS mother affect the fetus? Will the fetus be small for gestational age (SGA) (diminished placental perfusion and superimposed maternal hypertension) or large for gestational age (LGA) secondary to maternal gestational diabetes or hyperlipidemia? Given the adverse milieu of maternal PCOS, what mechanisms does the fetus use to accommodate to this array of maternal constraints to maximize its nutritional and metabolic status prenatally?

The fetus must develop a strategy to maximize its in utero status as well as prepare for survival as a newborn. This fetal "best match" strategy is achieved through epigenetic modifications of the fetal metabolic homeostatic set points [137] (Fig. 11.17).

Fetal epigenetic "best match" intra-uterine strategies

All cells of the body possess the same DNA genetic code. Epigenetics is the "software" that modifies the genetic hard drive by selective activation, modification, and silencing of gene activity to differentiate, develop, and specify organ, tissue, and cell development and function during embryonic development and throughout adult life [138]. It provides stable propagation of cell-specific gene expression during mitotic division and due to incomplete meiotic "erasure" allows transfer of some epigenetic modifications from one generation to their progeny.

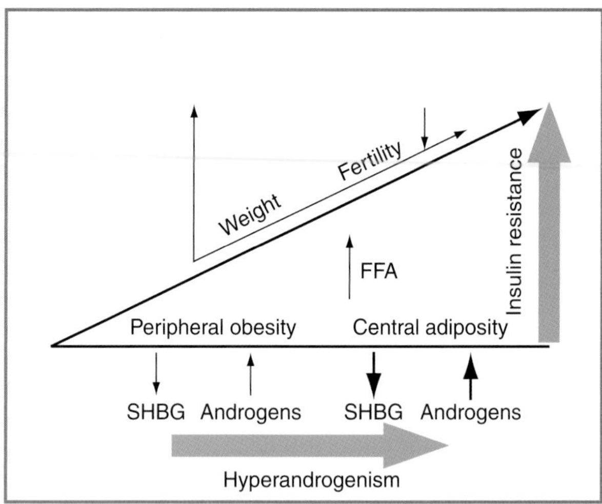

Fig. 11.16. Effects of obesity, adiposity, and hyperandrogenism in PCOS. The combination of increasing androgen, visceral adiposity, and hyperinsulinemia secondary to insulin resistance leads to the full pathophysiological and clinical expression of the PCOS.

Two major mechanisms among others are used to induce epigenetic "identity:" histone modification of nucleosomes and direct genome DNA methylation. Epigenetic modifications occur during intra-uterine development, during cell differentiation and/or cell proliferation, in a mature cell during renewal (plasticity) or at a point in adult life when "adverse" internal and external conditions or exposures require or induce modifications (resiliency).

Accordingly, the fetus of a PCOS mother will construct a "best match" epigenetic modification of homeostatic set points to accommodate to the imposed maternal constraints which it confronts. However, because of their "permanence" these epigenetic strategies, while appropriate for intra-uterine conditions, may present a serious *mismatch* in the post-natal adult environment. Fetal accommodations to a too poor or too rich intra-uterine developmental environment will replicate (although by different mechanisms) the PCOS phenotype during infancy, childhood, adolescence, and into adulthood.

Epigenetics in action

Reaction to *in utero* under-nutrition

For the PCOS mother, "under-nutrition" does not suggest lack of maternal nutrient intake or reserve [139,140]. Rather it reflects the extent to which occult vascular disease, extant hypertension, or vasoconstriction secondary to an excess systemic inflammatory state by a stressed relatively small underperfused placenta leads to diminished nutrient delivery to the fetus. In this scenario, the most urgent "accommodation" the fetus must make to restricted nutrient and oxygen availability is to divert maximum available glucose to its brain. Accordingly, the fetus must optimize its own insulin resistance as well as induce further maternal insulin resistance to maximize the maternal glucose supply (almost entirely by increased ROS from a distressed placenta). Among many epigenetic modifications undertaken to achieve fetal preferential glucose sparing redirection, skeletal muscle growth and development is decreased and its glut 4 glucose transfer capacity diminished.

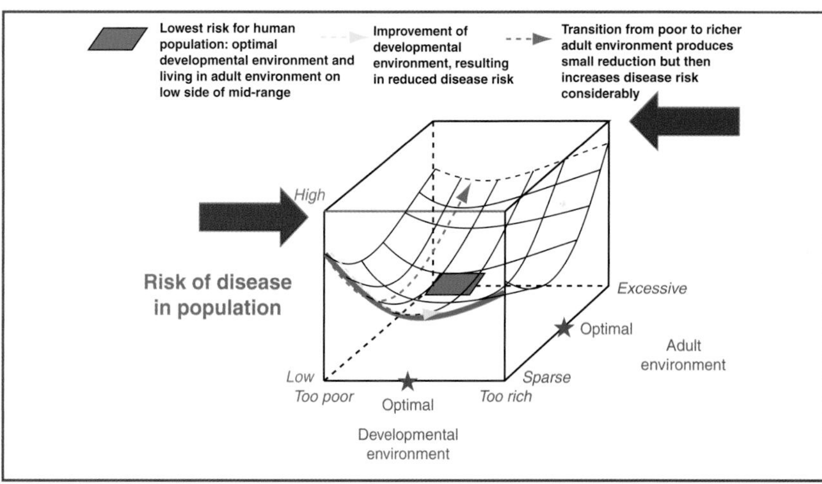

Fig. 11.17. Correlation between adolescent and adult obesity and disease and the fetal developmental environment. Maternal effects on an offspring's risk of developing metabolic disease: unbalanced maternal diet or body composition ranging from poor to rich intra-uterine environments adversely influences the offspring's response to later challenges such as high fat and high carbohydrate diet, and/or physical inactivity leading to increased risk of disease. Adapted from reference [140]. Reproduced from: Godfrey K, Gluckman PD, and Hanson MA. Developmental origins of metabolic disease: life course and intergenerational perspectives. Trends Endocrinol Metab, 2010;**21**(4):199-205. With permission from Elsevier.

This combination of effects reduces the size of the major organ of glucose usage (muscle) and diminishes glucose entry. In addition, the induction of the PI3 kinase insulin signaling transduction pathway is also diminished, further limiting non-neural glucose usage by reducing usage of whatever glucose is delivered to the cell.

These altered homeostatic set points, while affording the best match for fetal brain development, will lead to an SGA or IUGR growth-retarded neonate (Fig. 11.18). Furthermore, once delivered and entered into the nutrition rich extra-uterine environment of developed societies, the resulting dramatic mismatch of the fixed fetal insulin resistance leads to incremental, accelerating, irreversible, pubertal, and adult insulin resistance with emergence of the MetS and its various cardiac, endocrine, and metabolic consequences [140]. Similar mismatch disease outcomes have been reported following famines experienced during WWII in Europe, UK, and Russia [141] and following the Biafran civil war [142].

In summary:

- As a result of diminished placental perfusion in PCOS, fetal epigenetic reprogramming sustains the glucose requirements of the fetal brain by deflecting energy use from non-neural tissues through the effects of imposed fetal insulin resistance. In addition, maternal insulin resistance is maximized to increase glucose availability to the fetus.
- This epigenetic reprogramming persists postnatally and into adulthood where the insulin resistance mechanisms and its organ system consequences induced *in utero* are mismatched for the prevailing energy-rich environment encountered in extra-uterine life.
- The glucotoxicity, lipotoxicity, and systemic inflammatory state of the resulting MetS, compounded by additional epigenetic environmental stresses in infancy, childhood, adolescence, and adulthood lead to emergence or worsening of metabolic disease as an adult and development of the PCOS phenotype [143].

Reaction to maternal over-nutrition [131]

On the other hand, maternal obesity and excess weight gain during pregnancy lead to fetal over-nutrition. Under these circumstances both fetal and escalating maternal insulin resistance also prevails resulting in post-natal, persistent reactive hyperinsulinemia, obesity, and elements of the MetS manifested early in childhood and worsening into adulthood.

Maternal hyperglycemia driven by nutritional excess before and during pregnancy with or without MetS or PCOS, or pregnancies complicated by maternal gestational diabetes are likely to be associated with adverse pregnancy outcomes for the mother and her LGA baby [144,145]. However, the majority of large for gestational age births (and the associated adverse consequences) occurs in mothers with "normal" glucose levels in pregnancy as demonstrated in the large Hyperglycemia and Adverse Pregnancy Outcomes (HAPO) study [146]. In this report the risk of adverse outcomes increased progressively as a function of glucose levels at mid-gestation *that were within ranges below the OGTT standards thought to be "normal" for pregnancy*. An alternative explanation is that hyperlipidemia before and during pregnancy can also be a significant factor in adverse pregnancy outcomes for the fetus and offspring.

The evidence for the adverse effects of maternal hyperlipidemia during pregnancy

- *Excess maternal weight gain* in pregnancy leads to LGA offspring who develop obesity and type 2 DM in adolescence and adulthood [147]
- *During pregnancy*, despite well-controlled gestational diabetes (GDM) elevated fasting triglycerides and FFAs are associated with LGA and neonatal adiposity. Maternal lipid levels are strong determinants of fetal growth in pregnancy with and without GDM, i.e., "normal" glucose tolerance [148]
- *Pre-pregnancy* BMI and triglyceride levels significantly correlate with fetal growth in utero in neonates, and predict development of obesity in children at 8 years of age [149].

Maternal–fetal lipid dynamics and metabolism in pregnancy [150]

In normal pregnancy, like glucose, lipid is essential for normal fetal development, cell, tissue, organ structure, and function. Accordingly a variety of mechanisms are used to maximize maternal lipid transport across the placenta including diffusion (a maximum gradient to the fetus is achieved in late gestation), fatty acid carrier proteins and specific FFA transporters. Placental lipase hydrolyzes maternal triglycerides, chylomicrons, and VLDL particles into transferable FFAs. As a result fetal fat accretion is normal and significant and becomes maximal in the 3rd trimester.

These fetal requirements are met by significant increases in maternal lipid concentrations (serum triglycerides increase 200% and cholesterol by 50%) driven by insulin, cortisol, and the elevated estrogen and progesterone of pregnancy. Initially in early pregnancy, enhanced lipogenesis (increased lipoprotein lipase and triglyceride) are held in reserve in maternal adipose tissue storage. As normal pregnancy-associated maternal insulin resistance increases, a switch from anabolic storage to a catabolic state takes place with increased lipolysis and elevated circulating FFA. At the same time LPL is inhibited [151]. The resulting increase in FFAs and VLDL is available for passive and active lipid transport to the fetus. It must be emphasized here that the factors driving this essential lipid catabolic state are normal elements of pregnancy: human placental lactogen, increased maternal systemic inflammatory reaction, and "normal" pregnancy-induced maternal insulin resistance.

In the case of the PCOS mother (and even more so if she is obese), both the pre-gravid MetS and the insulin resistance developed during pregnancy act both independently and synergistically to create a marked hyperlipidemic state in both mother and fetus. This effect is worsened when the PCOS

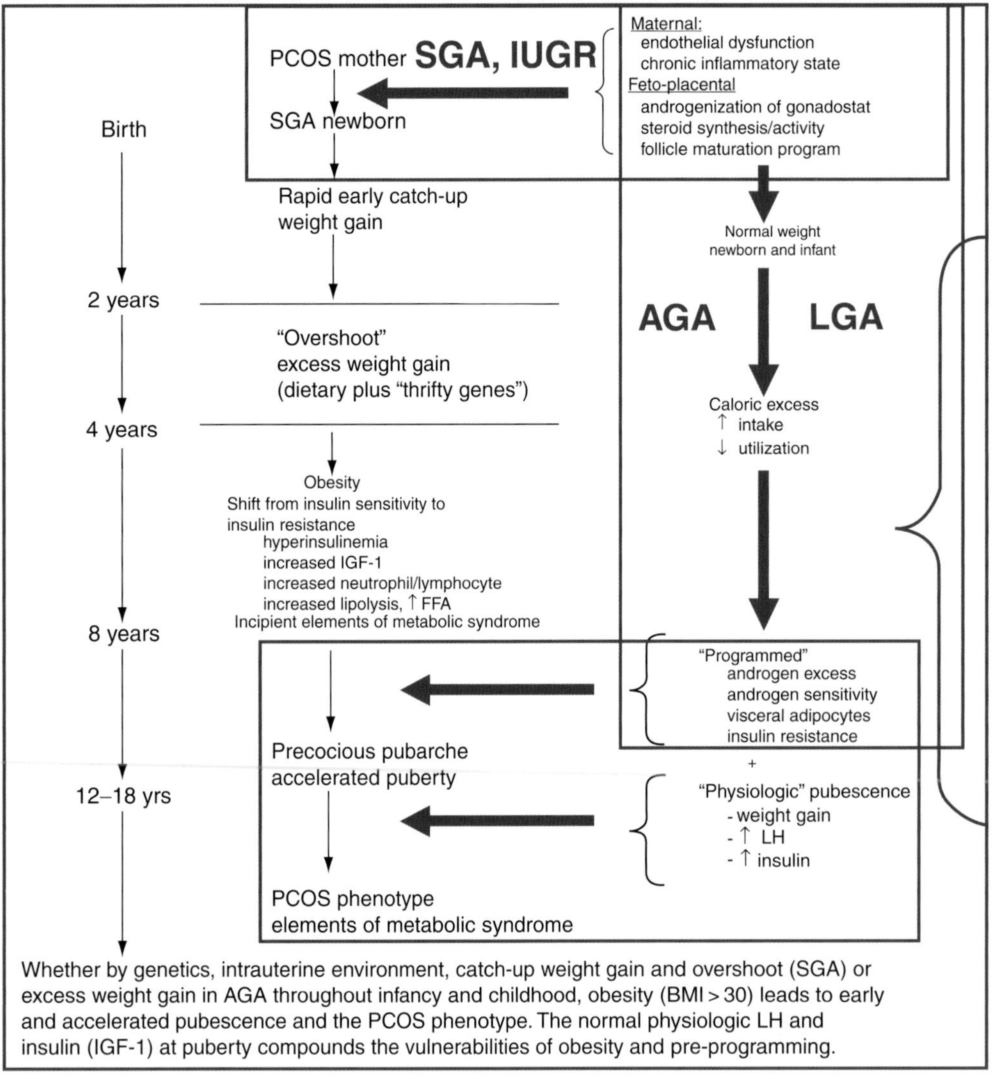

Fig. 11.18. Epigenetics in the developmental origin of disease.

mother (obese to begin with) gains excess weight during pregnancy. The result is combined maternal and fetal fat overload, fetal generalized and visceral adiposity, and fatty liver leading to fetal insulin resistance and long-term metabolic endocrine and cardiovascular consequences in adult life (Fig. 11.18) (Fig. 11.19) [131].

Excess maternal lipid transfer with fetal deposition affects critical fetal metabolic gene pathways influencing how the fetus stores energy, how it uses energy (mitochondrial injury), develops a systemic inflammatory state, and incurs an altered cell growth and apoptosis imbalance:

- Mitochondrial injury leads to reduced oxidation of FFAs and increased reactive oxygen species (ROS). The result is partition of fat to storage in muscle and liver and usage of glucose for energy production [152].
- Excess FFA and accumulation of triglyceride precursors (diacylglycerols) as well as ROS-induced pro-inflammatory cytokines inactivate insulin receptor substrate function by increased IRS-1 serine phosphorylation, impaired insulin receptor function, and fetal insulin resistance [25,153].

Increased fetal fat storage and an impaired cellular oxidation state impose effects beyond the neonate; the offspring faces a marked increased risk of insulin resistance, diabetes, obesity and cardiovascular disease.

This fetal state of impaired oxidation, mitochondrial injury and generalized fat accumulation may also:

- affect the quality of gonadal development, zygote development and the resulting mitochondrial dysfunction may affect the female oocyte [154]
- favor formation of adipocytes over myocytes from myeloid cell precursors in early organogenesis [155]
- alter hypothalamic "satiation" thresholds [156,157].

As a result the offspring faces the additional burdens of a larger number of pre-adipocytes, greater subcutaneous and visceral fat accumulation capacity and increased caloric intake with fatty food preferences.

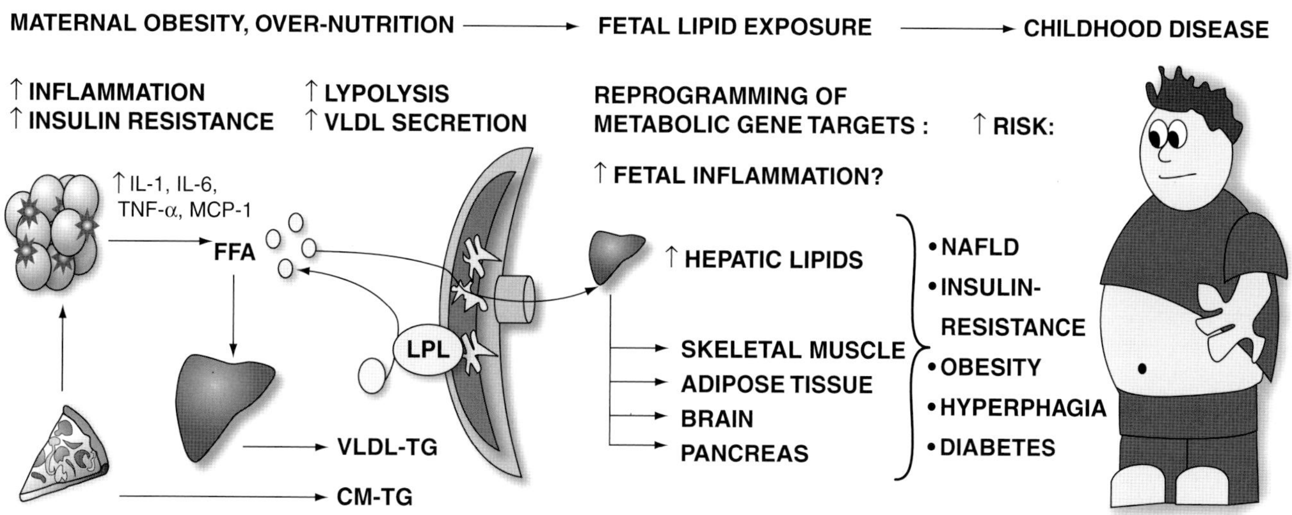

Fig. 11.19. Maternal PCOS, obesity, over-nutrition in pregnancy and induction of increased childhood and adult disease in her offspring. In PCOS, significant level of systemic inflammation and insulin resistance may exist before pregnancy. However the incremental effects of pregnancy related insulin resistance, hyperglycemia and hyperlipidemia lead to increased fetal lipid transfer and uptake with reprogramming of its metabolic gene targets (liver, muscle adipose tissue, brain β cells) and accumulation of lipid stores. The result is an increased life-long risk of non-alcoholic fatty liver disease, insulin resistance, obesity, cardiovascular disease and diabetes in progeny. Reproduced from reference [131], with permission.

Summary

When pregnant, PCOS women face *triple* the risk of developing gestational diabetes and 3.5 times the risk of developing hypertension/preeclampsia.

The life-cycle trajectory of long-term morbidity in PCOS

SGA, LGA, and even AGA (average for gestational age) daughters of PCOS mothers demonstrate early endocrine and metabolic derangements preceding the evolution of the full "mature" phenotype of PCOS [110,120,158,159]. In infancy and childhood early antral follicle AMH levels increase and remain elevated [160]. Ovarian mass, as follicles and stroma accumulate, also increases. Serum leptin and triglyceride levels are elevated and correlate with birth weight, current weight and reflect maternal BMI [161]. During late childhood, as puberty approaches insulin resistance, hyperinsulinemia and androgen excess emerge [162]. At puberty androgen, insulin, and LH increase significantly. In some cultures premature adrenarche [163], increased DHAS, and hyperinsulinemia is demonstrated in offspring of PCOS mothers – 30% of prepubertal daughters of Chilean mothers with PCOS develop exaggerated adrenarche accompanied by higher serum DHAS and insulin concentrations than age-matched BMI-matched girls born to women without PCOS [164]. Obesity amplifies hyperinsulinemia and hyperandrogenism as puberty evolves [165].

Diabetes mellitus (Fig. 11.20)

PCOS women are insulin resistant with reactive hyperinsulinemia compounded by the presence of obesity [110,120,166]. Insulin resistance occurs in about 50–70% of all women with PCOS and in 95% of obese women with PCOS [169]. The resulting impaired glucose tolerance defined in abnormal fasting glucose and oral glucose tolerance test presages the eventual increased risk of T2DM and premature CVD morbidity seen in PCOS women. Definitive T2DM will develop in classic PCOS women by the fourth decade of life; conversely, women with PCOS face a five-fold increased risk of developing T2DM within 8 years of PCOS diagnosis compared with ages- and weight-matched "healthy" women without PCOS [170]. As BMI increases, the risk of appearance of T2DM increases proportionally. A systematic Met analysis of 35 studies found that PCOS is associated with a 2.5-fold increased prevalence of IGT and a four-fold increased prevalence of T2DM [171].

Cardiovascular disease

Throughout this chapter the increased risk of cardiovascular events in PCOS women has been emphasized. Risk factors for CVD increase as obesity and dyslipidemia increase in PCOS women [110,120,172,173]. In the US the prevalence of dyslipidemia in PCOS is 70% (particularly hypertriglyceridemia, increased small, dense LDL-cholesterol and decreased HDL-C) [174]. These and other elements of the metabolic syndrome correlate with visceral adiposity [175]. Overall 33–47% of PCOS US women fulfill the diagnostic criteria for MetS and the incidence increases proportional to an increase in BMI (the MetS is 13.7-fold more likely in PCOS women with BMI > 30) [176]. As the MetS progresses, the combination of glucotoxicity, lipotoxicity, and systemic inflammatory state leads to impaired endothelial function, reduced vaso-reactivity, impaired endothelial integrity, and progressive atherogenesis (Fig. 11.21).

As a result PCOS women display:

- Increased carotid intima media thickness [178]
- Increases coronary artery calcium scores [179]
- Increased pre-event subclinical vascular disease [180]

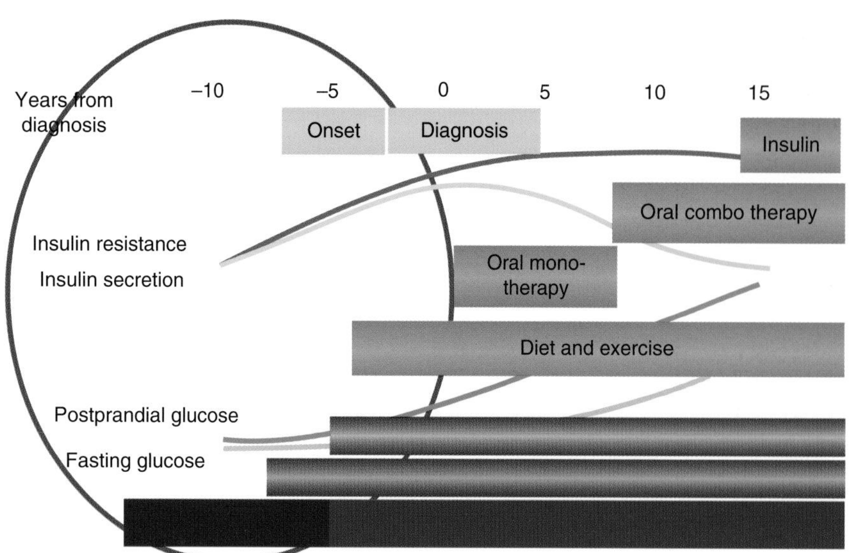

Fig. 11.20. Natural history of type 2 diabetes; typical progression of disease and treatment. In the decade before the formal diagnosis of type 2 DM, increasing insulin resistance and reactive hyperinsulinemia define the "silent" evolution of the prediabetic state. During this period however macro- and micro-vascular changes typical of overt diabetes are already under way. Once diagnosed various incremental steps in treatment are required beginning with diet and exercise.

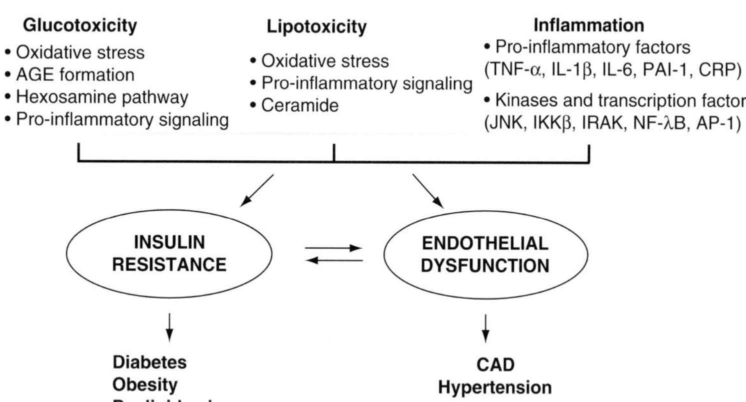

Fig. 11.21. Combined "toxic" effects of the metabolic syndrome on general cell function. Shared and interacting mechanisms of glucotoxicity, lipotoxicity, and inflammation underlie reciprocal relationships between insulin resistance and endothelial dysfunction that contribute to the linkage between metabolic and cardiovascular diseases. CAD, coronary artery disease. Reprinted from reference [177] with permission of Lippincott Williams & Wilkins.

- Eventually as Shaw et al. have shown [172], PCOS women experience more cardiovascular events and less event-free survival (fatal and non-fatal events) than women without PCOS.

Psychiatric disorders

Women with PCOS are burdened by an increased prevalence of mood disorders including depression (26–40%), anxiety (11.6%) and binge-eating (22.3%) [110,120,181], presumably, in part related to decreased quality of life imposed by obesity and hirsutism [182]. But metabolic elements also lead to psychiatric changes. Treatment of depression improves adiposity-dependent insulin resistance by 28%.

Any association between the presence of mood disorders and elevated systemic inflammation markers such as CRP, IL-6 or leukocyte number has been postulated [180].

There is evidence linking PCOS and bipolar disorder by self-identification questionnaire and linkages with hyperandrogenism [184]. Conversely treatments for bipolar disorder may induce POCS [11].

Malignancy

Although the relation between pre-menopausal PCOS, chronic anovulation, endometrial hyperplasia, and carcinoma is well established (sustained estrogen production, hyperinsulinemia) the possibility of increased breast and ovarian cancer (the presence of similar growth-promoting, apoptosis inhibiting factors) has been hypothesized [185]. However, the disproportionate excess prevalence of these cancers in post-menopausal women and the genetic basis for breast and ovarian cancer in premenopause (BRCA1 and BRCA2) make statistical assessment of a direct PCOS breast and ovarian cancer cause and effect relationship (as in endometrial disease) difficult to achieve.

Diagnosis of PCOS

A clinically valid differential diagnostic algorithm can be applied to all women who present with the suggestive but common combination of oligoamenorrhea and hirsutism [2].

The first step involves confirmation of the cardinal signs of the syndrome – anovulatory oligoamenorrhea and clinical evidence of androgenization. Thereafter, the step-wise evaluation devised by

Ehrmann is followed [31] (Table 11.5). It distinguishes possible PCOS as a "rule out" from other disorders which may cause anovulatory menstrual dysfunction combined with androgenicity and/or impaired metabolic function (Table 11.3).

Initially, all women of reproductive age who present with irregular menstrual function, regardless of the presence or absence of androgen excess, must be evaluated for the two most common disruptors of hypothalamic–pituitary–ovarian (HPO) function: thyroid disease [2] and hyperprolactinemia. Serum TSH and prolactin concentrations are assessed to rule out these common causes of menstrual dysfunction.

Thyroid-stimulating hormone (TSH). The normal range of TSH by immuno-metric assay is 0.4–4.2 mU/L. The lower limit of 0.4 is too high for pregnant individuals (lesson: rule out pregnancy by hCG testing in any amenorrheic female). Patients with *hyperthyroidism* will demonstrate sub-normal levels of TSH.

Patients with primary *hypothyroidism* show serum TSH concentrations that range from minimally elevated to 1000 mU/L. In general the degree of TSH elevation correlates with the clinical severity of hypothyroidism. Patients with TSH values between 5–15 have few if any symptoms and serum free T4 or free T4 index are typically low-normal with normal T3.

Prolactin excess [11]: The normal range of prolactin in non-pregnant (pregnancy testing required in amenorrhea!) non-lactating ovulatory women is 12–20 µg/L. If serum prolactin rises above 35 µg/L, FSH and LH oscillations are dampened and are fully suppressed when prolactin exceeds 50 µg/L.

Once these diagnostic possibilities are eliminated, the step-wise exclusion of disorders associated with androgen excess proceeds. Together, late-onset non-classical adrenal hyperplasia (NCAH), androgen-secreting tumors, Cushing's syndrome, severe insulin resistance syndromes and idiopathic hirsutism account for at most 10–30% of hyperandrogenism in women. Whereas all must be considered and excluded, few warrant detailed pursuit after initial clarifying assessment. Fritz and Speroff [2] have provided a detailed analysis of these uncommon diagnostic possibilities, particularly the infrequent but useful application of ACTH testing for presumptive late onset congenital adrenal hyperplasia using the 17α-OH progesterone responses in the 21 hydroxylase deficiency forms of the disease.

Once other entities are excluded and the diagnosis of presumptive PCOS made, it is essential to establish baseline markers to assess the presence of the metabolic syndrome. Thereafter annual follow-up studies to determine absence, emergence, or progression of the syndrome elements. Management decisions would respond according to these findings (Table 11.6).

Management of PCOS (Fig. 11.22)

The PCOS patient poses several management challenges and opportunities [108]. These include hyperandrogenism, anovulation, and infertility and metabolic dysfunction.

General approach to management

Three principles govern the development and usage of any management strategy:

Table 11.5. The core metabolic risk factors and the expression of their underlying components comprising the metabolic syndrome

Central obesity (↑waist circumference, ↑waist: hip ratio)
↑ circulating FFA
↓ adiponectin
↑ pro-inflammatory cytokines
↑ TNF_{α}
↑ IL-1, ↑IL-6,↑IL-10↑IL-18
↑ acute phase reactants: ↑CRP, ↑sialic acid
↑ plasminogen activator inhibitor 1 (PAI-1)
Atherogenic dyslipidemia
↑ triglycerides (TGs)
↑ apolipoprotein B (apoB)
↑ small low-density lipoproteins particles (LDL)
↓ high density lipoproteins (HDL)
Insulin resistance and hyperglycemia
↑ fasting insulin
↑ fasting glucose
Impaired glucose tolerance
Type 2 diabetes mellitus
Vascular dysfunction and inflammation
Hypertension
Endothelial dysfunction – atherogenesis
↑ carotid intimia – media thickness (IMT)
↑ coronary artery calcium (CAC)
↑ left ventricular hypertrophy

- The approach must be comprehensive and multifaceted, not limited to one identified pathophysiologic feature; treatment regimens in PCOS are rarely monotherapeutic.
- As a clinical syndrome, PCOS may present with one dominant element such as amenorrhea, but over time will progress to androgenization or insulin resistance.
- Sustained effective lifestyle initiatives (increased exercise and caloric restriction) modify all aspects of the syndrome even in those without elevated BMI.

Management of androgenization

Specific goals

The aims are to reduce the secretion, production, bioavailability, and activity of androgens expressed as biologic or biochemical evidence (hyperandrogenemia). Reduction of the androgen burden realizes several benefits: (1) control and stabilization of hirsutism, reduction of acne, and limited progression of alopecia; (2) relieve the intra-gonadal inhibition of follicle maturation by excess androgen; (3) reduces the misdirecting feedback of androgen on GnRH pulse frequency and theca-stimulating concentrations of LH; (4) modulates the influence of excess androgen on visceral adipocyte expansion, proliferation, inflammatory reaction, and dysfunctional secretions abetting insulin resistance and reactive hyperinsulinemia; (5) reduces substrate availability for extra-gonadal tissue aromatase conversion to chronic estrone concentrations; (6) reverses androgen-induced alterations in hepatic SHBG synthesis.

Table 11.6. Management decisions

Family history
Parents with DM, CVD, HTN
Metabolic syndrome in either parent
Gestational diabetes, gestational hypertension
PCOS, androgenicity, or PCOM in first degree relatives
Personal history
Anovulation, amenorrhea
Androgenization
Low birth weight
Childhood obesity
Physical exam
Hirsutism, acne, alopecia, acanthosis
Hypertension
Abdominal obesity (>35 inch waist)
BMI ≥30 kg/m^2
Laboratory
Assess for insulin resistance
Fasting and 1 or 2 hour OGTT as required
SHBG, triglycerides
Liver function tests
Assess for metabolic syndrome
Fasting cholesterol, HDL-C, LDL-C
Triglycerides
CHECK ANNUALLY
TREAT EMERGING POSITIVE SIGNS

Management strategy

Low-dose combined monophasic steroid oral contraceptive (OCs) are first-line therapy to control androgen excess [108].

(A) OCs reduce secretion and production of androgens: Combined OCs induce negative feedback and suppress circulating LH levels. As a result theca cell synthesis of testosterone is reduced and ovarian secretion of testosterone diminished. OCs also alter production (gonadal and extra-gonadal) of testosterone because androstenedione, secreted by both adrenal cortex and the LH-activated theca of polycystic ovaries is converted to testosterone at a variety of metabolic clearance sites and returned to the circulation as testosterone.

(B) OCs reduce biologic availability and target tissue activity of testosterone: Elevated testosterone and hyperinsulinemia combine to decrease SHBG production by 50%. The pharmacologic levels of estrogen in OCs reverse that deficiency. Decreasing the biologically available free testosterone reduces direct stimulation of androgen receptors (AR) by ligands T, 5α-reduced T, and androstenediol and limits the available molecular substrates for the 5α-reductase system production of ligands. In addition, depending on the progestin involved, the progestin content of the OC may also provide competitive inhibition of active androgen ligands at the AR and reduce 5α-reductase system activity.

(C) Together with OCs [186] (but on occasion separately) spironolactone confers incremental positive effects on the androgen burden of PCOS. In doses of 100–200 mg/d it controls androgen by:
- reduction of androgen synthesis in the adrenal cortex and theca cells of the ovary
- similar to progestin it competitively inhibits testosterone/androgen receptor interactions and inhibits 5α-reductase activity.

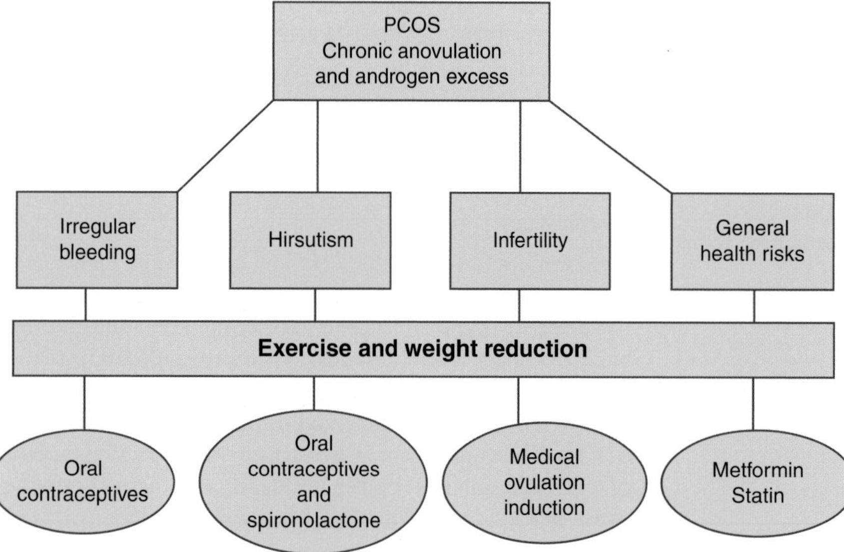

Fig. 11.22. Management of PCOS. For all PCOS women regardless of the array of clinical manifestations they present with, exercise and weight reduction is the primary management step. Thereafter, specific strategies are implemented to address the problems of dysfunctional uterine bleeding, infertility, androgen excess, and metabolic derangements.

As a result both OCs and spironolactone act to stabilize the current androgen-induced hirsutism. The likelihood of regression, if any, is slow.

(D) Some clinicians have questioned the safety of estrogen-progestin contraceptives in women with PCOS, primarily because of possible adverse effects on blood pressure or weight gain. However, substantial evidence supports OC safety in women with PCOS, with and without insulin resistance or hypertension.

(E) Combinations of OCs containing the spironolactone derivative drospirenone (an anti-androgen progestin) and anti-androgens such as flutamide, 62.5–250 mg/d or finasteride 2.5–5 mg/d control androgenization. [187]. Adding metformin to this combination results in reduced insulin resistance and reduced general body fat, but particularly visceral fat [188]. Given the possible toxicity and teratogenicity necessitating contraception with use of these modalities, OC alone and in combination with spironolactone remains the preferred approach.

(F) For PCOS women in whom administration of pharmacologic estrogen at any level is unacceptable or considered risky, Depo-Provera may be used. The progestin impact is two-fold: reduction of LH-driven androgen synthesis and competitive inhibition by the progestin at the androgen receptor. Contraceptive efficacy and compliance are additional advantages of this therapeutic tactic. However, the hypoestrogenicity of this regimen requires monitoring effects on bone density and lipid concentrations.

Alternative approaches

(a) Ablative procedures may be necessary for swifter cosmetic effect in established hirsutism [189]. Inhibition of hair growth by topical application of 13.5% eflornithine hydrochloride or direct attack on the hair follicle by electrolysis, laser, or even chemical depilatories may be required. These ablative procedures may be necessary for maximal cosmetic effect in established hirsutism.

(b) Androgenic alopecia is a difficult, therapeutically resistant burden in PCOS. It may require androgen suppression combined with androgen blockade and a topical means of stimulating hair re-growth, using minoxidil. Optimally this should be combined with an OC to prevent pregnancy on this therapy.

(c) Finally, in addition to their important effects on dyslipidemia, statins have been reported to reduce androgen concentrations as well as salutary effects on insulin resistance and abnormal lipids. However, the long-term effects (these benefits appear to plateau and stabilize at 6 months of application) have not been fully elucidated in PCOS. Use of statins in PCOS must be accompanied by effective contraception because statin use in pregnancy is an FDA assigned X category [190].

Although other insulin sensitizing agents such as thiazoladinediones decrease circulating insulin and androgen levels in women with PCOS, guidelines have been issued by the Endocrine Society against their use for the treatment of hirsutism [189].

Recommendation

In non-smoking, non-hypertensive PCOS women the low dose (20 μg ethinylestradiol) combined OC preparations which reduce or eliminate the hormone-free interval or reduce cycle frequency are recommended for stabilization and possibly over time modification of hirsutism and control of acne as well as providing the added benefit of contraception. The addition of spironolactone at 100 mg–200 mg/d is useful in accelerating cases of cutaneous androgenization. In this regard rapidly progressive virilization or failure to control testosterone levels with standard therapy demands evaluation for the presence of an androgen-secreting tumor or late-onset adrenal hyperplasia.

Anovulation, dysfunctional uterine bleeding, and infertility control of endometrial dysfunction and disease

Goals

Treatment is intend to avoid the excess endometrial proliferation, hyperplasia, and adenomatous hyperplasia that underlies dysfunctional uterine bleeding and polymenorrhea [2,110,120]. In addition, protect the endometrium from further abnormal growth to atypical adenomatous hyperplasia, endometrial carcinoma in situ, and endometrial carcinoma.

The endometrium in chronic anovulation/amenorrhea

The prolonged amenorrhea typical of PCOS does not reflect inactivity or atrophy of the endometrium. Rather, in contrast to the organized predictable pattern of sequential estrogen progesterone stimulation and withdrawal menses characteristic of the ovulatory menstrual cycle, in PCOS the anovulatory endometrium is fixed in the estrogen proliferative phase without the modulating structural and growth-restraining influences of corpus luteum progesterone. Furthermore, in the absence of programmed luteolysis the signal that induces regular controlled tissue shedding is lost. Over a period of time unrestrained estrogen-stimulated growth yields a thickened, glandular, highly vascularized, fragile tissue prone to intermittent, sometimes heavy and prolonged recurrent vaginal bleeding (dysfunctional uterine bleeding). With sustained chronic mitogenic stimuli such as estrogen and insulin [185], an increased risk of adenomatous endometrial hyperplasia and *premature* appearance of endometrial carcinoma may emerge in young adult PCOS women.

The goal of therapy is to reinstitute the protective benefits of progesterone before dysfunctional uterine breakthrough bleeding occurs let alone before the emergence of precancerous changes. Progestins at adequate doses and duration are antimitotic and anti-estrogenic at the endometrium. They stimulate conversion of estradiol to the weaker rapidly cleared estrone sulfate. Progestin also antagonizes estrogen action by inhibiting estrogen induction of its own receptor and thus reduces estrogen-abetted transcription of oncogenes. In addition, the progestin effect on the endometrial stroma – the pseudodecidual reaction – converts an unstable, hyperglandular, hypervascular easily fragmented tissue to a mechanically rigid endometrium which resists the asynchronous random breakdown underlying DUB. Furthermore prolonged OC virtually eliminates development of endometrial cancer not only during use but for a prolonged period after discontinuation. These goals can be achieved by administering either cyclic progestins or a combined monophasic OC.

Recommendations

Two considerations direct therapeutic decisions in this area: (1) the patient's desire for contraception, and (2) the willingness, particularly of the PCOS adolescent, to adhere to efficacious therapy. As the method of choice cyclic monophasic combined oral contraceptive provides contraception, reduces androgenization, and protects, repairs, and induces controlled "shedding" of the pseudodecidual endometrium.

Less patient-dependent methodologies such as the Depo-Provera injections, 150 mg every 3 months, are readily used and with the exception of BTB/amenorrhea in the early months of use, are well tolerated. The combined steroid vaginal contraceptive ring or patch is a less used and unproven but probably useful alternative.

When contraception is not required, oral medroxy progesterone acetate, 5–10 mg daily, or norethindrone acetate 2.5–10 mg/d for 2 weeks before anticipated menses or every 4–6 weeks in the absence of spontaneous menses are effective in achieving control of endometrial development and inducing synchronous growth, development, and shedding of a structurally stable endometrium. A progestin-releasing intrauterine device avoids systemic absorption and can be used to antagonize the mitotic actions of estrogen over a sustained period of time. Whatever method will be reliably used is the determining issue; all strategies that are progestin based and provide adequate dose and duration of the progestin are effective.

A note of caution: the longer the duration of anovulatory amenorrhea, the greater the possibility of *occult* endometrial malignancy. This can occur as early as the third decade of life. Accordingly, in newly diagnosed PCOS women who present with a history of prolonged amenorrhea, before starting any corrective therapy, either a transvaginal ultrasound assessment of endometrial thickness or an endometrial biopsy should be undertaken. The preferred choice of an endometrial biopsy is based on the patient's age and the duration of presumed exposure to unopposed estrogen stimulation. The validity of U/S measurements is also a factor; whereas a grossly thickened endometrium (≥12 mm) strongly suggests the possibility of endometrial hyperplasia a "normal" thickness does not exclude pathologic changes.

Anovulatory infertility

Goals and management strategy

The aim is to induce ovulation and pregnancy in anovulatory infertile PCOS women with maximum efficacy, safety, and the avoidance of multiple gestations [191]. In addition, intra-pregnancy complications must be addressed by minimizing metabolic dysfunction before ovulation induction and before pregnancy.

PCOS women displaying menstrual cycle frequencies of less than 4–6 per year or irregular intervals in excess of 7–8 weeks with or without DUB are likely to be chronically anovulatory and seek correction of infertility. In this circumstance a prolonged period of "observation" or a complex, costly excessively detailed "infertility work-up" is unnecessary. After assurance that endometrial histology is normal withdrawal bleeding should be induced and a trial of clomiphene citrate (Clomid) (50–150 mg/d for 5 days (beginning menstrual day 3–5) initiated. Clomiphene citrate alters GnRH secretion and reinduces adequate follicle-developing FSH release. The cumulative pregnancy rate achieved with Clomid is approximately 50% after three induced ovulatory cycles and approaches 75% within 6–9 cycles of treatment. The risk of multiple pregnancies is 5–8% [192].

PCOS anovulatory infertility refractory to clomiphene includes severely hirsute and/or obese women. In these individuals metformin in combination with clomiphene is the second tier choice. A 2008 meta-analysis including 17 randomized trials concluded that combined treatment with metformin and clomiphene achieves higher ovulation and pregnancy rates than treatment with clomiphene alone [193].

Failing in that approach, after more complete assessment (male factor, tubal pathology) the next strategy would be either ovarian drilling or if as is likely age is a pressing issue (≥ 35 years) a short course of gonadotropin induction of ovulation and/or IVF is warranted [194].

Induction of ovulation with exogenous gonadotropins is highly effective, but requires careful monitoring to avoid the risks of multiple pregnancy and ovarian hyperstimulation syndrome (OHSS). Curiously, PCOS women are highly sensitive to low doses of medication and exhibit a relatively narrow therapeutic range [195]. Whether metformin treatment can improve outcomes for women with PCOS in gonadotropin-stimulated or in vitro fertilization (IVF) cycles remains unclear, but evidence indicates the risk for ovarian hyperstimulation syndrome may be decreased.

Recommendations

Gonadotropins and laparoscopic ovarian drilling are third-line interventions if clomiphene (or combined clomiphene and metformin) fail to induce ovulation. In vitro fertilization is the fourth-line intervention, except with age, with associated pathologies (for example, severe endometriosis, male factor infertility, tubal damage) when it may be the only option and should be used sooner.

Control of metabolic dysfunction

Goals

The aims are to recognize, control, and reverse the presence or evolution of emerging markers of the metabolic syndrome, thereby addressing incipient hypertension, progressive glucose intolerance, and dyslipidemia to retard atherogenesis [2,110,120]. Emphasis is on achieving sustained lifestyle corrections (diet, exercise, smoking cessation) is imperative.

Control of metabolic dysfunction

While the PCOS woman's initial motivation is to seek medical evaluation of oligoamenorrhea or hirsutism and acne, or infertility, the associated compounding complications of PCOS – dyslipidemia, insulin resistance, and hypertension, are the more important indices of long-term health prospects. These cannot be overlooked even in the initial assessment. The metabolic derangements associated with PCOS cluster about the metabolic syndrome and are associated with increased risk of cardiovascular disease and diabetes mellitus later in life. The core metabolic risk factors are atherogenic dyslipidemia, elevated blood pressure, and elevated fasting plasma glucose, a pro-thrombotic state, and a pro-inflammatory state (Table 11.5) (Fig. 11.23).

The definition of the metabolic syndrome was promulgated by the International Diabetes Federation (IDF) in 2005 and revised in 2009 [196]. Central obesity (defined by increased waist circumference) is viewed as an essential component of the metabolic syndrome because of (a) the strength of evidence linking waist circumference with cardiovascular disease and (b) indication that central obesity may be the first and only physical indication of the initiation of the silent pathophysiologic cascade leading to the eventual full expression of the syndrome and its consequences. The elements of the metabolic syndrome are also associated with the presence of non-alcoholic fatty liver and sleep apnea. Physical inactivity and/or acceleration of obesity aggravate the syndrome.

Recommendations

The metabolic syndrome is evident at an early age in PCOS and appears irrespective of race and ethnicity. *Hyperinsulinemia* is both a central factor in the "vicious cycle" pathogenesis of PCOS and the critical link between PCOS-associated metabolic syndrome and the long-term risks of diabetes mellitus and cardiovascular disease. Strategies that attenuate insulin resistance address both PCOS and metabolic syndrome and reduce progression of endothelial dysfunction, atherogenesis, fatty liver disease, β-cell dysfunction and the prothrombotic state. These regimens include the use of insulin sensitizers, specific or combination therapies for metabolic syndrome or its individual elements. As noted but worthy of repetitive emphasis, lifestyle changes are essential for all PCOS patients including weight loss, exercise, and for all women with or without PCOS, smoking cessation.

Metformin

The recognition of the central role of insulin resistance in the pathophysiology of PCOS and knowledge of its potential longer-term health consequences have focused attention on the benefits of insulin-sensitizing medications and other drugs aimed at reducing the risks of developing diabetes and cardiovascular disease [2].

Metformin is an oral insulin-sensitizing agent and is the most widely used drug for the treatment of type 2 diabetes mellitus [198]. Metformin decreases hepatic glucose production, decreases intestinal glucose uptake, and increases peripheral insulin sensitivity. It also inhibits lipolysis, resulting in decreased circulating concentrations of insulin resistance inducing free fatty acids, and reduces hepatic gluconeogenesis. Metformin's mechanism of action is not entirely clear, but involves activation of the adenosine monophosphate-activated protein kinase pathway in liver and skeletal muscle.

Metformin is available in both a regular and sustained-release form that may be associated with fewer gastrointestinal side effects (nausea, vomiting, diarrhea, constipation, bloating,

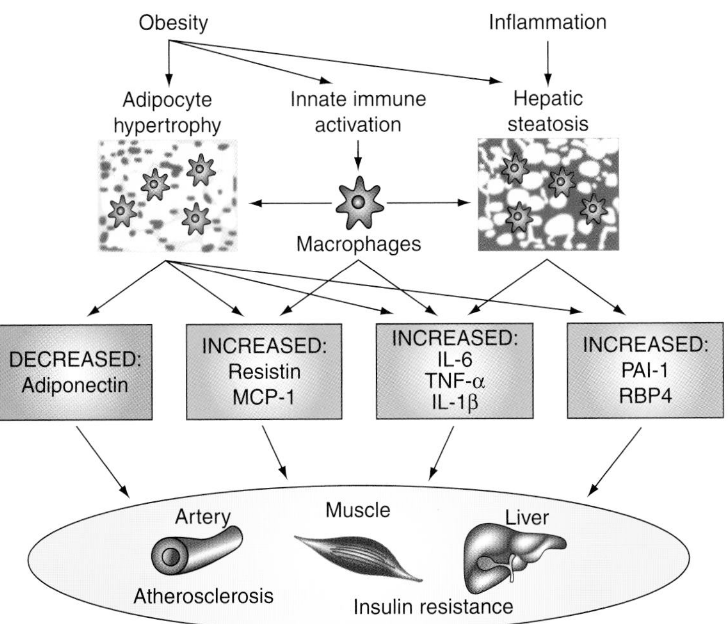

Fig. 11.23. PCOS, obesity, insulin resistance, and the metabolic syndrome. Insulin resistance results from pathophysiologic levels of circulating factors derived from several different cell types. The potential role of adipocytes, macrophages (in adipose tissue, liver, and elsewhere), hepatocytes and the secreted factors which modulate insulin action at the cellular level are shown. Reproduced from reference [197], with permission from Macmillan Publishers Ltd.

flatulence, heartburn, indigestion, unpleasant metallic taste). To improve tolerance and decrease side effects, metformin treatment should begin with a low dose (250–500 mg daily), and increase gradually over an interval of 4–6 weeks until the desired dose is attained. Lactic acidosis is a rare complication of metformin treatment, and for that reason, the drug should not be administered to those with renal insufficiency, liver disease, or alcohol abuse [199].

A large number of trials have observed beneficial effects of metformin in women with PCOS; in most, the dose has ranged between 1,500 and 2,000 mg daily. At these dose ranges Metformin does increase insulin sensitivity, decreases weight and BMI, and decreases blood pressure and LDL-cholesterol. A meta-analysis of 31 trials concluded that metformin increases insulin sensitivity up to 20%, decreases weight and BMI by 3–5%, decreases fasting glucose by about 5%, and increases HDL-cholesterol and decreases triglycerides by approximately 10% in patients at increased risk for developing diabetes [200]. No matter how severe, insulin resistance improves during metformin treatment and does so in lean and overweight women with PCOS as well as in those who are obese. Weight loss enhances the effects of metformin.

Oral contraceptive, metformin, and anti-androgen combinations

Combination therapies aimed at more comprehensive treatment, include estrogen-progestin contraceptives and metformin, and low doses of metformin (850 mg daily) and an anti-androgen (flutamide, 62.5 mg daily), with or without an estrogen–progestin contraceptive [201]. In women receiving an estrogen–progestin contraceptive, the addition of metformin improves insulin resistance and further reduces hyperandrogenism. The combination of low doses of metformin (850 mg daily) and an anti-androgen (flutamide, 62.5 mg daily) improves body composition (loss of fat and gain in lean mass) and lipid levels and increases levels of adiponectin, an anti-inflammatory adipokine released from adipose tissue that modulates glucose regulation and fatty acid metabolism.

Overall, these observations demonstrate that the spectrum of metabolic abnormalities that accompanies PCOS can be improved significantly by treatment with metformin and anti-androgens even in adolescents, and by their addition to estrogen-progestin contraceptives in young women.

Recommendations

The most logical candidates for treatment with metformin (aimed at preventing or slowing progression to type 2 diabetes and at reducing longer-term risks for cardiovascular disease) are women with impaired glucose tolerance or diabetes, those with obvious evidence of severe insulin resistance (acanthosis nigricans), and women having clear features of the metabolic syndrome, such as central obesity, hypertension, and dyslipidemia. All women with PCOS should therefore be screened with an oral glucose tolerance test at the time of presentation, and even 2 years thereafter. Those with impaired glucose tolerance warrant annual screening. There is good evidence from the Diabetes Prevention Trial that metformin treatment can decrease the risk for progression to diabetes in those with impaired glucose intolerance by approximately 30% (although better results were observed in those receiving intensive lifestyle interventions).

Anovulatory adolescent girls are another group that warrants periodic screening for glucose intolerance, and specific screening for insulin resistance, particularly if they are obese or had low birth weight. Both characteristics are associated with premature adrenarche and the development of PCOS during adolescence

Life-style changes

Lifestyle interventions including diet, weight loss, and increased physical exercise have beneficial effects on the health status of all populations studied [2,110,120]. These measures decrease insulin resistance, improve endothelial function, decrease the acute and chronic systemic inflammatory state, and have relevance to both PCOS adolescent or adult women. *Lifestyle modification*, such as *diet re-calibration* and *increased physical activity*, are considered the first-line treatment for PCOS women [202], particularly when BMI exceeds 25 kg/m^2.

Anovulation is a sentinel signal of PCOS. Reinitiation of ovulatory function reflects overall metabolic correction. Overweight infertile women with PCOS were randomized to either clomiphene citrate alone, the insulin sensitizer metformin alone, the combination of both, or a lifestyle modification program (low-calorie diet and risk-free exercise for 30 min/d) [203]. The lifestyle group women did better than the medicated groups with regard to waist circumference, LDL and insulin levels, while SHBG was improved equally in the lifestyle and metformin groups. Pregnancy rates were higher in the lifestyle group (20%) than in the combination group (14.8%), although this difference did not reach statistical significance. In a clinical trial randomizing obese, insulin-resistant PCOS women to lifestyle modification with the addition of metformin or placebo for 4 months, a small decrease in body weight through lifestyle changes was enough to improve menstrual cycles in these PCOS women. Thus, a modest weight loss in obese PCOS women of only 5% of initial body weight can result in pregnancy while a weight loss of 5–10% can reduce hyperandrogenism and insulin levels [204].

There are no conclusive data regarding the optimal composition of the diet which will reverse the clinical consequences of PCOS. Overweight PCOS women were randomized to a low or high protein diet for 12 weeks. Diet decreased both weight (7.5%) and abdominal fat (12.5%), and improved pregnancy rates, menstrual cyclicity, lipid profile, and insulin resistance. However diet composition had *no* differential effects on these beneficial results. Similarly, a randomized-controlled trial comparing high-protein and low-carbohydrate diets did not find significant differences in weight loss and clinical or biochemical improvement between diets.

At least 50% of women with PCOS are obese. It is important to stress that even a small reduction in weight can result in significant improvement in metabolic and reproductive function. The loss of abdominal fat may be the best predictor of the effects of weight loss.

Recommendations

Weight reduction by diet and exercise is the first and best treatment for obese PCOS women. Weight loss increases SHBG concentrations, thereby reducing free androgen levels and decreasing androgen stimulation of the pilosebaceous skin. Weight loss also improves ovulatory function, thereby increasing conception rates and probably decreasing the risk of miscarriage. A significant overall decrease in caloric intake is more important than the specific composition of the diet; there is no compelling evidence that a low-carbohydrate diet is better than a low-fat diet. Although treatment with metformin can facilitate weight loss primarily by suppressing appetite, the overall effect is modest and inconsistent. Consequently, metformin should not be used primarily for the purpose of weight reduction.

The benefits of exercise for improving diabetes and cardiovascular health have been demonstrated in the general population. Incorporation of moderate activity into daily activities appears as effective for reducing the risk of developing diabetes and cardiovascular disease as that achieved with vigorous physical activity, is more likely to be sustained, and is essential for maintaining weight loss over time.

A final thought

PCOS causes pain and impairment. It is syndromal, characterized by the presentation of a cluster of signs and symptoms and without a single identified lesion or causation. However, it progresses in the manner of a disease. Untreated, the burdens of PCOS become more diverse and less responsive to treatment. On the other hand, for some the syndrome disappears as menopause approaches. It affects the young, runs in families, and is found in every culture. It can affect multiple systems – reproductive and non-reproductive. But as many causes and effects link PCOS to the central organ from which it derives its name – the polycystic ovary – a return to almost normal function occurs once the ovary is relieved of the stultifying stresses that inhibit it. This happy outcome is not limited to application of "high-tech" assisted reproductive therapeutics or technologies – just weight loss and exercise! The ovary is resilient and can become "unstuck." But if the ovary is resilient, the metabolic consequences of the syndrome are not. The role of the physician is to identify and intercept these processes before irreversibility takes hold. What is needed is recognition; the corrective strategies are waiting to be implemented. Furthermore, the possibility of intercepting transgenerational epigenetic vulnerability is a legitimate prospect for current, effective intra-generational correction.

References

1. Oktem O. Understanding follicle growth in vivo. Hum Reprod. 2010;**25**:2944–54.
2. Fritz MA, Speroff L. Clinical gynecologic endocrinology and infertility. Chronic Anovulation and the Polycystic Ovary Syndrome, 8th edn. Baltimore, MD: Williams and Wilkins; 2011. p 495–531.
3. Dorn LD, Chrousos GP. The neurobiology of stress: understanding regulation of affect during female biological transitions. Semin Reprod Endocrinol. 1997;**15**(1):19–35.
4. Ahima RS. Body fat, leptin, and hypothalamic amenorrhea. N Engl J Med. 2004;**351**(10):959–62.
5. Marcus MD, Loucks TL, Berga SL. Psychological correlates of functional hypothalamic amenorrhea. Fertil Steril. 2001;**76**(2):310–16.
6. Frisch RE. Body fat, menarche, fitness and fertility. Hum Reprod. 1987;**2**(6):521–33.
7. Loucks AB. Energy availability, not body fatness, regulates reproductive function in women. Exerc Sport Sci Rev. 2003;**31**(3):144–8.
8. Welt CK, Chan JL, Bullen J, et al. Recombinant human leptin in women with hypothalamic amenorrhea. N Engl J Med. 2004;**351**(10):987–97.
9. Freda PU, Wardlaw SL, Post KD. Unusual causes of sellar/parasellar masses in a large transsphenoidal surgical series. J Clin Endocrinol Metab. 1996;**81**(10):3455–9.
10. Danziger J, Wallace S, Handel S, et al. The sella turcica in primary end organ failure. Radiology. 1979;**131**(1):111–15.
11. Melmed S, Casanueva FF, Hoffman AR, et al. Diagnosis and treatment of hyperprolactinemia: an Endocrine Society clinical practice guideline. J Clin Endocrinol Metab. 2011;**96**(2):273–88.
12. Seppälä M, Ranta T, Hirvonen E. Hyperprolactinaemia and luteal insufficiency. Lancet. 1976;**1**(7953):229–30.
13. Nieman LK, Biller BM, Findling JW, et al. The diagnosis of Cushing's syndrome: an Endocrine Society Clinical Practice Guideline. J Clin Endocrinol Metab. 2008;**93**(5):1526–40.
14. Melmed S. Medical progress: Acromegaly. N Engl J Med. 2006;**355**(24):255–8.
15. De Bellis A, Ruocco G, Battaglia M, et al. Immunological and clinical aspects of lymphocytic hypophysitis. Clin Sci (Lond). 2008;**114**(6):413–21.
16. Durodoye OM, Mendlovic DB, Brenner RS, et al. Endocrine disturbances in empty sella syndrome: case reports and review of literature. Endocr Pract. 2005:**11**(2);120–4.
17. Hu X, Wang J, Dong W, Fang Q, Hu L, Liu C. A meta-analysis of polycystic ovary syndrome in women taking valproate for epilepsy. Epilepsy Res. 2011;**97**:73–82.
18. Faddy MJ, Gosden RG. A model conforming the decline in follicle numbers to the age of menopause in women. Hum Reprod. 1996;**11**(7):1484–6.

19. Knight PG, Glister C. TGF-beta superfamily members and ovarian follicle development. Reproduction. 2006;**132**(2):191–206.
20. Ehrmann DA, Barnes RB, Rosenfield RL. Polycystic ovary syndrome as a form of functional ovarian hyperandrogenism due to dysregulation of androgen secretion. Endocr Rev. 1995;**16**(3):322–53.
21. Lin L, Ercan O, Raza J, et al. Variable phenotypes associated with aromatase (CYP19) insufficiency in humans. J Clin Endocrinol Metab. 2007;**92**(3):982–90.
22. Bakalov VK, Anasti JN, Calis KA, et al. Autoimmune oophoritis as a mechanism of follicular dysfunction in women with 46, XX spontaneous premature ovarian failure. Fertil Steril. 2005;**84**(4):958–65.
23. Cardozo E, Pavone ME, Hirshfeld-Cytron JE. Metabolic syndrome and oocyte quality. Trends Endocrinol Metab. 2011;**22**(3):103–9.
24. Siiteri PK, MacDonald PC. Role of extraglandular estrogen in human endocrinology. In: Geyer SR, Astwood EB, Greep RO (Eds.). *Handbook of Physiology, Section 7, Endocrinology*. Washington, DC: American Physiology Society; 1973, p 615.
25. Baptiste CG, Battista MC, Trottier A, et al. Insulin and hyperandrogenism in women with polycystic ovary syndrome. J Steroid Biochem Mol Biol. 2010;**122**(1–3):42–52.
26. Heinrichsdorff J, Olefsky JM. Fetuin-A: the missing link in lipid induced inflammation. Nat Med. 2012;**18**:1182–3.
27. Zawadzki JK, Dunaif A. Diagnostic criteria for polycystic ovary syndrome: towards a rational approach. In: Dunaif A, Givens JR, Haseltine FP, Merriam GR (Eds.). *Polycystic Ovary Syndrome*. Boston: Blackwell Scientific; 1992, p 377–84.
28. Rotterdam ESHRE/ASRM-Sponsored PCOS Consensus Workshop Group. Revised 2003 consensus on diagnostic criteria and long-term health risks related to polycystic ovary syndrome. Fertil Steril. 2004;**81**(1):19–25.
29. Azziz R, Carmina E, Dewailly D, et al. The Androgen Excess and PCOS Society criteria for the polycystic ovary syndrome: the complete task force report. Fertil Steril. 2009;**91**(2):456–88.
30. Johnstone EB, Rosen MP, Neril R, et al. The polycystic ovary post-Rotterdam: a common, age-dependent finding in ovulatory women without metabolic significance. J Clin Endocrinol Metab. 2010;**95**(11):4965–72.
31. Ehrmann DA. Polycystic ovary syndrome. N Engl J Med. 2005;**352**(12):1223–36.
32. Venturoli S, Porcu E, Fabbri R, et al. Episodic pulsatile secretion of FSH, LH, prolactin, oestradiol, oestrone, and LH circadian variations in polycystic ovary syndrome. Clin Endocrinol (Oxf). 1988;**28**(1):93–107.
33. Wajchenberg BL, Achando SS, Mathor MM, et al. The source(s) of estrogen production in hirsute women with polycystic ovarian disease as determined by simultaneous adrenal and ovarian venous catheterization. Fertil Steril. 1988;**49**(1):56–61.
34. Fauser BC. Observations in favor of normal early follicle development and disturbed dominant follicle selection in polycystic ovary syndrome. Gynecol Endocrinol. 1994;**8**(2):75–82.
35. Huang A, Brennan K, Azziz R. Prevalence of hyperandrogenemia in the polycystic ovary syndrome diagnosed by the National Institutes of Health 1990 criteria. Fertil Steril. 2010;**93**(6):1938–41.
36. Yildiz BO, Bolour S, Woods K, et al. Visually scoring hirsutism. Hum Reprod Update. 2010;**16**(1):51–64.
37. Rosner W, Auchus RJ, Azziz R, et al. Position statement: utility, limitations, and pitfalls in measuring testosterone: an Endocrine Society position statement. J Clin Endocrinol Metab. 2007;**92**(2):405–13.
38. Bardin CW, Lipsett MB. Testosterone and androstenedione blood production rates in normal women and women with idiopathic hirsutism or polycystic ovaries. J Clin Invest. 1967;**46**(5):891–902.
39. Longcope C. Adrenal and gonadal androgen secretion in normal females. Clin Endocrinol Metab. 1986;**15**(2):213–28.
40. Pasquali R. Obesity and androgens: facts and perspectives. Fertil Steril. 2006;**85**(5):1319–40.
41. Lasley BL, Santoro N, Randolf JF, et al. The relationship of circulating dehydroepiandrosterone, testosterone, and estradiol to stages of the menopausal transition and ethnicity. J Clin Endocrinol Metab. 2002;**87**(8):3760–7.
42. Puurunen J, Piltonen T, Jaakkola P, et al Adrenal androgen production capacity remains high up to menopause in women with polycystic ovary syndrome J Clin Endoocrinol Metab. 2009;**94**(6):1973–8.
43. Payne AH, Hales DB. Overview of steroidogenic enzymes in the pathway from cholesterol to active steroid hormones. Endocr Rev. 2004;**25**(6):947–70.
44. Jamnongjit M, Hammes SR. Ovarian steroids: the good, the bad, and the signals that raise them. 2006;**5**(11):1178–83.
45. Mendelson CR, Kamat A. Mechanisms in the regulation of aromatase in developing ovary and placenta. J Steroid Biochem Mol Biol. 2007;**106**(1–5):62–70.
46. Vinson GP. Adrenocortical zonation and ACTH. Microsc Res Tech. 2003;**61**(3):227–39.
47. Endoh A, Kristiansen SB, Casson PR, et al. The zona reticularis is the site of biosynthesis of dehydroepiandrosterone and dehydroepiandrosterone sulfate in the adult human adrenal cortex resulting from its low expression of 3 beta-hydroxysteroid dehydrogenase. J Clin Endocrinol Metab. 1996;**81**(10):3558–65.
48. Gilling-Smith C, Willis DS, Beard RW, et al. Hypersecretion of androstenedione by isolated thecal cells from polycystic ovaries. J Clin Endocrinol Metab. 1994;**79**(4):1158–65.
49. Tee MK, Dong Q, Miller WL. Pathways leading to phosphorylation of p450c17 and to the posttranslational regulation of androgen biosynthesis. Endocrinology. 2008;**149**(5):2667–77.
50. Yalamanchi SK, Sam S, Cardenas MO, et al. Association of fibrillin-3 and transcription factor-7-like 2 gene variants with metabolic phenotypes in PCOS. Obesity (Silver Spring). 2012;**20**:1273–8.
51. Goodarzi MO, Jones MR, Li X, et al. Replication of association of DENND1A and THADA variants with polycystic ovary syndrome in European cohorts. J Med Genet. 2012;**49**(2):90–5.

52. Brock BJ, Waterman MR. Biochemical differences between rat and human cytochrome P450c17 support the different steroidogenic needs of these two species. Biochemistry. 1999;**38**(5):1598–606.

53. Hyatt PJ, Bhatt K, Tait JF. Steroid biosynthesis by zona fasciculata and zona reticularis cells purified from the mammalian adrenal cortex. J Steroid Biochem. 1983;**19**(1C):953–9.

54. Sasano H, Okamoto M, Mason JI, et al. Immunolocalization of aromatase, 17 alpha-hydroxylase and side-chain-cleavage cytochromes P-450 in the human ovary. J Reprod Fertil. 1989;**85**(1):163–9.

55. Cedars MI, Steingold KA, de Ziegler D, et al. Long-term administration of gonadotropin-releasing hormone agonist and dexamethasone: assessment of the adrenal role in ovarian dysfunction. Fertil Steril. 1992;**57**(3):495–500.

56. Gilling-Smith C, Story H, Rogers V, et al. Evidence for a primary abnormality of thecal cell steroidogenesis in the polycystic ovary syndrome. Clin Endocrinol (Oxf). 1997;**47**(1):93–9.

57. Nestler JE, Powers LP, Matt DW, et al. A direct effect of hyperinsulinemia on serum sex hormone-binding globulin levels in obese women with the polycystic ovary syndrome. J Clin Endocrinol Metab. 1991;**72**(1):83–9.

58. Rittmaster RS, Thompson DL. Effect of leuprolide and dexamethasone on hair growth and hormone levels in hirsute women: the relative importance of the ovary and the adrenal in the pathogenesis of hirsutism. J Clin Endocrinol Metab. 1990;**70**(4):1096–102.

59. Nestler JE, Jakubowicz DJ. Decreases in ovarian cytochrome P450c17 alpha activity and serum free testosterone after reduction of insulin secretion in polycystic ovary syndrome. N Engl J Med. 1996;**335**(9):617–23.

60. Nestler JE, Jakubowicz DJ. Lean women with polycystic ovary syndrome respond to insulin reduction with decreases in ovarian P450c17 alpha activity and serum androgens. J Clin Endocrinol Metab. 1997;**82**(12):4075–9.

61. Romualdi D, Giuliani M, Draisci G, et al. Pioglitazone reduces the adrenal androgen response to corticotropin-releasing factor without changes in ACTH release in hyperinsulinemic women with polycystic ovary syndrome. Fertil Steril. 2007;**88**(1):131–8.

62. Taylor AE, McCourt B, Martin KA, et al. Determinants of abnormal gonadotropin secretion in clinically defined women with polycystic ovary syndrome. J Clin Endocrinol Metab. 1997;**82**(7):2248–56.

63. Wildt L, Häusler A, Marshall G, et al. Frequency and amplitude of gonadotropin-releasing hormone stimulation and gonadotropin secretion in the rhesus monkey. Endocrinology. 1981;**109**(2):376–85.

64. Fauser BC, Pache TD, Lamberts SW, et al. Serum bioactive and immunoreactive luteinizing hormone and follicle-stimulating hormone levels in women with cycle abnormalities, with or without polycystic ovarian disease. J Clin Endocrinol Metab. 1991;**73**:811.

65. Imse V, Holzapfel G, Hinney B, et al. Comparison of luteinizing hormone pulsatility in the serum of women suffering from polycystic ovarian disease using a bioassay and five different immunoassays. J Clin Endocrinol Metab. 1992;**74**(5):1053–61.

66. Soules MR, Steiner RA, Clifton DK, et al. Progesterone modulation of pulsatile luteinizing hormone secretion in normal women. J Clin Endocrinol Metab. 1984;**58**(2):378–83.

67. Wardlaw SL, Wehrenberg WB, Ferin M, et al. Effect of sex steroids on beta-endorphin in hypophyseal portal blood. J Clin Endocrinol Metab. 1982;**55**(5):877–81.

68. Chang RJ, Mandel FP, Lu JK, et al. Enhanced disparity of gonadotropin secretion by estrone in women with polycystic ovarian disease. J Clin Endocrinol Metab. 1982;**54**(3):490–4.

69. Pastor CL, Griffin-Korf ML, Aloi JA, et al. Polycystic ovary syndrome: evidence for reduced sensitivity of the gonadotropin-releasing hormone pulse generator to inhibition by estradiol and progesterone. J Clin Endocrinol Metab. 1998;**83**(2):582–90.

70. Berga SL. Polycystic ovary syndrome: a model of combinational endocrinology? J Clin Endocrinol Metab. 2009,**94**(7):2250–1.

71. Eagleson CA, Gingrich MB, Pastor CL, et al. Polycystic ovarian syndrome: evidence that flutamide restores sensitivity of the gonadotropin-releasing hormone pulse generator to inhibition by estradiol and progesterone. J Clin Endocrinol Metab. 2000;**85**(11):4047–52.

72. Adams JM, Taylor AE, Crowley WF Jr. Polycystic ovarian morphology with regular ovulatory cycles: insights into the pathophysiology of polycystic ovarian syndrome. J Clin Endocrinol Metab. 2004;**89**(9):4343–50.

73. Yildiz BO, Knochenhauer ES, Azziz R. Impact of obesity on the risk for polycystic ovary syndrome. J Clin Endocrinol Metab. 2008;**93**(1):162–8.

74. Apridonidze T, Essah PA, Iuorno MJ, et al. Prevalence and characteristics of the metabolic syndrome in women with polycystic ovary syndrome. J Clin Endocrinol Metab. 2005;**90**(4):1929–35.

75. Hotamisligil GS, Peraldi P, Budavari A, et al. IRS-1-mediated inhibition of insulin receptor tyrosine kinase activity in TNF-alpha- and obesity-induced insulin resistance. Science. 1996;**271**(5249):665–8.

76. Poretsky L, Cataldo NA, Rosenwaks Z, et al. The insulin-related ovarian regulatory system in health and disease. Endocr Rev. 1999;**20**(4):535–82.

77. Svendsen PF, Nilas L, Nørgaard K, et al. Obesity, body composition and metabolic disturbances in polycystic ovary syndrome. Hum Reprod. 2008;**23**(9):2113–21.

78. Yildirim B, Sabir N, Kaleli B. Relation of intra-abdominal fat distribution to metabolic disorders in nonobese patients with polycystic ovary syndrome. Fertil Steril. 2003;**79**(6):1358–64.

79. Gambineri A, Pelusi C, Vicennati V, et al. Obesity and the polycystic ovary syndrome. Int J Obes Relat Metab Disord. 2002;**26**(7):883–96.

80. Michelmore KF, Balen AH, Dunger DB, et al. Polycystic ovaries and associated clinical and biochemical features in young women. Clin Endocrinol (Oxf). 1999;**51**(6):779–86.

81. Alvarez-Blasco F, Botella-Carretero JI, San Millán JL, et al. Prevalence and characteristics of the polycystic ovary syndrome in overweight and obese women. Arch Intern Med. 2006;**166**(19):2081–6.

82. Kahn CR, Flier JS, Bar RS, et al. The syndromes of insulin resistance and

acanthosis nigricans. Insulin-receptor disorders in man. N Engl J Med. 1976;**294**(14):739–45.

83. Dunaif A. Insulin resistance and the polycystic ovary syndrome: mechanism and implications for pathogenesis. Endocr Rev. 1997;**18** (6):774–800.

84. DeUgarte CM, Bartolucci AA, Azziz R. Prevalence of insulin resistance in the polycystic ovary syndrome using the homeostasis model assessment. Fertil Steril. 2005;**83**(5):1454–60.

85. Tok EC, Ertunc D, Evruke C, et al. The androgenic profile of women with non-insulin-dependent diabetes mellitus. J Reprod Med. 2004;**49**(9):746–52.

86. Book CB, Dunaif A. Selective insulin resistance in the polycystic ovary syndrome. J Clin Endocrinol Metab. 1999;**84**(9):3110–16.

87. Moller DE, Flier JS. Insulin resistance–mechanisms, syndromes, and implications. N Engl J Med. 1991;**325**(13):938–48.

88. Baillargeon JP. Insulin action in polycystic ovary syndrome: in vivo and in vitro. In Azziz R (Ed.). The Polycystic Ovary Syndrome: Current Concepts in Pathogenesis and Clinical Care. New York: Springer; 2007, p 43.

89. Nelson-Degrave VL, Wickenheisser JK, Hendricks KL, et al. Alterations in mitogen-activated protein kinase kinase and extracellular regulated kinase signaling in theca cells contribute to excessive androgen production in polycystic ovary syndrome. Mol Endocrinol. 2005;**19** (2):379–90.

90. Willis D, Mason H, Gilling-Smith C, et al. Modulation by insulin of follicle-stimulating hormone and luteinizing hormone actions in human granulosa cells of normal and polycystic ovaries. J Clin Endocrinol Metab. 1996;**81**(1):302–9.

91. Smith S, Ravnikar VA, Barbieri RL. Androgen and insulin response to an oral glucose challenge in hyperandrogenic women. Fertil Steril. 1987;**48**(1):72–7.

92. Nestler JE, Barlascini CO, Matt DW, et al. Suppression of serum insulin by diazoxide reduces serum testosterone levels in obese women with polycystic ovary syndrome. J Clin Endocrinol Metab. 1989;**68**(6):1027–32.

93. Barbieri RL, Makris A, Ryan KJ. Insulin stimulates androgen accumulation in incubations of human ovarian stroma and theca. Obstet Gynecol. 1984;**64**(3 Suppl):73S–80S.

94. Czech MP, Corvera S. Signaling mechanisms that regulate glucose transport. J Biol Chem. 1999;**274**(4):1865–8.

95. Dunaif A, Xia J, Book CB, et al. Excessive insulin receptor serine phosphorylation in cultured fibroblasts and in skeletal muscle. A potential mechanism for insulin resistance in the polycystic ovary syndrome. J Clin Invest. 1995;**96**(2):801–10.

96. Tanti JF, Gual P, Grémeaux T, et al. Alteration in insulin action: role of IRS-1 serine phosphorylation in the retroregulation of insulin signalling. Ann Endocrinol (Paris). 2004;**65**(1):43–8.

97. Li M, Youngren JF, Dunaif A, et al. Decreased insulin receptor (IR) autophosphorylation in fibroblasts from patients with PCOS: effects of serine kinase inhibitors and IR activators. J Clin Endocrinol Metab. 2002;**87**(9):4088–93.

98. Zhang LH, Rodriguez H, Ohno S, et al. Serine phosphorylation of human P450c17 increases 17,20-lyase activity: implications for adrenarche and the polycystic ovary syndrome. Proc Natl Acad Sci U S A. 1995;**92** (23):10619–23.

99. Marshall JC. Obesity in adolescent girls: is excess androgen the real bad actor? J Clin Endocrinol Metab. 2006;**91**(2):393–5.

100. Dieudonne MN, Pecquery R, Boumediene A, et al. Androgen receptors in human preadipocytes and adipocytes: regional specificities and regulation by sex steroids. Am J Physiol. 1998;**274**(6 Pt 1):C1645–52.

101. Coviello AD, Legro RS, Dunaif A. Adolescent girls with polycystic ovary syndrome have an increased risk of the metabolic syndrome associated with increasing androgen levels independent of obesity and insulin resistance. J Clin Endocrinol Metab. 2006;**91**(2):492–7.

102. Janssen I, Powell LH, Crawford S, Lasley B, Sutton-Tyrrell K. Menopause and the metabolic syndrome: the study of women's health across the nation. Arch Intern Med. 2008;**168**:1568–75.

103. Katz M, Carr PJ, Cohen BM, et al. Hormonal effects of wedge resection of polycystic ovaries. Obstet Gynecol. 1978;**51**(4):437–44.

104. Kaaijk EM, Hamerlynck JV, Beek JF, et al. Clinical outcome after unilateral oophorectomy in patients with polycystic ovary syndrome. Hum Reprod. 1999;**14**(4):889–92.

105. Pache TD, Fauser BC. Polycystic ovaries in female-to-male transsexuals. Clin Endocrinol (Oxf). 1993;**39**(6):702–3.

106. Copperman AB. Polycystic ovarian syndrome. In Altchek A, Deligdisch L, Kase N (Eds.). Altchek's Diagnosis and Management of Ovarian Disorders. Elsevier; USA; 2003. p 337–55.

107. Maciel GA, Baracat EC, Benda JA, et al. Stockpiling of transitional and classic primary follicles in ovaries of women with polycystic ovary syndrome. J Clin Endocrinol Metab. 2004;**89** (11):5321–7.

108. ACOG Committee on Practice Bulletins – Gynecology. ACOG Practice Bulletin No. 108: Polycystic ovary syndrome. Obstet Gynecol. 2009;**114**(4):936–49.

109. Lass A. The role of ovarian volume in reproductive medicine. Hum Reprod Update. 1999;**5**:256–66.

110. Pasquali R. PCOS Forum: research in polycystic ovary syndrome today and tomorrow. Clin Endocrinol (Oxf). 2011;**74**(4):424–33.

111. Nagamani M, Hannigan EV, Dinh TV, et al. Hyperinsulinemia and stromal luteinization of the ovaries in postmenopausal women with endometrial cancer. J Clin Endocrinol Metab. 1988;**67**(1):144–8.

112. Greenblatt EM, Casper RF. Laparoscopic ovarian drilling in women with polycystic ovarian syndrome. Prog Clin Biol Res. 1993;**381**:129–38.

113. Erickson GF, Magoffin DA, Garzo VG, et al. Granulosa cells of polycystic ovaries: are they normal or abnormal? Hum Reprod. 1992;**7**(3):293–9.

114. Mason HD, Willis DS, Beard RW, et al. Estradiol production by granulosa cells of normal and polycystic ovaries: relationship to menstrual cycle history and concentrations of gonadotropins and sex steroids in follicular fluid. J Clin Endocrinol Metab. 1994;**79** (5):1355–60.

115. Driancourt MA, Reynaud K, Cortvrindt R, et al. Roles of KIT and KIT LIGAND in ovarian function. Rev Reprod. 2000;**5**(3):143–52.

116. Pellatt L, Hanna L, Brincat M, et al. Granulosa cell production of anti-Müllerian hormone is increased in polycystic ovaries. J Clin Endocrinol Metab. 2007;**92**(1):240–5.

117. Pigny P, Merlen E, Robert Y, et al. Elevated serum level of anti-mullerian hormone in patients with polycystic ovary syndrome: relationship to the ovarian follicle excess and to the follicular arrest. J Clin Endocrinol Metab. 2003;**88**(12):5957–62.

118. Lowe P, Kovacs G, Howlett D. Incidence of polycystic ovaries and polycystic ovary syndrome amongst women in Melbourne, Australia. Aust N Z J Obstet Gynaecol. 2005;**45**(1):17–19.

119. Hassan MA, Killick SR. Ultrasound diagnosis of polycystic ovaries in women who have no symptoms of polycystic ovary syndrome is not associated with subfecundity or subfertility. Fertil Steril. 2003;**80**(4):966–75.

120. Goodarzi MO, Dumesic DA, Chazenbalk G, et al. Polycystic ovary syndrome: etiology, pathogenesis and diagnosis. Nat Rev Endocrinol. 2011;**7**(4):219–31.

121. Kahsar-Miller MD, Nixon C, Boots LR, et al. Prevalence of polycystic ovary syndrome (PCOS) in first-degree relatives of patients with PCOS. Fertil Steril. 2001;**75**(1):53–8.

122. Vink JM, Sadrzadeh S, Lambalk CB, et al. Heritability of polycystic ovary syndrome in a Dutch twin-family study. J Clin Endocrinol Metab. 2006;**91**(6):2100–4.

123. Leibel NI, Baumann EE, Kocherginsky M, et al. Relationship of adolescent polycystic ovary syndrome to parental metabolic syndrome. J Clin Endocrinol Metab. 2006;**91**(4):1275–83.

124. Yildiz BO, Yarali H, Oguz H, et al. Glucose intolerance, insulin resistance, and hyperandrogenemia in first degree relatives of women with polycystic ovary syndrome. J Clin Endocrinol Metab. 2003;**88**(5):2031–6.

125. Sam S, Legro RS, Essah PA, et al. Evidence for metabolic and reproductive phenotypes in mothers of women with polycystic ovary syndrome. Proc Natl Acad Sci U S A. 2006;**103**(18):7030–5.

126. Goodarzi MO. Looking for polycystic ovary syndrome genes: rational and best strategy. Semin Reprod Med. 2008;**26**(1):5–13.

127. Petry CJ, Ong KK, Michelmore KF, et al. Association of aromatase (CYP 19) gene variation with features of hyperandrogenism in two populations of young women. Hum Reprod. 2005;**20**(7):1837–43.

128. Kase N. *The Polycystic Ovary Syndrome – Challenges and Opportunities in Adolescent Medicine, Chap 31*. New York: John Wiley and Sons; 2009, p 316–39.

129. Yalamanchi SK, Sam S, Cardenas MO, et al. Association of fibrillin-3 and transcription factor-7-like 2 gene variants with metabolic phenotypes in PCOS. Obesity (Silver Spring). 2012;**20**(6):1273–8.

130. Goodarzi, MO. Replication of association of DENND1A and THADA variants with polycystic ovary syndrome in European cohorts. J Med Genet. 2012;**49**:90–5.

131. Heerwagen MJ, Miller MR, Barbour LA, et al. Maternal obesity and fetal metabolic programming: a fertile epigenetic soil. Am J Physiol Regul Integr Comp Physiol. 2010;**299**(3): R711–22.

132. Kjerulff LE, Sanchez-Ramos L, Duffy D. Pregnancy outcomes in women with polycystic ovary syndrome: a metaanalysis. Am J Obstet Gynecol. 2011;**204**(6):558.e1–6.

133. Fritz MA, Speroff L. In: Clinical Gynecologic Endocrinology and Infertility, 8th edition, Chap 8. *Endocrinology of Pregnancy*. Baltimore, MD: Williams & Wilkins; 2011, p 269–328.

134. McIntyre HD, Chang AM, Callaway LK, et al. Hormonal and metabolic factors associated with variations in insulin sensitivity in human pregnancy. Diabetes Care. 2010;**33**(2):356–60.

135. Houstis N, Rosen ED, Lander ES. Reactive oxygen species have a causal role in multiple forms of insulin resistance. Nature. 2006;**440**(7086):944–8.

136. Herrera E. Metabolic adaptations in pregnancy and their implications for availability of substrates for the fetus. Eur J Clin Nutr. 2000;**54**(Suppl 1):S47–51.

137. Chmurzynska A. Fetal programming: link between early nutrition, DNA methylation, and complex diseases. Nutr Rev. 2010;**68**(2):87–98.

138. Jaenisch R, Bird A. Epigenetic regulation of gene expression: how the genome integrates intrinsic and environmental signals. Nat Genet. 2003;**33**(Suppl):245–54.

139. Barker DJ. The origins of the developmental origins theory. J Intern Med. 2007;**261**(5):412–17.

140. Gluckman PD, Hanson MA, Buklijas T, et al. Epigenetic mechanisms that underpin metabolic and cardiovascular diseases. Nat Rev Endocrinol. 2009;**5**(7):401–8.

141. Ahmed F. Epigenetics: tales of adversity. Nature. 2010;**468**(7327):S20.

142. Hult M, Tomhammar P, Ueda P, et al. Hypertension, diabetes and overweight: looming legacies of the Biafran famine. PLoS One. 2010;**5**(10):e13582.

143. Park JH, Stoffers DA, Nicholls RD, et al. Development of type 2 diabetes following intrauterine growth retardation in rats is associated with progressive epigenetic silencing of Pdx1. J Clin Invest. 2008;**118**(6):2316–24.

144. Catalano PM. The hyperglycemia and adverse pregnancy outcome study: associations of GDM and obesity with pregnancy outcomes. Diabetes Care. 2012;**35**(4):780–6.

145. Ouzilleau C, Roy MA, Leblanc L, et al. An observational study comparing 2-hour 75-g oral glucose tolerance with fasting plasma glucose in pregnant women: both poorly predictive of birth weight. CMAJ. 2003;**168**(4):403–9.

146. HAPO Study Cooperative Research Group. Hyperglycemia and adverse pregnancy outcomes. N Engl J Med. 2008;**358**:1991–2002.

147. Brion MJ, Ness AR, Rogers I, et al. Maternal macronutrient and energy intakes in pregnancy and offspring intake at 10 y: exploring parental comparisons and prenatal effects. Am J Clin Nutr. 2010;**91**(3):748–56.

148. Catalano PM, Farrell K, Thomas A, et al. Perinatal risk factors for childhood obesity and metabolic dysregulation. Am J Clin Nutr. 2009;**90**(5):1303–13.

149. Khan NA. Role of lipids and fatty acids in macrosomic offspring of diabetic pregnancy. Cell Biochem Biophys. 2007;**48**(2–3):79–88.

150. Duttaroy AK. Transport of fatty acids across the human placenta: a review. Prog Lipid Res. 2009;**48**(1):52–61.

151. Herrera E, Amusquivar E, López-Soldado I, et al. Maternal lipid metabolism and placental lipid transfer. Horm Res. 2006;**65**(Suppl 3:)59–64.

152. Yokota T, Kinugawa S, Hirabayashi K, et al. Oxidative stress in skeletal muscle impairs mitochondrial respiration and limits exercise capacity in type 2 diabetic mice. Am J Physiol Heart Circ Physiol. 2009;**297**(3):H1069–77.

153. Dresner A, Laurent D, Marcucci M, et al. Effects of free fatty acids on glucose transport and IRS-1-associated phosphatidylinositol 3-kinase activity. J Clin Invest. 1999;**103**(2):253–9.

154. Thouas GA, Trounson AO, Jones GM. Developmental effects of sublethal mitochondrial injury in mouse oocytes. Biol Reprod. 2006;**74**(5):969–77.

155. Kirchner S, Kieu T, Chow C, et al. Prenatal exposure to the environmental obesogen tributyltin predisposes multipotent stem cells to become adipocytes. Mol Endocrinol. 2010;**24**(3):526–39.

156. Bouret SG. Early life origins of obesity: role of hypothalamic programming. J Pediatr Gastroenterol Nutr. 2009;**48**(Suppl 1):S31–8.

157. Chang GQ, Gaysinskaya V, Karatayev O, et al. Maternal high-fat diet and fetal programming: increased proliferation of hypothalamic peptide-producing neurons that increase risk for overeating and obesity. J Neurosci. 2008;**28**(46):12107–19.

158. Sir-Petermann T, Hitchsfeld C, Maliqueo M, et al. Birth weight in offspring of mothers with polycystic ovarian syndrome. Hum Reprod. 2005;**20**(8):2122–6.

159. Legro RS, Roller RL, Dodson WC, et al. Associations of birthweight and gestational age with reproductive and metabolic phenotypes in women with polycystic ovarian syndrome and their first-degree relatives. J Clin Endocrinol Metab. 2010;**95**(2):789–99.

160. Crisosto N, Codner E, Maliqueo M, et al. Anti-Müllerian hormone levels in peripubertal daughters of women with polycystic ovary syndrome. J Clin Endocrinol Metab. 2007;**92**(7):2739–43.

161. Sir-Petermann T, Codner E, Pérez V, et al. Metabolic and reproductive features before and during puberty in daughters of women with polycystic ovary syndrome. J Clin Endocrinol Metab. 2009;**94**(6):1923–30.

162. Rosenfield RL. Clinical review: Identifying children at risk for polycystic ovary syndrome. J Clin Endocrinol Metab. 2007;**92**(3):787–96.

163. Ibáñez L, Potau N, Francois I, et al. Precocious pubarche, hyperinsulinism, and ovarian hyperandrogenism in girls: relation to reduced fetal growth. J Clin Endocrinol Metab. 1998;**83**(10):3558–62.

164. Maliqueo M, Sir-Petermann T, Pérez V, et al. Adrenal function during childhood and puberty in daughters of women with polycystic ovary syndrome. J Clin Endocrinol Metab. 2009;**94**(9):3282–8.

165. McCartney CR, Blank SK, Prendergast KA, et al. Obesity and sex steroid changes across puberty: evidence for marked hyperandrogenemia in pre- and early pubertal obese girls. J Clin Endocrinol Metab. 2007;**92**(2):430–6.

166. Ramlo-Halsted BA, Edelman SV. The natural history of type 2 diabetes. Implications for clinical practice. Prim Care. 1999;**26**:771–89.

167. Nathan DM. Initial management of glycemia in type 2 diabetes mellitus. N Engl J Med. 2002;**347**:1342–9.

168. Moran LJ. Impaired glucose tolerance, type 2 diabetes and metabolic syndrome in polycystic ovary syndrome: a systematic review and meta-analysis. Hum Reprod Update. 2010;**16**(4):347–63.

169. Ehrmann DA, Barnes RB, Rosenfield RL, et al. Prevalence of impaired glucose tolerance and diabetes in women with polycystic ovary syndrome. Diabetes Care. 1999;**22**(1):141–6.

170. Boudreaux MY, Talbott EO, Kip KE, et al. Risk of T2DM and impaired fasting glucose among PCOS subjects: results of an 8-year follow-up. Curr Diab Rep. 2006;**6**(1):77–83.

171. Wild RA. Long-term health consequences of PCOS. Hum Reprod Update. 2002;**8**(3):231–41.

172. Shaw LJ, Bairey Merz CN, Azziz R, et al. Postmenopausal women with a history of irregular menses and elevated androgen measurements at high risk for worsening cardiovascular event-free survival: results from the National Institutes of Health–National Heart, Lung, and Blood Institute sponsored Women's Ischemia Syndrome Evaluation. J Clin Endocrinol Metab. 2008;**93**(4):1276–84.

173. Talbott EO, Zborowski JV, Rager JR, et a Evidence for an association between metabolic cardiovascular syndrome and coronary and aortic calcification among women with polycystic ovary syndrome. J Clin Endocrinol Metab. 2004;**89**(11):5454–61.

174. Rizzo M, Berneis K. Lipid triad or atherogenic lipoprotein phenotype: a role in cardiovascular prevention? J Atheroscler Thromb. 2005;**12**(5):237–9

175. Cascella T, Palomba S, De Sio I, et al. Visceral fat is associated with cardiovascular risk in women with polycystic ovary syndrome. Hum Reprod. 2008;**23**(1):153–9.

176. Dokras A, Bochner M, Hollinrake E, et al. Screening women with polycystic ovary syndrome for metabolic syndrome. Obstet Gynecol. 2005;**106**(1):131–7.

177. Kim J, Montagnani M, Kon KK, Quon MJ. Reciprocal relationships between insulin resistance and endothelial dysfunction. Circulation. 2006;**133**:1888–904.

178. Luque-Ramírez M, Mendieta-Azcona C Alvarez-Blasco F, et al. Androgen exces is associated with the increased carotid intima-media thickness observed in young women with polycystic ovary syndrome. Hum Reprod. 2007;**22**(12):3197–203.

179. Christian RC, Dumesic DA, Behrenbeck T, et al. Prevalence and predictors of coronary artery calcification in women with polycystic ovary syndrome. J Clin Endocrinol Metab. 2003;**88**(6):2562–8.

180. Krentz AJ, von Mühlen D, Barrett-Connor E. Searching for polycystic ovary syndrome in postmenopausal women: evidence of a dose-effect association with prevalent cardiovascular disease. Menopause. 2007;**14**(2):284–92.

181. Hollinrake E, Abreu A, Maifeld M, et a Increased risk of depressive disorders i women with polycystic ovary syndrome Fertil Steril. 2007;**87**(6):1369–76.

182. Guyatt G, Weaver B, Cronin L, et al. Health-related quality of life in women with polycystic ovary syndrome, a self-administered questionnaire, was validated. J Clin Epidemiol. 2004;**57**(12):1279–87.

183. Benson S, Janssen OE, Hahn S, et al. Obesity, depression, and chronic low-grade inflammation in women with

polycystic ovary syndrome. Brain Behav Immun. 2008;**22**(2):177–84.

184. Rasgon NL, Altshuler LL, Fairbanks L, et al. Reproductive function and risk for PCOS in women treated for bipolar disorder. Bipolar Disord. 2005;7(3):246–59.

185. Chittenden BG, Fullerton G, Maheshwari A. Polycystic ovary syndrome and the risk of gynaecological cancer: a systematic review. Reprod Biomed Online. 2009;**19**(3):398–405.

186. Cibula D, Fanta M, Vrbikova J, et al. The effect of combination therapy with metformin and combined oral contraceptives (COC) versus COC alone on insulin sensitivity, hyperandrogenaemia, SHBG and lipids in PCOS patients. Hum Reprod. 2005;**20**(1):180–4.

187. Ibáñez L, de Zegher F. Low-dose flutamide-metformin therapy for hyperinsulinemic hyperandrogenism in non-obese adolescents and women. Hum Reprod Update. 2006;**12**(3):243–52.

188. Ibáñez L, De Zegher F. Flutamide-metformin therapy to reduce fat mass in hyperinsulinemic ovarian hyperandrogenism: effects in adolescents and in women on third-generation oral contraception. J Clin Endocrinol Metab. 2003;**88** (10):4720–4.

189. Martin KA, Chang RJ, Ehrmann DA, et al. Evaluation and treatment of hirsutism in premenopausal women: an Endocrine Society Clinical Practice Guideline. J Clin Endocrinol Metab. 2008;**93**(4):1105–20.

190. Banaszewska B, Pawelczyk L, Spaczynski RZ, et al. Comparison of simvastatin and metformin in treatment of polycystic ovary syndrome: prospective randomized trial. J Clin Endocrinol Metab. 2009;**94**(12):4938–45.

191. Thessaloniki ESHRE/ASRM-Sponsored PCOS Consensus Workshop Group. Consensus on infertility treatment related to polycystic ovary syndrome. Fertil Steril. 2008;**89**(3):505–22.

192. Imani B, Eijkemans MJ, teVelde ER, et al. Predictors of chances to conceive in ovulatory patients during clomiphene citrate induction of ovulation in normogonadotropic oligoamenorrheic infertility. J Clin Endocrinol Metab. 1999;**84**(5):1617–22.

193. Creanga AA, Bradley HM, McCormick C, et al. Use of metformin in polycystic ovary syndrome: a meta-analysis. Obstet Gynecol. 2008;**111**(4):959–68.

194. Costello MF, Chapman M, Conway U. A systematic review and meta-analysis of randomized controlled trials on metformin co-administration during gonadotrophin ovulation induction or IVF in women with polycystic ovary syndrome. Hum Reprod. 2006;**21**(6):1387–99.

195. Tummon I, Gavrilova-Jordan L, Allemand MC, et al. Polycystic ovaries and ovarian hyperstimulation syndrome: a systematic review. Acta Obstet Gynecol Scand. 2005;**84**(7):611–16.

196. Alberti KG, Eckel RH, Grundy SM, et al. Harmonizing the metabolic syndrome: a joint interim statement of the International Diabetes Federation Task Force on Epidemiology and Prevention; National Heart, Lung, and Blood Institute; American Heart Association; World Heart Federation; International Atherosclerosis Society; and International Association for the Study of Obesity. Circulation. 2009;**120**(16):1640–5.

197. Lazar MA. The humoral side of insulin resistance. Nat Med. 2006;**12**:43–4.

198. Bailey CJ, Turner RC. Metformin. N Engl J Med. 1996;**334**(9):574–9.

199. Nestler JE. Metformin for the treatment of the polycystic ovary syndrome. N Engl J Med. 2008;**358**(1):47–54.

200. Salpeter SR, Buckley NS, Kahn JA, et al. Meta-analysis: metformin treatment in persons at risk for diabetes mellitus. Am J Med. 2008;**121**(2):149–57.

201. Ibáñez L, De Zegher F. Flutamide-metformin plus an oral contraceptive (OC) for young women with polycystic ovary syndrome: switch from third- to fourth-generation OC reduces body adiposity. Hum Reprod. 2004;**19**(8):1725–7.

202. Bruner B, Chad K, Chizen D. Effects of exercise and nutritional counseling in women with polycystic ovary syndrome. Appl Physiol Nutr Metab. 2006;**31**(4):384–91.

203. Karimzadeh MA, Javedani M. An assessment of lifestyle modification versus medical treatment with clomiphene citrate, metformin, and clomiphene citrate-metformin in patients with polycystic ovary syndrome. Fertil Steril. 2010;**94**(1):216–20.

204. Glueck CJ, Aregawi D, Agloria M, et al. Sustainability of 8% weight loss, reduction of insulin resistance, and amelioration of atherogenic-metabolic risk factors over 4 years by metformin-diet in women with polycystic ovary syndrome. Metabolism. 2006;**55** (12):1582–9.

Chapter 12

Endometriosis of the ovary

Luciano G. Nardo, MD, MRCOG, Ioannis Gryparis, MD, and Sree Durga Patchava, MD, MRCOG

Introduction

Endometriosis is a common gynecological disease that affects 6% to 44% of all women of reproductive age [1]. It is defined as the presence of endometrial tissue, consisting of both glandular epithelium and stroma outside the uterus. The most frequent sites of implantation are the pelvic viscera and the peritoneum. Three different clinical entities of endometriosis can be distinguished: peritoneal endometriosis, ovarian endometriosis, and deep invasive (or infiltrating) endometriosis. They vary in appearance from a few minimal lesions on otherwise intact pelvic organs to large ovarian endometriotic cysts that affect tubo-ovarian anatomy and extensive adhesions often involving the bowel, bladder, and ureters. It is associated with pelvic pain and subfertility, and has a detrimental impact on quality of life [2,3].

Etiology

Although signs and symptoms of endometriosis have been described since 1896 by von Recklinghausen, its widespread occurrence was acknowledged during the 20th century. Even 120 years after its first description, the pathogenesis of this condition remains poorly understood.

Endometriosis is an estrogen-dependent disease. Three main theories have been proposed to explain the histogenesis.

1. Ectopic transplantation of endometrial tissue
2. Coelomic metaplasia
3. Induction.

No single theory can account for the location of endometriosis in all cases.

The *transplantation theory*, originally proposed by Sampson in 1927, is based on the assumption that endometriosis is caused by the seeding or implantation of endometrial tissue by transtubal regurgitation during menstruation [4]. Retrograde menstruation occurs in 70% to 90% of women, and it may be more common in women with endometriosis than in those without the disease. Endometriosis is most often found in dependent portions of the pelvis: the ovaries, the anterior and posterior cul-de-sac, the uterosacral ligaments, the posterior surface of the uterus, and the broad ligaments.

Ovarian endometriosis may be caused by either retrograde menstruation or by lymphatic flow from the uterus to the ovary [5]. Extra-pelvic endometriosis, although rare (1–2%), may possibly result from vascular or lymphatic dissemination of endometrial cells to gynecologic (vulva, vagina, and cervix) and non-gynecologic (bowel, lungs and pleural cavity, skin, lymph glands, nerves, and brain) sites [6].

If we accept the theory of retrograde menstruation as the main cause for the initiation of endometriosis, the ovaries are the most frequently involved organs because of the unique characteristics of their site. The ovaries are adjacent to the opening of the tube in the pelvic cavity, and that location alone will make them more prone to contamination by regurgitated menstrual flow. Another reason that contributes to the fact that the ovaries are a common site of implantation of the endometrial cells is that they have the highest level of steroid hormone compared with any other organ and, hence, represent an ideal environment for implantation and growth of ectopic endometrial tissue. In different studies, the involvement of the ovaries (either unilaterally or bilaterally) has been reported in up to 75% of the cases.

The *coelomic metaplasia theory* is as follows. The transformation (metaplasia) of coelomic epithelium to endometrial tissue has been proposed as a mechanism for the origin of endometriosis by Robert Meyer in 1919.

The *induction theory* is in principle an extension of the coelomic metaplasia theory. It proposes that an endogenous (undefined) biochemical factor can induce undifferentiated peritoneal cells to develop into endometrial tissue.

Ovarian endometriosis probably starts as a surface lesion. The process becomes invasive and the endometriotic lesion internalizes into the ovarian tissue. Once the menstrual flow and debris collect at the site of endometriosis in the ovaries, endometriotic cysts form filled with chocolate-color fluid. These are commonly called "chocolate cysts" or endometriomas and are nothing more than cysts that contain debris from prolonged cyclic menstruation. These cysts may continue to grow, with some documented as large as a baseball or grapefruit that completely replace the normal ovary. Usually there is a well-demarcated separation between the cyst wall and the normal adjacent ovarian tissue.

Diagnosis

Although women with endometriosis may be asymptomatic, symptoms are common and typically include dysmenorrhoea, pelvic pain, and infertility. Endometriosis is a disease of

Altchek's Diagnosis and Management of Ovarian Disorders, ed. Liane Deligdisch, Nathan G. Kase, and Carmel J. Cohen. Published by Cambridge University Press.

symptoms and clinical signs which are difficult to assess. The current revised American Fertility Society (r-AFS) classification describes the extent of the disease, but the correlation between symptoms and the diagnosis is rather poor.

The average delay between onset of pain symptoms and surgically confirmed endometriosis is approximately 8 years [7]. Over the past 2 decades, there has been a steady decrease in the delay in diagnosis and decline in the prevalence of advanced endometriosis at first diagnosis [8].

Clinical signs

Pelvic endometriosis is a disease confined to the pelvis. Accordingly, there are often no abnormalities on visual inspection of the patient.

Speculum examination of the vagina and cervix often reveals no signs of endometriosis. Occasionally, bluish or red powder burn lesions may be seen on the cervix or the posterior fornix of the vagina. Bimanual pelvic examination may reveal an enlarged cystic adnexal mass representing endometrioma that may be mobile or adherent to other pelvic structures. Pelvic organs may be fixed from adhesions, with the uterus often fixed in a retroverted position. The physical examination should be performed during early menses because implants are more likely to be large and tender at this time in the cycle.

Cancer antigen (CA) 125

Levels of CA125, a marker found on derivatives of coelomic epithelium, have been shown to positively correlate with the severity of endometriosis [9]. Unfortunately, although demonstrating adequate specificity, the assay has poor sensitivity in detecting endometriosis. A meta-analysis of studies evaluating CA125 in the diagnosis of endometriosis has revealed a sensitivity of only 28% and a specificity of 90% [10]. Several other serum markers like cancer antigen (CA19–9) have been studied, with limited diagnostic accuracy.

Ultrasonography

Non-invasive imaging techniques are becoming increasingly important to determine preoperatively the presence and extent of the surgical pathology. Whenever possible with the use of non-invasive techniques, the decision to operate or not should be based on accurate preoperative diagnosis and proper assessment of the extent of the disease.

Imaging techniques currently and commonly used to diagnose endometriosis of the pelvis are ultrasound scan (USS) and magnetic resonance imaging (MRI).

The ultrasonographic findings most commonly associated with endometriosis are endometriotic cysts of the ovary. Endometriomas can be unilateral or bilateral in up to half of the cases. Unilateral endometriomas occur more frequently in the left ovary [11]. They rarely exceed 15 cm in diameter and can be unilocular or multilocular. The cyst wall is usually thick and fibrotic.

Transabdominal (TA) and more so transvaginal (TV) USS performs well in detecting endometriomas. In a systematic review using gray scale TV ultrasound imaging, both the positive (7.6–29.8) and negative (0.1–0.4) likelihood ratios suggested that ultrasound can accurately confirm or exclude the diagnosis, although the 95% confidence intervals were wide. In these studies, the diameters of the endometriomas were greater than 18 mm. Therefore, the diagnosis of smaller endometriomas with conventional gray scale imaging has not been validated [11].

The use of high-frequency transducers in TV sonography and the advancement in the technology of ultrasonographic equipment resulted in improved differentiation of pelvic structures. As endometriomas can mimic sonographically different structures, there can be pitfalls and diagnostic challenges. The typical image of an endometrioma has been described as demonstrating diffuse low level homogeneous internal echoes with a "ground glass" texture (Fig. 12.1). In one study, 95% of the endometriomas had this appearance [12], whereas in other studies, slightly different definitions for the "classic" appearance of an endometrioma have been used.

Patel et al. [12] in an original study analyzed the sonographic features associated with endometriomas, giving specific consideration to the features in the cyst wall. The single highest predictor for the presence of an endometrioma was *hyperechoic wall foci* within the cyst wall, which were observed in approximately one-third of the cases. These foci should be discriminated from wall nodularity as they are more echogenic and smaller. It is speculated that these arise from the accumulation of cholesterol deposits in the endometriotic cyst wall over time. They can help in estimating the age of the cyst as they are very rarely seen in newly formed endometriomas.

Wall nodularity is characterized as solid masses protruding from the endometrioma wall into the cyst lumen.

Wall thickness has not been shown to be helpful in distinguishing between endometriomas and other ovarian masses.

Multilocularity with the presence of internal septations as a feature, in addition to low-level echoes, in the absence of malignant characteristics strongly suggests the diagnosis of an endometrioma.

Hemorrhagic cysts need to be differentiated from endometriomas as they can also demonstrate diffuse low-level internal echoes. However, they usually appear more heterogeneous with fibrinous strands and retracting clots suggesting recent hemorrhage, a feature not common in endometriomas. The hemorrhagic area will tend to be more central in location [12]. Fibrin strands when compared with septations are thinner and weaker reflectors giving a fishnet appearance and do not traverse the entire cyst [13]. The strongest feature to enable the differentiation of a hemorrhagic cyst from an endometrioma is the evolution over time of its internal structure, thus necessitating a follow-up examination scan [14].

Sometimes endometriomas can be atypically located in the pelvis as adhesions are usually formed in the disease process. The "sliding organ signs" when there is absence of free movement of the pelvic organs following gentle pressure with the vaginal probe can reveal adhesions. This may also produce deep dyspareunia. Bilateral endometriomas can be found adherent to each other in the pouch of Douglas or even above the uterus (known as kissing ovaries) (Fig. 12.2) [15].

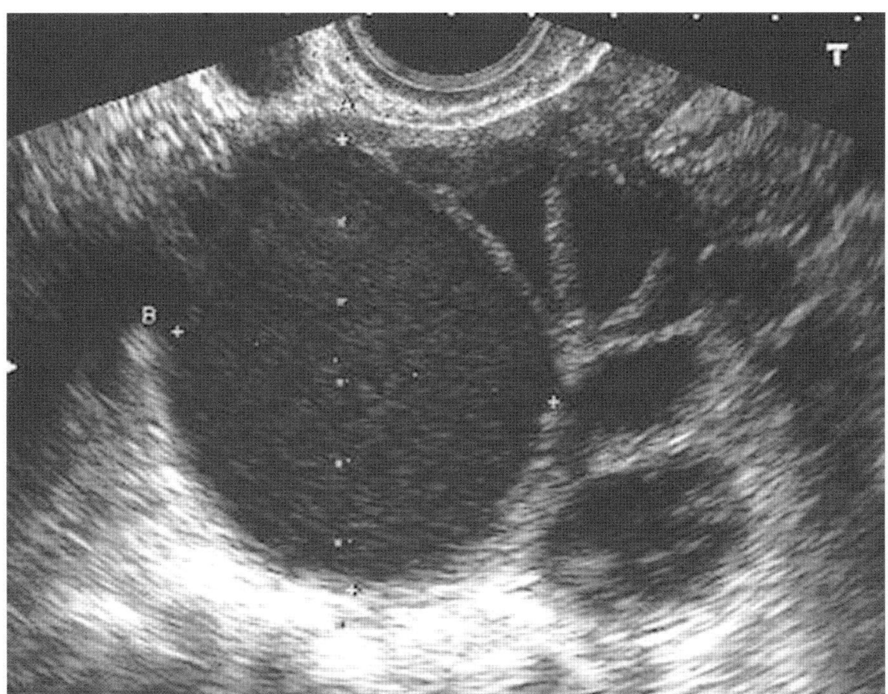

Fig. 12.1. Ultrasound appearance of an endometrioma and some developing follicles.

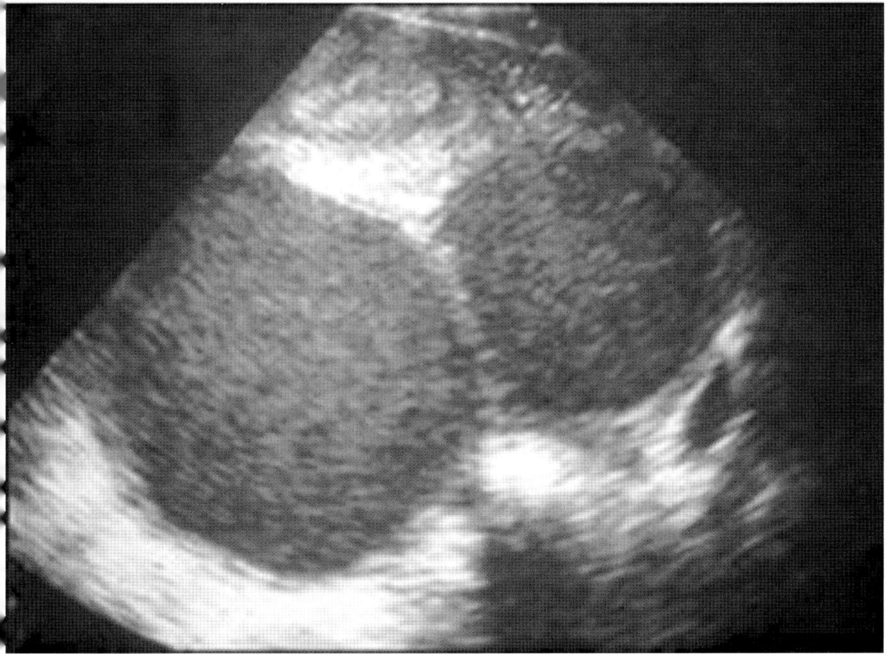

Fig. 12.2. Ultrasound appearance of bilateral endometriomas also known as "kissing ovaries."

The value of Doppler ultrasound in the diagnosis of endometriomas is still not well established. Guerriero et al. [16] suggested that color Doppler energy imaging or power Doppler imaging could be a useful "secondary test" for the characterization of adnexal masses in pre-menopausal women. Endometriomas are relatively avascular, whereas other adnexal masses, particularly malignant tumors are characterized by vascularization or the presence of color flow in the internal septations or the papillary projections of the cyst wall. Typically, a pattern of vascular distributions in the endometrioma showed vessels at the level of the ovarian hilus.

MR imaging

USS differentiation of endometriotic cyst from other adnexal masses may be difficult at times. MR imaging has been shown to have greater specificity for the diagnosis of endometriomas than other non-invasive imaging techniques. It affords a larger field of view than USS, and the effect of adhesions on surrounding anatomic structures is better depicted. Therefore, MR imaging can be a helpful adjunct for evaluation of adnexal masses. If available, MR imaging should be performed using a dedicated pelvic coil. The external multicoil arrays provide a higher signal-to-noise ratio, which improves spatial resolution and enhances visualization of anatomic detail. Imaging planes can include all three standard projections (axial, sagittal, and coronal). In addition to using routine T1-weighted and T2-weighted pulse sequences, a T1-weighted fat-suppressed sequence should always be performed. Fat suppression narrows the dynamic signal range, thereby accentuating differences in tissue signal. Endometriomas have a relatively homogeneous high signal intensity (similar to or greater than that of fat) on T1-weighted images. With the high signal intensity of surrounding fat removed, lesion conspicuity is improved.

Administration of gadolinium-based contrast material is not particularly useful in the evaluation of endometriomas. A false-positive diagnosis may be made when normally enhancing parametrium is misinterpreted as endometriotic foci [17]. Use of gadolinium should be reserved for those cases in which there is a concern for ovarian carcinoma.

A common and important feature of an endometrioma is "shading" (i.e., loss of signal within the lesion), which can be seen on T2-weighted images. This shading reflects the chronic nature of an endometrioma and helps differentiate it from other blood-containing lesions. These chronic lesions are very viscous, with extremely high concentrations of iron and proteins. Shading is present when a cyst that is hyperintense on a T1-weighted image becomes hypointense on a T2-weighted image. Although the T2-weighted image often shows mixed high and low signal intensity, findings can be quite variable. Shading can range from faint, dependent layering to complete signal void, reflecting the concentration of blood products [18]. Hemosiderin-laden macrophages combined with the fibretic nature of the cyst wall give it a low-signal intensity appearance on both T1- and T2-weighted images.

Looking at both the multiplicity and signal intensity of lesions, Togashi et al. (1991) found that a "definitive" diagnosis of an endometrioma was made when a cyst was hyperintense on T1-weighted images and shading was observed on T2-weighted images. The diagnosis was also "definitive" when multiple hyperintense cysts were seen on T1-weighted images regardless of their signal intensity on T2-weighted images. In their study, MR imaging yielded an overall sensitivity, specificity, and accuracy of 90%, 98%, and 96%, respectively. Because these cysts contain blood products of different ages and concentrations, cyst appearances can be variable. Those lesions that are not hyperintense on T1-weighted images can be difficult to distinguish from other adnexal masses. Other lesions that appear with high signal intensity on T1-weighted images include dermoids, mucinous cystic neoplasms, and hemorrhagic masses.

The most challenging lesions to differentiate are hemorrhagic corpus luteum cysts, whose MR imaging appearance can be similar to that of endometriomas. Hemorrhagic cysts are usually unilocular as opposed to endometriomas, which can be multilocular and bilateral. In addition, hemorrhagic cysts do not exhibit shading on T2-weighted images and will resolve with time [19]. A follow-up examination with ultrasound scan can confirm the diagnosis.

Laparoscopy

Laparoscopy is the standard technique for visual inspection of the pelvis and establishment of definitive diagnosis. The diagnosis of ovarian endometriosis is facilitated by careful inspection of the ovaries. With superficial ovarian endometriosis, lesions can be both typical and subtle. Large ovarian endometriotic cysts (endometriomas) (Fig. 12.3) are usually located on the

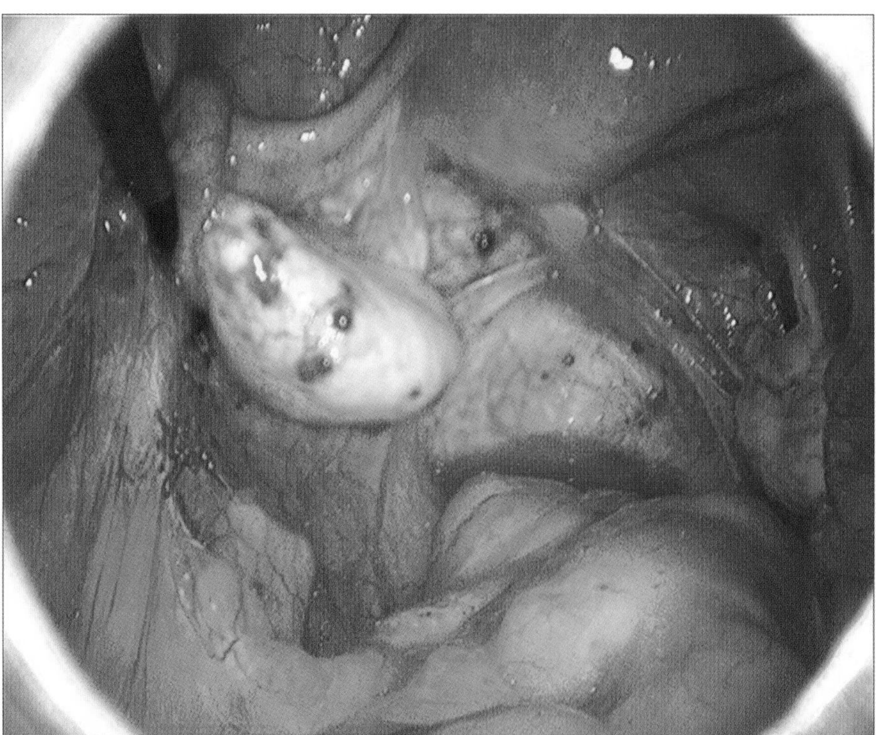

Fig. 12.3. Endometriosis deposits on the ovary.

anterior surface of the ovary and are associated with retraction, pigmentation, and adhesions to the posterior surface of the uterus. Vercellini and colleagues [20] have studied the visual diagnostic parameters of ovarian endometriomas. The gross characteristics that established the diagnosis included a size smaller than 12 cm in diameter, adhesions to pelvic side wall, to posterior broad ligament or both, the presence of powder burn lesions, superficial endometriosis with adjacent puckering on the surface of the ovary, and tarry, thick, chocolate-color fluid content. These criteria yielded a sensitivity of 97% and a specificity of 95%. Because this fluid may also be found in other conditions such as hemorrhagic corpus luteum, cyst biopsy is recommended with removal of the ovarian cyst for histological diagnosis. Ovarian endometriosis appears to be a signal for more extensive pelvic and intestinal disease.

Treatment

Treatment must be individualized, taking into consideration the clinical problem in its entirety. It is also important to involve the patient in all decisions, to be flexible in considering diagnostic and therapeutic approaches. There is insufficient evidence that any strategy to prevent endometriosis recurrence is uniformly successful.

Although there is reasonable evidence confirming an association between endometriosis and subfertility, a causal relationship has not yet been established. The anatomical insults to reproductive function due to endometriosis, such as tubal damage and severe adnexal adhesions, might be irreversible or not completely reparable. Measuring the magnitude of the effect of surgery is of utmost importance to define a therapeutic balance between benefits, harms, and costs in various clinical conditions.

Management of endometriosis must be tailored according to the desired treatment outcome, whether it is relief of pain, improvement of fertility, or the prevention of recurrence.

Surgical treatment

In most women with endometriosis, preservation of reproductive function and potential is desirable. Therefore, the least invasive and least expensive but most effective approach should be recommended. Depending on the severity of disease and diagnosis, removal of endometriosis should be performed at the time of surgery, provided that preoperative consent has been obtained. The goal of surgery is to excise all visible endometriotic lesions and associated adhesions and to restore normal anatomy of the pelvis.

Ovarian endometriomas (<3 cm in diameter) can be aspirated, irrigated, and inspected for intra-cystic lesions: the internal wall must be vaporized to destroy the mucosal lining of the cyst. Large ovarian endometriomas (>3 cm in diameter) should be aspirated, followed by incision and removal of the cyst wall from the ovarian cortex (Fig. 12.4). To prevent recurrence, the cyst wall must be removed while preserving normal ovarian tissue (Fig. 12.5).

Although as little as one-tenth of the ovary is enough to preserve function and fertility, there is increasing concern that ovarian cystectomy with concomitant removal or destruction of primordial follicles may reduce ovarian volume and reserve, and diminish fertility. In some cases, the ovarian cystectomy involves resection of healthy ovarian cortex with follicles and might not be the most appropriate approach for function-preserving surgery.

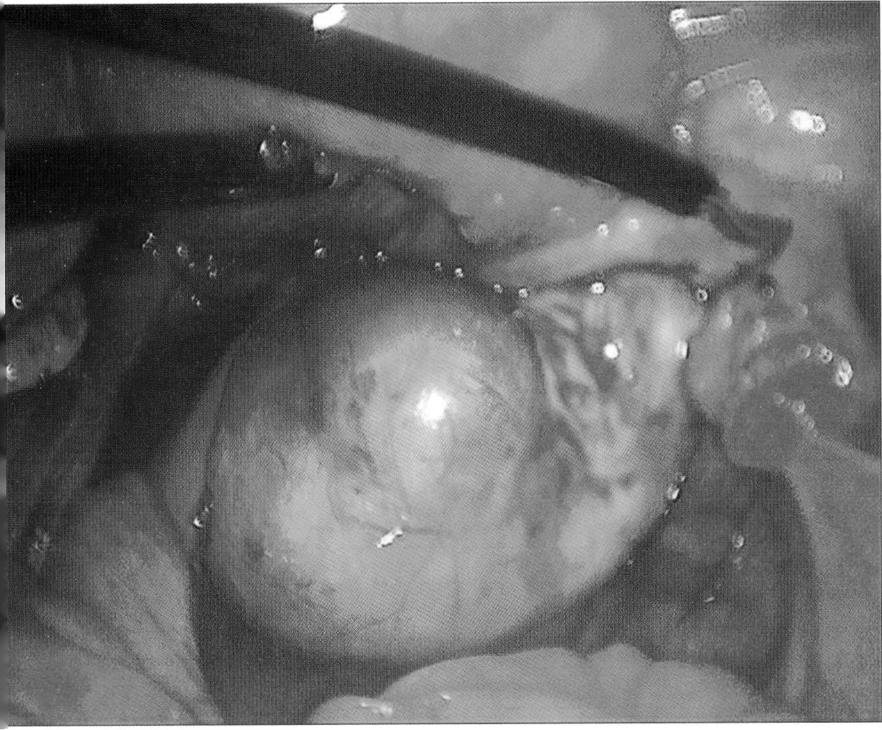

Fig. 12.4. Right endometrioma stuck to the posterior uterine wall and ovarian fossa.

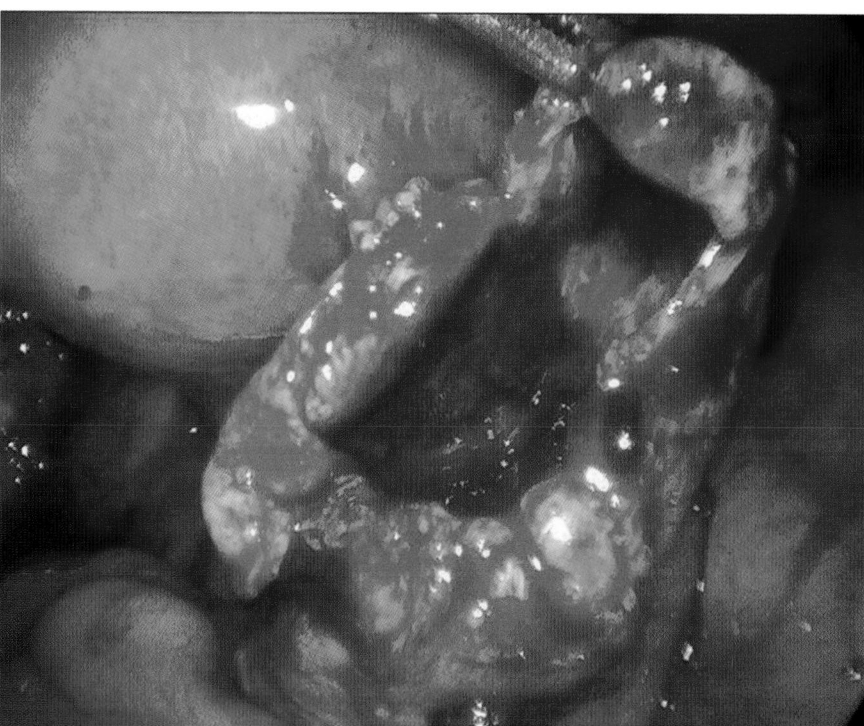

Fig. 12.5. Right endometrioma opened at the time of laparoscopy for ovarian cystectomy.

The main concern of ovarian surgery is the risk of destruction of healthy ovarian tissue, which can result in poor ovarian response during IVF. Some authors believe that surgery does not have any adverse effect on ovarian reserve in subsequent IVF cycles [21–23]. There is some evidence that laparoscopic surgery should be performed before assisted conception treatment not only for making a decision about the treatment course but also for establishing a good pelvic environment for pregnancy [24].

It has been shown that pre-treatment of endometrioma reduces the number of retrieved oocytes and that severe ovarian damage, occurring after surgery for ovarian endometriomas, is not a rare event [25]. The presence of endometriomas may be associated with a reduced responsiveness to gonadotropins [26], consequently a higher amount of follicle-stimulating hormone (FSH) is needed to achieve an acceptable ovarian response after surgery.

It is important to note that the vast majority of authors agree that, although ovarian surgery elicits longer stimulation, higher FSH requirement, and lower oocyte number, however fertilization, pregnancy, and implantation rates remain within acceptable levels [27]. To reduce time to pregnancy, to avoid potential surgical complications, and to limit costs, surgery should be offered only in the presence of large cysts (balancing the threshold to operate with the cyst location within the ovary), or to treat concomitant pain symptoms which are refractory to medical treatments, or when malignancy cannot reliably be ruled out [28].

Of interest, surgery remains the commonest treatment for endometriomas before IVF, a procedure which is in line with the recommendations of the European Society for Human Reproduction and Embryology (ESHRE) guidelines [29].

Postoperative hormone therapy with estrogen is required after bilateral oophorectomy; however, there is a rather negligible risk for renewed growth of residual endometriosis. To reduce this risk, hormone therapy should be withheld until [illegible] months after surgery. The addition of progestins to this regimen protects the endometrium. However, the decision to start hormone therapy with a combination of estrogen and progestin should be balanced against the increased risks associated with hormone therapy.

Results of surgical treatment

There is a significant placebo response to surgical therapy. Diagnostic laparoscopy without complete removal of endometriosis may alleviate pain in 50% of patients with superficial endometriosis. Hormonal therapy before surgery improves endometriosis scores, but there is insufficient evidence that it has any effect on pain relief after the operation.

Regarding fertility, surgical management of subfertile women with minimal to mild endometriosis is controversial. Laparoscopic cystectomy for ovarian endometriomas greater than 4 cm in diameter improves fertility compared with drainage and coagulation [30]. Surgery is currently proposed as the more appropriate therapeutic approach to most of the problems caused by, or associated with, endometriosis. Subfertile women with endometriosis constitute a paradigmatic situation in which the therapeutic approach should be 'problem-oriented' and not 'lesion-oriented', and before suggesting systematic resection, one should be reasonably confident that the chances of overcoming the main clinical problem would be substantially increased. Pregnancy is the main outcome of interest, independently of other variables.

By weighing the pros and cons of surgery, a balance should always be defined between the absolute benefit increase of a procedure and its related morbidity. The overall balance of surgery might appear advantageous in subfertile women with endometriomas, but unfavorable in those with deeply infiltrating lesions. It is important to realize that the first attempt at surgical treatment for ovarian endometriosis in a young woman might determine her reproductive potential. The effect of surgery seems reduced in women with relapsing disease, not to mention that the time to pregnancy is significantly delayed if laparoscopy has been done before IVF. Consequently, there is no convincing evidence that surgery before IVF enhances pregnancy rates. The choice of performing laparoscopy before assisted reproduction treatment (ART) is based essentially on physical considerations rather than on definite improvement of results [31].

Medical treatment

If the patient desires relief of pain symptoms suggestive of endometriosis in the absence of a definitive diagnosis, a therapeutic trial of hormonal medication to reduce menstrual flow is appropriate. Empirical treatment for pain presumed to be due to endometriosis includes counseling, analgesia, nutritional therapy, progestins, or combined oral contraceptives. Considering that endometriosis is a chronic inflammatory disease, anti-inflammatory drugs would appear to be effective for treatment. Non-steroidal anti-inflammatory drugs may be effective in reducing endometriosis-associated pain.

Hormonal medical treatment

Because estrogen is known to stimulate the growth of endometriosis, hormonal therapy has been designed to suppress estrogen synthesis, thereby inducing atrophy of ectopic endometrial implants or interrupting the cycle of stimulation and bleeding. There is evidence that suppression of ovarian function for 6 months reduces pain associated with endometriosis. Combined oral contraceptives, danazol, gestrinone, medroxyprogesterone acetate, and GnRH agonists are all equally effective but their side-effect and cost profiles differ [32–34].

The treatment of endometriosis with continuous low-dose monophasic combination contraceptives (one pill per day for 6–12 months) was originally used to induce pseudo-pregnancy caused by the resultant amenorrhea and decidualisation of endometrial tissue. The induction of a pseudo-pregnancy state with the combined oral contraceptive pill has been shown to be effective in reducing dysmenorrhea and pelvic pain. Oral contraceptives are less costly than other treatments and may be helpful in the short-term management of endometriosis with potential long-term benefits in some women.

Progestins may exert an anti-endometriotic effect by causing initial decidualization of endometrial tissue followed by atrophy. They can be considered as the first choice for the treatment of endometriosis because they are as effective as danazol or GnRH analogs and have a lower cost and a lower incidence of side effects than these agents. Medroxyprogesterone acetate given intra-muscularly every 3 months is also effective for the treatment of pain associated with endometriosis, but is not indicated in subfertile women because it induces profound amenorrhea and anovulation, and a varying length of time is required for ovulation to resume after discontinuation of therapy.

Local progesterone treatment of endometriosis-associated dysmenorrhea with a levonorgestrel-releasing intra-uterine system for 12 months has resulted in a significant reduction in dysmenorrhea, pelvic pain, and dyspareunia, a high degree of patient satisfaction, and a significant reduction in the volume of rectovaginal endometriotic nodules.

Progesterone antagonists and progesterone receptor modulators may suppress endometriosis based on their anti-proliferative effects on the endometrium, without the risk for hypoestrogenism or bone loss that occurs with GnRH treatment.

Danazol is not more effective than other available medications to treat endometriosis. Recognized pharmacologic properties of danazol include suppression of GnRH or gonadotropin secretion, direct inhibition of steroidogenesis, increased metabolic clearance of estradiol and progesterone, direct antagonistic and agonistic interaction with endometrial androgen and progesterone receptors, and immunologic attenuation of potentially adverse reproductive effects. The multiple effects of danazol produce a high-androgen, low-estrogen environment (estrogen levels in the early follicular to post-menopausal range) that does not support the growth of endometriosis, and the amenorrhea that is produced prevents new seeding of implants from the uterus into the peritoneal cavity.

Gonadotropin-releasing hormone agonists bind to pituitary GnRH receptors and stimulate LH and FSH synthesis and release. The agonists have a much longer biologic half-life (3–8 hours) than endogenous GnRH (3–5 minutes), resulting in the continuous exposure of GnRH receptors to GnRH agonist activity. This exposure causes a loss of pituitary receptors and down-regulation of GnRH activity, resulting in low FSH and LH levels. Consequently, ovarian steroid production is suppressed, providing a medically induced and reversible state of pseudomenopause. Various GnRH agonists have been developed and used in treating endometriosis (leuprolide, buserelin, nafarelin, goserelin, and triptorelin). Their results are similar to those of danazol or progestin therapy. Treatment of 3 months with a GnRH agonist is effective in improving pain for 6 months. However, some concerns remain about the long-term effects of GnRH analogs on bone loss. Therefore, GnRH agonists should not be prescribed to girls who have not yet attained their maximal bone density.

Medical treatment with progestins, danazol, gestrinone, or GnRH agonists is effective in treating pain associated with endometriosis. Postoperative medical therapy may be required in patients with incomplete surgical resection and persistent pain. Treatment should be continued at least 3 to 6 months and pain relief may be of shorter duration, presumably because endometriosis recurs.

Conception is unlikely during medical treatment of endometriosis. There is no evidence that medical treatment of minimal to mild endometriosis leads to better chances of pregnancy than expected management.

Assisted reproduction and endometriosis

The treatment of endometriosis-related subfertility is dependent on the age of the woman, the duration of subfertility, the stage of endometriosis, the involvement of ovaries, tubes, or both in the endometriosis process, previous therapy, associated pain symptoms, the priorities of the patient, the costs of treatment, and the expected results. Assisted reproduction including controlled ovarian hyperstimulation with intra-uterine insemination or in vitro fertilization and embryo transfer may be options for subfertility treatment in addition to surgical reconstruction and expectant management for early stage endometriosis. IVF is the method of choice when distortion of the tubo-ovarian anatomy contraindicates the use of superovulation with intra-uterine insemination.

The administration of GnRH agonists for a period of 3 to 6 months before IVF in women with pelvic endometriosis increases the odds of clinical pregnancy by four-fold [35]. It has been demonstrated that prolonged use of GnRH agonist before IVF in patients with endometriosis resulted in significantly higher ongoing pregnancy rates than did standard controlled ovarian hyperstimulation regimens [36]. Considering the implantation and clinical pregnancy rates, controlled ovarian hyperstimulation with either GnRH antagonist and GnRH agonist protocols may be equally effective in patients with mild-to-moderate endometriosis and endometriomas who did or did not undergo ovarian surgery [37].

In patients with severe endometriosis, IVF represents an effective treatment option for subfertility. The prognostic parameters of IVF are identical to those of other patients. However, the risks related to the severity of endometriosis, particularly the risk of suboptimal ovarian performance, need to be considered. Because of this issue, often compounded by endometriosis-related pain, IVF treatment should be initiated as early as possible, using appropriate protocols and after having fully informed the patient about the specific oocyte retrieval-related risks [38].

Fertility preservation in patients with severe endometriosis

Ovarian endometriomas have been reported to be associated with reduced ovarian reserve. This may be due in part to the endometrioma per se or to surgical removal of the endometrioma, causing loss of normal ovarian tissue and follicles [39]. Among the various indirect tests evaluating ovarian follicular reserve, the antral follicle count (AFC) is considered very accurate [40].

Recently, serum anti-Mullerian hormone (AMH) levels have been introduced as a novel measure of ovarian reserve. AMH is a product of granulosa cells of the preantral and antral follicles. Serum AMH levels decline with age and are related to the number of antral follicles and to the ovarian response after ovarian hyperstimulation [41,42].

Fertility preservation is offered mainly to women undergoing treatment with gonadotoxic agents due to malignancy or autoimmune disease. Among the various available fertility preservation options offered are embryo, ovarian tissue and oocyte cryopreservation. Embryo cryopreservation is the most conventional fertility preservation treatment. Another alternative is ovarian tissue cryopreservation, which offers the special benefit of providing estrogen activity after ovarian auto transplantation. This option requires two surgical procedures: one to excise the ovarian tissue and the second for autografting. Moreover, the survival time of the ovarian graft after transplantation is limited [43].

An alternative for oocyte cryopreservation is vitrification. This technique appears to be more effective than the slow freezing procedure [44]. Several investigators have reported marked improvement in oocyte survival, implantation, and clinical pregnancy rates [45]. Vitrification is indeed a promising method for oocyte cryopreservation and it offers a good opportunity for young women requiring fertility preservation because of recurrence of large endometriomas.

References

1. Vercellini P, Crosignani PG. Epidemiology of endometriosis. In. Brosens IA, Donnez J (Eds.). The Current Status of Endometriosis Research and Management. Proceedings of the World Congress on Endometriosis, Brussels, June 1992. Carnforth: CRC Press-Parthenon Publishing; 1993.
2. Olive DL, Schwartz LB. Endometriosis. N Engl J Med. 1993;**328**:1759–69.
3. Brosens IA. Endometriosis. Current issues in diagnosis and medical management. J Reprod Med. 1998;**43**:281–6.
4. Sampson JA. Peritoneal endometriosis due to menstrual dissemination of endometrial tissue into the pelvic cavity. Am J Obstet Gynecol. 1927;**14**:422–69.
5. Ueki M. Histologic study of endometriosis and examination of lymphatic drainage in and from the uterus. Am J Obstet Gynecol. 1991;**165**:201–9.
6. Rock JA, Markham SM. Extra pelvic endometriosis. In: Wilson EA (Ed.). Endometriosis. New York: AR Liss; 1987. p 185–206.
7. Hadfield RM, Mardon H, Barlow D, et al. Delay in the diagnosis of endometriosis: a survey of women from the USA and the UK. Hum Reprod. 1996;**11**:878–80.
8. Dmowski WP, Lesniewicz R, Rana N, et al. Changing trends in the diagnosis of endometriosis: a comparative study comparative study of women with endometriosis presenting with chronic pain or infertility. Fertil Steril. 1997;**67**:238–43.
9. Hornstein MD, Harlow BL, Thomas PP, et al. Use of new CA125 assay in the diagnosis of endometriosis. Hum Reprod. 1995;**10**:932.
10. Mol BW, Bayram N, Lijmer JG, et al. The performance of CA 125 measurement in the detection of endometriosis: a meta-analysis. Fertil Steril. 1998;**70**:1101.

11. Vercellini P, Aimi G, De Giorgi O, et al. Is cystic ovarian endometriosis an asymmetric disease? Br J Obstet Gynaecol. 1998;**105**:1018–21.
12. Patel MD, Feldstein VA, Chen DC, Lipson SD, Filly RA. Endometriomas: diagnostic performance of US. Radiology. 1999;**210**:739–45.
13. Brown DL, Dudiak KM, Laing FC. Adnexal masses: US characterization and reporting. Radiology. 2010;**254**:342–54.
14. Derchi LE, Serafini G, Gandolfo N, Gandolfo NG, Martinoli C. Ultrasound in gynecology. Eur Radiol. 2001;**11**:2137–55.
15. Savelli L. Transvaginal sonography for the assessment of ovarian and pelvic endometriosis: how deep is our understanding? Ultrasound Obstet Gynecol. 2009;**33**:497–501.
16. Guerriero S, Ajossa S, Mais V, et al. The diagnosis of endometriomata using colour Doppler energy imaging. Hum Reprod. 1998;**13**:1691–95.
17. Bis KG, Vrachliotis TG, Agrawal R, et al. Pelvic endometriosis: MR imaging spectrum with laparoscopic correlation and diagnostic pitfalls. RadioGraphics. 1997;**17**:639–55.
18. Togashi K, Nishimura K, Kimura I, et al. Endometrial cysts: diagnosis with MR imaging. Radiology. 1991;**180**:73–8.
19. Siegelman ES, Outwater EK. Tissue characterization in the female pelvis by means of MR imaging. Radiology. 1999;**212**:5–18.
20. Vercellini P, Vendola N, Bocciolone L, et al. Reliability of visual diagnosis of ovarian endometriosis. Fertil Steril. 1991;**56**:1198.
21. Shimizu Y, Takashima A, Takahashi K, et al. Long-term outcome, including pregnancy rate, recurrence rate and ovarian reserve, after laparoscopic laser ablation surgery in infertile women with endometrioma. J Obstet Gynaecol Res. 2010;**36**(1):115–18.
22. Tsoumpou I, Kyrgiou M, Gelbaya TA, Nardo LG. The effect of surgical treatment for endometrioma on in vitro fertilization outcomes: a systematic review and meta-analysis. Fertil Steril. 2009;**92**(1):75–87.
23. Marconi G, Vilela M, Quintana R, Sueldo C. Laparoscopic ovarian cystectomy of endometriomas does not affect the ovarian response to gonadotropin stimulation. Fertil Steril. 2002;**78**(4):876–8.
24. Nakagawa K, Ohgi S, Kojima R, et al. Impact of laparoscopic cystectomy on fecundity of infertility patients with ovarian endometrioma. J Obstet Gynaecol Res. 2007;**33**(5):671–6.
25. Benaglia L, Somigliana E, Vighi V, et al. Rate of severe ovarian damage following surgery for endometriomas. Hum Reprod. 2010;**25**(3):678–82.
26. Somigliana E, Infantino M, Benedetti F, et al. The presence of ovarian endometriomas is associated with a reduced responsiveness to gonadotropins. Fertil Steril. 2006;**86**(1):192–6.
27. Demirol A, Guven S, Baykal C, Gurgan T. Effect of endometrioma cystectomy on IVF outcome: a prospective randomized study. Reprod Biomed Online. 2006;**12**(5):639–43.
28. Garcia-Velasco JA, Somigliana E. Management of endometriomas in women requiring IVF: to touch or not to touch. Hum Reprod. 2009;**24**(3):496–501.
29. Gelbaya TA, Gordts S, D'Hooghe TM, Gergolet M, Nardo LG. Management of endometrioma prior to IVF: compliance with ESHRE guidelines. Reprod Biomed Online. 2010;**21**(3):325–30.
30. Chapron C, Vercellini P, Barakat H, et al. Management of ovarian endometriomas. Hum Reprod Update. 2002;**8**:6–7.
31. Vercellini P, Somigliana E, Vigano P, et al. Surgery for endometriosis-associated infertility: a pragmatic approach. Hum Reprod. 2009:**24**(2);254–69.
32. Moore J, Kennedy SH, Prentice A. Modern combined and oral contraceptives for pain associated with endometriosis (Cochrane Review). In: The Cochrane Library, Issue 3. Chichester, UK: John Wiley & Sons; 2004.
33. Prentice A, Deary AJ, Goldbeck WS, et al. Gonadotropin-releasing hormone analogues for pain associated with endometriosis. In: The Cochrane Library, Issue 3. Chichester, UK: John Wiley & Sons; 2004.
34. Prentice A, Deary AJ, Bland E. Progestagens and anti-progestagens for pain associated with endometriosis. In: The Cochrane Library, Issue 3. Chichester, UK: John Wiley & Sons; 2004.
35. Sallam HN, Garcia-Velasco JA, Dias S, Arici A. Long-term pituitary down-regulation before in vitro fertilization (IVF) for women with endometriosis. Cochrane Database Syst Rev. 2006;(1):CD004635.
36. Surrey ES, Silverberg KM, Surrey MW, Schoolcraft WB. Effect of prolonged gonadotropin-releasing hormone agonist therapy on the outcome of in vitro fertilization-embryo transfer in patients with endometriosis. Fertil Steril. 2002;**78**(4):699–704.
37. Pabuccu R, Onalan G, Kaya C. GnRH agonist and antagonist protocols for stage I-II endometriosis and endometrioma in in vitro fertilization/intracytoplasmic sperm injection cycles. Fertil Steril. 2007;**88**(4):832–9.
38. Dechaud H, Dechanet C, Brunet C, et al. Endometriosis and in vitro fertilisation: a review. Gynecol Endocrinol. 2009;**25**(11):717–21.
39. Busacca M, Riparini J, Somigliana E, et al. Postsurgical ovarian failure after laparoscopic excision of bilateral endometriomas. Am J Obstet Gynecol. 2006;**195**:421–5.
40. Broekmans FJ, Kwee J, Hendriks DJ, Mol BW, Lambalk CB. A systematic review of tests predicting ovarian reserve and IVF outcome. Hum Reprod Update. 2006;**12**:685–718.
41. de Vet A, Laven JSE, de Jong FH, Themmen APN, Fauser BCJM. Anti-Mullerian hormone serum levels: a putative marker for ovarian aging. Fertil Steril. 2002;**77**:357–62.
42. Van Rooij IA, Broekmans FJ, te Velde ER, et al. Serum anti-Mullerian hormone levels: a novel measure of ovarian reserve. Hum Reprod. 2002;**17**:3065–71.
43. Meirow D, Levron J, Eldar-Geva T, et al. Monitoring the ovaries after autotransplantation of cryopreserved ovarian tissue: endocrine studies, in vitro fertilization cycles, and live birth. Fertil Steril. 2007;**87**:418.e7–15.
44. Kuleshova LL, Lopata A. Vitrification can be more favorable than slow cooling. Fertil Steril. 2002;**78**:449–54.
45. Kuwayama M, Vajta G, Kato O, Leibo SP. Highly efficient vitrification method for cryopreservation of human oocytes. RBM Online. 2005;**11**:300–8.

Chapter 13

New advances and new horizons in assisted reproduction

Yuval Bdolah, MD, MSc, and Neri Laufer, MD

Induction: an ovulation overview

The goal of controlled ovarian hyperstimulation (COH) in assisted reproductive technologies (ART) is ovulation induction and achievement of several mature eggs in the hope that at least one will result in fertilization and pregnancy [1]. This aim can be accomplished in several ways using medications, either as single agents or in combination.

Clomiphene citrate (CC) binds to the estrogen receptor and exhibits both agonist and antagonist properties [2]. Patients using CC require little monitoring. It is given orally for 5 days in the early follicular phase, and generally causes ovulation 7 days after the last dose by means of a spontaneous luteinizing hormone (LH) surge in a "closed loop" feedback. CC is usually used in anovulatory patients, in an ovulation induction cycle, and is hardly used in in vitro fertilization (IVF) cycles.

Human menopausal gonadotropins (hMG) are drugs which contain equal concentrations of LH and follicle-stimulating hormone (FSH) or highly purified FSH alone. Until recently, all available human FSH pharmaceutical preparations were extracted from post-menopausal urine. However, biotechnology has made available a recombinant preparation of FSH (rFSH) for medical use.

Recombinant LH (rLH) preparations are also available and are sometimes added to rFSH preparations, in the course of ovulation induction cycles [3,4]. Novel preparations containing both rFSH and rLH are allowing the clinicians additional flexibility [5].

Intra-muscular or subcutaneous injection of hMG or rFSH begins in the early follicular phase and is continued daily until follicular development is judged to be adequate. Human chorionic gonadotropin (hCG), either biological or recombinant, is then administered to mimic the native LH surge and cause ovulation. HMG causes direct stimulation of follicular development on the ovary itself. HMG can be administered in excess. This is an example of an "open loop" feedback system where the body cannot control or limit further ovarian stimulation because it is being administered exogenously. To avoid excessive ovarian stimulation the growth and development of ovarian follicles are carefully monitored by serial transvaginal ultrasonography, and frequent serum E2 sampling. Progesterone and LH levels are sometimes measured as well to assist in controlling the cycle.

Gonadotropin releasing hormone (GnRH), also referred to as luteinizing hormone releasing hormone (LHRH), can be used to induce follicular development given intravenously or subcutaneously in a pulsatile manner. It stimulates the synthesis and release of LH and FSH from the anterior pituitary gland [6]. This is used rarely, when patients lack native pulsatile GnRH activity or lack a functional hypothalamic–pituitary portal system, which prevents delivery of endogenous GnRH to the pituitary.

Native GnRH is a decapeptide with a half-life of 2 min; however, it can be manipulated chemically to produce long-acting agonists. When GnRH agonists are first administered, the pituitary responds by releasing both LH and FSH (flare-up effect). However, continued administration over time causes GnRH receptor down-regulation, pituitary desensitization, and a fall in gonadotropin levels, and the ovary becomes dormant [7–9]. Thus, a pharmacologic yet reversible hypophysectomy can be achieved [10]. GnRH agonists are commonly used with hMG or rFSH for COH in an ART cycle. The agonists can be administered either by intra-muscular long-acting preparations, by subcutaneous injection, or by intra-nasal spray [11].

GnRH antagonists are compounds that directly inhibit the release of pituitary gonadotropins and do not cause release of hormone stores before suppression. They have become a useful tool in short ovulation induction protocols, thus preventing premature ovulation and allowing avoidance of ovarian hyperstimulation syndrome in ART.

Other adjuvant preparations are available for use in ovulation induction. One is growth hormone (GH), which increases ovarian levels of insulin-like growth factor-1 (IGF-1), that may enhance the action of gonadotropins on the developing follicle [12].

Each medication regimen also imparts a different set of risks and benefits that can be tailored to the situation at hand.

Medical induction of ovulation can be performed for any of several indications. When the ovaries of women with oligo/anovulation, or those of women undergoing empiric therapy are stimulated for ovulation induction, the physician cannot control the actual number of oocytes that are released for potential fertilization.

The approach to COH for in vitro fertilization (IVF) differs markedly from ordinary ovulation induction, based on the degree of ovarian stimulation and number of follicles set as

Altchek's Diagnosis and Management of Ovarian Disorders, ed. Liane Deligdisch, Nathan G. Kase, and Carmel J. Cohen. Published by Cambridge University Press.

optimum. Patients undergoing COH as of anovulation will benefit from ovulation of a single follicle. Patients undergoing IVF can have large numbers of oocytes recruited with undue fear of high-order pregnancies because the number of oocytes or embryos returned to them can be controlled. However, ovarian hyperstimulation syndrome (OHSS) should be avoided. The physician can choose the number of embryos to transfer the patient and cryopreserve the remaining embryos for transfer at a later date. Moreover, oocytes can be vitrified and fertilized after thawing them, allowing fertility preservation in single patients.

Whereas ordinary medical induction of ovulation in an unexplained infertility patient is, therefore, directed toward developing a few mature oocytes, COH for ART begins with the goal of developing a larger number of mature oocytes.

Clomiphene citrate

Clomiphene citrate (CC), an orally active, nonsteroidal triphenylethylene derivative [13,14], was approved for clinical use in 1967 (Fig. 13.1). CC alone was commonly prescribed for ovulation induction in the early and mid-1980s [15–17]. CC acts by binding to the estrogen receptor; in some tissues this results in a pro-estrogenic effect, and in others, it exhibits a distinctly anti-estrogenic effect. However, serum LH elevation may occur during the early follicular phase [18], which may impair fertilization [19–21] and cause subclinical pregnancy loss [22]. Approximately 80% of those receiving the drug can be expected to ovulate [23]. Adding human menopausal gonadotropin to CC resulted in an increase of follicles and oocytes retrieved; however, the anti-estrogenic effects persisted on mucus production [24–28]. Furthermore, this combination is often used as a second-line treatment, for low responders in assisted reproduction [29].

One other persistent problem was the occurrence of an LH surge before the achievement of adequate follicular development

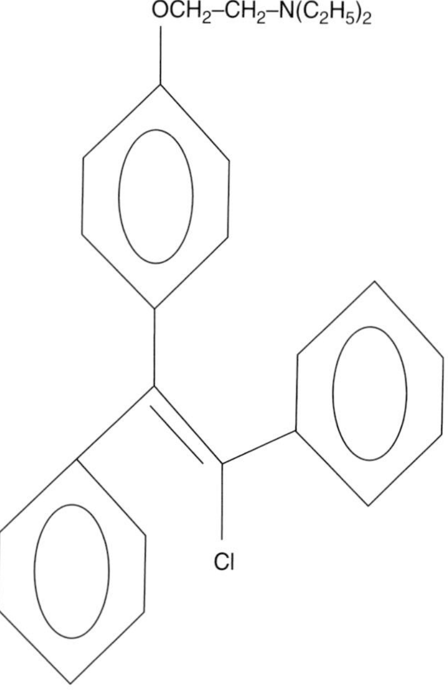

Fig. 13.1. The molecular structure of clomiphene.

resulting in resumption of meiosis [30] and granulosa and theca cell luteinization [31,32] with production of progesterone [33] and endometrial transformation. Inadequate oocyte development prevents the gamete from being fertilized; therefore, a "premature" LH surge cancels the cycle. CC/hMG was used in only 8.5% of all stimulation protocols for ART in 1990 [34].

On the basis of the theory that hyperinsulinemia impedes ovulation and may be an important contributor to the pathophysiology of polycystic ovarian syndrome (PCOS), the use of insulin sensitizers (metformin, and possibly rosiglitazone and pioglitazone) with or without CC was suggested. It is postulated that insulin sensitizers might improve the endocrine imbalances associated with PCOS, resulting in an increase in ovulatory menstrual cycles and pregnancy. Recent research shows conflicting results regarding the effectiveness of metformin to increase the number of ovulatory cycles in women with PCOS especially in conjunction with clomiphene [35,36]. The role of metformin in IVF is also debatable. Recent reviews found no evidence that metformin treatment before or during ART cycles improves live birth or pregnancy rates [37,38], although the risk of OHSS in women with PCOS and undergoing IVF or ICSI cycles was reduced with metformin [37,39].

Human menopausal gonadotropins

HMG, sometimes called menotropins, are available in ampules containing 75 IU of LH and 75 IU of FSH or as purified FSH. HMG acts to stimulate follicular development directly. Intramuscular or subcutaneous injection of hMG usually begins on menstrual cycle day 5 in ordinary ovulation induction and on day 3 in UVF cycles and is continued daily until follicular development is judged to be adequate by serial serum E2 levels and repeated measurement of mean follicular diameter by transvaginal ultrasonography (at least one follicle 14–18 mm) [40–44]. A dose of 5,000–10,000 IU of hCG should be administered to mimic the native LH surge and cause ovulation once the patient's serum E2 reaches an adequate level with one or more follicles ≥17 mm.

Use of hMG routinely drives the serum E2 concentration well above the natural cycle peak. Those with a low serum E2 response (≤50 pg/mL) after 5 days of hMG therapy, which routinely corresponds to cycle day 8, had a lower fertilization rate than patients with an initial E2 of 51–150 pg/mL [45]. A decline in serum E2 following hCG administration is predictive of a poor cycle outcome [24,46,47]. The predictive value does not apply when GnRH agonist is added to regimens containing hMG [48].

Transvaginal ultrasonography demonstrates the endometrium during monitoring of follicular development. Endometrial thickness on the day after hCG administration of patients who conceived by means of IVF found no differences in pregnancy rates between thickness of 8.6 mm or thickness ≥13 mm [40,49,50]. Serum E2 and progesterone (P) levels were not predictive of endometrial thickness [51].

The most serious complication associated with the use of hMG is the ovarian hyperstimulation syndrome (OHSS). OHSS encompasses a spectrum from mild ovarian enlargement and supraphysiologic serum E2 and P to potentially lethal disease marked by massive extra-vascular exudate accumulation combined with severe intra-vascular volume depletion, hemoconcentration, increased blood viscocity, coagulation abnormalities, and diminished renal function [52]. Fortunately, the severe form is a rare occurrence, largely due to well-established risk factors. Of foremost concern are the presence of multiple small (2–8 mm) and intermediate sized (9–15 mm) follicles and elevated serum E2 concentration above 1500 pg/mL.

Development of the full-blown syndrome is dependent upon either exogenously administered hCG or endogenous pregnancy-derived hCG stimulation. Exogenous hCG administration may be avoided. Endogenous, pregnancy-derived hCG can also be avoided by advising the patient to abstain from conception during this cycle. Moderate and mild disease can occur even within acceptable guidelines of E2 concentration and follicle number. The peak effects are seen 7–10 days after hCG administration and generally abate with menses. If pregnancy is achieved, the syndrome may worsen initially and persist for several weeks.

Prevention of OHSS has become a major goal in IVF programs. Withholding hCG and cycle cancellation is considered the safest option. Another option is withholding treatment for several days (coasting). It has been shown to diminish the incidence and severity of OHSS, but whether it is compromising pregnancy rates it is still debatable [53–55]. Freezing all of the embryos and refraining from fresh embryo transfer has also been suggested as an option to prevent OHSS, although some authors have shown that the process of freezing and thawing might carry the toll of impaired embryo survival [56,57]. The alternative of triggering final oocyte maturation with GnRHa in a GnRH antagonist cycle is a relatively new attractive one [58,59]. The ovulation-inducing agent commonly used so far in COS cycles is hCG. Its administration results in a prolonged luteotrophic effect and supraphysiologic levels of vascular endothelial growth factor [60], which may be pivotal to the development of OHSS by means of the enhancement of capillary leak [61]. The beneficial effect of the GnRHa approach is that it virtually eliminated OHSS in high-risk patients [62], although there have been claims associating it with lower ongoing pregnancy rates [63] because of inadequate endometrial receptivity. The way to overcome this reduction in receptivity is to add an adequate luteal phase support with either repeated low-dose hCG or intensive estradiol (E_2) and an intensive progesterone administration from the time of oocyte retrieval [64,65].

Although the pathophysiology of this syndrome remains unclear, it seems likely that the release of vasoactive substance secreted by the ovaries under hCG stimulation plays a key role in triggering this syndrome. The underlying mechanism responsible for the clinical manifestations of OHSS appears to be an increase in capillary permeability of the ovarian vessels and other mesothelial surfaces. Because the pathogenesis of OHSS has not been clearly elucidated, management is generally empiric. Pharmacologic therapies have had little effect on its clinical course. Patients with moderate ascites and mild hemoconcentration may be treated with bedrest and copious liquid intake while monitoring their urine output, hematocrit, and serum electrolytes, and may be candidates for paracentesis and/or plasma expanders if respiratory or renal function is compromised.

The debate whether hMG are inferior or superior to recombinant FSH in ovulation induction has been going on for more than a decade. Recent studies have established that highly purified hMG are at least as effective as rFSH in GnRH antagonist cycles [66].

Recombinant FSH

hMG may be used as a source of FSH as well as other urine-derived FSH preparations (urofollitropin and highly purified urofollitropin), which contain significantly reduced or negligible quantities of LH. Nevertheless, all urinary-derived preparations have the drawback of requiring the collection of large quantities of urine from multiple donors, leading to variability in supply and, perhaps most importantly, batch-to-batch inconsistency [67].

Recently, by using recombinant DNA technology, pure recombinant human FSH preparations were produced by inserting the genes encoding for α- and β-subunits of FSH into expression vectors that are transfected into a Chinese hamster ovary cell line. The use of mammalian cells for this purpose is necessary because glycosylation is required to ensure full biological activity of the protein. This technology has three advantages: FSH production is independent of urine collection, a constant FSH supply is ensured, and batch-to-batch consistency can be guaranteed. The highly effective purification process yields FSH preparations with a specific activity of 10,000 IU FSH/mg protein, thus these recombinant products are the most biochemically pure for clinical use, which confer safety and tolerability advantages [68].

There are two rFSH preparations currently available for clinical use: follitropin alpha and follitropin beta, which are devoid of any LH activity and extraneous human protein. Although both preparations have been developed using the same technique, the posttranslation glycosylation process and purification procedures are not identical. The purification procedure used for follitropin alpha includes the use of immunochromatographic methods, whereas purification of follitropin beta does not involve immunological methods.

Clinical studies in IVF established the efficacy and safety of rFSH in stimulating follicular development, with or without concurrent GnRH agonists, and showed that rFSH was at least as effective as uFSH or hMG. Pregnancy rates were not found to differ significantly between recombinant and urinary FSH. Some authors have claimed that in intra-uterine insemination cycles, rFSH was associated with higher per cycle pregnancy rates compared with highly purified FSH, when used at the same dose [69]. A recent Cochrane systematic review included 42 trials, comparing rFSH to any of the other gonadotropins irrespective of the down-regulation protocol used. The study did not result in any evidence of a statistically significant difference in live birth rate or in the OHSS rate [70].

Gonadotropin-releasing hormone agonist

Use of a GnRH agonist can achieve a pharmacologic and reversible hypophysectomy [7–9]. The use of GnRH agonists in superovulation protocols was first described in 1984. GnRH agonists prevent the untimely pituitary gonadotropin surge in response to rising serum estradiol levels from the multiple ovarian follicles, thereby reducing the chance of spontaneous ovulation and cycle cancellation and allowing continuation of stimulation in cases of asynchronous follicular growth. Other advantages of using a GnRH agonist in ovarian stimulation protocols include improved timing and convenience with regard to oocyte collection and embryo transfer, and simplification of planning for the patient, laboratory staff, and physician [71].

Pituitary suppression typically requires a minimum of 10 days of agonist administration, which may be given on either day 21 or day 3 [72–75]. The GnRH agonist is given until suppression down to serum E2 < 40 pg/mL, and then hMG is started electively.

The term "long protocol" with a GnRH agonists given on the preceding day 21 implies the existence of a "short protocol." The "flare-up" or short protocol differs from its long counterpart in that pituitary desensitization is not achieved before initiating hMG. In the flare-up protocol, a GnRH agonists is initiated on cycle day 1, or day 2, and hMG is either co-administered from the onset, or begun within the ensuing 2 or 3 days [76–78]. The initial response of the pituitary to the GnRH agonists administration, is the release of its stored LH and FSH. Co-administration of hMG during this phase causes the ovary to perceive an intense stimulatory signal. Continued GnRH agonists administration, however, is inhibitory and protects against an inopportune spontaneous LH surge.

The choice of a long protocol versus a flare-up protocol for patients entering an IVF program is controversial [79,80]. Several prospective randomized studies have compared short and long protocols, and have shown significantly better results with the long protocol. Results of these studies have been confirmed in a recent meta-analysis, which also confirmed the superiority of the long protocol over the ultrashort protocol. However, evidence suggests that the short protocol may be superior to the long protocol for women who were low responders to ovarian stimulation in previous treatment cycles.

A third variant of GnRH agonists administration exists. This is the so-called "ultrashort protocol." The GnRH agonists is administered in only the first 3–4 days of the menstrual cycle and then discontinued. The effect of this brief exposure to the GnRH agonists may be enough to protect against a premature spontaneous LH surge [81,82].

Gonadotropin-releasing hormone antagonists

In parallel with the development of GnRH agonists, other analogs were synthesized which also bind to pituitary GnRH receptors but are not functional in inducing the release of gonadotropins. These compounds, the GnRH antagonists, are far more complex than GnRH agonists, with modifications in the molecular structure not only introducing n-amino acids at positions 6 and 10, but also at positions 1, 2, 3, and 8 (Table 13.1).

Significant advantages of GnRH antagonists to GnRH agonists involve their ability to immediately suppress the pituitary gonadotropins by GnRH receptor competition and permit flexibility in the degree of pituitary–gonadal suppression. Moreover, discontinuation of GnRH antagonist treatment leads to a rapid and predictable recovery of the pituitary–gonadal axis. In women undergoing ovarian stimulation, GnRH antagonist treatment is required for only a few days when a premature LH surge is imminent. Also, in GnRH antagonist treatment protocols, a GnRH agonist may be used to trigger ovulation instead of hCG, thus decreasing significantly the cancellation rate and minimizing the risk for developing OHSS [83].

Studies have shown that cetrorelix has proven to be reliable in preventing the onset of premature LH surges during hMG stimulation, by daily injections (0.25 mg) from 5 or 6 days of stimulation onward or by a single injection (3 mg) on stimulation day 7 (Fig. 13.2). Pregnancy rates of about 30% per transfer were initially reported [84]. Clinical experience in IVF treatment thus far has proven that the use of GnRH antagonist compared with long GnRH agonist protocols was associated with a large reduction in OHSS, and there was no evidence of a difference in live-birth rates [85]. Furthermore, in an update to the Cochrane review they had published earlier, Al-Inany et al. stressed that the relative likelihood of OHSS with GnRH antagonist treatment was 50% of that with GnRH agonist treatment, while the ongoing pregnancy rate was nearly the same.

As mentioned before, the alternative of triggering final oocyte maturation with GnRHa in a GnRH antagonist cycle is an attractive one and allows the physician to avoid OHSS without compromising the clinical results [58,59]. That is the reason why a growing number of IVF units adopt the GnRH antagonist as the default protocol for young, high responder patients, especially the PCOS patients, as well as for ovum donors.

The question whether recombinant LH should be added to rFSH when GnRH antagonist is initiated has been addressed and recent evidence suggests that exogenous LH does not

Table 13.1. Structure of the GnRH antagonists cetrorelix and ganirelix compared with the native GnRH

	1	2	3	4	5	6	7	8	9	10
GnRH	Pyro-GLU	HIS	TRP	SER	TYR	GLY	LEU	ARG	PRO	Gly-NH2
Cetrorelix	Ac-D-Nal(2)	D-Phe(4Cl)	D/PAL	SER	TYR	D/CIT	LEU	ARG	PRO	D-Ala-NH2
Ganirelix	Ac-D-Nal(2)	D-Phe(4Cl)	D/PAL	SER	TYR	D-hArg(Et2)	LEU	L-hArg(Et2)	PRO	D-Ala-NH2

Note: Amino acid substitutions have been made at positions 1, 2, 3, 6, 8, and 10.

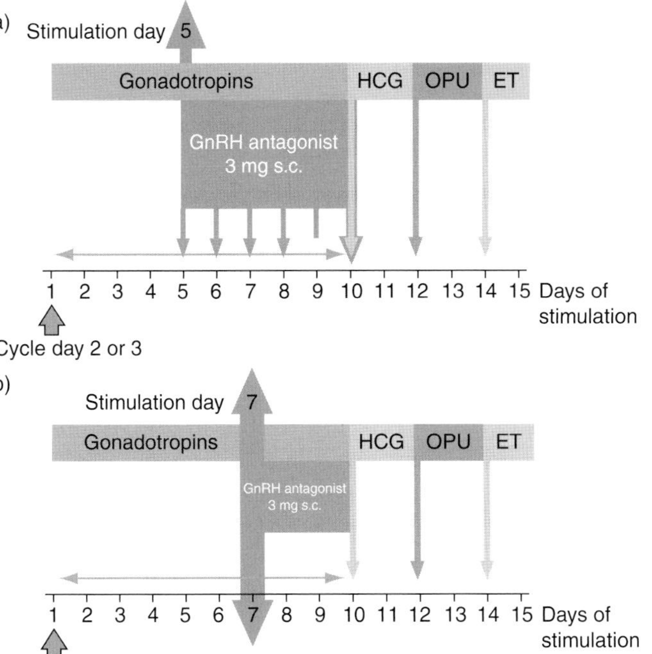

Fig. 13.2. (a) Multiple dose schedule of GnRH antagonist. (b) Single dose schedule of GnRH antagonist.

confer any significant benefit in women undergoing treatment with GnRH antagonist regimens [86].

Additional medications used for ovulation induction: GH and more

Growth-promoting peptides such as insulin, GH, and insulin-like growth factor might have a role in normal follicular development. Isolated GH deficiency can delay the onset of puberty [87]. The effect of GH on the ovaries is mediated by somatomedin C, which is similar to insulin (also termed insulin-like growth factor I) and produced by ovarian granulosa cells [88]. Ovarian IGF-1, in addition to FSH and LH, may play an important role in follicular development [88–93]. GH might act by direct action on GH receptors, by a systemic increase in IGF-1 levels, or by increasing intra-ovarian IGF-1. The finding that GH may have a direct gonadotropic effect on human granulose cells independent of FSH or IGF-1 suggests that physiologic GH seems to be a helpful adjunct in ovulation induction [94–98].

Lately the issue was re-visited: A recent meta-analysis provided evidence that GH addition does increase the probability of clinical pregnancy and live birth in poor responders undergoing ovarian stimulation with GnRH analogs and gonadotropins for IVF. However, the total number of patients analyzed was small [99]. A Cochrane review, including 10 studies, demonstrated a statistically significant difference in both live birth rates and pregnancy rates favoring the use of adjuvant growth hormone in in vitro fertilization protocols in women who are considered poor responders without increasing adverse events: odds ratio (OR) 5.39 (95% confidence interval (CI), 1.89–15.35) and OR 3.28 (95% CI, 1.74–6.20), respectively. However, the authors were unable to identify which subgroup of poor responders would benefit the most from adjuvant growth hormone and stated that the result needs to be interpreted with caution [100].

Dehydroepiandrosterone (DHEA) supplementation in women with diminished ovarian reserve is another adjuvant therapy sometimes used in IVF cycles of patients who are "low responders." One recent study reviewed previous literature and thought that it showed increasingly convincing clinical and experimental support for the use of DHEA, and possibly other androgens, in women with diminished ovarian reserve [101,102].

Summary

The understanding of human reproduction has advanced exponentially during the past 3 decades. The development of IVF techniques by Edwards & Steptoe, acknowledged and awarded the Nobel Prize in 2011, has enabled clinicians to assist infertile couples, using a variety of medications and protocols. This variability was reviewed. No doubt further understanding of the physiology of oocyte maturation combined with advances in pharmaceuticals will lead to improved treatment options.

References

1. Birmingham A. Ovulation Drugs: A Guide for Patients. Birmingham, AL: The American Fertility Society; 1990, p 8.
2. Adashi EY. Clomiphene citrate: mechanism(s) and site(s) of action – a hypothesis revisited. Fertil Steril. 1984;**42**(3):331–44.
3. Caglar GS, Asimakopoulos B, Nikolettos N, et al. Recombinant LH in ovarian stimulation. Reprod Biomed Online. 2005;**10**(6):774–85.
4. Balasch J, Fabregues F. LH in the follicular phase: neither too high nor too low. Reprod Biomed Online. 2006;**12**(4):406–15.
5. Buhler K, Naether O. A 2:1 formulation of follitropin alfa and lutropin alfa in routine clinical practice: a large, multicentre, observational study. Gynecol Endocrinol. 2011;**27**(9):650–4.
6. Schriock ED, Jaffe RB. Induction of ovulation with gonadotropin-releasing hormone. Obstet Gynecol Surv. 1986;**41**(7):414–23.
7. Dodson WC. Role of gonadotropin releasing hormone agonists in ovulation induction. J Reprod Med. 1989;**34**(1 Suppl):76–80.
8. Moghissi KS. Gonadotropin releasing hormones. Clinical applications in gynecology. J Reprod Med. 1990;**35**(12):1097–107.
9. Santen RJ, Bourguignon JP. Gonadotropin-releasing hormone: physiological and therapeutic aspects, agonists and antagonists. Horm Res. 1987;**28**(2–4):88–103.
10. Filicori M, Flamigni C. GnRH agonists and antagonists. Current clinical status. Drugs. 1988;**35**(1):63–82.

11. Penzias AS, Shamma FN, Gutmann JN, et al. Nafarelin versus leuprolide in ovulation induction for in vitro fertilization: a randomized clinical trial. Obstet Gynecol. 1992;**79**(5 Pt 1):739–42.
12. Davoren JB, Hsueh AJ. Growth hormone increases ovarian levels of immunoreactive somatomedin C/ insulin-like growth factor I in vivo. Endocrinology. 1986;**118**(2):888–90.
13. Allen RE, Palopoli FP, Schumann EL, et al. US Patent 2,914,563. 1959.
14. Ernst S, Hite G, Cantrell JS, et al. Stereochemistry of geometric isomers of clomiphene: a correction of the literature and a reexamination of structure-activity relationships. J Pharm Sci. 1976;**65**(1):148–50.
15. Edwards RG, Steptoe PC, Purdy JM. Establishing full-term human pregnancies using cleaving embryos grown in vitro. Br J Obstet Gynaecol. 1980;**87**(9):737–56.
16. Fritz MA, Speroff L. The endocrinology of the menstrual cycle: the interaction of folliculogenesis and neuroendocrine mechanisms. Fertil Steril. 1982;**38**(5):509–29.
17. Gronow MJ. Ovarian hyperstimulation for successful in vitro fertilization and embryo transfer. Acta Obstet Gynecol Scand Suppl. 1985;**131**:1–80.
18. Shoham Z, Borenstein R, Lunenfeld B, et al. Hormonal profiles following clomiphene citrate therapy in conception and nonconception cycles. Clin Endocrinol (Oxf). 1990;**33**(2):271–8.
19. Stanger JD, Yovich JL. Reduced in-vitro fertilization of human oocytes from patients with raised basal luteinizing hormone levels during the follicular phase. Br J Obstet Gynaecol. 1985;**92**(4):385–93.
20. Homburg R, Armar NA, Eshel A, et al. Influence of serum luteinising hormone concentrations on ovulation, conception, and early pregnancy loss in polycystic ovary syndrome. BMJ. 1988;**297**(6655):1024–6.
21. Howles CM, Macnamee MC, Edwards RG, et al. Effect of high tonic levels of luteinising hormone on outcome of in-vitro fertilisation. Lancet. 1986;**2**(8505):521–2.
22. Bateman BG, Kolp LA, Nunley WC Jr, et al. Subclinical pregnancy loss in clomiphene citrate-treated women. Fertil Steril. 1992;**57**(1):25–7.
23. Induction of ovulation. Ch. 31 in Speroff L, Glass RH, Kas NG (Eds.). Clinical Gynecologic Endocrinology and Infertility, 8th edition. Baltimore, MD: Williams & Wilkins; 2011. p 1293.
24. Lopata A. Concepts in human in vitro fertilization and embryo transfer. Fertil Steril. 1983;**40**(3):289–301.
25. Marrs RP, Vargyas JM, Shangold GM, et al. The effect of time of initiation of clomiphene citrate on multiple follicle development for human in vitro fertilization and embryo replacement procedures. Fertil Steril. 1984;**41**(5):682–5.
26. Quigley MM, Maklad NF, Wolf DP. Comparison of two clomiphene citrate dosage regimens for follicular recruitment in an in vitro fertilization program. Fertil Steril. 1983;**40**(2):178–82.
27. Quigley MM, Schmidt CL, Beauchamp PJ, et al. Enhanced follicular recruitment in an in vitro fertilization program: clomiphene alone versus a clomiphene/ human menopausal gonadotropin combination. Fertil Steril. 1984;**42**(1):25–33.
28. Diamond MP, Maxson WS, Vaughn WK, et al. Antiestrogenic effect of clomiphene citrate in a multiple follicular stimulation protocol. J In Vitro Fert Embryo Transf. 1986;**3**(2):106–9.
29. Fasouliotis SJ, Simon A, Laufer N. Evaluation and treatment of low responders in assisted reproductive technology: a challenge to meet. J Assist Reprod Genet. 2000;**17**(7):357–73.
30. Birkenfeld A, Mor-Joseph S, Ezra J, et al. Preovulatory luteinization during induction of follicular maturation with menotrophin and menotrophin-clomiphene combination. Hum Reprod. 1990;**5**(5):561–4.
31. World Health Organization. Temporal relations between ovulation and defined changes in the concentration of plasma estradiol-17 beta, luteinizing hormone, follicle-stimulating hormone, and progesterone. I. Probit analysis. WHO Task Force on Methods for the Determination of the Fertile Period. Am J Obstet Gynecol. 1980;**138**:383–90.
32. Collins W, Jurkovic D, Bourne T, et al. Ovarian morphology, endocrine function and intra-follicular blood flow during the peri-ovulatory period. Hum Reprod. 1991;**6**(3):319–24.
33. Yen SCC. The human menstrual cycle: neuroendocrine regulation. In: Yen SCC, Jaffe RB (Eds.). Reproductive Endocrinology, 3rd edition. Philadelphia, PA: WB Saunders; 1991. p 273–308.
34. In vitro fertilization-embryo transfer (IVF-ET) in the United States: 1990 results from the IVF-ET registry. Medical Research International. Society for Assisted Reproductive Technology (SART), The American Fertility Society. Fertil Steril. 1992(**57**):15–24.
35. Kim LH, Taylor AE, Barbieri RL. Insulin sensitizers and polycystic ovary syndrome: can a diabetes medication treat infertility? Fertil Steril. 2000;**73**(6):1097–8.
36. Johnson N. Metformin is a reasonable first-line treatment option for non-obese women with infertility related to anovulatory polycystic ovary syndrome – a meta-analysis of randomised trials. Aust N Z J Obstet Gynaecol. 2011;**51**(2):125–9.
37. Tso LO, Costello MF, Albuquerque LE, et al. Metformin treatment before and during IVF or ICSI in women with polycystic ovary syndrome. Cochrane Database Syst Rev. 2009(**2**):CD006105.
38. Swanton A, Lighten A, Granne I, et al. Do women with ovaries of polycystic morphology without any other features of PCOS benefit from short-term metformin co-treatment during IVF? A double-blind, placebo-controlled, randomized trial. Hum Reprod. 2011;**26**(8):2178–84.
39. Palomba S, Falbo A, Carrillo L, et al. Metformin reduces risk of ovarian hyperstimulation syndrome in patients with polycystic ovary syndrome during gonadotropin-stimulated in vitro fertilization cycles: a randomized, controlled trial. Fertil Steril. 2011;**96**(6):1384–90.
40. Jones GS. Update on in vitro fertilization. Endocr Rev. 1984;**5**(1):62–75.
41. Haning RV Jr, Levin RM, Behrman HR, et al. Plasma estradiol window and urinary estriol glucuronide determinations for monitoring menotropin induction of ovulation. Obstet Gynecol. 1979;**54**(4):442–7.
42. Seibel MM, McArdle CR, Thompson IE, Berger MJ, Taymor ML. The role of ultrasound in ovulation induction: a critical appraisal. Fertil Steril. 1981;**36**(5):573–7.

43. Navot D, Margalioth EJ, Laufer N, et al. Periovulatory 17 beta-estradiol pattern in conceptional and nonconceptional cycles during menotropin treatment of anovulatory infertility. Fertil Steril. 1987;**47**(2):234–7.

44. Shapiro SS. Clinical parameters influencing success in IVF. In: Wolf DP (Ed.). In Vitro Fertilization and Embryo Transfer, a Manual of Basic Techniques. New York: Plenum Press; 1988. p 397–8.

45. Hershlag A, Asis MC, Diamond MP, et al. The predictive value and the management of cycles with low initial estradiol levels. Fertil Steril. 1990;**53**(6):1064–7.

46. Laufer N, DeCherney AH, Tarlatzis BC, et al. The association between preovulatory serum 17 beta-estradiol pattern and conception in human menopausal gonadotropin-human chorionic gonadotropin stimulation. Fertil Steril. 1986;**46**(1):73–6.

47. Jones HW Jr, Acosta A, Andrews MC, et al. The importance of the follicular phase to success and failure in in vitro fertilization. Fertil Steril. 1983;**40**(3):317–21.

48. Penzias AS, Shamma FN, Gutmann JN, et al. Luteinizing response to human chorionic gonadotropin does not predict outcome in gonadotropin releasing hormone agonist-suppressed/ human menopausal gonadotropin-stimulated in vitro fertilization (IVF) cycles. J Assist Reprod Genet. 1992;**9**(3):244–7.

49. Fleischer AC, Herbert CM, Sacks GA, et al. Sonography of the endometrium during conception and nonconception cycles of in vitro fertilization and embryo transfer. Fertil Steril. 1986;**46**(3):442–7.

50. Gonen Y, Casper RF, Jacobson W, et al. Endometrial thickness and growth during ovarian stimulation: a possible predictor of implantation in in vitro fertilization. Fertil Steril. 1989;**52**(3):446–50.

51. Rabinowitz R, Laufer N, Lewin A, et al. The value of ultrasonographic endometrial measurement in the prediction of pregnancy following in vitro fertilization. Fertil Steril. 1986;**45**(6):824–8.

52. Navot D, Bergh PA, Laufer N. Ovarian hyperstimulation syndrome in novel reproductive technologies: prevention and treatment. Fertil Steril. 1992;**58**(2):249–61.

53. Garcia-Velasco JA, Isaza V, Quea G, et al. Coasting for the prevention of ovarian hyperstimulation syndrome: much ado about nothing? Fertil Steril. 2006;**85**(3):547–54.

54. Delvigne A, Rozenberg S. A qualitative systematic review of coasting, a procedure to avoid ovarian hyperstimulation syndrome in IVF patients. Hum Reprod Update. 2002;**8**(3):291–6.

55. Moreno L, Diaz I, Pacheco A, et al. Extended coasting duration exerts a negative impact on IVF cycle outcome due to premature luteinization. Reprod Biomed Online. 2004;**9**(5):500–4.

56. Queenan JT Jr. Embryo freezing to prevent ovarian hyperstimulation syndrome. Mol Cell Endocrinol. 2000;**169**(1–2):79–83.

57. Manzanares MA, Gomez-Palomares JL, Ricciarelli E, et al. Triggering ovulation with gonadotropin-releasing hormone agonist in in vitro fertilization patients with polycystic ovaries does not cause ovarian hyperstimulation syndrome despite very high estradiol levels. Fertil Steril. 2010;**93**(4):1215–19.

58. Gonen Y, Balakier H, Powell W, et al. Use of gonadotropin-releasing hormone agonist to trigger follicular maturation for in vitro fertilization. J Clin Endocrinol Metab. 1990;**71**(4):918–22.

59. Bodri D, Guillen JJ, Galindo A, et al. Triggering with human chorionic gonadotropin or a gonadotropin-releasing hormone agonist in gonadotropin-releasing hormone antagonist-treated oocyte donor cycles: findings of a large retrospective cohort study. Fertil Steril. 2009;**91**(2):365–71.

60. McClure N, Healy DL, Rogers PA, et al. Vascular endothelial growth factor as capillary permeability agent in ovarian hyperstimulation syndrome. Lancet. 1994;**344**(8917):235–6.

61. Lesterhuis WJ, Rennings AJ, Leenders WP, et al. Vascular endothelial growth factor in systemic capillary leak syndrome. Am J Med. 2009;**122**(6):e5–7.

62. Humaidan P, Bredkjaer HE, Bungum L, et al. GnRH agonist (buserelin) or hCG for ovulation induction in GnRH antagonist IVF/ICSI cycles: a prospective randomized study. Hum Reprod. 2005;**20**(5):1213–20.

63. Griesinger G, Diedrich K, Devroey P, et al. GnRH agonist for triggering final oocyte maturation in the GnRH antagonist ovarian hyperstimulation protocol: a systematic review and meta-analysis. Hum Reprod Update. 2006;**12**(2):159–68.

64. Engmann L, DiLuigi A, Schmidt D, et al. The use of gonadotropin-releasing hormone (GnRH) agonist to induce oocyte maturation after cotreatment with GnRH antagonist in high-risk patients undergoing in vitro fertilization prevents the risk of ovarian hyperstimulation syndrome: a prospective randomized controlled study. Fertil Steril. 2008;**89**(1):84–91.

65. Humaidan P, Kol S, Papanikolaou EG. GnRH agonist for triggering of final oocyte maturation: time for a change of practice? Hum Reprod Update. 2011;**17**(4):510–24.

66. Devroey P, Pellicer A, Nyboe Andersen A, Arce JC; Menopur in GnRH Antagonist Cycles with Single Embryo Transfer (MEGASET) Trial Group. A randomized assessor-blind trial comparing highly purified hMG and recombinant FSH in a GnRH antagonist cycle with compulsory single-blastocyst transfer. Fertil Steril. 2012;**97**:561–71.

67. Out HJ, Bennink HJ, de Laat WN. What are the clinical benefits of recombinant gonadotrophins?: the development of recombinant FSH (Puregon): a scientific business. Hum Reprod. 1999;**14**(9):2189–90.

68. Group RHFs. Clinical assessment of recombinant human follicle stimulating hormone in stimulating ovarian follicle developement before in vitro fertilization. Fertil Steril. 1995;63:77–86.

69. Matorras R, Osuna C, Exposito A, et al. Recombinant FSH versus highly purified FSH in intrauterine insemination: systematic review and metaanalysis. Fertil Steril. 2011;**95**(6):1937–42, 1942.e1–3.

70. van Wely M, Kwan I, Burt AL, et al. Recombinant versus urinary gonadotrophin for ovarian stimulation in assisted reproductive technology cycles. Cochrane Database Syst Rev. 2011;**2**:CD005354.

71. Laufer N, Simon A, Hurwitz A, et al. In vitro fertilization. In: Seibel MM (Ed.). Infertility: a Comprehensive Text. Stamford, CT: Appelton & Lange; 1996, p 703–49.

72. Porter RN, Smith W, Craft IL, et al. Induction of ovulation for in-vitro fertilisation using buserelin and gonadotropins. Lancet. 1984;**2**(8414):1284–5.

73. Pellicer A, Simon C, Miro F, et al. Ovarian response and outcome of in-vitro fertilization in patients treated with

gonadotrophin-releasing hormone analogues in different phases of the menstrual cycle. Hum Reprod. 1989;**4**(3):285–9.

74. Rosen GF, Cassidenti DL, Stone SC, et al. Comparing mid-luteal and early follicular phase down regulation with Leuprolide acetate. In: 40th Annual Meeting of the Pacific Coast Fertility Society; 1992 April 8–12; Indian Wells, CA; 1992. (abstract P-19).

75. Seifer DB, Thornton KL, DeCherney AH, et al. Early pituitary desensitization and ovarian suppression with leuprolide acetate is associated with in vitro fertilization-embryo transfer success. Fertil Steril. 1991;**56**(3):500–4.

76. Howles CM, Macnamee MC, Edwards RG. Short term use of an LHRH agonist to treat poor responders entering an in-vitro fertilization programme. Hum Reprod. 1987;**2**(8):655–6.

77. Owen EJ, Davies MC, Kingsland CR, et al. The use of a short regimen of buserelin, a gonadotrophin-releasing hormone agonist, and human menopausal gonadotrophin in assisted conception cycles. Hum Reprod. 1989;**4**(7):749–53.

78. Matthews CD, Warnes GM, Norman RJ, et al. The leuprolide flare regime for in-vitro fertilization/gamete intra-fallopian transfer and embryo cryopreservation. Hum Reprod. 1991;**6**(6):817–22.

79. Acharya U, Small J, Randall J, et al. Prospective study of short and long regimens of gonadotropin-releasing hormone agonist in in vitro fertilization program. Fertil Steril. 1992;**57**(4):815–18.

80. Tan SL, Kingsland C, Campbell S, et al. The long protocol of administration of gonadotropin-releasing hormone agonist is superior to the short protocol for ovarian stimulation for in vitro fertilization. Fertil Steril. 1992;**57**(4):810–14.

81. Martikainen H, Ronnberg L, Tapanainen J, et al. Endocrine responses to gonadotrophins after LHRH agonist administration on cycle days 1–4: prevention of premature luteinization. Hum Reprod. 1990;**5**(3):246–9.

82. Macnamee MC, Howles CM, Edwards RG, et al. Short-term luteinizing hormone-releasing hormone agonist treatment: prospective trial of a novel ovarian stimulation regimen for in vitro fertilization. Fertil Steril. 1989;**52**(2):264–9.

83. Mannaerts B, Gordon K. Embryo implantation and GnRH antagonists: GnRH antagonists do not activate the GnRH receptor. Hum Reprod. 2000;**15**(9):1882–3.

84. Felberbaum R, Diedrich K. Use of GnRH antagonists in ovulation induction. In: Filicori M, Flamigni C (Eds.). Treatment of Infertility: The New Frontiers. New Jersey: Communications Media for Education; 1998, p 135–8.

85. Al-Inany HG, Youssef MA, Aboulghar M, et al. Gonadotrophin-releasing hormone antagonists for assisted reproductive technology. Cochrane Database Syst Rev. 2011;(**5**):CD001750.

86. Griesinger G, Shapiro DB. Luteinizing hormone add-back: is it needed in controlled ovarian stimulation, and if so, when? J Reprod Med. 2011;**56**(7–8):279–300.

87. Sheikholislam BM, Stempfel RS Jr. Hereditary isolated somatotropin deficiency: effects of human growth hormone administration. Pediatrics. 1972;**49**(3):362–74.

88. Adashi EY, Resnik, CE, Hernandez ER, et al. Potential relevance of insulin-like growth factor I to ovarian physiology: from basic science to clinical application. Semin Reprod Endocrinol. 1989;7:94–9.

89. Adashi EY, Resnick CE, D'Ercole AJ, et al. Insulin-like growth factors as intraovarian regulators of granulosa cell growth and function. Endocr Rev. 1985;**6**(3):400–20.

90. Adashi EY, Resnick CE, Svoboda ME, et al. Follicle-stimulating hormone enhances somatomedin C binding to cultured rat granulosa cells. Evidence for cAMP dependence. J Biol Chem. 1986;**261**(9):3923–6.

91. Adashi EY, Resnick CE, Svoboda ME, et al. Somatomedin-C synergizes with follicle-stimulating hormone in the acquisition of progestin biosynthetic capacity by cultured rat granulosa cells. Endocrinology. 1985;**116**(6):2135–42.

92. Jia XC, Kalmijn J, Hsueh AJ. Growth hormone enhances follicle-stimulating hormone-induced differentiation of cultured rat granulosa cells. Endocrinology. 1986;**118**(4):1401–9.

93. Erickson GF, Garzo VG, Magoffin DA. Insulin-like growth factor-I regulates aromatase activity in human granulosa and granulosa luteal cells. J Clin Endocrinol Metab. 1989;**69**(4):716–24.

94. Mason HD, Martikainen H, Beard RW, et al. Direct gonadotrophic effect of growth hormone on oestradiol production by human granulosa cells in vitro. J Endocrinol. 1990;**126**(3):R1–4.

95. Homburg R, Eshel A, Abdalla HI, Jacobs HS. Growth hormone facilitates ovulation induction by gonadotrophin. Clin Endocrinol (Oxf). 1988;**29**(1):113–17.

96. Owen EJ, West C, Torresani T, et al. Insulin-like-growth factors in women receiving growth hormone on addition to clomophene and human menopausal gonadotropines for IVF-ET. In: 6th World Congress of In Vitro Fertilization and Alternate Assisted Reproduction; 1989 April 2–7; Jerusalem, Israel; 1989, p 28.

97. Volpe A, Coukos G, Barreca A, et al. Ovarian response to combined growth hormone-gonadotropin treatment in patients resistant to induction of superovulation. Gynecol Endocrinol. 1989;**3**(2):125–33.

98. Menashe Y, Lunenfeld B, Pariente C, et al. Effect of growth hormone on ovarian responsiveness II. In: Joint meeting of the European Society of Human Reproduction and Embryology; 1990 August 29; Milan, Italy; 1990. (abstract 190).

99. Kolibianakis EM, Venetis CA, Diedrich K, et al. Addition of growth hormone to gonadotrophins in ovarian stimulation of poor responders treated by in-vitro fertilization: a systematic review and meta-analysis. Hum Reprod Update. 2009;**15**(6):613–22.

100. Duffy JM, Ahmad G, Mohiyiddeen L, et al. Growth hormone for in vitro fertilization. Cochrane Database Syst Rev. 2010;(**1**):CD000099.

101. Gleicher N, Barad DH. Dehydroepiandrosterone (DHEA) supplementation in diminished ovarian reserve (DOR). Reprod Biol Endocrinol. 2011;**9**:67.

102. Wiser A, Gonen O, Ghetler Y, et al. Addition of dehydroepiandrosterone (DHEA) for poor-responder patients before and during IVF treatment improves the pregnancy rate: a randomized prospective study. Hum Reprod. 2010;**25**(10):2496–500.

Chapter 14

Endometriosis and ovarian cancer

Douglas N. Brown, MD, FACOG, Tanja Pejovic, MD, PhD, and Farr R. Nezhat, MD, FACOG, FACS

Introduction

Endometriosis has been traditionally defined as the presence of endometrial glands and stroma in ectopic locations. This disease affects approximately 6 to 10% of reproductive-aged women, resulting in dysmenorrhea, dyspareunia, chronic pelvic pain, and/or infertility [1]. Endometriosis is a debilitating condition, posing quality-of-life issues for the individual patient. The prevalence of endometriosis in women experiencing pain, infertility, or both can be as high as 50%. The disorder represents a major cause of gynecologic hospitalization in the United States resulting in over $3 billion in inpatient health care costs in 2004 alone [2,3]. The significant individual and public health concerns associated with endometriosis are paramount to understanding its pathogenesis. The first recorded description of pathology consistent with endometriosis was provided by Shroen in 1690 [4,5]. Despite decades of extensive clinical and scientific investigation, the exact pathogenesis of this enigmatic disorder still remains largely unknown.

Theories regarding pathogenesis of endometriosis

Numerous theories detailing the development of endometriosis have been described. These theories can generally be classified into two groups: (1) Nonendometrial, those that propose that implants arise from tissues other than the endometrium, and (2) Endometrial, those that propose that implants arise from uterine endometrium (Table 14.1).

Nonendometrial origin

Central to the theory of a nonendometrial origin is the concept of metaplasia of coelomic epithelium. According to this theory, normal peritoneal tissue transforms by means of metaplastic transition to ectopic endometrial tissue [6,7]. Merrill et al. proposed a closely related induction theory that holds that an endogenous inductive stimulus, such as a hormonal or immunologic factor, promotes the differentiation of undifferentiated cells in the peritoneal lining into endometrial cells [7,8]. This induction theory is further supported by the finding of totipotent mesothelial serosal cells in the coelomic lining [9]. Moreover, when ovarian surface epithelium (OSE) is co-cultured with endometrial stromal cells in a collagen lattice and exposed to supraphysiologic levels of 17β-estradiol, endometriosis appears to arise by means of a metaplastic transformation of the mesothelium [10]. Finally, the theory of embryonic Mullerian cell rests postulates that cells residual from embryologic Mullerian duct migration maintain the capacity to develop into endometriotic lesions under the influence of estrogen [11,12].

Support for a nonendometrial origin is further lended in clinical reports of histologically confirmed endometriotic tissue developing in patients without menstrual endometrium. Endometriosis has been documented in a patient with Rokitansky–Kiister–Hauser syndrome who did not have functioning endometrium [13]. Perhaps the most compelling evidence for a non-endometrial etiology comes from cases of men with prostate cancer undergoing high-dose estrogen treatment who were subsequently diagnosed with endometriosis and evidence of urinary system endometriosis in men [14,15].

Endometrial origin

Benign metastasis

Originally proposed in the 1920s, the theory of benign metastasis holds that ectopic endometrial implants are the result of lymphatic or hematogenous dissemination of endometrial cells [9,16–19]. Evidence for this mechanism is considerable. Microvascular studies have demonstrated the presence of lymph flow from the uterus to the ovary, alluding to a possible mechanistic role for the lymphatic system in the etiology of ovarian endometriosis [19]. Moreover, endometriosis has been documented in 6.5% of women at lymphadenectomy and 6.7% of women at autopsy [20]. The most compelling evidence for the theory of benign metastasis is derived from reports of histologically proven endometriotic lesions occurring in sites distant from the uterus or pelvis, including bone, brain, and lung [21].

Retrograde menstruation

Perhaps most widely accepted is the theory of retrograde menstruation. Initially proposed by Sampson in the 1920s, the theory of retrograde menstruation is both intuitively attractive and supported by multiple lines of scientific evidence [22]. According to this theory, eutopic endometrium is sloughed into the peritoneal cavity by means of patent fallopian tubes

Altchek's Diagnosis and Management of Ovarian Disorders, ed. Liane Deligdisch, Nathan G. Kase, and Carmel J. Cohen. Published by Cambridge University Press. © Cambridge University Press 2013.

Table 14.1. Classification of theories regarding the pathogenesis of endometriosis

Theory	Proponent(s)
Non-endometrial origin	
Coelomic metaplasia	Iwanoff, 1898 [6]
Induction	Levander and Normann, 1955 [7]; Merrill, 1966 [8]
Endometrial origin	Russell, 1899 [9]; Batt and Smith, 1989 [10]
Endometrial origin	
Benign metastasis	Halban, 1924 [11]
Retrograde menstruation/ implantation	Sampson, 1927 [12]

during menstruation. The mechanism of this proposed phenomenon is supported by the finding of menstrual blood in the peritoneal fluid of up to 90% of healthy women with patent fallopian tubes undergoing laparoscopy during the perimenstrual period of the cycle [23]. The incidence of bloody peritoneal fluid was only 15% in the patients with bilaterally occluded tubes. Further support for this etiology is derived from studies of obstructed or compromised outflow tracts. In adolescent girls with congenital outflow obstruction, there is a high prevalence of endometriosis [24]. Abuzeid et al. demonstrated a higher prevalence of endometriosis in women with a uterine septum, suggesting that even a slight compromise of antegrade menstruation may predispose to the formation of endometriosis [25]. Moreover, iatrogenic obstruction of the outflow tract in baboons resulted in endometriotic lesions within the peritoneal cavity [26]. The viability of these peritoneal endometrial cells is of paramount importance for the plausibility of the retrograde transplantation theory. This has been most elegantly addressed by the experiments of Ridley and Edwards, who injected menstrual effluent into the subcutaneous adipose layer of women scheduled to undergo laparotomy [27]. The site of injection was excised at the time of surgery, and histologic review demonstrated viable endometrial glands and stroma up to 180 days post-injection.

The anatomic distribution of endometriotic lesions also favors the retrograde menstruation theory. Superficial implants are more often located in the posterior compartment of the pelvis and in the left hemipelvis [28,29]. Primary and recurrent ovarian endometriomas are also more often located on the left ovary in contrast to the distribution of nonendometriotic benign ovarian cysts which do not display a predilection for sidedness [30–32]. In one large observational study, deep infiltrating endometriosis also exhibited a predilection for the posterior compartment and the left side of the pelvis [33]. The propensity for lesions to implant into the posterior cul-de-sac is best explained by the accumulation of regurgitated menstrual effluent in the most dependent portion of the peritoneal cavity. The presence of a retroverted uterus, by allowing flow from the anterior to posterior compartment in the upright or supine position, has been correlated with the finding of posterior deeply infiltrating lesions [34]. The propensity for the left hemipelvis to be affected by superficial, ovarian, and deeply infiltrating endometriosis is thought to be a function of the close anatomic relationship between the sigmoid colon and the le adnexa. By acting as an obstacle to the diffusion of menstru effluent from the left fallopian tube, the sigmoid colon pro motes stasis of this effluent, thereby extending the interval fc regurgitated endometrial cells to implant to the left pelvic side wall, the left uterosacral region, and the left ovary.

In 2005, Dinulescu et al. proposed a murine model c endometriosis that has provided insight into the pathogenes of peritoneal endometriosis [35]. The conditional activation c the *K-ras* oncogene in endometrial cells deposited into th peritoneum resulted in histologically confirmed peritone endometriotic implants in nearly 50% of mice within 8 month Similar activation of the *K-ras* oncogene in peritoneal cel showed no progression to endometriosis. These results furthe support the theory of retrograde menstruation in the develop ment of peritoneal endometriosis as well as the role of *K-ra* oncogene in endometriosis initiation.

Logically, it would follow that situations that decreas the available endometrium or that occlude the tubal condu for retrograde deposition should reduce the propensity fo the establishment of endometriosis. Interestingly, the rate o endometriosis recurrence is significantly reduced whe endometrial ablation is coupled with the treatment of endo metriosis [36]. Moreover, in women with known endome triosis who have undergone tubal sterilization, retrograd menstruation into the proximal tubal segment has bee demonstrated to result in histopathologic implantation which may result in tuboperitoneal fistulization or sever dysmenorrhea [37,38].

Retrograde menstruation may explain the physical displace ment of endometrial fragments into the peritoneal cavity, bu additional steps are clearly necessary for the development o these implants. Attachment of endometrial fragments to th mesothelium of the peritoneum, invasion of the mesothelium establishment of a vascular supply, and circumvention of th immune response are all necessary if endometriosis is t develop from retrograde passage of sloughed endometrium Perhaps it is this propensity for implantation that best account for the disparity between the 90% prevalence of retrograd menstruation and the approximately 10% prevalence of th disease. Hereditary or acquired properties of the endometrium hereditary or acquired defects of the peritoneal epithelium and/or defective immune clearance of sloughed endometriu are areas of active investigation in the search for the factor o factors that influence predisposition toward implantation of th displaced endometrial cells.

Evidence for an endometrial factor in the predisposition to disease

The evidence for an endometrial genetic predisposition towar endometriosis implantation is compelling. Endometrial stro mal cells (ESCs) appear to be the critical cells vital to implanta tion into the mesothelium. Lucidi et al. developed a nove in vitro model using ESCs and peritoneal mesothelial cell (PMCs) from various sources in demonstrating that the sourc of the ESCs and not the source of the PMCs had the greates

Table 14.2. Candidate genes implicated in the pathogenesis of endometriosis

Gene	Function	Reference(s)
MMP-3, -7	Matrix metalloproteinases	Bruner-Tran et al., 2002 [47]
KRAS	Oncogene	Dinulescu et al., 2005 [36]
PTEN	Tumor suppressor gene	Dinulescu et al., 2005 [36]
CYP19	Aromatase enzyme	Noble et al., 1996 [48]
17f3HSD-2	Hydroxysteroid dehydrogenase	Zeitoun et al., 1998 [49]
BCL-2	Antiapoptosis	Jones et al., 1998 [50]

impact on the rate of implantation [39]. Additionally, the risk for the development of endometriosis is six times higher in first-degree relatives of women with severe endometriosis than for relatives of unaffected women [40]. Studies of monozygotic twins also demonstrate high concordance rates for histologically confirmed endometriosis [41,42]. Familial aggregation implicating a genetic predisposition has been linked in population studies and in a nonhuman primate model [43,44]. Perhaps the most compelling evidence comes from linkage analysis studies that have attempted to identify candidate gene loci. Treloar et al. in one of the largest studies to date, involving more than 1,100 families with two or more affected sib-pairs, identified a significant susceptibility locus for endometriosis on chromosome locus 10q26 [45]. Further research on the identification of other possible genetic loci is ongoing. A partial list is provided in Table 14.2.

The concept of endometriosis as an estrogen-dependent disorder is well supported by molecular evidence [46]. Genetic or acquired hormonal receptor alterations may influence the ability of endometrial cells to proliferate, attach to the mesothelium, and/or evade immune-mediated clearance. An interesting finding in ectopic endometrial tissue relative to eutopic endometrium is the increased expression of aromatase enzyme and decreased expression of 17β-hydroxysteroid dehydrogenase (17β-HSD) type 2 [47,48]. This differential expression profile leads to a marked increase in the locally bioavailable estradiol concentration. This alteration in hormonal regulation provides molecular evidence that further supports endometriosis as an estrogen-dependent disease, and validates therapeutic treatments aimed at promoting a hypoestrogenic microenvironment.Moreover, there is evidence to support the characterization of endometriosis as a progesterone-resistant condition [49]. Kitawaki et al. have demonstrated an overall reduction of progesterone receptors in ectopic endometrial lesions relative to eutopic endometrium, and an absence of progesterone receptor-B (PR-B) in ectopic endometrial lesions [46]. Additionally, Osteen et al. have demonstrated reduced progesterone action during endometrial maturation alluding to a potential risk factor for the development of endometriosis [50].

Acquired aberrations of the endometrium have also been postulated to result in predisposition toward implantation of refluxed endometrial cells. The acquired aberration may be a random genetic event or consequent to an environmental exposure. Dioxin has received considerable attention as an environmental factor associated with endometriosis. Rhesus monkeys exposed to daily dioxin (5 to 25 ppm) for 4 years developed endometriosis of dose-dependent severity [51]. Dioxin, also known as 2,3,7,8 tetrachlorodibenzo-*p*-dioxin (TCDD), is a ubiquitous environmental by-product of combustion [52]. Dietary or occupational exposure to this lipophilic compound may result in adipose accumulation. When bound to the aryl hydrocarbon receptor, the resulting complex may act as a transcription factor. Dioxin has been documented to exert carcinogenic and immuno-suppressive effects in animal studies [53]. Although biologically plausible, a direct causal link between dioxin exposure and the development of endometriosis remains equivocal [54]. Interestingly, TCDD has been demonstrated to selectively down-regulate stromal PR-B expression and increase matrix metalloproteinase (MMP) expression in cultured endometrial cells, providing a potential mechanism for both predisposition to implantation and the observed progesterone resistance associated with this disorder [55].

Furthermore, it is well established that the endometrium undergoes an extraordinary cell turnover rate, and is therefore consequently, vulnerable to errors of genetic recombination. Any acquired or inherent genetic alteration represents a potential increased survival advantage to sloughed endometrial cells and in the establishment of endometriotic implants. Guo et al. propose that the occurrence of this type of genomic alteration in eutopic endometrium may be consequent to repetitious oxidative stress [56]. Genomic alterations within endometriotic implants have been described using the comparative genomic hybridization (CGH) microarrays [57]. These specific genomic alterations may hold promise in determining the types of genetic alteration necessary in the implantation, survival, and proliferation of endometriosis.

Evidence for a peritoneal factor in the predisposition to disease

As an intact mesothelium is likely to act as a protective barrier against the implantation of regurgitated endometrial tissue, it holds that a heritable or acquired condition of the peritoneal surface may also predispose to the attachment and invasion of endometrial fragments. Indeed, in vitro studies have shown that endometrial fragments adhere to the peritoneum only at locations where the basement membrane or extracellular matrix was exposed because of mesothelial damage [58]. Menstrual effluent has been shown to induce a toxic effect on the mesothelium, alluding to a potential mechanistic predisposition for sloughed endometrial attachment [59]. Gene expression profiling of the peritoneum from subjects with and without endometriosis has demonstrated up-regulation of MMP-3 during the luteal phase and up-regulation of intracellular adhesion molecule-l (I CAM-1), transforming growth factor-β (TGF-β), and interleukin-6 (IL-6) during the menstrual phase [60]. The differential expression of these cytokines and growth factors may provide the biochemical microenvironment that protects against immune-mediated clearance thereby permitting endometrial implantation.

Evidence for an immune factor in the predisposition to disease

Under normal conditions, refluxed endometrial tissue is cleared from the peritoneum by the immune system. The dysregulation of this immuno-regulation has been implicated in the predisposition to the implantation, survival, and progression of endometriosis (Table 14.3). Larger tissue fragments as opposed to individual cells demonstrate an increased capacity to implant [61]. Additionally, eutopic endometrium from women with endometriosis was found to be more resistant to lysis by natural killer (NK) cells than was the eutopic endometrium from women without disease [62]. Further studies have identified the constitutive shedding of ICAM-1 by ESCs from patients with endometriosis as the potential mechanism by which these cells escape NK cell-mediated clearance [63].

Gene expression profiling of menstrual phase endometrium in women with endometriosis demonstrated up-regulation of tumor necrosis factor-α (TNF-α), interleukin-8 (IL-8), and MMP-3 as compared with the corresponding profile in women without the condition [60]. IL-8 and TNF-α both promote angiogenesis and cell proliferation of endometrial cells. Increases in the production may therefore predispose to the development of invasive endometriotic lesions. Compared with disease-free controls, the eutopic endometrium of women with endometriosis has also been shown to exhibit increased production of IL-6 [64]. IL-6 plays a significant role in many chronic inflammatory conditions. IL-6 is secreted by macrophages as well as epithelial endometrial cells and has been shown to significantly stimulate aromatase expression in cultured endometriotic and adipocyte stromal cells [65]. Proteomics has identified a unique protein structurally similar to haptoglobin in the peritoneal fluid of patients with endometriosis that essentially bind to macrophages, reducing their phagocytic capacity, and increasing their production of IL-6 [66,67]. Other cytokines or chemokines expressed differentially in the peritoneal fluid of patients with endometriosis include IL-l, regulated on activation, normal T expressed and secreted (RANTES), and monocyte chemoattractant protein-l (MCP-I) [68–72]. These cytokines act as chemo-attractants and facilitate the recruitment of additional macrophages further increasing the inflammatory response. The resultant cytokine milieu is a complex system in which these cytokines may induce or repress their own synthesis thereby inducing unregulated mitotic division, growth and differentiation, and migration or apoptosis similar to malignant transformation mechanisms.

Table 14.3. Immune factors implicated in the pathogenesis of endometriosis

Factor	Reference(s)
Increased activated macrophage fraction	Halme et al., 1984 [24]
Increased IL-8	Ryan et al., 1995 [76]
Increased RANTES	Khorram et al., 1993 [77]
Increased MCP-I	Akoum et al., 1996 [78]
Decreased NK cell activity	Oosterlynck et al., 1991 [68]
Increased TGF-α activity	Oosterlynck et al., 1994 [79]
Increased ICAM-I	Somigliana et al., 1996 [69]
Altered macrophage function-haptoglobin	Sharpe-Timms et al., 2002 [75]
Altered Thl: Th2 cell balance	Hsu et al., 1997 [80]
Increased IL-6 secretion	Tsenget al., 1996 [70]

The relationship of endometriosis and ovarian malignancy

It is clear that endometriosis has mixed traits of both benign and malignant disease. The pathogenesis involves loss of control of cell proliferation and is associated with local and distant spread. Endometriosis, however, does not cause catabolic disturbance, metabolic consequences, or death in humans [73]. Although endometriosis is not termed a premalignant condition, epidemiologic, histopathologic, and molecular data suggest that endometriosis does have malignant potential. Ovarian carcinogenesis may involve precursor lesions arising from endometriosis or those arising from Mullerian metaplasia of the ovarian surface epithelium (OSE) as well as de novo carcinogenesis.

The theories on the histogenesis of endometriosis can be categorized into five major categories: coelomic metaplasia, retrograde menstruation, embryonic cell rests, induction, and lymphatic and vascular dissemination [74–77]. Ovarian carcinoma, likewise, has been theorized to be caused by genetic alteration of damaged ovarian epithelium during ovulation, elevated gonadotropins, androgen excess with progesterone deficiency, retrograde menstruation with pelvic contamination, and chronic inflammation [78,79] (Table 14.4).

Table 14.4. An overview of common factors of both endometriosis and ovarian cancer

Similar theories on etiology	Protective factors	Risk factors	Common pathogenic mechanisms
Damaged ovarian epithelium	Oral contraceptives	Early menarche	Familial predisposition
Elevated gonadotropins	Tubal ligation	Late menarche	Immuno-biological factors
Androgen excess	Hysterectomy		Cell adhesion factors
Retrograde menstruation	Pregnancy		Angiogenic factors
Chronic Inflammation			

Epidemiology

The exact incidence of endometriosis is unknown, because accurate diagnosis requires surgical intervention and ultimately depends upon the indication for surgery, the type of surgical procedure, and the thoroughness and familiarity of the surgeon with the various appearances of endometriosis. The specific correlation of endometriosis and ovarian malignancy regarding their epidemiologic patterns has been extensively studied. There is suggestion of a common mechanism based on similar disease responses, such as the protective effects of tubal ligation, hysterectomy, oral contraceptives, and pregnancy, increased risks with infertility, and early menarche, late menopause, and nulliparity for both ovarian cancer and endometriosis [78] (Table 14.4).

The prevalence of ovarian cancer developing in women with endometriosis is higher than sporadic ovarian cancer in the general population (Table 14.5). Several studies have specifically addressed the ovarian cancer risk in patients with endometriosis. Brinton et al. reviewed 20,686 women hospitalized with endometriosis identified through the Swedish Inpatient Registry from 1969 to 1983 with a mean follow-up of 11.4 years [78]. The cases of all incident cancers in this cohort were garnered through the National Swedish Cancer Registry, identifying 738 overall malignancies and 29 ovarian malignancies. Standardized incidence ratios (SIRs) with 95% confidence intervals (CIs) from this study showed an increased overall cancer risk of 1.2 (1.1–1.3), 1.9 (1.3–2.8) for ovarian cancer, 1.3 (1.1–1.4) for breast cancer, and 1.8 (1.0–1.8) for hematopoietic cancers. The incidence ratio for those with follow-up of $\geq$ 10 years increased to 2.5, and the highest cancer risk was among women with the longest history of endometriosis: SIR 4.2 (95% CI 2.0–7.7). This analysis may overestimate the cancer risk, because only hospitalized endometriosis patients were accounted for. Borgfeldt and Andolf also identified a cohort of 28,163 endometriosis patients born before 1970 from the National Swedish Hospital Discharge Registry from 1969 to 1996 and matched each case with three controls [79]. The cohort of endometriosis patients had an increased risk for ovarian cancer of 1.3 (95% CI 1.0–1. 8) with a significantly lower mean age at diagnosis of 49 years versus 51.6 years in the control population.

The significance of this relationship was further confirmed by Brinton et al. in 2004 [80] with a retrospective cohort study conducted in the United States, analyzing the correlation of endometriosis causing primary infertility and ovarian cancer, resulting in an SIR of 4.19 (95% CI 2.0–7.7) and a risk ratio of 2.72 (95% CI 1.1–6.7) compared with patients with secondary infertility and no endometriosis. Further analysis within the cohort of primary infertility patients with endometriosis in 2005 by Brinton et al. again revealed elevated relative risks (95% CI) of 2.9 (1.2–7.1) for ovarian cancer, 2.4 (0.7–8.4) for colon cancer, 4.65 (0.8–25.6) for thyroid cancer, and 2.3 (0.8–6.7) for melanomas [81]. These Swedish cohort studies were expanded by Melin et al. in 2006 to evaluate if risk ratios were consistent with longer follow-up [82]. The cohort was 64,492 endometriosis patients discharged from hospitalization identified through the Swedish Inpatient Registry from 1969 to 2000. When cross-referenced with the National Swedish Cancer Registry, 3,349 patients were identified to have developed ovarian cancer. With extended follow-up and calculation of updated standardized incidence ratios, there was no risk for overall cancer (1.04), but an increase was noted in ovarian cancer (1.43 [95% CI 1.2–1.7]), endocrine tumors (1.36 [95% CI 1.2–1.6]), non-Hodgkin lymphoma (1.24 [95% CI 1.0–1.50]), and brain tumors (1.22 [95% CI 1.0–1.4]). Importantly, the risk for women with early diagnosis and long-standing endometriosis was most pronounced, with SIRs of 2.01 and 2.23, respectively [83]. Of note, women with a history of hysterectomy at or before the time of endometriosis diagnosis did not show an elevated risk [84]. Again, both studies of the Swedish cohorts may be skewed to reflect malignant incidence ratios for cases of more severe endometriosis, because the cohorts were hospitalized patients with more advanced stages of endometriosis. Also, because records of hospitalized patients were retrospectively cross-referenced with a separate cancer patient registry, there is the possibility of negating or including cases erroneously.

Olsen et al. completed the largest study that did not support the increased ovarian cancer risk in endometriosis patients [84]. Analyzing a group of 37,434 post-menopausal women, a cohort of 1,392 post-menopausal patients who self-reported the diagnosis of endometriosis was isolated. After an average 13-year follow-up, no significant increased risk was found for all cancers, breast cancer, or ovarian cancer, but there was a significant association with increased risk of non-Hodgkin lymphoma, with an age-adjusted risk ratio of 1.8 (95% CI 1.0–3.0). This study involved acceptable long-term follow-up; however, several factors must be taken into account. The study was underpowered as the cohort was smaller and included only three ovarian cancer cases. Furthermore, the endometriosis was not histologically confirmed and, because all of the patients were post-menopausal, it is possible that younger patients may have already developed ovarian cancer and died. Table 14.5 summarizes the epidemiologic studies of ovarian cancer risk in endometriosis patients.

Reciprocal analysis of the prevalence of endometriosis found in ovarian cancer patients also supports the clinical correlation. In a review of 29 studies from 1973 to 2002 on the prevalence of endometriosis in epithelial ovarian cancers organized by location of disease, the following three groups were compiled: (1) histologic proof of transition from ovarian endometriosis to cancer as defined by Sampson, (2) ovarian cancers with endometriosis in the same ovary, and (3) ovarian cancers with concomitant pelvic endometriosis [76]. The second category was considered to be the best estimation of endometriosis in the different histologic subtypes, yielding a prevalence of 4.5% in serous, 1.4% in mucinous, 35.9% in clear-cell, and 19% in endometrioid carcinomas [77,85].

These data were further corroborated by Valenzuela et al. in 2007; among 22 cases of ovarian endometrioid adenocarcinomas of the ovary, three patients were found to have concomitant endometriosis as defined by the Sampson criteria [86]. The review by Van Gorp et al. calculated an ovarian cancer prevalence of 0.9% in all cases of endometriosis, 2.5% when present in the same ovary, and 4.5% when coexistent with any

Table 14.5. Epidemiologic studies assessing ovarian cancer risk in endometriosis patients

Author	Study type	Cohort size	Mean follow-up (Years)	Ovarian malignancies identified	Ovarian cancer in endometriosis patients (SIR/OR)	
Brinton et al., 1997 [78]	Cohort	20,686	11.4	29	Overall cancer risk	1.2
		endometriosis			Ovarian cancer	1.9
		patients			Ovarian cancer with ≥ 10 yrs	2.5
					follow-up	4.2
					Ovarian cancer with long-standing endometriosis	
Brinton et al., 2004 [80]	Cohort	12,193		45	Ovarian cancer	2.5
		Infertility patients				
Brinton et al., 2005 [81]	Cohort			2,491	2.53 (1.19–5.38)	
Ness et al., 2000 [90]	Case control			66	Ovarian cancer	1.7
Borgfeldt et al., 2004	Nested case control	28,163		81	Ovarian cancer	1.3
Modugano et al., 2006	Case control			177	1.3 (1.1–1.6)	
Melin et al., 2006 [82]	Cohort	64,492	12.7	122	Overall cancer risk	1.04
					Ovarian cancer	1.43
					Ovarian cancer early diagnosed	2.0
					endometriosis	2.2
					Ovarian cancer with long-standing endometriosis	
Olsen et al., 2002 [84]	Cohort	1,392	13	3	No increased risk for overall or ovarian cancer	
Kobayashi et al., 2007	Cohort	6,398	12.8	46	Ovarian cancer	8.95
					Ovarian cancer > 50 yrs old	13.2

pelvic endometriosis [77]. Malignant extra-ovarian endometriosis is estimated to account for 25% of all malignant transformations of endometriosis and 80% of the endometrioid subtype [87–89].

Looking at the trend of ovarian cancer in endometriosis is more difficult, because endometriosis is not always aggressively resected and confirmed by histopathologic studies. Only a limited number of the studies controlled for confounding factors for both diseases, such as parity, infertility, tubal ligation, ovarian hyperstimulation, and duration of endometriosis. Ness et al. completed two case–control studies confirming the association between endometriosis and ovarian cancer [90,91]. In a group of 767 women with ovarian cancer and 1,367 control subjects, with adjustments made for age, parity, family history of ovarian cancer, race, oral contraceptive use, tubal ligation, hysterectomy, and breast-feeding, overall women with breast cancer were 1.7-fold more likely to report an endometriosis history [90]. Furthermore, in a pooled study of 13,000 women, ovarian cancer was more likely among subfertile women, especially with infertility resulting from endometriosis, showing an odds ratio of 1.9 (95% CI 1.2–2.9) [91].

The relationship of endometriosis and ovarian cancer was further explored in terms of bias versus causality using the nine criteria proposed by Austin Bradford Hill which serve as fundamentals of causal inference: strength of association, consistency, biologic gradient, specificity, temporality, biologic plausibility, experimental evidence, analogy, and coherence [92]. The criterion of strength was not fulfilled, and data on the association was insufficient or mixed for biologic gradient, plausibility, analogy, and coherence. Consistency, temporality, specificity, and experimental evidence, however, all fulfilled the criteria in animal models. The article concluded that a causal relationship between endometriosis and ovarian cancer should be recognized, but that the low degree of risk observed could be attributed to the possibility that ectopic and eutopic endometrium undergo malignant transformation at similar rates [92].

Molecular pathogenesis

Common pathogenetic factors of both endometriosis and ovarian malignancy include familial predisposition, genetic alterations, immuno-biologic, cell adhesion, angiogenic, and hormonal factors (Table 14.4).

Genomic instability and mutations

Although there are reports of mendelian inheritance patterns of endometriosis, such as an increased risk in first-degree relatives and twins, there is increasing evidence that endometriosis is inherited as a complex genetic trait involving the interaction of multiple genes and environmental factors conferring disease susceptibility and malignant behaviors [93].

Genomic instability is a known characteristic of cancer cells. Ovarian cancer occurs as a result of numerous genetic and epigenetic changes that successively alter benign ovarian surface epithelium into malignant. The hypothesis has been put forth that inflammation acts as an intermediary between an extrinsic factor such as infection or physical or chemical stimuli, and carcinogenesis has been linked to inflammatory mediators and cytokines, eicosanoids, and immune cells (Fig. 14.1). Prolonged exposure to these factors that aim to degrade noxious stimuli may lead to increased oxidative stress, disruption of homeostasis, genomic instability, and consequently to abnormal proliferation.

Endometriosis demonstrates somatically acquired genetic alterations similar to those found in cancer, leading to clonal expansion of genetically abnormal cells, as demonstrated in several studies [94,95]. Endometriotic cysts are monoclonal and characterized by the loss of heterozygosity in 75% of endometriotic cyst cases with associated adenocarcinoma, and even in 28% of cases without accompanying carcinoma [96,97]. The most commonly affected chromosome arms are 9p, 11q, and 22q [98]. Comparative genomic hybridization studies of endometriosis have revealed loss of DNA copy numbers on 1p, 22q, and X, and gain on 6p and 17q [99,100]. Fluorescent in situ hybridization analyses confirmed that gain of 17q includes amplification of the proto-oncogene *HER-2neu* [101]. Loss of heterozygosity at 5q, 6q, 9p, 1 lq, 22q, p16, and p53, indicating loss of tumor suppression genes, has been identified in endometriosis and endometriosis-derived cell lines [102]. Ovarian cancers and adjacent endometriotic lesions have shown common genetic alterations, such as *PTEN* gene mutations, suggesting a possible malignant genetic transition spectrum. Loss of heterogenicity at 10q23.3 occurs with high frequency in solitary endometrial cysts (56.5%), endometrioid carcinoma of the ovary (42.1%), and clear cell carcinoma of the ovary (27.3%), and a concentration of mutations in the *PTEN* gene encoding the phosphatase domain has been demonstrated in endometrial cysts and clear cell carcinomas of the ovary [103]. In a mouse model of endometrioid ovarian cancer, *PTEN* deletion in the background of oncogenic *K-ras* activation within the OSE gives rise to endometriosis-like precursor lesions which developed invasive endometrioid ovarian carcinoma within 7–12 weeks [104]. These studies demonstrate that benign endometriosis-like lesions can develop within the normal OSE after expression of oncogenic *K-ras;* however, progression to endometrioid ovarian cancer necessitates inactivation of *PTEN*. Additional data provided by Dinulescu et al. show activition of PI3K (phosphatidylinositol 3' kinase)-AKT-mTOR (mammalian target of rapamycin) and MAP kinase pathways in this model, suggesting potential utility of the model in therapeutic protocols [104]. Based on these data, Matzuk proposed that activation of β-catenin may be involved in endometrioid or clear cell carcinoma of the ovary [105]. Several lines of investigation exploring the genetic modifications of mouse ovarian surface epithelial cells necessary for tumorigenic transformation delineate that inactivation of p53 and activation of *c-myc, Kras*, or *AKT* contribute to early tumorigenesis [106]. Cheng et al. demonstrated in an explant model of epithelial ovarian cancer that aberrant *Hoxa10* expression along with *Hoxa7* and *Hoxa9* confer early endometrioid differentiation [107]. The authors speculated that deregulated expression of *HOX* genes "tip the balance toward tumorigenicity" in "phenotypically uncommitted" OSE undergoing neoplastic transformation.

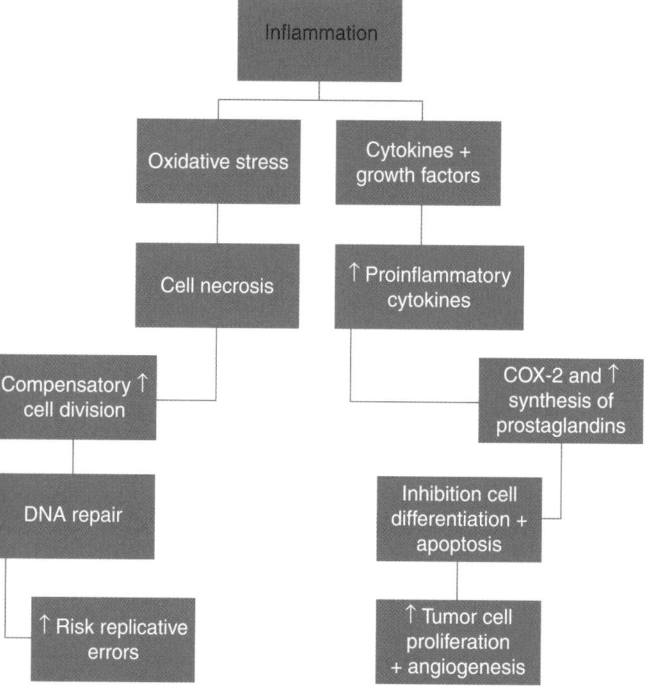

Fig. 14.1. Flow chart from inflammation to cancer.

Moreover, abnormal gene expression of the tumor suppression gene *PTEN* and DNA mismatch repair gene *hMLHl* was identified in endometrial and ovarian cancers and has been similarly recognized in advanced-stage endometriosis. A 2002 study by Martini et al. analyzed the methylation status of *hMLHl* and *p16* and the protein expression of *PTEN* and *hMLHl* in 46 cases of endometriosis stages III and IV [108]. Hypermethylation resulting in absence of the hMLHl protein was noted in 8.6% of endometriotic lesions, and reduced protein expression of PTEN was noted in 15% of cases [109]. Frequent mutations of the *PTEN* gene are seen in endometrioid ovarian tumor compared with eutopic endometrium counterparts, but not in serous or mucinous epithelial ovarian tumors

[110]. Overexpression of p53 and bcl-2 proteins involved in apoptosis and matrix metalloproteinase 9 involved in basement membrane dissolution has been reported in cancers and associated endometriosis compared with benign control samples [111,112].

Phenotypic transition

Malignant transformation of endometriosis was first reported by Sampson with the following criteria: (1) coexistence of carcinoma and endometriosis of the same ovary; (2) a similar histologic relationship; and (3) exclusion of another primary site [75]. Later, Scott added that benign endometriosis should be contiguous with malignant tissue, but this has rarely been found, owing to sampling technique and possible destruction of benign tissue by tumor invasion [113]. Studies have confirmed, however, histologic transition from endometriosis in direct continuity with tumor and malignant transformation of extra-ovarian endometriosis and cytologically "atypical" endometriosis. Malignant progression of the ovary to endometrioid and clear cell carcinoma in the background of atypical endometriosis is a biologically plausible phenomenon of multidimensional molecular complexity. About 60–80% of cases of endometrioid endometriosis-associated ovarian cancers (EAOCs) arise in the presence of atypical endometriosis. Of these cases, 25% show direct continuity with the atypical ovarian endometriosis [114,115]. Okamura and Katabuchi presented evidence of direct transition from endometriotic gland to atypia to carcinoma in endometrioid carcinoma arising from an ovarian endometriotic cyst [109,116].

In larger studies involving up to 1,000 cases, ovarian cancer was present in 5–10% of ovarian endometriotic lesions [117]. In this study, the ovarian cancers associated with endometriosis were approximately 60% endometrioid and approximately 15% clear cell, proportions much greater than the general make-up of the ovarian cancer population. Interestingly, 40% of 79 women with stage I ovarian cancer had associated endometriosis: 41% of the cases were endometrioid, 31% clear cell, and 18% mixed endometrioid-clear cell. This histologic pattern was corroborated with a combination of clinical and histologic data by Deligdisch et al. [118]. Of the 76 stage I ovarian carcinomas, 54 cases (71%) were nonserous types (endometrioid and clear cell) and 22 (29%) were serous pathology. Ovarian endometriosis was present in 40 of the 76 cases, 39 of which were nonserous carcinomas. Moll et al. reported the occurrence of clear cell carcinoma in a patient with cytologic atypia in the presence of endometriosis within 3 years [119].

Immunogenic modulation

The implantation of ectopic endometriosis on OSE induces a distinct microenvironment in which regulatory signals from multiple cell types affect both intra- and intercellular signal transduction pathways, thereby altering the physiologic homeostasis under which these cells are normally regulated. The principal biologic modulators localized within this microenvironment are growth factors inducing proliferation, cytokines promoting cell activation and proliferation, hormones inducing nuclear factors and inflammatory mediators, and chemokines inducing chemotaxis and cell migration. Based on previous observations, it is increasingly evident that within the endometriosis–ovarian cancer entity, these molecular mediators, along with genetic factors, confer cellular capabilities toward the acquisition of a malignant phenotype. The features of the malignant phenotype were outlined by the landmark publication of Hanahan and Weinberg on the hallmarks of cancer [120]. Accordingly, a cancer cell must have self-sufficiency in growth signals, insensitivity to anti-proliferative signals, resistance to apoptosis, sustained angiogenesis, tissue invasion and metastasis, and genomic instability. Green and Evan theorized that "deregulation of proliferation, together with a reduction of apoptosis, creates a platform that is both necessary and sufficient for cancer" [121]. The subsequent molecular aberrations of endometriosis may explain the possibility of malignant transformation at the ovarian endometriosis foci. Furthermore, it is widely accepted that the OSE harbors pleuripotential embryonic properties, including a capacity to undergo an epithelial–mesenchymal conversion as well as differentiation along the Mullerian duct pathway with characteristics of metaplasia [122].

Cheng et al. offered a molecular explanation for the emergence of Mullerian differentiation in ovarian cancer, including expression of epithelial membrane antigens such as mucins and E-cadherin [107]. The mucin MUC1, used frequently as a marker for preneoplastic lesions and many chronic inflammatory diseases, is present in ovarian endometriosis and is overexpressed and deficiently glycosylated in endometrioid and clear cell carcinoma as well as other ovarian tumors [123]. Expression of E-cadherin emerges in OSE of inclusion cysts and may render OSE cells more susceptible to neoplastic transformation [124]. The frequency of Mullerian differentiation may be a factor in initiation of transformation of the OSE. Molecular aberrations, however, characteristic of the inflammatory processes in endometriosis, may contribute with several survival and growth signals toward malignant transformation of OSE. Endometriosis at the ovary confers an imbalance in the cytokine milieu, inducing surges of immuno-modulatory and growth-stimulating cytokines similar to those observed in ovarian malignancy [125]. In addition, endometriosis drastically changes the hormonal milieu at the ovarian epithelial surface. Thus, endometriosis generates growth signals to which ovarian cancer cells have demonstrated dependency. In theory, the propensity of endometriotic cells to expand clonally, as a result of intrinsic signal pathway anomalies and advanced inflammation mediators, generates an abundant flux of several stimulatory signals, which OSE cells persistently exploit. This results in the induction of progressive transcriptional changes that drive sustained cellular proliferation, increasing the rate of DNA synthesis and repair, and thereby increasing the likelihood of accumulation of mutations in these cells.

Inflammation is central to tumorigenesis. Balkwill and Mantovany offer an elegant description of this link: "If genetic damage is the 'match that lights a fire' of cancer, some types of inflammation may provide 'the fuel that feeds the flames'" [126]. Inflammation is considered to be a hallmark of endometriosis, with local and systemic implications [125]. Local inflammatory reactions at the endometriotic implant site elicit pro-inflammatory protein secretions by associated immune cells as well as cells integral to the implant. The orchestrated aberrant expression of pro-inflammatory IL-l, IL-6, IL-8, and TNF-α alter several physiologic processes leading to cell survival at the endometriosis–ovarian junction. Chronically activated innate immune cells within this microenvironment can regulate intracellular signaling pathways through nuclear factor NF-kB, thus directly promoting transformation by means of paracrine modulation. Indirectly, chronically activated innate immune cells suppress anti-tumor adaptive immune responses. The central role of NF-kB and its activating kinases IKKα and IKKβ in linking cancer to inflammation by differential regulation of cell survival and production of pro-inflammatory cytokines has recently been established [127,128]. In the subsequent sections we will discuss the potential role of the pro-inflammatory interleukins (IL-1, IL-6), transforming growth factor α TGF-α, tumor necrosis factor α TNF-α, the chemokine IL-8, hormones, and growth factors within the endometriosis–ovarian microenvironment.

Interleukin-1

High concentrations of IL-1, produced by macrophages, are found in the peritoneal fluid of women with endometriosis [129]. Interleukin-1β can up-regulate the cyclooxygenase (COX-2) promoter activity in ectopic endometriotic tissue, and, compared with eutopic endometrium, ectopic endometriotic implants from patients with ovarian endometrioma show much higher COX-2 mRNA, possibly contributing to sustained elevation of COX-2 and concomitant prostaglandin-E2 production [130]. This induction of COX-2 expression by IL-1β in ectopic implants is 100 times more sensitive compared with eutopic loci [131]. COX-2 is up-regulated in several cancers and premalignant conditions, and it is thought to contribute to tumor cell proliferation, survival, and angiogenesis. In the ovary, COX-2 is implicated in early events of neoplastic transformation, because it is rarely found in normal OSE but is present in ovarian inclusion cysts (considered to be premalignant). Furthermore, expression levels of COX-2 increase progressively in malignant ovarian tumors [132]. Microarray analysis of cultured ovarian epithelium shows that IL-1 can up-regulate the steroidogenic gene expressing 11β-HSD-1 and suppress the GnRH receptor, thus inducing glucocorticoids and progesterone irresponsiveness, respectively, which may trigger proliferation [132].

Interleukin-6

Inflammation-mediated activation of the transcription factor NF-kB in myeloid cells within the endometriosis–ovarian junction microenvironment leads to up-regulation of many proinflammatory cytokines, including IL-6. Interleukin-6 is secreted by endometriotic peritoneal macrophages as well as ectopic implant cells [133, 134]. Interleukin-6 in conjunction with interferon-γ (IFN-γ) may up-regulate soluble intracellular adhesion molecule 1 (ICAM-1) production by macrophages in patients with endometriosis. Expression of soluble ICAM-l is also up-regulated in ectopic endometrium compared with eutopic endometrium [135], and has been detected at increased levels in the peritoneum of women with endometriosis [136]. High concentrations of soluble ICAM-1 may affect the function of immune cells involved in tumor surveillance by blocking the interaction of lymphocyte function-associated antigen 1 (LFA-I)-positive immune cells, resulting in impaired immune response, thus enabling malignant cells to evade immune surveillance. An increase of serum levels of IL-6 is also noted in women with endometriomas as well as women with malignant ovarian cancer [137].

TGF-α

The peritoneal fluid of women with endometriosis shows increased TGF-α activity that correlates with the stage of endometriosis [138]. TGF-α has been implicated in ovarian tumorigenesis. TGF-α down-regulates c-Myc in normal OSE cells, inhibiting their growth. Ovarian cancer cells lose their responsiveness to TGF-α. It has been postulated that ovarian cancer cells acquire selective advantage by expressing a functional tumor-promoting TGF-α signaling pathway leading to the inherent loss of c-Myc down-regulation and loss of the growth inhibition by means of p 15 INK4b [139].

TNF-α

Tumor necrosis factor alpha is produced by peritoneal macrophages and endometriotic lesions. It has been shown to promote endometrial cell proliferation, adhesion, and angiogenesis. Concentrations of TNF-α are elevated in the serum of women with endometriomas and those with ovarian malignancy. The TNF-α levels are increased in the fluid of malignant ovarian cysts compared with endometriomas and benign ovarian tumors [140]. Recent studies allude to the importance of the TNF-α/IKKα signaling pathway in linking inflammation to cancer by inducing evasion of apoptosis and insensitivity of anti-growth signals [128]. TNF-α has been implicated in the promotion and progression of premalignant cells by activation of the NF-kB-dependent anti-apoptotic pathway in magnitude and duration. In vitro studies by Kulbe et al. [141] show that TNF-α, produced in an autocrine manner by ovarian cancer cell lines, leads to the stimulation of the angiogenic vascular endothelial growth factor (VEGF), IL-6, the chemokine CCL2, and the chemokine CXCLl2. These mediators form a close network of interactions, where TNF-α acts as an inducer of VEGF, which induces the chemokine CXCL12, all contributing to stimulation of neovascularization in ovarian cancer. Clearly, inflammatory mediators such as TNF-α can up-regulate VEGF; however, VEGF in itself is shown to affect the inflammatory process by inducing peripheral blood mononuclear cells to produce increased levels of TNF-α and IL-6, as well as by augmenting the TH1 phenotype leading to an increase in IL-2 and IFN-γ [142]. The peritoneal fluid of patients with endometriosis contains increased VEGF concentrations compared with normal subjects [143], consistent with the finding that peritoneal T cells of women with endometriosis express predominantly IL-2 and IFN-γ.

Moreover, stimulation of ovarian epithelial cells and ovarian cancer cell lines with TNF-α leads to the up-regulation of CXCR4, the receptor for CXCLl2. The expression of the chemokine receptor CXCR4 is thought to increase survival and metastatic potential of epithelial ovarian cells by means of NF-kB, resulting in increased proliferation under suboptimal conditions [141]. Clearly, ovarian cancer cells are dependent on a constitutive network of tumor-promoting cytokines and angiogenic factors sustained by TNF-α. Within the endometriosis–ovarian milieu, high TNF-α levels could be maintained by the endometriotic implant, contributing and perhaps in some instances promoting growth in OSE cells.

Furthermore, TNF-α differentially modulates the expression of adhesion molecule CD44 in ovarian cancer cells in vitro [144]. CD44 is a membrane receptor, with many isoforms playing differential roles in cell proliferation, adhesion, motility, and metastasis by means of the PAKI signaling pathway. CD44 is found associated with HER2/neu in ovarian cancer cells, and signaling derived through this association is considered to be important in the development of ovarian malignancies [145]. *HER2/neu* is overexpressed in most ovarian cancers [146,147].

Interleukin-8

IL-8 is a proinflammatory chemokine unique to humans. It is a macrophage-derived protein that triggers rapid migration of neutrophils. Ectopic endometrial cells express high concentrations of IL-8 [148]. Peritoneal fluid of women with endometriosis contains high concentrations of IL-8, derived largely from peritoneal macrophages [133]. Although peripheral blood concentrations of IL-8 are not related to the presence of endometriosis, this cytokine shows increased levels in the cyst fluid of endometriomas and ovarian carcinomas, with highest concentrations observed in the fluid of malignant ovarian cysts [137]. It has been demonstrated that activation of the *RAS* proto-oncogene can up-regulate IL-8, resulting in inflammatory activity at tumor sites, angiogenesis, and tumor growth [149]. Furthermore, IL-8 has been shown to increase soluble Fas ligand in endometriotic lesions, thus inducing apoptosis of T cells relevant to immune-mediated cell death, consequently increasing the chance of malignant cells to evade immune surveillance within the ovarian endometriosis foci [150].

Endocrine factors

Both endometriotic cell components and ovarian surface epithelium have the capacity to undergo proliferation in response to endocrine and growth factors. In that respect, an important aberration of ectopic endometrial cells, namely, the pathologic expression of P450 aromatase, triggers constitutive expression of estradiol (E2) [151]. A second anomaly of this tissue is the lack of the enzyme 17β-HSD-2, which converts E2 to estrone, leading to further accumulation of E2. Elevated estrogen levels stimulate COX-2 production in these cells, leading to an increase of prostaglandin-E production, which in turn stimulates further aromatase activity contributing to the constitutive production of E2. Prostaglandin-E2 is itself implicated in tumor progression, and ovarian tumors are shown to contain increased levels of this prostaglandin [152]. Additionally, ectopic endometriotic cells express low levels of the progesterone receptor isoform A and none of isoform B, rendering these cells unresponsive to progesterone and prone to proliferation, thus increasing levels of E2 in the microenvironment [152]. A marked reduction in expression of the two progesterone receptor isoforms is also noted in ovarian carcinoma specimens, leading to unresponsiveness of those cells to progesterone and thus increasing the possibility for proliferation [153,154]. The estrogen-rich environment created by endometriotic cells may also trigger increased responsiveness to E2 in malignant ovarian epithelia by means of altered expression of estrogen receptors in those cells, thus further propagating the growth of malignant cells [155]. Estradiol has also been shown to regulate the production of IL-6 in malignant human OSE cells, promoting growth of these cells in an autocrine manner [156]. Importantly, in vitro studies of immortalized OSE cells demonstrate estrogen-mediated up-regulation of hTERT by means of direct and indirect stimulation of the hTERT promoter, enabling these cells to achieve malignancy [157]. Clearly, high estrogen levels persist in the microenvironment created by the presence of an endometriotic implant at the ovary, generating a highly altered physiologic milieu surrounding the OSE. This suggests proliferative pressure with an enhanced level of DNA synthesis and repair and thus a higher chance of DNA damage and mutations. Specific changes in hormone receptors and enzyme expressions in transformed OSE cells continually exposed to nonphysiologic hormonal conditions may lead to further progression to malignancy.

Growth factors

Increased estrogen levels associated with the proximity of endometriotic cells may trigger up-regulation of insulin-like growth factor (IGF)-binding proteins in OSE cells, leading to estrogen-induced growth [158]. IGF-1 signaling in these cells may be altered by the higher levels of plasma IGF-1 shown in severe cases of endometriosis and the higher levels of IGF-l in the peritoneal fluid of women with endometriosis [159,160]. Up-regulation of IGF-l has been shown to inhibit apoptosis in normal human OSE cells after hCG exposure [161]. Thus, in the presence of endometriosis, dysregulation of IGF-l–mediated signaling may also be a potential factor in the induction of proliferative activity of OSE.

In addition to IGF-l, the peritoneal fluid of women with endometriosis contains significantly higher levels of several other growth factors compared with patients without endometriosis. In severe endometriosis, high levels of hepatocyte growth factor (HGF) in the peritoneal fluid have been reported [162]. During normal OSE development, a paracrine interaction between HGF and its receptor, Met, is necessary in ovarian physiology; however, this balance is perturbed in ovarian cancer cells, and the generation of an autocrine HGF-Met loop confers malignant transformation of the OSE. High peritoneal levels of HGF in the presence of endometriosis may trigger a similar imbalance, resulting in mitogenic activity of OSE.

This is supported by the fact that high levels of HGF are also present in the fluid of malignant ovarian cysts compared with benign cysts and that Met is expressed in high levels in 28% of epithelial ovarian cancer and levels of expression increase in differentiated ovarian carcinomas compared with normal OSE [163,164,165]. In addition, in patients with hereditary ovarian cancer, enhanced stability of c-Met and HGF secretion are implicated as early factors in ovarian carcinogenesis [166]. Platelet-derived growth factor has also been identified in the peritoneal fluid of women with endometriosis, and this growth factor significantly enhances the proliferation of human OSE cells in a dose-dependent manner [167,168].

In summary, these key inflammatory modulators, hormones, and growth factors are maintained at high levels by immune and endometriotic cells at the ovarian endometriosis foci. The resulting microenvironment is similar to that found in ovarian cancer, and malignant OSE cells are shown to use these modulators for proliferation, evasion of apoptosis, and evasion of immune surveillance. It is reasonable to surmise that sustained elevation of these biologic modulators in the ovarian endometriosis microenvironment may promote malignant transformation in susceptible OSE cells (Fig. 14.1).

Clinical implications

Diagnosis of endometriosis

Owing to its malignant potential, endometriosis requires particular vigilance during diagnosis and treatment. Routine imaging studies have not been able to diagnose either endometriosis or malignant transformation of endometriotic disease. However, recently, magnetic resonance imaging evidence of malignant transformation within an endometrioma has been suggested. The finding that was most important for a diagnosis of malignant change was the presence of one or more contrast material-enhanced mural nodules within a cystic mass. Enlargement of the endometrioma and the disappearance of shading within the mass on T_2-weighted images may be suggestive of malignant transformation [169].

Diagnosis has thus far been limited to direct observation through surgery; the appearance of endometriosis has been described as having a protean, or widely varied, appearance, making a gold standard for diagnosis difficult. Proteomic techniques are now being used to identify proteins that are potential biomarkers for the disease. This strategy uses mass spectrometry to identify, purify, and sequence proteins directly rather than through mRNA and complementary DNA intermediates. Identifying an accurate marker will be challenging, owing to the likely multifactorial etiology of endometriosis and the variations between individuals and varying influences of steroid hormones during the menstrual cycle. However, proteomic profiling in combination with bioinformatics software has the potential for major diagnostic contributions for the endometriosis disease process [170]. These updated techniques may have a complementary role in diagnosing patients with endometriosis, and thus a population with an increased cancer risk.

Treatment of endometriosis

The correlation of endometriosis and malignancy may require earlier and more meticulous surgical intervention for complete disease treatment. Currently, there are no established recommendations for women with endometriosis who have completed childbearing. Special consideration should be given toward bilateral oophorectomy in women with endometriosis undergoing hysterectomy near the age of menopause, especially those with a history of infertility, a family history of ovarian and breast cancer, or ovarian hyperovulation stimulation. Endometriosis should be treated by surgical intervention in conjunction with hormone suppression. Surgical approaches for pelvic pain consist of either conservative or extirpative management. Efficacy of surgical treatment of endometriosis for chronic pelvic pain and infertility is well established [171–174]. A literature review in 2007 by Bosteels et al. accepted that enough evidence exists to incorporate the use of diagnostic laparoscopy in the current fertility practice [175].

Conservative surgical techniques may be used for reproductive preservation to restore anatomic relationships by division of adhesions, excision of peritoneal implants, resection of ovarian lesions, restoration of the cul-de-sac, uterosacral nerve ablation, and/or presacral neurectomy. Because endometriosis appears to be estrogen dependent, any kind of oral hormonal therapy will improve pain and can be used as adjuvant therapy after surgical resection of endometrial implants. The extirpative approach to surgical management consists of hysterectomy and bilateral salpingo-oophorectomy in cases of failed conservative therapy or undesired fertility. Retention of any ovarian tissue continues estrogen stimulation of endometrial implants and shows increased rates of symptom recurrence or further surgery. Postoperative hormone replacement therapy in patients with endometriosis after extirpative surgical management remains controversial, particularly in severe cases and those with residual endometriosis after resection. Unopposed estrogen in posthysterectomy patients may still hold a risk due to possible degeneration of endometrial foci from normal to hyperplastic, atypical, or malignant epithelium. Therefore, postoperative hormone replacement in women with known residual endometriosis may benefit from the addition of progestins. Hormone replacement therapy after radical surgery can be initiated with progestins followed by combined estrogen-progesterone. Although use of progestins has not been shown to increase the risk of malignant transformation in endometriosis foci, it must be noted that multiple lines of evidence do suggest that regimens with both estrogen and progesterone versus estrogen alone are associated with greater risk of breast cancer [176]. Therefore, patient counseling and treatment individualization is highly recommended. There are also case reports of endometrioid carcinomas arising from ovarian endometriosis in women on tamoxifen therapy [177]. Therefore, women with endometriosis on tamoxifen may benefit from increased surveillance. Aromatase inhibitors have also shown significant benefit in reducing pelvic pain due to endometriosis. One pilot study showed laparoscopic evidence of eradication of pelvic implants and pelvic pain reduction. Phase II clinical trials have concluded that aromatase inhibitors: (1) effectively treat endometriosis-induced pelvic pain resistant to first-line therapies; (2) are the agent of choice for post-menopausal endometriosis; (3) should be used in combination with a GnRH analog progestin, or combination oral contraceptive for ovarian suppression; and (4) have side effect profiles that are favorable and, for most regimens, do not include bone loss [178,179].

Causal relationship and clinical patterns

In a clinical and histologic correlation study of endometriosis and ovarian cancer by Deligdisch et al., ovarian endometriosis was present in 40 out of 76 ovarian carcinoma cases [118]. Of the 54 patients with non-serous carcinomas, 100% had associated endometriosis. Two recent studies have addressed in a systematic manner the published reviews on association between endometriosis and ovarian cancer [180,181]. The results revealed that seven of eight studies suggest a modest increase in ovarian cancer risk with an odds ratio of 1.32–1.90 [180]. This current evidence may not be sufficient to establish a cancer relationship between the two; however, there is substantial evidence to demonstrate the transformation of endometriotic foci to the endometrioid and clear-cell type of ovarian cancer. Most recently, Wiegland et al. found mutations in the tumor-suppressor gene ARID1A in endometrioid and clear cell carcinomas and none in serous ovarian cancer and showed the same mutation to be present in atypical endometriosis and associated ovarian carcinomas in two patients [182].

While none of these findings are sufficient to recommend mutations screening test in patients with endometriosis and changing the treatment to aggressive surgical debulking of mutation positive endometriotic lesions, gynecologists as well as general practitioners must be mindful of the apparently increased risk of ovarian cancer among endometriosis patients. At the present time, in the absence of sensitive imaging and tumor markers for preoperative diagnosis, vigilant follow-up of these patients is warranted and recommended. Moreover, with recent advancements in ovarian cancer understanding a dualistic model of ovarian cancer pathogenesis has emerged. This model divides ovarian carcinomas into high-grade, serous carcinomas presenting at advanced stage, possibly developing from tubal epithelium and harboring *TP53* mutations and low grade serous, endometrioid and clear cell carcinomas that present as early stage, indolent tumors characterized by PTEN and/or ARID1A mutation likely arising from endometriosis. Therefore, women with endometriosis-associated cancer most likely represent a unique subgroup of ovarian cancer patients, perhaps requiring a different screening approach and different therapy. For example, in this group of women screening strategies may allow for early detection of cancer, while the group of high-grade serous ovarian carcinomas developing from tubal epithelium always presents as advanced stage disease and early detection is not feasible. Likewise, the treatment of these two subgroups of ovarian carcinomas should be directed toward different molecular targets.

Conclusions

Although not yet fully delineated, there is a strong relationship between endometriosis and ovarian cancer. Gynecologists as well as general practitioners must be mindful of the apparently increased risk of ovarian cancer among endometriosis patients. Special attention should be paid to patients with early endometriosis diagnosis, a long-standing history of disease, and associated infertility and/or infertility treatment as these patients seem to be at the highest risk. Advancements in more precise diagnostic analysis into the pathogenesis of endometriosis and the possibility of malignant transformation may help to provide new insights into diagnostic and treatment modalities. Specifically, further elucidation of the involved genetic and immune mechanisms of endometriosis is necessary. Overall once the transition from benign endometriosis to atypical and malignant tissue is clearly elucidated, marker expression can be analyzed to guide clinical management and outcome. Genomics and proteomics may facilitate the development of these diagnostic tools. At this time, however, surgical resection followed by medical treatment remains the primary method of treatment of endometriosis. With the correlation of endometriosis and ovarian cancer continuing to strengthen over time, appropriate and timely resection and elimination of disease should be practiced.

References

1. Eskenazi B, Warner ML. Epidemiology of endometriosis. Obstet Gynecol Clin North Am. 1997;**24**:235–58.
2. Zhao SZ, Wong JM, Davis MB, et al. The cost of inpatient endometriosis treatment: an analysis based on the Healthcare Cost and Utilization Project Nationwide Inpatient Sample. Am J Manag Care. 1998;**4**:1127–34.
3. Barrier BF, Kendall BS, Ryan CE, et al. HLA-G is expressed by the glandular epithelium of peritoneal endometriosis but not in eutopic endometrium. Hum Reprod. 2006;**21**:864–69.
4. Shroen D. Disputatio inauguralis medica de ulceribus uteri. Lena: Krebs; 1690. p 6–17.
5. Knapp VJ. How old is endometriosis? Late 17th- and 18th-century European descriptions of the disease. Fertil Steril. 1999;**72**:10–14.
6. Iwanoff NS. Dusiges cystenhaltigesuterusfibromyom compliciert durch sarcom und carcinom. (Adenofibromyoma cysticum sarcomatodes carcinomatosum). Monatsch Geburtshilfe Gynakol. 1898;7:295–300.
7. Levander G, Normann P. The pathogenesis of endometriosis. An experimental study. Acta Obstet Gynecol Scand. 1955;**34**:366–98.
7. Merrill JA. Endometrial induction of endometriosis across Millipore filters. Am J Obstet Gynecol. 1966;**94**:780–90.
8. Russell WW. Aberrant portions of the mullerian duct found in an ovary. Ovarian cysts of mullerian origin. Bull Johns Hopkins Hosp. 1899;**10**:8.
9. Suginami H. A reappraisal of the coelomic metaplasia theory by

reviewing endometriosis occurring in unusual sites and instances. Am J Obstet Gynecol. 1991;**165**:214–18.

10. Matsuura K, Ohtake H, Katabuchi H, Okamura H. Coelomic metaplasia theory of endometriosis: evidence from in vivo studies and an in vitro experimental model. Gynecol Obstet Invest. 1999;**47**(Suppl I):18–22.

11. Batt RE, Smith RA. Embryologic theory of histogenesis of endometriosis in peritoneal pockets. Obstet Gynecol Clin North Am. 1989;**16**:15.

12. Halban J. Metastatic hysteroadenosis. Wien Klin Wochenschr. 1924;**37**:1205–6.

13. Rosenfeld DL, Lecher BD. Endometriosis in a patient with Rokitansky-Kuster-Hauser syndrome. Am J Obstet Gynecol. 1981;**139**:105.

14. Schrodt GR, Alcorn MO, Ibanez J. Endometriosis of the male urinary system: a case report. J Urol. 1980;**124**:722–3.

15. Oliker AI, Harris AE. Endometriosis of the bladder in a male patient. J Urol. 1971;**106**:858–9.

16. Sampson JA. Metastatic or embolic endometriosis, due to menstrual dissemination of endometrial tissue into venous circulation. Am J Pathol. 1927;**3**:93.

17. Iavert CT. Observations on the pathology and spread of endometriosis based on the theory of benign metastasis. Am J Obstet Gynecol. 1951;**62**:477–87.

18. Ueki M. Histologic study of endometriosis and examination of lymphatic drainage in and from the uterus. Am J Obstet Gynecol. 1991;**165**:201–9.

19. Iavert CT. The spread of benign and malignant endometrium in the lymphatic system with a note of coexisting vascular involvement. Am J Obstet Gynecol. 1952;**64**:780–806.

20. Iubanyik KI, Comite F. Extrapelvic endometriosis. Obstet Gynecol Clin North Am. 1997;**24**:411–40.

21. Sampson JA. Perforating hemorrhagic (chocolate) cysts of the ovary; their importance and especially their relation to pelvic adenomas of endometrial type (adenomyoma of the uterus, rectovaginal septum, sigmoid, etc.). Arch Surg. 1921;**3**:245–323.

22. Sampson JA. Peritoneal endometriosis due to menstrual dissemination of endometrial tissue into the peritoneal cavity. Am J Obstet Gynecol. 1927;**14**:442–69.

23. Halme I, Hammond MG, Hulka JF, et al. Retrograde menstruation in healthy women and in patients with endometriosis. Obstet Gynecol. 1984;**64**:151–4.

24. Sanflilippo JS, Wakim NG, Schikler KN, et al. Endometriosis in association with uterine anomaly. Am J Obstet Gynecol. 1986;**154**:39–43.

25. Abuzeid M, Sakhel K, Ashraf M, et al. The association between uterine septum and infertility. Fertil Steril. 2005;**84** (Suppl l):S472.

26. D'Hooghe TM, Bambra CS, Suleman MA, et al. Development of a model of retrograde menstruation in baboons (*Papio anubis*). Fertil Steril. 1994;**62**:635–8.

27. Ridley JH, Edwards IK. Experimental endometriosis in the human. Am J Obstet Gynecol. 1958;**76**:783–90.

28. Dmowski WP, Radwanska E. Current concepts on pathology, histogenesis and etiology of endometriosis. Acta Obstet Gynecol Scand. 1984;**123** (Suppl):29–33.

29. Al-Fozan H, Tulandi T. Left lateral predisposition of endometriosis and endometrioma. Obstet Gynecol. 2003;**10**(1):164–6.

30. Vercellini P, Aimi G, de Giorgi O, et al. Is cystic ovarian endometriosis an asymmetric disease? Br J Obstet Gynaecol. 1998;**105**:1018–21.

31. Vercellini P, Busaca M, Aimi G, et al. Lateral distribution of recurrent ovarian endometriotic cysts. Fertil Steril. 2002;**77**:848–9.

32. Vercellini P, Pisacreta A, Vicentini S, et al. Lateral distribution of non endometriotic benign ovarian cysts. Br J Obstet Gynaecol. 2000;**107**:556–8.

33. Chapron C, Chopin N, Borghese B, et al. Deeply infiltrating endometriosis: pathogenetic implications of the anatomical distribution. Hum Reprod. **21**:1839–45.

34. Jenkins S, Olive DL, Haney AF. Endometriosis: pathogenetic implications of the anatomic distribution. Obstet Gynecol. 1986;**67**:335–8.

35. Dinulescu DM, Ince TA, Quade BI, et al. Role of K-ras and Pten in the development of mouse models of endometriosis and endometrioid cancer. Nat Med. 2005;**1**:63–70.

36. Bulletti C, de Ziegler D, Stefanetti M, et al. Endometriosis: absence of recurrence in patients after endometrial ablation. Hum Reprod. 2001;**16**:2676–9.

37. Rock JA, Parmley TH, King TM, et al. Endometriosis and the development of tuboperitoneal fistulas after tubal ligation. Fertil Steril. 1981;**35**:16–20.

38. Morrissey K, Idriss N, Nieman L, et al. Dysmenorrhea after bilateral tubal ligation: a case of retrograde menstruation. Obstet Gynecol. 2002;**100**:1065–7.

39. Lucidi RS, Witz CA, Chrisco MS, et al. A novel in vitro model of the early endometriotic lesion demonstrates that attachment of endometrial cells to mesothelial cells is dependent on the source of endometrial cells. Fertil Steril. 2005;**84**:16–21.

40. Simpson JL, Elias S, Malinak LR, Buttram VC Jr. Heritable aspects of endometriosis, I: genetic studies. Am J Obstet Gynecol. 1980;**137**:327–31.

41. Hadfield RM, Mardon HI, Barlow DH, Kennedy SH. Endometriosis in monozygotic twins. Fertil Steril. 1997;**68**:941–2.

42. Treloar SA, O'Connor DT, O'Connor VM, et al. Genetic influences on endometriosis in an Australian twin sample. Fertil Steril. 1999;**71**:701–10.

43. Stefansson H, Geirsson RT, Steinthorsdottir V, et al. Genetic factors contribute to the risk of developing endometriosis. Hum Reprod. 2002;**17**:555–9.

44. Zondervan KT, Weeks DE, Colman R, et al. Familial aggregation of endometriosis in a large pedigree of rhesus macaques. Hum Reprod. 2004;**19**:448–55.

45. Treloar SA, Wicks I, Nyholt DR, et al. Genomewide linkage study in 1,176 affected sister pair families identifies a significant susceptibility locus for endometriosis on chromosome 10q26. Am J Hum Genet. 2005;**77**:365–76.

46. Kitawaki I, Kado N, Ishihara H, et al. Endometriosis: the pathophysiology as an estrogen-dependent disease. Steroid Biochem Mol Biol. 2003;**83**:149–55.

47. Noble A, Simpson SE, Johns A, et al. Aromatase expression in endometriosis. J Clin Endocrinol Metab. 1996;**81**:174–9.

48. Zeitoun K, Takayma K, Sasano H, et al. Deficient 17fJhydroxysteroid dehydrogenase type 2 expression in

endometriosis-derived stromal cells. J Clin Endocrinol Metab. 1998;**83**:4474–80.

49. Bulun SE, Cheng YH, Yin P, et al. Progesterone resistance in endometriosis: link to failure to metabolize estradiol. Mol Cell Endocrinol. 2006;**248**:94–103.
50. Osteen KG, Bruner-Tran KL, Eisenberg E. Reduced progesterone action during endometrial maturation: a potential risk factor for the development of endometriosis. Fertil Steril. 2005;**83**:529–37.
51. Rier SE, Martin DC, Bowman RE, et al. Endometriosis in rhesus monkeys (*Maccaca mulatta*) following chronic exposure to 2,3,7,8tetrachlorodibenzo-p-dioxin. Pundam Appl Toxicol. 1993;**21**:431–41.
52. Birnbaum LS. The mechanism of dioxin toxicity: relationship to risk assessment. Environ Health Perspect. 1994;**102** (Suppl 9):157–67.
53. Hinsdill RD, Couch DL, Speirs RS. Immunosuppression in mice induced by dioxin (TCDD) in feed. J Environ Pathol Toxicol. 1980;**4**:401–25.
54. Guo SW. The link between exposure to dioxin and endometriosis: a critical reappraisal of primate data. Gynecol Obstet Invest. 2004;**57**:157–73.
55. Igarashi TM, Bruner-Tran KL, Yeaman GR, et al. Reduced expression of progesterone receptor-B in the endometrium of women with endometriosis and in cocultures of endometrial cells exposed to 2,3,7,8-tetrachlorodibenzo-p-dioxin. Fertil Steril. 2005;**84**:67–74.
56. Guo SW, Wu Y, Strawn E, et al. Genomic alterations in the endometrium may be a proximate cause for endometriosis. Eur J Obstet Gynecol Reprod Biol. 2004;**116**:89–99.
57. Wu Y, Strawn E, Basir Z, et al. Genomic alterations in ectopic and eutopic endometrial of women with endometriosis. Gynecol Obstet Invest. 2006;**62**:148–59.
58. Demir Weusten AY, Groothuis PG, Dunselman GA, et al. Morphological changes in mesothelial cells induced by shed menstrual endometrium in vitro are not primarily due to apoptosis or necrosis. Hum Reprod. 2000;**15**:1462–8.
59. Groothuis PG, Koks CA, De Goeij AF, et al. Adhesion of human endometrial fragments to peritoneum in vitro. Fertil Steril. 1999;**71**:1119–24.
60. Kyama CM, Overbergh L, Debrock S, et al. Increased peritoneal and endometrial gene expression of biologically relevant cytokines and growth factors during the menstrual phase in women with endometriosis. Fertil Steril. 2006;**85**:1667–75.
61. Nap AW, Groothuis PG, Demir AY, et al. Tissue integrity is essential for ectopic implantation of human endometrium in the chicken chorioallantoic membrane. Hum Reprod. 2003;**18**:30–4.
62. Oosterlynck DJ, Cornillie FJ, Waer M, et al. Women with endometriosis show a defect in natural killer activity resulting in a decreased cytotoxicity to autologous endometrium. Fertil Steril. 1991;**56**:45–51.
63. Somigliana S, Vigano P, Gaffuri B, et al. Human endometrial stromal cells as a source of soluble intercellular adhesion molecule (ICAM)-l molecules. Hum Reprod. 1996;**11**:1190–4.
64. Tseng JF, Ryan IP, Milam TD, et al. Interleukin-6 secretion in vitro is up-regulated in ectopic and eutopic endometrial stromal cells from women with endometriosis. J Clin Endoerinol Metab. 1996;**81**:1118–22.
65. Velasco I, Rueda J, Acien P. Aromatase expression in endometriotic tissues and cell cultures of patients with endometriosis. Mol Hum Reprod. 2006;**12**:377–81.
66. Sharpe-Timms KL, Piva M, Ricke EA, et al. Endometriosis synthesizes and secretes a haptoglobinlike protein. Biol Reprod. 1998;**58**:988–94.
67. Sharpe-Timms KL, Zimmer RL, Ricke EA, et al. Endometriotic haptoglobin binds to peritoneal macrophages and alters their function in women with endometriosis. Fertil Steril. 2002;**78**:810–19.
68. Ryan IP, Tseng JF, Schriock ED, et al. Interleukin-8 concentrations are elevated in peritoneal fluid of women with endometriosis. Fertil Steril. 1995;**63**:929–32.
69. Khorram O, Taylor RN, Ryan IP, et al. Peritoneal fluid concentrations of the cytokine RANTES correlate with the severity of endometriosis. Am J Obstet Gynecol. 1993;**169**:1545–9.
70. Akoum A, Lemay A, McColl S, et al. Elevated concentration and biologic activity of monocyte chemotactic protein-1 in the peritoneal fluid of patients with endometriosis. Fertil Steril. 1996;**66**:17–23.
71. Oosterlynck D, Meuleman M, Waer M, et al. Transforming growth factor-B activity is increased in peritoneal fluid from women with endometriosis. Obstet Gyneeol. 1994;**83**:287–92.
72. Hsu CC, Yang BC, Wu MH, Huang KE. Enhanced interleukin-4 expression in patients with endometriosis. Fertil Steril. 1997;**67**:1059–64.
73. Gazvani R, Templeton A. New considerations for the pathogenesis of endometriosis. Int J Gyn Obstet. 2002;**76**:117–26.
74. Olive DL, Schwartz LG. Endometriosis. N Engl J Med. 1993;**328**:1759–69.
75. Sampson JA. Peritoneal endometriosis due to the menstrual dissemination of endometrial tissue into the peritoneal cavity. Am J Obstet Gynecol. 1927;**14**:422–69.
76. Sampson JA. Endometrial carcinoma of ovary arising in endometrial tissue in that organ. Arch Surg. 1925;**10**:1–72.
77. Van Gorp T, Amant F, Vergote NP. Endometriosis and the development of malignant tumors of the pelvis. A review of literature. Best Pract Res Clin Obstet Gynaecol. 2004;**18**:349–71.
78. Brinton LA, Gridley G, Persson I, Baron J, Bergqvist A. Cancer risk after a hospital discharge diagnosis of endometriosis. Am J Obstet Gynecol. 1997;**176**:572–9.
79. Borgfeldt C, Andolf E. Cancer risk after hospital discharge diagnosis of benign ovarian cysts and endometriosis. Acta Obstet Gynecol Scand. 2004;**83**:395–400.
80. Brinton LA, Lamb EJ, Moghissi KS, et al. Ovarian cancer risk associated with varying causes of infertility. Fertil Steril. 2004;**82**:405–14.
81. Brinton LA, Westhoff CL, Scoccia B, et al. Causes of infertility as predictors of subsequent cancer risk. Epidemiology. 2005;**16**:500–7.
82. Melin A, Sparen P, Persson I, Bergqvist A. Endometriosis and the risk of cancer with special emphasis on ovarian cancer. Hum Reprod. 2006;**21**:1237–42.
83. Melin A, Sparen P, Bergqvust A. The risk of cancer and the role of parity among women with endometriosis. Hum Reprod. 2007;**22**:3021–6.
84. Olson JE, Cerhan JR, Janney CA, et al. Postmenopausal cancer risk after self-

reported endometriosis diagnosis in the Iowa Women's Health Study. Cancer. 2002;**94**:1612–18.

85. Kondi-Pafiti A, Papakoulantinou E, Iavazzo C, et al. Clinicopathologic characteristics of ovarian cancer associated with endometriosis. Arch Gynecol Obstet. 2012;**285**:479–83.

86. Valenzuela P, Ramos P, Redondo S, et al. Endometrioid adenocarcinomas of the ovary and endometriosis. Eur J Obstet Gynaecol Reprod Biol. 2007;**134**:83–6.

87. Heaps JM, Nieberg RK, Berek JS. Malignant neoplasms arising in endometriosis. Obstet Gynecol. 1990;**75**:1023–8.

88. Modessit SC, Tortoleo-Luna G, Robinson JB, et al. Ovarian and extraovarian endometriosis-associated cancer. Obstet Gynecol. 2002; **100**:788–95.

89. Benoit L, Arnould L, Cheynel N, et al. Malignant extraovarian endometriosis: a review. Eur J Surg Oncol. 2006;**32**:6–11.

90. Ness RB, Grisso JA, Cottreau, Klapper J, et al. Factors related to inflammation of the ovarian epithelium and risk of ovarian cancer. Epidemiology. 2000; **II**:111–17.

91. Ness RB, Cramer OW, Goodman MT, et al. Infertility, fertility drugs, and ovarian cancer: a pooled analysis of case-control studies. Am J Epidemiol. 2002;**155**:217–24.

92. Vigano P, Somigliana E, Parazzini F, et al. Bias versus causality: interpreting recent evidence of association between endometriosis and ovarian cancer. Fertil Steril. 2007;**88**:588–93.

93. Bischoff FZ, Simpson JL. Heritability and molecular genetic studies of endometriosis. Hum Reprod Update. 2000;**6**:37–44.

94. Wu Y, Basir Z, Kajdacsy-Balla A, et al. Resolution of clonal origins for endometriotic lesions using laser capture microdissection and the human androgen receptor assay (HUMARA). Fertil Steril. 2003;**79**:710–17.

95. Varma R, Rollason T, Gupta JK, Maher E. Endometriosis and the neoplastic process. Reproduction. 2004;**127**:293–304.

96. Nilbert M, Pejovic T, Mandahl N, et al. Monoclonal origin of endometriotic cysts. Int J Cancer. 1995;**5**:61–3.

97. Wells M. Recent advances in endometriosis with emphasis on pathogenesis, molecular pathology, and neoplastic transformation. Int J Gynecol Pathol. 2004;**23**:316–20.

98. Taylor RN, Lundeen SG, Giudice LC. Emerging role of genomics in endometriosis research. Fertil Steril. 2002;**78**:694–8.

99. Gogusev J, Bouquet de Jolinière J, Telvi L, et al. Detection of DNA copy number changes in human endometriosis by comparative genomic hybridization. Hum Genet. 1999;**105**(5):444–51.

100. Veiga-Castelli LC, Silva JC, Meola J, et al. Genomic alterations detected by comparative genomic hybridization in ovarian endometriomas. Braz J Med Biol Res. 2010;**43**(8):799–805.

101. Uzan C, Darai E, Valent A, et al. Status of HER1 and HER2 in peritoneal, ovarian and colorectal endometriosis and ovarian endometrioid adenocarcinoma. Virchows Arch. 2009;**454**(5):525–9.

102. Bisdroff FZ, Heard M, Simpson JL. Somatic DNA alterations in endometriosis: high frequency of chromosome 17 and p53 loss in late stage endometriosis. J Reprod Immunol. 2002;**55**:49–64.

103. Sato N, Tsunoda H, Nishida M, et al. Loss of heterozygosity on 10q23.3 and mutations of the tumor suppressor gene PTEN in benign endometrial cyst of the ovary: possible sequence progression from benign endometrial cyst to endometriod carcinoma and clear cell carcinoma of the ovary. Cancer Res. 2000;**60**:7052–6.

104. Dinulescu OM, Ince TA, Quade BJ, et al. Role of K-ras and PTEN in the development of mouse models of endometriosis and endometrioid ovarian cancer. Nat Med. 2005;**11**:63–70.

105. Matzuk MM. Gynecologic diseases get their genes. Nat Med. 2005;**II**:24–6.

106. Orsulic S, Li Y, Soslow R, et al. Induction of ovarian cancer by defined multiple genetic changes in a mouse model. Cancer Cell. 2002;**1**:53–62.

107. Cheng W, Lui J, Yoshida H, et al. Lineage infidelity of epithelial ovarian cancers is controlled by HOX genes that specify regional identity in the reproductive tract. Nat Med. 2005;**11**:531–7.

108. Martini M, Ciccarone M, Garganese G, et al. Possible involvement of hMLHJ, pJ6(INK4a) and PTEN in the malignant transformation of endometriosis. Int J Cancer. 2002;**102**:398–406.

109. Okamura H, Katabuchi H. Pathophysiological dynamics of human ovarian surface epithelial cells in epithelial ovarian carcinogenesis. Int Rev Cytol. 2005;**242**:1–54.

110. Ogawa S, Kaku T, Amada S, et al. Ovarian endometriosis associated with ovarian carcinoma: a clinicopathological and immunohistochemical study. Gynecol Oncol. 2000;**77**:298–304.

111. Nezhat F, Cohen C, Rahaman J, et al. Comparative immunocytochemical studies or bcl-2 and p53 proteins in benign and malignant ovarian endometriotic cysts. Cancer. 2002;**94**:2935–40.

112. Chung H, When Y, Chun S, et al. Matrix metalloproteinase-9 and tissue inhibitor of metalloproteinase-3 mRNA expression in ectopic and eutopic endometrium in women with endometriosis: a rationale for endometriotic invasiveness. Fertil Steril. 2001;**75**:152–9.

113. Scott RB. Malignant change in endometriosis. Obstet Gynecol. 1953;**2**:283–9.

114. Stern RC, Dash R, Bentley RC, et al. Malignancy in endometriosis: frequency and comparison of ovarian and extraovarian types. Int J Gynecol Pathol. 2001;**20**:133–9.

115. Erzen M, Kovacic J. Relationship between endometriosis and ovarian cancer. Eur J Gynaecol Oncol. 1998;**19**:553–5.

116. Okamura H, Katabuchi H. Detailed morphology of the human ovarian surface epithelium focusing on its metaplastic and neoplastic capability. Ital J Anat Embriol. 2001;**106**(Suppl 2):263–76.

117. Sainz de la Cuesta R, Eichhorn JH, Rice LW, et al. Malignant neoplasms arising in endometriosis to early epithelial ovarian cancer. Gynecol Oncol. 1996;**60**:238–44.

118. Deligdisch L, Penault-Llorca F, Schlosshauer P, et al. Stage I ovarian carcinoma: different clinical pathologic patterns. Fertil Steril. 2007;**88**:906–10.

119. Moll UM, Chumas JC, Challas E, Mann WJ. Ovarian carcinoma arising in

atypical endometriosis. Obstet Gynecol. 1990;**75**:537–9.

120. Hanahan D, Weinberg RA. The hallmarks of cancer. Cell. 2000;**100**:57–70.

121. Green DR, Evan GI. A matter of life and death. Cancer Cell. 2002;**1**:19–30.

122. Ahmed N, Thompson EW, Quinn MA. Epithelial–mesenchymal interconversions in normal ovarian surface epithelium and ovarian carcinomas: an exception to the norm. J Cell Physiol. 2007;**213**:581–7.

123. Vlad MA, Diaconu I, Gant KR. MUCI in endometriosis and ovarian cancer. Immunol Res. 2006;**36**:229–36.

124. Karlan BY, Jones J, Greenwald M, Lagasse LD. Steroid hormone effects on the proliferation of human ovarian surface epithelium. Am J Obstet Gynecol. 1995;**173**:97–104.

125. Ness RB, Modugno F. Endometriosis as a model for inflammation–hormone interactions in ovarian and breast cancers. Eur J Cancer. 2006;**42**:691–703.

126. Balkwill F, Montovani A. Inflammation and cancer: back to Virchow? Lancet. 2001;**357**:539–45.

127. Affara NI, Coussens LM. IKKa at the crossroads of inflammation and metastasis. Cell. 2007;**129**:25–6.

128. Lee D-F, Kuo HP, Chen CT, et al. IKK/3 suppression of TSCI links inflammation and tumor angiogenesis via the mTOR pathway. Cell. 2007;**130**:440–5.

129. Ho HN, Wu MY, Yang YS. Peritoneal cellular immunity and endometriosis. Am J Reprod Immunol. 1997;**38**:400–12.

130. Wu MH, Wang CA, Lin CC, et al. Distinct regulation of cyclooxygenase-2 by interleukin-Izi in normal and endometriotic stromal cells. J Clin Endocrinol Metab. 2005;**90**:286–95.

131. Rask K, Zhu Y, Wang W, et al. Ovarian epithelial cancer: a role for PGET synthesis and signaling in malignant transformation and progression. Mol Cancer. 2006;**5**:62–75.

132. Rae MT, Niven D, Forster T, et al. Steroid signaling in human ovarian surface epithelial cells: the response to interleukin la determined by microarray analysis. J Endocrinol. 2004;**183**:19–28.

133. Rana N, Brown DP, House R, et al. Basal and stimulated secretion of cytokines by peritoneal macrophages in women with endometriosis. Fertil Steril. 1996;**65**:925–30.

134. Harada T, Iwabe T, Terakawa N. Role of cytokines in endometriosis. Fertil Steril. 2001;**76**:1–10.

135. Vigano P, Gafuri B, Somigliana E, et al. Expression of intracellular adhesion molecule ICAM-I mRNA and protein is enhanced in endometriosis versus endometrial stromal cells in culture. Mol Hum Reprod. 1998;**4**:1150–6.

136. Fukaya T, Sugawara J, Yoshida H, et al. Intracellular adhesion molecule 1 and hepatocyte growth factor in human endometriosis: original investigation and a review of literature. Gynecol Obstet Invest. 1999;**47**:11–6.

137. Darai E, Detchev R, Hugot D, et al. Serum and cyst fluid levels of interleukin (IL)-6, IL-8 and tumor necrosis factor-alpha in women with endometriomas and benign and malignant cystic ovarian tumors. Hum Reprod. 2003;**18**:1681–5.

138. Oosterlinck DJ, Meuleman C, Waer M, et al. Transforming growth factor 3 activity is increased in peritoneal fluid from women with endometriosis. Obstet Gynecol. 1994;**83**:287–92.

139. Baldwin RL, Tran H, Karlan BY. Loss of c-myc repression coincides with ovarian cancer resistance to transforming growth factor beta growth arrest independent of transforming growth factor beta/Smad signaling. Cancer Res. 2003;**63**:1413–9.

140. Artini PG, Cristello F, Monti M, et al. Vascular endothelial growth factor and its soluble receptor in ovarian pathology. Gynecol Endocrinol. 2005;**21**:50–6.

141. Kulbe H, Thompson R, Wilson JL, et al. The inflammatory cytokine tumor necrosis factor-α generates an autocrine tumor promoting network in epithelial ovarian cancer. Cancer Res. 2007;**67**:585–92.

142. Mor F, Quintana FJ, Cohen IR. Angiogenesis-inflammation cross-talk: vascular endothelial growth factor is secreted by activated T cells and induces TEl polarization. J Immunol. 2004;**172**:4618–23.

143. Bourlev V, Volvkov N, Pavlovich S, et al. The relationship between microvessel density, proliferative activity and expression of vascular endothelial growth factor-A and its receptors in eutopic endometrium and endometriotic lesions. Reproduction. 2006;**132**:501–9.

144. Muthukumaran M, Miletti-Gonzalez KE, Ravindranath AK, et al. Tumor necrosis factor-a differentially modulates CD44 expression in ovarian cancer cells. Mol Cancer Res. 2006;**4**:511–20.

145. Bourguignon LYW, Zhu H, Diedrich F et al. Hyaluronan promotes CD44v3-Vav2 interactions with Grb2-p1851HER2 and induces rael and ras signaling during ovarian tumor cell migration and growth. J Biol Chem. 2001;**276**:48679–92.

146. Mayr D, Kanitz V, Amann G, et al. HER-21new gene amplification in ovarian tnmors: a comprehensive immunohistochemical and FISH analysis on tissue microarrays. Histopathology. 2006;**48**:149–56.

147. Rodriguez-Rodriguez L, Sancho-Tores L, Leakey P, et al. CD44 splice variant expression in clear cell carcinoma of th ovary. Gynecol Oncol. 1998;**71**:223–39

148. Akoum A, Lawson C, McColl S, et al. Ectopic endometrial cells express high levels of (IL)-8 in vivo regardless of the menstrual cycle phase and respond to oestradiol by up-regulating IL-I induce IL-8 expression in vitro. Mol Hum Reprod. 2001;**7**:859–66.

149. Karin M. Inflammation and cancer: the long reach of ras. Nat Med. 2005;**11**:20–1.

150. Garcia-Velasco J, Mulaim N, Kayisli U, et al. Elevated levels of soluble Fas ligand may suggest a role for apoptosis in women with endometriosis. Fertil Steril 2002;**78**:855–9.

151. Bulun SE, Fang Z, Imir G, et al. Aromatase and endometriosis. Semin Reprod Med. 2004;**22**:45–50.

152. Tariverdian N, Theoharides TC, Siedentopf F, et al. Neuroendocrine-immune disequilibrium and endometriosis: an interdisciplinary approach. Semin Immunopathol. 2007;**29**:193–210.

153. Lau KM, Mok Sc, Ho SM. Expression of human estrogen receptor-alpha and -beta, progesterone receptor, and androgen receptor mRNA in normal and malignant ovarian epithelial cells. Proc Natl Acad Sci U S A. 1999;**96**:5722–7.

154. Mukherjee K, Syed V, Ho SM. Estrogen induced loss of progesterone expression in normal and malignant ovarian surface epithelial cells. Oncogene. 2005;**24**:4388–400.

55. Li AJ, Baldwin RL, Karlan BY. Estrogen and progesterone receptor subtype expression in normal and malignant ovarian epithelial cells in cultures. Am J Obstet Gynecol. 2003;**189**:22–7.

56. Sayed V, Ulinski G, Mok SC, Ho SM. Reproductive hormone induced, STAT3-mediated interleukin 6 action in normal and malignant human ovarian surface epithelial cells. J Natl Cancer Inst. 2002;**94**:617–29.

57. Kyo S, Takakura M, Kanaya T, et al. Estrogen activates telomerase. Cancer Res. 1999;**59**:5917–21.

58. Kalli KR, Falowo OI, Bale LK, et al. Functional insulin receptors on human epithelial ovarian carcinoma cells: implication for IGF-II mitogenic signaling. Endocrinology. 2002;**143**:3259–67.

59. Druckmann R, Rohr UD. IGF-l in gynaecology and obstetrics: update 2002. Maturitas. 2002;**41**(Suppl 1): S65–83.

60. Kim JG, Suh CS, Kim SH, et al. Insulin like growth factors, IGF binding proteins (IGFBPs) and IGFBP-3 protease activity in the peritoneal fluid of patients with and without endometriosis. Fertil Steril. 2000;**73**:996–1000.

61. Kuroda H, Mandai M, Konishi I, et al. Human ovarian surface epithelial cells (OSE) express LHI hCG receptors, and hCG inhibits apoptosis via up-regulation of insulin like growth factor-I. Int J Cancer. 2001;**92**:309–15.

62. Osuga Y, Tsutsumi O, Okagage R, et al. Hepatocyte growth factor concentrations are elevated in the peritoneal fluid of women with endometriosis. Hum Reprod. 1999;**14**:1611–13.

63. Baykal C, Demirtas E, Ai A, et al. Comparison of hepatocyte growth factor levels of epithelial ovarian cancer cyst fluids with benign ovarian cysts. Int J Gynecol Cancer. 2004;**14**:152–6.

164. Di Renzo MF, Olivero M, Katsaros D, et al. Overexpression of the MetlHGF receptor in ovarian cancer. Int J Cancer. 1994;**58**:658–62.

165. Huntsman D, Resau JH, Klineberg E, et al. Comparison of c-met expression in ovarian epithelial tumors and normal epithelia of' the female reproductive tract by quantitative laser scan microscopy. Am J Pathol. 1999;**155**:343–8.

166. Wong AS, Pelech SL, Woo MM, et al. Coexpression of hepatocyte growth factor-Met: an early step in ovarian carcinogenesis? Oncogene. 2001;**20**:1318–28.

167. Halme J, White C, Kauma SS, et al. Peritoneal macrophages from patients with endometriosis release growth factor activity in vitro. J Clin Endocrinol Metab. 1988;**66**:1044–9.

168. Dabrow MB, Francesco MR, McBrearty FX, et al. The effects of platelet derived growth factor and receptor on normal and neoplastic human ovarian surface epithelium. Gynecol Oncol. 1998;**71**:29–37.

169. Takeuchi M, Matsuzaki K, Uehara H, et al. Malignant transformation of pelvic endometriosis: MR imaging findings and pathologic correlation. Radiographies. 2006;**26**:407–17.

170. Poliness A, Healey MG, Brennecke SP, et al. Proteomic approaches in endometriosis research. Proteomics. 2004;**4**:1897–902.

171. Nezhat C, Crowgey S, Nezhat F. Videolaparoscopy for the treatment of endometriosis associated with infertility. Fertil Steril. 1989;**51**:237–40.

172. Fuch F, Raynal P, Salama S, et al. Reproductive outcome after laparoscopic treatment of endometriosis in the infertile population. J Gynecol Obstet Biol Reprod. 2007;**36**:354–9.

173. Nakagawa K, Oghi S, Horikawa T, et al. Laparoscopy should be strongly considered for women with unexplained infertility. J Obstet Gynecol Res. 2007;**33**:665–700.

174. Littman E, Giudice L, Lathi R, et al. Role of laparoscopic treatment of endometriosis in patients with failed in vitro fertilization cycles. Fertil Steril. 2005;**84**:1574–8.

175. Bosteels J, Van Herendael B, Weyers S, et al. The position of diagnostic laparoscopy in current fertility practice. Hum Reprod Update. 2007;**13**:477–85.

176. Ahmad G, Watson A, Vanderckhove P, et al. Techniques for pelvic surgery in subfertility. Cochrane Database Syst Rev. 2006;(2):CD00022I.

177. Cohen I, Altaras MM, Lew S, et al. Ovarian endometrioid carcinoma and endometriosis developing in postmenopausal breast cancer patient during tamoxifen therapy: a case report and review of the literature. Gynecol Oncol. 1994;**55**:172–4.

178. Laschke MW, Elitzsch A, Scheuer C, et al. Rapamycin induces regression of endometriotic lesions by inhibiting neovascularization and cell proliferation. Br J Pharmacol. 2006;**149**:137–44.

179. Attar E, Bulun S. Aromatase inhibitors: the next generation of therapeutics for endometriosis? Fertil Steril. 2006;**85**:1307–18.

180. Sayasneh A, Tsivos D, Crawford R. Endometriosis and ovarian cancer: a systematic review. ISRN Obstet Gynecol. 2011;**2011**:140310.

181. Munksgaard PS, Blaakaer J. The association between endometriosis and ovarian cancer: a review of histological, genetic and molecular alterations. Gynecol Oncol. 2012;**124**:164–9.

182. Wiegand KC, Shah SP, Al-Agha OM, et al. ARID1A mutations in endometriosis-associated ovarian carcinomas. N Engl J Med. 2010;**363**:1532–43.

Chapter 15

Laparoscopic surgery of the benign ovary and new laparoscopic developments

Michel Canis, MD, Revaz Botchorishvili, MD, Gerard Mage, MD, Antoine Maurice Bruhat, MD, Nicolas Bourdel, MD, and Benoit Rabischong, MD

Introduction

During the past 10 years of the previous century, laparoscopic surgery became both the key step in the diagnosis and the gold standard in the treatment of benign adnexal masses. This period clearly emphasized the limits and the potential pitfalls of any surgical approach. National survey and case reports demonstrated that tumor dissemination might occur if an ovarian tumor is punctured and or biopsied and not removed entirely and immediately [1–6]. However, this complication also occurred previously when the patients were managed by laparotomy [7,8]. This situation should be avoided, as it is the main risk of the surgical management of an adnexal mass.

Every effort should be made to prevent this potential risk including a careful and cautious surgical diagnosis, and cautious use of the conclusions of frozen sections. A malignant tumor, diagnosed as benign during surgery, may be mistakenly managed conservatively thus inducing a risk of postoperative dissemination. To avoid false negative diagnosis of malignancy, one should accept some false positives and the unnecessary adnexectomies performed to removed macroscopically suspicious tumors eventually diagnosed as benign on permanent sections [9,10]. If an apparently benign mass which has not been entirely removed is later found to be malignant, the delay between the laparoscopic diagnosis and the staging procedure should be as short as possible, ideally less than 8 or 17 days according to Kinderman et al. [5] and Wenzl et al. [6], respectively. The restaging should be considered as a true "oncologic emergency." To keep this delay as short as possible, it is essential when the macroscopic diagnosis of an adnexal mass was doubtful to first inform the pathologist that the situation is at risk and you need the result as soon as possible and second to inform the patient that a reoperation may be necessary very soon. She should be informed immediately after the operation. When she is informed very early, she generally accepts the reoperation more easily than when she is informed several days or weeks after the first procedure. When the diagnosis of cancer was not suspected during the operation, it is essential to inform the patient as soon as the diagnosis of cancer is available and to organize the restaging as soon as possible. A delayed staging after a unilateral adnexectomy is acceptable even if the delay should be as short as possible to minimize the potential growth of lymph node or distant metastases.

Diagnosis is and will remain for some years the key step in the management of adnexal masses. The surgical treatment is considered an easy procedure, however this procedure should be performed according to the guidelines proposed by Winston, Gomel, and Swolin for the treatment of tubal infertility [11]. It has been shown that a simple stripping technique may damage the ovary of patients operated for ovarian endometrioma thus emphasizing the importance of a perfect surgical technique [12]. The goal of surgery is complete and immediate treatment of the mass. Benign tumors should be treated using ovarian preserving procedures; malignant tumors should be removed entirely and immediately [2], and staged as soon as possible. However in young patients, if only one adnexa is involved, an adnexectomy followed by a restaging appears adequate. Indeed stage I ovarian grade 1 and 2 invasive cancers may be safely treated conservatively [13]. As tumor grading is impossible on frozen sections, an adequate treatment of contralateral adnexa is impossible during the first surgical step and a two-step surgical approach should be preferred. According to the patient's age, desire for pregnancy, and to the pathologic diagnosis of the mass, an IVF procedure may even be organized between the two surgical steps.

The management of adnexal masses involves two steps: diagnosis and treatment. These two steps should be distinguished; obviously a laparotomy may be decided after a laparoscopic diagnosis. In our department all adnexal masses are currently diagnosed laparoscopically.

Preoperative work-up

Unfortunately a perfect preoperative selection, which would diagnose all the cancers and avoid any laparotomy for the diagnosis of benign adnexal masses, is not yet possible. Even using a nomogram, Lachance et al. recently reported a specificity of 75% and a sensitivity of 90% [14]. In Table 15.1, we show that according to the incidence of adnexal cancer in the population, in a group of 1000 patients the number of cancers that would be first evaluated by laparoscopy and the number of unnecessary laparotomies would range from 10 to 40 and from 150 to 220 respectively. Consequently, it appears that the best preoperative evaluation cannot be used to select the surgical approach (laparoscopy, laparotomy by a Pfannenstiel or a midline incision). This recent study confirmed previous

Altchek's Diagnosis and Management of Ovarian Disorders, ed. Liane Deligdisch, Nathan G. Kase, and Carmel J. Cohen. Published by Cambridge University Press.

Table 15.1. Number of cancer cases diagnosed adequately and of benign cases diagnosed as malignant in a group of 1,000 patients, when using a diagnostic method which has 90% sensitivity and 75% specificity

Incidence of cancer	10%*	20%	30%	40%
Positive test among cancer (n, laparoscopy for invasive cancer)	90	180	270	360
Positive test among benign masses (n, laparotomy for benign masses)	225	200	175	150
Patients operated by oncologists	315	380	445	510

studies by others [15]. Moreover, it is well known that expert systems such as ultrasound scores or neural networks are less effective when used by a team not involved in the initial design of the model [16]. Therefore, the surgical diagnosis is still essential, and laparoscopy appears as the best way to achieve this essential step [9,10].

However, the preoperative work-up is essential, it may first help to refer patients with obvious cancer to a tertiary care oncological center and second help the surgeon to decide the intra-operative management. The intra-cystic examination begins before the surgical procedure using vaginal ultrasound and other imaging techniques, particularly MRI. Although its value has not been prospectively established in patients who had a vaginal ultrasound, we recommend an MRI for each patient with a suspicious adnexal mass. This MRI should include an examination of the upper abdomen and of the kidneys. In patients diagnosed with a peritoneal carcinomatosis, CT scan is probably a better staging tool, but MRI is more accurate to evaluate the content of the ovarian tumor in the pelvis.

In our group, one or two pelvic ultrasonographic examinations are performed before deciding the surgical management, and vaginal ultrasound is repeated in the department, the day before surgery by a member of the surgical team. This step is essential to check that the adnexal mass has not disappeared during the days before surgery, to teach ultrasonographic appearances of adnexal masses to residents and fellows who have the opportunity to see the mass at laparoscopy the following day, and to guide the surgeon during the procedure. When the surgeon has to decide whether or not the puncture of the mass is safe, this evaluation is often checked again in the operating room.

Timmerman et al. recently showed that adding a single CA125 measurement to ultrasound imaging performed by an experienced examiner does not improve preoperative discrimination between benign and malignant adnexal masses [17,18]. Therefore, tumor markers are only sampled the day before surgery to be available for the postoperative follow-up of patients diagnosed with an ovarian cancer, but they are not used preoperatively to decide which surgical approach is used.

Again we emphasize that the preoperative evaluation is a key step which will probably in the future allow an accurate preoperative diagnosis of malignancy. Obviously, national recommendations will soon propose routine management of patients with suspicious adnexal masses in oncology departments, to avoid inadequate management of ovarian cancers. However, we are convinced that oncological teams will have to include infertility surgeons so as to avoid unnecessary adnexectomies and other inadequate surgical managements in young women operated for highly complex masses induced by endometriosis and or pelvic inflammatory disease. A recent survey in the United States showed that when presented with a patient with a suspicious ovarian mass, the majority of primary care physicians do not self-report direct referral to a gynecologic oncologist [19]. This surprising result may contribute to the high rates of non-comprehensive surgery for ovarian cancer patients [20]. It should be improved to improve the survival rates of patients with advanced ovarian cancers, but the knowledge of infertility surgeons is mandatory to allow optimal care of young patients with complex masses.

To puncture or not to puncture is the question

In 2001, Vergote et al. published a multicentric retrospective study which demonstrated that pre and or intra-operative rupture of a stage I ovarian cancer worsens the prognosis [21]. However, many of these patients had not been staged adequately. Recently, four additional studies were published on the consequences of surgical rupture [22–25]. Bakkum et al. concluded that intra-operative capsule rupture portends a higher risk of disease recurrence; however, this difference was not statistically significant when excluding stage IC patients with rupture and positive cytology (before the rupture) and patients with positive cytology without rupture [22]. These authors hypothesized that an occult infiltration of the cyst wall may predispose to rupture and may be difficult to identify after the rupture. Paulsen et al. found better disease-free tumor survival in patients without intra-operative rupture in both uni- and multi-variate analysis, but found no influence of a laparoscopic approach which was used in a selected group of patients [23]. Two other studies found no influence of surgical rupture; particularly, Higashi et al. found no influence of intra-operative rupture in clear cell carcinoma [24,25].

From these results, we cannot conclude that laparoscopic puncture should never be performed and or that the prognosis of patients whose adnexal mass is punctured is significantly worsened. Indeed most surgeons try to avoid surgical rupture; consequently, it probably occurs more often in larger tumors, particularly if they are fixed by adhesions, poorly differentiated, or with an occult infiltration of the cyst wall. As a result, independently of the consequences of the rupture, the prognosis of tumors that rupture during surgery is probably worse than that of tumors remaining intact. Surgical rupture cannot be evaluated in a randomized trial and this bias will never be avoided.

As a puncture will never improve the prognosis of an early ovarian cancer, it should be avoided whenever possible. Examples shown in Fig. 15.1 clearly demonstrate that in many adnexal masses a puncture can be avoided as an adnexectomy is indicated from the suspicious ultrasonographic appearance of the cyst content. Moreover, a puncture carefully performed, taking care to minimize spillage, as described below, does not

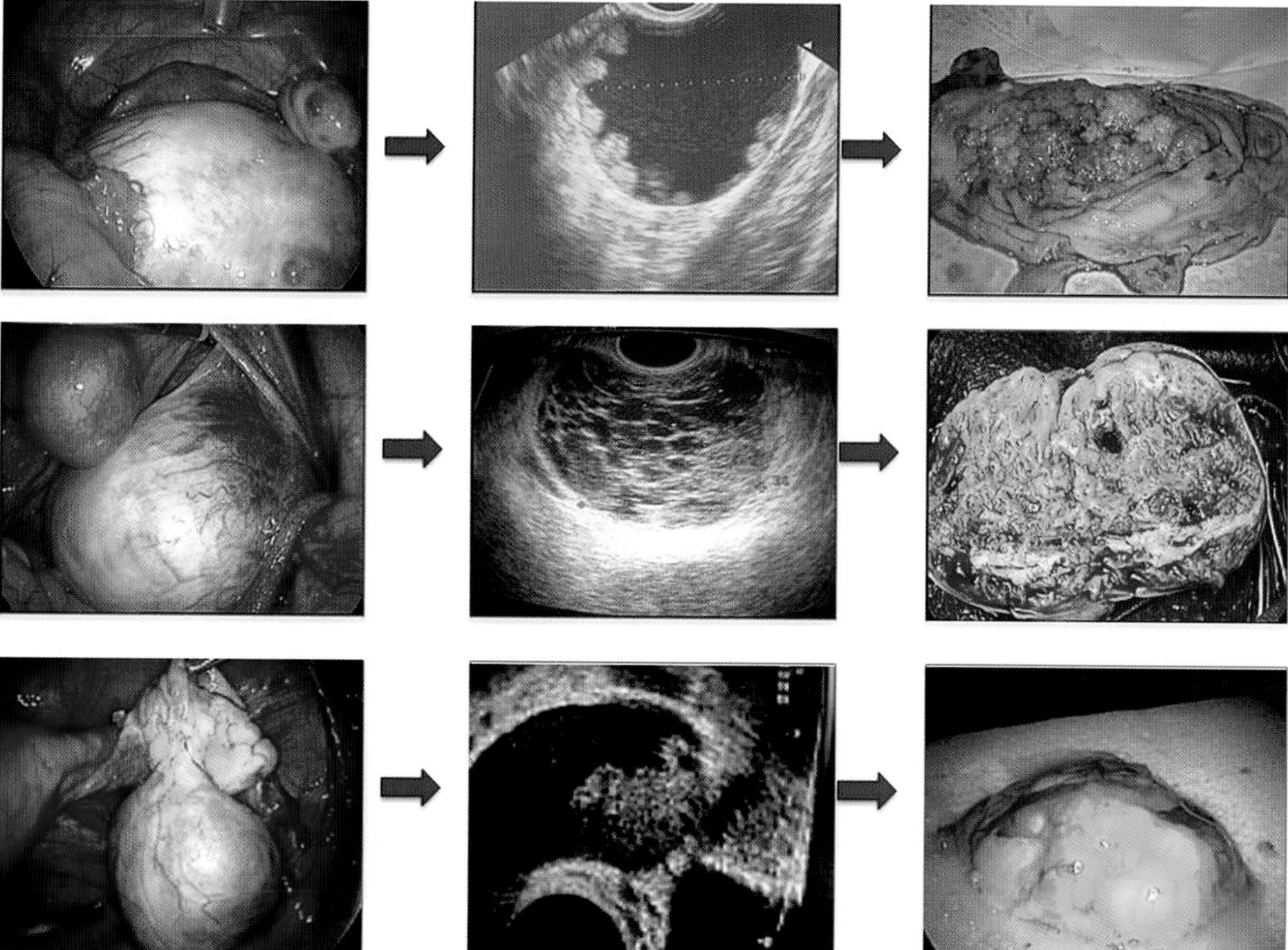

Fig. 15.1. In some adnexal masses, a puncture is obviously contraindicated.

have the same risks and potential consequences as an accidental and unplanned surgical rupture.

In contrast, it seems impossible and not reasonable to manage every patient to avoid a puncture of any early ovarian cancer. Indeed two approaches may be proposed to achieve complete treatment of the mass without any risk of puncture or rupture. The first is to perform an adnexectomy for all masses that are suspicious at ultrasound. This approach is acceptable in patients who are more than 40 years old, but it is unacceptable in younger patients. Indeed many adnexal masses found to be suspicious at ultrasound are benign and may be treated while preserving the ovary. The potential consequences of a careful puncture do not justify the functional consequences of so many unnecessary adnexectomies. Cystectomy without puncture is the other theoretical approach. But this surgical approach is unrealistic. Indeed a cancer invades the cleavage plane, so that it is impossible to do a cystectomy without rupture of the mass.

Puncture should always be decided carefully accounting for all clinical ultrasonographic and imaging data. This surgical decision is often difficult and sometimes stressful. The technique, described below, should minimize the potential consequences. A completely leak-proof puncture is impossible, but using bags, conical instruments, and effective aspiration lavage devices, the peritoneal contamination will be minimal.

"Informed" consent

It is difficult to explain all the different situations that may be encountered, especially in a young woman. Nevertheless, it is essential to have the patient's agreement to carry out laparotomy, a supra- and sub-umbilical midline laparotomy, adnexectomy which may be bilateral, hysterectomy, omentectomy, and lymph node dissection, and even a restaging procedure within a few days after the initial surgical procedure. In a young patient with a unilateral mass, it is essential to explain that restaging may be necessary a few days after an adnexectomy. This second surgical procedure is much easier to organize when the patients are informed before the first operation; this is essential, as too long a delay should be avoided.

Organization of the surgical procedure

A purely liquid cyst can be handled very easily. Conversely, there are situations when it must be possible to use frozen sections and when expertise in oncology and medically assisted reproduction should be available if needed.

Frozen sections are often used in the management of adnexal masses. It should be emphasized that this intra-operative pathological examination is often difficult and that false negative diagnosis of malignancy may occur. Therefore, the surgeons must decide the management of the tumor and of the adnexa, accounting for the limits and the difficulties of this technique.

Surgeons should also be aware that most false negative diagnoses of malignancy in frozen sections are the consequences of inadequate sampling of the tumor [26–28]. As sampling is the most difficult step, it should be performed by the pathologist rather than by the surgeon; therefore, if the mass is macroscopically suspicious, the "entire adnexa" should be removed and sent to the pathologist. The only exception to this rule concerns adnexal masses with a small (<5 mm) solitary vegetation, when the local conditions (diameter of the mass, pelvic adhesions, etc.) allow satisfactory macroscopic inspection of the inner cyst wall. In such cases, with only one suspicious area, the sampling is easy and the incidence of malignancy is less than 20% [29]. Some young patients (< 40 years old) will be treated by cystectomy, despite a small intra-cystic vegetation. This approach should be used very cautiously, and if there is any doubt and or if dissection is difficult, an adnexectomy should be performed.

Frozen section is mandatory during surgery for the following:

- bilateral suspicious lesion in a young woman or a suspicious lesion in a young patient who has already had an adnexectomy
- suspicious lesion in a post-menopausal patient
- obvious or very probable cancer.

Installation of the patient and of the laparoscopic trocars and instruments

The patient is positioned in a modified dorso-lithotomy position with legs semi-flexed and apart, and with both arms by her side. The buttocks of the patient should project slightly beyond the edge of the operating table to allow for effective uterine manipulation. When setting up for laparoscopy, blind puncture of the lesion should be avoided. The approach depends on the size of the lesion and morphology of the patient (weight, height, and umbilical–pubic distance).

- For lesions < 5 cm, the pneumoperitoneum needle and optical trocar can be inserted in the umbilicus. But, to reduce the risk of large vessel injury, in our department we no longer insert the pneumoperitoneum needle in the umbilicus; we routinely use the Palmer's point in the left hypochondrium.
- For lesions between 5 and 10 cm, the pneumoperitoneum should be created in the left upper quadrant and the trocar inserted in the umbilicus.
- For lesions > 10 cm, the pneumoperitoneum needle and a 5 mm trocar are inserted in the left upper quadrant, after which we use a 5 mm laparoscope or a 10 mm laparoscope subsequently inserted in the umbilicus.
- If the lesion is over 10 or 15 cm, laparoscopy is implemented by performing open laparoscopy if necessary in the left upper quadrant.

An open laparoscopy may be used in all situations, but we reserve it for very large lesions to achieve a puncture under visual control using a technique which decreases the peritoneal contamination.

Again the site of insertion of operative trocars depends on the lesion size and morphology of the patient. The larger the lesion, the higher the trocars should be inserted in the anterior abdominal wall. The operative trocar sites must be located between the optical trocar and the lesion. It is not possible to work comfortably and efficiently if the trocars are inserted very low on the abdominal wall. A low insertion may be chosen for purely esthetic reasons, but this should be reserved for very simple situations (i.e., entirely cystic lesion of less than 4 cm).

We use three 5 mm suprapubic trocars almost systematically (Fig. 15.2). Active participation by the assistant helps with the surgical skills learning process. When it is the senior surgeon who operates, residents who control an instrument and thus participate actively will learn more than by simple observation. If the resident carries out the procedure, which should often be the case, the senior surgeon can then use his instrument to guide the resident's movements.

The trocars must be inserted perpendicular to the abdominal wall to ensure that excision of the trocar path will be efficient if indicated during a restaging operation. Finally, if the mass is suspicious at ultrasound, trocars should be inserted higher on the abdominal wall to allow an easier dissection of the para aortic area and omentectomy if a complete staging was required.

Surgical treatment

Although the choice between laparotomy and laparoscopy appeared as the key question from the debates published over the past 20 years, the main choice for the surgeon is to decide between an oophorectomy and a surgical procedure that preserves the ovary. Obviously, this choice depends on the ultrasonographic and macroscopic appearances, on the age of the patient and on her past medical history including previous surgical procedures and desire for future fertility.

The intra-operative management of adnexal masses should be to avoid any risk of postoperative dissemination, which may occur when a malignant tumor is biopsied or punctured and not removed immediately. Importantly, this is the same aim as when the surgical diagnosis is derived by laparotomy.

Techniques

Conservative procedures

Puncture techniques

There is no way to ensure a perfectly sealed puncture, but peritoneal contamination should be minimal. Lesions under 12 cm are placed in a bag before puncture. This requires a bag

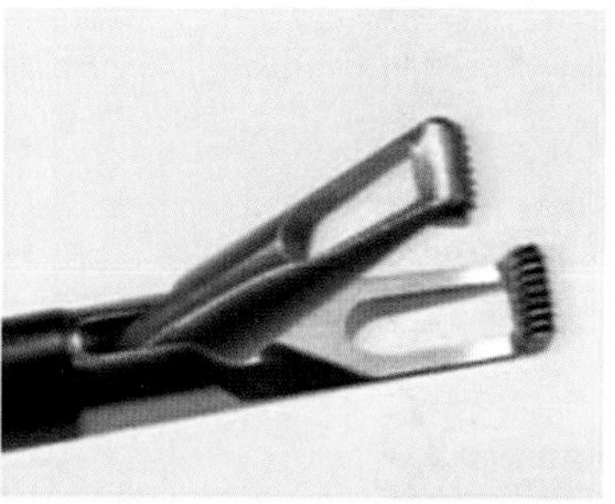

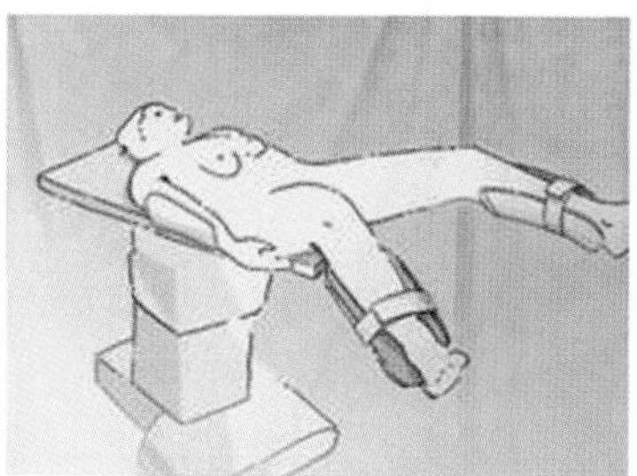

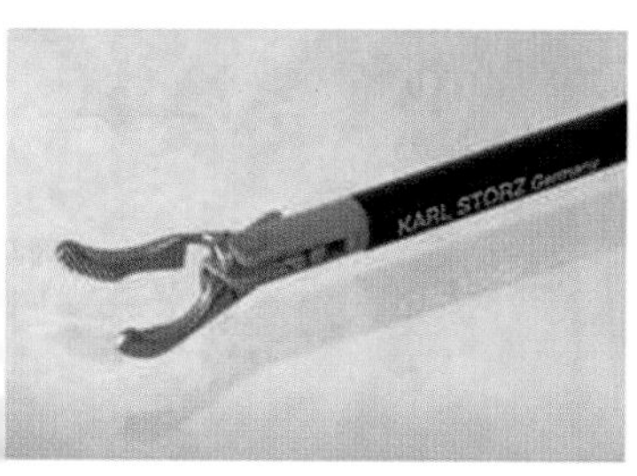

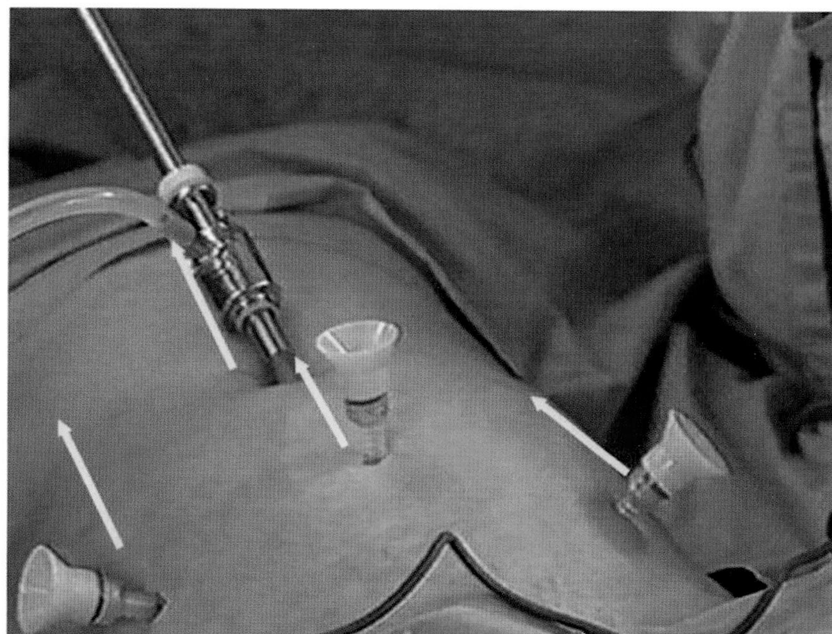

Fig. 15.2. Patient installation, trocar sites, and instruments used.

with a large opening. It must be transparent and should not be attached to any trocar site by a suture. We use this system for suspicious cysts that we decide to puncture and dermoid cysts whose contents may cause peritoneal irritation and postoperative adhesions [9].

Puncture must take place (Fig. 15.3):

- under direct vision, inside a bag
- perpendicular to the surface of the ovary
- with a conical instrument.

Indeed a puncture tangential to the surface of the cyst would create a hole wider than the diameter of the instrument. Moreover, with a conical instrument, penetration is achieved by cutting the cyst wall and, because of the elasticity of tissues, the puncture is more leak-proof.

If a cystectomy is planned, the puncture must be performed on the anti-mesenteric edge of the ovary where the ovarian incision allows spontaneous approximation of the ovarian tissue without any suture at the end of the procedure. Lesions less than 8 cm are punctured with a 5 mm diameter needle, introduced by means of an operative trocar. The anti-mesial edge of the ovary is exposed using atraumatic forceps applied on the utero-ovarian ligament to rotate the ovary outward. The liquid is aspirated with a syringe and then sent for cytological examination.

For lesions larger than 8 cm, we use a 5 mm conical tip trocar that can be inserted through operative trocars 5.5 mm in diameter or directly through the abdominal wall. Thus, a 5 mm suction-irrigation system is introduced into the cyst. Leakage of small amounts of fluid often occurs when the trocar is removed and the suction cannula is inserted. This leakage is usually minimal, but a bag should be placed under the ovary whenever possible. Once the suction starts, the puncture site is grasped and raised with atraumatic forceps to prevent spillage (Fig. 15.3). A suction-irrigation procedure is performed using small volumes. After draining and irrigation, the puncture site can be enlarged with scissors to carry out cystoscopy and/or closed with one or two endoloops to allow surgery to continue without any leaks.

Special cases

Endometriotic cysts are almost always ruptured during ovarian adhesiolysis at the point where they adhere to the broad ligament. A puncture should never be performed before the adhesiolysis, as it would generally pass through the hilum of the ovary.

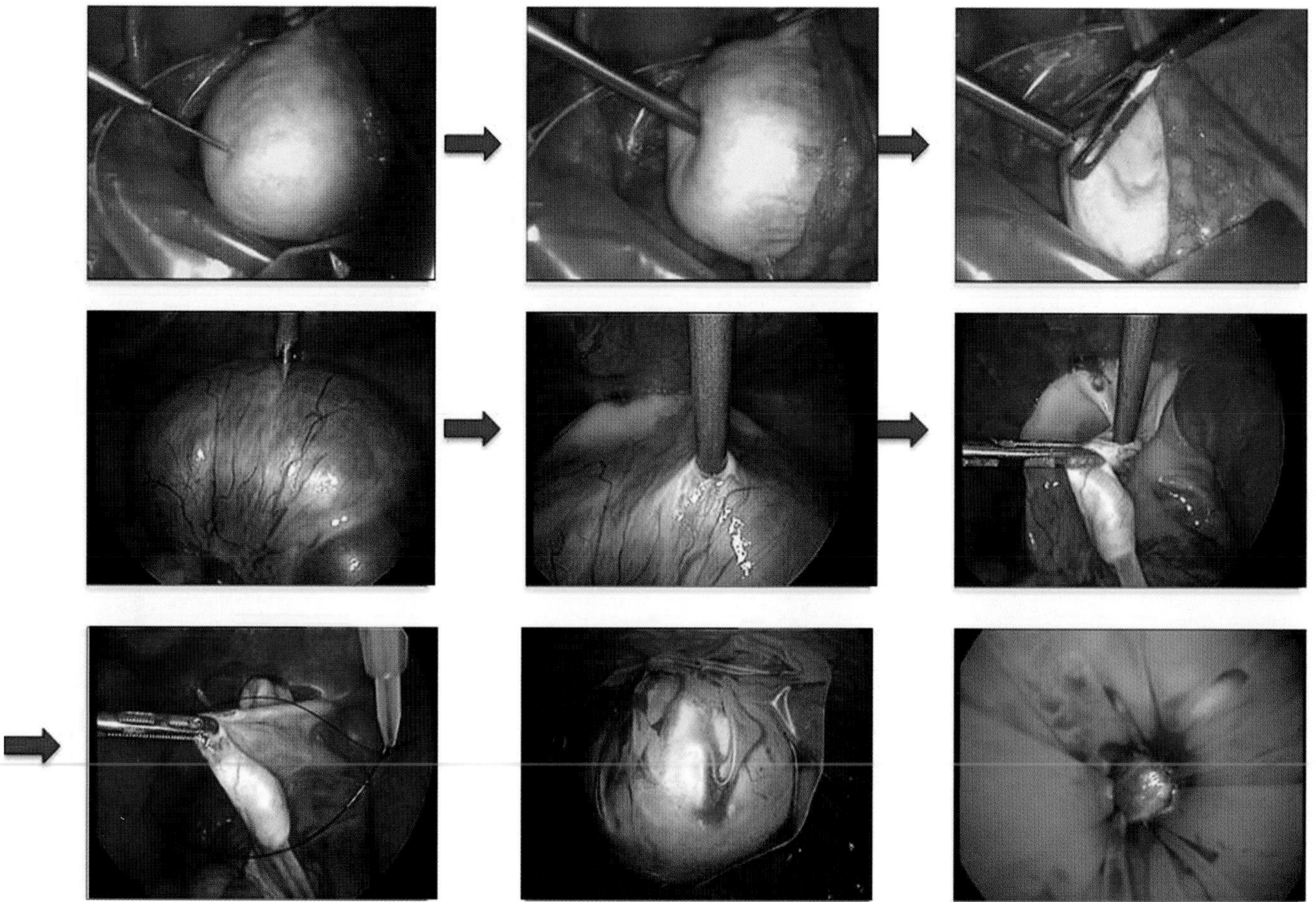

Fig. 15.3. Punctures.

Dermoid cysts under 7 cm in size are not punctured before dissection. They are placed in a bag and punctured at the end of treatment. Very large dermoid cysts are punctured with an aspiration cannula measuring 10 mm or more, introduced along the path of the mini laparotomy which is often used for their treatment.

If treatment of the cyst or adnexa is carried out without prior puncture, the cyst is punctured in a bag inside the peritoneum, or after extraction of the bag either transparietally or transvaginally. Once again direct vision must be used to ensure that puncture is made inside the bag and not through the bag! It may be difficult to ensure this precaution is achieved, especially when making a transabdominal puncture in an obese patient. The incision should in this case be enlarged to obtain reliable visual control of the puncture procedure (Fig. 15.3).

Treatment techniques

Biopsy

The biopsy should be broad and representative of the rest of the cyst wall. For this reason, it must be preceded by careful extra-cystic and a complete intra-cystic inspection. A biopsy should always be performed with laparoscopic scissors; samples obtained with biopsy forceps currently available are too small to allow a reliable pathologic diagnosis. This technique is used to confirm that a cyst is functional when there is no doubt (Fig. 15.4). It should also be performed in patients diagnosed with an ovarian endometrioma before starting a vaporization or a 3-month post-operative medical treatment if a three-step approach is planned [30].

Cystectomy after puncture (Fig. 15.5)

The puncture site, located on the anti-mesial edge of the ovary, will serve as a starting point for the ovarian incision which must take place on this side of the ovary. Because of gravity, locating the incision here allows for self-healing of the ovary after surgery. The incision must be large enough to allow reliable examination of all sides of the cyst in search of vegetations. To facilitate this step a small amount of saline can be injected into the cyst. After cystoscopy, the incision is inspected to find the cleavage plane which usually opens spontaneously. The ovarian tissue and ovarian cyst wall retract differently and separate spontaneously after the incision. Dissection begins by positioning a grasping forceps on each side of the cleavage plane. The forceps must provide a strong yet atraumatic grip on the tissues. In our experience, it was only once Hubert Manhes had produced his grasping forceps (the so-called "grip forceps") that we were able to develop intra-peritoneal cystectomy in 1986 (Fig. 15.2). Traction on the two forceps will begin the dissection. The forces that are applied must be moderate, and the tissue must not be torn. Dissection is correct in the following.

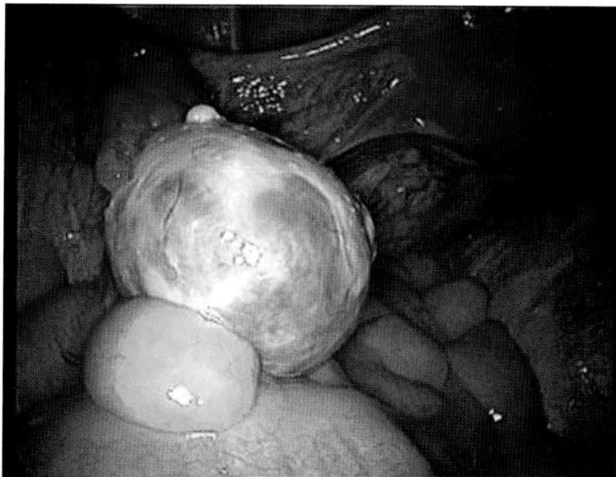

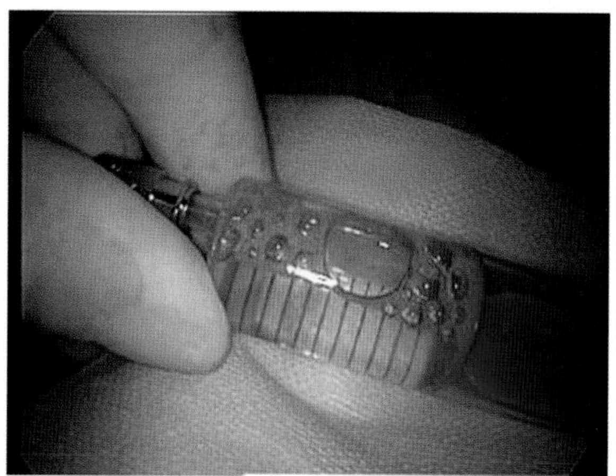

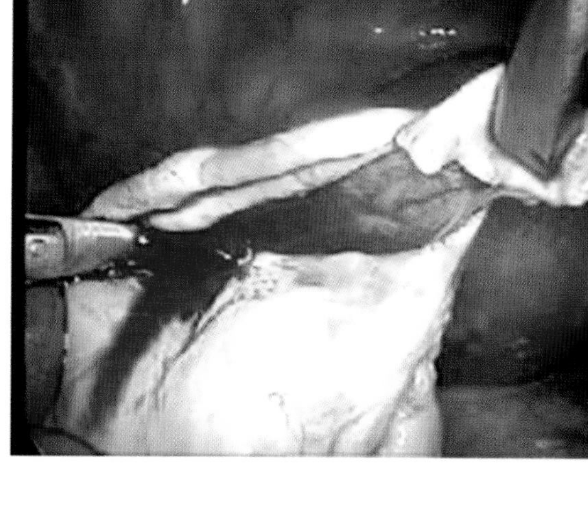

Fig. 15.4. Large biopsy of a functional cyst.

- The procedure consists of short pulls applied with moderate force, which often involves moving the grasping forceps because traction is more effective if instruments are close to the cleavage plane.
- Dissection takes place under constant vision, which makes sure that the cyst is not torn, leaving tissue in place which it was intended to remove. Therefore, perfect exposure of the cleavage plane is required and is achieved by frequent adjustments to the position of the forceps and careful hemostasis.
- The surface of the cyst must be white, without any red fibers. If any red tractus is visible on the surface of the cyst, the dissection plane is probably too far from the cyst wall and a better plane will be found by moving closer to the cyst.
- Bleeding should be minimal or nil. Hemostasis, if necessary, is performed during dissection when the bleeding is easy to see and control thanks to the exposure obtained by the tractions applied. These precautions are all the more important when the cyst is large and the procedure more difficult.
- Dissection does not enlarge the ovarian incision and does not tear the remaining ovarian tissues.

Two grasping forceps are usually used for cystectomy. But the third trocar is a big advantage because it allows bipolar coagulation or a third grasping forceps to be used. Indeed, to position a forceps on or near the cleavage plane once dissection has progressed several inches, it is important not to release the tissue to which traction has just been applied and then try to take it up again. If the tissue is released, it will shrink back, it will be difficult to grasp the same area again and temporarily impossible to expose the next area. Instead, a third forceps should be brought into play, placing it at the desired location before leaving go of the tissues currently held. This point is mandatory for large cysts.

In case of difficulty, bleeding, or when repeated traction movements have little effect, the following can be done:

- bring the active grasping forceps closer to the cleavage plane to make them more effective
- search for the cleavage plane closer to the surface of the cyst particularly if its surface is pink or red
- resume cystoscopy to look for an area of vegetations not recognized during the first inspection
- resume dissection in another part of the cyst, leaving the most difficult part for the end of the intervention when exposure will be better.

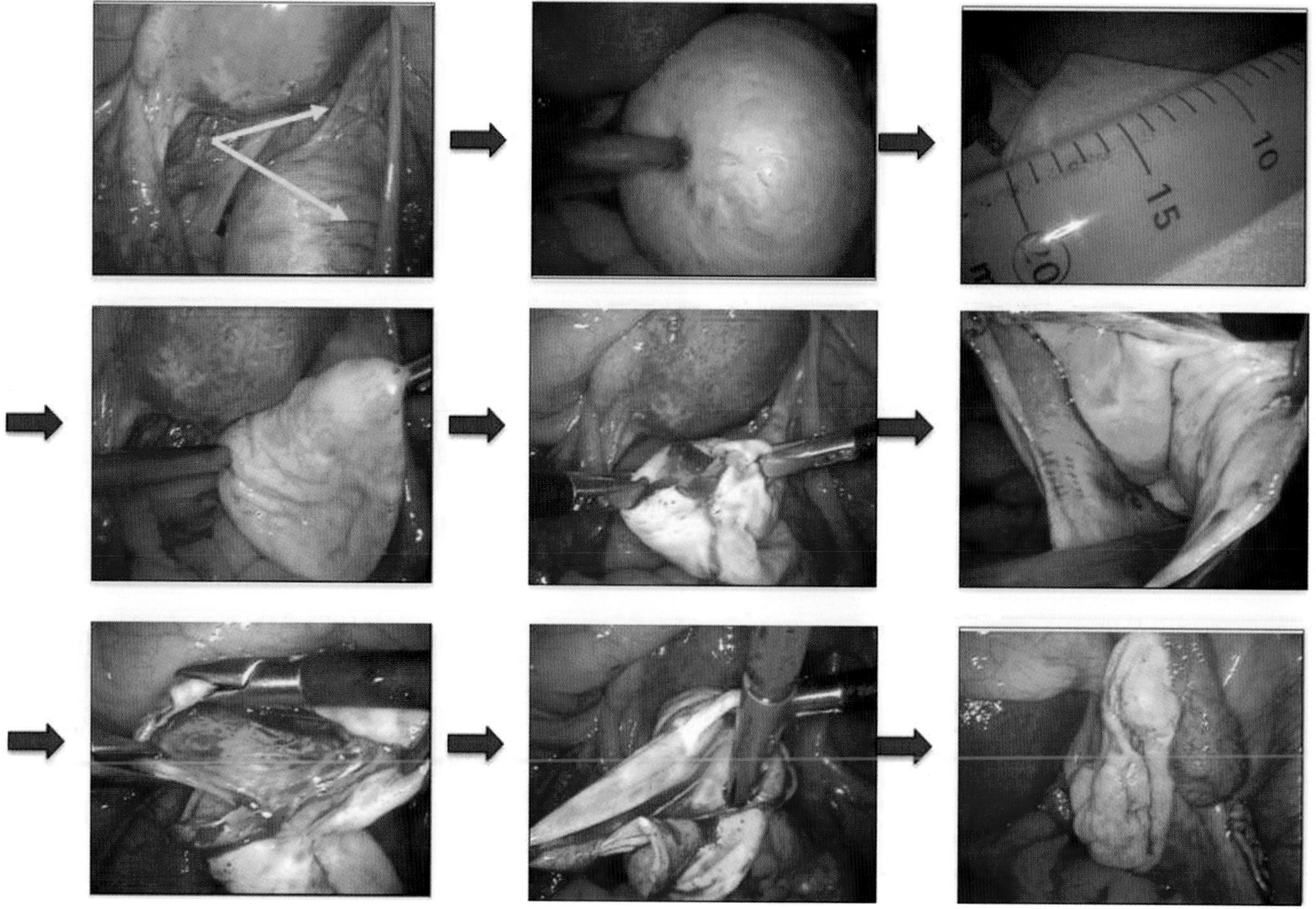

Fig. 15.5. Cystectomy after a puncture.

At the end of cystectomy, complete hemostasis must be achieved. We describe the techniques for ovarian repair and removal of the ovarian cyst later.

Cystectomy without puncture

Ovarian cysts (Fig. 15.6) Cystectomy without puncture is not always successful, and accidental rupture during dissection is common, occurring in about 50% of cases in our experience. So, the ovary must be placed in a bag before beginning dissection.

The incision should again be situated on the anti-mesial edge of the ovary. It is more or less easy to perform depending on how distended the normal ovarian parenchyma is around the cyst. If possible, the surface of the ovary is grasped and the fold thus obtained incised carefully for a few millimeters with scissors. The scissors are inserted slowly then opened inside the incision. When the incision is long enough (1–2 cm), a grasping forceps is placed on each edge and it is enlarged after dissection of the plane with scissors or by hydro dissection. The incision should be as long as the diameter of the cyst.

This phase of extending the incision once the cleavage plane is identified for a few millimeters requires special attention because the cyst is often ruptured at this point of the procedure when the most difficult part seems to be over. Again, the cleavage plane is satisfactory if the surface of the cyst is white or yellow with no red fibers, and if dissection results in no or minimal bleeding. Once the incision is complete, a grasping forceps is placed on each edge and the cyst can be dissected using these two forceps pulling in opposite directions, helped by the pelvic sidewall which becomes a third dissection instrument as the ovary is pressed against it.

If this method is effective, it should be continued slowly. If it is ineffective, dissection must continue using the grasping forceps and scissors. The gestures used for dissection are essential: the instruments should press against the remaining ovary, work should proceed away from the cyst, and the instruments should be applied tangentially to the surface of the cyst. Dissection becomes easier once more than half the cyst surface has been dissected. At this point, it is possible to continue by lifting the remaining ovarian parenchyma and using gravity, which makes the cyst fall away.

Three actions must be avoided:

- moving the instruments toward the cyst, especially with active instruments perpendicular to the surface of the cyst
- direct traction on the surface of the cyst, the wall of which is thin, fragile and easily torn with endoscopic instruments.

Cystectomy without puncture is complicated or even impossible for lesions larger than 8 cm in diameter.

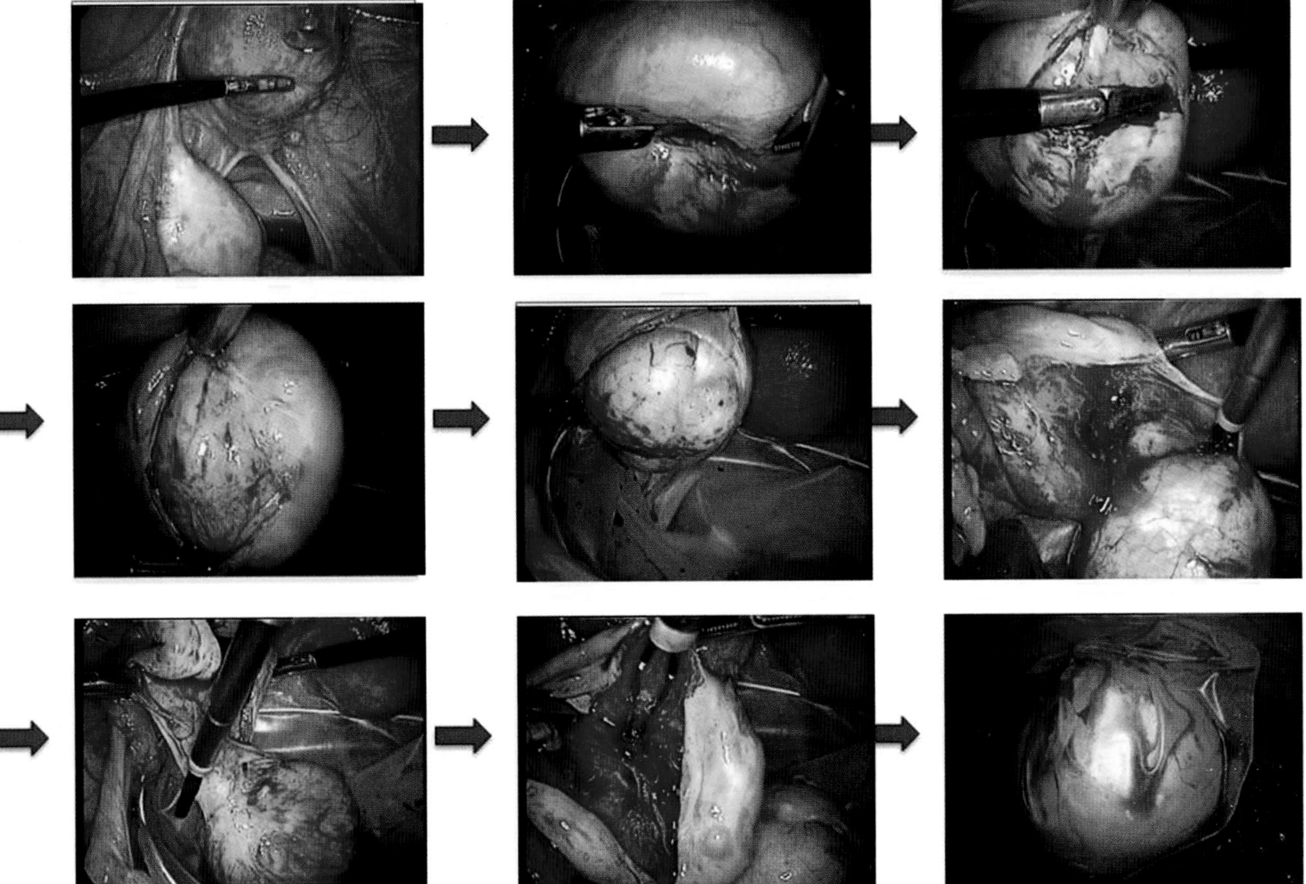

Fig. 15.6. Cystectomy without puncture.

Once the procedure has been completed, the techniques for hemostasis, repair of the ovary and extraction of the cyst are identical to those used in the techniques for cystectomy after puncture. More attention must be paid to the shape of the ovary because the incision is larger (Figs. 15.5, 15.6).

Para-tubal cyst (Fig. 15.7) These cysts are not always benign: in our series and in the literature the frequency of malignancies is 2.2% [31]. They are covered only by peritoneum, so the cyst contents can be seen through the peritoneum and the cyst wall. The usual fluid content appears bluish through these two membranes. Conversely, if the cyst wall contains intra-cystic vegetations, it appears whitish. Cystectomy should always start before puncture, especially for small cysts, which, once emptied, are difficult to identify between the peritoneal layers.

The incision site must be chosen carefully to avoid compromising the function of the fimbria. Dissection begins with the peritoneum, which is easy to grasp with forceps and incise with scissors. The plane is correct if the surface of the cyst appears bluish without red fibers. The incision is enlarged until it is equal to the diameter of the cyst. Similar to the method for dissection of ovarian cysts, two grasping forceps are placed on either side of the incision and then pulled in opposite directions while pressing the cyst against the pelvic wall. This initial phase of the dissection is simple. As it progresses closer to the ovary, the cleavage plane often becomes more difficult to follow, and vascular fibrous tractus become visible on the surface of the cyst. At this point, it is important to get closer to the cyst to avoid the section of these tractus. It is important to preserve the peritoneum of the mesosalpinx found around the cyst. If it is excised to "facilitate" the dissection, the mobility of the tube becomes abnormal and increases the risk of postoperative infertility.

Puncture is performed with a needle inside the bag or through the abdominal wall after externalizing the bag. At the end of the dissection, it is very important to check the anatomy of the tube and of the fimbria which may be buried in the retroperitoneal space due to inversion of the region induced by the dissection. It is imperative to restore normal tubal anatomy by replacing the fimbria in an intra-peritoneal position.

Transparietal cystectomy This technique is also known as cystectomy by mini laparotomy [32]. A 3- to 4-cm skin incision is used for this technique, which can be qualified as endoscopic because the postoperative course is almost the same as that of pure endoscopic techniques. This method of cystectomy, assisted by endoscopy, combines laparoscopic diagnosis and

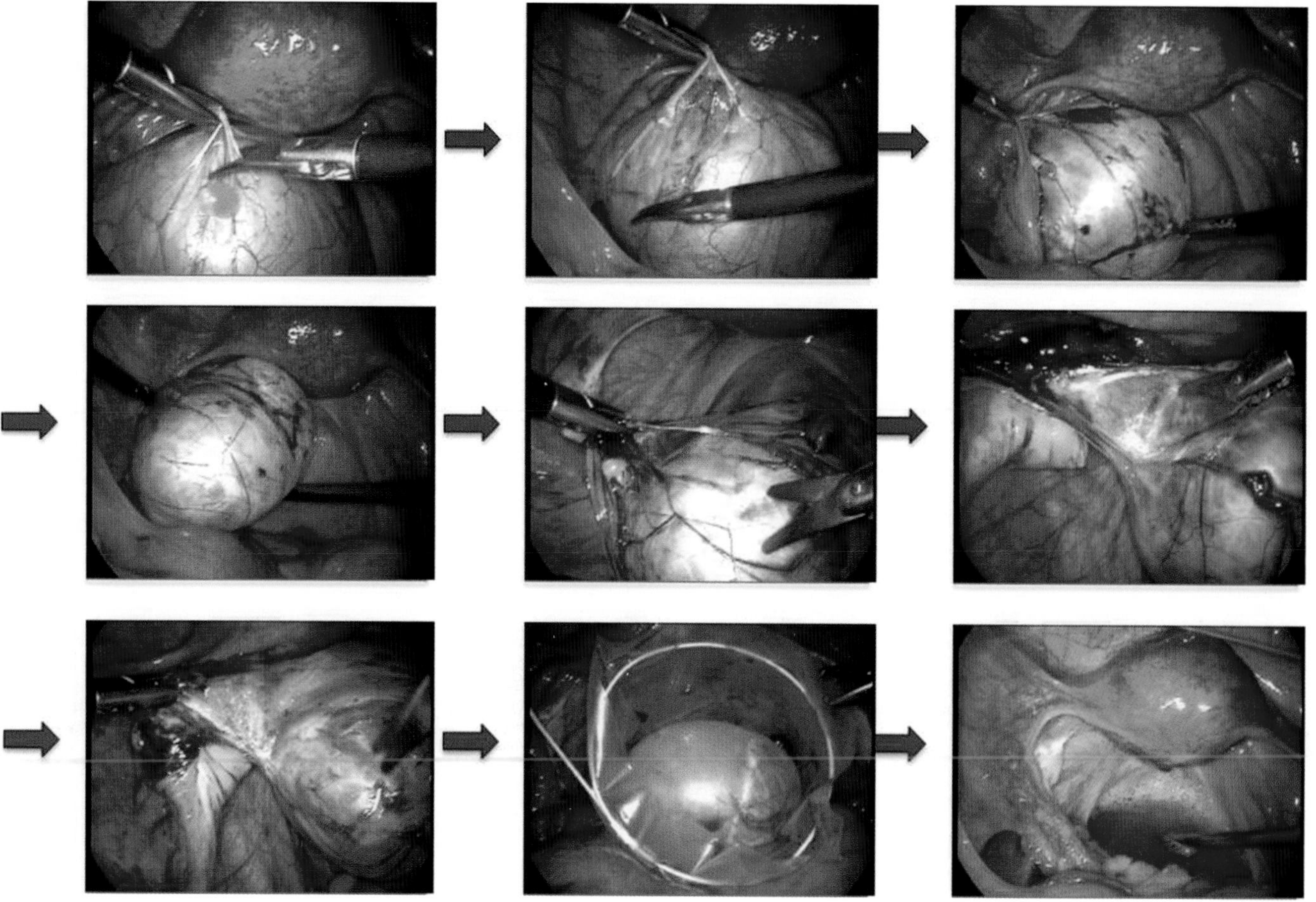

Fig. 15.7. Treatment of a para ovarian cyst.

puncture with extraction and treatment of the cyst by means of mini-laparotomy. This approach is currently reserved for conservative treatment of large dermoid cysts whose contents are difficult to extract using laparoscopic suction–irrigation systems and are more easily dealt with using a mini-laparotomy incision.

After the usual diagnostic steps, the cyst is punctured with a 5 mm or 10 mm trocar and aspirated at least partially. Then the mini-laparotomy takes place. The incision site is selected depending on which side the cyst is located, taking care to avoid the epigastric vessels. The incision is placed either along the line of a Pfannenstiel or toward the bottom of a median incision, after checking the bladder is empty. The skin and fascial incision are identical to a laparotomy. However, incision of the peritoneum should be performed "over" the cyst.

To do this, a standard surgical atraumatic forceps is inserted into the incision through the peritoneum under direct vision. To minimize peritoneal contamination, this forceps is used to grasp the puncture site. The cyst is pulled up against the wall and the peritoneum is incised "over" the cyst through the mini-laparotomy incision. This method of peritoneal incision ensures that extraction and loss of pneumoperitoneum are simultaneous, and allows the size of the incision to be adjusted to the diameter of the tissues to be extracted. This trick makes extraction of the cyst and repositioning of the ovary at the end of the intervention much easier.

Once the puncture hole is externalized, drainage of the cyst is completed, if necessary with laparotomy instruments, then the whole ovary is extracted and cystectomy performed, as it would be by laparotomy. Again, it is essential to work in an avascular plane, following by laparotomy all the principles of a good endoscopic dissection.

Just as with standard endoscopic cystectomy, hemostasis and suture of the ovary are generally not necessary. If the compression exerted on the ovarian veins by the edges of the incision gives the impression of increased bleeding, after hemostasis of the larger vessels, the ovary should be put back into the peritoneal cavity and laparoscopic vision used to assess and treat if necessary the bleeding. This technique is more difficult in obese patients and it is not a suitable method for suspicious lesions. The risks of contamination of the abdominal wall are greater than with purely endoscopic techniques. However, it can make it easier to complete conservative treatment of a non-suspicious but very large cyst.

Finally, this method is possible even in hospitals with minimal endoscopic equipment, meaning that all patients can benefit from the advantages of endoscopy in an operating room where the endoscopic equipment is limited to that required for tubal sterilization [32].

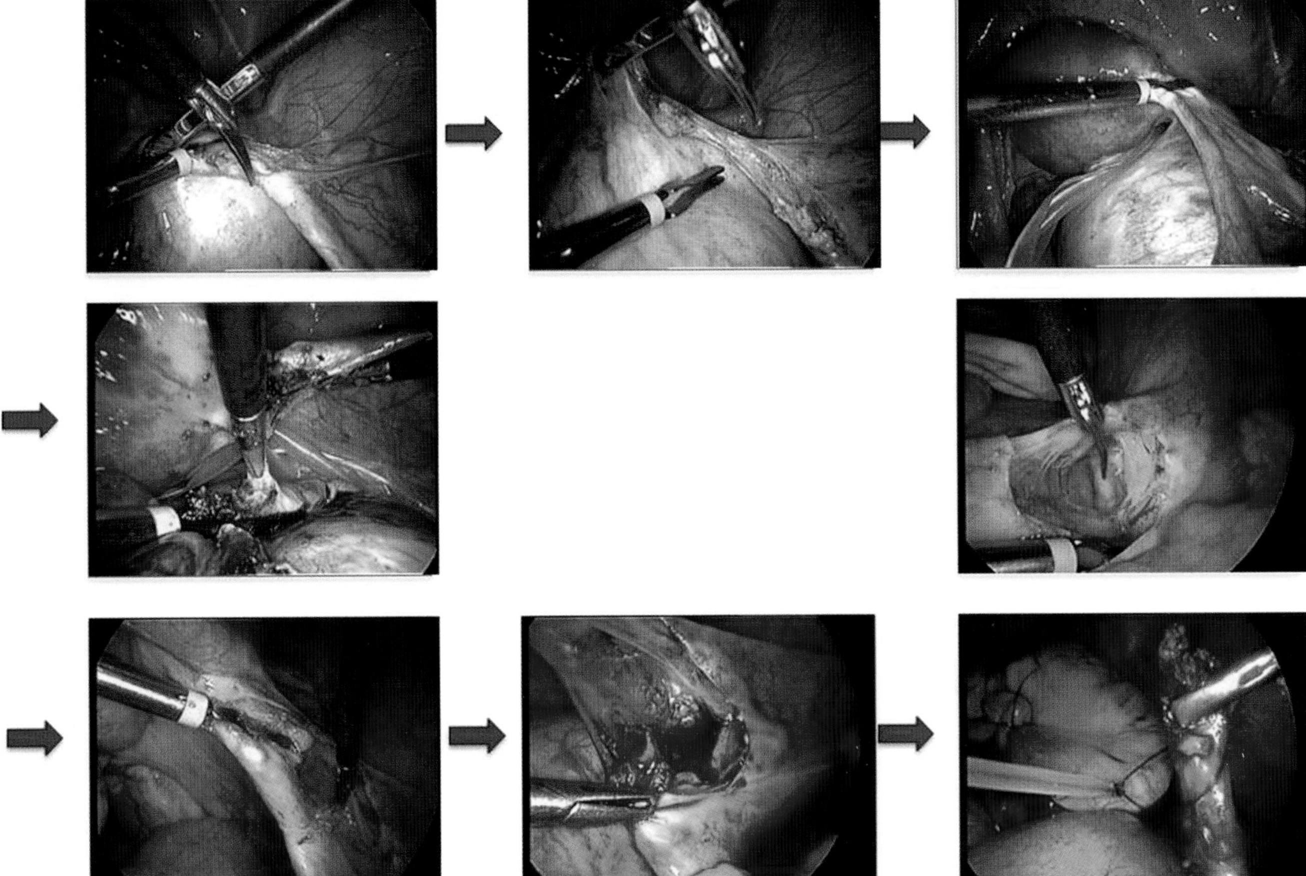

Fig. 15.8. Adnexectomy.

Adnexectomy (Fig. 15.8) To remove the ovary, we routinely perform an adnexectomy, as this approach allows a more reliable complete excision of all the ovarian tissue than an oophorectomy. Before beginning the procedure, it is important to look for any ovarian adhesions to the peritoneum of the broad ligament. If dense adhesions are found, the adnexectomy should remove the peritoneum of the broad ligament and a retroperitoneal approach is necessary to dissect the ureter up to the uterine vessels. The manipulation of the ovary should be kept to minimal to minimize the risks of tumor dissemination.

If there are no adhesions, adnexectomy is easy as the ovarian ligaments that are lengthened by the ovarian tumor are easily exposed, dissected, and treated. We generally use the fenestration of the broad ligament as described in our technique of laparoscopic hysterectomy [33]. The peritoneum of the anterior leaf of the broad ligament is opened after a meticulous coagulation of peritoneal capillaries to maintain an optimal vision of the operating field. This incision is stopped 1 cm short of midline and extended dorsolaterally to the infundibulopelvic ligament up to the pelvic sidewall. The wide opening of the anterior leaf of the broad ligament dorsally thus allows clear access to the posterior leaf of the broad ligament. This facilitates the detection of bowel behind this layer. The intention is to make a window in this posterior aspect of the broad ligament to separate the infundibulopelvic ligament from the ureter which is thus pushed laterally away from the vessels.

Once the window is enlarged, the ureter may be identified as being separate and distant from the infundibulopelvic ligament. However a ureteral dissection is not routinely necessary and/or performed. It should be used only when necessary in patients with extensive adhesion, severe endometriosis or myoma of the broad ligament.

After the fenestration, the infundibulopelvic ligament is coagulated and divided safely, avoiding any possible ureteric injury. To achieve safe coagulation of these vessels, it is essential to apply the bipolar coagulation on the vessels after dissection of the peritoneum. If the coagulation is applied on the peritoneum, which covers the vessels, it would retract and prevent the electrical current effectively coagulating the vessels. It is necessary to coagulate the infundibulopelvic ligament approximately twice to three times the width of the bipolar forceps to ensure reliable hemostasis.

If bleeding from the infundibulopelvic ligament occurs after its section, it is essential to grasp it and to dissect it again before using another method of hemostasis. Indeed when it retracts the distal end of the ligament is very close to the ureter and cannot be coagulated or ligated safely (Fig. 15.8).

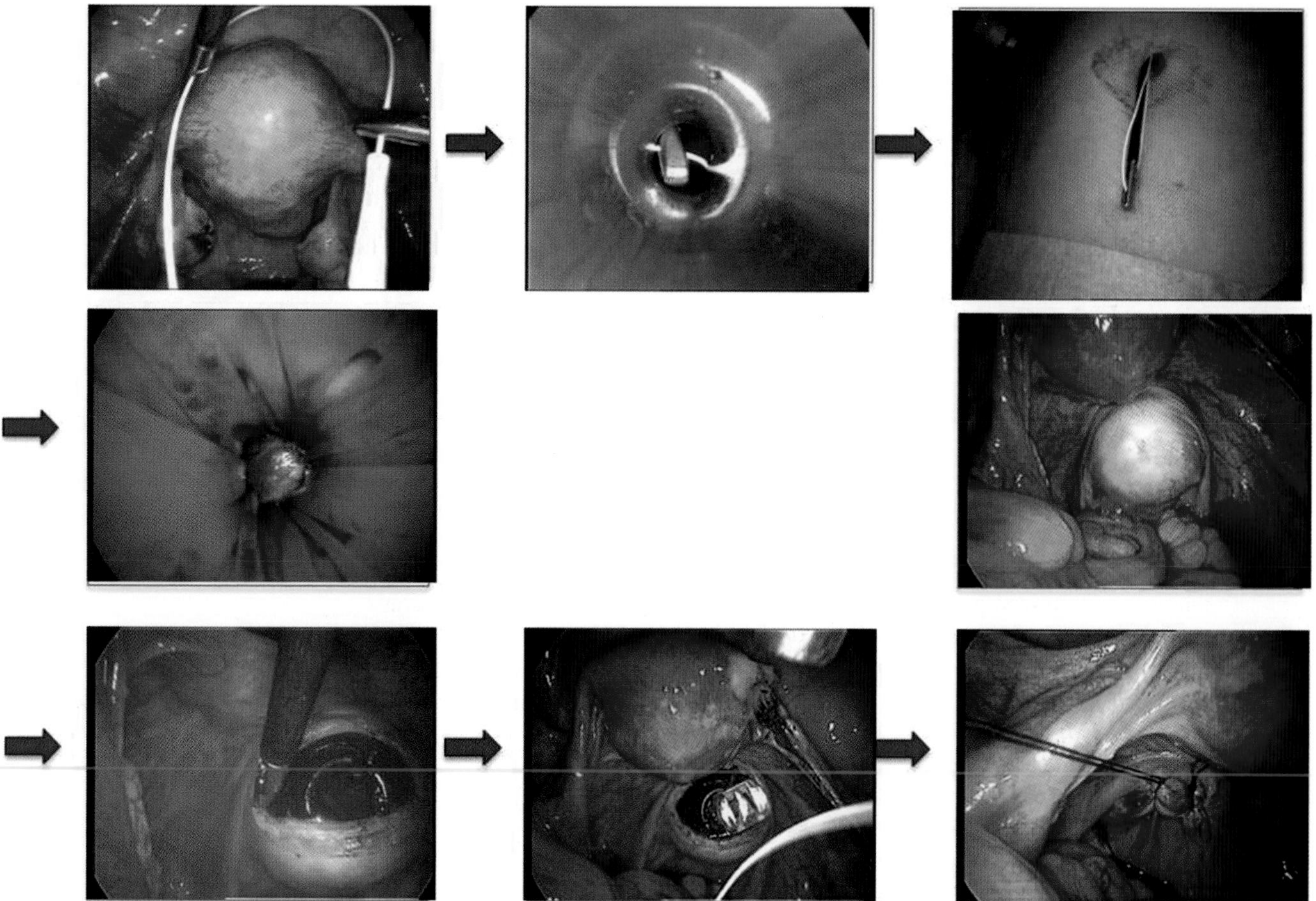

Fig. 15.9. Extraction of the mass.

Then the adnexal vessels are coagulated and cut gradually beginning by the treatment of the tube, of the utero-ovarian ligament, and of the adnexal vessels. Pulling the ovary posteriorly exposes these vessels. Again, it is important to grasp the ligament not the ovary itself. As cyst or tumor rupture may occur during an adnexectomy, the adnexa should be placed in an endobag before the procedure.

If the ovary is fixed to the broad ligament, the fenestration is impossible. The peritoneum is opened laterally to the infundibulo pelvic ligament. The retroperitoneal tissue is dissected to identify and dissect the ureter. The infundibulopelvic ligament is coagulated and cut. Then the ureter is dissected and the peritoneum adherent to the ovary excised. Dissection of the ureter may be difficult in patients previously operated for severe endometriosis, but it is mandatory to allow safe and complete excision of the ovary. Obviously, the risks of rupture are higher when the adhesions are severe. However, difficulties would be similar if the procedure was performed by laparotomy.

Laparotomy When laparoscopy proves to be too difficult to continue, it should be borne in mind that laparotomy is not contraindicated, nor a failure, nor indeed a complication of endoscopy. Moreover a laparotomy is mandatory, whenever an ovarian morcellation would be necessary for the extraction of the ovarian mass. Finally, in a young patient treated for a benign cyst, conservative treatment by laparotomy should be preferred to an adnexectomy by laparoscopy if the adnexectomy was only indicated because of a too difficult conservative laparoscopic procedure!

Extraction of the cyst or mass (Fig. 15.9)

Peritoneal and abdominal grafts may occur after treatment of benign lesions as well as after the treatment of malignant lesions [8,9,31]. This complication occurred before endoscopic bags became available, and confirms the need to protect the path of incision when extracting all surgical specimens. This rule also applies to the vagina.

A bag needs to have several qualities. It must be:

- suited to the size of the cyst: large enough to allow puncture for an 8- to 10-cm cyst, small enough for extraction of small cysts without enlarging the incision
- easy to open in the abdomen where it must remain open spontaneously, the orifice must be kept open thanks to a material that is rigid enough to make handling easier [6,12]
- long enough, so that extraction of tissues is easy and possible in obese patients
- strong enough to withstand the repeated traction applied by the surgeon without breaking: *the force applied is always too strong*

transparent to allow work under direct vision, both at the time of the puncture in the bag and also during extraction of the specimen.

If no endoscopic bag is available, small cystic lesions can be extracted after puncture using a 10 mm trocar with a reducing sleeve and a 5 mm instrument. The trocar and instrument can be removed once the cyst has been pulled inside the trocar. The difference in diameter between trocar and instrument allows the cyst to slip inside the trocar, avoiding the "guillotine" effect that would occur if both devices were of the same diameter. However, this method should be reserved for small lesions.

There are several ways to extract lesions placed in a bag. For patients with a previous appendectomy, the same skin incision can be used for extraction. However, in our department, extraction generally makes use of the umbilical trocar. For this, the bag is guided into the umbilical port using a suprapubic instrument under direct visual control. (Fig. 15.9) The lens is removed gradually as the suprapubic instrument moves into the umbilical trocar. When the lens has been completely removed from the trocar, the umbilical trocar is removed.

At this point, the end of the handle of the bag and the suprapubic instrument holding it are outside the abdomen. The bag is grasped, and the suprapubic grasping forceps withdrawn by means of its own trocar. Then the bag is opened using two or three abdominal surgery forceps and the cyst is extracted under visual control. It may be necessary to enlarge the umbilical incision around the bag.

If colpotomy is chosen, there are two possible techniques. The first applies in case of concomitant hysterectomy, when the vaginal opening is used for extraction. For the second technique, a colpotomy is made under endoscopic control using a special instrument (the "Spulher" ball), which enables a bulge to be produced in the posterior vaginal fornix while introducing a grasping forceps in a leak-proof manner [34] (Fig. 15.9). Colpotomy is convenient to extract large lesions. However it is not certain that the functional consequences of a vaginal incision are always preferable to the esthetic consequences of an abdominal incision.

For solid lesions, the rule is to enlarge the incision so that the cyst can be removed without morcellation and without adverse effects on the pathological examination. The only exception is fibrous lesions that resemble uterine fibroids, which can be incised in a bag by means of the vagina in the same manner as for uterine fibroids. The procedure must be stopped immediately if the lesion appears friable. Morcellation of ovarian fibroma is never acceptable unless the lesion is in a bag that fully protects the abdominal wall and peritoneal cavity.

Repairing the ovary

Ovarian suture is not necessary to prevent postoperative adhesions. In our experience, adnexal adhesions after treatment of non-endometriotic adnexal cysts have been observed only after treatment of benign teratomas and never after treatment of serous or mucinous cysts [31]. These adhesions were more likely caused by the contents of the cyst than by the procedure. Two experimental studies have shown that suturing the ovary induced more adhesions [35,36]. In these animal models, the ovary was incised and split in two along its largest diameter so that it returned to its normal shape spontaneously at the end of the intervention.

It is important to ensure that the ovary will gradually return to its normal shape at the end of the intervention. The technique should include:

- incision at the anti-mesial edge of the ovary, so that gravity closes the ovary when it falls back into the pouch of Douglas
- incision long enough to avoid tearing the ovary
- initial steps of ovarian reconstruction are patience and irrigation. Indeed, after dissection, if the ovary is given 5 to 10 minutes to recover, it is amazing how quickly the ovarian parenchyma recovers, retracts and "spontaneously reconstructs" the ovary
- if this is not quite good enough, "inversion" of the ovarian parenchyma after surgery is achieved using bipolar coagulation with low power densities on the surface of the cyst bed.

No sutures are needed in more than 90% of cases. However, if at the end of surgery the ovary is torn in many places, its shape should be restored using minimum suturing, to minimize ischemia in the remaining tissue. We use absorbable sutures placed only inside the ovary, as the ovarian cortical tissue is much more prone to adhesions than the peritoneum.

Intra-operative indications (Table 15.2)

Functional cyst

Preoperatively, every effort should be made to avoid surgical management of functional cysts. However, a functional cyst may be encountered in patients who are operated for another indication, such as infertility work-up or hysterectomy. The surgeon should be able to distinguish during the procedure a functional cyst from an organic cyst. This difference is essential because an organic cyst has to be entirely and immediately removed, whereas a functional cyst may only be biopsied to confirm the diagnosis and will disappear spontaneously a few weeks later. Despite the description of very precise macroscopic signs (Table 15.3), it is our experience that it can difficult to distinguish functional and organic cysts during surgery [9]. As a cystectomy is not indicated for the treatment of functional cyst, some organic ovarian cyst may be undertreated when diagnosed as functional. To avoid this, we recommend performing a cystectomy whenever technically feasible even for cysts diagnosed as functional. In functional cysts, the cystectomy may be impossible when the cyst wall is torn by any attempt of dissection thus confirming the diagnosis. However, this additional sign is pathognomonic of the diagnosis, only when malignancy can be excluded without any doubt.

Table 15.2. Intra-operative indications

Histology	Benign cyst	Condition	Method of treatment
Functional	Certain Certain	Reliable cystoscopy Doubtful diagnosis	Puncture biopsy Cystectomy after puncture if possible
Serous	Certain Uncertain: single vegetation Uncertain: multiple vegetations	No vegetation Negative frozen section	Cystectomy after puncture whatever the diameter Cystectomy after puncture if easy Adnexectomy without prior frozen section
Mucinous	Certain Certain Uncertain: vegetations	Single cyst or number < 3 Multiple cysts	Cystectomy after puncture whatever the diameter Adnexectomy whenever cystectomy appeared impossible despite the patient's age and careful dissection of all the cyst Adnexectomy without prior frozen section
Dermoid	Certain Certain Certain	Cyst < 7 cm Cyst from 7 to 10 cm Cyst > 10 cm	Cystectomy without puncture whatever the diameter Cystectomy after puncture whatever the diameter Transparietal cystectomy whatever the diameter
Para-tubal	Certain	No vegetation	Cystectomy without puncture whatever the diameter
Endometrioma	Certain Certain Certain Certain	< 4 cm 4 to 10 cm > 10 cm Multiple cysts	Destruction by CO_2 laser or bipolar coagulation Cystectomy after rupture and adhesiolysis Partial cystectomy and destruction or treatment in 3 steps Cystectomy or treatment in 3 steps

Table 15.3. Comparison between functional cyst and organic cyst

	Organic	Functional
Utero-ovarian ligament	Elongated	Normal
Cyst wall	Thick	Fine
Vessels	Comb at the hilum	Coralliform
Appearance of fluid	Variable	Saffron
Inside of cyst wall	Smooth	Retinoid
Cystectomy	Possible	"Impossible"

We emphasize that the diagnosis of functional cysts should be routinely confirmed by a large biopsy performed with scissors as shown in Fig. 15.3. A diagnosis based only on the inspection of the cyst is not reliable enough, indeed some serous cysts which are close to the surface of the ovary also appear blue when inspecting the ovarian surface. In the same way, chocolate cysts should be routinely biopsied to confirm the diagnosis of endometrioma; indeed it is well established that one-third of them are functional [37].

Ovarian neoplasms

Surgical indications currently used in our department are summarized in Table 15.2. Infertility surgeons initially designed operative laparoscopy. One of the main progresses of this approach was the conservative management of most benign ovarian and adnexal cysts. In our experience, we found that a vast majority of ovarian cysts of more than 8 centimeters can be managed with ovarian preserving procedures [31]. We and others demonstrated that high numbers of follicles and oocytes can be found in the ovarian tissue stretched by large cysts [38,39]. Therefore, this tissue should be preserved. If a cyst is benign a cystectomy is always the first choice, and resection of a part of the ovarian parenchyma found around the cyst is a mistake.

However, as emphasized above an adnexectomy should be done in macroscopically suspicious masses.

Conclusion

The development of laparoscopic surgery was a revolution in the treatment of adnexal masses. It also helped surgeons to improve the management of these patients. We learned from laparoscopic mistakes that complications also occurred before when patients were managed by laparotomy. As laparotomy was the only approach, these complications were rarely reported and discussed as consequences of inadequate surgical management. While developing safe laparoscopic management, we established simple rules to avoid these complications, making surgery of adnexal masses safer than before the endoscopic revolution. Finally, this revolution appears to be major progress as it allowed the utmost importance of ovarian-preserving procedures to be reiterated. Within the next 10 years, further technological revolutions, such as robotics, enhanced reality, and single port surgery, will be introduced. For simple procedures, such as the management of adnexal masses, the cost will be essential as this clinical problem is very common, and managed in small hospitals and in developing countries who will not be able to pay for highly expensive technologies which do not represent an obvious benefit for the patients.

References

1. Kruitwagen RF, Swinkels BM, Keyser KG, et al. Incidence and effect on survival of abdominal wall metastases at trocar or puncture sites following laparoscopy or paracentesis in women with ovarian cancer. Gynecol Oncol. 1996;**60**:233–7.
2. Maiman M, Seltzer V, Boyce J. Laparoscopic excision of ovarian neoplasms subsequently found to be malignant. Obstet Gynecol. 1991;77:563–5.
3. Blanc B, Boubli L, D'Ercole C, et al. Laparoscopic management of malignant ovarian cysts: a 78-case national survey part 1: preoperative and laparoscopic evaluation. Eur J Obstet Gynecol Reprod Biol. 1994;**56**:177–80.
4. Blanc B, D'Ercole C, Nicoloso E, et al. Laparoscopic management of malignant ovarian cysts: a 78-case national survey part 2: Follow up and final treatment. Eur J Obstet Gynecol Reprod Biol. 1994;**61**:147–50.
5. Kinderman G, Maassen V, Kuhn W. Laparoscopic management of ovarian malignomas. Geburtshilfe Frauenheilkd. 1995;**55**:687–94.
6. Wenzl R, Lehner R, Husslein P, et al. Laparoscopic survey in cases of ovarian malignancies: an Austria-wide survey. Gynecol Oncol. 1996;**63**:57–61.
7. Young RC, Decker DG, Wharton JT, et al. Staging laparotomy in early ovarian cancer. JAMA. 1983;**250**:3072–6.
8. Helawa ME, Krepart GV, Lotocki R. Staging laparotomy in early epithelial ovarian carcinoma. Am J Obstet Gynecol. 1986;**154**:282–6.
9. Canis M, Mage G, Pouly JL, et al. Laparoscopic diagnosis of adnexal cystic masses: a 12 years experience with long-term follow-up. Obstet Gynecol. 1994;**5**:707–12.
10. Canis M, Pouly JL, Wattiez A, et al. Laparoscopic management of adnexal masses suspicious at ultrasound. Obstet Gynecol. 1997;**89**:679–83.
11. Gomel V. The impact of microsurgery in gynecology. Clin Obstet Gynecol. 1980;**23**:1301–10.
12. Somigliana E, Benaglia L, Vigano' P, et al. Surgical measures for endometriosis-related infertility: a plea for research. Placenta. 2011;**32**(Suppl 3): S238–42.
13. Zanetta G, Chiari S, Rota S, et al. Conservative surgery for stage I ovarian carcinoma in women of childbearing age. Br J Obstet Gynaecol. 1997;**104**:1030–5.
14. Lachance JA, Choudhri AF, Sarti M, et al. A nomogram for estimating the probability of ovarian cancer. Gynecol Oncol. 2011;**121**:2–7.
15. Boll D, Geomini PM, Brölmann HA, et al. The pre-operative assessment of the adnexal mass: the accuracy of clinical estimates versus clinical prediction rules. BJOG. 2003;**110**:519–23.
16. Mol BW, Boll D, De Kanter M, et al. Distinguishing the benign and malignant adnexal mass: an external validation of prognostic models. Gynecol Oncol. 2001;**80**:162–7.
17. Timmerman D, Van Calster B, Jurkovic D, et al. Inclusion of CA-125 does not improve mathematical models developed to distinguish between benign and malignant adnexal tumors. J Clin Oncol. 2007;**25**:4194–200.
18. Valentin L, Jurkovic D, Van Calster B, et al. Adding a single CA125 measurement to ultrasound imaging performed by an experienced examiner does not improve preoperative discrimination between benign and malignant adnexal masses. Ultrasound Obstet Gynecol. 2009;**34**:345–54.
19. Goff BA, Miller JW, Matthews B, et al. Involvement of gynecologic oncologists in the treatment of patients with a suspicious ovarian mass. Obstet Gynecol. 2011;**118**:854–62.
20. Bristow RE. Predicting "unresectable" ovarian cancer: taking aim at a moving target. Gynecol Oncol. 2006;**100**:449–50.
21. Vergote I, De Brabanter J, Fyles A, et al. Prognostic importance of degree of differentiation and cyst rupture in stage I invasive epithelial ovarian carcinoma. Lancet. 2001;**357**:176–82.
22. Bakkum-Gamez JN, Richardson DL, Seamon LG, et al. Influence of intraoperative capsule rupture on outcomes in stage I epithelial ovarian cancer. Obstet Gynecol. 2009;**113**:11–17.
23. Paulsen T, Kærn J, Tropé C. Improved 5-year disease-free survival for FIGO stage I epithelial ovarian cancer patients without tumor rupture during surgery. Gynecol Oncol. 2011;**122**:83–8.
24. Higashi M, Kajiyama H, Shibata K, et al. Survival impact of capsule rupture in stage I clear cell carcinoma of the ovary in comparison with other histological types. Gynecol Oncol. 2011;**123**:474–8.
25. Goudge CS, Li Z, Downs LS Jr. The influence of intraoperative tumor rupture on recurrence risk in stage Ic epithelial ovarian cancer. Eur J Gynaecol Oncol. 2009;**30**:25–8.
26. Twaalfhoven FCM, Peters AAW, Trimos JB, et al. The accuracy of frozen section diagnosis of ovarian tumors. Gynecol Oncol. 1990;**41**:189–92.
27. Obiakor I, Maiman M, Mittal K, et al. The accuracy of frozen section in the diagnosis of ovarian neoplasms. Gynecol Oncol. 1991;**43**:61–3.
28. Canis M, Mashiach R, Wattiez A, et al. Frozen section in laparoscopic management of macroscopically suspicious ovarian masses. J Am Assoc Gynecol Laparosc. 2004;**11**:365–9.
29. Granberg S, Wikland M, Jansson I. Macroscopic characterization of ovarian tumors and the relation to the histological diagnosis: criteria to be used for ultrasound evaluation. Gynecol Oncol. 1989;**35**:139–44.
30. Donnez J, Nisolle M, Gillet N, et al. Large ovarian endometriomas. Hum Reprod. 1996;**1**:641–6.
31. Canis M, Botchorishvili R, Manhes H, et al. Management of adnexal masses: role and risk of laparoscopy. Semin Surg Oncol. 2000;**19**:28–35.
32. Mage G, Canis M, Manhes H, et al. Laparoscopic management of adnexal cystic masses. J Gynecol Surg. 1990;**6**:71–9.
33. Canis M, Botchorishvili R, Ang C, et al. When is laparotomy needed in hysterectomy for benign uterine disease? J Minim Invasive Gynecol. 2008;**15**:38–43.
34. Spuhler SC, Sauthier PG, Chardonnens EG, De Grandi P. A new vaginal extractor for laparoscopic surgery. J Am Assoc Gynecol Laparosc. 1994;**1**:401–4.
35. Wiskind AK, Toledo AA, Dudley AG, et al. Adhesion formation after ovarian wound repair in New Zealand white rabbits: A comparison of microsurgical closure with ovarian non closure. Am J Obstet Gynecol. 1990;**163**:1674–8.

36. Brumsted JR, Deaton J, Lavigne E, et al. Postoperative adhesion formation after wedge resection with and without ovarian reconstruction in the rabbit. Fertil Steril. 1990;**53**:723–6.

37. Martin DC, Berry JD. Histology of chocolate cysts. J Gynecol Surg. 1990;**6**:43–6.

38. Schubert B, Canis M, Darcha C, et al. Human ovarian tissue from cortex surrounding benign cysts: a model to study ovarian tissue cryopreservation. Hum Reprod. 2005;**20**:1786–92.

39. Maneschi F, Marasa L, Incandela S, et al. Ovarian cortex surrounding benign neoplasms: a histologic study. Am J Obstet Gynecol. 1993;**169**:388–93.

Chapter 16

Ultrasound, MRI, CT, and PET imaging of ovarian cancer

William L. Simpson, Jr., MD, and Lale Kostakoglu, MD MPH

Introduction

The ovaries are paired almond-shaped organs located along each pelvic sidewall. Normal ovarian volumes range up to 20 mL and 8–10 mL in pre-menopausal and post-menopausal women, respectively [1]. Each ovary is covered by surface epithelium and encloses numerous follicles, containing germ cells (eggs), within the ovarian stromal tissue [2]. With each menstrual cycle, a follicle matures and releases its ovum into the fallopian tube and then becomes a corpus luteum, which in the absence of pregnancy involutes to form a corpus albicans.

Ovarian cancer is the ninth most common cancer among women worldwide. It is the fifth most common cause of female cancer-related death. Ovarian cancer causes more deaths than any other cancer of the female reproductive tract. In 2013, in the United States there will be an estimated 22,240 new cases of ovarian cancer diagnosed and 14,030 deaths from the disease [3]. Risk factors for the development of ovarian cancer include advanced age, nulliparity, early menarche, late menopause, and long-term hormone replacement therapy [4]. Furthermore, approximately 10% of ovarian cancers are related to genetic mutations with the breast and ovarian cancer genes, *BRCA1* and *BRCA2*, and Lynch II syndrome accounting for the majority of these cases [3–5].

Approximately 85–90% of ovarian neoplasms originate in the surface epithelium, whereas 10% originate in the germ cells or stroma and 5% are metastatic lesions to the ovary [6,7]. Ovarian neoplasms are categorized as benign, borderline, or malignant. At the time of diagnosis, approximately 65% of women are advanced stage (stage III or IV) [3] with an estimated 5-year survival of 23–73% [8]. This is due to the fact that early ovarian cancer is often asymptomatic. When confined to the ovary (stage 1), the 5-year survival increases to 92% [8]. Borderline tumors often occur in pre-menopausal women, and 75% are diagnosed at stage 1 leading to a favorable prognosis [9].

Positron emission tomography imaging

Positron emission tomography (PET) is based on functional rather than morphological characterization of tissues. The principal radiolabeled molecule for PET imaging, 18-fluorodeoxyglucose (FDG; T1/2:110 min) is a glucose analog and transported by the glucose transporter proteins across the cell membranes of tumor cells that preferentially accumulate FDG on the basis of their greater glucose metabolic rates compared with normal cells. Following entry into the cell, FDG is instantly phosphorylated by the enzyme hexokinase, whose expression is increased in tumor cells, and is trapped within the cell without further metabolism.

Over the past decade, the advent of dedicated PET and computer tomography (PET/CT) scanners has allowed the integration of anatomic and functional data in cancer imaging, which is conducive to increased lesion detection with metabolic tracing and simultaneously obtained anatomic reference. This metabolic modality has proved to be useful and more accurate than conventional techniques in staging and restaging of various malignancies. Although the data on the utility of FDG PET imaging in ovarian cancer are relatively limited, there is mounting evidence that PET is increasingly used in imaging ovarian cancer, particularly in the post-therapy setting to identify disease relapse. At present, there is a growing interest in assessing the incremental value of FDG PET/CT when combined with conventional tests with an intention of its integration into the diagnostic algorithm.

Patient preparation for imaging and FDG PET/CT protocols

The patients should be prepared for PET imaging to increase the test accuracy. The bladder should be voided to prevent the urinary excretion of FDG into the bladder from obscuring pelvic findings. It is advisable to use a urinary catheter for continuously emptying the bladder during the imaging procedure. Patient hydration is encouraged with 1,000 mL of 0.9% isotonic saline given intravenously starting from 30 min after injection of FDG. Furosemide should be considered (20 mg intravenously), 45 min after FDG injection. Patients should drink approximately 250 mL of water to distend the stomach before their undergoing imaging to avoid stomach wall uptake. There are various approaches with respect to the CT technique that can be adopted for PET/CT imaging:

1. Use of low-dose unenhanced CT for attenuation correction and co-registration;
2. Use of a dedicated CT protocol that uses intravenous contrast, such that the CT data are used for attenuation correction, co-registration, and diagnosis [10];

Altchek's Diagnosis and Management of Ovarian Disorders, ed. Liane Deligdisch, Nathan G. Kase, and Carmel J. Cohen. Published by Cambridge University Press.

3. Combined approach, with low-dose CT performed first primarily to obtain attenuation information for PET data, followed by diagnostic standard-dose contrast material – enhanced CT.

Whole-body PET is performed with the patient's arms raised to cover between the orbitomeatal line and the proximal third of the femurs. In addition, a separate one- or two-bed prone pelvic view is recommended to ensure separation of the bladder and the prerectal space for better evaluation of the presacral structures and the relation of the mass with respect to the bladder and the rectum to guide the surgeon. Helical CT of the abdomen and pelvis is performed according to the institutional protocol. Depending on the capability of the scanner, sections of 2.5–5.0 mm may be obtained to optimize visualization of the cervix and parametrial tissues.

Adnexal mass characterization; benign versus malignant lesions

Ovarian cancer most commonly presents as an ovarian mass. An adnexal mass is a common finding occurring in 10% of both pre- and post-menopausal women [11,12]. Diagnosis can be challenging because benign and malignant imaging features may overlap [13]. The majority of adnexal masses are usually benign [12] with only 13–21% of adnexal masses that go to surgery revealing malignancy [14]. Ultrasound is the first-line imaging modality for the evaluation of the gynecologic organs and a suspected adnexal mass due to its low cost, wide availability, and lack of ionizing radiation. Clinical information such as the patient's age and pregnancy status must be considered in the differential diagnosis.

Both transabdominal and transvaginal ultrasound (TVU) is used to evaluate the ovaries. The transabdominal approach has the advantage of a larger field of view which can facilitate imaging of large masses which extend up into the abdomen from the pelvis. Disadvantages of the transabdominal approach include interposed bowel gas (which can obscure visualization of the ovaries), diminished penetrance of ultrasound in obese patients, its operator dependability, and variable results based on the presence of an optimal acoustic imaging window which uses a full urinary bladder. Transvaginal ultrasound has higher resolution allowing for a more detailed evaluation of ovarian architecture at the expense of a smaller field of view limiting assessment of large masses.

Both morphologic gray scale and color Doppler findings should be used to optimally assess an adnexal mass [15–19]. Imaging features that favor malignancy in an ovarian mass are listed in Table 16.1 (Fig. 16.1a). Early signs of malignancy include an ovary that is enlarged for the patient's age or one that is more than twice the volume of the contralateral ovary [18]. The most important feature for malignancy is the presence of a solid component in an ovarian mass [15]. Benign lesions tend to have peripheral vascular flow, whereas their malignant counterparts demonstrate central flow in the solid components [20]. On spectral Doppler analysis, ovarian carcinoma commonly demonstrates low-resistance waveforms due to the lack

Table 16.1. Imaging findings suggestive of malignancy

1. Solid mass
2. Solid component (mural nodule, papillary projections) in a cystic lesion that is not hyper-echoic
3. Septations more than 3 mm in thickness
4. Central color or power Doppler flow within the solid component of a mass
5. Ascites (any in post-menopausal women and more than the physiologic amount in a pre-menopausal woman)

of smooth muscle in tumor neo-vascularity [18]. However, there is insufficient evidence to support a specific resistive index threshold value because several benign lesions can also demonstrate low resistance vascular flow [21,22].

Some adnexal masses remain indeterminate after ultrasound. Magnetic resonance imaging (MRI) is then used as a problem solving tool. A meta-analysis showed that contrast enhanced MRI when compared with CT or combined gray scale and color Doppler ultrasound resulted in the highest probability of malignancy in an indeterminate adnexal mass [23]. Tissue characterization based on MR signal characteristics can confidently diagnose several benign adnexal masses. This is the predominant contribution of MRI in adnexal mass characterization [24].

A pelvic MRI examination directed to adnexal mass assessment should include T1-weighted and T2-weighted images to delineate pelvic anatomy, fat saturated T1-weighted images for differentiation of fat and hemorrhage, and gadolinium enhanced T1-weighted images to demonstrate the internal structure of cystic lesions and improve detection of solid components [7, 11]. Imaging features suggestive of malignancy are similar to those for ultrasound (Table 16.1) and include a mixed solid and cystic mass or a predominantly cystic mass with enhancing thick (>3 mm) septations, mural nodules, or papillary projections (Fig. 16.1b). An irregular or thickened cyst wall and necrosis within a solid mass are additional findings suspicious for malignancy. Ancillary findings that increase confidence in a malignant diagnosis include involvement of the pelvic side wall, peritoneal disease, ascites, and adenopathy [7,24,25].

CT is not used specifically for characterization of adnexal masses due to its poor tissue contrast. However, with increasing usage of CT, incidental ovarian lesions are frequently detected. CT is often the first-line imaging examination in patients presenting with vague abdominal pain or distention, which can be the non-specific presentation of ovarian cancer [13]. Imaging features suggestive of malignancy are similar to those for MRI (Table 16.1) and include mixed solid and cystic masses with thick or irregular walls, enhancing thick septations (Fig. 16.1c), mural nodules or papillary projections, and necrosis in a solid tumor [24]. In addition, size larger than 4 cm and bilateral solid masses on CT also raise suspicion for malignancy [11]. Again, ancillary findings such as pelvic organ or side wall invasion, ascites, peritoneal carcinomatosis, and lymphadenopathy increase diagnostic confidence [7,24,25].

In screening of asymptomatic adnexal masses, FDG PET has not proved superior to morphologic modalities with a

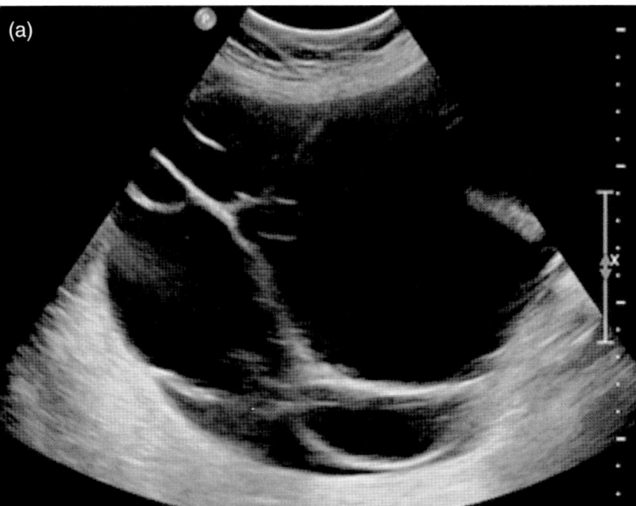

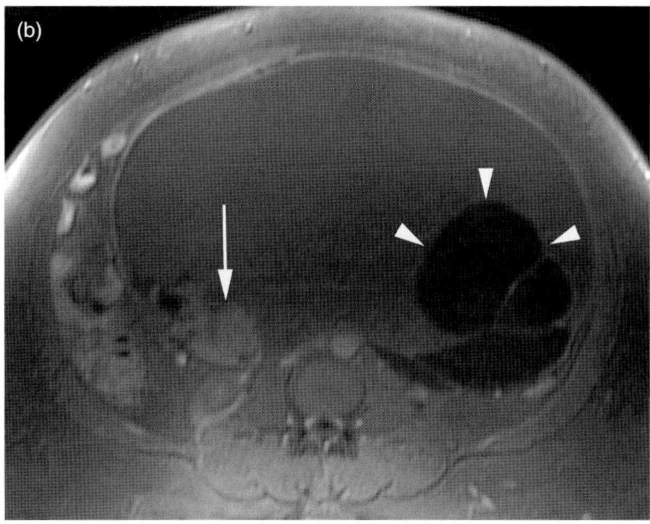

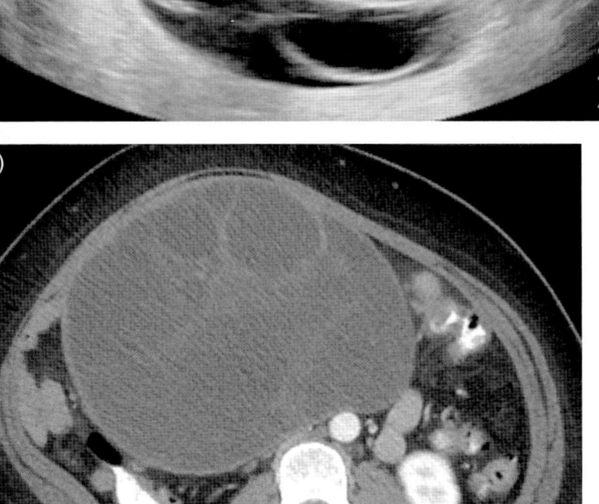

Fig. 16.1. (a) Longitudinal gray scale ultrasound image of a large right ovarian mass demonstrating findings suspicious for malignancy including multiple thickened septations measuring more than 3 mm in a predominantly cystic mass. (b) Axial T1-weighted post gadolinium image through the lower abdomen shows a large predominantly cystic mass with loculations demonstrating lower signal than the remainder of the fluid (arrowheads) as well as an enhancing mural nodule (arrow). (c) Axial contrast-enhanced CT image demonstrates a large cystic ovarian mass extending up into the abdomen with several thickened and enhancing septations.

reported sensitivity of only 60% and a specificity of 75% [26,27]. However, with the introduction of integrated PET/CT imaging, promising results were obtained in the characterization of asymptomatic adnexal masses. In a study of 50 patients presenting with a pelvic lesion, Castellucci et al. found a FDG PET/CT sensitivity, specificity, negative predictive value (NPV), and positive predictive value (PPV) of 87, 100, 81, and 100%, respectively, compared with 90, 61, 78, and 80%, respectively, for transvaginal ultrasound (TVU). It is noteworthy to state that FDG PET/CT was true negative in all patients (n = 18) with histologically proven benign ovarian masses [28]. In patients presenting with a pelvic mass, an FDG PET/CT sensitivity of as high as 100% and a specificity of 85–93% were reported in two studies designed to discriminate benign and borderline ovarian tumors from malignant ovarian tumors [29,30]. A focally and significantly increased FDG uptake with a standardized uptake value (SUV) of 3.0 or higher was considered positive for ovarian malignancy [28] (Fig. 16.2a,b). Similarly, in a more recent study ($n = 30$), the degree of FDG uptake in a benign mass was found to be significantly lower than that of malignant tumors (SUVmax 1.7 vs. 9.3; $P = 0.005$), however, the SUVs were not helpful in discriminating between benign and borderline tumors [31]. More recently, pretreatment metabolic parameters such as metabolic tumor volume showed a statistically significant association ($P = 0.022$, hazard ratio 5.57) with recurrence in patients with epithelial ovarian cancer in a preliminary study [31]. Further prospective, confirmatory data are warranted to define a cut-off SUV for the differentiation of malignant from benign processes. US and MRI are the mainstay for the diagnosis of borderline ovarian tumors and combining MRI PET may facilitate the identification of some borderline tumors.

In summary, PET/CT has a high specificity for lesions within its resolution limits (6–7 mm), but its sensitivity is lower than that of TVU, which continues to be the test of choice for screening of pelvic masses to rule out ovarian cancer. However, because of its high specificity FDG PET/CT imaging can be used as a problem-solving tool to confirm the diagnosis of ovarian cancer in borderline cases before surgical intervention.

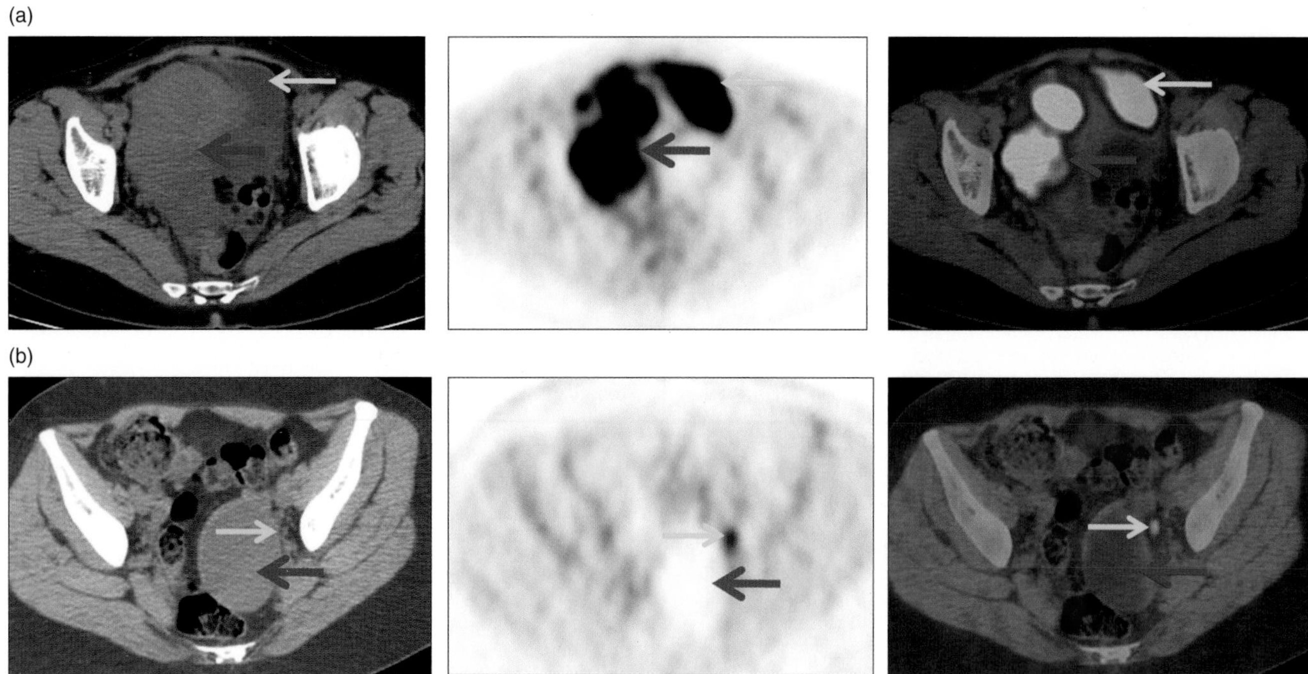

Fig. 16.2. (a) A 55-year-old woman recently diagnosed with serous papillary adenocarcinoma of the ovary, referred for evaluation of extent of disease. Axial images of PET/CT (left CT, middle PET, right fusion PET/CT) demonstrate intensely increased FDG uptake in the right pelvis corresponding to an irregular mass in the region of the right ovary (red arrow) displacing the bladder to the left (yellow arrow). The subsequent surgery revealed an advanced stage disease with involvement of the bladder wall. (b) A 56-year-old woman with a history of lymphoma, referred for evaluation of disease status after completion of chemotherapy. Axial images of PET/CT demonstrate a large cystic mass in the left pelvis (red arrow) displacing the ureter (yellow arrow) with no FDG uptake typical for a benign ovarian cyst. However, caution should be exercised in that copious mucin in some malignant lesions may be falsely positive on FDG PET imaging. Thus, pelvic ultrasound examination should be recommended in patients with large ovarian cystic lesions, particularly in the post-menopausal population.

Staging of ovarian cancer

Tumor stage represents the most important prognostic factor in ovarian cancer with a 5-year survival rate of 93, 70, 37, and 25% for stage I, stage II, stage III, and stage IV cancers, respectively [32]. Thus, accurate staging is crucial for determining the appropriate therapeutic strategy in ovarian cancer.

Traditionally, ovarian cancer has been staged surgically. A full staging laparotomy includes hysterectomy, bilateral salpingo-oophorectomy, pelvic and retroperitoneal lymph node biopsies, omentectomy, peritoneal biopsies, and peritoneal washings [33]. The most widely used staging classification is the International Federation of Obstetrics and Gynecology (FIGO) system (Table 16.2) [34]. Pre-operative cross-sectional imaging has gained acceptance as a complimentary noninvasive staging tool to provide surgeons with potential targets for biopsy. The goals of pre-operative staging are (a) confirm a malignant adnexal mass, (b) assess tumor burden and map location of metastatic disease, (c) diagnose complications such as bowel or ureteral obstruction, and (d) exclude a metastatic primary gastrointestinal malignancy that mimics ovarian cancer [35].

Knowledge of the typical pattern of spread for ovarian cancer is necessary for optimal pre-operative staging. Ovarian cancer spreads by local extension, peritoneal dissemination, lymphatic dissemination, and hematogenous dissemination.

As a mass in the ovary grows, it can directly invade local structures such as the uterus, rectum, or bladder. Obliteration of the fat plane between the tumor and the bladder or rectum can be a sign of direct invasion. Pelvic sidewall invasion is considered to be present if there is less than 3 mm between the tumor and the pelvic sidewall [36].

The most common pathway of ovarian cancer spread is peritoneal dissemination, which is found in 70% of patients at diagnosis [37]. Because the majority of ovarian cancers arise from the surface epithelium, tumor cells can easily shed into the peritoneum. The cells then follow the circulation of the peritoneal fluid up the paracolic gutters to the diaphragm. Metastases appear as enhancing nodular masses or plaque-like thickening of the peritoneum (Fig. 16.3). They commonly occur at peritoneal reflections where the fluid tends to stay longer such as the cul-de-sac, paracolic gutters, liver surface, subdiaphragmatic regions, and bowel surfaces; less frequently seen sites of metastases include the mesentery, porta hepatis, gastrohepatic, and gastrosplenic ligaments [7]. However, the omentum is the most common site of abdominal peritoneal spread [11]. Early omental involvement can appear as a fine net-like or reticulonodular pattern (Fig. 16.4a), which can then progress to soft tissue nodules and conglomerate masses known as "omental caking" [4] (Fig. 16.4b). The presence of ascites makes the detection of peritoneal metastases easier and is a positive predictor of peritoneal disease.

Lymphatic dissemination occurs by means of three routes. The main lymphatic drainage of the ovaries is along the gonadal vessels to the para-aortic retroperitoneal nodes (Fig. 16.5a). Alternate routes of drainage are along the broad ligament to the external iliac (Fig. 16.5b) and obturator nodes and less

Table 16.2. FIGO staging of ovarian cancer

Stage	Description
Stage I	Tumor limited to ovaries
IA	Tumor limited to one ovary, capsule intact, no tumor on ovarian surface, no malignant cells in ascites or peritoneal washings
IB	Tumor limited to both ovaries, capsule intact, no tumor on ovarian surface, no malignant cells in ascites or peritoneal washings
IC	Tumor limited to one or both ovaries with any of the following: capsular rupture, tumor on ovarian surface, malignant cells in ascites or peritoneal washings
Stage II	Tumor involves one or both ovaries with pelvic extension or implants
IIA	Extension and/or implants on uterus and/or tubes, no malignant cells in ascites or peritoneal washings
IIB	Extension and/or implants on other pelvic tissues, no malignant cells in ascites or peritoneal washings
IIC	Pelvic extension and/or implants with malignant cells in ascites or peritoneal washings
Stage III	Tumor involves one or both ovaries with microscopically confirmed peritoneal metastasis outside the pelvis
IIIA	Microscopic peritoneal metastasis beyond pelvis without macroscopic tumor
IIIB	Macroscopic peritoneal metastasis beyond pelvis ≤ 2 cm in greatest dimension
IIIC	Macroscopic peritoneal metastasis beyond pelvis > 2 cm in greatest dimension
Stage IV	Distant metastasis (excludes peritoneal metastasis)

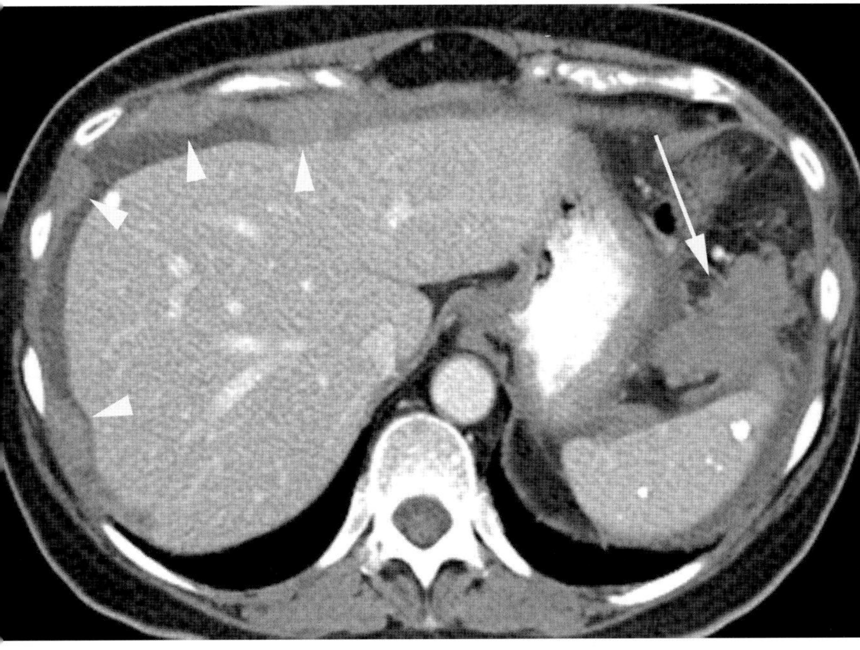

Fig. 16.3. Axial contrast-enhanced CT image through the upper abdomen demonstrates multiple enhancing masses along the peritoneum lining the right hemidiaphragm (arrowheads) consistent with peritoneal metastases. An additional enhancing mass is seen between the stomach and spleen (arrow) consistent with a gastro-splenic ligament metastasis. Ascites is also present around the liver and spleen.

ommonly along the round ligament to the inguinal odes [7,11]. Cardiophrenic lymph nodes can be clinically ignificant because they are along the main drainage route f the peritoneal cavity [38]. If the lymphatics of the iaphragm become occluded with malignant cells, it will lead o the accumulation of ascites. On cross-sectional imaging, ymph nodes larger than 1 cm in short axis are considered bnormal. Using this threshold, pre-operative CT has sensitivty and specificity of 50% and 92%, respectively, while that of IRI is 83% and 95% [26].

Hematogenous dissemination refers to abdominal visceral arenchymal involvement or spread outside the peritoneal cavty. It is rare at the time of initial diagnosis [7,11,38]. Common sites of hematogenous metastasis include the liver, lung, pleura, adrenal glands, and spleen [7,11] (Fig. 16.6). It is important to differentiate between a liver surface metastasis (stage III) and a parenchymal metastasis (stage IV). The presence of a pleural effusion can suggest pleural involvement; however, cytologic evaluation is required to confirm malignant dissemination because pleural effusions are common findings on imaging studies of the abdomen and pelvis.

Although US and/or MRI are the preferred imaging modalities for the initial diagnosis of a malignant ovarian mass, CT is the modality of choice for staging ovarian cancer. It provides coverage of the entire abdomen and pelvis in a short amount of time and is widely available. Intravenous contrast enhancement in the

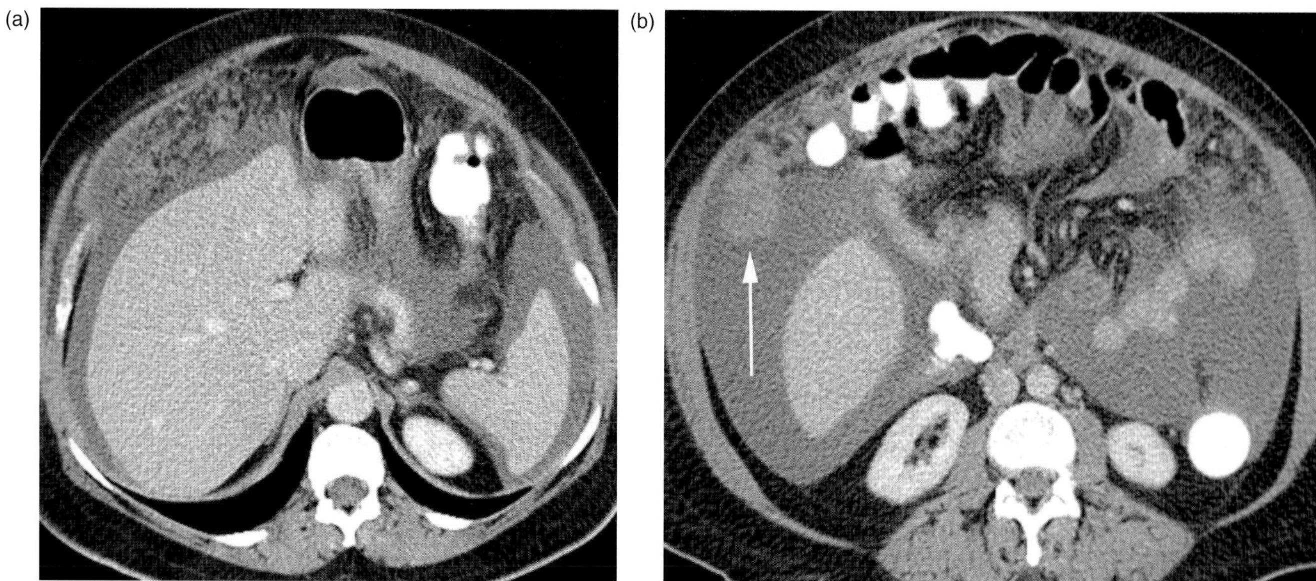

Fig. 16.4. (a) Reticulonodular infiltration is noted in the omentum anterior to the liver consistent with early omental metastasis. Ascites is also present. (b) More inferiorly in the same patient there is a solid mass in the omentum (arrow) on the right side of the abdomen consistent with a more advanced and solid metastasis, tl so-called "omental cake."

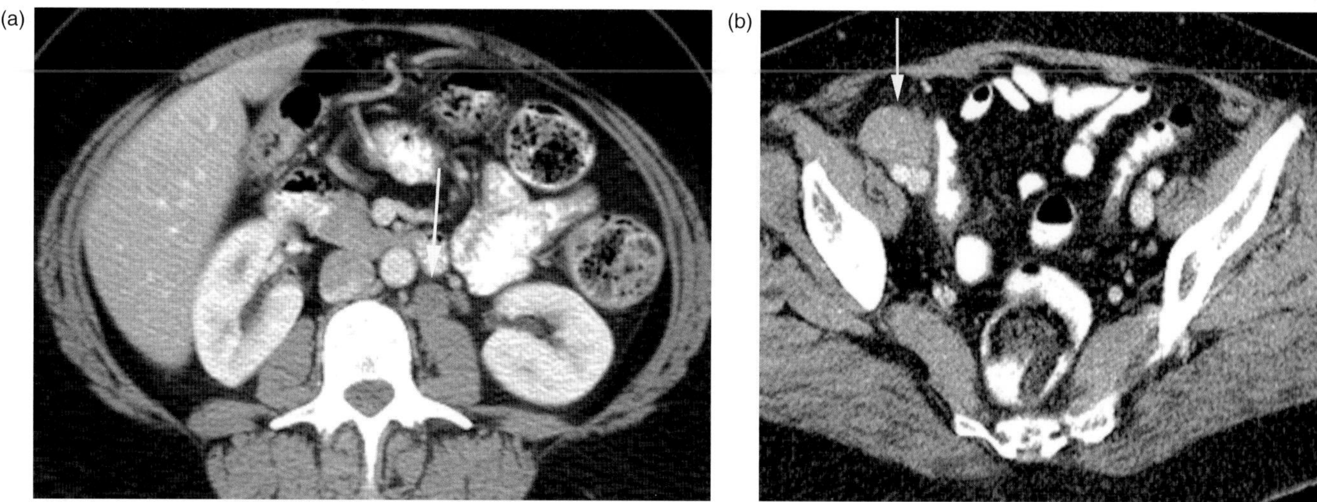

Fig. 16.5. (a) Enlarged left para-arotic lymph node (arrow) proven to be metastatic disease in a woman with ovarian cancer. (b) Enlarged and enhancing right extern iliac chain node (arrow) in a patient with known ovarian cancer.

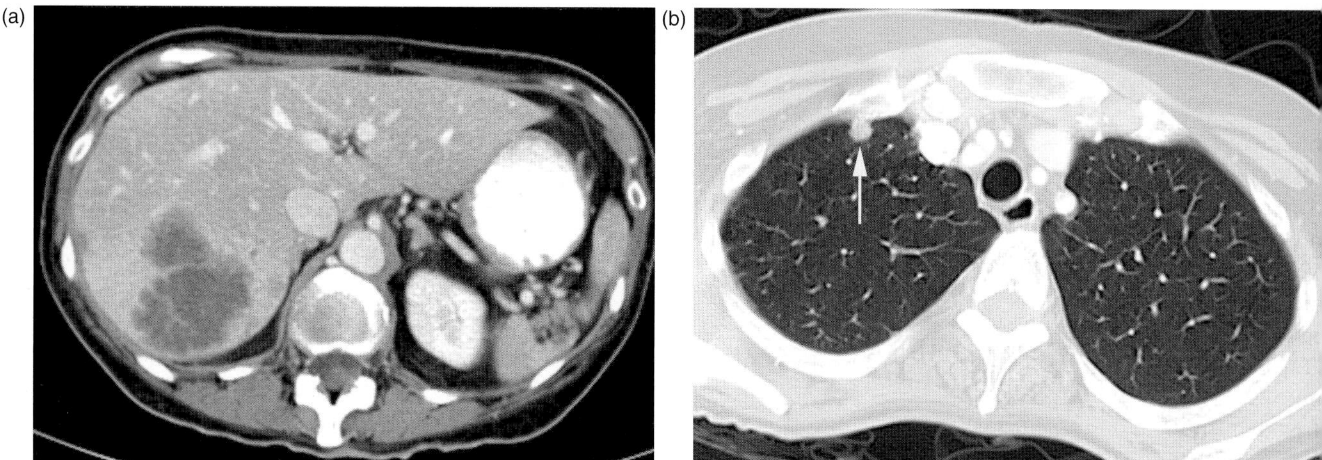

Fig. 16.6. (a) A single bilobed versus two adjacent irregularly bordered, low density masses in the right lobe of the liver consistent with parenchymal metastasis. (Well-defined non-calcified subpleural nodule anteriorly in the right upper lobe (arrow) proven to be metastatic ovarian carcinoma.

ɜnous phase is typically performed to detect solid enhancing ɔmponents in complex adnexal masses and peritoneal implants. owel opacification with oral contrast helps differentiate owel loops from lymphadenopathy and peritoneal/omental nplants. It can also aid in the detection of bowel wall thickening condary to serosal implants. Rectal contrast can be used to cilitate detection of bowel involvement at the rectosigmoid gion. The accuracy of CT in staging ovarian cancer ranges om 70–90% [4,26,39].

As in ovarian cancer detection, MRI is used primarily as a roblem solving tool for staging. Although it is not the modality of noice for staging ovarian cancer, studies have shown no differ-nce in the accuracy of staging between CT and MRI [36,40]. /hen used for staging, MR examination should include T1-eighted and T2-weighted sequences through the pelvis in at ast two planes, T2-weighted sequences through the abdomen, nd contrast-enhanced T1-weighted fat-saturated sequences rough the abdomen and pelvis. Bowel opacification is not typ-ally used. MR imaging has the advantage of improved soft tissue ontrast over CT. It can also be used in patients with an allergy to dinated contrast and in pregnant patients. Disadvantages of RI include difficulty covering the entire abdomen and pelvis ith adequate resolution, long examination time and high cost. ecent studies have shown that a diffusion-weighted sequence can crease reader confidence and identify metastatic lesions that can e difficult to visualize on standard sequences [41].

Although ultrasound is particularly useful for the detection f an ovarian mass, it is not used for ovarian cancer staging. his is due to its relatively small field of view, operator depend-nce, and technical limitations due to patient obesity and bowel as. Ultrasound, however, is useful for the detection and local-ation of ascites.

In one of the preliminary studies (n = 15), Yoshida et al. und that CT staging correlated with postoperative staging in 3% of the patients, whereas FDG PET provided additional formation improving accuracy to 87% [42]. More recently, DG PET/CT proved useful in evaluating for distant metastases s well as equivocal lesions [28,43]. PET/CT particularly has a igh sensitivity in identifying peritoneal deposits and meta-atic lymph nodes that are greater than 1.0 cm. In a series of 2 patients contrast-enhanced CT results were concordant with ostsurgical pathologic stage in 53% of patients, whereas FDG ET/CT was concordant in 69% proving a higher accuracy than T alone [28]. Moreover, the improved staging accuracy btained with the use of PET/CT was most striking in distin-uishing patients with stages III C–IV from those with stages I–IB cancer. For this classification, the specificity, sensitivity, nd accuracy of FDG PET/CT was 91, 100, and 98%, respec-vely, in comparison with 64, 97, and 88% for CT. In a later udy of 40 patients studied for staging before primary debulk-g surgery, the results of contrast-enhanced CT and FDG PET/T performed with intravenous contrast enhancement were oncordant with the final pathologic staging in 55% and 75% f patients, respectively [43]. Moreover, the combined use of DG PET with contrast-enhanced CT increased the overall sion-based sensitivity from 37.6% to 69.4% ($P < 0.001$), and pecificity from 97.1% to 97.5% (not significant), in comparison with CT alone [43]. Thus, integrated PET/CT with contrast enhancement may be helpful in the identification of patients for whom optimal debulking is not possible without undergoing neoadjuvant chemotherapy.

Detection of extra-pelvic spread is of prime importance for patient management in ovarian cancer. In a significant number of advanced stage patients, adequate cytoreduction may not be achieved due to failure in debulking sizeable masses, especially when they involve the hepatic hilum or root of the mesentery [44]. Several studies reported the distant metastatic sites that were missed by CT when FDG PET demonstrated true positive results in the liver, pleura, mediastinum, and supraclavicular lymph nodes [28,45]. In another study, PET/CT revealed unpredicted extra-abdominal lymph node metastases in 15% of cases in a series of 95 patients [46].

In summary, FDG PET/CT in the staging of ovarian cancer may increase the staging accuracy when combined with contrast-enhanced CT, however, further studies with larger patient populations are warranted to definitively prove its clinical value. The niche for FDG PET/CT lies in its ability to identify extra-pelvic spread and distant metastases. FDG PET/CT should be used as a staging tool in selected cases presenting with high risk for extra-pelvic spread, mainly, those in whom neoadjuvant chemotherapy would be considered the first-choice treatment before surgery.

Restaging and response to therapy

The treatment of ovarian cancer is based on surgical staging. The staging procedure includes tumor debulking where an attempt is made to remove all macroscopic tumor deposits. This cytoreductive surgery is then followed by chemotherapy. However, not all patients have disease burden amenable to optimal cytoreduction. After the stage of disease, residual tumor following cytoreduction is an important prognostic factor. Optimal cytoreduction is generally considered to be residual lesion size of less than 1 cm [47].

Criteria for suboptimal cytoreduction or non-resectability include: lymph node enlargement above the renal hilum, abdominal wall invasion, parenchymal liver metastasis (Fig. 16.6a), presacral disease, and implants measuring > 2 cm in any of the following locations: diaphragm (Fig. 16.3), lesser sac, porta hepatis, falciform ligament, gallbladder fossa, gastrosplenic ligament (Fig. 16.3), gastrohepatic ligament, or small bowel mesentery [48]. The role of imaging is in selecting patients that would benefit from neoadjuvant chemotherapy and interval debulking surgery instead of primary cytoreduction. Pre-operative CT and MRI have been shown to be accurate in the prediction of non-resectable tumor. In one study, the sensitivity, specificity, PPV, and NPV for suboptimal debulking were 76, 99, 94, and 96%, respectively [48]. The same study showed no difference in accuracy between the two imaging modalities (96% CT vs. 95% MRI). Again similar to staging, ultrasound has no role in restaging of ovarian cancer.

Several studies reported that neoadjuvant chemotherapy followed by interval debulking surgery was comparable to primary debulking surgery followed by chemotherapy as a treatment option for patients with bulky stage IIIC or IV ovarian carcinoma [49–51]. However, patients not responding to neoadjuvant chemotherapy seem to have a poorer prognosis and reduced overall survival compared with patients who are sensitive to chemotherapy [52]. Although the advantage of evaluating metabolic response using FDG PET/CT is debatable until the role of neoadjuvant therapy is established, FDG PET has shown promising preliminary results as a response assessment tool in ovarian cancer. Avril et al. reported that sequential FDG PET yielded more accurate results than those obtained with clinical or histopathologic response criteria in patients undergoing carboplatin-based chemotherapy [53]. A significant correlation was observed between FDG-PET metabolic response after the first and third cycle of chemotherapy and overall survival. With a threshold of 20% decrease in SUVmax after the first cycle, median overall survival was 38.3 months in metabolic responders compared with 23.1 months in metabolic nonresponders. There was no correlation between clinical response criteria or CA125 response criteria and overall survival. Contrasting with these data, Sassen et al. [54] reported that scattered solitary tumor cells intermixed with foamy macrophages, and foreign-body giant cells did not allow the differentiation of responding from nonresponding patients due to high false-positive findings. However, the residual tumor size after neoadjuvant chemotherapy significantly correlated with treatment response and subsequent overall survival [54]. Further studies are warranted to prove its role in clinical management.

Surveillance of ovarian cancer

After primary definitive therapy, the National Comprehensive Cancer Network (NCCN) guidelines recommend monitoring disease status in all stages with visits every 2–4 months in the first 2 years, visits every 3–6 months for the next 3 years, then annually for 5 years. The recommended tests consist of blood tests including CA125 or other markers, physical and pelvic examinations, and contrast-enhanced CT, MRI, and/or FDG PET/CT imaging, as clinically indicated [55]. The tumor marker CA125 is a very good predictor of epithelial tumor activity [56]. In patients with a complete response to therapy, three consecutive elevations of CA125 values, even within the normal range, at 1–3 month intervals is highly predictive of tumor recurrence [57]. Moreover, the tumor marker elevation can be detected months before radiologic or clinical recurrence manifests [58]. Despite high PPVs (> 95%) associated with CA125, the NPV is undesirably low at 50–60% [59,60].

Imaging is used to assess treatment response and to evaluate suspected recurrence based on elevated tumor markers or clinical symptoms. The majority of tumor recurrence occurs in the pelvis either at the vaginal cuff or pelvic sidewall [7] (Fig. 16.7). CT is the modality of choice for surveillance as in staging. In cases of pelvic sidewall recurrence, MRI is preferred for surgical planning due to its ability to better delineate fat planes as well as its multiplanar imaging capability.

In the appropriately selected patient subset, secondary cytoreduction is associated with a survival benefit in patients with recurrent ovarian cancer [61]. The administration of chemotherapy and radiation therapy is largely determined b the extent of disease [62]. There is an unfulfilled need fo accurate diagnostic methods to timely determine the presenc of residual or recurrent disease to serve as a clinically relevan surrogate marker [63]. FDG-PET may be a good candidate as useful diagnostic tool before second-look surgery particularl when the conventional imaging techniques are negative o equivocal. In a pilot prospective study, 22 patients wit advanced stage ovarian cancer, who had achieved a complet biochemical, clinical, and radiographic response after six cycle of chemotherapy, underwent FDG PET before second-loo laparotomy. Persistent disease was found in 59% at surgery but FDG PET without the association of CT demonstrated onl 10% sensitivity and 42% specificity [64]. In a more recent stud using integrated PET/CT technology, Sironi et al. found higher sensitivity and specificity at 78 and 75%, respectively for identifying malignant lesions, even in lesions as small a 5 mm, before second-look surgery [65].

Imaging of recurrent ovarian cancer

Despite high clinical remission rates after optimal debulkin and combination chemotherapy, 50–75% of ovarian cance patients will present with a relapse [66]. The objective of post therapy imaging is to identify specific disease sites and deter mine the extent of recurrent disease. Thus, diagnostic imagin is highly relevant to clinical management in the selection o potentially effective therapeutic modalities [67]. The early diag nosis of recurrence is challenging because metastases from ovarian cancer primarily involve the peritoneum rather tha parenchymal sites. Consequently, small volume recurrence and metastatic deposits on the visceral surfaces pose diffi culties for anatomic imaging with CT and MRI [48,68] Notwithstanding the current standard of care approach wit the use of CT as the imaging modality of choice to detec ovarian cancer recurrences, distortion of anatomic plane after surgical intervention may result in a significant numbe of equivocal or false positive CT results [48]. The detection an site localization of recurrent lesions are critical to guide man agement for a proper therapy strategy. FDG PET/CT is a usefu imaging modality to detect recurrent or residual ovarian cance owing to its higher sensitivity and specificity compared wit conventional imaging techniques in the post therapy setting However, small-size disease or necrotic, mucinous, cystic, an low-grade tumors may yield false negative findings Additionally, in the post-therapy setting inflammatory/infec tious processes can result in false positive PET/CT interpreta tions. With the recent development of targeted biologica therapies for the management of recurrent cases, PET/C imaging, particularly when performed with intravenous con trast, may play a crucial role for early detection of small volum disease and for the selection of patients for secondary surgica cytoreduction.

The sensitivity and specificity of FDG PET/CT for detectin recurrent ovarian cancer ranges between 80% and 100% an 42% and 100%, respectively [10,69–71], based on various stud ies. Considering that PET has a spatial resolution o

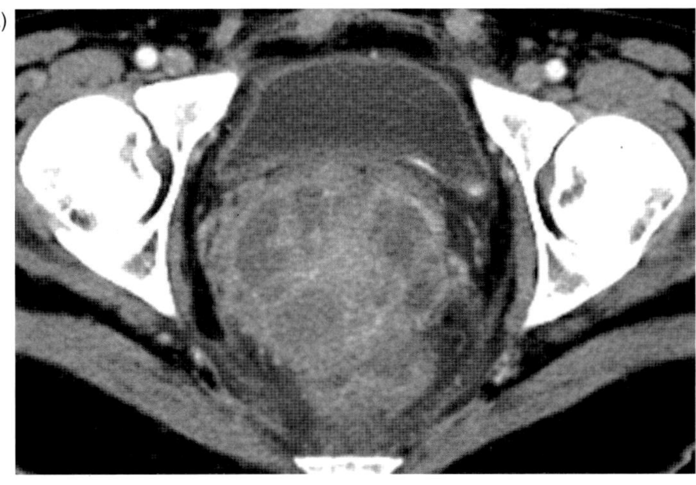
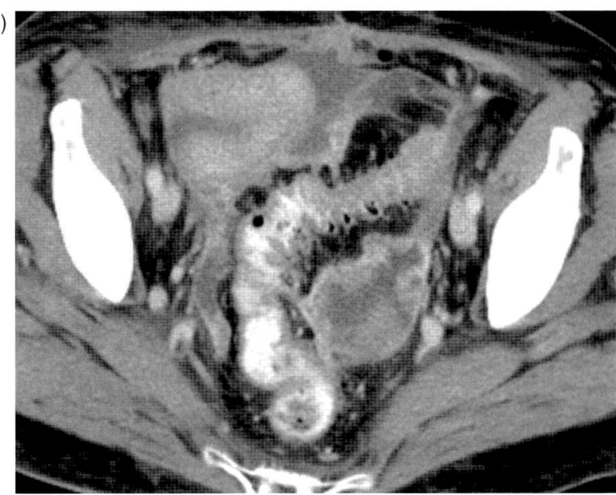

Figure 16.7. (a) Recurrent ovarian cancer in the midline of the pelvis likely originating at the vaginal cuff. It manifests as a large heterogeneously enhancing mass with areas of low density suggesting necrosis. (b) Pelvic side wall recurrence in a different patient manifests as a solid and cystic mass with irregular nodular enhancement of the wall.

approximately 6–7 mm, its detection rate for lesions measuring less than 7 mm in size is not clinically relevant [69]. Hence, omental carcinomatosis of multiple coalescing subcentimeter lesions may not be detected by PET imaging, even if the disease process is suggested at CT [70]. Sebastian et al. reported a favorable interobserver variability for FDG PET compared with CT in detecting ovarian cancer recurrence. Additionally, the accuracy of PET/CT exceeded that of CT alone particularly in the abdomen, at 91% versus 79%, respectively [72].

Although the elevation of CA125 titer is not specific to a malignant cause, its progressive rise is often an indication of recurrent epithelial ovarian cancer. Nonetheless, in these cases conventional imaging modalities may fail in identifying the site of recurrence, especially when the recurrence is in the abdomen [57,58,73]. In patients with rising CA125 levels FDG PET not only had a high sensitivity at 96% in localizing recurrent disease but also PET evidence of recurrent ovarian cancer preceded CT findings by 6 months, which allowed for earlier reintroduction of salvage therapy [74]. Combination of FDG PET evaluation and CA125 titers in monitoring epithelial ovarian cancer was found to increase the sensitivity of detection to above 95% when conventional imaging studies were negative or equivocal [75,76]. FDG-PET/CT imaging also allowed for a change in clinical management strategy by revealing a different disease distribution in at least one-third of patients presenting with suspicion of ovarian cancer recurrence, based on the increased CA125 levels [77].

Kitajima et al. reported a higher accuracy for the integrated PET performed with contrast-enhanced CT for detection of recurrent ovarian cancer compared with PET performed with low-dose CT and contrast-enhanced CT alone ($n = 132$) [78]. Patient-based analysis demonstrated that the sensitivity and specificity of combined PET/contrast-enhanced CT were 79% and 91%, respectively, compared with 74% and 91%, respectively, for PET/low-dose CT and 61% and 85%, respectively, and for CT alone. PET/CT findings resulted in a change in clinical management in 39% of the cases. These authors proved that the integration of contrast-enhanced CT with FDG PET into a single study is technically feasible for evaluation of the abdomen and pelvis.

Similar findings were reported in a study of 32 patients with suspected recurrent ovarian cancer. Upon comparison of laparoscopy with imaging findings, Mangili et al. reported that integrated PET/contrast-enhanced CT may detect tumor relapse in a higher percentage of patients than could CT alone leading to a management change in 44% of patients [79]. These results proved the hypothesis that performing contrast-enhanced CT with PET in the same session increases detection accuracy. It remains to be proven, however, whether the anatomical information provided by contrast-enhanced CT significantly improves the overall diagnostic PET accuracy and leads to a survival benefit.

In a systematic review, Gu et al. showed that CA125 and PET/CT had the highest pooled specificity at 93% and the highest pooled sensitivity at 91% [80]. Comparison between each of the modalities showed that the accuracy for PET with or without the integration of CT was higher than that of CT or MRI (93–96% vs. 80–88%) in identifying recurrent ovarian cancer [80]. However, this study failed to show a significant difference between PET results interpreted with and without the use of CT. This thought-provoking finding is likely a result of the inability of CT to localize the diffuse nature of disease involvement within the peritoneum. Because of surgically introduced anatomic distortions, the uptake in the bowel loops can be interpreted as physiologic uptake rather than serosal tumor implants, unless there are discrete nodules appreciated on the accompanying CT study. A recent retrospective study in 175 patients with treated ovarian cancer reported that PET/CT was able to detect active disease at relatively low levels of CA125, thereby facilitating the early diagnosis of recurrence or residual disease. The optimal cut-off point of CA125 after treatment to reflect active disease on PET/CT was 18 U/mL, achieving a detection rate of 85.6%. Also in patients with low

CA125 levels (<30 U/mL), PET/CT had a relatively high detection rate (53%) [81]. In the early detection of recurrent disease in patients with low-level increases in serum CA125, the detection rate of PET/CT for recurrent ovarian cancer was 91–100%. FDG-PET/CT affected the clinical management by localizing recurrent lesions and creating a specific treatment plan for each patient, especially patients who demonstrated a low-level CA125 increase [82].

In summary, in the post-therapy setting, there is convincing evidence to support the use of FDG PET/CT in patients with suspected recurrence with rising CA125 levels and negative or inconclusive CT or MR imaging for the diagnosis of early recurrent ovarian cancer. Although there is evidence that FDG PET/CT has the ability to demonstrate disease recurrence in the absence of elevated CA125 titers, this application is still evolving and the benefits of its use in a surveillance setting should be justified by further studies. FDG PET/CT may be used as a guide in the optimization of the patient selection process for site-specific treatment, including radiation treatment planning, and may aid in the selection of surgical candidates. Consequently, as alluded above, PET/CT findings may result in significant management changes in 40–60% of patients with suspected ovarian cancer recurrence [78,79,82,83].

Imaging pitfalls

An awareness of the various pitfalls in the imaging of ovarian cancer is important. Most relate to the imperfect detection and/or characterization of an ovarian tumor.

Peritoneal implants

The detection of peritoneal implants is dependent on lesion size and the increased conspicuity in the presence of ascites. Small peritoneal implants can be difficult to detect. CT has reported sensitivity of 85–93% and specificity of 91–96% for the detection of implants > 1 cm in size outside the pelvis [84]. In contrast, the sensitivity decreased to 25–50% for detection of implants less than 1 cm in size in that study. There is no difference in the accuracy of CT or MR in the detection of peritoneal implants [40]. Diffusion-weighted MR imaging may prove helpful in detecting small peritoneal implants [41].

Peritoneal implants can be identified as FDG avid nodular soft tissue masses [85]. Omental thickening and nodularity with diffuse FDG uptake are characteristics of omental involvement (Fig. 16.8). The impairment of lymphatic drainage of the peritoneum by the tumor implants plays a significant role in development of ascites which demonstrate minimal FDG uptake as evidence of malignant ascites (Fig. 16.8c). In detecting peritoneal lesions, the overall lesion-based sensitivity of FDG PET/CT and MRI was 43% and 75%, respectively. Thus, combination of PET and MRI may increase detection sensitivity for peritoneal lesions [86]. The involved sites follow an expected pattern spanning from the posterior cul-de-sac, bladder serosa, paracolic gutters, small bowel mesentery, the ileo-cecal junction, the diaphragmatic surface, particularly in the right subphrenic space and along the convexity of the liver (Fig. 16.3 and Fig. 16.9) and the pleura (Fig. 16.9). Gravitational accumulation of tumor cells in mesenteric recesses leads to seeding of malignant cells on small bowel serosal surfaces and the ileo-cecal junction in almost 50% of patients who present with FDG avid mesenteric masses inseparable from bowel loops. Importantly, however, the inability to detect small volume disease (<7 mm) and miliary peritoneal involvement should be recognized by image interpreters (Fig. 16.8b) and should not preclude surgical staging which is the gold standard for the evaluation of small peritoneal implants.

Liver metastasis

It is important to differentiate between a liver surface serosal metastasis (stage III) and a parenchymal metastasis (stage IV). This distinction can be problematic when a liver parenchymal metastasis is located in a subcapsular location. A liver serosal implant tends to be well defined, round or oval, and scallops the liver contour. Parenchymal metastases tend to be round, have ill-defined borders, and are surrounded by liver parenchyma (Fig. 16.6a). On rare occasions, a serosal implant can progress to invade the liver. Also, an implant in the falciform ligament can be mistaken for an intra-parenchymal location. PET/CT can be helpful in these situations.

Lymph nodes

Detection of lymph node metastases by CT and MRI is dependent on the size of the node in short axis. Lymph nodes with a short axis greater than 1 cm are considered suspicious for malignant involvement. Using this threshold, preoperative imaging had a sensitivity and specificity of 50% and 92% for CT and 83% and 95% for MR, respectively [36]. It is important to note that lymph nodes smaller than 1 cm can harbor metastatic disease; conversely, lymph nodes larger than 1 cm can be reactive with no metastatic disease present.

The lymph node involvement at initial surgery occurs in one-quarter of patients with stage I, 50% in patients with stage II, and three-quarters of patients with stage III–IV disease [87]. Approximately 30% of patients with peritoneal metastases harbor visceral or extra-peritoneal metastases involving pelvic, paraaortic or inguinal lymph nodes. The number rather than size of the nodal metastasis is related to survival. Actuarial 5-year survival rates of stage III patients with one and more than one positive lymph node were 58% and 28%, respectively [87].

In advanced ovarian cancer, pelvic lymph node metastases are common (>50%) and detectable by FDG PET in nodes usually measuring >7 mm (Fig. 16.10a). Approximately 50% of patients with positive pelvic nodes will have paraaortic spread [88,89] (Fig. 16.10b,c). Nonetheless, the paraaortic lymph nodes can be the sites for skip metastases without the involvement of pelvic lymph nodes in up to 15% of patients. FDG PET has shown worse results in the detection of lymph node metastases compared with CT and MRI, that could be attributed to an FDG avid ovarian mass obscuring the neighboring lymph nodes similar to that seen in colorectal cancer. FDG-excretion through the ureters or into the urinary bladder

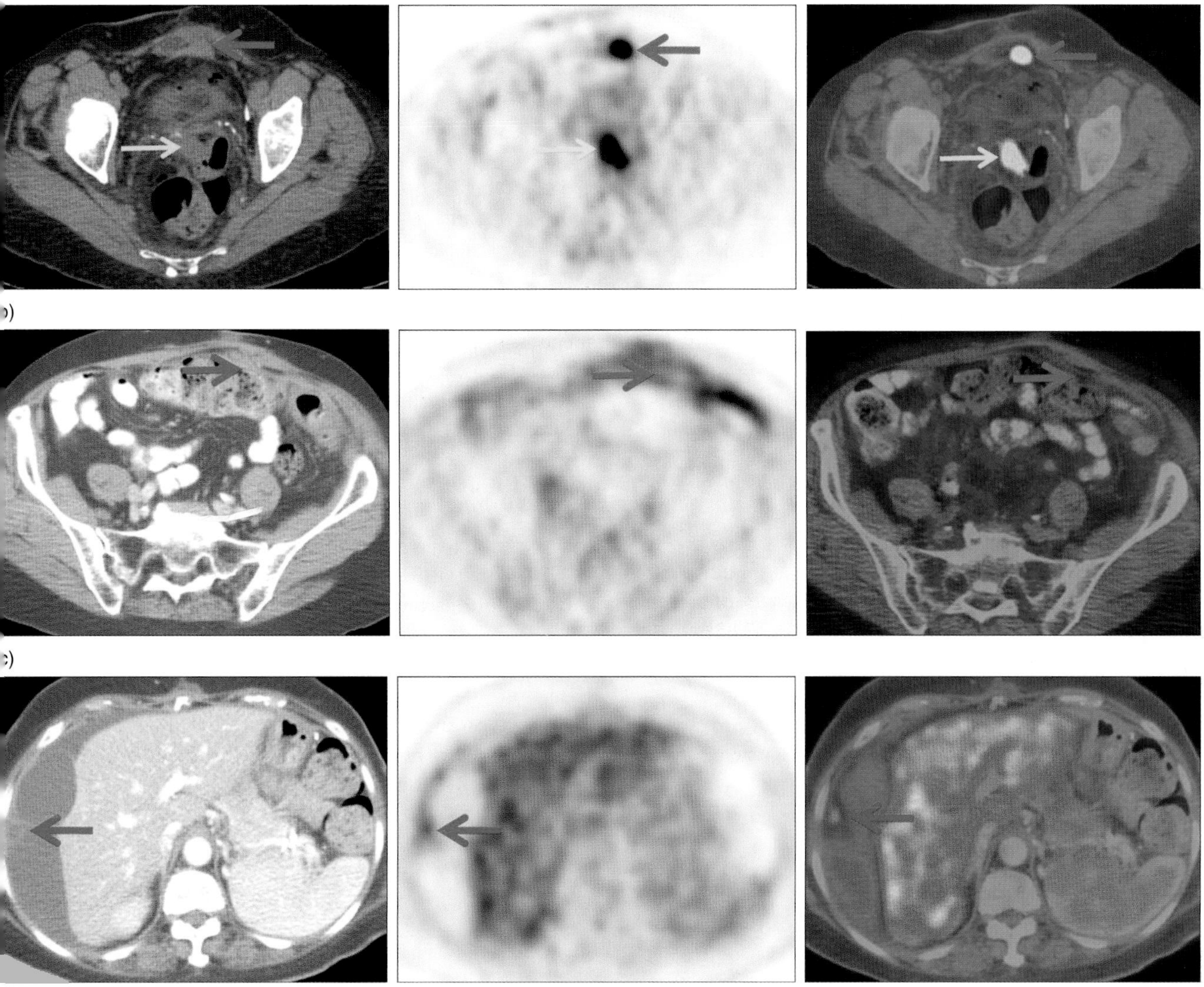

a)

b)

c)

ig. 16.8. Three different patients with a history of stage IIIC ovarian serous papillary adenocarcinoma who underwent surgery and chemotherapy now present with evated CA125 during follow-up. (a) Axial images of CT and PET/CT demonstrate markedly increased FDG uptake corresponding to an irregular soft tissue density in the nterior pelvic wall, probably representing a peritoneal implant (red arrow) as well as in a hypodense nodule adjacent to the distal sigmoid colon probably representing serosal tumor implant. The patient subsequently underwent chemotherapy. Both findings are consistent with peritoneal metastases. (b) Peritoneal stranding anterior the transverse colon with evidence of linear soft tissue fullness and nodularity which abuts the anterior abdominal wall which is characteristic for peritoneal volvement by tumor. (c) A non-FDG-avid collection of perihepatic ascites along the peritoneal surface of the hepatic convexity compressing the liver parenchyma, but iere is mild FDG uptake (SUVmax 2.8) corresponding to a soft tissue density within the fluid collection (red arrow). These findings are consistent with peritoneal arcinomatosis. An FDG PET/CT study is limited in detecting cystic or mucinous components of the neoplasm; however, FDG accumulates in solid parts of the tumor.

a) (b) (c)

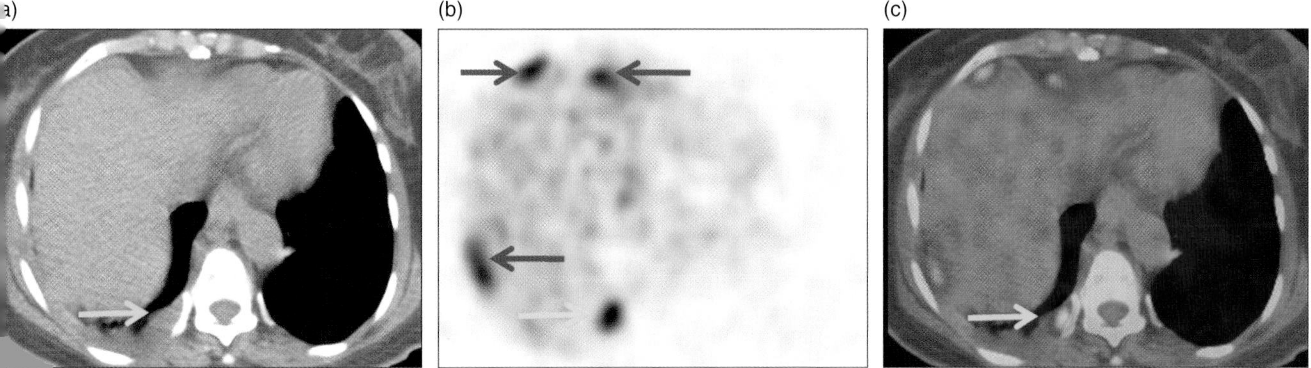

ig. 16.9. A 65-year-old patient with a history of stage II serous papillary cystadenocarcinoma, status post debulking surgery and chemotherapy, who presents with evated CA125. PET/CT and CT were performed for evaluation of extent of recurrent disease. Axial images of CT and PET/CT demonstrate diffuse thickening of the eura at the right lung base with focally increased uptake corresponding to a pleural nodule (yellow arrow). There are also multiple other foci of focally increased FDG ptake corresponding to nodular densities around the convexity of the liver, all representing peritoneal metastases on the diaphragmatic surface (red arrows). PET/CT is useful tool to demonstrate additional sites of disease that are otherwise unnoticed.

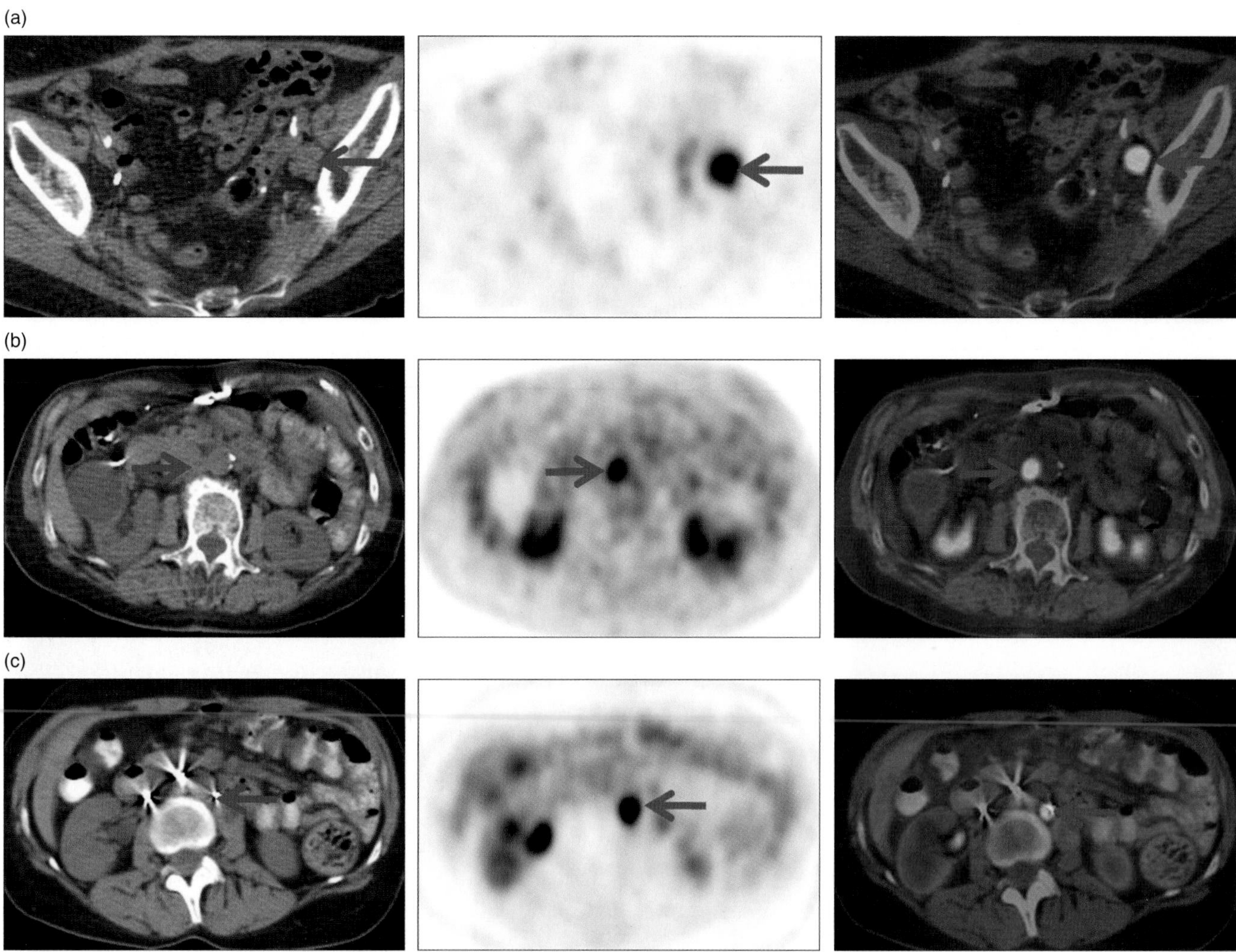

Fig. 16.10. Three different patients who underwent TAH and BSO and chemotherapy for stage IIIC ovarian carcinoma presented with elevated CA125 during follow-up. Axial images of CT and PET/CT demonstrate increased metabolic activity. (a) A 1.2-cm enlarged left external iliac lymph node (arrow). (b) A sub-centimeter right paraaortic lymph node (arrows). (c) A sub-centimeter left paraortic lymph node adjacent to a surgical clip. Note that the corresponding slice of the CT does not reveal a definitive mass lesion adjacent to the surgical clip, probably due to the small volume of disease and metallic artifacts. All are consistent with lymph node metastases.

may also further mask nearby lymph node metastases [90]. In a series of ovarian cancer patients with rising CA125 levels and negative CT scan, even the combined use of PET and CT failed to identify 60% of pathologically positive lymph nodes [91]. It may be hypothesized that tumor infiltration may be present in normal-sized nodes which may show FDG uptake despite a negative CT or MRI (Fig. 16.10B,C). However, for small sized or necrotic lymph nodes or early nodal involvement, PET/CT also falls short with high false-negative rates [92].

Although rare, unexpected spread through the retroperitoneal and the diaphragmatic drainage into the internal mammary, supraclavicular or superior mediastinal lymph nodes can be detected by FDG PET imaging (Fig. 16.11).

Pleural effusion

In general, the lung bases are included in an abdominal/pelvic CT or MR which facilitates the identification of pleural effusions. Any pleural effusion must be sampled to confirm cytologic malignancy and stage IV disease. The presence of pleural nodularity or pleural-based masses signifies metastasis and is better visualized when pleural fluid is present. Chest CT is not indicated in the routine staging of ovarian cancer because distant hematogenous spread is rare at presentation [7].

Benign ovarian lesions

Several benign physiologic ovarian lesions, such as hemorrhagic cysts and endometriomas, can have similar imaging characteristics as malignancy [7,11]. However, these lesions will change and/or resolve with time. These lesions, particularly in pre-menopausal women where they are more common, should receive follow-up in a different portion of the menstrual cycle to exclude any transient physiologic change. Only lesions that persist and show no change should be considered abnormal.

In pre-menopausal women, the frequently present physiologic accumulation of FDG within the ovaries, particularly in the early luteal phase, should be recognized as a pitfall to be able to discern from a malignant cause (Fig. 16.12). Thus, special attention should be given to the timing of PET and the menstrual

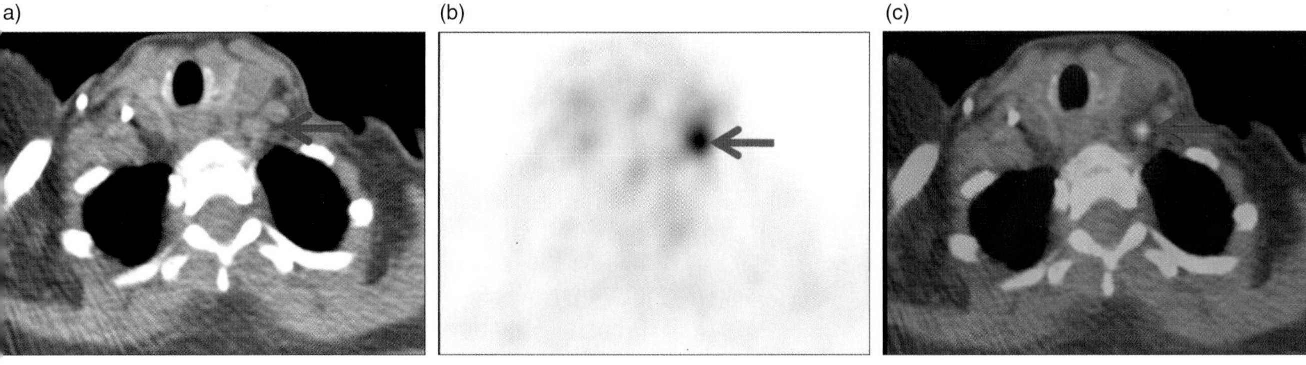

Fig. 16.11. A 52-year-old woman with a history of stage IV serous papillary adenocarcinoma status post chemotherapy with elevated CA125 during follow-up. PET/CT and CT were performed to evaluate for disease extent during follow-up. Axial images of CT and PET/CT demonstrate a large hypermetabolic left supraclavicular lymph node (arrow), consistent with distant metastatic disease. Spread through the lymphatic channels of the retroperitoneal lymph nodes and the diaphragm can lead to dissemination of disease into the superior mediastinal and supraclavicular lymph nodes.

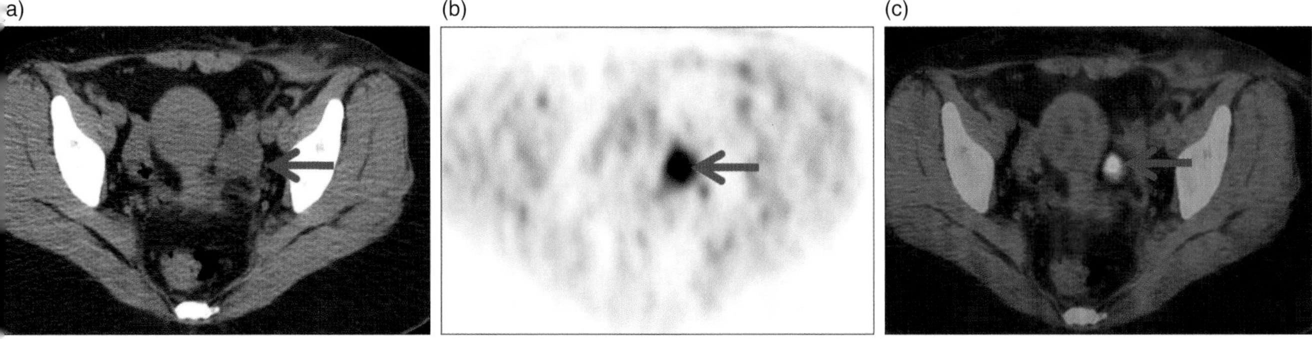

Fig. 16.12. A 42-year-old female with a history of Hodgkin lymphoma, referred for PET/CT imaging for restaging following chemotherapy. Axial images of CT and PET/CT demonstrate an increased radiotracer uptake corresponding to a cystic structure in the left pelvic wall in the region of the left adnexa (red arrow). This finding is most consistent with uptake in a corpus luteum cyst in a pre-menopausal woman. Query of the date of last menstrual cycle would adequately resolve the questions related to such a finding. However, a similar finding in post-menopausal women should require further investigation with pelvic ultrasound to rule out a malignant cause.

cycle, if necessary imaging should be scheduled immediately after the time of menstruation. The characteristic benign appearance usually consists of diffuse or focal but homogeneous uptake in a smoothly marginated ovary, in the adnexal region with a characteristic contrast-enhanced CT appearance of a small rim-enhancing cyst, as well as the absence of any locoregional lymphadenopathy [93]. In post-menopausal women, however, any grade of FDG uptake in the ovaries should be treated as suspicious until it is proven benign with definitive test results.

Ovarian cancer mimics

Primary peritoneal carcinoma is histologically similar to ovarian cancer. It diffusely involves the peritoneal surfaces resulting in carcinomatosis, but there is no associated ovarian mass. Peritoneal carcinomatosis and ascites can be associated with Meig's syndrome as well as with peritonitis due to actinomycosis and tuberculosis. Lymph node metastases without peritoneal spread are rare in ovarian cancer and suggest an alternate diagnosis such as fallopian tube cancer, dysgerminoma, or lymphoma [38].

PET/CT imaging

The main pitfalls of FDG PET/CT imaging include normal physiologic activity in the bowel loops or bowel peristalsis or focal-retained activity in the urinary system and, sometimes, within arteries with atherosclerotic plaques [93,94]. FDG PET/CT can also be falsely negative in cystic or necrotic lesions or lesions with copious mucinous collections (Fig. 16.8c). Knowledge of prior surgeries and of surgical complications is essential for proper interpretation of PET imaging. Asymmetric FDG uptake along the surgical bed or site in a variable period induced by increased glucose transporter is commonly demonstrated, sometimes mimicking malignancy [95].

Future prospects

Ultrasound

Contrast-enhanced ultrasound has been investigated as a tool to differentiate benign from malignant ovarian masses [96–98]. Various contrast parameters have shown statistical significance in differentiating masses, including peak enhancement, wash-out time, and area under the curve [97]. Contrast-enhanced sonography is currently a research tool but is very promising as another tool in the imaging armamentarium if approved for clinical use by the FDA.

PET

An important hallmark of cancer is tumor growth and dissemination through increased proliferative signaling capacity. The 3′-deoxy-3′-^{18}F-fluorothymidine (FLT) is a pyrimidine analog and reflects the activity of a thymidine kinase-1 during the S phase of DNA synthesis [99]. FLT PET has become the most extensively investigated probe for non-invasive measurement of cancer cell proliferative capacity [100], which provided grounds for the future selection of patients for individualized treatment. In a recent pilot study, FLT uptake was found higher in malignant (mean) compared with benign (4.8 vs. 1.6) and normal ovarian control tissue (1.1). An increasing trend between FLT uptake and Ki67 mitotic index is seen in malignant tissue. Additional studies will determine whether FLT PET/CT is specific enough to distinguish between cancerous and non-cancerous cells and to assess its role in ovarian carcinoma patient management [101]. Targeting the mammalian target of rapamycin (mTOR) pathway is a potential means of overcoming cisplatin resistance in ovarian cancer patients. Because mTOR inhibition affects cell proliferation, a study showed that reduction in FLT uptake correlated well with the level of mTOR inhibition by everolimus in ovarian cell lines. These data suggest that early treatment monitoring by FLT PET may be of use in future preclinical or clinical trials evaluating treatment of cisplatin-resistant ovarian tumors by mTOR inhibitors [102].

Recently introduced effective therapy agents targeting specific molecular pathways have also stimulated the development of labeled molecules defining hypoxia, angioneogenesis, and apoptosis. There is a plethora of ongoing preclinical and clinical trials using these specific imaging probes with a common prospect of improving diagnostic and prognostic accuracy [103].

References

1. Coakley FV, Hricak H. Imaging of peritoneal and mesenteric disease: key concepts for the clinical radiologist. Clin Radiol. 1999;**54**:563–74.
2. Standing S (Ed.). Grays Anatomy: The Anatomic Basis of Clinical Practice. Philadelphia: Elsevier; 2008. p 1293–7.
3. Siegel R, Naishadham, Jemal A. Cancer statistics 2013. CA Cancer J Clin. 2013;**63**(1):1–30.
4. Woodward PJ, Hosseinzadeh K, Saenger JS. From the archives of the AFIP: radiologic staging of ovarian carcinoma with pathologic correlation. Radiographics. 2004;**24**:225–46.
5. Holschneider CH, Berek JS. Ovarian cancer: epidemiology, biology and prognostic factors. Semin Surg Oncol. 2000;**19**:3–10.
6. Travassoli FA, Devilee T. (Eds.). Pathology and genetics. In: Tumours of the Breast and Female Genital Organs: WHO Classification of Tumour. Geneva: World Health Organization; 2003, p 12.
7. Mironov S, Akin O, Pandit-Tasker N, Hann LE. Ovarian cancer. Radiol Clin North Am. 2007;**45**:149–66.
8. Howlader N, Noone AM, Krapcho M, et al. SEER Cancer Statistics Review, 1975–2008. National Cancer Institute website. 2011. http://seer.cancer.gov. (accessed August 15, 2011).
9. Suh-Burgmann E. Long term outcomes following conservative surgery for borderline tumor of the ovary: a large population based study. Gynecol Oncol. 2006;**13**:841–7.
10. Pannu HK, Bristow RE, Cohade C, Fishman EK, Wahl RL. PET-CT in recurrent ovarian cancer: initial observations. Radiographics. 2004;**24**:209–23.
11. Shaaaban A, Rezvani M. Ovarian cancer: detection and radiologic staging. Clin Obstet Gynecol. 2009;**52**:73–93.
12. McDonald JM, Modesitt SC. The incidental post menopausal adnexal mass. Clin Obstet Gynecol. 2006;**49**:506–16.
13. Jeong YY, Outwater EK, Kang HK. Imaging evaluation of ovarian masses. Radiographics. 2000;**20**:1445–70.
14. NIH Concensus Conference. Ovarian cancer: screening, treatment and follow-up. NIH Concensus Development Panel on Ovarian Cancer. JAMA. 1995;**273**:491–7.
15. Brown DL, Doubilet PM, Miller FH, et al. Benign and malignant ovarian masses: selection of the most discriminating grayscale and color Doppler sonographic features. Radiology. 1998;**208**:103–10.
16. Kinkel L, Hricak H, Ying L, et al. US characterization of ovarian masses: a meta-analysis. Radiology. 2000;**217**:803–11.
17. Cohen LS, Escobar PF, Scharm C, et al. Three-dimensional power Doppler ultrasound improves accuracy for ovarian cancer prediction. Gynecol Oncol. 2001;**82**:40–8.
18. Salem S, Wilson SR. Gynecologic ultrasound. In: Rumack CM, Wilson SR, Charboneau JW, et al. (Eds.). Diagnostic Ultrasound, 4th edition. Philadelphia: Mosby; 2011. p 572–93.
19. Funt SA, Hann LE. Detection and characterization of adnexal masses. Radiol Clin North Am. 2002;**40**:591–608.
20. Guerriero S, Alcazar JL, Coccia ME, et al. Complex pelvic mass as a target of evaluation of vessel distribution by color Doppler sonography for the diagnosis of adnexal malignancy: results of a multicenter European study. J Ultrasound Med. 2002;**21**:1105–11.
21. Brown DL, Frates MC, Liang FC, et al. Ovarian masses: can benign and malignant lesions be differentiated with color and pulsed Doppler US? Radiology. 1994;**190**:333–6.
22. Levine D, Feldstein VA, Babcock CJ, et al. Sonography of ovarian masses: poor sensitivity of resistive index for

identifying malignant lesion. AJR Am J Roentgenol. 1994;**162**:1355–9.

23. Kinkel K, Lu Y, Mehdizade A, et al. Indeterminate ovarian mass at US: incremental value of a second imaging test for characterization-meta-analysis and Bayesian analysis. Radiology. 2005;**236**:85–94.
24. Iyer VR, Lee SI. MRI, CT and PET/CT for ovarian cancer detection and adnexal lesion characterization. AJR Am J Roentgenol. 2010;**194**:311–21.
25. Sohaib SA, Reznek RH. MR imaging in ovarian cancer. Cancer Imaging. 2007;**7**:S119–29.
26. Grab D, Flock F, Stohr I, et al. Classification of asymptomatic adnexal masses by ultrasound, magnetic resonance imaging, and positron emission tomography. Gynecol Oncol. 2000;**77**:454–9.
27. Fenchel S, Grab D, Nuessle K. Asymptomatic adnexal masses: correlation of FDG PET and histopathologic findings. Radiology. 2002;**223**:780–8.
28. Castellucci P, Perrone AM, Picchio M. Diagnostic accuracy of 18F-FDG PET/CT in characterizing ovarian lesions and staging ovarian cancer: correlation with transvaginal ultrasonography, computed tomography, and histology. Nucl Med Commun. 2007;**28**:589–95.
29. Risum S, Høgdall C, Loft A, et al. The diagnostic value of PET/CT for primary ovarian cancer – a prospective study. Gynecol Oncol. 2007;**105**:145–9.
30. Yamamoto Y, Oguri H, Yamada R, et al. Preoperative evaluation of pelvic masses with combined 18F-fluorodeoxyglucose positron emission tomography and computed tomography. Int J Gynecol Obstet. 2008;**102**:124–7.
31. Chung HH, Kwon HW, Kang KW, et al. Prognostic value of preoperative metabolic tumor volume and total lesion glycolysis in patients with epithelial ovarian cancer. Ann Surg Oncol. 2012;**19**:1966–72.
32. Pignata S, Vermorken JB. Ovarian cancer in the elderly. Crit Rev Oncol Hematol. 2004;**49**:77–86.
33. Marsden DE, Friedlander M, Hacker NF. Current management of epitheal ovarian carcinoma: a review. Semin Surg Oncol. 2000;**19**:11–19.
34. Benedet JL, Bender H, Jones H, Ngan HY, Pecorelli S. FIGO staging classifications and clinical practice guidelines in the management of gynecologic cancers. FIGO Committee on Gynecologic Oncology. Int J Gynaecol Obstet. 2000;**70**:209–62.
35. Forstner R, Sala E, Kinkel K, Spencer JA. ESUR guidelines: ovarian cancer staging and follow-up. Eur Radiol. 2010;**20**:2773–80.
36. Forstner R, Hricak H, Occhipinti KA, et al. Ovarian cancer: staging with CT and MRI. Radiology. 1995;**197**:619–26.
37. Buy JN, Moss AA, Ghossain MA, et al. Peritoneal implants from ovarian tumors: CT findings. Radiology. 1988;**169**:691–4.
38. Forstner R. Radiological staging of ovarian cancer: imaging findings and contribution of CT and MRI. Eur Radiol. 2007;**17**:3223–46.
39. Shiels RA, Peel KR, MacDonald HN, Thorogood J, Robinson PJ. A prospective trial of computed tomography in the staging of ovarian malignancy. Br J Obstet Gynaecol. 1985;**92**:407–12.
40. Tempany CM, Zou KH, Silverman SG, et al. Staging of advanced ovarian cancer: comparison of imaging modalities – report from the Radiological Diagnostic Oncology Group. Radiology. 2000;**205**:761–7.
41. Low RN, Sebrechts CP, Barone RB, Muller W. Diffusion weighted MRI of peritoneal tumors: comparison with conventional MRI and surgical and histiopathologic findings – a feasibility study. AJR Am J Roentgenol. 2009;**193**;461–70.
42. Yoshida Y, Kurokawa T, Kawahara K, et al. Incremental benefits of FDG positron emission tomography over CT alone for the preoperative staging of ovarian cancer. AJR Am J Roentgenol. 2004;**182**:227–33.
43. Kitajima K, Murakami K, Yamasaki E. Diagnostic accuracy of integrated FDG-PET/contrast-enhanced CT in staging ovarian cancer: comparison with enhanced CT. Eur J Nucl Med Mol Imaging. 2008;**35**:1912–20.
44. Heinz AP, Hacker NF, Berek JS. Cytoreductive surgery in ovarian carcinoma: feasibility and morbidity. Obstet Gynecol. 1986;**67**:783–8.
45. Fanti S, Nanni C, Castellucci P, et al. Supra-clavicular lymph node metastatic spread in patients with ovarian cancer disclosed at 18F-FDG-PET/CT: an unusual finding. Cancer Imaging. 2006;**6**:20–3.
46. Nam EJ, Yun MJ, Oh YT, et al. Diagnosis and staging of primary ovarian cancer: correlation between PET/CT, Doppler US, and CT or MRI. Gynecol Oncol. 2010;**116**:389–94.
47. Eisenkop SM, Spirtos NM. What are the current surgical objectives, strategies, and technical capabilities of gynecologic oncologists treating advanced epithelial ovarian cancer? Gynecol Oncol. 2001;**82**:489–97.
48. Quayyum A, Coakley FV, Westphalen AC, et al. Role of CT and MRI in predicting optimal cytoreduction of newly diagnosed primary epithelial ovarian cancer. Gynecol Oncol. 2005;**96**:301–6.
49. Vergote I, Tropé CG, Amant F, et al. Neoadjuvant chemotherapy or primary surgery in stage IIIC or IV ovarian cancer. N Engl J Med. 2010;**363**:943–53.
50. Park TW, Kuhn WC. Neoadjuvant chemotherapy in ovarian cancer. Expert Rev Anticancer Ther. 2004;**4**:639–47.
51. Kuhn W, Rutke S, Spathe K, et al. Neoadjuvant chemotherapy followed by tumor debulking prolongs survival for patients with poor prognosis in International Federation of Gynecology and Obstetrics stage IIIC ovarian carcinoma. Cancer. 2001;**92**:2585–91.
52. Fanfani F, Ferrandina G, Corrado G, et al. Impact of interval debulking surgery on clinical outcome in primary unresectable FIGO stage IIIc ovarian cancer patients. Oncology. 2003;**65**:316–22.
53. Avril N, Sassen S, Schmalfeldt B, et al. Prediction of response to neoadjuvant chemotherapy by sequential F-18-fluorodeoxyglucose positron emission tomography in patients with advanced-stage ovarian cancer. J Clin Oncol. 2005;**23**:7445–53.
54. Sassen S, Schmalfeldt B, Avril N, et al. Histopathologic assessment of tumor regression after neoadjuvant chemotherapy in advanced-stage ovarian cancer. Hum Pathol. 2007;**38**:926–34.

55. NCCN Clinical Practice Guidelines in Oncology. National Comprehensive Cancer Network. http://www.nccn.org/professionals/physician_gls/f_guidelines.asp (accessed February 15, 2012).

56. Bast RC, Xu FJ, Yu YH, et al. CA 125: the past and the future. Int J Biol Markers. 1998;**13**:179–87.

57. Santillan A, Garg R, Zahurak ML, et al. Risk of epithelial ovarian cancer recurrence in patients with serum CA-125 levels within the normal range. J Clin Oncol. 2005;**23**:9338–43.

58. Gadducci A, Cosio S. Surveillance of patients after initial treatment of ovarian cancer. Crit Rev Oncol Hematol. 2009;**71**:43–52.

59. Potter ME, Moradi M, To AC, Hatch KD, Shingleton HM. Value of serum 125Ca levels: does the result preclude second look? Gynecol Oncol. 1989;**33**:201–3.

60. Van der Burg ME, van Lent M, Buyse M, et al. The effect of debulking surgery after induction chemotherapy on the prognosis in advanced epithelial ovarian cancer. 1995;**332**:629–34.

61. Bristow RE, del Carmen MG, Pannu HK, et al. Clinically occult recurrent ovarian cancer: patient selection for secondary cytoreductive surgery using combined PET/CT. Gynecol Oncol. 2003;**90**:519–28.

62. Amendola MA. The role of CT in the evaluation of ovarian malignancy. Crit Rev Diagn Imaging. 1985;**24**:329–68.

63. Petru E, Lück HJ, Stuart G, et al. Gynecologic Cancer Intergroup (GCIG). Gynecologic Cancer Intergroup (GCIG) proposals for changes of the current FIGO staging system. Eur J Obstet Gynecol Reprod Biol. 2009;**143**:69–74.

64. Rose PG, Faulhaber P, Miraldi F, Abdul-Karim FW. Positive emission tomography for evaluating a complete clinical response in patients with ovarian or peritoneal carcinoma: correlation with second-look laparotomy. Gynecol Oncol. 2001;**82**:17–21.

65. Sironi S, Messa C, Mangili G, et al. Integrated FDG PET/CT in patients with persistent ovarian cancer: correlation with histologic findings. Radiology. 2004;**233**:433–40.

66. Gadducci A, Cosio S, Zola P, et al. Surveillance procedures for patients treated for epithelial ovarian cancer: a review of the literature. Int J Gynecol Cancer. 2007;**17**:21–31.

67. von Georgi R, Schubert K, Grant P, Munstedt K. Post-therapy surveillance and after-care in ovarian cancer. Eur J Obstet Gynecol Reprod Biol. 2004;**114**:228–33.

68. Kim Hj, Kim JK, Cho KS. CT features of serous surface papillary carcinoma of the ovary. AJR Am J Roentgenol. 2004;**183**:1721–4.

69. Torizuka T, Nobezawa S, Kanno T, et al. Ovarian cancer recurrence: role of whole-body PET using 18-FDG. Eur J Nucl Med Mol Imaging. 2002;**29**:797–803.

70. Cho SM, Ha HK, Byun JY, et al. Usefulness of FDG PET for assessment of early recurrent epithelial ovarian cancer. AJR Am J Roentgenol. 2002;**179**:391–5.

71. Yen RF, Sun SS, Shen YY, Changlai SP, Kao A. Whole body positron emission tomography with 18F-fluoro-2-deoxyglucose for the detection of recurrent ovarian cancer. Anticancer Res. 2001;**21**:3691–4.

72. Sebastian S, Lee SI, Horowitz NS, et al. PET-CT vs. CT alone in ovarian cancer recurrence. Abdom Imaging. 2008;**33**:112–18.

73. Hogberg T, Kagedal B. Long-term follow-up of ovarian cancer with monthly determinations of serum CA 125. Gynecol Oncol. 1992;**46**:191–8.

74. Zimny M, Siggelkow W, Schroder W, et al. 2-[Fluorine-18]-fluoro-2-deoxy-D-glucose positron emission tomography in the diagnosis of recurrent ovarian cancer. Gynecol Oncol. 2001;**83**:310–15.

75. Thrall MM, DeLoia JA, Gallion H, Avril N. Clinical use of combined positron emission tomography and computed tomography (FDG-PET/CT) in recurrent ovarian cancer. Gynecol Oncol. 2007;**105**:17–22.

76. Sheng XG, Zhang XL, Fu Z, et al. Value of positron emission tomography-CT imaging combined with continual detection of CA125 in serum for diagnosis of early asymptomatic recurrence of epithelial ovarian carcinoma. Zhonghua Fu Chan Ke Za Zhi. 2007;**42**:460–3.

77. Soussan M, Warski M, Cherel P, et al. Impact of FDG PET-CT imaging on the decision making in the biologic suspicion of ovarian carcinoma recurrence. Gynecol Oncol. 2008;**108**:160–5.

78. Kitajima K, Murakami K, Yamasaki E, et al. Performance of integrated FDG-PET/contrast-enhanced CT in the diagnosis of recurrent ovarian cancer: comparison with integrated FDG-PET/non-contrast-enhanced CT and enhanced CT. Eur J Nucl Med Mol Imaging. 2008;**35**:1439–48.

79. Mangili G, Picchio M, Sironi S, et al. Integrated PET/CT as a first-line re-staging modality in patients with suspected recurrence of ovarian cancer. Eur J Nucl Med Mol Imaging. 2007;**34**:658–66.

80. Gu P, Pan LL, Wu SQ, Sun L, Huang G. CA 125, PET alone, PET-CT, CT and MRI in diagnosing recurrent ovarian carcinoma: a systematic review and meta-analysis. Eur J Radiol. 2009;**71**:164–74.

81. Palomar A, Nanni C, Castellucci P, et al. Value of FDG PET/CT in patients with treated ovarian cancer and raised CA125 serum levels. Mol Imaging Biol. 2012;**14**:123–9.

82. Peng NJ, Liou WS, Liu RS, et al. Early detection of recurrent ovarian cancer in patients with low-level increases in serum CA-125 levels by 2-[F-18]fluoro-2-deoxy-D-glucose-positron emission tomography/computed tomography. Cancer Biother Radiopharm. 2011;**26**:175–81.

83. Fulham MJ, Carter J, Baldey A, et al. The impact of PET-CT in suspected recurrent ovarian cancer: a prospective multi-centre study as part of the Australian PET Data Collection Project. Gynecol Oncol. 2009;**112**:462–8.

84. Coakley FV, Choi PH, Gougoutas CA, et al. Peritoneal metastases: detection with spiral CT in patients with ovarian cancer. Radiology. 2002;**223**:495–9.

85. Panagiotidis E, Datseris IE, Exarhos D, et al. High incidence of peritoneal implants in recurrence of intra-abdominal cancer revealed by 18F-FDG PET/CT in patients with increased tumor markers and negative findings on conventional imaging. Nucl Med Commun. 2012;**33**:431–8.

86. Kim CK, Park BK, Choi JY, Kim BG, Han H. Detection of recurrent ovarian cancer at MRI: comparison with

integrated PET/CT. J Comput Assist Tomogr. 2007;**31**:868–75.

87. Burghardt E, Girardi F, Lahousen M, Tamussino K, Stettner H. Patterns of pelvic and paraaortic lymph node involvement in ovarian cancer. Gynecol Oncol. 1991;**40**:103–6.
88. Harter P, Gnauert K, Hils R, et al. Pattern and clinical predictors of lymph node metastases in epithelial ovarian cancer. Int J Gynecol Cancer. 2007;**17**:1238–44.
89. Morice P, Joulie F, Camatte S, et al. Lymph node involvement in epithelial ovarian cancer: analysis of 276 pelvic and paraaortic lymphadenectomies and surgical implications. J Am Coll Surg. 2003;**197**:198–205.
90. Drieskens O, Stroobants S, Gysen M, et al. Positron emission tomography with FDG in the detection of peritoneal and retroperitoneal metastases of ovarian cancer. Gynecol Obstet Invest. 2003;**55**:130–4.
91. Bristow RE, Giuntoli RL Jr, Pannu HK, et al. Combined PET/CT for detecting recurrent ovarian cancer limited to retroperitoneal lymph nodes. Gynecol Oncol. 2005;**99**:294–300.
92. Choi HJ, Roh JW, Seo SS, et al. Comparison of the accuracy of magnetic resonance imaging and positron emission tomography/computed tomography in the presurgical detection of lymph node metastases in patients with uterine cervical carcinoma: a prospective study. Cancer. 2006;**106**:914–22.
93. Liu Y. Benign ovarian and endometrial uptake on FDG PET-CT: patterns and pitfalls. Ann Nucl Med. 2009;**23**:107–12.
94. Lerman H, Metser U, Grisaru D, et al. Normal and abnormal 18F-FDG endometrial and ovarian uptake in pre- and postmenopausal patients: assessment by PET/CT. J Nucl Med. 2004;**45**:266–71.
95. Subhas N, Patel PV, Pannu HK, et al. Imaging of pelvic malignancies with in-line FDG PET-CT: case examples and common pitfalls of FDG PET. Radiographics. 2005;**25**:1031–43.
96. Veyer L, Marret H, Bleuzen A, et al. Preoperative diagnosis of ovarian tumors using pelvic contrast-enhanced sonography. J Ultrasound Med. 2010;**29**(7):1041–9.
97. Fleischer AC, Lyshchik A, Andreotti RF, et al. Advances in sonographic detection of ovarian cancer: depiction of tumor neovascularity with microbubbles. AJR Am J Roentgenol. 2010;**194**(2):343–8.
98. Fleischer AC, Lyshchik A, Jones HW, et al. Diagnostic parameters to differentiate benign from malignant ovarian masses with contrast-enhanced transvaginal sonography. J Ultrasound Med. 2009;**28**(10):1273–80.
99. Rasey JS, Grierson JR, Wiens LW, Kolb PD, Schwartz JL. Validation of FLT uptake as a measure of thymidine kinase-1 activity in A549 carcinoma cells. J Nucl Med. 2002;**43**:1210–17.
100. Bading JR, Shields AF. Imaging of cell proliferation: status and prospects. J Nucl Med. 2008;**49**(Suppl 2):64S–80S.
101. Richard SD, Bencherif B, Edwards RP, et al. Noninvasive assessment of cell proliferation in ovarian cancer using [18F] 3'deoxy-3-fluorothymidine positron emission tomography/computed tomography imaging. Nucl Med Biol. 2011;**38**:485–91.
102. Aide N, Kinross K, Cullinane C, et al. 18F-FLT PET as a surrogate marker of drug efficacy during mTOR inhibition by everolimus in a preclinical cisplatin-resistant ovarian tumor model. J Nucl Med. 2010;**51**:1559–64.
103. Dunphy MP, Lewis JS. Radiopharmaceuticals in preclinical and clinical development for monitoring of therapy with PET. J Nucl Med. 2009;**50**(Suppl 1):106S–21S.

Chapter 17

Ovarian cysts and tumors of the fetus, child, adolescent, and young adult

Albert Altchek, MD, FACS, FACOG, and Liane Deligdisch, MD

Introduction

The subject of ovarian cysts and tumors in the young patient has often been overlooked. Our house staff–resident teaching programs in gynecology teach the traditional gynecologic problems of the mature woman. Training of pediatricians also has overlooked gynecologic problems.

The young patient in all aspects is completely different from the mature woman. The young patient has frequent functional physiologic benign cysts (simple follicle cysts; complex corpus luteum cysts), most of which are asymptomatic and self-limited. They are often discovered by coincidence when a pelvic or abdominal ultrasound examination is done on a child for other purpose, usually pain. It takes clinical judgment and experience to decide whether the pain is due to the cyst or perhaps due to another cause, such as a gastrointestinal problem.

Ovarian cysts are often a normal developmental occurrence in neonates, children, and adolescents. They are common, frequently regress, and are seldom associated with malignancy [1].

Benign mature teratoma (dermoid cyst) is the most common cystic ovarian neoplasm in the adolescent. They are solid masses which are often palpable and with symptoms of pressure, increased abdominal girth, and with or without pain. About one-third of solid neoplasms may be malignant.

The goal of surgical treatment of the young patient aside from preserving her health is to preserve fertility if at all possible. The latter is often possible because the malignant ovarian tumors including germ cell cancer (MOGC) usually do not involve the opposite ovary.

The word "complex" ovarian cyst in a pelvic sonogram report suggests fluid and solid portions. Unfortunately, "complex" is used to suggest a corpus luteum cyst but also is used for the suspicion of a malignancy. The radiologist should give a more precise description or impression.

Because the adolescent often has more ovarian tumors and cysts than the prepubertal child, from the viewpoint of the clinician, it would be helpful in a large series to separate the groups. Unfortunately, most series combine both groups.

Retrospective reviews of surgery for ovarian masses are not reliable because many are reports of previous practice, and certain hospitals have biased types of patient selection. Thus, there are no reliable estimates of the incidence of cysts and tumors of ovaries because the retrospective reviews were only of cases who underwent surgery. With time, surgery for functional physiologic cysts has been reduced.

In general, ovarian cysts in the fetus are managed only by observation. Needle aspiration is usually not done. Surgical removal or detorsion would require delivery of the fetus and problems of prematurity.

The conservative observational management of the fetus changes after delivery with options of needle aspiration, and laparoscopy or laparotomy to attempt to salvage a torsed ovary, for symptoms, for suspicion of malignancy, and for persistent large cysts.

Background

The young patient presents unique problems including the following.

1. Preservation of fertility as much as possible
2. Diagnosis and management of ovarian malignancies which is completely different from that of the traditional mature woman patient
3. Understanding that functional physiologic cysts usually spontaneously disappear with time and usually do not require surgery; follicular cysts are unilocular and "simple" with thin walls and clear fluid whereas corpus luteal cysts are "complex" by ultrasound with liquid and solid parts
4. Because of long pedicles associated with migration of the adnexa from the level of the 10th thoracic vertebra into the true pelvis, there may be torsion of the normal ovary, of the ovary with a functional cyst or containing a dermoid cyst. Malignant cysts usually do not undergo torsion because they are large and have a snug tight fit in the pelvis. Torsion causes sudden severe right or left lower abdominal cramps followed by nausea and vomiting. Pelvic ultrasound is not reliable regarding torsion. The diagnosis is clinical. Prompt surgery is advised to preserve the torsed ovary by detorsion.

Pediatric and adolescent gynecology is often not taught adequately, because it requires a multidisciplinary approach. Nevertheless, it is important for patient care.

Europe has been in advance of the United States. In 1939, a Hungarian pediatrician Laszlo von Dobszay wrote the first

Altchek's Diagnosis and Management of Ovarian Disorders, ed. Liane Deligdisch, Nathan G. Kase, and Carmel J. Cohen. Published by Cambridge University Press.

monograph on pediatric gynecology published in German by Barth, Leipzig [2].

In 1953, the Charles University of Prague appointed Rudolph Peter to the position of Chair of Obstetrics and Adult and Pediatric Gynecology, the first in the world.

In 1956, Denys Seriron at the Hôpital Bretonneau in Paris started the first consultation in pediatric and adolescent gynecology in France.

The International Federation of Infantile and Juvenile Gynecology was founded in 1971. Professor R. Contamin was elected President, Professor John Huffman (Chicago) was Vice President and Irmi Rey-Stocker, Secretary General (University of Lausanne, Switzerland).

By the middle of the 20th century, three main centers had been established for the study, practice, and teaching of gynecology and adolescence: one in Eastern Europe based in Prague, one based in Chicago (J.W. Huffman, North Western University), and another in New York (Albert Altchek, Mount Sinai Hospital).

The national group of the FIGIJ in France is Groupement Français, de Gynécologie de L'Enfant et de L'Adolescente since 1972.

The North American Society of Pediatric and Adolescent Gynecology (NASPAG) was founded in 1956 [2].

In the United States, the American Board Specialists Examination Tests in Obstetrics and Gynecology and Pediatrics now have questions on pediatric and adolescent gynecology. The tests are required to be repeated every 6 years.

Imaging

The review of Contemporary Pediatric Gynecology Imaging indicated that ultrasound is the screening modality for pediatric gynecology. Magnetic resonance imaging (MRI) is used for additional information of complex ovarian masses and congenital anomalies and gives better visualization than computed tomography (CT). MRI may require sedation. CT involves radiation, and it is used for tumor staging [3].

The standard and preferred imaging is the pelvic sonogram done with a full bladder. Sonograms usually give better ovarian images than magnetic resonance imaging (MRI), which is frightening and may require sedation. Sonograms are better than CT, which includes radiation to image the ovary [3].

For the young non-virginal adult, a transvaginal ultrasound is recommended, because it is closer to the ovary than the pelvic sonogram and gives a more precise picture.

Pelvic and lower abdominal ultrasound is helpful for the prepubertal child before the migration of the adnexa from the abdomen to the pelvis.

If there is a large tumor mass extending into the abdomen from the pelvis in the adolescent, then a pelvic lower abdominal sonogram is recommended.

Sonograms are relatively reliable when done by experts in differentiating a benign from a malignant lesion in an enlarged ovary.

In general, simple cysts with thin walls and low echogenicity contrast and ≤ 2 cm are considered variations of normal (Fig. 17.1).

Corpus luteum cysts are echogenic and may be complex with solid and liquid areas and may contain fresh and/or old bleeding residue (Fig. 17.2). A report of a physiologic cyst should be followed by a repeat ultrasound in 6–8 weeks.

Doppler flow study with ultrasound theoretically should detect malignant tumors which have a large volume of blood but slow circulation because of increase of new irregular thin walled blood vessels. It is not always reliable. Malignancies may have normal Doppler flow, and benign ones might have an abnormal Doppler test.

Malignancies usually have liquid and solid or only solid contents with thick walls and papillations or irregularities on the inner or outer surface. Internal septa were previously con-

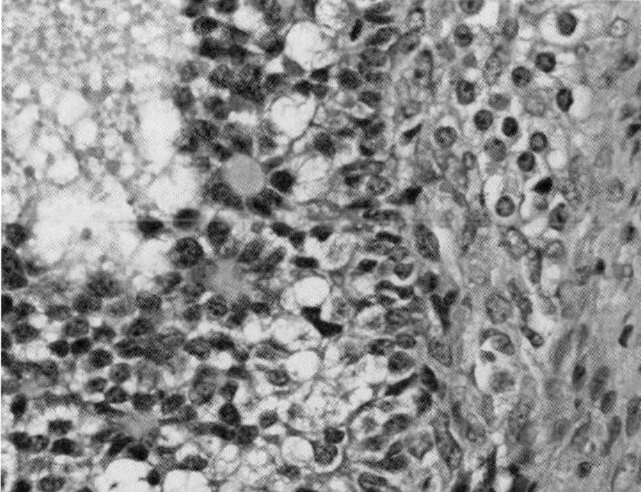

Fig. 17.1. Ovarian follicle cyst lined by granulosa cells with Call–Exner bodies Hematoxylin and eosin stain; original magnification, ×400.

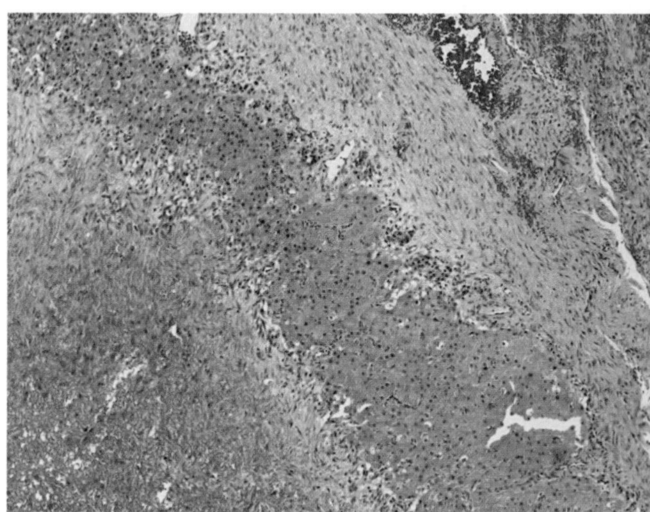

Fig. 17.2. Hemorrhagic luteal cyst lined by luteinized granulosa cells. Hematoxylin and eosin stain; original magnification, ×100.

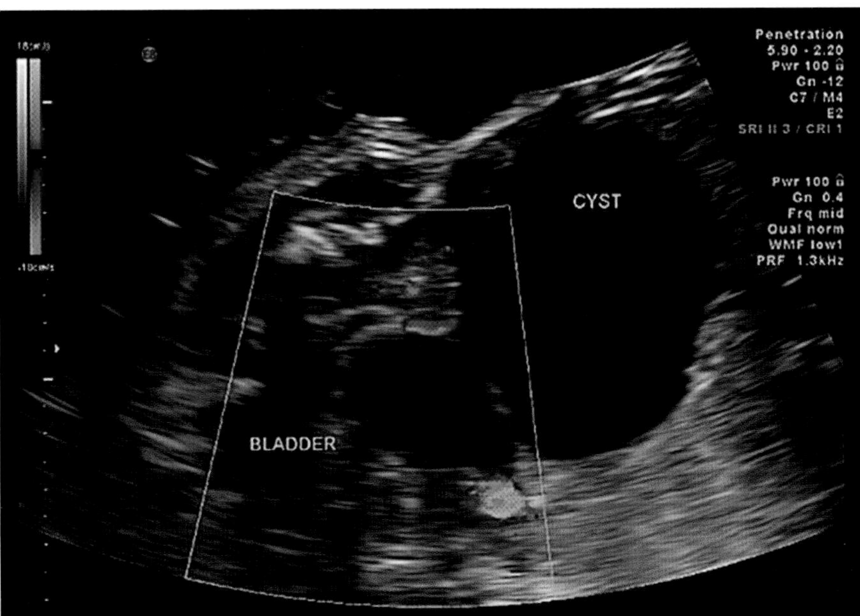

Fig. 17.3. Thin walled ovarian fetal cyst. Reprinted with permission from Contemp Ob/Gyn, Vol. 55, No. 7, July 2010, p 24. © Advanstar Communications Inc. All rights reserved.

sidered a mark of malignancy but may also be seen in corpus luteum benign cysts.

Fetal and neonatal ovarian cysts

With the advent of almost routine ultrasound in pregnancy of the fetus, ovarian cysts have occasionally been discovered. One of the problems is identification of the origin of the cyst. Most publications recommend simple serial observation by ultrasound and searching for other unusual findings.

After birth, the ultrasound is repeated and the infant observed. In most cases the ovarian cysts of the fetus and neonate spontaneously resolve over a few months (Fig. 17.3).

Aspiration of fetal cysts is usually not done.

Ultrasound guidance of aspiration of large fetal simple ovarian cysts is usually avoided because the cyst may not be ovarian and nearby structures or blood vessels may be injured [4].

Complex fetal cysts are not aspirated [5].

Ovarian cysts when present usually appear in the second and third trimester. Internal cyst echoes or fluid levels may be caused by torsion or hemorrhage. Nevertheless, most authors recommend simple observation with repeated ultrasound. Most cysts get smaller or remain the same size. Rupture is very rare. Fetal surgery is usually not done because of the need for delivery and prematurity.

Differential diagnosis of cysts in females includes gastroenterological or urinary tract cysts or dilatations. Other causes include multicystic dysplastic kidney.

Follicular ovarian cysts are common in the fetus and neonates. There is an increase with maternal diabetes mellitus, preeclampsia, rhesus isoimmunization, placentomegaly, and fetal hyperparathyroidism. Clinically significant ovarian cysts of the fetus occur 1 in 2,500. Small simple cysts (2 cm) are variations of normal due to hormonal stimulation. They are usually unilateral and are observed by ultrasound at 3–4 week intervals. Complications of fetal ovarian cysts include intracystic hemorrhage, rupture, torsion with necrosis, becoming calcified or sessile or "wandering," incarceration in an inguinal hernia, urinary or gastrointestinal obstruction, and respiratory distress at birth [5].

In 2008, 79 pregnant women were reported who had 82 ovarian cysts in the fetus (three with bilateral cysts). The fetal cysts were discovered between 26 and 39 weeks (average 32). In the 79 cases with one cyst, there were 48 on the right and 26 on the left. None had a neoplasm. The size of the cyst did not correlate with the risk of torsion. The authors conclude that "it is unnecessary to operate on simple cysts" [6].

In a 2002 retrospective series of 64 fetuses with an ovarian cyst, it was concluded that fetal ovarian cysts should undergo serial ultrasound monitoring and that the delivery should be in a perinatal center. After delivery, surgery revealed one teratoma [4].

In a series of 21 fetuses, there were 11 with simple ovarian cysts and 12 with complex ovarian cysts. Significantly higher rates of ovarian loss were diagnosed when the sonographic appearances of the ovarian cyst was simple on the prenatal scan and complex on the postnatal scan (in 6 of 7) compared with when the ovarian cyst was simple in both scans [7].

The most common complication in the fetal ovarian cyst is torsion which is difficult to determine. Even after delivery, diagnosis of ovarian torsion is difficult. The best clue is lower quadrant abdominal pain. There may also be vomiting, elevated white blood cells, and low-grade fever. The ultrasound with torsion may show (in the fetus and adult) septation, debris, and homogeneous low level "ground glass" echoes.

The fetal cyst is thought to develop due to gonadotropin stimulation. Most cysts are lined by granulosa cells. There are also theca-luteal or simple cysts of unknown origin [7].

There was a case report of a newborn laparotomy who had a large ovarian cyst as a fetus. The cyst showed hemorrhage and calcification and had adhesions which had caused a bowel volvulus requiring resection of 30 cm of necrotic jejunum [8].

Presumably, there was hemorrhagic rupture of the fetal large ovarian cyst.

In a case report, unexplained ascites in a newborn girl could have been due to a ruptured ovarian cyst. At 29 weeks, the fetus had an 11-cm distended anechoic cyst. After delivery, the abdomen was distended. Sonography on day 1 revealed a large amount of diffuse ascites containing septa and debris [9].

The histology of the cysts may be that of a follicular (graafian) or of a luteal cyst (Fig. 17.2).

Large cysts, however, cannot always be reliably assigned a histology or definite etiology based on sonographic findings alone [10].

Some think that a large fetal cyst has an increased chance of torsion. Torsion may cause ovarian infarction, adhesion, necrosis, infection, and sepsis [10].

A case report described on ultrasound an abdominal cyst in a 30-week fetus. Postnatal ultrasound showed a right pelvic cyst of 3.2 cm. Computed tomography and magnetic resonance imaging revealed cyst wall calcification and intra-cystic hemorrhage. At laparotomy at age 3 weeks, a free-floating "wandering" brown round smooth cystic lesion 3.3 cm without a stalk was removed from the peritoneal cavity. It was the result of ovarian cyst autoamputation. The histology was hemorrhagic necrotic autolytic tissue with dystrophic calcification ("but did not contain any ovarian tissue"). (Comment: Autoamputation is usually caused by torsion necrosis.)

Autoamputation of ovarian cysts under 1 year is extremely rare. This was the 13th report. Only one had symptoms.

The MRI detected the hemorrhage and calcification. Autoamputated ovarian teratomas may be reimplanted as omental masses.

If there is no regression early removal of an autoamputated ovarian cyst of the neonate is recommended [10].

Most fetal ovarian cysts have no echo. Echoes may indicate hemorrhage or torsion [11].

Occasionally, there may be bilateral fetal ovarian cysts. A 3,910-gram newborn with an Apgar score of 9 had bilateral unilocular cysts lined by benign theca–luteal cells [12].

Another case of bilateral ovarian cysts occurred in a neonate with salt-wasting congenital adrenal hyperplasia [13].

For neonatal ovarian cysts, there is a similar differential diagnosis as for the fetus. About 50% disappear in the first 3 months, and almost all by 6 months. If the cyst persists consider malignancy, torsion, or misdiagnosis. Cyst aspiration of the neonate is safer than in the fetus and some do it to prevent torsion which can occur with any size of cyst. The authors indicated that 30 to 40% present with torsion or another complication. Some believe that this is an overestimation because of patient selection. The symptoms of torsion are sudden lower abdominal pain, nausea, vomiting, and low-grade fever. Surgery is done to detorse the ovary to salvage it. At the time of detorsion, if the ovary continues to have a dark blue–black color the authors recommend a "bivalve" technique to incise the detorsed ovary to reduce its internal pressure which reduced blood flow. (Note: most surgeons do not do the "bivalve" incision to avoid tissue injury. It is difficult to make a clinical decision during surgery to estimate the viability of the ovary.)

Laufer and Growdon recommend the following neonatal cyst management:

1. Serial ultrasound at intervals of 4 to 6 weeks until the cyst resolves
2. Aspiration of simple cysts over 4 to 5 cm
3. Surgery (laparoscopy) for complex cysts, increasing size of cyst, symptomatic cysts, cysts which last for more than 4 to 6 months [14].

A review of ovarian masses in the newborn indicated that in about 6 months there is usually spontaneous resolution of simple ovarian cysts less than 5 cm, presumably the result of hormonal changes. Simple asymptomatic cysts less than 5 cm are observed with ultrasound. Symptomatic cysts should have surgery. If simple cysts are larger than 5 cm, there is a difference of opinion whether to continue observation or intervene because of the possibility of later torsion. Possible approaches include aspiration and/or laparoscopy. On ultrasound, a complex cyst may indicate torsion and surgery should be done to attempt to save the ovary and avoid complications of hemorrhage, peritonitis, intestinal obstruction, or a wandering tumor. The emphasis is to preserve fertility [15].

Ovarian cysts of children and adolescents

Helmrath et al. wrote a clinical review of ovarian cysts in children. They observed that "the ovary is dynamic, and undergoes constant change from the fetal stage until the onset of puberty" [16].

The ovary is initially an abdominal organ at the level of the 10th thoracic vertebra and migrates into the true pelvis before puberty. It has a large pedicle which predisposes to torsion, which may be intermittent with mild pain in the lower abdomen or periumbilical.

Pelvic ultrasound is recommended. Unfortunately, pelvic Doppler flow ultrasound is not reliable regarding torsion. Prompt surgery is mandatory to detorse the ovary.

Management of the prepubertal child depends on the ultrasound finding, clinical status, and symptoms. Even if the cyst persists, if it is simple and asymptomatic, it should still be observed.

Usually rupture and bleeding of physiologic cysts is self-limited, and the patient may be observed. If there is significant bleeding, surgery is done (laparoscopic or laparotomy).

For torsion, prompt surgery is done to save the ovary. There is no consensus regarding whether pexy of the detorsed ovary and other ovary should be done [15]. (See section on torsion.)

When menses start, up to 20% of adolescents will have multicystic and enlarged ovaries.

Large ovarian cysts tend to occur in the first year of life and at the time of menarche. Development of a large ovarian cyst in between suggests abnormal hormone release with a specific endocrine syndrome or a neoplasm [16].

With adolescence, there is an increase of simple follicular cysts and complex corpus luteum cysts. There may or may not be symptoms such as pain, pressure, rupture, torsion, or menstrual disturbances. Most cysts are asymptomatic and usually resolve in 6–8 weeks, when the ultrasound is repeated.

Corpus luteum cysts are complex by ultrasound, with increased echoes (Fig. 17.2). If they are asymptomatic and less than 10 cm, they are usually observed by ultrasound and usually disappear within 3 months. Complications include torsion, and intra-cystic or peritoneal bleeding.

In 66% of torsion cases, there may be a unilateral enlarged ovary with dilated peripheral small cysts.

With torsion, the necrotic ovary may adhere to the intestine and cause obstruction.

Pelvic sonography may not be adequate for a diagnosis of hemorrhage into an ovarian cyst, ovarian tumor, or adnexal torsion.

Rupture of a hemorrhagic cyst is unusual and self-limited and usually resolves by itself. Very rarely there may be sudden significant hemoperitoneum.

True precocious puberty with increased gonadotropins may cause bilateral multiple small ovarian cysts. It may be treated by gonadotropin-releasing-hormone analogs or antagonists.

Pseudo-puberty may be caused by a unilateral large independent follicular ovarian cyst. Follicle-stimulating hormone (FSH) and luteinizing hormone (LH) are low and estrogen is elevated and gonadotropin-releasing hormone analog therapy does not help. This may occur with McCune–Albright syndrome of fibrous dysplasia of bone with café-au-lait skin pigmentation. It is treated by removal of the cysts, although sometimes it recurs. It is associated with mosaic mutations [16].

Most girls with hypothyroidism have a delayed puberty. Some with severe hypothyroidism have an overlap from thyroid-stimulating hormone (TSH) which also stimulates prolactin because TSH shares a common gonadotropin 2 (alpha) subunit. This may cause large multicystic ovaries, galactorrhea and precocious puberty. It is treated with oral thyroid hormone.

Asymptomatic simple follicular cysts up to 10 cm are observed by repeat ultrasound after 6 to 8 weeks at which time the cyst usually has disappeared or become smaller. Previous reports of oral contraceptives to reduce the size of cysts are now considered to be coincidental. High-dose oral contraceptives may reduce the chance of new recurrent simple cysts.

Aspiration of cysts is discouraged because of uncertain diagnosis and recurrence of cysts.

If with observation the simple cyst persists, grows larger, or causes symptoms then ovarian cystectomy is considered. If there are small follicular cysts, they are left alone to avoid surgery and adhesions.

In all surgical procedures, preservation of fertility is critical [16].

A case report described a 13-year-old postmenarchal girl with a pituitary macroadenoma secreting large amounts of FSH, which caused 6 months of amenorrhea and bilateral ovarian tumors with multiple giant cysts due to ovarian hyperstimulation. The ovarian masses filled the entire lower hemi-abdomen. Trans-sphenoidal resection of the adenoma caused the disappearance of the ovarian masses [17].

It is difficult to differentiate ovarian cysts from para-ovarian cysts with sonography. The latter is suggested by the finding of an ovary on the same side.

With the migration of the adnexa into the true pelvis, the infundibulopelvic ligament stretches and becomes long and loose. This predisposes to torsion of the ovary. The chance of ovarian torsion might be increased if there was a previous torsion, or a family history of torsion.

The child adnexal torsion may occur with normal adnexa, whereas with the adolescent and young adult, there is a greater chance that there is a cyst or mass in the ovary.

Polycystic ovary syndrome in adolescents

Polycystic ovary syndrome (PCOS) is associated with menstrual disturbances, hyperinsulinism, hyperandrogenism, insulin resistance, acanthosis nigricans, and increased LH with normal FSH. There may be enlarged bilateral polycystic ovaries [16].

A literature review suggests that PCOS is a heterogeneous disorder associated with increased androgens and insulin resistance. It is a genetic disorder of ovarian function causing increased secretion of androgens perhaps present in the fetus and manifestation in early puberty. Obesity amplifies the problem [18].

PCOS may start to develop in adolescents and is associated with chronic anovulation, hyperandrogenism (clinical and biochemical), and polycystic ovaries.

Previously, it was assumed that PCOS presented in the young adult with oligomenorrhagia and infertility. When PCOS presents in the adolescent, there may be anovulatory dysfunctional uterine bleeding manifested by completely irregular bleeding or the characteristic 3 months of amenorrhea followed by 1 month of continuous bleeding. Such patients tend to have anovulation and PCOS in young adulthood.

The risk of metabolic syndrome may vary in adolescent PCOS with different phenotypes and lipid profiles.

"Longitudinal follow-up studies are needed to determine whether an early intervention, such as in adolescence, reducing androgen and improving metabolic profile may effectively result in a decrease of the metabolic complication of PCOS later in life" [19].

Adolescents with primary amenorrhea and PCOS have increased features of the metabolic syndrome and higher androstenedione than those with secondary amenorrhea and PCOS. Primary amenorrhea is an unusual manifestation of PCOS.

Metabolic syndrome in PCOS includes anovulation, hyperandrogenism, acne, hirsutism, obesity, and polycystic ovaries. The prevalence of metabolic syndrome in adolescents in the United States is between 4.2% and 8.4%. It is 28% to 39% in obese adolescents.

PCOS is rarely listed as a differential diagnosis for primary amenorrhea [20].

A 2008 review notes that adolescent obesity contributes to the pathophysiology of polycystic ovarian syndrome and increases the chance of associated metabolic and cardiovascular morbidities [21].

A 6-year follow-up from the Karolinska Institute, Stockholm, of adolescents with menstrual disturbances (amenorrhea or oligomenorrhea) states that menstrual disturbances were still present in 62% (of 87 women) of which 59% had PCOS. Persistent menstrual disturbances were more common in those with previous oligomenorrhea rather than secondary amenorrhea [22].

In 2006, a study from China proposed a hypothesis of "epigenetic abnormality underlying the fetal origin of PCOS." Fetal exposure to hyperandrogenism may disturb the epigenetic reprogramming in fetal reproduction resulting in postnatal PCOS phenotype in women of reproductive age. Incomplete epigenetic abnormality in the germ cells after fertilization may promote the transgenerational inheritance of PCOS [23].

Polycystic ovarian syndrome may cause irregular menstrual bleeding for 12–18 months after menarche and 5–6 years before menopause begins.

(Comment: irregular bleeding is present at the start [in adolescence] and end of menstruation cycles [menopausal]. It is probably due to lack of ovulation. About half of girls do not ovulate with the first menses. The question is: is this the cause of irregular bleeding or is it due to PCOS, as the authors suggest.)

The Wnt gene family has been found in ovaries with PCOS [24].

The Wnt 4 gene family has an important role in the development of the embryo of almost all present animals from *Drosophila* to humans and has been conserved over 500 million years of evolution from the time of the common ancestor [25].

Ovarian torsion in the young patient

Ovarian torsion is one of the leading causes of emergency gynecologic surgery [14].

It may occur at any age. The symptoms are not specific.

In previous years, there was fear of untwisting a torsed ovary because of the theoretical possibility that it might dislodge a blood clot in the twist and cause a pulmonary embolism. In the past 20 years, it is now recognized that the twisted ovarian pedicle does not have clots and untwisting is not dangerous.

The authors point out that previous attacks of unexplained abdominal pain are common because of partial recurrent torsion. Sonography may show an enlarged dishomogeneous ovary with small peripheral cysts and some free peritoneal fluid. Sonography is not precise.

The chance of torsion is increased in pregnancy and in ovarian hyperstimulation for in-vitro fertilization (IVF). The highest incidence of ovarian torsion is in reproductive age women because of neoplasms and pregnancy [26].

In adult females, ovarian cysts and neoplasms cause 94% of torsion.

In prepubertal children, torsion may occur with ovarian cysts or neoplasm but also with normal ovaries. In children, at least 50% of torsion cases have normal ovaries. Children have an increased risk for torsing normal ovaries. It has been suggested that a long uterine ovarian and/or infundibulopelvic ligament may predispose to increase ovarian torsion. Torsion occurs more in the right ovary than the left.

With torsion vein and lymph outflow is reduced or obstructed resulting in edema, enlargement of the ovary, and a dark blue–black color. The arterial inflow is less obstructed because of the arterial muscular wall and higher blood pressure.

Sometimes the torsed ovary may have an ultrasound picture of peripheral small cysts presumably representing distended cystic primordial Graafian follicles.

Diagnosis of ovarian torsion

The symptoms are sudden severe lower quadrant abdominal pain with nausea and vomiting. Sometimes, a tender adnexal mass is palpable. The newborn refuses to feed, and has vomiting, abdominal distention, and irritability. There may be a low-grade fever and leukocytosis.

The diagnosis is difficult. In a citation of 115 cases who had surgery for the preoperative diagnosis of torsion, only 38 patients had torsion [14]. (Comment: There may have been some biased selection because most authors report better results.)

Ultrasound can detect enlargement of the ovaries, but it is not reliable regarding torsion, including the use of Doppler flow ultrasound. "... we have not found either the presence or absence of Doppler flow to be diagnostically useful in children" [14].

CT and MRI are not reliable regarding torsion. Usually CT and MRI are not done.

Suggestive laboratory tests include complete blood count, serum interleukin-6 (IL-6), and serum electrolytes [14]. (Comment: serum IL-6 is not a usual test.)

If there is suspicion of ovarian carcinoma, then serum tumor markers should be tested.

The differential diagnosis of torsion includes ectopic pregnancy, ruptured ovarian cyst, appendicitis, pelvic inflammatory disease, degenerating fibroid, endometriosis, and ovarian neoplasm.

Therapy

Diagnosis and treatment is accomplished by surgery which should be done as an emergency to detorse and save the ovary. The decision to operate is essentially clinical depending on experience, clinical examination, and judgment concerning an enlarged painful and tender ovary often with a heterogeneous ultrasound appearance.

Because of lack of adequate and long-term reports there are differences of opinion regarding further surgery. These include: (1) intra-operative watching for undefined length of time to see if color returns to the detorsed ovary; (2) the inability during surgery to evaluate the detorsed ovary, that is, whether it is a rue hemorrhagic necrotic ovary or whether it is still viable; (3) f the ovary is left in place, should it be fixed using an absorbable r non-absorbable ligature?; (4) removal of ovarian cyst or eoplasm in the detorsed retained ovary; (5) whether to pex he opposite ovary.

Detorsed ovary has been incised and bivalved with the ssumption that it would reduce internal ovarian pressure. Comment: The vast majority of surgeons believe bivalving auses more harm than good [14].)

Intra-operative fluorescein injection of an ovarian blood essel and examination with ultraviolet light has been recommended. This is not usually done because of lack of preparation nd lack of other reports [14].

With the bivalve technique, the surgeon must be certain that here is no malignancy. If there is suspicion of malignancy on ppearance or by frozen section or if the ovary looks nonviable, unilateral salpingo-oophorectomy is done and serum tumor narkers are drawn.

Some recommend ovarian pexy in all torsion cases in children with normal ovaries, but not if there is an ovarian cyst which is removed. They also recommend pexy if there has been previous oophorectomy for torsion [5,14].

Isolated fallopian tube torsion is rare. It may occur with normal tubes, hydrosalpinx, infection, in pregnancy, paraovarian cyst, neoplasm, anomaly, ectopic pregnancy, and endometriosis.

Bilateral torsions are not unusual. Doppler ultrasound is not eliable. Ovariectomy is done for non-resectable tumors and for gangrenous necrosed ovaries that did not bleed on incising hem 15 minutes after detorsion.

In a review of 40 cases of ovarian torsion in 38 children for he 10 cases operated within the first 24 hours, 80% had conservative ovarian surgery. For the 15 operated between 24 and 72 hours, 47% had conservative surgery. For the 11 operated more than 3 days after onset, there was only 9% salvage of the ovary. When the ovarian torsion (OT) occurred in a normal ovary, the ratio right/left was 7:2 or 78% [27].

The overall OT was 23/40 (57.5%) on the right side, and 17/40 (42.5%) on the left side. The median size of the ovaries with OT was 7.78 cm (3–15 cm). There were 29 ovarian neoplasms associated with OT, 15 mature teratomas, 11 cystadenomas, and 2 malignant tumors (dysgerminoma, carcinoma).

Five of the 38 (13%) had bilateral synchronous ovarian lesions.

There was no torsion in any mass larger than 15 cm, because arge tumors are fixed in the pelvis [27].

The average age was 11 years (range 3–14); 23 girls were prepubescent and 12 were pubescent. The usual clinical presentation was acute abdominal or pelvic pain and vomiting in more than two-thirds. Simple puncture or partial resection of the cyst is not done because of recurrence.

There is no consensus regarding oophoropexy after detorsion nor of preventive pexy in the opposite side.

A case report describes a recurrent torsion after an ovarian cyst had been fixed with an absorbable suture. Therefore, a nonabsorbable suture is recommended. An alternative to fixation of the detorsed salvaged ovary to the peritoneal or uterine fixation is shortening the utero-ovarian ligament but this might disturb the vascularization and function of the ovary and tubes [27].

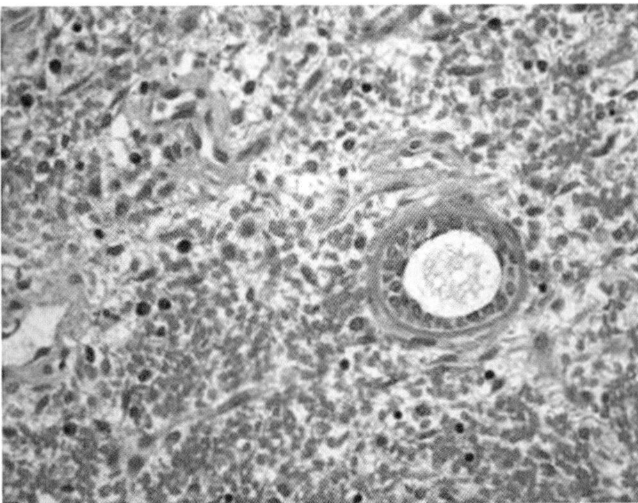

Fig. 17.4. Normal oocyte in ovary with clinical "hemorrhagic necrotic torsed ovary."

New concepts

The standard custom is to remove a detorsed ovary with "hemorrhagic necrosis" based on a clinical dark blue–black appearance which persists after detorsion.

Nevertheless, new observations create an option of leaving the detorsed "hemorrhagic necrotic" ovary in situ, especially if the opposite ovary had been removed previously. Even if the opposite ovary is present, with preoperative informed consent, it is reasonable to leave the detorsed ovary in situ.

The problem is that during surgery it is not possible to judge the viability of the ovary and its oocytes.

We had a prepubertal patient with a persistent black–blue color and enlarged ovary after detorsion and it was removed. Pathology showed necrotic stroma but normal primary oocytes (Fig. 17.4). Perhaps the "resting" primordial oocytes are truly resting and need less blood supply. The premeiotic oocyte does not have blood vessels until it is prepared for ovulation. Fluid circulation comes from channels between the surrounding granulosa cells.

There may not be an association of duration of symptoms and ovarian necrosis, which may be due to partial or intermittent torsion [28].

A 6 year old with a previous oophorectomy for ovarian torsion who developed torsion of her remaining ovary was treated by detorsion and oophoropexy. Postoperative serial ultrasound confirmed viability of the ovary "... despite the severely necrotic appearance of the ovarian tissue" [29].

Cohen et al. examined 102 torsed ovaries which were detorsed and not observed for restoration of color: a large percentage were still functional ovaries. The authors wrote "we suggest, based on our experience with 102 patients, that even gangrenous-appearing adnexa should not be removed because it is not possible to estimate during surgery what the chances are for recuperation and most patients with these adnexa do indeed recuperate" [30].

Kodama et al. reported whole ovarian autotransplantation in a patient age 34 without vascular anastomosis. The ovaries had been out of the body 30 minutes by accident after a cesarean hysterectomy. The ovaries were replaced in the retroperitoneum. Subsequently, there were biphasic hormonal cycles with elevations of progesterone. This suggests that the oocytes can survive without blood supply for 30 minutes [31].

In a review of surgical management of an incidentally identified ovarian mass, the advice for ovarian torsion is "Excision of blu–black or frankly necrotic-appearing ovaries is no longer recommended." This was based on a review in which 58 patients with mean age 25 ± 8 years of which 3 were premenarchal had laparoscopic detorsion of black–blue colored or frankly necrotic-appearing ovaries. There were no oophorectomies. Six weeks later, sonography showed ovarian function in 39 of 42 patients. Cystectomy should not be done at the time of detorsion if there is no solid component because it may lead to loss of functional ovarian tissue. There is a need for large, long-term evidence-based data. Para-ovarian cysts should be resected with preservation of the tube [32].

There is a difference of opinion about whether a cyst if present should be removed at that time. Most surgeons do cystectomy to verify a diagnosis and to prevent recurrent torsion should the detorsed preserved ovary torse again. Some surgeons do not remove a benign functional cyst to avoid further injury to the ovary.

Regarding the possibility of overlooking an ovarian tumor, if there is no ultrasound evidence or no intra-operative evidence it is safe to leave the ovary in place. In addition, the sonogram should be repeated in 6–8 weeks [15].

If there had been a previous ovarian torsion, a family history of torsion, or if the other ovary had been removed previously, the ovary is usually pexed.

There is also difference of opinion of whether the ovary should be fixed (pexy) by suture to the uterus or lateral pelvic wall to prevent repeat torsion. Some surgeons do not do pexy because of concern of further trauma to the ovary.

There are differences of opinion whether absorbent or non-absorbent sutures should be used because absorbent sutures may allow recurrent torsion.

A 6-year-old presented with a persistent adnexal mass (4.5 cm) and a highly elevated serum CA125 but with no other tumor markers. Laparotomy revealed an enlarged adherent ovary filled with necrotic material which was excised. The ovary was spared. The frozen section did not show any mali nancy. The ovarian cortex was of unknown viability. The path ology was consistent with some necrosis after ovarian torsio The CA125 became normal. Follow-up sonography showe normal ovaries [33].

There are differences of opinion regarding a pexy of th remaining normal ovaries by sewing it to the back of the uteru by shortening the round ligament of the ovary without blockin the blood vessels, or by attaching the ovary to the lateral pelv wall. Care is taken to avoid creating an intra-peritoneal herni Some surgeons use non-absorbable ligatures because later su gery reveals the original absorbent sutures had dissolved an the ovary was not fixed.

Wandering cyst

Torsion of an ovarian cyst may result in necrosis, and the cy may become amputated. Serial ultrasound may show a "wan dering cyst."

There was a case report of an abdominal cyst in a 30-wee fetus which on repeat ultrasound after birth showed a righ pelvic cyst, 3.2 cm in diameter. CT and MRI revealed cyst wa calcification and intra-cystic hemorrhage. At surgery, a fre autoamputated right ovarian cyst was removed. This would b the mechanism of a wandering cyst [10].

A long infundibulopelvic ligament pedicle may also allo an ovarian cyst to "wander."

Avni reported torsion of a fetal 4-cm cyst. Ultrasoun observation was continued until 3 months after birth to hav a satisfactory body weight for surgery. The follow-up ultra sounds showed a wandering ovarian cyst [34].

Lee et al. reported a left pelvic cyst discovered by ultrasoun in a 34 week fetus. After delivery ultrasound and CT sca showed a right pelvic cyst with a fluid-debris level. At age days, surgery revealed a left ovarian cyst with torsion and salpingo-oophorectomy was done. The pathology was a rar benign ovarian epithelial serous cystadenoma. The author wrote "we suggest that a wandering cystic mass in a femal fetus and newborn should be considered an indication fo surgical intervention due to its high risk of torsion. (Comment: This suggests that there may have been a lon pedicle to allow "wandering" which they believe predispose to torsion. It is uncertain when the torsion occurred [35] Conclusion: The wandering cyst could indicate a long pedicl or previous torsion and amputation.)

References

1. Strickland JL. Ovarian cysts in neonates, children and adolescents, Curr Opin Obstet Gynecol. 2002;**14**(5):459–65.
2. Irmi Rey-Stocker I. In: Altchek A, Deligdisch L (Eds.). Pediatric, Adolescent and Young Adult Gynecology, Chapt 32. Oxford: Wiley-Blackwell; 2009, p 487–91.
3. Servaes S, Victoria T, Lovrenski J, et al. Contemporary pediatric gynecologic imaging. Semin Ultrasound CT MR. 2010;**31**(2):116–40.
4. Heling KS, Chaoui R, Kirchmair F, et al. Fetal ovarian cysts: prenatal diagnosis, management and postnatal outcome. Ultrasound Obstet Gynecol. 2002;**20**(1):47–50.
5. Laufer MR. In: Trochia MM (Ed.). Ovarian cysts and neoplasms in infants children and adolescents. Waltham, MA: Up To Date; 2010.
6. Galinier P, Carfagna L, Juricic M, et al. Fetal ovarian cysts management and ovarian prognosis: a report of 82 cases. J Pediatr Surg. 2008;**43**(11):2004–9.

7. Ben-Ami I, Kogan A, Fuchs N, et al. Long-term follow-up of children with ovarian cysts diagnosed prenatally. Prenat Diagn. 2010;**30**(4):342–7.
8. Zachariou Z, Roth H, Boos R, et al. Three years' experience with large ovarian cysts diagnosed in utero. J Pediatr Surg. 1989;**24**(5):478–82.
9. Gallagher TA, Lim-Dunham JE, Vade A, et al. Sonographic appearance of ruptured ovarian cyst in the neonatal period. J Clin Ultrasound. 2007;**36**(1):53–5.
10. Koike Y, Inoue M, Uchida K, et al. Ovarian autoamputation in a neonate: a case report with literature review. Pediatr Surg Int. 2009;**25**(7):655–8.
11. Alexander CD, Kuller JA. Fetal ovarian cyst. J Diagn Med Sonogr. 2004;**20**(6):431–5.
12. Jouppila P, Kirkinen P, Tuononen S. Ultrasonic detection of bilateral ovarian cysts in the fetus. Eur J Obstet Gynecol Reprod Biol. 1982;**13**(2):87–92.
13. Shankar R, Mahajan JK, Khanna S, et al. Bilateral ovarian cysts in a neonate with salt-wasting congenital adrenal hyperplasia. J Pediatr Surg. 2010;**45**(5):e19–21.
14. Laufer MR, Growdon WB. Ovarian and Fallopian Tube Torsion. Waltham, MA: Up To Date; 2010.
15. Dolgin SE, Lublin M, Shlasko E. Maximizing ovarian salvage when treating idiopathic adnexal torsion. J Pediatr Surg. 2000;**35**(4):624–6.
16. Helmrath MA, Shin CE, Warner BW. Ovarian cysts in the pediatric population. Semin Pediatr Surg. 1998;**7**(1):19–28.
17. Gryngarten MG, Braslavsky D, Ballerini MG, et al. Spontaneous ovarian hyperstimulation syndrome caused by a follicle-stimulating hormone-secreting pituitary macroadenoma in an early pubertal girl. Horm Res Paediatr. 2010;**73**(4):293–8.
18. Franks S. Polycystic ovary syndrome in adolescents. Int J Obes (Lond). 2008;**32**(7):1035–41.
19. Fruzzetti F, Perini D, Lazzarini V, et al. Adolescent girls with polycystic ovary syndrome showing different phenotypes have a different metabolic profile associated with increasing androgen levels. Fertil Steril. 2009;**92**(2):626–34.
20. Rachmiel M, Kives S, Atenafu E, et al. Primary amenorrhea as a manifestation of polycystic ovarian syndrome in adolescents: a unique subgroup? Arch Pediatr Adolesc Med. 2008;**162**(6):521–5.
21. Stanley T, Misra M. Polycystic ovary syndrome in obese adolescents. Curr Opin Endocrinol Diabetes Obes. 2008;**15**(1):30–6.
22. Wiksten-Almströmer M, Hirschberg AL, Hagenfeldt K. Prospective follow-up of menstrual disorders in adolescence and prognostic factors. Acta Obstet Gynecol Scand. 2008;**87**(11):1162–8.
23. Li Z, Huang H. Epigenetic abnormality: a possible mechanism underlying the fetal origin of polycystic ovary syndrome. Med Hypotheses. 2008;**70**(3):638–42.
24. Jansen E, Laven JS, Dommerhold HB, et al. Abnormal gene expression profiles in human ovaries from polycystic ovary syndrome patients. Mol Endocrinol. 2004;**18**:3050–63.
25. Altchek A, Deligdisch L. The unappreciated Wnt-4 gene. J Pediatr Adolesc Gynecol. 2010;**23**(3):187–91.
26. Mashiach S, Bider D, Moran O, et al. Adnexal torsion of hyperstimulated ovaries in pregnancies after gonadotropin therapy. Fertil Steril. 1990;**53**(1):76–80.
27. Rousseau V, Massicot R, Darwish AA, et al. Emergency management and conservative surgery of ovarian torsion in children: a report of 40 cases. J Pediatr Adolesc Gynecol. 2008;**21**(4):201–6.
28. Anders JF, Powell EC. Urgency of evaluation and outcome of acute ovarian torsion in pediatric patients. Arch Pediatr Adolesc Med. 2005;**159**(6):532–5.
29. Eckler K, Laufer MR, Perlman SE. Conservative management of bilateral asynchronous adnexal torsion with necrosis in prepubescent girl. J Pediatr Surg. 2000;**35**(8):1248–51.
30. Cohen SB, Wattiez A, Seidman DS, et al. Laparoscopy versus laparotomy for detorsion and sparing of twisted ischemic adnexa. JSLS. 2003;**7**:295–9.
31. Kodama Y, Sameshima H, Ikenoue T, et al. Successful fresh whole ovarian autotransplantation without vascular anastomosis. Fertil Steril. 2010;**94**(6):2330.e11–12.
32. Hayes-Jordan A. Surgical management of the incidentally identified ovarian mass. Semin Pediatr Surg. 2005;**14**(2):106–10.
33. McCarthy JD, Erickson KM, Smith YR, et al. Premenarchal ovarian torsion and elevated CA-125. J Pediatr Adolesc Gynecol. 2010;**23**(1):e47–50.
34. Avni EF, Godart S, Israel C, et al. Ovarian torsion cyst presenting as a wandering tumor in a newborn: antenatal diagnosis and post natal assessment. Pediatr Radiol. 1983;**13**(3):169–71.
35. Lee JH, Tang JR, Wu MZ, et al. Ovarian cyst with torsion presenting as a wandering mass in a newborn. Acta Paediatr Taiwan. 2003;**44**(5):310–12.

Chapter 18

Should the ovaries be removed during a hysterectomy?

Michael S. Broder, MD, MSHS, and Wendy C. Hsiao, BS

ntroduction

n the United States, bilateral salpingo-oophorectomy (BSO) at ıe time of hysterectomy for benign disease is commonly done ɔ prevent the subsequent development of ovarian cancer. lmost all BSOs (87%) are done at the time of hysterectomy 1]. Oophorectomy rates appear to have peaked recently, with 5% of hysterectomies accompanied by the procedure in 1999 ompared with 39–45% in more recent years [2–4]. Recent data how age remains the strongest predictor of elective BSO, with 0% of women 40–44 years old, 78% of women 50–54 years old, nd 68% of women 55 years or older having had BSO at ysterectomy [5].

Despite the common practice of "risk-reducing" or prophy- ıctic oophorectomy at the time of hysterectomy for benign isease, an increasing body of evidence suggests removal of ormal ovaries has minimal overall benefit for those women vho are not at an increased risk of breast or ovarian cancer. everal large cohort studies suggest that, while removing nor- nal ovaries reduces the risk of ovarian cancer to almost zero, rophylactic oophorectomy does not appear to increase overall urvival. This chapter will address the history of risk-reducing ophorectomy, assess the evidence for the practice, and con- ider its appropriateness in light of recent studies.

listory

'he development of modern abdominal surgery and the search or safe surgical treatments for ovarian tumors are closely ntertwined. In 1806, Ephraim McDowell removed an ovarian umor, and made history when the patient survived. Forty- even years later, Walter Burnham performed the first success- ul hysterectomy [6]. The ensuing 100 years saw a substantial ncrease in oophorectomy resulting from better anesthesia, the ntroduction of aseptic techniques and effective antibiotics, and he widespread use of exogenous replacements for ovarian ormones. Advances in anesthesia and reductions in infection ncreased oophorectomy indirectly by contributing to the more videspread use of hysterectomy, while the synthetic estrogens emoved a major barrier to incidental BSO: the reluctance to nduce surgical menopause and its concomitant risks.

In the second half of the 19th century, the use of ether and hloroform allowed physicians to experiment with surgical rocedures that previously could not be attempted. In 1867, Joseph Lister published his treatise "On the Antiseptic Principle of the Practice of Surgery," and not long after, the "hand-washing fool," Ignaz Semmelweis, dramatically reduced rates of puerperal sepsis by introducing hand-washing to Vienna General Hospital's obstetric service. Halsted introduced the sterilized medical glove in 1890, but even with these infection-reducing innovations, the mortality rate for hysterectomy was 30% in the late 19th century [6]. The modern antibiotic era began with mass production of penicillin (driven by the needs of U.S. troops in World War II). By 1950, penicillin was reported to reduce morbidity after vaginal hysterectomy. As the mortality fell, it became more appropriate to consider hysterectomy for non–life-threatening conditions, and in 1984 more than a third of women could expect to have a hysterectomy by age 60 [7].

Although hysterectomy rates rose steadily in the late 20th century, rates of BSO remained fairly constant. A multi-center study showed hysterectomy was accompanied by BSO at a rate of between 9% and 15% over the 25 years from 1928 to 1953 [8]. This began to change when, in the 1950s, a series of publications raised concern among gynecologists about ovarian cancer in "residual" ovaries – those not removed at hysterectomy [9,10]. Case series of women who developed ovarian cancer years after hysterectomy were extrapolated to calculate the number of women who could have been "saved" had all such procedures been accompanied by BSO [11,12]. As a result, by the 1960s, gynecologists were enthusiastically recommending BSO at hysterectomy after age 40, or younger if childbearing was complete [8].

The primary disadvantage of BSO before natural menopause was considered to be the combination of symptoms caused by lack of ovarian hormones and osteoporosis. In 1941, the newly established Food and Drug Administration approved diethylstilbestrol (DES) to treat menopausal symptoms, and approval of conjugated equine estrogens followed the year after. Several books published over the next 25 years, most notably "Feminine Forever" by gynecologist Robert Wilson, depicted menopause as the enemy of youth [13]. As estrogen therapy (ET) began to be seen as the cure for the scourge of menopause, the number of women using it to treat menopausal symptoms rose: from about 2.5 million women in 1966 to over 4.7 million women in 1975. After unopposed estrogen was linked to endometrial cancer, the number dropped to 2.3

ltchek's Diagnosis and Management of Ovarian Disorders, ed. Liane Deligdisch, Nathan G. Kase, and Carmel J. Cohen. Published y Cambridge University Press.

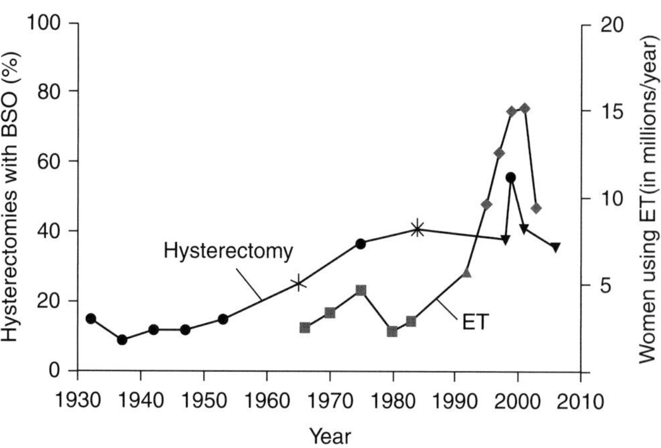

Fig. 18.1. Estrogen therapy (ET) use and BSO at hysterectomy in US women. Sources: †see Ref. 2; ▼see Ref. 3; *see Ref. 7; ●see Ref. 8; ■see Ref. 14; ◆see Ref. 15; ◆see Ref. 19; ▲see Ref. 20.

million in 1980. The introduction of combination estrogen/progestin therapy (E+P) negated this risk, and by 1995, 10 million US women were using exogenous estrogen. A proposed cardiovascular benefit helped drive this up to approximately 15 million by 2001 [14–16].

Following the publication of data from the Women's Health Initiative (WHI) in 2002, faith in hormone therapy drastically declined [17]. This large randomized placebo-controlled trial of E+P in post-menopausal women was terminated prematurely when the overall health risks were demonstrated to exceed the benefits [18]. By 2003, fewer than 10 million women were taking exogenous estrogen, a level not seen since the mid-1990s [15].

With no reliable tools to screen for or prevent ovarian cancer, oophorectomy has been seen as the best form of prevention, with hormone deprivation its primary downside. Thus, when faith in estrogen was high, the oophorectomy rate climbed; when faith declined, so did the rate of BSO. The figure shows this relationship. In 1965, 25% of hysterectomies in the United States were accompanied by BSO. By 1975, the proportion had increased to almost 40% [7,19]. The percentage of hysterectomies with BSO peaked in 1999 at 55%, but by 2006 was estimated at only 36% [2,3] (Fig. 18.1).

Recent evidence

Two recent large prospective cohort studies have provided new evidence concerning the benefits and risks of BSO. These studies, together involving more than 50,000 U.S. women, estimated the health effects of BSO compared with ovarian conservation at hysterectomy on mortality and a variety of other outcomes. Taken together, they represent the best evidence currently available to estimate the influence of BSO on overall health.

The Nurses' Health Study (NHS) is a large, prospective cohort study of female nurses aged 30–55 in 1976. In 2009, we published a study of 29,380 women enrolled in the NHS who had hysterectomy for benign disease [21]. Of these, 55.6% had BSO and 44.4% had ovarian conservation. The mean age at enrollment was 51 years, and the cohort consisted mostly of white women with relatively uniform education, socioeconomi status, and access to health care. These women were followed fo an average of 24 years, from 1980 through 2004, and the reported new diagnoses and health conditions every 2 years b mail-in survey. Survey data were confirmed in interviews and b review of medical records. We stratified the cohort into thos <45, 45–54, and 55 years or older at the time of hysterectom The study analyzed the incidence of breast, epithelial ovaria lung, or colorectal cancer; hip fracture; coronary heart diseas (CHD); stroke; pulmonary embolism (PE); cause-specific deat for each of these causes; and death due to all causes.

The second large cohort study was published in 2011 an followed 25,448 post-menopausal women from the Women' Health Initiative (WHI) Observational Study who had hyste ectomy [22]. The WHI Observational Study is a prospectiv cohort study of women aged 50–79 years at enrollment wh were invited to participate in a randomized controlled tri (RCT) comparing dietary modification to exogenous hor mones, but who were ineligible or declined to participat Study participants were contacted yearly and reported an hospitalizations or events related to outcomes of interes Survey data were confirmed by medical record review. Mea follow-up time was slightly less than 8 years, compared with 2 years in the NHS analysis. Like the NHS, 56% had BSO and 44% had ovarian conservation. The mean age at enrollment was 6 years, compared with 51 in the NHS, but the cohorts wer otherwise similar. Study subjects were stratified into thos < 40, 40–49, and 50 years or older at the time of hysterectom Outcome measures included incident ovarian, breast, lung or colorectal cancer; hip fracture; cardiovascular events includ ing CHD, stroke, and total cardiovascular disease events; an all-cause death. The study did not report cause-specific deat Both studies performed separate analyses among women wh did not use ET. We summarize the study results by outcom below.

Cancer

Breast cancer

The NHS demonstrated a statistically significantly reduced risk o breast cancer in women who had BSO compared with those wh had ovarian conservation (all women, hazard ratio [HR] 0.75; 95% confidence interval [CI] 0.68–0.84; women < 45 years old a hysterectomy, HR 0.62, 95% CI 0.53–0.74). In women wh never used ET, BSO reduced the point estimate for breast cance risk, but the difference was not statistically significant (all wome HR 0.85, 95% CI 0.61–1.20; women < 50 years old at hysterec tomy, HR 0.66, 95% CI 0.43–1.03). There was no difference in th risk of death from breast cancer between BSO and ovarian con servation (all women, HR 0.94, 95% CI 0.70–1.26) [21].

The WHI data showed a statistically significant protectiv effect of BSO on breast cancer in women < 40 at time o hysterectomy with no history of ET use (HR 0.36, 95% C 0.14–0.95). The authors did not attempt to estimate the risk o death from breast cancer [22]. Both studies suggest BSO reduces breast cancer risk, particularly in younger wome but it may not reduce risk of death from breast cancer. Powe

Table 18.1. Impact of oophorectomy on cancer outcomes[a]

	Hazard ratio (95% confidence interval)					
	Breast cancer		Ovarian cancer		All cancers	
	Incidence	Death	Incidence	Death	Incidence	Death
Younger women						
< 45 years	0.62 (0.53–0.74)	0.74 (0.47–1.18)	0.03 (0.01–0.14)	0.06 (0.01–0.43)	0.83 (0.75–0.92)	1.08 (0.91–1.27)
< 40 years[b]	0.72 (0.51–1.02)	–	–	–	0.97 (0.81–1.17)	–
No ET use, < 50 years old	0.66 (0.43–1.03)	–	–	–	–	–
No ET use, < 40 years old[b]	0.36 (0.14–0.95)	–	–	–	0.93 (0.62–1.39)	–
Older women						
≥ 55 years old	1.05 (0.71–1.55)	1.28 (0.46–3.54)	0.07 (0.01–0.60)	–	1.01 (0.79–1.29)	1.50 (0.91–2.45)
≥ 50 years old[b]	1.11 (0.80–1.55)	–	–	–	1.08 (0.89–1.32)	–
No ET use, ≥ 50 years old	1.88 (0.66–5.32)	–	–	–	–	–
No ET use, ≥ 50 years old[b]	0.77 (0.41–1.45)	–	–	–	0.92 (0.63–1.33)	–
All women						
All ages	0.75 (0.68–0.84)	0.94 (0.70–1.26)	0.04 (0.01–0.09)	0.06 (0.02–0.21)	0.90 (0.84–0.96)	1.17 (1.04–1.32)
All ages[b]	0.96 (0.81–1.13)	–	–	–	0.96 (0.87–1.05)	–
No ET use, all ages	0.85 (0.61–1.20)	–	–	–	–	–
No ET use, all ages[b]	0.72 (0.49–1.05)	–	–	–	0.90 (0.74–1.10)	–

Et, estrogen therapy.
[a] See Ref. 21, unless otherwise noted.
[b] See Ref. 22.

calculations suggest that, if the actual reduction in mortality were equal to that observed in the NHS (0.94), an RCT of over 400,000 patients would be required to have 80% power to detect such a difference (Table 18.1).

Ovarian cancer

The NHS showed that BSO statistically significantly reduced the risk of ovarian cancer in all women (HR 0.04, 95% CI 0.01–0.09) and reduced the risk of death from ovarian cancer (all women, HR 0.06, 95% CI 0.02–0.21) [21]. In the WHI study, there was a 0.02% incidence of ovarian cancer in women who received both BSO and hysterectomy, compared with 0.33% incidence in women with hysterectomy alone. BSO reduced the risk of ovarian cancer in women who did not use ET (0.04% vs. 0.23%) [22]. There is some evidence from other studies that hysterectomy alone reduces the risk of ovarian cancer, but BSO at hysterectomy clearly reduces both the risk of ovarian cancer and the risk of death from this disease.

Lung cancer

BSO was associated with a statistically significantly increased risk of lung cancer (HR 1.26, 95% CI 1.02–1.56) and an increased risk of death from lung cancer in the NHS (HR 1.31, 95% CI 1.02–1.68) in all women. Risk of lung cancer was further increased in women who had never used ET (HR 2.09, 95% CI 1.01–4.33) [21]. There was no association of BSO with lung cancer in the WHI study (all women, HR 0.96, 95% CI 0.72–1.27) [22]. There is no agreed-upon biological explanation of the observations from the NHS, although some theories have been proposed [23,24].

Total cancer

In the NHS, BSO was associated with a statistically significantly reduced risk of total cancer (all women, HR 0.90, 95% CI 0.84–0.96), consistent with the reduction in breast and ovarian cancer. However, the risk of death from all cancers was statistically significantly increased in all women who had BSO (HR 1.17, 95% CI 1.04–1.32) [21]. The WHI study found a similar point estimate for the risk of total cancer, but the result was not statistically significant (all women, HR 0.96, 95% CI 0.87–1.05) [22]. The study did not report cancer-specific mortality.

Cardiovascular disease

In the NHS, BSO was associated with a statistically significantly increased risk of CHD (all women, HR 1.17, 95% CI 1.02–1.35). BSO was associated with increased point estimates of risk for stroke among all women, although the results were not statistically significant (HR 1.14, 95% CI 0.98–1.33). The effect of BSO on cardiovascular disease risk was greater in women who had not used ET: in the group of never users, BSO statistically significantly increased the risk of stroke (HR 1.85, 95% CI 1.09–3.16). Women younger than 50 who did not use ET had increased risk of both CHD (HR 1.98, 95% CI 1.18–3.32) and stroke (HR 2.19, 95% CI 1.16–4.14). BSO was associated with a statistically significantly increased risk of death from CHD (HR 1.28, 95% CI 1.00–1.64) and an increased point estimate of the risk of death from stroke (HR 1.11, 95% CI 0.82–1.51), although this last finding did not reach statistical significance [21].

Table 18.2. Impact of oophorectomy on non-cancer health outcomes[a]

	Hazard ratio (95% confidence interval)				
	Coronary heart disease		Stroke		
	Incidence	Death	Incidence	Death	All-cause mortality
Younger women					
< 45 years	1.26 (1.04–1.54)	1.14 (0.81–1.61)	1.19 (0.96–1.49)	0.85 (0.54–1.34)	1.06 (0.95–1.18)
< 40 years[b]	0.98 (0.72–1.35)	–	1.13 (0.81–1.58)	–	0.90 (0.72–1.13)
No ET use, < 50 years old	1.98 (1.18–3.32)	–	2.19 (1.16–4.14)	–	1.40 (1.01–1.96)
No ET use, < 40 years old[b]	1.33 (0.77–2.30)	–	1.44 (0.78–2.65)	–	1.15 (0.78–1.70)
Older women					
≥ 55 years old	1.31 (0.73–2.36)	4.10 (0.41–41.06)	1.51 (0.86–2.64)	2.26 (0.85–5.95)	1.14 (0.85–1.52)
≥ 50 years old[b]	1.02 (0.74–1.41)	–	0.98 (0.68–1.41)	–	1.07 (0.84–1.35)
No ET use, ≥ 50 years old	0.70 (0.34–1.44)	–	1.21 (0.48–3.00)	–	2.05 (0.87–4.79)
No ET use, ≥ 50 years old[b]	1.00 (0.56–1.78)	–	1.37 (0.62–3.00)	–	0.97 (0.62–1.52)
All women					
All ages	1.17 (1.02–1.35)	1.28 (1.00–1.64)	1.14 (0.98–1.33)	1.11 (0.82–1.51)	1.12 (1.03–1.21)
All ages[b]	1.00 (0.85–1.18)	–	1.04 (0.87–1.24)	–	0.98 (0.87–1.10)
No ET use, all ages	1.42 (0.93–2.16)	–	1.85 (1.09–3.16)	–	1.20 (0.91–1.57)
No ET use, all ages[b]	1.24 (0.92–1.68)	-	1.31 (0.92–1.87)	–	0.99 (0.80–1.23)

Et, estrogen therapy.
[a] See Ref. 21, unless otherwise noted.
[b] See Ref. 22.

In contrast, the WHI study found no difference in the risk of cardiovascular disease between women who had BSO compared with those with ovarian conservation (all women, HR 0.99, 95% CI 0.91–1.09). Among women who did not use ET, the point estimate for risks of CHD (HR 1.24, 95% CI 0.92–1.68), stroke (HR 1.31, 95% CI 0.92–1.87), and total cardiovascular disease (HR 1.05, 95% CI 0.89–1.25) were increased, but these findings were not statistically significant. The WHI findings are limited by short follow-up (~8 years), especially because CHD may take approximately 15 years to develop following oophorectomy [22,25].

Overall, the evidence suggests that BSO at the time of hysterectomy increases the risk of cardiovascular disease and cardiovascular-disease-related mortality. Lack of ET use further increases risk. Inconsistencies between studies may be due to lower power in the WHI study (Table 18.2) [22].

Hip fracture

In both the NHS and WHI studies, there was no statistically significant association between BSO and hip fracture (all women, HR 0.89, 95% CI 0.71–1.12 in the NHS; all women, HR 0.83, 95% CI 0.63–1.10 in the WHI), and these findings were consistent whether or not there was a history of ET use [21,22].

Survival

The NHS found that BSO statistically significantly increased all-cause mortality (all women, HR 1.12, 95% CI 1.03–1.21), related in part to the increased risk of death from lung cancer, all cancers and CHD. Risk of all-cause mortality was statistically significantly increased in women less than 50 at hysterectomy who had never used ET (HR 1.40, 95% CI 1.01–1.96) [21]. The WHI study found no statistically significant difference in mortality among all women (HR 0.98, 95% CI 0.87–1.10). In women less than 40 who had not used ET, the point estimate for mortality was increased, but this was not statistically significant (HR 1.15, 95% CI 0.78–1.70) [22]. Neither study reported a survival benefit for BSO at any age or in any subgroup (Table 18.1).

Other evidence

While these two studies represent the largest and best-controlled studies to examine the impact of oophorectomy compared with conservation of the ovaries at hysterectomy, other studies have addressed various aspects of the question. A recent systematic review of the impact of BSO on CHD found oophorectomy did not increase the risk of CHD overall, but most of the trials were low quality. The review found no benefit of BSO [26]. A large cohort study published in 2011 investigated cardiovascular disease risk in 184,441 hysterectomized women in the Swedish Inpatient Register, showing statistically significantly increased risks of both CHD and stroke in women younger than 50 who had BSO at hysterectomy compared with those who had neither hysterectomy nor BSO [27]. A retrospective cohort study of 4,748 women in Olmsted County, MN, found an increase in all-cause mortality in women < 45 who had oophorectomy, but observed no such increase in older women [28]. Using the same cohort, an association between oophorectomy and increased risk of neurologic conditions (Parkinsonism, dementia, and anxiety or depression) was identified, but the findings await confirmation in other populations [29,30]. Finally, a Markov model estimated that overall mortality was increased in women who had oophorectomy before age 65. At no age was there a survival advantage with oophorectomy [31].

Recommendations

Oophorectomy at the time of hysterectomy has become a common operation, primarily as a prophylactic measure to reduce the risk of ovarian cancer. There are several reasons why this traditional practice should be reconsidered for women who do not have a clearly elevated risk of breast or ovarian cancer due to BRCA mutation or family or personal history.

First, a major driver of the increase in oophorectomy rates was the availability of exogenous estrogen therapy. As recent studies have shown, however, encouraging long-term drug therapy without long-term outcome studies is fraught with potential dangers. Fewer women are willing to begin taking estrogen, and among those who do, the continuation rate is low. Even if women could be persuaded to stay on therapy, long-term estrogen has not been shown to lengthen life, nor does it completely mitigate the risks of oophorectomy. Second, while oophorectomy does dramatically reduce the risk of ovarian cancer in all women and reduces the risk of breast cancer in younger women, there is no evidence that it prolongs life. In fact, the best available evidence suggests either a net harmful effect or, at best, a neutral effect. Current evidence indicates this lack of overall benefit likely relates to the relatively low incidence of ovarian cancer in contrast to the relatively common nature of CHD, the risk of which is increased with oophorectomy.

The data on which these conclusions are based derive from observational studies. However, the data supporting prophylactic oophorectomy were based on even lower quality evidence – namely, theoretical considerations and case series. Considering the weight of the evidence, if "prophylactic oophorectomy" was a new drug or device, regulatory agencies would be unlikely to approve it. Waiting for evidence for RCTs before deciding whether to recommend BSO for a woman having hysterectomy might be reasonable (although given the necessary size of such a trial, analysis of patient outcomes would entail a long wait), but in the meantime, it might be wise to consider the admonition to "first, do no harm."

References

1. Melton LJ III, Bergstralh EJ, Malkasian GD, et al. Bilateral oophorectomy trends in Olmsted County, Minnesota, 1950–1987. Epidemiology. 1991;**2**(2):149–52.
2. Keshavarz H, Hillis SD, Kieke BA, Marchbanks PA. Hysterectomy surveillance – United States, 1994–1999. MMWR Surveill Summ. 2002;**51**(SS05):1–8.
3. Asante A, Whiteman MK, Kulkarni A, et al. Elective oophorectomy in the United States: trends and in-hospital complications, 1998–2006. Obstet Gynecol. 2010;**116**(5):1088–95.
4. Lowder JL, Oliphant SS, Ghetti C, et al. Prophylactic bilateral oophorectomy or removal of remaining ovary at the time of hysterectomy in the United States, 1979–2004. Am J Obstet Gynecol. 2010;**202**(6):538.e1–9.
5. Jacoby VL, Vittinghoff E, Nakagawa S, et al. Factors associated with undergoing bilateral salpingo-oophorectomy at the time of hysterectomy for benign conditions. Obstet Gynecol. 2009;**113**(6):1259–67.
6. Rock JA. Historical development of pelvic surgery. In: Thompson JD, Rock JA (Eds.). Te Linde's Operative Gynecology, 7th edition. Philadelphia, PA: JB Lippincott Company; 1992, p 1.
7. Pokras R, Hufnagel VG. Hysterectomy in the United States, 1965–84. Am J Public Health. 1988;**78**(7):852–3.
8. Randall CL, Paloucek FP. The frequency of oophorectomy at the time of hysterectomy: trends in surgical practice, 1928–1953. Am J Obstet Gynecol. 1968;**100**(5):716–26.
9. Christ JE, Lotze EC. The residual ovary syndrome. Obstet Gynecol. 1975;**46**(5):551–6.
10. Speert H. Prophylaxis of ovarian cancer. Ann Surg. 1949;**129**(4):468–75.
11. Grundsell H, Ekman G, Gullberg B, et al. Some aspects of prophylactic oophorectomy and ovarian carcinoma. Ann Chir Gynaecol. 1981;**70**(1):36–42.
12. Sightler SE, Boike GM, Estape RE, et al. Ovarian cancer in women with prior hysterectomy: a 14-year experience at the University of Miami. Obstet Gynecol. 1991;**78**(4):681–4.
13. Stefanick ML. Estrogens and progestins: background and history, trends in use, and guidelines and regimens approved by the US Food and Drug Administration. Am J Med. 2005;**118**(Suppl 12B):64–73.
14. Kennedy DL, Baum C, Forbes MB. Noncontraceptive estrogens and progestins: use patterns over time. Obstet Gynecol. 1985;**65**(3):441–6.
15. Hersh AL, Stefanick ML, Stafford RS. National use of postmenopausal hormone therapy: annual trends and response to recent evidence. JAMA. 2004;**291**(1):47–53.
16. Wysowski DK, Golden L, Burke L. Use of menopausal estrogens and medroxyprogesterone in the United States, 1982–1992. Obstet Gynecol. 1995;**85**(1):6–10.
17. Wegienka G, Havstad S, Kelsey JL. Menopausal hormone therapy in a health maintenance organization before and after Women's Health Initiative hormone trials termination. J Womens Health (Larchmt). 2006;**15**(4):369–78.
18. Writing Group for the Women's Health Initiative Investigators, Rossouw JE, Anderson GL, et al. Risks and benefits of estrogen plus progestin in healthy postmenopausal women: principal results from the Women's Health Initiative randomized controlled trial. JAMA. 2002;**288**(3):321–33.

19. Pokras R, Hufnagel VG. Hysterectomies in the United States. Vital Health Stat. 1987;**13**(92):1–32.

20. Wysowski DK, Governale LA. Use of menopausal hormones in the United States, 1992 through June, 2003. Pharmacoepidemiol Drug Saf. 2005;**14**(3):171–6.

21. Parker WH, Broder MS, Chang E, et al. Ovarian conservation at the time of hysterectomy and long-term health outcomes in the Nurses' Health Study. Obstet Gynecol. 2009;**113**(5):1027–37.

22. Jacoby VL, Grady D, Wactawski-Wende J, et al. Oophorectomy vs ovarian conservation with hysterectomy: cardiovascular disease, hip fracture, and cancer in the Women's Health Initiative Observational Study. Arch Intern Med. 2011;**171**(8):760–8.

23. Brinton LA, Gierach GL, Andaya A, et al. Reproductive and hormonal factors and lung cancer risk in the NIH-AARP Diet and Health Study cohort. Cancer Epidemiol Biomarkers Prev. 2011;**20**(5):900–11.

24. Liu Y, Inoue M, Sobue T, et al. Reproductive factors, hormone use and the risk of lung cancer among middle-aged never-smoking Japanese women: a large-scale population-based cohort study. Int J Cancer. 2005;**117**(4):662–6.

25. Parrish HM, Carr CA, Hall DG, et al. Time interval from castration in premenopausal women to development of excessive coronary atherosclerosis. Am J Obstet Gynecol. 1967;**99**(2):155–62.

26. Jacoby VL, Grady D, Sawaya GF. Oophorectomy as a risk factor for coronary heart disease. Am J Obstet Gynecol. 2009;**200**(2):140.e1–9.

27. Ingelsson E, Lundholm C, Johansson AL, et al. Hysterectomy and risk of cardiovascular disease: a population-based cohort study. Eur Heart J. 2011;**32**(6):745–50.

28. Rocca WA, Grossardt BR, de Andrade M, et al. Survival patterns after oophorectomy in premenopausal women: a population-based cohort study. Lancet Oncol. 2006;7(10):821–8.

29. Rocca WA, Bower JH, Maraganore DM, et al. Increased risk of cognitive impairment or dementia in women who underwent oophorectomy before menopause. Neurology. 2007;**69**(11):1074–83.

30. Rocca WA, Bower JH, Maraganore DM, et al. Increased risk of parkinsonism in women who underwent oophorectomy before menopause. Neurology. 2008;**70**(3):200–9.

31. Parker WH, Broder MS, Liu Z, et al. Ovarian conservation at the time of hysterectomy for benign disease. Obstet Gynecol. 2005;**106**(2):219–26.

Chapter 19

The aging ovary

Norbert Gleicher, MD, FACOG, FACS, and David H. Barad, MD, MS, FACOG

Introduction

It is well recognized that female reproductive capacity declines with advancing female age. This decline in ability to conceive has mostly been attributed to changes in ovarian function. Lay public and scientists, alike, therefore, for the longest time have perceived ovaries as "aging." The subject of this book chapter will be the description of selected newly reported features of this ovarian aging process.

Among scientists, the definition of ovarian "age," actually, is mathematical rather than anatomic or histologic. It is defined by number of follicles in ovaries remaining available for procreation. The more follicles a woman retains in her ovaries, the better the so-called ovarian reserve (OR), and the "younger" the ovary; the fewer follicles ovaries contain, the poorer the OR, and the "older" the ovary.

Dogma still holds that females are born with a finite number of follicles/oocytes. Ovarian aging is, thus, perceived mediated by declines in ovarian follicles and available oocyte numbers [1] (Fig. 19.1). Dogma, however, also holds that oocytes age, as women age, defining aging by declines in follicle numbers/OR, as well as deterioration of follicle and oocyte quality. It is the decline in follicle/oocyte quality that has been suggested responsible for increasing oocyte and embryo aneuploidy with advancing female age (Fig. 19.2), clinically presenting by means of declining pregnancy rates [2] (Fig. 19.3) and increasing miscarriage rates [3] (Fig. 19.4).

This chapter presents a newly evolving concept of ovarian aging, which no longer is based on "aging" follicles and oocytes but, instead, assumes that unrecruited primordial follicles and their oocytes are "suspended in time," and do not age. What ages is the ovarian environment in which follicles, once recruited into follicle maturation, undergo folliculogenesis. It is then this aging ovarian environment that ages, as women age, and it is the aging ovarian environment that adversely affects the follicle maturation process, leading to poor quality oocytes and increased aneuploidy [4,5].

This conceptual distinction between "aging" follicles/oocytes versus ovarian environments is of major potential importance because, once damaged, oocytes only unlikely can be reverted to health. In contrast, a deteriorating ovarian environment, very likely, can be pharmacologically improved. Ovarian aging, defined by aging ovarian environments, therefore, promises the possibility of successful therapeutic interventions and improvements in treatment of diminished OR (DOR).

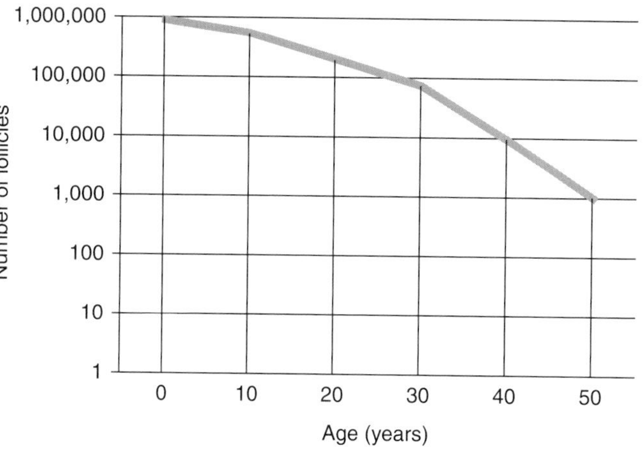

Fig. 19.1. Decline in ovarian follicles with advancing female age. The graph represents a schematic representation of approximate follicle numbers, remaining in ovaries at various ages in women with normal, physiologic ovarian aging. Women with premature ovarian aging (POA), at each age, demonstrate lower follicle numbers. The graph represents an approximation, based on data recently reported by Hansen et al. [1].

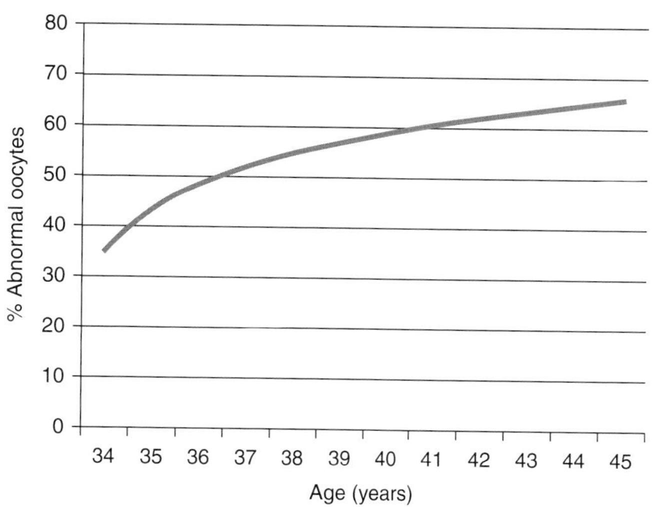

Fig. 19.2. Increasing aneuploidy with advancing female age. Several reports in the literature approximately represent aneuploidy rates in human oocytes/embryos at different female ages. The literature mildly varies in rates at different ages, likely representing shortcomings in technology used for most studies. Aneuploidy rates, however, undoubtedly increase with advancing female age.

Altchek's Diagnosis and Management of Ovarian Disorders, ed. Liane Deligdisch, Nathan G. Kase, and Carmel J. Cohen. Published by Cambridge University Press.

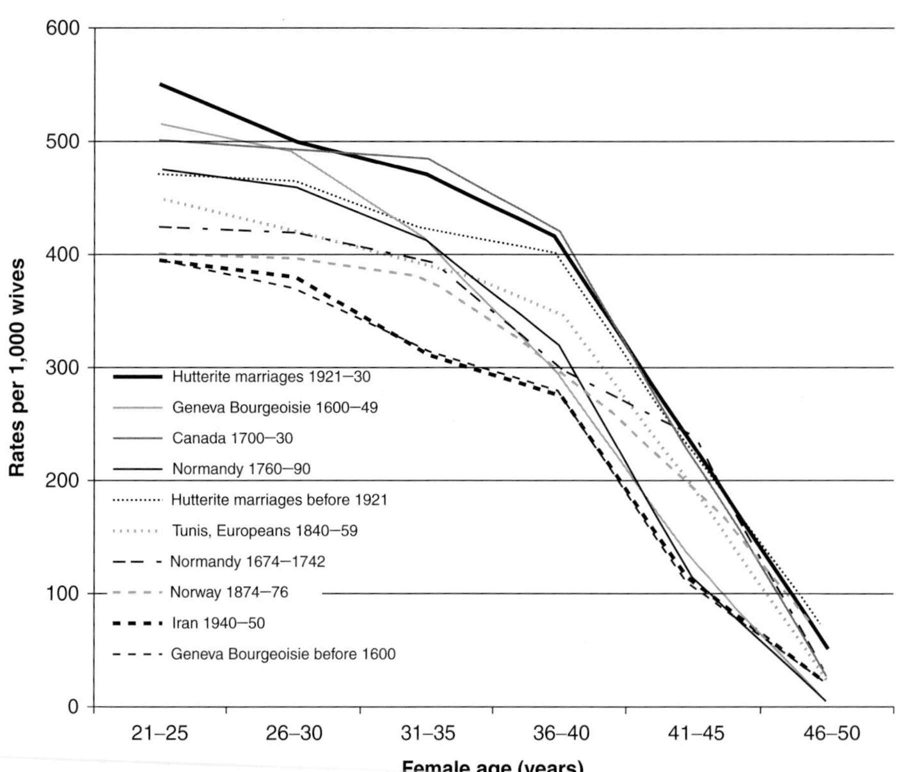

Fig. 19.3. Declining fertility rates with advancing female age. Fertility rates in different patient population, as reported in the classic study by Menken et al. [2], with permission from Science. While in the Menken graphs marital fertility rates were recorded, similar curves are also seen with fertility treatments, like in vitro fertilization.

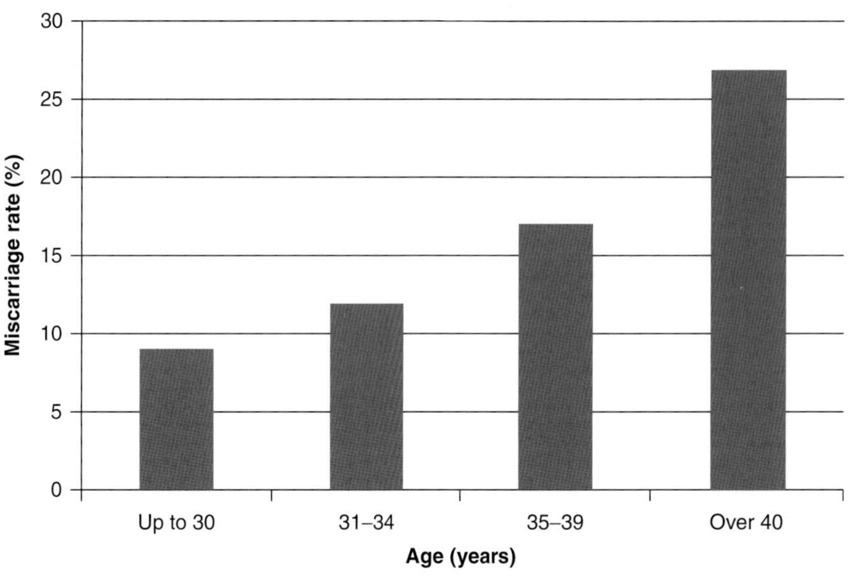

Fig. 19.4. Increasing miscarriage rates with advancing female age. The graph demonstrates increasing miscarriage rates in singleton IVF pregnancies with advancing female age. Modified from Spandorfer et al. [3] with permission.

As will be discussed later in this chapter, recent data, indeed, support the concept that follicle maturation in women with "older" ovaries can be therapeutically improved.

Background

Ovarian aging cannot be understood without a basic explanation of follicle recruitment and subsequent maturation. We noted above that current dogma still holds that women are born with a finite pool of follicles and oocytes. This pool mostly consists of so-called primordial follicles, the most immature stage of follicle development, containing oocytes arrested in meiotic prophase I. Primordial follicles remain quiescent until recruited into follicle maturation.

It is this pool of follicles that we now believe to be "suspended in time," and not aging. How they are activated to enter maturation is still largely unknown. It appears that the recruitment process involves complex bi-directional signals between oocytes and surrounding somatic cells [6]. In the mouse, deletion of Pten (phosphatase and tensin homolog, deleted on chromosome 10) results in premature recruitment of practically the whole pool of primordial follicles, causing premature ovarian failure (POF), now often called primary varian insufficiency (POI) [7]. Whether Pten plays a similar ole in humans is still undetermined.

As a consequence of recruitment, follicles become exposed environmental influences from the ovary, which, as we will iscuss later, indeed appear age-dependent.

As primordial follicles (also called resting or non-growing ollicles) are steadily recruited, large cohorts of follicles pass in ynchronized waves through different maturation stages, with ach wave resulting in spontaneous ovulation of usually only a ingle follicle. All other, originally recruited follicles degenerate nd undergo apoptosis.

Follicle recruitment appears to occur at random, although he "production line hypothesis," offered in 1968 by Henderson and Nobel laureate Robert Edwards suggested an rder [8]. Individually recruited follicles are then, however, rogressively aligned in generational cohorts of maturing ollicles. Individual recruitment is, thus, converted into epiodic maturation, ultimately leading toward a regular mentrual cycle pattern, characteristic of a normally ovulating emale.

Even when ovulation is not reached, like in women with olycystic ovarian (PCO) phenotype, by time of maturation rrest, follicle cohorts appear already mostly properly aligned n size and maturation. The importance of this development rom initially anarchical recruitment to episodic cycle maturaion has been widely overlooked. It is best documented by the bservation that young, normally functioning ovaries usually manage the process well. Older and more dysfunctional ovaries, owever, no longer do!

A clinically well-recognized feature of "older" ovaries is, herefore, the presence of increasingly inhomogeneous and multi-generational follicle cohorts in response to ovarian timulation. Older women and patients with dysfunctional varies, therefore, demonstrate significantly wider oocyte maturation ranges than women with normally functioning varies.

Folliculogenesis

Our understanding of the maturation process of follicles after recruitment (folliculogenesis) has recently undergone considerable change. For the longest time, androgens have been considered toxic to the process of egg maturation. A considerable volume of animal and human data now, actually, suggest otherwise.

This, of course, does not mean that excessive androgen levels may not exert toxic effects [4]. Indeed, they undoubtedly can [9]. Within therapeutic range, they, however, now have to be assumed to contribute significantly to normal follicle maturation.

Likely, the most impressive data come from exquisitely executed experiments with androgen receptor knock out (ARKO) mice, in which investigators were able to basically mimic almost any ovary-associated infertility phenotype in mice where androgen receptors (AR) were knocked out in granulosa cells but not where AR was knocked out in oocytes [10]. These data, beyond reasonable doubt, at least in the mouse, demonstrate how essential androgen effects on granulosa cells are to normal follicle maturation and, indeed, to female fertility [11].

Presence of AR is, however, mostly restricted to small follicles (Fig. 19.5). After small pre-antral stages, no more AR can be detected in follicles. These observations, therefore, suggest that androgen effects, leading to female infertility phenotypes, are induced at relatively early stages of follicle maturation, long before the stage of gonadotropin sensitivity of follicles, which in over 5 decades of research into infertility and ovulation induction has remained the exclusive purview of clinical interventions.

Recognizing this fact, it appears time to expand basic research and pharmacologic applications into earlier stages of follicle development. Such an approach, of course, would also go hand in hand with the above outlined concept of pharmacologically restituting aging ovarian environments in older women.

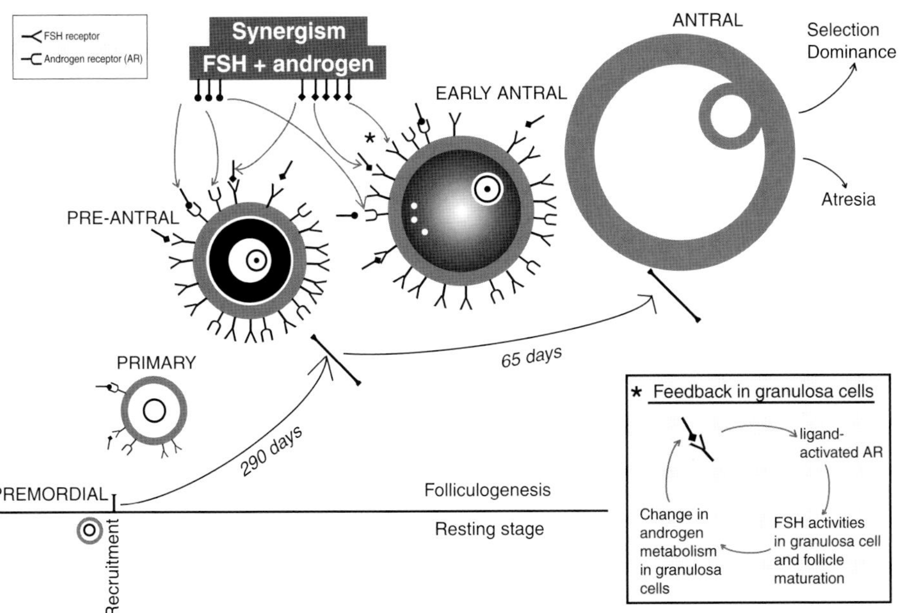

Fig. 19.5. Effects of androgens on follicle maturation. This figure depicts stages of follicle maturation and synergism of action between androgens and FSH at small follicle stages (primary, pre-antral and early antral). Of note is the high concentration of AR at these stages and their complete absence at antral follicle stage. Presence of AR is strongly supportive of essential functions of AR, and therefore androgens, at those developmental stages. Their absence thereafter suggests absence of androgen effects, starting at antral stage. The box in the right corner demonstrates reported synergistic effects between FSH and androgens in granulosa cells, based on Lenie and Smitz [11]. The figure is modified from Gleicher et al. [4], with permission.

Such an expanded treatment approach, however, mandates reassessment of what, currently, is considered a fertility treatment cycle. For any fertility treatment this, presently, is the time unit between two menstrual periods. Looking at such an expanded concept, a treatment cycle would, now, however, have to be considered the time period from recruitment to ovulation, a time period many months long, and including a good number of treatment cycles, as currently defined. It is reasonable to assume that reorientation of ovulation induction from the last 2 weeks of gonadotropin-sensitivity toward earlier follicle maturation stages, will allow for the next big improvement in fertility therapy, primarily benefiting women with "older" ovaries.

Definitions

As noted before, most investigators equate "ovarian age" with the size of a woman's remaining follicle pool, often also given the acronym OR. Unfortunately, neither the complete follicle pool nor OR really represents "ovarian age" accurately. Indeed, confusion abounds when it comes to usage of these terminologies [4].

While OR mathematically correctly describes a woman's remaining chance of conception by attempting to quantitate all remaining follicles, no tools really exist to currently achieve such a goal. A woman's total OR (TOR) is, in large majority, comprised of still unrecruited primordial follicles (non-growing follicles). Only a small minority of follicles, at any stage, has entered maturation (growing follicles). Non-growing follicles cannot currently be assessed accurately.

Because recruitment rates have been correlated to size of remaining primordial follicle pools, and because anti-Mullerian hormone (AMH) inversely relates to recruitment, AMH has been widely proposed as representative [12]. Such a conclusion has, however, to be questioned because ovaries, of even menopausal women, still contain primordial follicles, and even women with completely undetectable AMH levels can still conceive [13]. Even documentation by ultrasound of pre-antral follicles does not guarantee that those follicles are still capable of normal maturation [14]. Indeed, at least one rather well defined autoimmune condition affecting ovaries is typically characterized by large numbers of arrested small follicles, resistant to further maturation [15].

AMH, at best, is, therefore, of only limited value in determining the size of the non-growing follicle pool, and no current technology exists to really reliably quantitate this pool. All AMH can do is to quantitate growing follicles, what we have come to call functional ovarian reserve (FOR) [4]. FOR, however, represents, at any given moment, only a very small component of TOR. The suggestion of some investigators to make judgments about TOR (i.e., the mathematical expression of "ovarian age"), solely based on AMH levels, therefore, appears misleading.

These mostly theoretical considerations were also confirmed by clinical investigations in humans, when AMH, above age 42 years, was found to have lost its superiority at younger ages over follicle-stimulating hormone (FSH) in assessing ovarian responses to stimulation with gonadotropins [16]. The uncomfortable truth, therefore, is that the mathematical model, considering remaining follicle representative of "ovarian age," is theoretically correct but practically unusable.

Physiologic versus premature ovarian aging

Ovarian aging represents a natural phenomenon, which is predictable for approximately 90% of women. This means that in this large majority certain milestones are reached at predictable ages. Table 19.1 summarizes the phenotypic expression of ovarian aging.

For the lay public normal, physiologic ovarian aging is defined by the recognition that establishing a pregnancy gets "more difficult" as women age, with age 40 years, generally, considered a major milestone, age 42–43 representing the practical end of spontaneous conception for most, and age 45 representing ultimate loss of reproductive capacity. This, of course, means that functional reproductive menopause is reached ca. 6–7 years before cessation of menses, which for most women occurs at age 51–52 years.

As noted earlier, this physiologic aging pattern is also characterized by declining follicle numbers (TOR and FOR, Fig. 19.1), declining pregnancy rates, whether spontaneous or with infertility treatments (Fig. 19.3), increasing aneuploidy (Fig. 19.2), and increasing miscarriage rates (Fig. 19.4).

Approximately 10% of females, however, do not follow this physiologic ovarian aging pattern. We consider them, therefore, afflicted by premature ovarian aging (POA) [4]. As colleagues have started to use the acronym POI (primary ovarian insufficiency) in lieu of POF (premature ovarian failure), the term occult POI (OPOI) has increasingly also been used in lieu of POA.

Table 19.1. Phenotypic expression of ovarian aging

Characteristics of ovarian aging	References
Initial oocyte numbers at birth and menarche vary between individuals	[17,18]
Pace of follicle recruitment varies between individuals	[18]
Pace of follicle recruitment decreases with advancing female age, leading to:	[18]
Declining growing follicle numbers with advancing female age	
Declining oocyte quality with advancing female age	[19–21]
The effects lead on to:	
Decreasing embryo quality with advancing female age	
Decreasing fecundity with advancing female age	
Decreasing oocyte and embryo yields (with IVF) with advancing female age	
Decreasing pregnancy rates with IVF with advancing female age	[21,22]
Increasing embryo aneuploidy with advancing female age, resulting in increasing miscarriage rates	[23]
Modified from Gleicher et al. [4], with permission.	

POF/POI represents the end stage of POA/OPOI, reached by only 1 in 10 of 10% of women with POA/OPOI. Only approximately 1% of all women, therefore, ever reach the diagnosis of POF/POI, defined by persistent FSH levels above 40.0 mIU/mL before age 40 years. This conclusion is, however, somewhat misleading because it depends on the rather arbitrary definition of POF/POI.

Many more than 1% of women reach menopausal follicle-stimulating hormone (FSH) levels before the usual menopause age of 51–52 years, although after age 40. These women are currently within a definition vacuum and their number has remained undetermined. How to define the occurrence of menopause between ages 40 and 51 years, therefore, remains to be established.

It has been suggested that women with POA/OPOI may be at increased risk for POF/POI [24]. Because approximately 9% of females develop POA/OPOI, and because POF/POI is diagnosed in only approximately 1%, a large majority of POA women very obviously never develop a diagnosis of POF/OPI, suggesting their disproportional representation among women with "early" menopause between ages 40 and 51–52 years.

This fact, however, still needs to be confirmed. Recent data from our center suggest that some women with low OR at young ages may actually preserve OR into advanced ages (see later for more detail). In a zero-sum game, with a finite number of initial follicles, OR at advanced age appears not only affected by how many follicles a woman was born with or entered menarche with but also by how actively she recruits from her primordial non-growing follicle pool.

That follicle recruitment is genetically controlled has been suggested for quite some time [18]. We recently demonstrated in several studies that the *FMR1* gene, and especially its recently defined ovarian genotypes and sub-genotypes appear to play a significant role (for further detail, see below). Genetic control of recruitment is, however, very obviously multifactorial and, overall, still poorly understood.

In comparison with a large majority of women with normal physiologic aging, approximately 10% apparently, age their ovaries prematurely at different speeds. They are disproportionally represented among infertility patients, and especially among women with so-called unexplained infertility [25]. A principal reason is that, even in competent fertility centers, POA/OPOI is, still, often overlooked.

Accurate and timely diagnosis of ovarian aging

The diagnosis of age-dependent, physiologic ovarian aging is usually uncomplicated because almost all women above age 40 suffer from low OR. The problem is much more vexing in younger women, where low OR, as a consequence of POA, can occur at practically any age, and, usually, is unexpected.

Age-specific OR assessments

To combat this diagnostic problem, we proposed the concept of age-specific OR testing, established age-specific FSH levels for our center [26], and later added age-specific AMH levels [27] (Fig. 19.6). The concept of age-specific OR testing is based on the previously noted observation that OR declines with advancing female age. Consequently, what represents normal assessment levels has to vary with advancing female age.

A very obvious principle has, thus, paradoxically, historically not been applied to routine clinical practice. Indeed, until today most general gynecologists and reproductive endocrinologists, alike, still consider FSH 10.0 mIU/mL as the age-independent, general cut-off value, differentiating normal from abnormal OR. This, of course, makes neither physiologic nor clinical sense!

Figure 19.6 demonstrates age-specific FSH and AMH levels for our center, based on 95% confidence intervals (CIs) for all age groups (Fig. 19.6). As the figure demonstrates, what represents "normal" is, as women age, defined by increasing FSH and

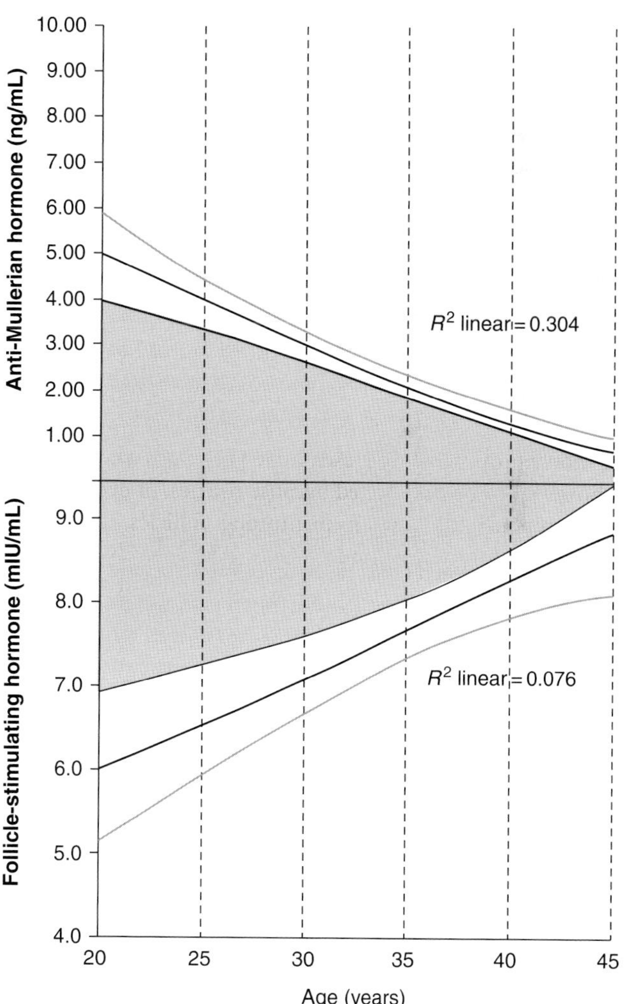

Fig. 19.6. Age-specific AMH and FSH levels. This figure demonstrates age-specific AMH (upper panel) and FSH levels (lower panel), based on 95% CI of our center's patient population. Because 95% CIs were established in an infertile population, it appears likely that normal ranges in a normally fertile population may demonstrate mildly lower FSH and mildly higher AMH levels than demonstrated in this graph. Normal age-specific values in normally fertile women have, however, so far not been established.

declining AMH levels (Fig. 19.6). The figure, however, also demonstrates that, unless age-specific levels replace age-independent cut-off values, a diagnosis of POA at young ages becomes, practically and clinically, impossible.

Timely diagnosis of POA, a very crucial step in successful treatment of POA (to be further discussed below), is, therefore, not achievable unless standard clinical practice moves from universal to age-specific OR assessments. This statement applies to any OR assessment, whether by FSH, AMH, antral follicle count (AFC), ovarian size/volume, clomiphene citrate-challenge test (CCT), or other methods.

Normal age-specific ranges in Figure 19.6 are based on data derived from infertile women. Ideally, normal ranges should, of course, be developed in normally fertile populations. To reach consensus, such studies are urgently needed. Final "normal" age-specific FSH levels, therefore, can be expected to be marginally lower than shown in the figure, while final AMH levels likely will be marginally higher.

What are the best tools to assess OR?

OR assessment has undergone considerable changes in recent years. Only approximately a decade ago, baseline FSH levels, obtained on cycle days 2–3, were considered the only practical tool to assess OR. Today, the ability to assess OR accurately has greatly improved, although it still lacks desirable specificity.

OR assessments are currently still primarily based on baseline FSH and estradiol levels on days 2–3 of the cycle. However, AMH levels, which can be drawn on any cycle day and AFCs, which also, preferably, should be obtained at cycle start, are increasingly used in parallel. Reproductive endocrinologists nowadays mostly rely on a combination of FSH and AMH, although some favor AFCs.

FSH and AMH, in principle, correlate. For example, an AMH of 0.5 ng/mL is predictive of a baseline FSH of 12.1 mIU/mL (95% CI 11.8–12.4) and an AMH value of 1.0 ng/mL of an FSH of 10.0 mIU/mL (95% CI 9.3–10.8) [28]. Similarly, AMH and AFCs have been demonstrated to correlate well [12]. These correlations are, however, far from perfect, and it, therefore, has become increasingly obvious that FSH and AMH are not interchangeable.

For example, at younger ages AMH appears better predictive of oocyte yields in in vitro fertilization (IVF) than FSH; yet above age 42, when such predictive abilities are most important, FSH appears superior [16]. Moreover, when we recently investigated ratios of retrieved oocytes per FSH (FSHo) and AMH (AMHo), FSHo but not AMHo at all ages proved predictive of pregnancy chances [29].

AMH also has very poor specificity at very low levels. Indeed, one can state that below 0.4–0.8 ng/mL, AMH is almost worthless in predicting pregnancy chances, as the establishment of many pregnancies, even in the absence of detectable AMH, well demonstrates [13]. So what is going on here?

What explains these discrepancies between independently very useful OR assessment tools are these aspects of ovarian physiology discussed above, with different OR parameters representing different stages of follicle maturation. For example AMH and AFCs correlate well because both reflect the same small growing follicle pool of mostly pre-antral and early antral stage follicles. In contrast, FSH and AMH correlate less well because FSH primarily represents large, gonadotropin-sensitive pre-ovulatory follicles, whereas AMH represents a much more immature pool of follicles.

These intricacies of OR assessment are not well understood yet, but have to be developed if OR assessments are to further improve. Accurate assessments of follicle maturation stage appear, of course, essential if the previously described concept of therapeutic improvements in ovarian environments is to be clinically pursued. Here are two examples: Even though AMH levels change with female age, an AMH of 1.05 ng/mL at all ages differentiates between poorer and better pregnancy chances [30], suggesting that, independent of age, a certain minimum amount of small growing follicles must still be present to offer a reasonable pregnancy chance in association with IVF. One, of course, also can assume this to be the case with spontaneous conception.

Maybe even more telling are the findings with above noted AMHo and FSHo. They very clearly demonstrate the overwhelming primacy of mature follicles over small growing follicles for pregnancy success, especially when very few follicles are present, as with severe DOR [29]; yet the dichotomy between AMH and FSH in these two examples well demonstrates the many challenges but also opportunities in attempting to understand FOR better.

A few final words on AMH

We previously noted that, among various OR assessment tools, many investigators now believe AMH levels to best reflect FOR [12]. Yet, we also pointed out obvious shortcomings for AMH in this function, especially at very low levels of the hormone and at very advanced female ages. In addition, we questioned the widely held assumption that AMH is really a good representation of the non-growing follicle pool of primordial follicles, which we consider "suspended" in time until recruitment.

We, however, failed to explain so far why AMH, nevertheless, reflects FOR so well in younger women, and especially at still reasonable AMH levels [12,16]. Basic to the answer is that, in various animal models, AMH has been well established as an antagonist to follicle recruitment. Produced by granulosa cells of small growing follicles (Fig. 19.5), it appears to be part of a feedback mechanism, controlling follicle recruitment: every time the recruitment spigot opens, small follicles enter the lengthy road toward maturation. As follicles develop, their granulosa expands, and several interesting activities initiate in granulosa cells in parallel at exactly the same developmental stages of follicles: (i) androgen receptors are induced; (ii) FSH receptors are induced; and (iii) AMH production increases (Fig. 19.5).

That all three events occur in parallel is interesting because ndrogens and FSH have been demonstrated to act synergisti- ılly in both recruitment and follicle maturation [5]. AMH, owever, acts in opposition by restraining recruitment and ıaturation of small growing follicles.

It, thus, appears that granulosa cells of small primary, pre- ntral, and early antral follicles represent the battle ground etween enhancing and restraining forces for follicle recruitment ıd maturation. As the recruitment spigot opens, AMH rises, in ttempt to shut down further recruitment. As recruitment falls, eed for AMH diminishes, and AMH production declines. The onsequence is that low AMH is characteristic of low recruitment tuation, such as DOR, pregnancy, oral contraceptive use, and ong-term agonist suppression, whereas high AMH levels are pical of high recruitment states, such as PCO [12].

How all of this, in synergism with FSH, interfaces with ndrogen activity is further discussed below. Here outlined me correlations, however, very likely explain why AMH is uch a valuable tool in assessing FOR: it is simply better than ny other parameters, defines ongoing follicle recruitment, and, ıerefore, the amount of small follicles entering maturation. 'his number, of course, as previously discussed, closely corre- ıtes with female age, is genetically controlled and is ultimately losely related to the number of available gonadotropin- ensitive follicles stimulated during ovulation induction.

Vhat controls ovarian aging genetically?

s Wallace and Kelsey recently reaffirmed, ovarian aging varies etween individuals. With the end point of age of menopause, hey determined that follicle numbers and speed of follicle ecruitment change with female age [18]. We reached similar onclusions in trying to elucidate the effects of the *FMR1* gene, nd its recently described ovarian genotypes and sub- enotypes, on ovarian aging [31–33].

Although for decades known to be associated with POF/POI n its premutation-range genotype (ca. 55–200 CGG repeats), the *'MR1* gene, until recently, was not perceived as a significant layer in ovarian physiology. This, however, changed with the ew description of ovarian genotypes and sub-genotypes, based n the newly determined "normal" range of CGG repeats of 26– 4. This range lies well within what, up to that point, had been onsidered a normal range, without determining phenotypes 34]. In analyzing distribution patterns of CGG repeats, this epeat length, however, jumped out as an obvious new "normal," vith a median of 30 CGG repeats, which, previously, had been eported as the switching point between normal and abnormal nessage and as the point of peak translation of message [35].

In absence of determining phenotypes below approximately 5 CGG repeats, no attention had been paid to the gene at such ow CGG repeat counts. All investigative attention had been xtended to expansions exceeding that range, and especially at remutation range genotype (55–200 CGG repeats) and at full nutation, the fragile X syndrome (at > 200 CGG repeats). 'remutation and full mutation genotypes were, of course, nown for associated severe neuropsychiatric phenotypes, vith POF/POI, in association with the premutation genotype, representing the only non-neuropsychiatric phenotype ever associated with the *FMR1* gene [34].

It was exactly this phenotypical POF/POI association that raised our interest in the gene, and, ultimately, led to the discovery of new ovarian genotypes and sub-genotypes of *FMR1*, which we initially thought were exclusively associated with ovarian phenotypes, relating to ovarian aging [31].

Since then, we discovered that these (by now likely misnamed) ovarian genotypes and sub-genotypes appear to serve major additional physiological functions, with little or no relevance to ovaries. Indeed, it increasingly appears that *FMR1* lies at the cross roads of many major physiological functions, with sub-genotypes associated with risk/protection toward autoimmunity [32] and cancer [36]. They, however, of course, also affect ovarian aging and female infertility to significant degrees [31,32].

It would exceed the framework of this chapter to go into too much detail. Therefore, only so much: Depending on whether both of a woman's alleles are in normal range (26–34 CGG repeats), her *FMR1* genotypes can be described as normal (norm, both in normal range), heterozygous (het, one inside and one allele outside range), or homozygous (hom, both alleles outside range). Heterozygous and homozygous genotypes can then be further divided into high (> 34 CGG repeats) or low (< 26 CGG repeats). Table 19.2 summarizes all possible ovarian *FMR1* genotypes and sub-genotypes.

It very quickly became apparent that norm, het, and hom women differed in ovarian aging patterns (Fig. 19.7). But, far more interesting were phenotypical observations in association with *FMR1* sub-genotypes. For example het-norm/low was found associated with a PCO-like phenotype at young age, which rapidly depleted the OR, resulting in DOR at relatively young age [32]. In contrast, het-norm/high appears associated with relatively low FOR at young ages, slow recruitment, and offers the best FOR at ages above 42 years [37].

Women with norm genotype demonstrate the highest and those with het-norm/low sub-genotype the lowest pregnancy

Table 19.2. Summary of all possible ovarian *FMR1* genotypes and sub-genotypes

Genotype/sub-genotype	Abbreviation	Definition based on CGG repeats
Normal	*norm*	Both alleles in normal range [26–34]
Heterozygous	*het*	One allele in and one outside range
normal/high	*-norm/high*	One allele in range and one > 34
normal/low	*-norm/low*	One allele in range and one < 26
Homozygous	*hom*	Both alleles outside normal range
high/high	*-high/high*	Both alleles > 34
high/low	*-high/low*	One allele > 34 and the other < 26
low/low	*-low/low*	Both alleles < 26

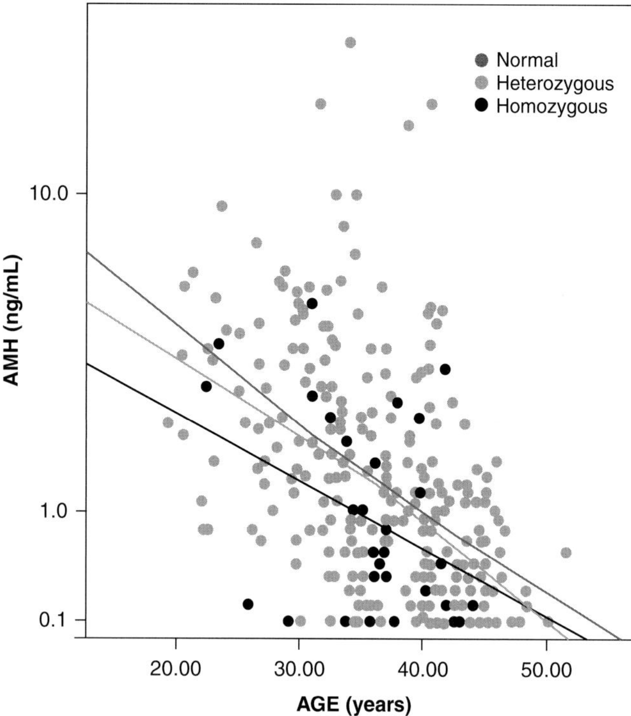

Fig. 19.7. Age-dependent declines in OR, based on ovarian *FMR1* genotypes. The figure depicts the age-dependent decline of OR in women with norm, het, and hom *FMR1* genotypes, modified from Gleicher et al. [31] with permission. Since these ovarian genotypes of *FMR1* were described, we discovered that het and hom genotypes could be further divided into sub-genotypes, depending on whether abnormal CGG counts were below (*low*) or above (*high*) the normal range of 26–34 repeats. Sub-genotypes, indeed, demonstrated some of the most remarkable differences in phenotypical expression, and were also found to have significance in defining autoimmune and cancer risks in women. For further detail see text.

rates in association with IVF, while het-norm/high women fall in between [32]. Women with het-norm/low sub-genotypes, especially if associated with PCO-like phenotypes, demonstrate almost universal evidence of autoimmunity, while het-norm/high appears almost protective of autoimmunity [32].

Finally, after all of these negative impacts, het-norm/low also appears to have an, at least conditionally, positive one on humanity: it appears to successfully combat embryo lethality of BRCA1/2 mutations. The consequence, of course, is that het-norm/low women (and women with low hom sub-genotypes), due to high BRCA1/2 prevalence likely are at increased risk for BRCA1/2 associated cancers [36].

How much of ovarian aging is under *FMR1* control remains to be established. *FMR1*, however, undoubtedly plays an important role. Its evolving importance to a broad array of medical processes very likely will turn it into a major target of investigation in the near future.

The importance of androgens

Figure 19.5 demonstrates a somewhat abbreviated illustration of follicle maturation. The figure, however, also demonstrates the only quite recently recognized importance of androgens for normal follicle maturation and, indeed, female fertility in general [5].

Until recently, androgens were viewed almost universally as enemies of normal follicle maturation. An important reason for this still widely held opinion has been the hyperandrogenism observed in many women with PCO phenotypes, often associated with anovulation and female infertility. Yet, it is actually somewhat surprising that such a hostile view toward androgens has been maintained for so long, considering that some of nature's own experiments for the longest time have hinted at important, and potentially positive, functions of androgens in folliculogenesis.

A few examples come to mind: While PCO, of course, mostly prevailed in causing negative interpretations of androgen effects, it, at minimum, should have suggested a potential beneficial effect on recruitment, demonstrated in explosive responses of women with PCO phenotypes to ovarian stimulation [38]. Further support comes from observations in female to male transgender patients, who after exposure to high androgen levels fairly typically develop ovaries with PCO phenotype. Finally, a widely used small animal model of PCO is dehydroepiandrosterone (DHEA) induced [5,39].

The most convincing evidence comes, however, from recent small animal experiments, especially with ARKO mice. Walters and associates summarized how ARKO mouse models are able to decipher AR-mediated female reproductive functions [40]. Using granulosa cell- and oocyte-specific ARKO mice, Sen and Hammes developed an elegant model, which allowed them to trace where androgen effects were located [10]. Almost all phenotypical infertility expressions observed in the animals reflected androgen effects by means of AR in granulosa cells only. This included POF, subfertility with prolonged estrous cycles and smaller ovulated follicle numbers, increases in pre-antral follicles, larger numbers of atretic follicles, fewer antral follicles, and fewer corpora lutea.

Overall, in vitro growth of follicles slowed in comparison to wild-type animals. While disruption in AR signaling also altered uterine development, this did not reduce the fertility of female mice. Observed fertility impairments in ARKO mice, therefore, appear primarily ovarian in nature. Moreover, because oocyte-specific ARKO mice did not demonstrate any of these infertility phenotypes, one can conclude that, at least in the mouse, androgen-associated female infertility is granulosa cell based, and, likely, induced at small follicle stages when follicles demonstrate AR (Fig. 19.5).

The androgen required by growing follicles is derived from theca cells. P450 aromatase then converts androgens in granulosa cells into estrone and 17β estradiol [41]. Androgens may, therefore, also exert effects by means of estrogen receptors, a point to be addressed further in the next section of this chapter.

Androgens are, however, dependent on gonadotropins: Wu et al. recently demonstrated in rat granulosa cells that, in the absence of gonadotropins, testosterone increases aromatase (Cyp 19) and P450scc side-chain cleavage expression, both enzymes of major importance for normal ovarian function. While Cyp 19 converts testosterone into estradiol, 5α-reductase converts it into the pure androgen 5α-dehydrotestosterone

Testosterone also directly affects gene expression in granulosa cell differentiation [42].

Sensitivity of these processes is, indeed, quite astonishing: Sanchez and associates reported that even as minimal changes in FSH concentrations such as 2.5-fold increases can change transcription levels in cumulus–oocyte complexes of mice [43]. These data suggest a rather remarkable sensitivity of androgen/FSH synergism at small follicle stages.

More importantly, however, with advancing female age, androgen and FSH levels go in opposite directions: while FSH increases, androgen levels decline. This divergence can, therefore, be assumed to affect granulosa cell function, and, very well may be reflective of a deteriorating ovarian environment for follicle maturation, as women age. As we will discuss in the next section of this chapter, infertile women who conceive after androgen supplementation are usually those who start with lowest, and end up with highest, androgen levels after supplementation.

Can we treat "old" ovaries?

We began this chapter with the suggestion that the ovarian aging process may have to be reassessed, by changing from the current dogma of aging oocytes to a concept of aging ovarian environments for follicle maturation. This idea arose from our experience with DHEA supplementation in women with DOR; i.e., women with either physiologically aging ovaries or younger women with POA. In both groups, DHEA supplementation has been proven highly effective.

It would exceed the framework of this chapter to offer too much detail. For this the reader is referred to a recent review [44]. Only so much: After initial, rather accidental discovery that DHEA has "rejuvenating" effects on "older" ovaries, studies have demonstrated that DHEA in women with DOR, indeed, improves egg and embryo numbers, oocyte and embryo quality, spontaneous pregnancy rates, pregnancy rates in association with IVF, and cumulative pregnancy rates. In addition, DHEA supplementation reduces embryo aneuploidy and, therefore, miscarriage rates in association with IVF (Table 19.3). Consequently, the usage of DHEA supplementation in women with DOR is quickly expanding worldwide.

Table 19.3. DHEA supplementation effects in women with DOR

Improves oocyte and embryo numbers
Improves oocyte and embryo quality
Shortens time to pregnancy
Improves pregnancy chances with IVF
Improves cumulative pregnancy chances
Decreases embryo aneuploidy
Decreases miscarriage rates

How, specifically, DHEA accomplishes its "rejuvenating" effects has remained unknown but several potential mechanisms have been suggested: The mere fact that DHEA reduces aneuploidy [45] in itself can be expected to improve pregnancy chances and to reduce miscarriage rates, as has been reported [46]. Moreover, DHEA, itself a mild androgen, is, of course, an important intermediate step of steroidogenesis, representing the substrate for conversion to testosterone as well as estradiol. As noted before, DHEA activities could, therefore, be mediated by means of AR and/or estrogen receptor.

Because a majority of DHEA is converted to androgens, it appears likely that most DHEA effects are, indeed, AR-mediated. Observed DHEA effects, therefore, are likely to be primarily directed at small, growing follicles (Fig. 19.5). In a recent study, this suspicion was confirmed when we were able to demonstrate that pregnancy chances in association with DHEA supplementation were the best in women with DOR who started with the lowest testosterone levels and, with DHEA supplementation, over time, reached the highest levels of free and total testosterone [47]. It, therefore, as of this point, appears reasonable to conclude that at least a majority of DHEA effects in women with DOR are AR-mediated.

It was our experience with DHEA supplementation that led us to conclude that the currently prevalent concept of aging oocytes likely is incorrect. We reached this conclusion after observing surprisingly high pregnancy and low miscarriage rates in women with the most severe forms of DOR [13]. Under a concept of slowly decaying oocytes, such outcomes are inconceivable because it appears extremely unlikely that any pharmacologic intervention would be able to restore to health already severely damaged oocytes. Especially in women with severe DOR, where follicle numbers are small, reasonable pregnancy rates and low miscarriage rates leave, however, no doubt about the presence of good-quality oocytes.

Our DHEA experience in women with DOR, therefore, left us with no choice but to seek another possible explanation for observed outcomes. The only explanation that made sense was to replace the concept of aging oocytes with a new concept of aging ovarian environments.

Under such a concept DHEA, likely, is only the first pharmacologic intervention among many more to come in the future, directed at ovarian environments in older women. It is reasonable to assume that many more will follow, once the aging process of ovarian environments is better understood.

The here-presented new concept of ovarian aging, therefore, has the potential of directing infertility treatment of aging ovaries into two radically new directions: First, from aging oocytes to aging ovarian environments; and, second, from concentration on the gonadotropin-sensitive, last 2 weeks of follicle maturation into much earlier stages of folliculogenesis. Both appear timely developments as ages of women seeking fertility care are increasing.

Conclusions

In many ways, the aging ovary represents the last frontier in an incredible success story of treating human infertility. In over 30 years since the birth of the first child conceived by means of IVF, over 4,000,000 children have been born using various forms of the IVF procedure. This almost unmatched accomplishment was in 2010, much too late, finally, recognized by the Swedish Nobel Committee by awarding, unshared, the Nobel Prize for Physiology and Medicine to Prof. Robert Edwards, PhD, the reproductive physiologist who, together with Patrick Steptoe, MD, was responsible for the world's first IVF birth.

The importance of IVF, however, goes far beyond just millions of births: IVF has opened human reproductive physiology to previously unachievable research opportunities. For very obvious reasons, much of this research has, however, almost exclusively concentrated on the final 2 weeks of follicle maturation, the gonadotropin-sensitive stage.

Now that IVF, in its various formats, indeed, has solved most female as well as male infertility problems, it appears time to take the next big step, which involves a better understanding of earlier stages of follicle maturation. It has been suggested that our ability to improve IVF outcomes may be plateauing [48]. Epidemiologically, this is the consequence of three demographic developments: (i) younger women now conceive quickly and efficiently; and (ii) in the developed world, the percentage of older women attempting fertility and going through pregnancy is very rapidly increasing, raising mean ages of infertile populations; and (iii) ages, even among older women trying to conceive, are getting older.

Oocyte donation, today in many countries a routine treatment in female infertility, therefore, now represents the quickest growing form of IVF in the U.S. Most women, however, of course, greatly prefer conception with use of their own oocytes. The aging ovary, therefore, for investigators in this field, very likely represents the last major challenge in research as well as clinical practice.

Potential conflicts of interest statement

Both authors have in the past received financial research grant support, travel funds, and speaker honoraria from a variety of pharmaceutical and medical device companies, none, however, related to the subjects covered in this book chapter. Both authors are listed as co-inventors of two US patents, which claim therapeutic benefits from supplementation with DHEA in women with DOR, and receive royalties from Fertility Nutraceuticals, LLC, a company that produces a DHEA supplement. N.G. is a shareholder in this company. Both authors are also listed as co-inventors on still pending US patent applications for DHEA supplementation and on US patent applications, which define new, so-called ovarian genotypes of *FMR1*, and claim various fertility- and non-fertility-related diagnostic benefits from determining ovarian genotypes and sub-genotypes of this gene. N.G. is owner of the Center for Human Reproduction.

Support

The work presented here was supported by the Foundation for Reproductive Medicine and intra-mural funds from the Center for Human Reproduction–New York.

References

1. Hansen KR, Craig LB, Zavy MT, et al. Ovarian primordial and nongrowing follicle counts according to the Stages of Reproductive Aging Workshop (STRAW) staging system. Menopause. 2012;**19**:164–71.
2. Menken J, Trussel J, Larsen U. Age and infertility. Science. 1986;**233**:1389–94.
3. Spandorfer SD, Davis OD, Barmat LI, et al. Relationship between maternal age and aneuploidy in in vitro fertilization pregnancy loss. Fertil Steril. 2004;**81**:1265–9.
4. Gleicher N, Weghofer A, Barad DH. Defining ovarian reserve to better understand ovarian aging. Reprod Biol Endocrinol. 2011;**9**:23.
5. Gleicher N, Weghofer A, Barad DH. The role of androgens in follicle maturation and ovulation induction: friend or foe of infertility treatment? Reprod Biol Endocrinol. 2011;**9**:116.
6. McLaughlin EA, McEver SC. Awakening the oocyte: controlling primordial follicle development. Reproduction. 2009;**137**:1–11.
7. Reddy P, Liu L, Adhikari D, et al. Oocyte-specific deletion of Pten causes premature activation of the primordial follicle pool. Science. 2008;**319**:611–13.
8. Henderson SA, Edwards RE. Chiasma frequency and maternal age in mammals. Nature. 1968;**218**:22–8.
9. Tarumi W, Tsukamoto S, Okutsu Y, et al. Androstenedione induces abnormalities in morphology and function of developing oocytes, which impairs oocyte meiotic competence. Fertil Steril. 2012;**97**:469–76.
10. Sen A, Hammes SR. Granulosa-cell specific androgen receptors are critical regulators of ovarian development and function. Mol Endocrinol. 2010;**24**:1393–403.
11. Lenie S, Smitz J. Functional AR signaling is evident in an in vitro mouse follicle culture bioassay that encompasses most stages of folliculogenesis. Biol Reprod. 2009;**80**:685–95.
12. Ledger WL. Clinical utility of measurement of anti-mullerian hormone in reproductive endocrinology. J Clin Endocrinol Metab. 2010;**95**:5144–54.
13. Weghofer A, Dietrich W, Barad DH, Gleicher N. Live birth chances in women with extremely low-serum anti-Mullerian hormone levels. Hum Reprod. 2011;**26**:1905–9.
14. Conway GS, Kaltsas G, Patel A, et al. Characterization of idiopathic premature ovarian failure. Feril Steril. 1996;**65**:337–41.
15. Hoek A, Schoemaker J, Drexhage HA. Premature ovarian failure and ovarian autoimmunity. Endocr Rev. 1997;**18**:107–34.
16. Gleicher N, Weghofer A, Barad DH. Discordance between follicle stimulating hormone (FSH) and anti-Müllerian hormone (AMH) in female infertility. Reprod Biol Endocrinol. 2010;**8**:64.
17. Hansen KR, Knowlton NS, Thyer A, et al. A new model for reproductive aging: the decline in ovarian non-growing follicle number from birth to

menopause. Hum Reprod. 2008;**23**:699–708.

18. Wallace WH, Kelsey TW. Human ovarian reserve from conception to the menopause. PLoS One. 2010;**5**:e8772.
19. Ireland JJ, Zielak-Steciwko AE, Jimenez-Krassel F, et al. Variation in ovarian reserve is linked to alterations in intrafollicular estradiol production and ovarian biomarkers of follicular differentiation and oocyte quality in cattle. Biol Reprod. 2009;**80**:954–64.
20. Broekmans FJ, Soules MR, Fauser BC. Ovarian aging: mechanisms and clinical consequences. Endocr Rev. 2009;**30**:465–93.
21. La Marca A, Sighinolfi G, Radi D, et al. Anti-Mullerian hormone (AMH) as predictive marker in assisted reproductive technology (ART). Hum Reprod Update. 2010;**16**:113–30.
22. Navot D, Bergh PA, Williams MA, et al. Poor oocyte quality rather than implantation failure as a cause of age-related decline in female fertility. Lancet. 1991;**337**;1375–7.
23. Wartburton D. Biological ageing and the etiology of aneuploidy. Cytogenet Genome Res. 2005;**111**:266–72.
24. Broer SL, Eijkemans MS, Scheffer GJ, et al. Anti-mullerian hormone predicts menopause: a long-term follow-up study in normoovulatory women. J Clin Endocrinol Metab. 2011;**96**:2532–9.
25. Gleicher N, Barad D. Unexplained infertility: does it really exist? Hum Reprod. 2006;**21**:1951–5.
26. Barad DH, Weghofer A, Gleicher N. Age-specific levels for basal follicle-stimulating hormone assessment of ovarian function. Obstet Gynecol. 2007;**109**:1404–10.
27. Barad DH, Weghofer A, Gleicher N. Utility of age-specific serum anti-Müllerian hormone concentrations. Reprod Biomed Online. 2011;**22**:284–91.
28. Singer T, Barad DH, Weghofer A, Gleicher N. Correlation of anti-müllerian hormone and baseline follicle-stimulating hormone levels. Fertil Steril. 2009;**91**:2616–9.
29. Gleicher N, Kim A, Weghofer A, Barad DH. Toward a better understanding of functional ovarian reserve: AMH (AMHo) and FSH (FSHo) hormone ratios per retrieved oocyte. J Clin Endocrinl Metab. 2012;**97**:995–1004.
30. Gleicher N, Weghofer A, Barad DH. Anti-Müllerian hormone (AMH) defines, independent of age, low versus good live-birth chances in women with severely diminished ovarian reserve. Fertil Steril. 2010;**94**:2824–7.
31. Gleicher N, Weghofer A, Barad DH. Ovarian reserve determinations suggest new function of *FMR1* (fragile X gene) in regulating ovarian ageing. Reprod Biomed Online. 2010;**20**:768–75.
32. Gleicher N, Weghofer A, Lee IH, Barad DH. *FMR1* genotype with autoimmunity-associated polycystic ovary-like phenotype and decreased pregnancy chances. PLoS One. 2010;**5**:e15303.
33. Gleicher N, Barad DH. The FMR1 gene as regulator of ovarian recruitment and ovarian reserve. Obstet Gynecol Surv. 2010;**65**:523–30.
34. Wittenberger MD, Hagerman RJ, Sherman SL, et al. The FMR1 premutation and reproduction. Fertil Steril. 2007;**87**:456–65.
35. Chen LS, Tassone F, Sahota P, Hagerman PJ. The (CGG)n repeat element within the 5' untranslated region of the FMR1 message provides both positive and negative cis effects on in vivo translation of a downstream reporter. Hum Mol Genet. 2003;**12**:3067–74.
36. Weghofer A, Tea MK, Barad DH, et al. BRCA1/2 are embryo lethal human gene mutations, rescued by low count (CGG n<26) FMR1 mutations, suggesting CGG <n<26 as a new target for female cancer screening. Submitted for publication.
37. Barad DH, Weghofer A, Kim A. The het-norm/high FMR1 sub-genotype increases oocyte yields at in vitro fertilization (IVF) with advanced female age. Fertil Steril. 2011;**96**(Suppl):S119.
38. Barnes RB. The pathogenesis of polycystic ovary syndrome: lessons from ovarian stimulation studies. J Endocrinol Invest. 1998;**21**:567–79.
39. Luchetti GC, Solano ME, Sander V, et al. Effects of dehydroepiandrosterone on ovarian cystogenesis and immune function. J Reprod Immunol. 2004;**64**:59–74.
40. Walters KA, Simanainen U, Handelsman FJ. Molecular insights into androgen actions in male and female reproductive function from androgen receptor knock out models. Hum Reprod Update. 2010;**16**:543–58.
41. Young JM, McNeilly AS. Theca: the forgotten cell of the ovarian follicle. Reproduction. 2010;**140**:489–504.
42. Wu YG, Bennett J, Talla D, Stocco C. Testosterone, not 5alpha-dihydrotestosterone stimulates LRH-1 leading to FSH-independent expression of Cyp 19 and P450scc in granulosa cells. Mol Endocrinol. 2011;**26**:656–8.
43. Sánchez F, Adriaenssens T, Romero S, Smitz J. Different follicle-stimulating hormone exposure regimens during antral follicle growth alter gene expression in the cumulus–oocyte complex in mice. Biol Reprod. 2010;**83**:514–24.
44. Gleicher N, Barad DH. Dehydroepiandrosterone (DHEA) supplementation in diminished ovarian reserve (DOR). Reprod Biol Endocrinol. 2011;9:67.
45. Gleicher N, Weghofer A, Barad DH. Dehydroepiandrosterone (DHEA) reduces embryo aneuploidy: direct evidence from preimplantation genetic screening (PGS). Reprod Biol Endocrinol. 2010;**8**:140.
46. Gleicher N, Ryan E, Weghofer A, et al. Miscarriage rates after dehydroepiandrosterone (DHEA) supplementation in women with diminished ovarian reserve: a case control study. Reprod Biol Endcrinol. 2009;**7**:108.
47. Weghofer A, Kim A, Barad DH, Gleicher N. The impact of androgen metabolism and FMR1 genotypes on pregnancy potential in women with dehydroepiandrosterone (DHEA) supplementation. Hum Repod. 2012;**27**:3287–93.
48. Brown S. ART success rates have "reached a plateau," EIM monitoring data show that both pregnancy- and multiple pregnancy-rates have not changed from the previous year. Focus Reprod. 2011;13–14.

Chapter 20

Menopause

Nathan G. Kase, MD

Introduction

Menopause is the "landmark" in a woman's life when she experiences permanent cessation of menstruation. The collective follicle capacity of the ovaries to secrete adequate estradiol diminishes to a level at which proliferation of an endometrium adequate to produce menstruation is no longer achievable. But menopause is justifiably more than simply loss of menses or even reproductive competence. Although some ovarian steroid secretion continues transiently beyond this critical point and limited extra-gonadal production of estrogen may persist, at menopause the ability of the ovaries to function as endocrine organs capable of providing sufficient hormone to sustain the estrogen-dependent biologic aspects of a wide variety of tissues has also ceased.

Reviewed in Chapter 2, estrogen modulates a broad array of non-reproductive functions including bone and mineral metabolism, cardiovascular function, fuel and metabolic homeostasis, neuropsychiatric balance, and the risk of progression of age-related neurodegenerative diseases.

The consequences of age combined with a prolonged hypoestrogenic state and the various reactive strategies available to meet these challenges will be reviewed in this chapter. It will deal with the definitions of the various phases surrounding menopause and the sometimes paradoxical endocrinology of each stage. In addition, the increased metabolic, endocrine, cardiovascular, and cancer risks accompanying aging and how these might be affected by a prolonged state of hypoestrogenism will be analyzed. The benefits–risks of hormonal replenishment and an individual-appropriate clinical management algorithm is provided. The effort will be inclusive but not exhaustive; it should encourage the reader to pursue more encyclopedic resources [1–6], which are emphasized in the text.

The dimensions of the challenge: an aging population

The 2010 U.S. Census [7] records more than 43.5 million women between 40 and 59 years of age and an additional 15.3 million age 60–69. This represents an increase of 37% and 10.5%, respectively, from the numbers of similar aged women in 2000 or almost a 20% increase in the entire age group. At close to 59 million women aged 40–69, this group constitutes 37% of the total U.S. female population.

Ovarian follicle endowment, attrition, and exhaustion

The *cause* of menopause reflects the fact that the ovary is endowed with a finite, non-renewable, post-mitotic pool of dormant primordial follicles [8]. Defined endocrinologically, menopause is the consequence of the irreversible depletion and final exhaustion of ovarian follicles, which results in permanent loss of gonadal estradiol secretion and the end of "physiologic" (ovarian follicle generated and controlled) menstruation.

The "timing" of menopause: factors controlling follicle reserve and attrition

Menopause is linked to the complete loss of the primordial follicle reserve. "Timing" of menopause therefore reflects the number of primordial follicles initially "stored" in the fetal ovary and the rate of attrition that follows. Certain genetic [9] and non-genetic [10] observations inform the understanding of these crucial processes.

Genetic factors

Mothers, daughters, and identical twins experience menopause at the same age. A study of 275 monozygotic and 353 dizygotic female twin pairs yielded a heritability (h^2) factor for age at menopause of 63%. After adjustment for confounders, early menopause was found to be significantly influenced by genetic factors [11].

Accelerated follicle atresia occurs in utero in 45x Turner's syndrome, suggesting both X chromosomes must be active in germ cells to avoid premature activation and atresia. The occurrence of premature ovarian failure in mosaicisms (45x/46xx; 46xx/47xxx) intensified interest in identifying factors on the X chromosome which govern normal ovarian follicle maintenance and control [12]. A review of 118 cases of balanced X-autosome translocations and 31 cases of balanced inversions revealed critical involvement of regions on the X chromosome (Xq13-q22, Xq22–26) [13]. At least eight different genes on Xq21 are involved in premature ovarian failure.

Not all gene defects which alter the initial number and attrition rate of the ovarian follicle pool are located on the X chromosome. Five genes significantly involved in this process have been studied: those for AMH, AMH type II receptor (AMH R2), BMP-15, FOXL2, and GDF9. In a population-based cross-sectional study of 3,600 Dutch women with natural menopause, two SNPs in the *AMHR2* gene were associated with later age of natural menopause (by approximately 1 year) and parity [9].

Meta-analyses of 22 genome wide association studies involving almost 40,000 women of European descent with replication in close to 15,000 women have expanded the identity and role of genes in the timing of menopause [14]. In addition to confirming earlier findings, candidate genes located at three newly associated loci include genes implicated in DNA repair, immune function, and genes effecting neuro-endocrine pathways. Impaired DNA damage, cell cycle and cell death controls, NF-κB signaling, mitochondrial dysfunction, autoimmune dysregulation, altered gonadotropin and steroid synthesis have been added to the heritability of age of menopause.

In summary, the process of ovarian aging involves both somatic and germ line aging.

Non-genetic factors

Multiple studies have consistently documented the age of menopause is earlier by an average of 1.5 years as a consequence of smoking [15]. In addition, evidence indicates body mass is a factor: under-nourished women, thin women, and vegetarians experience earlier menopause [5,16]. There is no correlation between age of menopause and age of menarche, race, height, or duration or intensity of physical labor.

Data on age of menopause are found in the Massachusetts Women's Health Study and the ongoing SWAN studies. The former observed 2,570 women aged 45–55 over a 4.5-year interval and showed the median age for menopause was 51.3 years [17]. Only current smoking was identified as a cause of earlier menopause (1.5 years). As opposed to median age, in the longitudinal study of Treloar, the average age of the menopause was 50.7 years with a 95% range of 44–56 years [18].

In the SWAN study of women's health across the nation, a longitudinal study of a community-based multiethnic sample representative of the female population in the United States the median age of menopause was 51.4 with earlier onset associated with current smoking, lower level of education, and socio-economic status [10]. On the other hand, later age of menopause was associated with increased parity and use of oral contraceptives (OCs). Premature menopause, defined as permanent cessation of menses under 40 years of age occurred in 1.1% [19].

Women who have undergone unilateral oophorectomy or chemotherapy do have an earlier onset of menopause, especially if these interventions occur later in reproductive life [20]. OC use marginally delays menopause and multiparity and/or prolonged breast feeding are also associated with a modest delay in menopause. Finally, follicle "over-usage," i.e., women who have undergone repeated cycles of gonadotropin induction of ovulation or delivered dizygotic twins, experience earlier menopause [21].

Unlike the earlier initiation of puberty seen in developed and developing societies associated with improved general health, sanitary living conditions, and nutritional status, most historical investigations indicate the age of menopause has changed very little since Greek times or the middle ages [1].

Definitions: peri-menopause, menopause, and the menopausal transition

According to the World Health Organization (WHO) [22], *menopause* is defined as the date "of the final menstrual period" retrospectively designated as 1 year without flow in appropriately aged women (over 40 years). *Peri-menopause* includes the period of years immediately before the menopause (when the endocrinologic, biologic, and clinical features of approaching menopause commence) and the first year after the menopause (Fig. 20.1) [5].

The possibly confusing inclusion of the 1 year of amenorrhea that at once ends the peri-menopause and begins menopause reflects a compromise that has reasonable biologic grounds. First, very few women abruptly end their menstrual life and enter menopause in a single month. The blurred transition is also appropriate because before complete exhaustion a limited number of active follicles do transiently exist at the time of menopause but collectively cannot secrete sufficient estradiol to induce menses.

On the other hand, it will be seen that peri-menopause is not simply the decade of intermittent but relentless withdrawal of ovarian function which blends imperceptibly into menopause and the years beyond. To the contrary, peri-menopause is a state of accelerated follicle activation and endocrine hyperactivity, initially shorter inter-cycle intervals, sporadic ovulations, the return or new appearance of acne and hirsutism as well as oligoamenorrhea and increased menstrual cycle instability (dysfunctional uterine bleeding, DUB) [5,23].

Peri-menopause

Although the definition of the end of peri-menopause is clear – 12 months of amenorrhea – the start of peri-menopause is less certain. Peri-menopause begins when previously normal ovulatory cycles become less frequent and cycle lengths change. Defined endocrinologically, peri-menopause begins when serum non-cyclic FSH levels begin permanent ascent to and beyond concentrations of 20 mIU/mL [5,23].

The initial shortening of cycle length reflects rising FSH-induced earlier recruitment and selection of the emerging follicle cohort. Thereafter, lengthening and marked irregularity reflects first luteal phase dysfunction and then anovulation. Nevertheless, estrogen secretion persists over longer intervals leading to unchecked endometrial proliferation and DUB. Despite the presence of mid-proliferative phase E2, FSH levels continue to rise, reflecting the loss of negative feedback by granulosa secreted Inhibin B [5,23] (Fig. 20.2). Both rising FSH and declining Inhibin B are the first signs of declining follicle "competence." The decline in follicle competence may begin even earlier. The reduction in fertility and fecundity in

	Menarche						FMP (0)			
Stage	−5	−4	−3b	−3a	−2	−1	+1 a	+1b	+1c	+2
Terminology	**REPRODUCTIVE**				**MENOPAUSAL TRANSITION**		**POSTMENOPAUSE**			
	Early	Peak	Late		Early	Late	Early			Late
					Per-imenopause					
Duration	*Variable*				*Variable*	1–3 years	2 years (1+1)		3-6 years	*Remaining lifespan*
PRINCIPAL CRITERIA										
Menstrual cycle	Variable to regular	Regular	Regular	Subtle changes in flow/ length	*Variable length* Persistent ≥7- day difference in length of consecutive cycles	Interval of amenorrhea of ≥60 days				
SUPPORTIVE CRITERIA										
Endocrine										
FSH			Low	Variable*	↑ Variable*	↑ >25 IU/L**	↑ Variable		Stabilizes	
AMH			Low	Low	Low	Low	Low		Very low	
Inhibin B				Low	Low	Low	Low		Very low	
Antral follicle count			Low	Low	Low	Low	Very low		Very low	
DESCRIPTIVE CHARACTERISTICS										
Symptoms						Vasomotor symptoms *likely*	Vasomotor symptoms *most likely*			*Increasing* symptoms of urogenital atrophy

* Blood draw on cycle days 2–5 ↑ = elevated

**Approximate expected level based on assays using current international pituitary standard

Fig. 20.1. Various stages of hormonal function, ovarian status, menstrual status, and reproductive status in women from menarche through post-menopause. Reproduced from reference [5], with permission.

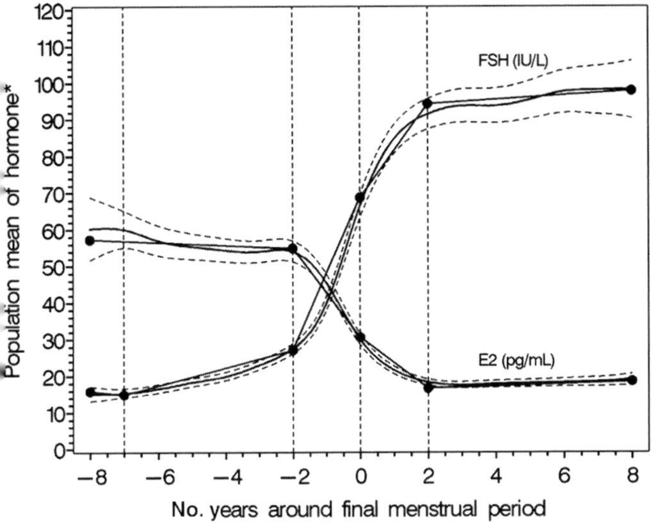

Fig. 20.2. Estradiol and gonadotropin (FSH and LH) levels correlated with the final menstrual period. Reproduced from reference [5], with permission.

pre-menopause begins at age 35, fully 13 or more years before formal menopause [24].

In summary, peri-menopause is characterized by average age of onset at 46 years (range for 95% of women between 39 and 51 years), with an average duration of 5 years (range 2–8 years for 95% of women).

Endocrinology of peri-menopause

Peri-menopause is a unique endocrinologic state [5]. During this 2- to 8-year interval, while anovulatory cycles become progressively more frequent, ovarian follicles undergo an increased rate of reactivation and loss before eventual total depletion. This acceleration appears to begin when the total number of remaining follicles reaches approximately 25,000 (at about 37–38 years of age) and correlates with increases in FSH and decreases in Inhibin B. As more follicles grow, collectively these follicles secrete higher levels of estradiol per cycle [23].

Initially, the rise in FSH reflects the reduced functional quality of the granulosa of aging follicles and their inability to produce Inhibin B. Local concentrations of AMH (the intracrine product of granulosa responsible for *repressing* follicle maturation) also decline. AMH levels define the number as well as quality of antral follicles present at any given time [25].

Clinical characteristics of peri-menopause

The endocrinologic changes across peri-menopause become clinical realities [26,27]. Because mean estradiol levels both in follicular and premenstrual phases are significantly higher than in younger women and 50% or more cycles are anovulatory, the resulting peri-menopausal "syndrome" of heavy prolonged unpredictable menses, DUB, meno-metrorrhagia, breast tenderness and enlargement, fluid retention, migraine headaches, and unpredictable mood swings are understandable.

Vasomotor symptoms in the peri-menopause

Vasomotor symptoms (VMS) occurs in 11–60% of menstruating peri-menopausal women [28]. How can VMS, the hallmark of declining estrogen, be such a frequent feature of the high estrogen state of peri-menopause? Several points only intensify this apparent contradiction of the received wisdom (i.e., VMS are "classic symptoms of estrogen deficiency").

(a) "Standard" hormone replenishment therapy, so effective in the post-menopause, frequently does not control peri-menopausal VMS satisfactorily particularly in younger women. However, the higher steroid content of standard birth control pills (combined E plus P) does control peri-menopausal VMS. If even higher hormone doses are required especially if their effectiveness seems to deteriorate, other concerns such as thyroid disease among other possibilities should be investigated.
(b) Variation of estrogen effect by agonist/antagonist therapy such as clomid or tamoxifen (reduction) or hyper stimulation with recombinant human FSH (rhFSH) ovulation induction (excess) can provoke VMS.
(c) Untreated estrogen-deficient Turner's syndrome patients do not experience VMS, but once given estrogen replacement and then withdrawn, VMS develops.
(d) Postpartum women do not usually experience VMS, despite the acute and dramatic withdrawal from exceedingly high steroid levels over the past 9 months.
(e) On the other hand, hormone-deficient hypophysectomized women do experience VMS.

Despite uncertainty two clinical points are clear: VMS occurs in peri-menopause and is associated with decreased quality of life especially when accompanied by sleep deprivation leading to the "domino effect" [26,27].

Menstrual flow and cycle-related symptoms

Excess, unpredictable menstrual flow is a major problem occurring in as many as 45% of peri-menopausal women. Thickened endometrial stripe by transvaginal ultrasound, the higher frequency of endometrial polyps, and the appearance and/or growth of sub-mucosal fibroids abets the oligo-anovulatory dysfunctional bleeding in these women.

Bone loss begins in peri-menopause [1,29,30]

After reaching peak bone mass in the early 20s and plateauing at age 35, bone loss begins slowly in the peri-menopause and dramatically accelerates after menopause. Evidence suggests the rise in FSH initiates and then adds to the dominant E2-related bone loss seen later. Many variables including hereditary proclivity and lifestyle factors are involved in the initiation of bone loss despite high levels of estradiol [1]. Equally important is the quantity and quality of bone mass set down and nourished from fetal life through late adolescence – the "reserve" available to resist the osteoporosis of menopause. A detailed discussion of the diagnosis and treatment of osteoporosis is offered in the section on osteoporosis.

Therapeutic considerations for peri-menopause

The morbidities associated with this phase of a woman's life include menorrhagia, mastalgia, increased PMS, migraine headaches, uterine fibroid symptomatology, DUB, and the inherent risks of operative interventions [31].

Dysfunctional uterine bleeding

Management of the variable, prolonged menstrual intervals, oligoamenorrhea, and menorrhagia, begins with a controlling regimen of 10–12 days of cyclic progestin before delayed menses. Short-term medroxyprogesterone acetate and/or a 19-norprogestin offer once-a-day administration as opposed to the multiple daily doses oral micronized progesterone requires. Physicians use monophasic low-dose combined OC regimens in non-smoking, non-hypertensive women in peri-menopause. OC confer substantial benefits beyond contraception in the peri-menopause. These include the following [2,32]: endometrial cancer protection; VMS control, reduced dysmenorrheal; prevention of bone loss; reduced ovarian cysts; improved lipoprotein profile and control of acne and hirsutism. Practitioners caring for the peri-menopausal woman must also consider dysfunctions beyond the reproductive system.

Accordingly, the primary "therapy" for peri-menopause is reinforcement of important lifestyle corrections (smoking cessation) and enhancements (diet and exercise). In addition to the "standard" complete medical history and physical performed annually, visits should include calculation of body mass index waist circumference measurement as well as baseline and follow-up TSH, lipid profile, and hemoglobin A1C.

Baseline abnormalities or at follow-up identify impending risk of later cardiovascular or endocrine/metabolic disease.

Menopause

The WHO definition of menopause is a clinically appropriate descriptor: permanent loss of menstrual function for 12 months in appropriately aged women. Longitudinal studies define an age range between 45 and 56 years but outliers invariably exist [5].

Unlike peri-menopause, menopause displays consistent interdependence between endocrinology and clinical manifestations (Fig. 20.1). The prolonged hypoestrogenic state presents short- and long-term consequences that extend beyond the reproductive system and includes multisystem dysfunctions which influence overall life expectancy and quality of life issues.

Endocrinology of menopause

Within a year after the final menstrual period (FMP), ovarian follicle exhaustion is complete (Fig. 20.2) [1,5,33]. FSH and LH continue to rise, achieving a 10- to 20-fold increase in FSH and tripling of LH by 3 years post-menopause. Hypergonadotropism persists at gradually diminishing levels but always in castrate range.

Estrogens

The total estrogen available in the post-menopause is derived from non-gonadal androgen conversion to estrogen (the production rate of estrogen in both intact and oophorectomized post-menopausal women is the same: 0.045 mg/day (45 μg/24 hr) (Tables 20.1 and 20.2) [33,34]. Estradiol concentrations are invariably below 30 pg/ml and usually in the 10–20 pg/mL range. This estradiol does not arise from gonadal secretion but is produced at extra-gonadal sites from estrone. At 30–70 pg/mL the circulating level of the biologically weaker estrone is the estrogen of the post-menopausal years.

Substrate availability at extra-gonadal sites increases circulating estrogen levels. Available estrogen will vary among women and in the same woman over time; for example, as the amount of fat and the inherent aromatase capacity of fat tissue increases circulating levels of total and free estrone and estradiol increase. With obesity, sex hormone-binding globulin (SHBG) levels decrease, thereby providing both greater androgen substrate availability and higher concentrations of free biologically active estrogens [34].

Precursor androgen may vary as a result of increased input or diminished clearance, i.e., increased ACTH or alterations in androgen clearance and metabolism as in liver disease. Chronic stress in an obese post-menopausal woman may increase and sustain estrogen sufficiently to cause endometrial proliferation and hyperplasia as well as dysfunctional uterine bleeding and cancer.

Androgens

Dehydroepiandrosterone (DHEA) and its sulfate (DHEAS) originate entirely from the adrenal cortex and decline markedly with aging [33–35]. In the decade after menopause, the circulating levels of these androgens decrease by 70–75%. Androstenedione decreases by 50%. The age-related decline in these steroids is called "adrenopause." As adrenarche appears to have no influence on the timing of puberty, neither does the adrenopause govern the timing of menopause.

While overall testosterone concentrations decrease in post-menopause by 25% due to reduced adrenal androstenedione secretion, the early post-menopausal ovary continues to secrete important quantities of this steroid. Elevated LH drives the remaining ovarian stromal tissue to sustained testosterone synthesis and secretion [36]. Testosterone availability in the virtual absence of estrogen induces facial hirsutism, scalp alopecia, and contributes to the post-menopausal increase in elements of the metabolic syndrome (MetS) [37].

Eventually, the ovarian stroma is exhausted, and despite persistent high levels of gonadotropins, ovarian secretion of androgen is lost and total estrogen availability diminishes to nadir levels. At this stage, circulating levels of estrogen no longer can sustain reproductive and non-reproductive system estrogen-dependent tissues.

Accordingly, the management of the post-menopausal woman is divided into early and late post-menopausal concerns and issues. "Early" corresponds to the approximately 5-year post-menopausal phase in which the slope of estrogen decline is acute and rapid; "late" is the prolonged remaining years in which a chronically hypoestrogen state prevails. Each poses unique manifestations and burdens.

Table 20.1. Blood production rates of steroids

	Reproductive age	Post-menopausal	Oophorectomized
Androstenedione	2–3 mg/day	0.5–1.5 mg/day	0.4–1.2 mg/day
Dehydroepiandrosterone	6–8	1.5–4.0	1.5–4.0
Dehydroepiandrosterone sulfate	8–16	4–9	4–9
Testosterone	0.2–0.25	0.05–0.18	0.02–0.12
Estrogen	0.350	0.045	0.045

After menopause the production of androstenedione, testosterone, and estrogens declines significantly. However, note that oophorectomy has no effect on post-menopausal estrogen production indicating the entire availability of estrogen is due to extra-gonadal conversion from androgen. The decline in dehydroepiandrosterone and its sulfate is dramatic (the "adrenopause") and is exclusively related to diminished adrenocortical secretion.

Table 20.2. Changes in circulating hormone levels at menopause

	Pre-menopause	Post-menopause
Estradiol	40–400 pg/mL	10–20 pg/mL
Estrone	30–200 pg/mL	30–70 pg/mL
Testosterone	20–80 ng/dL	15–70 ng/dL
Androstenedione	60–300 ng/dL	30–150 ng/dL

Concentrations of all steroids decline after menopause. However, testosterone levels remain relatively stable reflecting both continued gonadal secretion and extra-glandular conversion of precursors.

Clinical manifestations of menopause

The clinical manifestations of the post-menopause can be considered in three areas [1,5].

1. *Estrogen excess:* dysfunctional uterine bleeding, endometrial hyperplasia, and endometrial cancer.
2. *Estrogen loss:* VMS and atrophy of estrogen-dependent tissues (vagina, urethra, and bladder). Some cluster in the early post-menopausal years (VMS) and still others (atrophy) dominate the late post-menopause.
3. *The "menopausal transition"* (ages 35 through 65 and beyond): a combination of non-reproductive vascular, endocrine, and metabolic manifestations of aging, disadvantageous lifestyle compounded by loss of estrogen.

Problems of estrogen excess

Among the problems of early menopause is the frequency of dysfunctional uterine bleeding. Although the clinician is appropriately concerned about underlying neoplasia, the most common cause is endogenous estrogen stimulation of endometrial growth in the absence of progesterone. Whereas the bleeding problems of peri-menopause reflect anovulation, in post-menopause abnormal bleeding arises from sustained, not necessarily elevated concentrations of extra-gonadal production of estrogen in the total absence of endogenous progesterone.

Management and therapeutic considerations of estrogen excess

In all post-menopausal women who experience vaginal bleeding evaluation for specific organic causes (i.e., neoplasia) is mandatory. In addition to a careful history and physical examination to rule out general medical disease (thyroid, liver, and renal) and extra-uterine (vulva, vagina, urethra) sources of bleeding, a transvaginal ultrasound measurement of endometrial thickness, presence of polyps, or submucosal fibroids is essential [1,2]. In many instances, the clinician may choose direct histologic appraisal by biopsy and/or hysteroscopy.

The first sign of endometrial cancer is abnormal vaginal bleeding. However, carcinoma will be found in only 1–2% of post-menopausal endometrial biopsies [38]. Normal endometrium is retrieved in 50%, polyps in 3%, hyperplasia in 15%, and atrophic endometrium in 30%. The persistence of abnormal bleeding demands re-evaluation; approximately 10% of patients with benign findings initially will subsequently develop significant pathology in 2 years [38].

When dysfunctional uterine bleeding is associated with endometrial proliferation or hyperplasia, progestin therapy must be initiated or if currently in use the dosage and duration - increased. Consideration of a progestin eluting intra-uterine device may be the best and least symptomatic solution.

If hyperplasia is present, follow-up biopsy after 3 months of appropriate therapy is required to confirm the initial diagnosis and effectiveness of therapy. The presence of atypia or dysplasia at any time requires hysterectomy, because progestin will not inhibit progression or reverse these processes.

On the other hand, if atrophic endometrium is found either continuous combined hormone therapy (CEE plus MPA) or simple reassurance and observation for recurrence may be all that is necessary.

In all cases of dysfunctional uterine bleeding, ovarian cancer must be ruled out. Clinicians choose transvaginal ultrasound imaging of the pelvic organs in all such cases. Non-palpable otherwise asymptomatic ovarian cysts are common in post-menopause and are readily detected by ultrasound. Cysts less than 5 cm in diameter, without septations or solid components and a thin regular lining, have a low potential for malignant disease and can be managed with serial ultrasounds [39]. If growth occurs or solid elements emerge, then surgery must be done.

Estrogen deficiency: hormone therapy in early post-menopause

Low estrogen imposes adverse effects on most body systems. In some instances lack of estrogen leads to loss of "protection" or earlier appearance and/or acceleration of dysfunctional states usually attributable to aging. Hormone replenishment relieves many of these adverse consequences [1,2,5]. However, although the beneficial effects of estrogen replenishment may be substantial, a significant portion of recipients show limited or no salutary modification of system dysfunction. Depending on age, obesity, smoking status, and the presence of elements of MetS, estrogen plus a progestin may cause serious adverse reactions and complications [40].

A series of reports over the past decade recording findings from the large prospective randomized trials known as the Women's Health Initiative, while confirming most of the positive and negative results of observational studies (increased breast cancer, venous thrombophlebitis and embolism (VTE), cholecystitis, reduced hip fracture, reduced colon cancer) also disclosed unanticipated negative effects of therapeutic combinations of conjugated equine estrogen (CEE) plus medroxyprogesterone acetate (MPA). These included increased risk of cardiovascular events which had been previously thought to be dramatically reduced by hormone therapy in multiple large observational studies [3,4].

This stunning reversal of the prevalent clinical understanding necessitated re-examination of fundamental premises – research protocol design and interpretation, the populations studied, the timing, dosage, the nature of the steroids, and how they were administered – were all placed in question.

A carefully constructed benefit/risk stratification of possible hormone recipients is necessary; clinical need, availability of alternatives, and potential for adverse effects is mandatory.

The section on management (A clinical approach to post-menopausal hormone therapy) will return to these "when and whom, if at all" questions. It will be seen that, in the decade since the first report of the WHI (2002) [40], useful clinical answers to these pivotal questions have emerged and steps can be taken to stratify post-menopausal women into those who may benefit or be placed at risk using these regimens.

Early post-menopause: symptoms, signs, and system changes

Vasomotor symptoms (VMS)

The vasomotor flush or flash is experienced to some degree by most post-menopausal women especially in early post-menopause. It peaks in frequency and severity in the first years after the last menses, lasts for 4–5 years in 50% of women and in some even longer (>5 years 25%) and up to 15 years in 10% [41,42].

The experience involves the sudden onset of flushing of head, neck, chest, and back, accompanied by feeling of intense body heat and concluded by perfuse sweating. The event is variable in duration (seconds to minutes), in frequency, and in timing (day or night or both).

Standard estrogen replacement substantially relieves post-menopausal VMS and curtails the "domino" effects associated with them (i.e., sleep deprivation and mood swings).

The effectiveness of estrogen therapy is so consistent failure is a clinical sign of non–estrogen-related causes of VMS (thyroid disease, pheochromocytoma, carcinoid, leukemia, cancer) [43]. VMS may be a reaction to stress or a component of a psychosomatic disorder; a high (but transient) response to a placebo is part of the assessment of refractory VMS.

Skin

A decline in skin collagen content and skin thickness occurs with aging [44,45]. Low-dose estrogen replenishment leads to a clinically significant arrest or avoidance of skin wrinkling. This estrogen effect on collagen is evident in both skin and bone. Bone mass and collagen decline in parallel after menopause. Estrogen treatment reduces collagen turnover and improves collagen quality.

Psychophysiologic effects

According to "conventional" wisdom menopause does not impose a deleterious effect on women's mental health. Cited are surveys such as the Massachusetts Women's Health Study and the U.S. National Health Examinations Study which find no evidence that natural or surgically induced menopause lead to increased psychologic stress or depression [46,47]. Many of the problems are thought to be due to preceding and current stressful events occurring in a "vulnerable" population of women. According to this thesis, a segment of menopausal women confronted with stress or poor health (personal, family) identify the menopause as the cause of their problems and seek hormone therapy as a solution.

On the other hand, evidence has accumulated establishing estrogen as essential for normal brain development and maintenance of function. Estrogen (E) enhances rodent learning and memory, mood and behavior, and executive and cognitive function (see Chapter 2). E exerts these influences by generally supporting neurogenesis, neuronal protection, synaptic plasticity, and specific actions restricted to specialized nerve centers related to mood and behavior. With regard to women, The Pennsylvania Ovarian Aging Study followed over 400 women and correlated onset of depressive mood and hormonal changes: 50% of women developed increased measures of depression, and 26% met the criteria for clinical depression during the peri-menopausal transition when compared with their own pre-menopausal status [48].

In a prospective cohort study of women regardless of a prior history of depression, the Harvard Study of Moods and Cycles found women entering the peri-menopausal transition almost doubled their risk of new depression from pre-menopausal status [49]. The presence of VMS and a history of previous adverse life events significantly contributed to the increased risk of new depression. The SWAN studies demonstrated similar findings; in 16% of participants the first episode of diagnosed depression was associated with past anxiety disorders, stress, and VMS [50].

The benefits of E replenishment as anxiolytic and anti-depressant are not solely dependent on correction of sleep disturbance. Clinical studies have demonstrated a beneficial effect of E therapy alone and when added to standard anti-depressive therapies (SSRIs and SGAs) provided incremental efficacy over SSRIs and SGAs alone (independent of VMS) [51].

In summary, the frequency of depression does increase during the menopausal transition. It likely reflects the additive effects of sleep deprivation and estrogen deficiency on a group of women with previous diagnosis of depression or with "depression-suggestive" signs and symptoms earlier in life.

Osteoporosis

Osteoporosis, a silent rapidly progressive process, if detected early can be stabilized and possibly repaired. But with each year of post-menopause, the risk of fracture increases and the efficacy of therapy decreases (Figs. 20.3 and 20.4) [52,53].

The magnitude of the problem

Osteoporosis imposes burdens on the individual as well as major public health problems. The number of factures experienced in a single year exceeds the combined number of diagnosed invasive breast cancers or cardiovascular disease events.

Osteoporosis is a major and growing public health problem in the United States. But, as dramatic as the overall statistics are, the individual risks and costs are staggering (Table 20.3).

Hip fracture, for example, is associated with significant mortality and morbidity. Approximately 16% of patients with hip fracture die within the first 3 months after injury due to heart failure, pulmonary embolism, or pneumonia. But even with survival, the residual loss of personal integrity, dignity, and quality of life, i.e., loss of job, recreational opportunities, mobility, decreased independent living, and ability for self-care, problems with gait, bowel, and pulmonary function combined with reduction in sexual possibilities, taken together are a discouraging reality.

Pathogenesis

The risk of fracture depends on two factors: the bone mass achieved in teenage years and the subsequent rate of bone loss

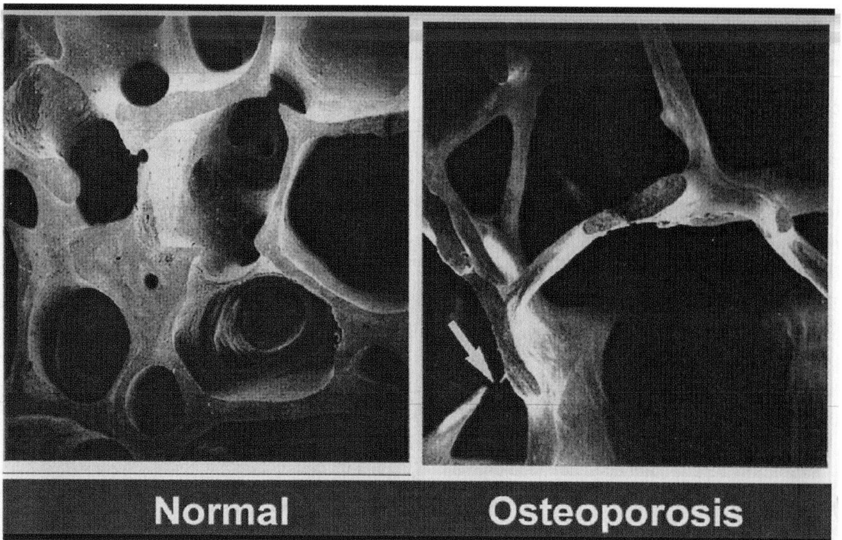

Fig. 20.3. Post-menopausal osteoporosis: bone resorption greater than bone formation. A skeletal disorder characterized by an imbalance of bone resorption and bone replacement. Loss of bone densit and discontinuity of trabecular bridges lead to loss of bone strength and risk of fracture.

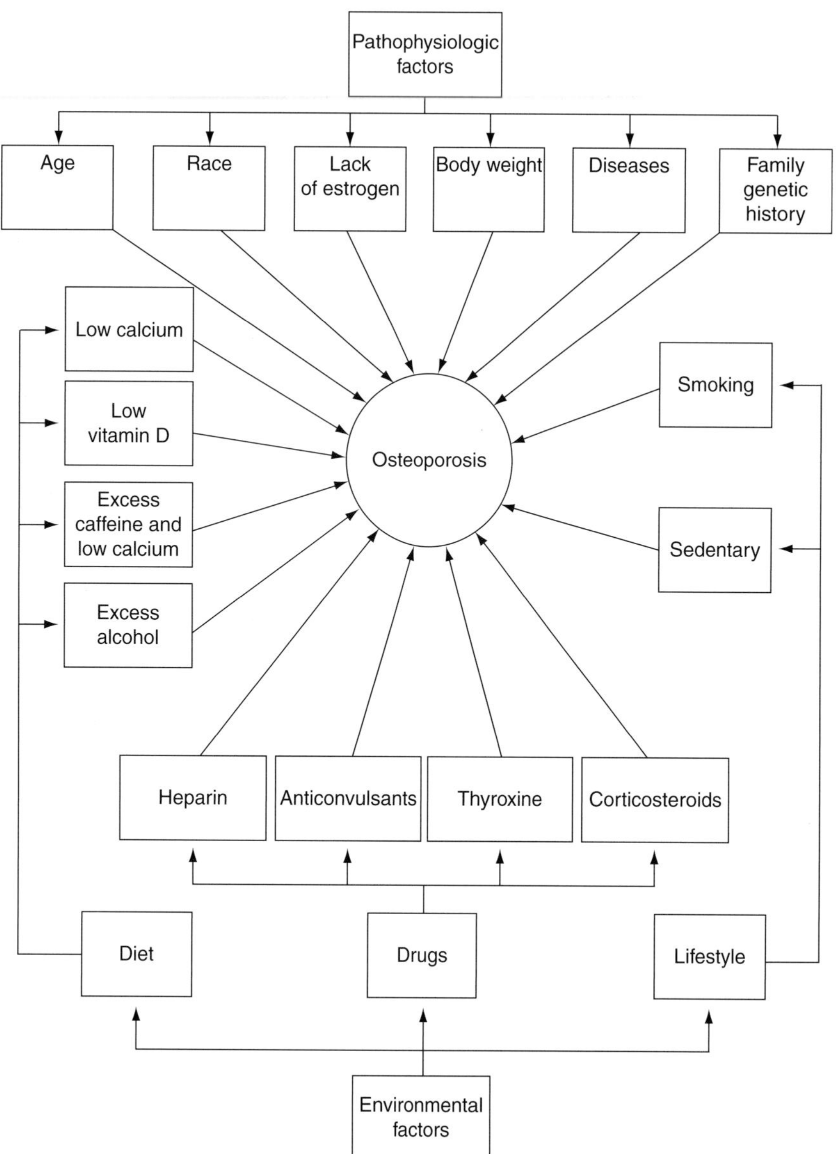

Fig. 20.4. The multiplicity of factors involved in osteoporosis including genetic, environmental, dietary, lifestyle, and hormonal elements, many of which may exist in combination in an individual patient. Smoking, diet, exercise, and hormone (estrogen) effects are emphasized. Not shown is development of maximal bone "reserve" during adolescence.

Table 20.3. National Osteoporosis Foundation data for the USA

10 million women with diagnosed osteoporosis
34 million women at risk (osteopenia, undiagnosed osteoporosis)
300,000 hip fractures/year
40,000/year mortality
Mortality rate in first year after hip fracture: 20–30%
Greater risk of hip fracture than risk of breast, uterine ovarian cancer *combined*
More than half of individuals with hip fracture are unable to return to previous lifestyle
15% lifetime risk of Colles' fracture (distal radius/ulna)
50% of women over 65 years of age have spinal compression fractures
2005: $19 billion costs of care for osteoporosis sufferers

Source: National Osteoporosis Foundation 2010.

xperienced over the remainder of life [1,52]. Five percent of rabecular bone (spine, hip) and 1–1.5% of cortical bone mass s lost per year after menopause. Post-menopause accelerated oss will continue for 10–15 years after which the rate dimin-shes but continues as age-related loss continues. Taken ogether, in the 20-year interval following menopause, there vill be a 50% loss in trabecular bone and a 30% reduction in ortical bone

Osteoporosis involves decreased bone mass but with reten-ion of a normal ratio of mineral to matrix. The bone loss haracteristic of osteoporosis reflects an imbalance in the com-onents of the bone remodeling process within each bone emodeling unit. Whereas localized bone loss (osteoclast activ-ty) is normally balanced by bone formation (osteoblast activ-ty), in osteoporosis new bone formation and repair do not keep ace with bone resorption.

tiology

The multiplicity of genetic, environmental, endocrinological, nd detrimental behavioral factors which promote imbalance of one homeostasis are shown in Fig. 20.4.

Longitudinal studies suggest that several factors regulate eak bone density, including dietary intake of specific nutrients, hysical activity, and genetic determinants. Among the most mportant risk factors are age, family or personal history of steoporotic fracture, diet (low calcium), hypoestrogenism, lcohol abuse, and chronic use of bone-depleting medications corticoids, thyroid hormone, SSRIs).

The challenge for research and clinical management is pro-ression of bone loss is silent until facture or symptoms and igns of vertebral compression emerge.

ites and frequency of fracture in women

a. *Spinal (vertebral) compression fracture.* Symptomatic spinal osteoporosis, causing pain, loss of height, kyphosis with consequent pulmonary, gastrointestinal, and bladder dysfunction, is five times more common in white women than men. Approximately 50% of women over 65 years of age incur spinal compression fractures; about two-thirds are clinically unrecognized (except for loss of height). The most common sites for vertebral fractures are the 12th thoracic and the first three lumbar vertebrae.
b. *Colles' fracture.* A 10-fold increase in distal forearm fractures occurs in white women as they age (approximately a 15% lifetime risk of a forearm fracture).
c. *Head of femur fracture.* The incidence of hip fractures rises from 0.3/1,000 to 20/1,000 from age 45 to 85 years. Eighty percent of all hip fractures are associated with osteoporosis. A woman at 50 faces a 14% lifetime risk of sustaining a hip fracture; a black 50-year-old woman is not spared but her risk is less, 6%. A total of 25% of patients over the age of 50 with hip fractures die due to the fracture or its complications (surgical, embolic, and cardiopulmonary) within 1 year. The survivors are frequently severely disabled and may become permanent invalids.
d. *Tooth loss.* Oral alveolar bone loss parallels osteoporosis; a correlation exists between spinal bone density and the number of teeth retained. Post-menopausal women who use hormone therapy lose fewer teeth.

Measuring bone density status and assessing the rate of bone loss

Given the public health impact and the burdens individual women incur from this initially silent disease, the presence of *any* risk factor demands baseline bone status measurement at menopause [1,3,4,53]. Cost is a factor; depending on the assess-ment of a patient's risk for osteoporosis and the necessity for establishing current and future risk, the least costly step is serial height measurements over the peri-menopausal transition. In more uncertain situations relatively low cost single photon single energy X-ray absorptiometry and/or ultrasonography of the heel, metacarpal bone, and distal radius may be used for initial assessment. When high precision is required, the best information is provided by dual energy X-ray absorptiometry (DEXA) measurements at lumbar spine, femoral neck, and total hip. Results are reported as bone mineral density (BMD) T- and Z- scores (for specific use of these measures, see References 1,3,4,53).

A *normal* BMD is defined as a T score of 0 to minus 1 SD from the reference standard (BMD of 84% of the population); a T score of minus 1 to minus 2.5 SD defines osteopenia and osteoporosis at T scores below minus 2.5 SD.

The Z score measures the SD between the patient and the average bone density for women of the same age and weight. A Z score lower than minus 2.0 requires evaluation of causes other than post-menopausal estrogen-related bone loss. The cumulative T score is a more useful measure of bone density loss post-menopause.

Biochemical markers of bone turnover

Many serum and urinary biochemical markers of bone turn-over are available. The most commonly used tests are NTX (N-terminal telopeptide) measured in serum or urine as a marker of bone turnover and the less variable serum CTX (carboxy-terminal collagen crosslinks) biomarker of bone resorption. These are not routinely applied clinically.

Prevention and treatment of osteopenia and osteoporosis

While both elements of bone are lost in osteoporosis, more critical is the erosion and final loss of continuity of the bony bridges of trabecular bone (lumbar spine, upper femur, distal radius), which combine mechanical strength with minimal skeletal weight. Once continuity of these bridges is lost, it cannot be re-united despite enhancement of bone mass. Repeated fracture despite anabolic/anti-resorptive strategies is predictable; improvement in bone density measurements or biochemical markers does not ensure reduced fracture risk at these sites.

Estrogen, anti-resorptive therapy, diet, and physical exercise can stabilize and, to a degree, even reverse some bone loss. What cannot be undone is the adverse impact of behavioral and dietary abuses in adolescence and early adulthood.

Non-hormonal approaches

Vitamin D maintains bone integrity and fracture resistance by maintaining blood calcium through increased dietary calcium absorption and reduced calcium loss by diminishing renal clearance [54]. Vitamin D level less than 20 ng/mL indicates deficiency requiring supplementation. This level is seen in women over age 60 and individuals living in the long winter season areas such as the northern United States. Doses of 1,000 to 2,000 IU of vitamin D3 daily maintain 25-hydroxyvitamin D above 30 ng/mL. Adequate vitamin D levels reduces fracture incidence providing adequate calcium intake is also undertaken (1200 mg/day).

Steroid hormone therapy

CEE or CEE+ MPA administration at menopause prevents bone loss and with continued use some bone is replaced [1–3,106,107]. After 1 year, BMD at the lumbar spine increased: relative risk (RR) of 5.39 (CI, 4.24–6.46) and after 2 years it was 6.76 (CI, 5.63–7.89). Similarly for femoral neck after 1 year RR was 2.50 (CI, 16–3.83) and after 2 years RR it was 4.12 (CI, 3.45–4.80).

A delay of 3 to 4 years stabilized and to a small extent reversed bone loss. However, further delay did not restore lost bone [55].

Improvement was equivalent to that seen with the bisphosphonate alendronate. The combination of CEE and alendronate has modest additive effects on bone mass density. However, while the gains achieved with alendronate persisted for at least 1 year after discontinuation, withdrawal of CEE led to the immediate return of bone loss at a rate equivalent to untreated early menopause [56].

The effect of estrogen on bone is exquisitely sensitive; transdermal 17β-estradiol in amounts as low as 0.025 μg as well as low-dose oral E preserves bone mass [57]. Following cessation of therapy rapid resumption of bone loss leads to a 7–10% increase in hip fractures within 5 years [56].

Other treatment modalities

Bisphosphonates

Available under a variety of names, dosages, frequencies (from daily oral to every 2 years by IV), bisphosphonates bind to bone mineral and inhibit bone resorption by inducing osteoclast apoptosis [1,2]. Three to 4 years of treatment reduce overall fractures by as much as 30% (vertebral by 50%) in women with T scores below minus 2.5. Despite efficacy, long-term compliance is limited by inconvenient use (oral), side effects (esophagitis, bone and joint pain), cost (IV), or the 2–3% incidence of atrial fibrillation. Because of prolonged retention in bone and recirculation, use beyond 3–5 years is unnecessary and possibly leads to bone brittleness.

The number of approved therapies for osteoporosis has doubled in 15 years, but the level of fracture-risk reduction is good but limited; current treatments reduce the risk of non-vertebral fractures by 30–40% at best. Adding to the sense of urgency are the perceived risks of long-term CEE or CEE+MPA (as per WHI) and the long-term safety of bisphosphonates. Reports of complications include osteonecrosis of the jaw and subtrochanteric femoral fractures.

Denosumab

Osteoclast maturation is dependent on RANKL, which is expressed on the surface of bone marrow stromal and/or osteoblast precursor cells, T cells, and B cells. RANKL binds its cognate receptor RANK on osteoclast lineage cells, and is neutralized by the soluble decoy receptor osteoprotegerin (OPG), which is also produced by osteoblastic lineage cells [59]. Denosumab is a human monoclonal antibody that binds to RANKL, thereby reducing osteoclast differentiation, activity, and survival, leading to decreased bone resorption [52,58]. Multiple trials using denosumab (two injections/year) have been carried out in humans. Denosumab treatment resulted in a 68% decrease in vertebral fractures, 40% decrease in hip fractures, and a 20% decrease in non-vertebral fractures. [59]. Compared with alendronate, women receiving denosumab treatment showed greater increase in BMD at all skeletal sites [60].

Post-menopausal women previously treated with alendronate and switched to denosumab increased total hip BMD by 1.90% compared with a 1.05% increase in subjects continuing on alendronate.

The FDA recently approved denosumab for the treatment of post-menopausal women with a high risk of osteoporotic fractures, previous fracture, multiple risk factors for fracture, or who have failed or are intolerant to other osteoporosis therapies.

Unfortunately, osteonecrosis of the jaw has been reported with denosumab.

Teriparatide, PTH 1–34

A recombinant version of human PTH, teriparatide, is approved for the treatment of post-menopausal osteoporosis [52,61]. PTH is secreted by the parathyroid glands in response to low circulating calcium levels. PTH acts directly on bone to mobilize calcium, at the kidney to promote calcium reabsorption, and in the gut to promote calcium absorption [61,62].

Paradoxically, in primary and secondary hyperparathyroidism, high levels of PTH are associated with cortical bone loss and fractures, whereas intermittent PTH administration enhances trabecular bone mass and reduces fractures.

A placebo-controlled clinical trial using teriparatide in post-menopausal women with severe osteoporosis, 20 μg per day of PTH, administered subcutaneously, reduced spinal and non-vertebral fractures (but not hip fractures) by more than 50% and substantially increased lumbar BMD by 8%/year [52,61,62].

The current recommendation is that PTH therapy be limited to individuals with moderate to severe osteoporosis, and continued for only 2 years (PTH effect on BMD plateaus after 2 years of treatment). PTH is also approved for the treatment of glucocorticoid-induced osteoporosis.

Unlike the bisphosphonates, discontinuation of PTH results in bone loss of up to 4% in the first year which is prevented by adding an anti-resorptive drμg after PTH is stopped [63].

The introduction of teriparatide raised expectations that a strategy could be formulated to recover lost bone and then stabilized at new (hopefully fracture limiting) levels by following with anti-resorptive medications. This hope has not materialized to any satisfactory degree.

A complicating factor: serotonin

Serotonin (5-hydroxytryptophan) is a neurotransmitter affecting behavioral and emotional activity. Unfortunately, it has unanticipated effects on bone homeostasis [52,64].

Antipsychotic agents (SSRIs and SGAs) have been widely prescribed to treat mood disturbance, depression, and psychosis. However, these agents have a deleterious effect on skeletal mass and have been implicated in bone loss and a higher fracture risk. At this point, chronic use of these agents mandates initial and repeat BMD assessments by DEXA.

Conclusion

Taken together, the diagnostic difficulties inherent in "silent" progression, the timing, and costs of diagnosis and therapy, the limited impact of current anti-resorptive and anabolic therapies and the guarded prospect for new stronger "anabolic" agents, and the global, public health, and individual burdens of bone loss demand assiduous application of what current medicine has to offer *including hormone replacement*. Osteoporosis is not curable and has limited potential for reversibility, but if detected early, it is treatable with expectations for stabilization and some reduction of fractures.

Degenerative arthritis

The progressive degradation of articular cartilage and overall joint structure characteristic of osteoarthritis leads to joint stiffness, pain, disability, and diminished loss of quality of life [3 (p. 16)]. Estrogen receptors (ERs) have been identified in articular cartilage in animals and humans. Through these, estrogen can elicit genomic and non-genomic effects on the regulation of cartilage metabolism [65].

Early hormone initiation can avoid the deleterious effects of estrogen deprivation on intervertebral discs. This protective effect on osteoarthritis is due to estrogen alone. In the WHI adherent recipients on CEE alone had lower rates (RR, 0.73 (CI, 0.58–0.93) of arthroplasty than the placebo group, a benefit not evident in the CEE+MPA arm [66].

Late post-menopause

Specific symptoms, signs, and system changes in late post-menopause

Manifestations of estrogen deprivation cluster in the early post-menopausal years (such as VMS) and still others (atrophy) predominate in the late post-menopause (Fig. 20.5).

Genitourinary atrophy [67]

Genitourinary atrophy (G-U) atrophy leads to a variety of symptoms that affect quality of post-menopausal life. Chronic lack of estrogen results in atrophy of the vaginal mucosa with the appearance of vaginitis, pruritus, dyspareunia, and eventually vaginal stenosis. The vaginal wall loses collagen, adipose tissue, and the ability to retain water. With loss of its outer squamous layer, the epithelium thins to a few layers of para-basal and basal cells. Blood flow diminishes and

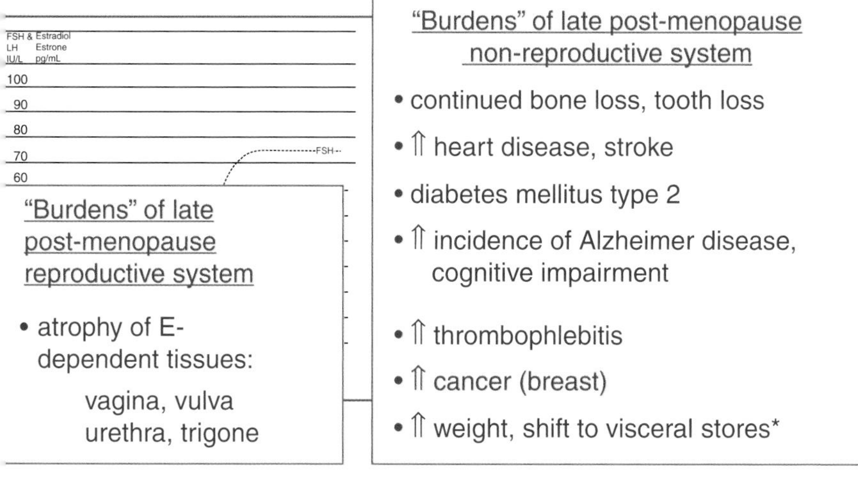

Fig. 20.5. The menopausal "transition" late post-menopause. Burdens affecting both the reproductive system and the emerging metabolic, endocrine, cardiovascular, skeletal, and cancer risks. See Carr [85].

vaginal lubrication is reduced. As pH changes reduced colonization with lactobacilli leads to greater susceptibility to infection.

E insufficiency causes *overactive bladder* (OAB) [68], inducing increased frequency, urge incontinence, increased sensation of need to void, reduced bladder capacity, and susceptibility to *recurrent urinary tract infections* (RUTI). The initial UTI prevalence rate in post-menopausal women is 8–10%/year and 5% recur within a year [69].

Low-dose local estrogen significantly corrects these problems: reinitiation of vaginal epithelial growth, squamous maturation, recolonization with lactobacilli as pH returns to 4.5. The vagina recovers elasticity and lubrication. Once stabilized, even intermittent very low-dose local E therapy diminishes recurrence rates. However, systemic E is needed to correct the overactive bladder symptoms of urgency and urge incontinence, and improve bladder capacity.

Whereas locally applied E in low doses (7.5–25 μg twice a week) has minimal to no systemic effects and does not induce endometrial hyperplasia or cancer, the need for systemic therapy to treat OAB does carry these risks.

Muscle mass and strength [70,71]

Both aging men and women experience a steady reduction in muscle strength and mass. Many factors other than diminished gonadal steroids contribute to this decline including human growth hormone and the limitation of physical activity imposed by frailty, disease, dysfunction, and socioeconomic factors. Lean body mass deficit leads to impaired balance and higher risk of falls. E repletion has been reported to increase post-menopausal women's strength, but confounding variables limit applicability of this information. This is an aging-, not an estrogen-related, change.

Cognition, dementia, and Alzheimer's disease

The evidence supporting E modulation of memory, mood, behavior, and cognitive function, the functional differences in ERα and ERβ receptor subtype stimulation by circulating and local E2, the local aromatase system, and its protective responses to injury of all types, toxic and traumatic, was reviewed in detail in Chapter 2. The benefit of E2 availability to the brain is limited to prevention and protection against damage or apoptosis. However, the inability of E to reverse existing damage has also been emphasized. This evidence suggests early E replenishment at menopause might be brain protective.

Cognition

Assessment of the degree to which estrogen deprivation is a factor in neuronal aging is complicated by a variety factors, most prominent is that the efficacy of E replenishment can only be tested in those sufficiently burdened by the menopausal syndrome to seek hormone therapy. Longitudinal studies across the menopausal transition show no change in cognitive performance, verbal memory, working memory, or perceptual speech [1,3–5,72]. On the other hand, menopausal women receiving estrogen do demonstrate higher scores on immediate and delayed recall, and better recall of proper names (but not word recall) [73,74].

However, these salutary results are not universal. Taken together, if there is any clinical benefit to E replenishment in preserving cognitive competence (verbal memory, vigilance, reasoning, and monitor speed), the intensity and durability of the effect is not known.

Alzheimer's disease

As women age, the incidence of Alzheimer's disease (AD) appears earlier and three times more frequently than in men (75).

Observational studies show AD and related dementia occurs less frequently (up to 60%) in E recipients, particularly in those with prolonged duration of use. While this protective effect was demonstrated in the Baltimore (54% decrease), NYC (60% decrease), and Italian (72% decrease) studies, the UK General Practice Study showed E had no impact [76–78].

These disparate findings bring up the recurrent issue in estrogen therapy; *timing of initiation*. Apparently CEE or CEE + MPA convey no benefit on established AD and may worsen the condition (WHI) [79,80].

However, a primary prevention effect may exist. The Cache County (Utah) report (81), a prospective cohort study (estrogen therapy vs. none) showed a positive impact on AD: 41% reduced risk of AD with *any* use, reduced risk of AD with 10 or more years of use, and improved cognitive performance in recipients. However, *no effect* was seen if E therapy was initiated within 10 years of the diagnoses of AD. The WHI CEE and CEE+ MPA treatment was initiated in women 65 years or older. Women on treatment suffered worsened cognition and an increased risk of developing dementia.

These findings sμggest that there may be a primary preventive effect of E therapy on AD incidence but only if administered early in the post-menopause. This is a recurrent theme echoing findings in osteoporosis and in cardiovascular disease; timing of initiation of hormone therapy proximate to menopause in younger women provides benefit, whereas delay yields either no benefit or induces deleterious effects [3,6].

The mid-life transition: women 35–65 years of age

The mid-life phase of the female life cycle spans the decades between the pre-menopause and extends beyond late post-menopause. During this prolonged interval several factors, including age, vascular, metabolic, as well as the endocrine changes combine in a progressive modification of health and for many women, the emergence of dysfunction and disease. As women age the incidence of cardiovascular disease (coronary artery events and stroke) and type 2 diabetes mellitus increases. However, the silent antecedent pathologic changes begin decades earlier. Therefore, neither can be categorized as early or late manifestations of age or hypoestrogenicity – these are matters that evolve over much of a woman's life (perhaps even as a fetus). Like osteoporosis, these changes evolve silently; but unlike osteoporosis without a clear relationship to any phase of the menopause and without signals of their entrainment until the abrupt appearance of clinical symptoms or signs of illness.

The following pages explore the health status of American women and modifications incurred across the mid-life transition. The effects imposed by the loss of endogenous estrogen in the post-menopause are discussed in detail.

Weight gain and re-distribution

Women gain weight across midlife at a rate of approximately 1 pound/year without deflection at menopause [82]. But many U.S. women enter pre- and peri-menopause already overweight or obese. The population prevalence of obesity in 2009–2010 and trends in the distribution of body mass index over the period 1999–2010 for adults and adolescents were reported in the latest National Health and Nutrition Examination Survey (NHANES) [83,84]. The mean body mass index (BMI) for women age 20 and older was 28.7 (CI, 28.4–29.0); the age adjusted prevalence of obesity 35.8% (CI, 34.0–37.7%). Obesity in women ages 40–59 (43.5 million women) is concerning; the prevalence of BMI > 30 in this age group was 31.8% in white, 62.7% in black, 48.0% in Hispanic and 53.9% in Mexican American women. A total of 17.6% of all women in this age group reached obesity grades 2 and 3 (BMI > 35) and 8.4% were grade 3 (BMI ≥ 40) level of obesity.

Visceral adiposity and the emergence of the MetS

The BMI data obscures a more serious implication of obesity. Even at stable BMI and unchanged total body weight, as women progress through mid-life a shift occurs in where fat is stored, from subcutaneous deposits to accumulations in abdominal visceral sites [85].

Visceral adiposity is the driving force in the emergence of the MetS and its cardiovascular, metabolic/endocrine, and carcinogenic consequences in mid-life women (Table 20.4). The combination of abdominal obesity (defined as waist circumference greater than 88 cm or 35 inches), physical inactivity, and consumption of a high-fat atherogenic diet leads to metabolic dysfunction regardless of BMI.

The expanded visceral adipose tissue differs from the simple storage cells that characterize subcutaneous fat. They are enlarged, compacted, highly vascularized, and populated by abundant activated macrophages (M-1). It is a metabolically active, innate immunity reactive tissue capable of autocrine, paracrine, and with time significant systemic metabolic and endocrine effects by increased secretion of pro-inflammatory cytokines (TNF-α, IL-6, IL-10, IL-18), coagulation factors (PAI-1, tissue factor), resistin (from macrophages), renin–angiotensin system factors (angiotensinogen, angiotensin II), acute phase reactants (hsCRP), lipid metabolic factors (LPL, CETP, APOE), chemotactic molecules (MCP1), and in particular excess non-esterified (FFAs) and fetuin-A. These adverse effects are compounded by chronic high-fat dietary intake. Portal absorption of the constituents of the high-fat diet (HFD), endocrine/vascular transport of FFAs, and pro-inflammatory signals from visceral adiposity to the liver leads to non-alcoholic fatty liver disease (NAFLD). Excess FFA and pro-inflammatory cytokines from three sources (visceral fat, NAFLD, and diet) combine to induce local changes and eventually insulin resistance (principally muscle). Activation of serine rather than tyrosine kinases and reduction of auto-phosphorylation of IRS-1 reduces insulin receptor function and impedes glucose entry into target tissues (Fig. 20.6) [86].

In summary, a state of systemic, tissue-specific insulin resistance with reactive hyperinsulinemia is initiated by excess visceral adiposity. The resulting glucotoxicity, lipotoxicity, and systemic inflammatory state underlies the clinical manifestations of the MetS and the subsequent development of atherosclerosis, diabetes, and cancer (Figs. 20.7 and 20.8).

Table 20.4. The metabolic syndrome

Women displaying these signs:	
Hypertension	130/85 mmHg or higher
Triglyceride	150 mg/dL or higher
HDL-cholesterol	Less than 50 mg/dL
Abdominal obesity	35 inch waist size or more
Fasting glucose	100 mg/dL or higher

Source: Grundy SM et al: American Heart Association/National Heart, Lung, and Blood Institute scientific statement: executive summary. Circulation. 2005;**112**; e285–90

Obesity is defined as BMI > 30 (overweight > 25). Metabolically "healthy" or unhealthy."

The MetS appears and worsens as age and weight increases

The MetS affects 32.6% of aging women. According to the National Health Statistics Reports using MetS prevalence of 15.6% at age 20–39 as a reference, MetS prevalence at 40–59 was 37.2%, OR = 3.20 (CI, 2.32–4.43) and at 60 years and older 54.4%, OR = 6.44 (CI, 4.75–8.72) [87].

Appearance and progression of the MetS with age was reported in the Study of Women's Health Across the Nation (SWAN) [37]. The odds for a typical community-based woman developing MetS were increased in pre-menopause (OR for MetS/yr = 1.45 (CI, 1.35–1.56) and post-menopause (OR of MetS/yr = 1.24 (CI, 1.18–1.30). A continuous linear increase over the transition period occurred without deflection at time of menopause. The MetS emerges and increases with age as concentrations of free testosterone increase.

MetS in normal weight "metabolically obese" women [88]

The prevalence rate of the MetS and its individual components were assessed in normal weight and slightly overweight women (BMI of 18.5–26.9 kg/m^2) using data from the Third National Health and Nutrition Examination Survey [87]. MetS increased in a stepwise manner; compared with reference point women with BMI of 18.5–20.9 the odds for the existence of the MetS increased dramatically: at 21–22.9, OR = 4.34 (CI, 2.08–9.07), at BMI 23–24.9, OR = 7.77 (CI, 3.95–15.26), and at the "normal" BMI of 25–26.9, OR = 17.34 (CI, 9.29–32.38). This relatively high prevalence and the increased risks imposed by the MetS at body

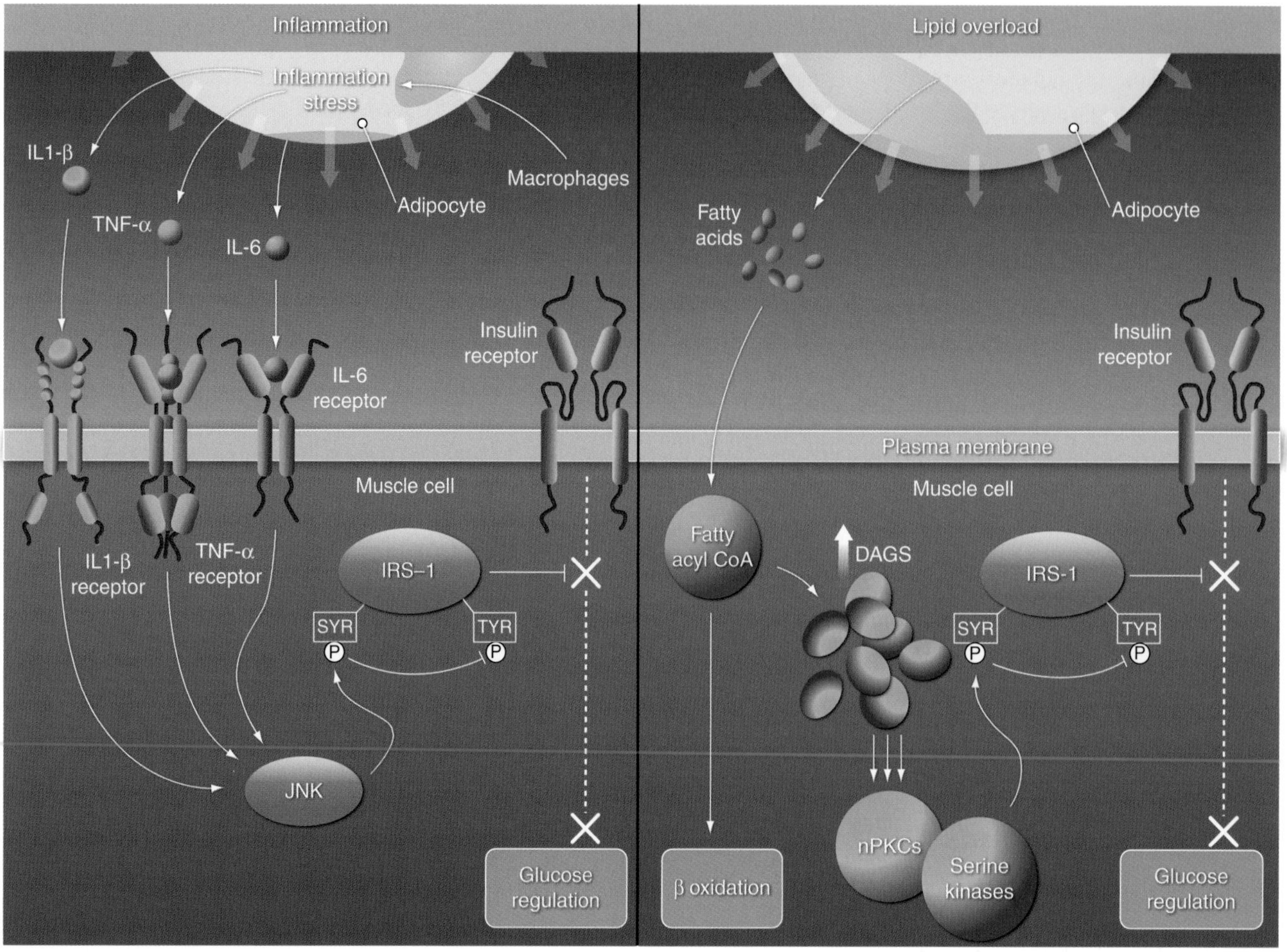

Fig. 20.6. The pathogenesis and pathophysiology of insulin resistance. Visceral adipose tissue releases pro-inflammatory cytokines and FFAs which alter insulin receptor substrate kinase activation leading to insulin receptor dysfunction. Glucose entry is impaired and reactive hyperinsulinemia results. Reprinted from: Taubes G. Insulin resistance: prosperity's plague. Science, 2009;**325**(5938):256–60. With permission from American Association for the Advancement of Science.

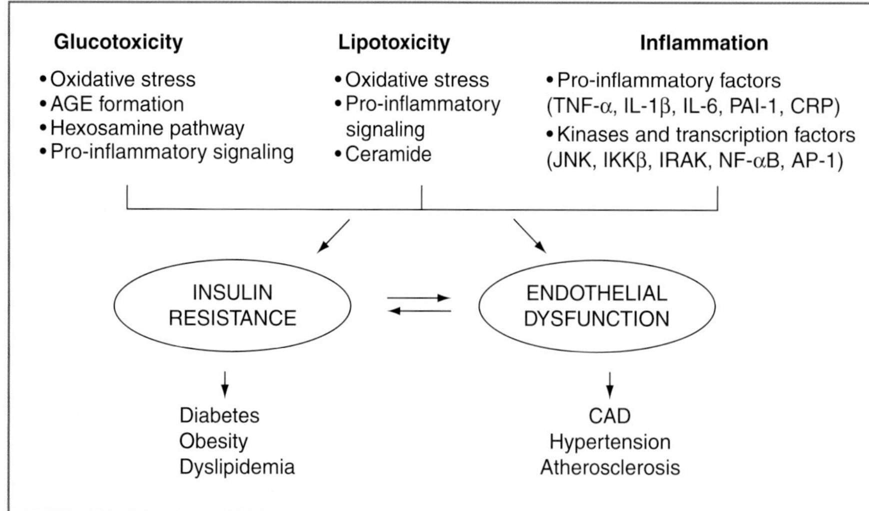

Fig. 20.7. The pathophysiology of the metabolic syndrome. The combined "toxic" effects of glucotoxicity, lipotoxicity, and a systemic inflammatory state lead to insulin resistance and endothelial dysfunction. Reprinted from: Kim JA, et al. Reciprocal relationships between insulin resistance and endothelial dysfunction: molecular and pathophysiological mechanisms. Circulation, 2006;**113**(15):1888–904.

eights and BMIs considered normal is the basis for adopting the escriptive term and acronym Normal Weight, Metabolically bese, NWMO. Regardless of what it is called, the existence of WMO points up the false reliance on BMI as a guide to physical ealth status principally in short, rotund individuals.

aist circumference: a sentinel sign of "silent" emerging MetS

he prevalence of the MetS increases with age and central besity as measured by waist circumference at the level of the ac crests. It is the earliest sign and displays the strongest rrelation with the appearance of MetS; 43% of women with aist circumference of > 88 cm or > 35 inches develop the agnosis of MetS within 5 years. This simple, low-cost, and producible procedure identifies individuals with silent evolvg increased risk of coronary heart disease, type 2 diabetes ellitus, and greater risk of developing cancer.

isks of cardiovascular and endocrine/metabolic isease associated with the menopausal transition

progressive deterioration of normal cardiovascular function ccurs during the menopausal transition (Table 20.5) (89):

- Vascular disease markers: coronary artery calcium scores and carotid artery interna/media thickness both increase with age as the MetS elements emerge and accelerate in the decade post-menopause.
- Hypertension: the prevalence of hypertension (≥140/90) increases with age, rising from 7% at ages 18–39 years to 67% in women 60 years and older.
- Diabetes [90]: According to the American Diabetes Association, 12.6 million or 10.8% of all U.S. women over age 20 have diagnosed DM II. However, the prevalence of DM II is 10 times higher in women over 60 than younger age groups. Increased insulin resistance and the compensating β cell increase in insulin secretion begin as much as 10 years before formal diagnosis and when macro- and micro-vascular complications are under way, and 5 years before levels of impaired glucose tolerance testing are sufficiently altered to meet current diagnostic criteria.

The cardiovascular lifetime risk pooling project [91] (Fig. 20.9)

The Lifetime Risks of Cardiovascular Disease report is an analysis of data from more than 250,000 male and female participants derived from reports of 18 cohorts during a period of more than 50 years of observation. It is the most comprehensive study establishing the critical relationships among age, smoking, elements of the MetS, and subsequent risk of cardiovascular morbidity and mortality. It projects lifetime risks of cardiovascular disease (fatal and non-fatal stroke and myocardial infarction) using the presence of designated risk factors, that is, blood pressure, cholesterol level, smoking status, and diabetes at specific ages (45, 55, 65, 75 years).

The presence of elevated levels of risk factors at all ages translates into markedly higher risks of cardiovascular disease as women age (Fig. 20.9). In women age 55 with an *optimal risk factor profile* (total cholesterol <180 mg; blood pressure <120 mmHg systolic and 80 mmHg diastolic; non-smoking;

Table 20.5. Metabolic syndrome and risk of CVD in women

2006	Age 35–44	1.0	20,637/year
	Age 45–54	2.8	64,220/year
	Age 55–64	6.7	126,507/year
	Age 65–74	12.3	61,921/year

CHD events (MI) begin 10 years later as women age compare to men. Framingham and AHA/NHS (206) CHD events data demonstrated moderate increase in incidence of MI age 45–54 (2.8 MI per 1,000 women/person years) to 6.7 MI age 55–64 and to 12.3 MI per 1,000 female person-years a more than 400% increase in the decades post-menopause.

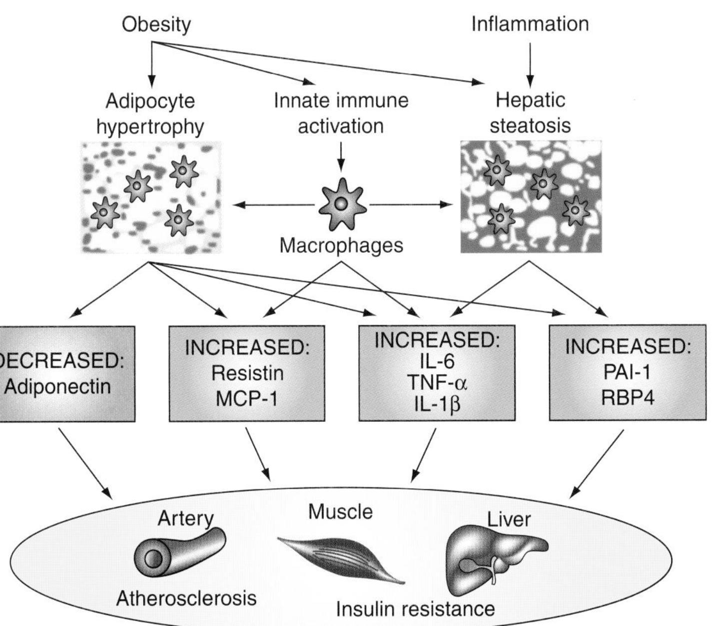

Fig. 20.8. Obesity, insulin resistance, and the metabolic syndrome. Insulin resistance results from pathophysiologic levels of circulating factors derived from several different cell types. The potential role of adipocytes, macrophages, hepatocytes, and the secreted factors which modulate insulin action at the cellular level. Reproduced from Lazar MA. The humoral side of insulin resistance. Nature Med, 2006;**12**(1):43–4. With permission from Macmillan Publishers Ltd.

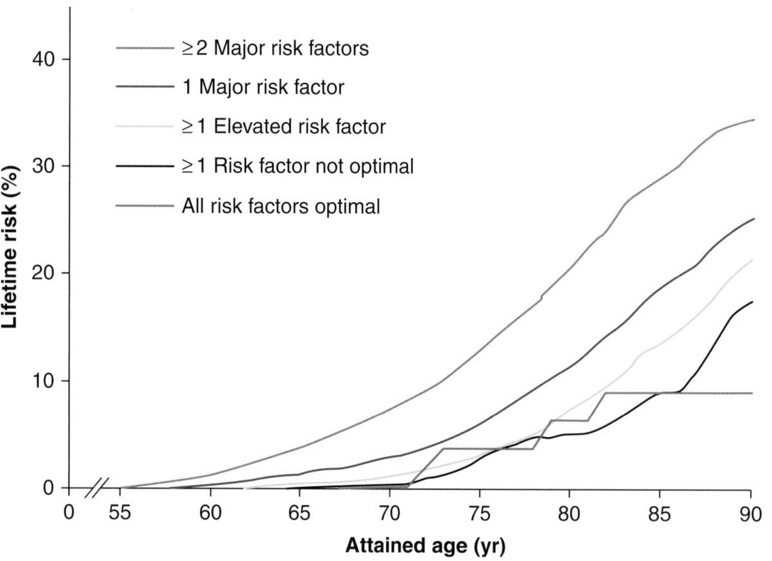

Fig. 20.9. Lifetime risk of death from cardiovascular disease among women at 55 years of age, according to the aggregate burden of risk factors and adjusted for competing risks of deat *Risk factors at age 55 (abnormal):* blood pressure *above* 120/80; total cholesterol *above* 180 mg/dL; smoking status = yes; diabet status = yes. *Risk of cardiovascular disease death by age 80:* women, optimal risk factors, 6.4%; two or more risk factors: 20.5 *Fatal/non-fatal myocardial infarction by age 80:* women, <1% vs 18.3%. *Fatal/non-fatal stroke by age 80:* women, 5.3% vs. 10.7%. Differences [of initial] risk factor burden translate into marked differences in the lifetime risk of CVD, and these differences are consistent across race and birth cohorts. Reproduced from reference [91], with permission.

non-diabetic status) had substantially *lower* risks of death from CVD through the age of 80 years than participants with two or more risk factors (6.4% vs. 20.5%). Women with optimal risk factor profiles had lower overall lifetime risks of fatal and nonfatal MI (<1% vs. 18%) and fatal and non-fatal stroke (5.3% vs. 10.7%). Two-thirds of all women placed in the two highest risk groups.

The study examined the effects of "birth cohort" and the possible confounding influence of therapy and lifestyle changes likely to have occurred during the 50-year study interval. Compared with women in NHANES I (1976–1980), women in NHANES III (1988–1994) had a lower 20-year adjusted risk of death from cardiovascular disease (12.2% dropping to 7.0%) accompanied by a reduced prevalence of two or more major risk factors (4.3% for older women vs. 23.0% for younger women). The beneficial effects of diet, exercise, and medication led to reduced risk factors and deaths.

However, the 20-year adjusted risk of death from cardiovascular disease was substantially greater across birth cohorts when risk factors were untreated and/or persisted. The findings were consistent across risk factor strata between both U.S. black and white women and across multiple birth cohorts.

The effect of menopause on cardiovascular function and disease [92,93]

Diseases of the cardiovascular system, particularly coronary artery heart disease (CHD) are the leading causes of death for U.S. women. In 2005, CHD caused 1 in 6 female deaths compared with 1 in 30 for breast cancer. CVD risk factors are the same in men and women; however, before the age of 40, men have twice the risk of CHD than women. With increasing age, this differential is gradually lost. CVD in general and CHD in particular remains the leading cause of death in both men and women; women incur higher rates than men after age 65 [1].

A correlation exists among estrogen biologic availability, age, and the presence of the MetS in women beyond menopause. HDL-cholesterol levels are 10 mg/dL higher in healthy women even beyond menopause. However, while total cholesterol and LDL-cholesterol are initially lower in women than men, these levels gradually increase with age and rise rapidly after menopause. After age 60, the risk of CHD doubles for women as the atherogenic lipid changes reach levels greater than in men.

Decades of "silent" progression

Coronary atherosclerosis is a lifelong process (Fig. 20.10). The Pathobiological Determinants of Atherosclerosis in Youth (PDAY) study documented the presence of fatty streaks in adolescents which increased with age [93]. The association of body mass index (BMI) at adolescence and progression of clinical diabetes and angiographic proven coronary heart disease (CHD) in adulthood is further evidence of the early initiation and progression of silent vascular dysfunction (94). However, women lag behind men in the incidence of CHD events by 10 years and for myocardial infarction and sudden death by 20 years. Is this "protection" due in part to positive estrogen effects on genomic and non-genomic factors which maintain endothelial function and resilience, fuel and metabolic homeostasis? (See Chapter 2.)

Estrogen and cardiovascular disease: evidence from basic science

Mendelssohn and Karas [95,96] have summarized the estrogen estrogen-regulated (E–ER) genes involved in maintaining "healthy" cardiovascular system (Table 20.6).

In rodent models E–ER gene-activated systems induce protective effects on normal or endothelium minimally affected by atherosclerotic changes by enhanced vasodilatation and decreased local inflammatory pathway activation (Fig. 20.11). E–ER actions promote healing of experimentally induced endothelial injury by recruiting circulating endothelial stem cells to the injury site. E–ER increases nitric oxide synthesis and action, decreases local inflammatory cell adhesion molecules, platelet activation, vascular smooth muscle proliferation, and decreases LDL-cholesterol oxidation/binding/entry.

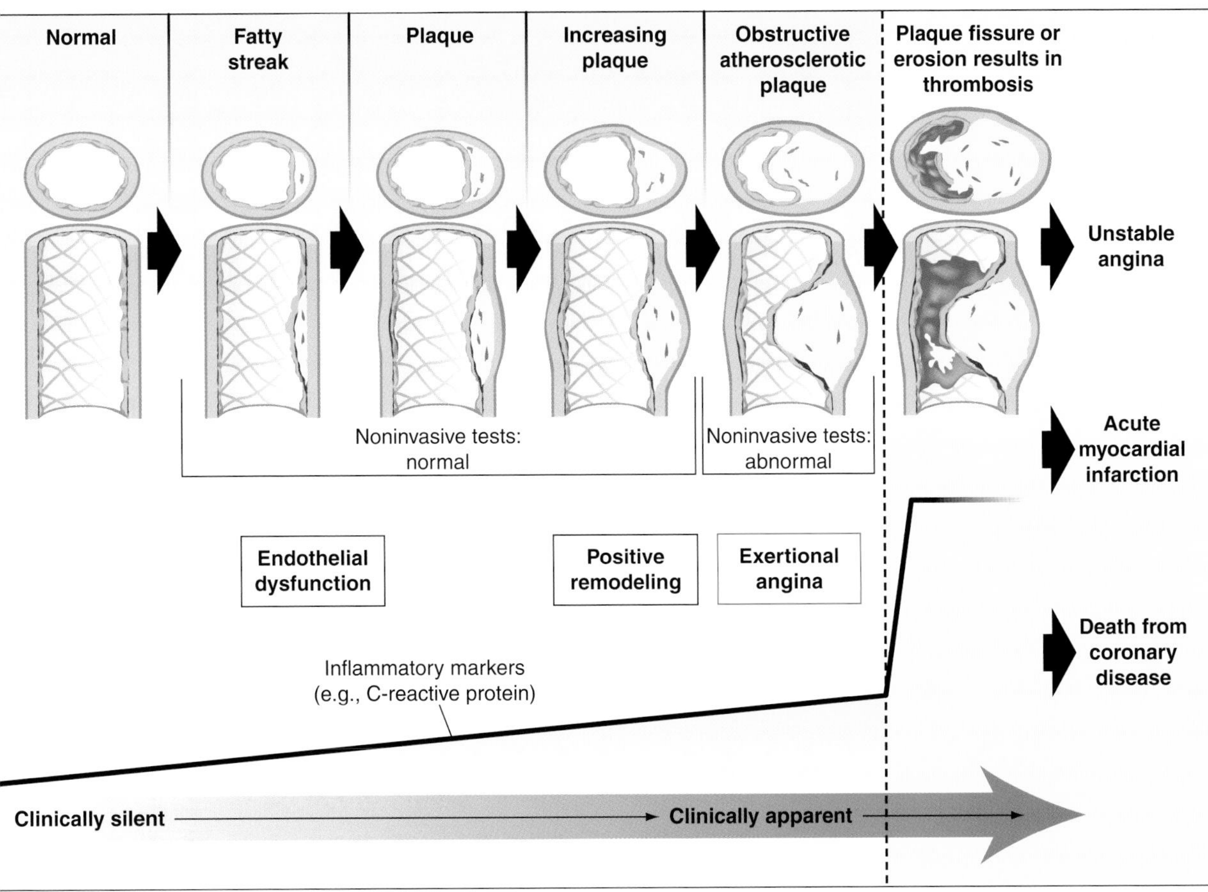

ig. 20.10. Silent progression of coronary atherosclerosis. Atherogenesis begins in childhood (perhaps in utero), silently progresses through dolescence and adulthood only to be identified by clinical events occurring post-menopause.

Critical to the subject of the *timing* of estrogen therapy, ER eactivity is lost when destructive atherosclerotic vascular disease is n place. Under these circumstances, ER concentrations and functions are reduced, eliminating the protective effects of E while the therogenic process progresses unabated. As matrix metalloproteinases (MMPs) increase and neo-vascularization invades the xpanding foam cell plaque, the plaque becomes unstable, and s fibrous cap becomes fragile and prone to fracture. As these lterations progress eventually an acute intra-luminal thrombus nay form and/or intra-plaque hemorrhagic expansion takes place. The result is coronary artery insufficiency and occlusion.

linical studies

s the basic scientific evidence of estrogen-induced gene activity elevant to the human disease process and its consequences? The "protective" effects of E in maintaining a "healthy" cardiovascular system have been validated in clinical studies [1].

favorable effect of estrogen on the vascular system

Direct anti-atherosclerotic effects include the following:

- Endothelium-dependent vasodilation and anti-platelet aggregation by increased NO and decreased endothelin-1
- Positive actions on the heart and large blood vessels by improved vascular compliance
- Inhibition of LDL-cholesterol oxidation by inherent processes and stimulation of anti-oxidant activity
- A favorable impact on fibrinolysis by lowering fibrinogen and plasminogen activator inhibitor-1 (PAI-1) and modulating MMPs activity
- Inhibition of intimal thickening by reduced proliferation and migration of vascular smooth muscle cells
- Inhibition of macrophage infiltration and foam cell formation
- Reduction of adhesion molecules by reducing macrophage attractant molecules
- A favorable impact on lipids and lipoproteins with reduction of LDL-cholesterol and increased HDL-cholesterol
- Improvement in metabolic dysfunction (Fig. 20.12)
  - Reduction of weight, waist circumference, waist to hip ratio
  - Reduced fasting glucose
  - Reduced hyperinsulinemia (reduced insulin resistance).

The consequences of hypoestrogenism independent of age

Untreated premature ovarian failure (POF) and untreated bilateral oophorectomy have been studied [3,11]. Young women with POF (under age 40 with a normal XX genotype) or women who

Table 20.6. E–ER regulates other, non-sex steroid nuclear receptors

Gene product	Physiologic or pathophysiologic role[a]
Candidate estrogen-regulated genes (vascular cells)	
Prostacyclin synthase	Vasodilatation
Endothelial nitric oxide synthase	Vasodilatation
Inducible nitric oxide synthase	Vasodilatation in response to vascular injury
Endothelin-I	Vasoconstriction
Collagen	Vascular, matrix formation
Matrix metalloproteinase 2	Vascular, matrix remodeling
E-selection	Cell adhesion
Vascular cell adhesion molecule	Cell adhesion
Vascular endothelial growth factor	Angiogenesis and endothelial-cell proliferation
Candidate estrogen-regulated genes (nonvascular cells)	
Growth- and development-related genes	
Transforming growth factor-β_1	Wound healing
Epidermal growth factor receptor	Cell growth in response to vascular injury
Platelet-derived growth factor	Cell growth in response to vascular injury
Fit-4 tyrosine kinase	Angiogenesis and endothelial cell proliferation
Coagulation- and fibrinolysis-related genes	
Tissue factor	Hemostasis in response to thrombosis
Fibrinogen	Hemostasis in response to thrombosis
Protein S	Hemostasis in response to thrombosis
Coagulation factor VII	Hemostasis in response to thrombosis
Coagulation factor XII	Hemostasis in response to thrombosis
Plasminogen-activator inhibitor I	Hemostasis in response to thrombosis
Tissue plasminogen activator	Fibrinolysis
Anti-thrombin III	Anti-coagulation
Signaling-related and miscellaneous genes	
Estrogen receptor α	Hormonal regulation and gene expression
Estrogen receptor β	Hormonal regulation and gene expression
Monocyte chemotactic protein 1	Monocyte recruitment and atherosclerosis
I_{sk} and HK2 (cardiac potassium channels)	Cardiac conductin
Connexin 43	Cardiac conductin
Leptin	Fat metabolism and obesity
Apolipoproteins A, B, D and E and Lp(a)	Lipid metabolism and atherosclerosis
Angiotensin-converting enzyme	Vasoconstriction
Angiotensin II receptor, type 1	Vasoconstriction

[a] Data from Mendelsohn, M. E. and Karas, R. H. (1999). N. Engl. J. Med. 340, Table 1 therein, p 1804.

received pre-menopausal bilateral oophorectomy lose bone mineral density and incur a 2.6-fold increased risk of hip fracture [97].

A survey of more than 19,000 women ages 25–100 years with POF incur significantly increased risk for overall mortality (OR = 2.14; CI, 1.15–3.9) [98].

In women with bilateral oophorectomy, the risks are significant [3]. Increases include total mortality RR = 1.12 (CI, 1.03–1.21), fatal and non-fatal CHD RR = 1.17 (CI, 1.02–1.35), stroke RR = 1.14 (CI, 0.98–1.56), and lung cancer RR = 1.26 (CI, 1.02–1.56). Whereas total cancer mortality increased in thi group, oophorectomy was associated with *decreased* risk o breast cancer, RR = 0.75 (CI, 0.68–0.84).

Age, the MetS, and cancer

Older women (74.1 ± 0.3 years) with MetS suffer a higher all cause mortality (63.4%) with almost 50% of deaths due to CVD but 15% are cancer related. The incidence of most cancer

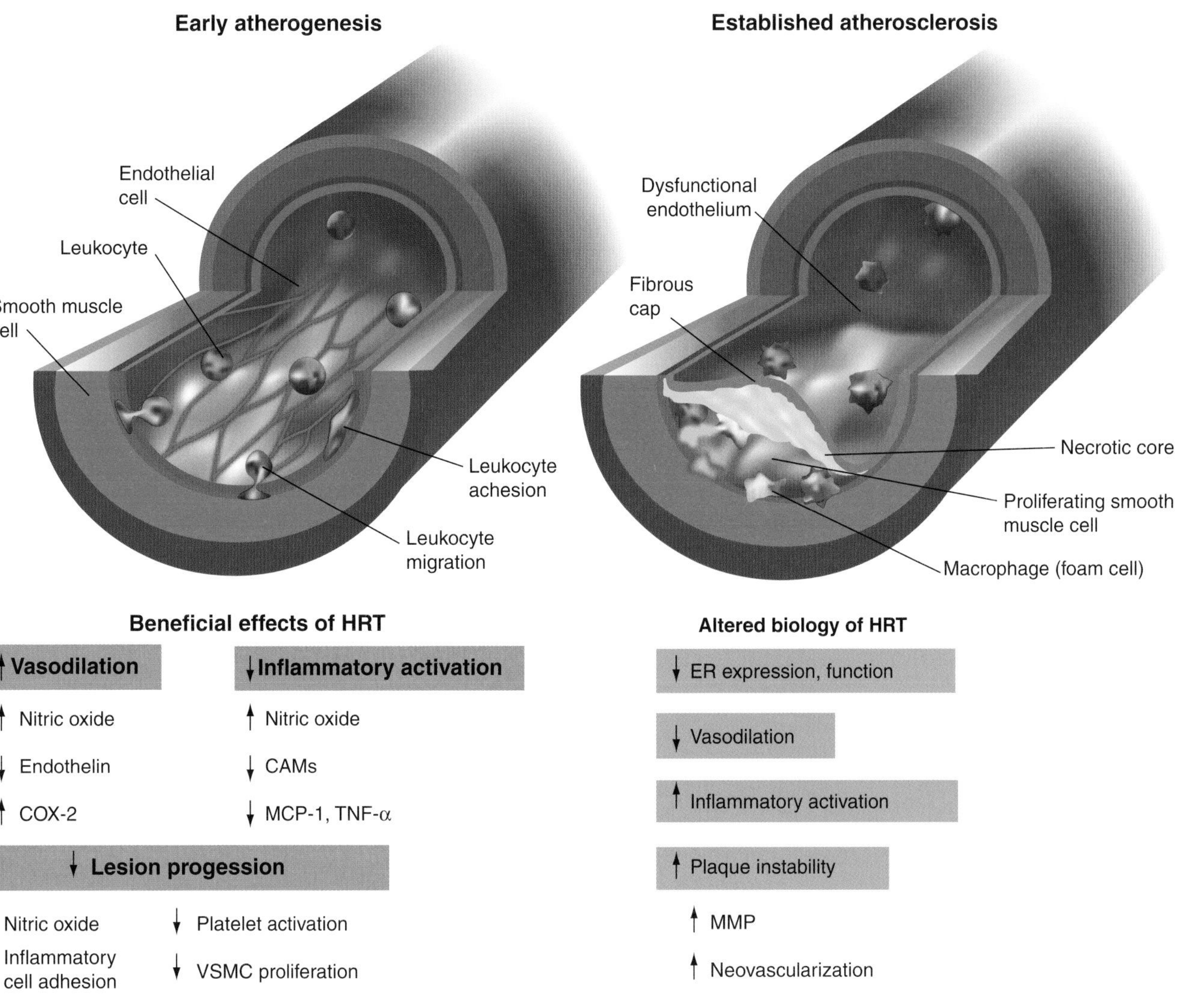

ig. 20.11. The effects of progression of atherosclerosis on E–ER biology. E–ER activation in healthy endothelium yields beneficial effects on vasodilation, flammatory reactivity, and endothelial healing. When endothelium is altered by atherosclerotic disease decreased ER expression leads to adverse vasomotor activity, flammatory activation, and plaque instability. Reproduced from reference [96], with permission.

ıcreases with age; for the purposes of this chapter, however, ıe substantial increase in acquired breast cancer in postıenopausal women will be the primary focus of discussion.

·reast cancer

·reast cancer is an important clinical issue in the magnitude of s scope; approximately 233,000 new cases of invasive breast ancer will be diagnosed in the United States in 2011 and close) 40,000 will succumb to the disease [1,3,6,99,100]. Incidence ıcreases with age with a sharp upward inflection at age 45 eaching a peak rate per 100,000 women at age 75–79, more ıan *triple* (3 times) higher than the rate in women ages 40–44 Fig. 20.13). Independent of any exogenous therapy, currently ıe woman in six will be diagnosed with breast cancer in her fetime (1 in 8 with invasive cancer). Her perception of the ıagnitude of that risk and its physical, emotional, and behavıral impact on self-image and self-confidence is at once an incentive to adopt a healthy life style but also a negative factor regarding hormone therapy.

This fear remains pervasive despite the fact that breast cancer incidence rates have decreased from 1999 to 2007 by 1.8% per year [101,102]. Although advances in technology and stabilization of mammography rates that reduced the pool of previously undiagnosed cancer may have contributed to this finding, the prevailing view is the decline reflects widespread discontinuation of hormone therapy after release of the WHI randomized trial report in 2002.

Whereas SEER data (1980–2008) recorded reduced incidence of ER/PR-negative cancer, ER/PR-positive disease increased [101]. SEER data also identified a two-fold higher proportion of lobular cancers between 1987 and 1999, an increase in tumor type thought to be secondary to hormone therapy.

That estrogen could stimulate a receptor-positive tumor in an estrogen-dependent organ is the biologically plausible basis

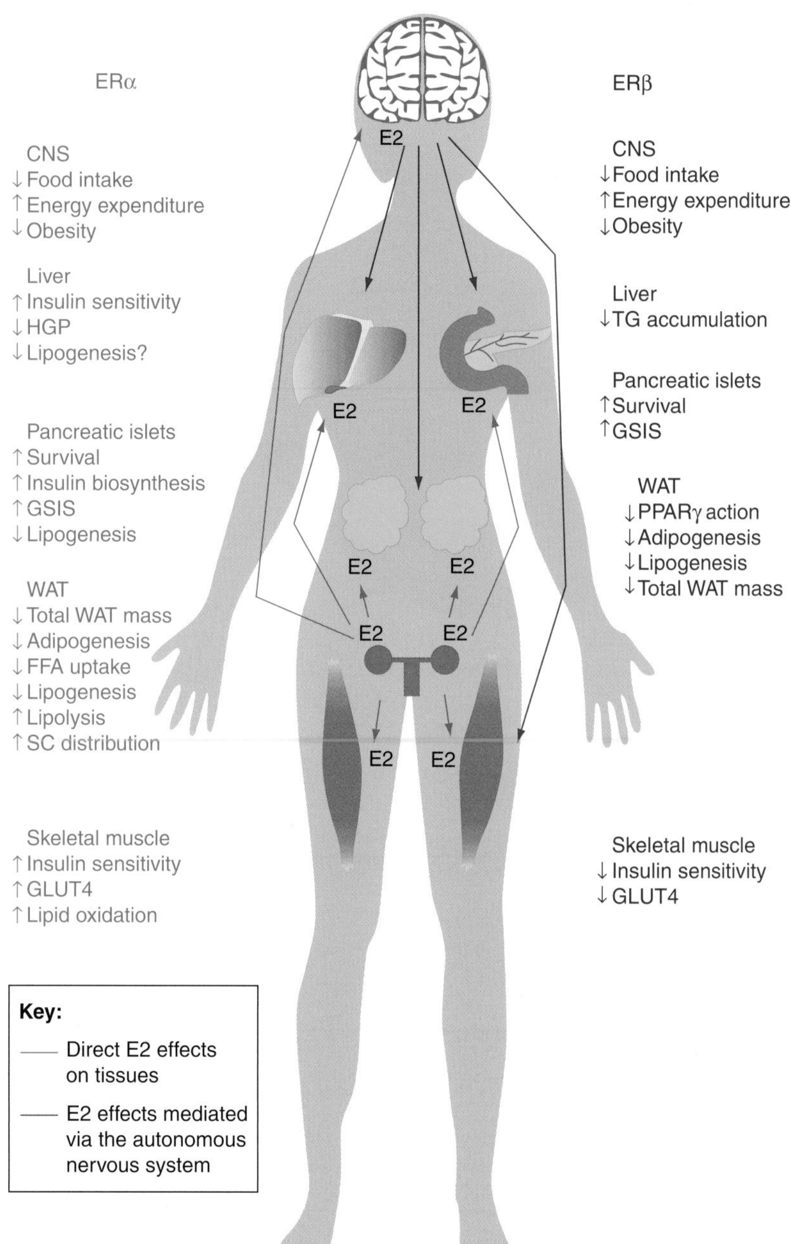

Fig. 20.12. E–ERα, ERβ: normal homeostatic maintenance. The metabolic, endocrine, and fuel homeostatic effects of estrogen and its ERα and ERβ subtype receptors. WAT, white adipose tissue. Reproduced from Mauvais-Jarvis F. Estrogen and androgen receptors: regulators of fuel homeostasis and emerging targets for diabetes and obesity. Trends Endocrinol Metab, 2011;**22**(1):24–38. With permission from Elsevier.

for some but not all of the SEER findings. Normal human mammary epithelial cells spontaneously escape senescence and with this potential for continued or resumed growth have the opportunity to acquire gain in function or loss of inhibition mutations and telomeric sequence erosion, opening the possibility for cancer transformation in previously clinically silent disease [103] (Fig. 20.14).

These observations beg the question: are there endogenous sources of stimulation such as increased estrogen production or other mammary gland growth factors which activate or renew mitotic activity and oncogenicity?

Endogenous estrogen and breast cancer incidence

Fritz and Speroff [2 (p. 819)] have summarized the evidence linking lifelong breast exposure to "excess" (but concentrations within normal range for post-menopause) of endogenous production of estrogen (principally E1) and increased risk of breast cancer:

- Significant difference in incidence between females versus males. Whereas males generate significant estrogen (although less than women) the massive anti-estrogen effect of endogenous testosterone production may explain this dramatic gender difference
- Small *decrease* in risk with late menarche
- Small *increase* in risk with early onset menarche
- Moderate increase with later onset of menopause
- Increased risk in obese post-menopausal women presumably reflecting a higher production rate of estrone

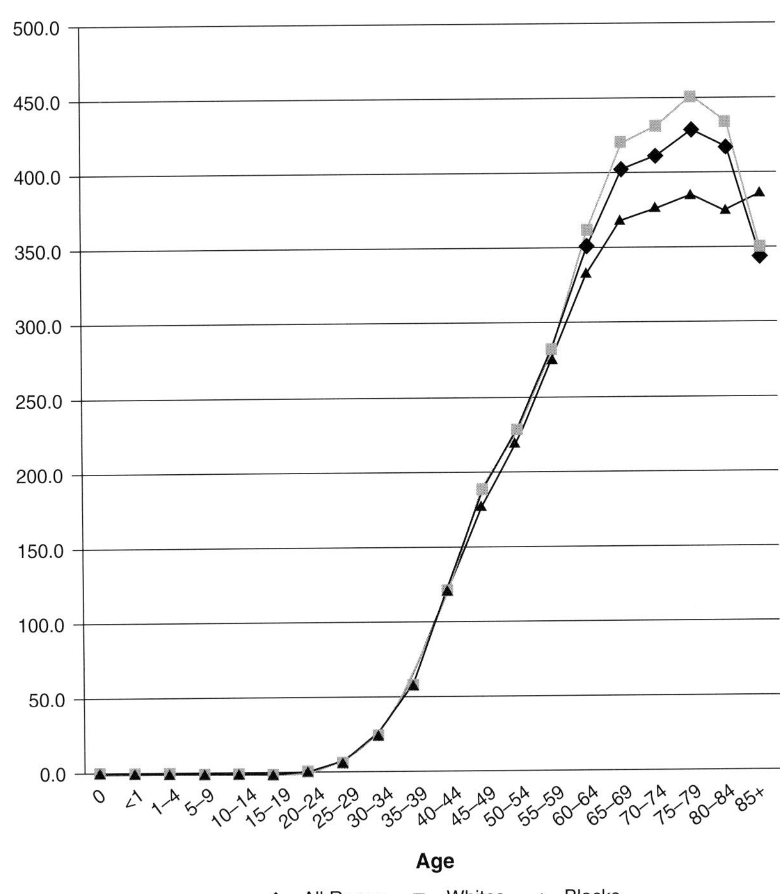

Fig. 20.13. National Cancer Institute SEER results for breast cancer: incidence and age at diagnosis 2004–2008. Note dramatic increase in acquired breast cancer throughout post-menopause. Drawn from data found in reference [100].

(androgen conversion) and higher *free* estrogen levels as obesity decreases sex hormone-binding globulin (SHBG)

However suggestive, these correlations do not clarify some contradictory clinical observations:

- Pre-menopausal bilateral oophorectomy without replacement estrogen *decreases* breast cancer incidence. Although their eventual overall risk is elevated, ovary intact obese pre-menopausal women experience a *decreased* risk of breast cancer compared with lean pre-menopausal subjects
- Pre-menopausal women are at *low risk* of breast cancer despite production of logarithmic increments of estradiol over at least 4 decades of full reproductive function compared with the post-menopause when breast cancer incidence risk rises exponentially.

Reviewed later in this chapter, it is important to note here that the CEE-alone arm of the WHI trial used therapeutic levels of this biologically active estrogen far exceeding the endogenous concentrations of the post-menopause. Nevertheless, CEE recipients showed a statistically significant *decrease* in the incidence of invasive breast cancer compared with the randomized placebo group [104].

In summary, returning to the potential link between obesity, endogenous estrogen production rates, and increased risk of post-menopausal breast cancer, although biologically plausible, the relationship in most studies is so marginal that reaching statistical significance is a struggle. Other stimulants of cancer progression must exist – either systemic or localized to the breast itself.

What other factor(s) might be responsible for stimulation and progression of occult disease or induce de novo initiation of ER- and PR-linked breast cancer in post-menopausal women?

The effect of weight, BMI, and diet on post-menopausal breast cancer

Although probably not associated with increased circulating estrogen production as the stimulant for breast cancer, increased BMI and greater weight gain over the menopausal transition is associated with a higher risk of the disease [105]. Weight loss due to caloric restriction and exercise reduces the risk of breast cancer (RR = 0.55; CI, 0.41–0.69) [106,107].

Dietary fat intake

There appears to be a greater risk of invasive breast cancer with higher dietary fat intake. In the prospective NIH/AARP Diet and Health Study, women in the highest quintile of fat intake (median 90 g/day, 40% of total calories from fat) experienced rates of invasive breast cancer 11–22% higher than those of women in the lowest quintile (median 24.2 g/day, or 20% of calories from fat) [108].

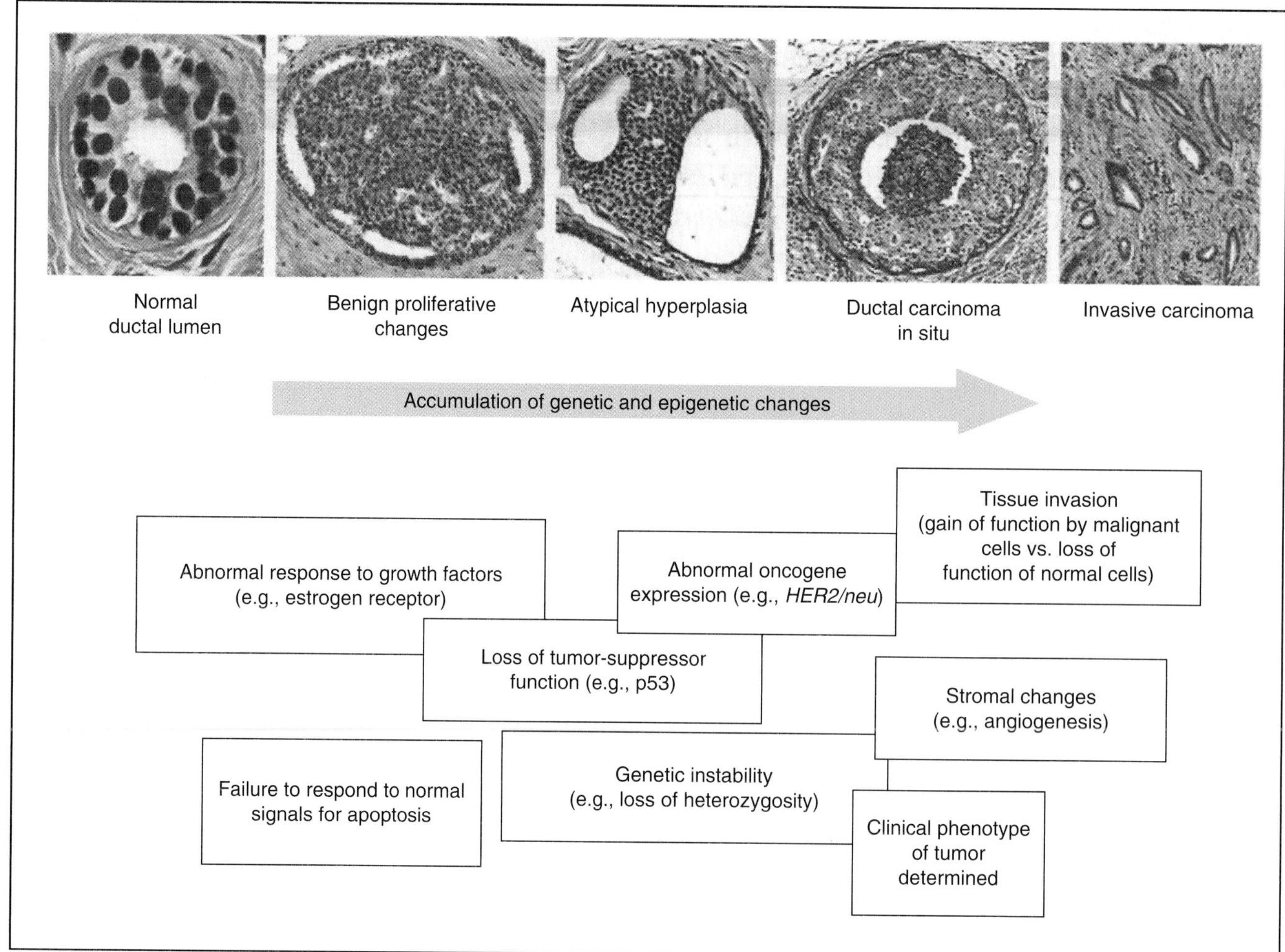

Fig. 20.14. "Silent" DCIS. Genetic changes, oncogene expression, and loss of normal cell cycle regulation occur before and during early DCIS. However, less than 50% of DCIS progress to invasive disease in 10 years. Reproduced from reference [103], with permission.

Physical activity

A more consistent protective effect on breast cancer incidence is achieved by regular strenuous exercise [109–112] as opposed to dietary caloric intake alone. Benefits accrue to women who engage in the equivalent of 10 hours or more per week of brisk walking, particularly if they were in the lowest tertile of BMI.

In summary and to varying degrees, obesity, the rate of increase and when weight gain occurs, diet, and physical activity contribute to the emergence of breast cancer in the post-menopause.

Post-menopausal breast cancer and the MetS

Insulin and insulin-like growth factors (IGF-1, IGF-2)

Historically, the linkage to carcinogenesis of the three growth-stimulating hormones insulin, IGF-1 and IGF-2 [113] was limited to studies correlating diet and calories with breast cancer incidence (Fig. 20.16) [114]. The positive impact of early and sustained lifestyle interventions suggested a role for chronic hyperinsulinemia and hyperglycemia in the promotion of breast cancer.

Epidemiologic findings re-opened a possibility of linkage: therapy with insulin and insulin secretagogues in individuals with type II diabetes were at a higher risk of dying from various cancers compared with individuals with normal body mass index and without diabetes [115,116].

IGF-1R is frequently over expressed during mammary cell transformation [117]. Consistent with these studies, a Nurses' Health Study cohort correlated IGF-1R expression levels in benign breast biopsies with subsequent risk of breast cancer [118]. Down-regulation of the insulin receptor (IR) in cancer cells reduced cell proliferation, angiogenesis, lymphangiogenesis, and metastases [117]. Finally, the insulin receptor isoform IR-A [119] specifically activates cancer cell proliferation and anti-apoptotic pathways in tumors.

Glucose levels also affect cancer biology. In vivo studies of colon, breast, prostate, and bladder cancer cells grown in hyperglycemic conditions show accelerated growth upon the addition of insulin [120].

Does *reducing* insulin levels or blocking insulin signaling inhibit tumor growth [121]? Observational studies suggest metformin may protect against cancer development. In a group of patients with type 2 diabetes mellitus,

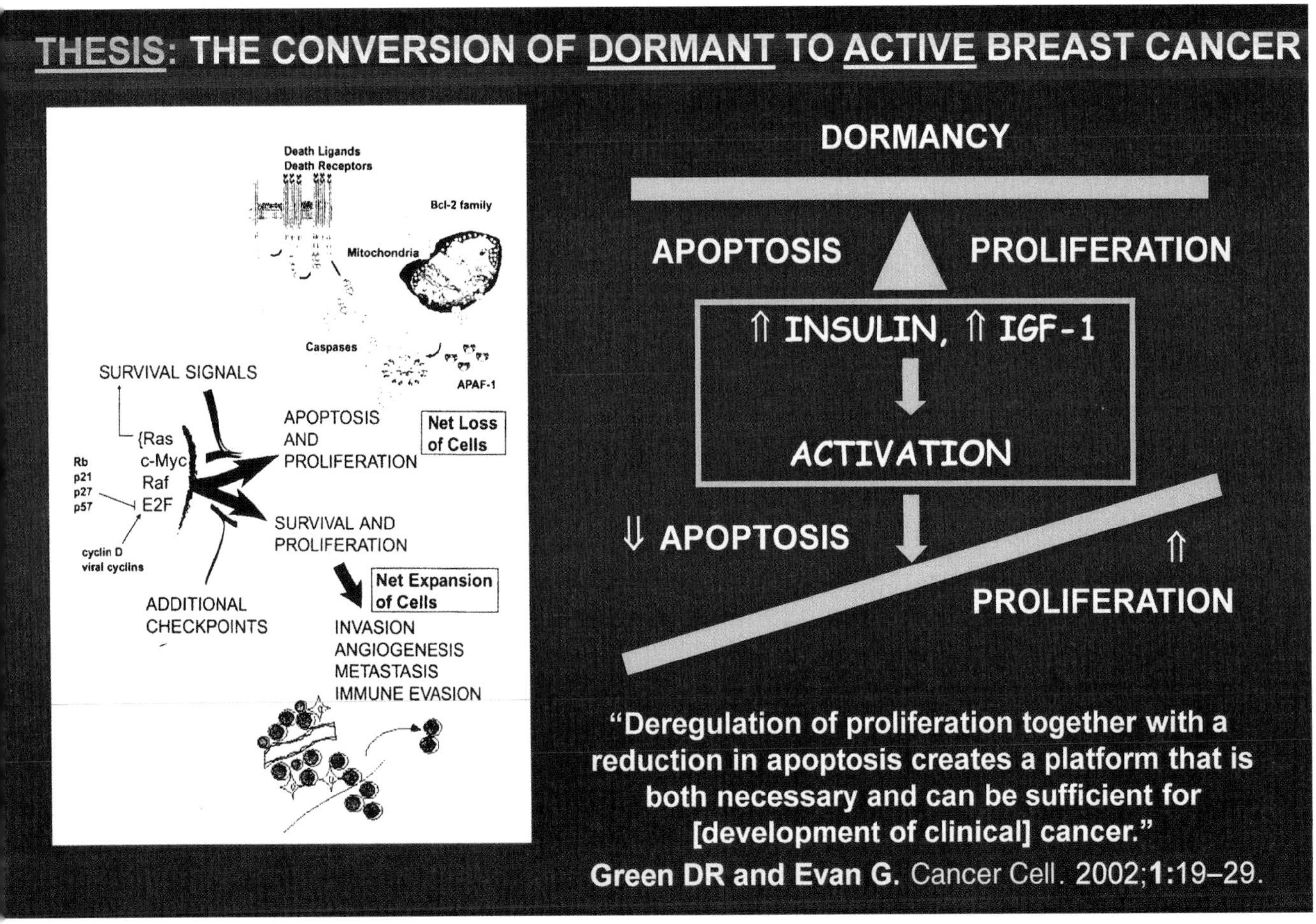

THESIS: THE CONVERSION OF DORMANT TO ACTIVE BREAST CANCER
Death Ligands
Death Receptors
Bcl-2 family
Mitochondria
Caspases
APAF-1
SURVIVAL SIGNALS
{Ras
c-Myc
Raf
E2F
Rb
p21
p27
p57
cyclin D
viral cyclins
APOPTOSIS
AND
PROLIFERATION
Net Loss
of Cells
SURVIVAL AND
PROLIFERATION
Net Expansion
of Cells
ADDITIONAL
CHECKPOINTS
INVASION
ANGIOGENESIS
METASTASIS
IMMUNE EVASION
DORMANCY
APOPTOSIS
PROLIFERATION
⇑ INSULIN, ⇑ IGF-1
ACTIVATION
⇓ APOPTOSIS
⇑
PROLIFERATION
"Deregulation of proliferation together with a reduction in apoptosis creates a platform that is both necessary and can be sufficient for [development of clinical] cancer."
Green DR and Evan G. Cancer Cell. 2002;1:19–29.

Fig. 20.15. Age, obesity, and breast cancer. Role of insulin and insulin-like growth factors. As growth factors and their cognate receptors increase and oncogene expression progresses, an imbalance between growth promotion (proliferation) and cell death (apoptosis) evolves. Reproduced from: Green DR and Evan GI. A matter of life and death. Cancer Cell, 2002;(1):19–29. With permission from Elsevier.

(a)
2.5
2.0
1.5
1.0
0.5
0.0
Relative risk
1%/year
0
5
10
15
20
25
Duration of use (years)
(b)
2.5
2.0
1.5
1.0
0.5
0.0
Relative risk
8%/year
0
5
10
Duration of use (years)

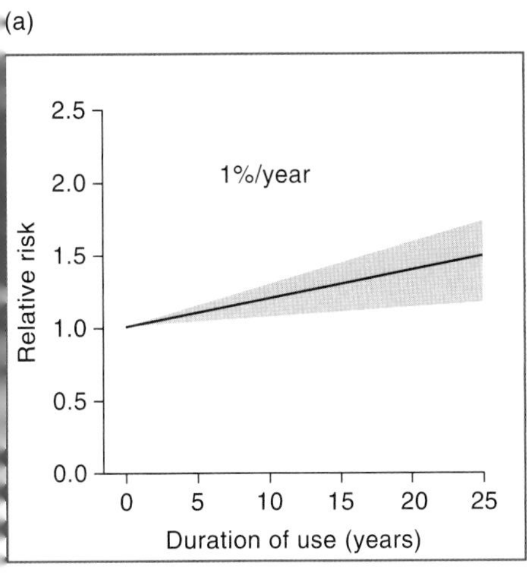

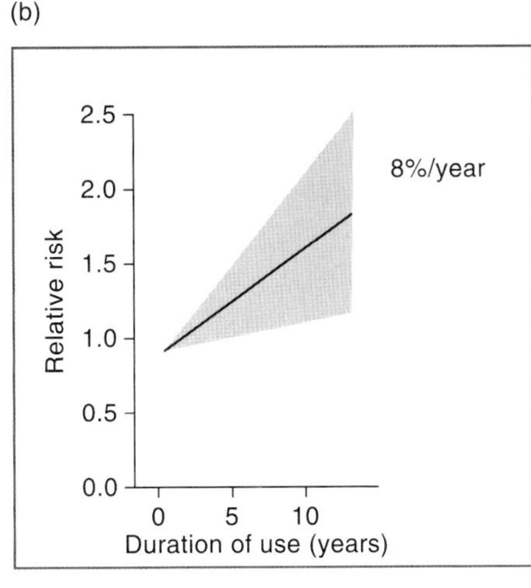

Fig. 20.16. Disparate impact of CEE only (a) and CEE+MPA (b) on the incidence of breast cancer with hormone therapy in the WHI trials. There was progestin-specific accelerating effect on breast cancer. Redrawn from: Schairer C, et al. Menopausal estrogen and estrogen-progestin replacement therapy and breast cancer risk. JAMA 2000;**283**(4):485–91, with permission.

those taking metformin had a lower risk of developing cancers of many types compared with those not taking metformin [122].

In summary, the combined effects of excess insulin stimulation of growth and nutritional support by hyperglycemia may stimulate neoplastic disease in general and breast cancer in post-menopausal women with MetS in particular.

Hypercholesterolemia and breast cancer

27-Hydroxycholesterol is an endogenous agonist at the breast [123]

Breast cancer incidence increases with age and obesity. The incidence accelerates unabated after menopause; up to 85% of human breast cancer occurs in the post-menopausal decades.

Despite the decline of circulating E2 in these women, ER⊕ and PR⊕ breast cancer is the prevalent form of this cancer in this age group. The main circulating metabolite of cholesterol is 27-OH cholesterol (27-OHC). 27-OHC displays *partial agonist* activity in cellular models of normal human breast and breast cancer cell lines, where it functions at physiologic concentrations (but with lower efficacy than E2). Both E2 and 27-OHC activate the transcriptional activity of ERα (the dominant ER subtype in breast epithelium) in target gene expression, recruit the ligand-ERα complex to the DNA ERE, and induce proliferation of ERα positive breast CA cells. 27-OHC, as an E2 agonist activates typical biologic estrogen function by increasing concentrations of progesterone receptor (PR) protein.

27-OHC is capable of inducing ERα activation as estrogen concentrations fall to low levels in post-menopause.

These observations may explain in part why obese/hypercholesterolemic women incur increased risk, progression, and worse prognosis of breast cancer. Furthermore, 27-OHC would be unaffected by aromatase inhibitor therapies.

Progesterone as an exogenous mammary gland agonist [124]

Mammary stem cells (MaSCs) give rise to all cells of the mammary gland including PR⊕ cancer cells. Progesterone activation of PR leads to cell proliferation. During pregnancy, in response to rising P levels PR⊕ mammary cells secrete RANKL which activates MaSC proliferation in preparation for adequate lactation capacity.

Could pharmacologic levels of progestin combined with other growth stimulators activate a malignant breast cancer clone or induce progression of clinical breast cancer?

The effects of hormone therapy in the menopause

Hormone therapy and cardiovascular disease: evidence from observational studies [1,3,4]

This massive literature, much still clinically informing, has been fully reviewed and assessed in the reports of The Endocrine Society [3] and the American Association of Clinical Endocrinologists [4]. Although replaced by prospective randomized trials (WHI) and subsequent iterations, by size and duration the Nurses Health Study (NHS) is worthy of specific mention [125]. With more than 20 years of follow-up the age-adjusted risk of CHD in current hormone users was reduced by 39% (RR = 0.61; CI, 0.52–0.71). Benefit was accrued at both 0.625 mg and 0.3 mg CEE doses. The benefit began to wane 3 years after discontinuation of therapy. Continuing users maintained a 37% reduced all cause mortality (due largely to less CHD) independent of diet, alcohol intake, aspirin use, or exercise. In this regard, in the WHI CAC scores were significantly lower in women on CEE [126].

Stroke

In contrast to the uniform results of the association between post-menopausal hormone therapy and coronary heart disease in observational studies, epidemiologic data over the past 30 years regarding estrogen use and stroke have not been consistent. This uncertainty is evident in studies in which either a small increase, no effect or a reduction in the risk of stroke associated with estrogen or estrogen-progestin use was observed [127–129].

Hypertension is both a risk factor for cardiovascular mortality and a common problem in older women. Studies have either shown no effect or a small statistically significant decrease in blood pressure due to estrogen treatment in both normotensive and hypertensive women. The addition of a progestin did not affect this response [130].

Cardiovascular disease: evidence from randomized, prospective clinical trials

The Women's Health Initiative

The Women's Health Initiative (WHI) was organized by the National Institutes of Health in 1992 to study the health of post-menopausal women [131]. From 1993 to 1998, the WHI enrolled 161,809 women ages 50 to 79 in 40 clinical centers. The major components of the WHI were: (1) two randomized trials of post-menopausal hormone therapy scheduled to conclude in 2005, (2) a dietary modification trial randomizing 48,000 women to either a sustained low-fat or self-determined diet, (3) a calcium/vitamin D supplementation trial, and (4) an observational study. One of the post-menopausal hormone therapy trials, the combined CEE plus MPA arm (daily 0.625 mg CEE and 2.5 mg medroxyprogesterone acetate), randomized 16,608 women to either treatment or placebo. The other arm of the hormone trial, an estrogen-only arm (daily 0.625 mg CEE) randomized 10,739 hysterectomized women to treatment or placebo.

The Estrogen plus progestin arm

In May 2002, the Data and Safety Monitoring Board (DSMB) made its periodic review of the data accumulated by the WHI. As a result in July 2002 the DSMB announced two recommendations: (1) discontinue the trial arm administering daily estrogen-progestin and (2) continue the daily unopposed estrogen trial arm. The combined estrogen–progestin arm was discontinued because the anticipated decrease in breast cancer was accompanied by an unexpected *increase* in cardiovascular events [131].

Estrogen-only arm

In 2004, the NHLBI also canceled the estrogen-only arm of the WHI. This arm included 10,739 hysterectomized, post--menopausal women who had completed an average of 6.8 years of follow-up [132].

Revision and reanalysis

The results of coronary heart disease (CHD) risk in the CEE+MPA arm were revised after reversal of the local diagnoses [133]. Central adjudication disagreed with 10% of the diagnoses for myocardial infarction and 3% for death due to coronary heart disease. This reduction changed the strength of the conclusions of the initial report. In the updated report, the overall results do not achieve statistical significance. Furthermore only the first year results were statistically significant in the year-by-year analysis, suggesting the WHI might have been a secondary prevention trial in which clinically silent but significant arteriosclerotic cardiovascular disease existed.

Age effects

In subgroup analyses, only the women in the estrogen-progestin arm who were 20 or more years distant from menopause incurred the statistically significant increased risk of coronary heart disease. Excluding this group from the analysis, an identical prevalence of coronary heart disease event in both the treated and placebo groups is observed [3,6]. As early as 2004, sub-analysis of the data from the estrogen-only arm indicated that younger women 50–59 years of age experienced a reduced risk of coronary heart disease [132].

Duration of use

Further uncertainty might have arisen from disparate dropout rates; 40.5% of the estrogen–progestin group were unblinded because of vaginal bleeding and left the study in contrast to only 6.8% of the placebo group [134]. The impact of this development blurs the assessment of CVD risk in the study; the high dropout rates influences any duration of use effect. For example, a case–control study in the United Kingdom found a significant reduction in the risk of myocardial infarction only with the use of hormone therapy for more than 5 years [135].

Women with significant menopausal symptoms had been excluded from the study to avoid a high drop-out rate in the placebo group. Women who had been on hormone therapy (about 25% of the initial pool of participants in the estrogen-progestin arm and 35% in the estrogen-only arm) underwent a 3-month "washout" period. Those that experienced menopausal symptoms were discouraged from participation. This exclusion left only a small number of participants in the WHI who were close to the age of menopause (16.5% of the participants in the estrogen-progestin arm were less than 5 years since their menopause) [134].

Dose effect

Clarkson and colleagues had studied the effects of a lower-dose estrogen in a monkey model of coronary atherosclerosis [136]. The monkeys were fed an atherogenic diet calculated to induce atherosclerosis comparable to that observed in post-menopausal women. After oophorectomy, the animals were randomized to treatment for 2 years with a placebo or a dose of CEE equivalent to 0.3 mg/day in women. This dose had no effect on circulating lipid levels; nevertheless the treated animals had an average 52% reduction in coronary atherosclerosis. The degree of protection was similar to studies in this model using a dose of CEE to 0.625 mg/day [136].

In the NHS prospective observational study of post-menopausal hormone therapy and primary prevention of cardiovascular disease, the risk of CHD in users versus never users on both 0.3 mg and 0.625 mg CEE was the same RR=0.61 (0.52–0.71) [137].

Stroke [138–140]

Stroke is the leading cause of prolonged adult disability and the third leading cause of death among women. The incidence increases steeply with age. As in CHD, the age-specific incidence is lower in women than men until late old age. Because of women's longer life expectancy, a woman's lifetime risk of stroke is about 1 in 5, higher than that of men.

Reviewed earlier in this chapter and extensively in Chapter 2, estrogen exerts positive effects in brain, vascular endothelium, lipids, inflammatory pathways, and relevant blood elements. Consequently, it would be expected to be as effective in stroke risk reduction as in CHD. However, both the randomized control trials of WHI and the large NHS cohort do not support this thesis; in the WHI CEE-alone or CEE +MPA arms non-fatal ischemic stroke risk increased by about 1/3; CEE with MPA (RR=1.31; 95% CI, 1.02–1.68); CEE without MPA (RR = 1.37; 95% CI, 1.09–1.73) [141,142]. The absolute excess risk was estimated as 4.5 additional strokes per 1,000 women per 5 years of use [3]. In these studies, there was no indication that risk or rate was modified by preparation type (see dose below).

In the original report, the increased risk was observed for all women initiating hormone therapy whether at young ages and near menopause or at older ages or more than 10 years after menopause. Re-analysis however, showed short-term (<5 years) hormone therapy initiated at menopause and younger ages was not associated with an increase in a stroke. However, this result was based on a small number of cases [6]. In the NHS, the attributable risk of stroke is relatively low in younger women [50–54] – 2 cases of stroke per 100,000 women/year on hormones [143].

The Nurses' Health Study reported an update of its data [142] adjusted for age, BMI, cholesterol levels, diabetes, hypertension, smoking, and family history of early coronary heart disease. The relative risks observed for ischemic stroke are virtually identical to the WHI results.

Current use of estrogen alone: RR = 1.39 (CI, 1.18–1.63)
Current use of estrogen-progestin: RR = 1.53 (CI, 1.21–1.95)

However, the NHS reported elimination of the increased risk of stroke with a decreased dose of estrogen (*P* for trend was < .001):

0.3 mg estrogen	25 cases	RR = 0.93 (95% CI, 0.62–1.40)
0.625 mg	268 cases	RR = 1.54 (95% CI, 1.31–1.81)
1.25 mg	60 cases	RR = 1.62 (95% CI, 1.23–2.14)

Furthermore, this possible dose-related benefit was not associated with a loss of CHD protection.

In a WHI reanalysis in which women with prior cardiovascular disease or older than 60 years of age were excluded, the risk of stroke was not significantly increased in women less than 10 years since their menopause [144].

In a nested case–control study deriving data from a cohort of women in the U.K. General Practice Research Database

(GPRD), current use of oral and transdermal hormone therapy based on recorded prescriptions was compared with no use in 15,710 cases and close to 60,000 controls. The adjusted rate risk ratio (RR) for stroke for current use of transdermal estrogens, with or without a progestin, was not increased (RR, 0.95; 95% CI, 0.75–1.20) compared with a significant increase associated with oral estrogen, with or without a progestin (RR, 1.28; 95% CI, 1.15–1.42). There was an indication of a dose–response relationship; a significant increase in risk was observed with transdermal estrogen doses greater than 50 μg but no increased risk with transdermal treatment at doses of 50 μg or less. The higher concentrations of circulating biologically active estrogen, not the route of administration or the type of estrogen, is implicated in stroke risk [145].

The timing hypothesis [3,6]

The importance of the timing of initiating hormone administration and the duration of the interval in availability of endothelial protection is a fundamental question in ongoing basic and clinical hormone research. In this respect, the timing hypothesis stipulates that estrogen can reduce the risk of coronary heart disease when administered to relatively young postmenopausal women before atherosclerosis has developed to the stage of unstable plaques (plaques with necrosis and inflammation). Timing hypothesis predicts that protection from CHD is evident only when hormone therapy is initiated proximal to the onset of menopause and before the development of advanced atherosclerosis.

The WHI investigators conducted a secondary analysis of the two canceled clinical trial arms [3,6,144]. The results in the estrogen-only arm, the combined estrogen–progestin arm, and with all participants combined were separated into age groups at randomization, 50–59, 60–69, and 70–79 and according to years since menopause (<10, 10–19 and 20 or more). An increased risk for coronary heart disease was present only in the oldest women in the trials. There were no increases for CHD, stroke, or total mortality in women aged 50–59. Only the increase in CHD events in women 20+ years since menopause reached statistical significance. On the other hand, a statistically significant reduced risk was present for total mortality in women aged 50–59.

Duration effects

A re-examination of data from the WHI suggests reduced coronary heart disease risk may appear only after 5 to 6 years of treatment. Risk ratios for coronary heart disease were calculated as 1.08 (95% CI, 0.86–1.36) in years 1 to 6 and 0.46 (95% CI, 0.28–0.78) in years 7 [146] in the CEE alone arm. Beneficial effects occur not only with early initiation but also prolonged exposure to estrogen.

Cancer and hormone therapy

Breast cancer and menopausal hormone therapy

As a result of over 50 case–control and cohort studies and at least seven meta-analyses, the Nurse's Health Study and in particular the more recent WHI trials have now provided sufficient explicit epidemiologic and disease incidence data on the relationship between hormone therapy and breast cancer to assemble a personal benefit/risk ratio which balances quality of life, CVD risk, and osteoporosis against hormone-related breast cancer risk [6,147].

The cancelled CEE+MPA arm of the WHI trial found an increased risk of breast cancer that rose rapidly and reached significance by the fifth year of exposure (Fig. 20.16) [148]. However, the cancelled CEE-only arm not only did not demonstrate increased risk over the duration of the study risk but on reanalysis *reached* statistical significance. Follow-up studies have indicated a reduced incidence of breast cancer in former uses [104].

An exploratory analysis of the updated WHI results reported a 33% reduction in invasive breast cancer (IBC) incidence in patients who strictly adhered to their estrogen only therapy (HR, 0.67; 95% CI, 0.47–0.97). In addition, a 31% lower incidence of localized breast cancer DCIS (HR, 0.69; 95% CI, 0.51–0.95) and a 29% reduction in ductal cancers (HR, 0.71; 95% CI, 0.52–0.99) were reported among women who used estrogen alone. Concurrent observational data from the Nurses' Health Study (NHS) suggested a 26% decrease in breast cancer risk in obese women (HR, 0.74; 95% CI, 0.55–1.00), and a non-significant 10% decrease in all study participants who took estrogen alone for 5–9 years [149]. Overall, these results are suggestive of a *beneficial* effect of exogenous estrogen on breast cancer risk over a *short-term* of 10 years. However, longer term use (>20 years) of therapeutic doses of exogenous estrogen increases breast cancer risk [150]. The Nurse's Health Study (NHS) evaluated post-menopausal women who used estrogen alone for > 20 years and found a slow, progressive increase in breast cancer incidence which became statistically significant compared with non-users at 15–18 years of use and beyond 20 years rose to a 42% increase in breast cancer risk in all women (HR, 1.42; 95% CI, 1.13–2.77) and a 77% increase in a subset of lean women (HR, 1.77; 95% CI, 1.26–2.48).

The WHI confirmed recipients with a positive family history of breast cancer do not incur an increased risk with CEE-alone therapy. Furthermore, all disease encountered on therapy was associated with better survival rates than non-users.

Most studies examining breast cancer mortality rates of women using post-menopausal hormone therapy at the time of diagnosis have documented improved survival rates. Tumors found in users were smaller, yet more easily detected by screening. There were more non-invasive DCIS and more well-differentiated lower grade and stage invasive tumors compared with nonusers, evidence consistent with stimulation of pre-existing undiagnosed tumors.

Surveillance/detection bias is not the only explanation for better survival. Lower grade tumors were diagnosed independent of the frequency of mammographic screening or the detection methodology used.

At least three elements underlie the paradoxical U shape relationship between estrogen and breast cancer incidence:

- The WHI reported an *overall* reduction in breast cancer incidence induced by exogenous estrogen therapy when administered in the first decade post-menopause. However, if hormone is initiated within 2–3 years of menopause no statistically significant reduction can be demonstrated. The reduction in breast cancer was seen in the recipients who began CEE-alone later beyond 2–3 years post-menopause and was responsible for the numeric shift that made the overall reported incidence statistically significant. This hiatus effect in hormone availability has become known as the "gap" period [3,6].
- A substantial reservoir of undiagnosed pre-existing occult breast cancers may exist in women who start hormone therapy at menopause. The brief initial "spike" in diagnosis of disease induced by CEE-alone possibly reflects acute stimulation of this previously occult pool of disease to a now diagnosable advanced DCIS or early invasive disease state.
- Several studies have assessed the frequency of occult malignant disease, primarily ductal carcinoma in situ (DCIS), found at autopsy in women aged 40 years to >70 years with no history of breast cancer [151]. The frequency of occult DCIS varied considerably among the studies (0–15%), undoubtedly reflecting methodological differences. Nevertheless, of the 952 total cases from these studies approximately 7% showed DCIS and 1% occult IBC. The fact that in some studies undiagnosed *multi-focal* lesions were found in one breast and *bilateral disease* in perhaps 25% of positive autopsies is concerning [151]. It is reasonable to assume, therefore, that 5–10% of the women who participated in the WHI had occult breast cancer at enrollment which might have been responsible for the acute appearance of breast cancer immediately after CEE administration at menopause. By contrast, increased long-term breast cancer risk as seen in the NHS might reflect initiation and promotion of de novo tumors [152].

The commonly accepted explanation for why long-term estrogen therapy increases breast cancer risk is that locally produced estrogen stimulates expression of breast cancer proliferation genes, increases the rate of breast cell division and enhances the chance of mutation [147].

These observations suggest that both direct genotoxic effects and E–ER-mediated promotional mechanisms might be responsible for the long-term carcinogenic effects of estrogen.

The estrogen-progestin arm of the WHI produced a substantially different outcome. CEE+MPA induced earlier appearance of increased numbers of breast cancers. That WHI participants included a large number of older, obese, current, and past smokers is evidence of the deleterious effect of lifestyle and diet not just in CVD risk but also cancer incidence. While the adverse impact of MPA is probably the inciting biologic factor in these observations, the susceptibility of the population studied and the likelihood of occult cancer being present in this group must also contribute to these findings [134].

These conclusions support the notion that CEE+MPA accelerates the growth of a malignant locus already in place but also leads to early detection, improved survival rates, lower frequency of late stage disease, and better differentiated lobular tumor [153–155].

The CEE+MPA increased risk disappears within 4 years of discontinuing therapy. Nevertheless, the impact of the progestin on breast cancer risk warrants alternative management strategies balancing competing breast cancer and endometrial cancer risks.

Other cancers

Endometrial cancer

Endometrial cancer is relatively common (40,000 cases annually). It announces its existence early by dysfunctional uterine bleeding; it can be diagnosed by transvaginal ultrasound endometrial stripe thickness measurement and readily confirmed by office aspiration biopsy [156,157].

Accordingly, it is diagnosed at early, well-differentiated stages and is a hormonally responsive cancer. Cure rates are high.

Endometrial cancers are rarely seen when repetitive ovulatory progesterone is available to opposed estrogen stimulation. Exogenous administration of estrogen in the absence of progestin induces progression to adenomatous hyperplasia and with time endometrial carcinoma in situ (ECIS) and finally invasive carcinoma. Estrogen therapy increases the incidence of endometrial cancer by a factor of 2–10 times over the baseline rate of 1:1000 in untreated post-menopausal women per year. The risk increases with duration and dose of estrogen is largely eliminated by the addition of progestin of adequate dose and duration (but not completely). Once established, ECIS may not respond to progestin intervention. For this reason, continuous progestin therapy for 3 years or more yields only a 76% reduction in risk but which persists after discontinuing therapy for at least 10 years. On the other hand, sequential therapies, i.e., continuous daily estrogen with 10–14 days of progestin every 3 months, increases risk 3 times greater than continuous combined therapy.

But as Taylor [6] points out, while continuous combined hormone regimens significantly but incompletely reduce endometrial cancer risks this benefit must be balanced with the less adverse effect of sequential regimens on the far more prevalent and dangerous breast cancer risk associated with continuous CEE+MPA. Sequential CEE+MPA has been shown to yield a smaller increase in relative risk of breast cancer compared with continuous progestin use. Norethisterone acetate (a 19-nor progestin) induces even higher risks than MPA [158].

These data profoundly influence therapeutic decisions. They link any synthetic progestin and by any route with the adverse effect on breast cancer incidence. The differences in the risk/benefit ratios governing the choice of regimens to reduce risk of endometrial cancer versus breast cancer is simple; to restrict progestin use to its only legitimate therapeutic target, i.e., the endometrium by means of a progestin-eluting IUD seems a mandatory component of all combined hormone therapy regimens in women with an intact uterus.

Ovarian cancer

Largely on the basis of the long-term reduction in ovarian cancer rates in recipients of combined OC [159], menopausal hormone use was not anticipated to be a risk factor for ovarian cancer in post-menopausal women. However, serial reports from the Cancer Prevention Study II of the American Cancer Society showed an increased risk of fatal ovarian cancer (RR, 2.20; 95% CI, 1.53–3.17) with CEE alone for 10 or more years. The annual age-adjusted ovarian cancer death rate per 100,000 women was 64.4 for users of 10 or more years compared with 26.4 for never users [1].

Data are also available on the risk of ovarian cancer in CEE+MPA users [160]. A population-based study involving a prospective cohort of Danish women aged 50–79 who used hormone therapy was followed from 1995 through 2005. Of the nearly 1 million women assessed for ovarian cancer, over 3,000 ovarian cancers were detected, of which 2,681 were epithelial cancers. Compared with women who never used hormone therapy, users had an increased risk for all ovarian cancers (RR, 1.38) and RR 1.44 (95% CI, 1.30–1.51) for epithelial cancers. The risk declined to baseline by 2 years after discontinuation of therapy and further significant decrease below baseline after 6 years.

Although ovarian cancer is increased by use of hormones the absolute risk is quite small; approximately one extra-ovarian cancer for every 8,300 women on hormone therapy per year [159,160]. Given the low lifetime risk for ovarian cancer (1.7%), benefit/risk analysis in the individual context is essential. The small incremental risk of ovarian cancer should not materially influence prescribing decisions.

Lung cancer

A similar benefit/risk question arises considering the impact of E + P therapy on lung cancer incidence and mortality [161]. The WHI showed a non-significant trend toward an increase in lung cancer in women receiving CEE + MPA compared with placebo. More concerning however, more CEE + MPA recipients died of NSC lung cancer and continued to incur increased mortality in the 2.7 years of follow-up after stopping hormones (HR = 1.71; 95% CI, 1.16–2.52). While the overall treatment with CEE+MPA may not increase the incidence of NSCLC, it does increase death from the disease and that risk continues after cessation of therapy.

Given all the incremental risks of smoking demonstrated in many studies, past and certainly current smoking should be a strong contraindication to all types of hormone replenishment therapy in menopausal women.

Colon cancer

A more positive picture emerges when colon cancer and menopausal hormone therapy is studied [162,163]. Observational studies and three metanalyses reported that colon cancer was decreased in current and past users of hormone therapy (E and E+P of various types and regimens) with persistent reduction more than 5 years after cessation of therapy. A metanalysis reported a 20% reduction in colon cancer incidence in ever users of E+P (RR = 0.80; 95% CI, 0.70–0.86) and a 34% reduc tion in current users compared with non-users.

Randomized controlled trials provide more detailed infor mation. The WHI CEE+MPA trial reported a decrease in inva sive colorectal cancer compared with placebo RR = 0.5 (95% CI, 0.38–0.81). Specifically for colon cancer RR = 0.5 (CI, 0.36–0.82) and for rectal cancer RR = 0.66 (95% CI, 0.26–1.64). Further analysis revealed that while the incidence wa different, invasive colo-rectal cancers were similar for both th CEE+MPA and placebo groups with respect to location, tumo grade, and histologic features. However, there was more lymph node involvement, and more advanced stage at diagnosis in th CEE+MPA cancers than placebo tumors. More regional an metastatic disease was found. CEE alone showed no statisticall different colon cancer incidence than placebo (RR 1.12 ([95% CI, 0.77–1.63]).

Planning routine colonoscopy beginning at 50 is manda tory, regardless of hormone treatment decision.

A clinical approach to post-menopausal hormone therapy

The challenges encountered by women as they traverse th menopausal transition have been examined in detail. Even fo "healthy" women the issues imposed by age and estrogen los can be significant: but in addition to those burdens, man women incur the compounding complications of viscera adiposity, evolving hypertension, increasing dyslipidemia impaired glucose tolerance, vascular endothelial dysfunction – an assembly of dysfunctions encapsulated in the complex o glucotoxicity, lipotoxicity, and the systemic inflammatory stat know as the MetS. Individually and collectively, these advers vascular, endocrine, and metabolic disturbances lead to th emergence of atherosclerotic cardiovascular disease, diabete mellitus, and cancer. It has also been shown (Chapter 2) tha estradiol acting through ERα and ERβ receptors materiall protects precisely those physiologic systems threatened by ag and the various elements of the MetS. However, the salutar effects of endogenous and/or exogenous estrogen depend on th presence of healthy, resilient tissues capable of responding t protective, function enhancing signals. In those circumstance estrogen does protect endothelial cells, neurons, and β cells. Bu once pathologic processes are under way, these E-related bene fits are lost and reversibility unlikely. The problem become acute when one appreciates the prolonged multi-decade sub clinical "silent" period all these disabling, life-threatening pro cesses pursue.

The dimensions and variety of these problems ar significant:

- The prolonged evolution of subclinical atherosclerosis
- Multi-decade insulin resistance precedes the micro and macro vascular changes of impaired glucose tolerance and final β cell exhaustion
- The presence of silent, indolent breast DCIS which slowl becomes diagnostically recognized by mammography a decade or more later

- Bone loss, presaged by inadequate bone deposition early in adolescence and in young adulthood, silently progresses until fracture, pain, and disability announces extreme skeletal fragility
- The still mystifying but prolonged incubation of neural tissue degeneration before serious cognitive loss and Alzheimer's disease is diagnosed.

Unfortunately, the dilemma facing women and their physicians is that paradoxically hormones thought to be protective when administered too late in the silent period leads not to benefit but exacerbation of vascular disease, acceleration of breast cancer, and probably dementia. The opportunities for "primordial" prevention, except by early in life and sustained positive lifestyle interventions (prudent diet, sufficient exercise, abstaining from smoking) exist but are unrealistic given current behavioral preferences. For epidemiologists, primary prevention is too simply "before an event occurs"; for clinicians primary prevention approaches the primordial pre-condition phase with decisive reaction to the first signs of emerging risk. For all women, immediate if not life-long institution of dietary and exercise programs is necessary.

All well and good – but is there a place for hormone replenishment in primary prevention? If so, this set of questions – "who, when, what, how, how much, and for how long" must be addressed. These are not idle questions. There are many valid reasons to offer hormone therapy to appropriate recipients because real benefits do accrue from prudent hormone administration:

- Improvement of the quality of life in the relief of hot flashes
- Protection against osteoporotic fractures, less osteoarthritis
- Reduction in colon cancer
- Reduction of new onset diabetes mellitus
- Maintenance of skin turgor and elasticity
- With appropriate timing, primary prevention of coronary artery events.

Furthermore, contrary to current public views, in many important respects the WHI results essentially support decades of observational research [1,3]:

- Coronary heart disease; protection in the recipient less than 10 years past menopause
- Stroke: no increase in early post-menopausal [50–54] healthy women
- Stabilization of bone mass density and reduction in osteoporotic fractures
- Reduction in overall mortality
- Reduction in type II diabetes mellitus.

Any yet:

- Contrary to the reduction in colon cancer, a small increase in ovarian cancer and lung cancer
- Increase in breast cancer on CEE+MPA but reduced risk in CEE-only recipients
- A two-fold increase risk of venous thromboembolism (VTE) in the first year of use, concentrated in those with recognized risk factors
- Increased cholecystitis on both CEE-only or CEE+MPA
- *Stroke*: increase estimated at a 0–5 excess risk/1,000 women using CEE-alone or CEE+MPA for 5 years or longer.

The following analysis should not detract from the need for application of specific therapies. Heeding the birth cohort effect emphasized in Berry et al. [90], in addition to life-style remedies, appropriately chosen statins, metformin, aspirin, angiotensin-converting enzyme (ACE) inhibitors, angiotensin receptor blockers (ARBs), and diuretics are essential elements of good medical practice.

Management decisions: hormone replenishment in the post-menopause

Who?

The Berry report confirms what observational studies and WHI have suggested; the presence of risk factors does stratify patients into groups who will most benefit or be at greatest risk for the cardiovascular effects of either CEE-alone or CEE+MPA therapy. In the original WHI study, 50% were past or current smokers and more than 1/3 were clinically obese, BMI (>30 kg/m^2). Guidance comes from Berry; at age 55, women with an optimal risk factor profile (the MetS elements and smoking not present) had longer survival and lower lifetime risks of myocardial infarction or stroke than women with two or more adverse factors. Taken together a combination of signs indicative of the clinically silent presence of atherosclerotic cardiovascular disease represents absolute exclusion criteria for either CEE only or CEE+MPA replenishment therapy.

When?

The "timing hypothesis" predicts that protection from cardiovascular events is evident when hormone therapy is initiated in younger women proximal to the onset of menopause [3,6]. Treatment remote from menopause on the other hand was either not beneficial or harmful. A retrospective review of this subject by the NHS investigators, defining proximity as within 4 years of menopause and distance from menopause as greater than 10 years, confirmed the validity of the timing hypothesis. In the WHI, CEE-alone initiated in young women (mean age 56) and within 10 years of menopause showed significantly lower CAC scores than placebo recipients. It is worth emphasizing here that the observational studies which had indicated as much as a 40–60% reduction in CHD events were performed in women who received CEE-alone or CEE+ MPA for VMS in the peri-menopause, at menopause, or shortly thereafter.

In summary, metabolically healthy women who begin hormone therapy at or shortly after menopause and are 50–54 years of age accrue CHD protection. Women 10 years or longer beyond menopause do not share such benefit.

The Endocrine Society Panel [3] dealt with the "CHD protection" issue correctly; "the major implication of these findings is that whereas menopausal hormone therapy is not recommended for [primary] CHD risk reduction, its use for other indications should not be hampered by fear of increasing CHD in younger, newly menopausal women."

In an unanticipated finding, the WHI trials showed no increase in breast cancer in the CEE-alone group over an average of 7 years, RR = 0.80 (95% CI, 0.62–1.04). In a subsequent sub-group analysis [104], women who were medication compliant had a significant reduction in breast cancer (which has persisted after discontinuation of CEE compared with placebo recipients).

What?

For all practical purposes, the bulk of evidence on which an estrogen product might be assessed for efficacy is based almost entirely on the multi-decade use of orally active CEE. However, the issue is not what estrogen is administered but by what route (oral or transdermal) and in what dose. Even more important is whether the commonly used orally active MPA is the correct choice, if any, of synthetic progestin.

The oral administration of MPA is solely intended to inhibit estrogen-induced endometrial hyperplasia and cancer. Although this intention was in part realized (there was no increase in endometrial cancer compared with non-recipients, as shown in Table 20.7), in every instance, MPA either worsened or did not add beneficial outcomes.

For most women, the issue of yes or no to any hormone use is whether it will increase breast cancer risk. MPA cannot be reassuring in this regard. There is more to the MPA story.

Other effects of MPA

MPA differs from progesterone in its effects on the brain [164,165]. Whereas E2 and progesterone sustain and enhance brain mitochondrial energy transduction capacity, MPA inhibits E2 clearance of accumulated lipid peroxides. MPA, unlike progesterone, induces a decline in glycolytic and oxidative phosphorylation activity. MPA is potentially detrimental to neuronal health.

With respect to mood, anxiety, or depression, serotonin regulation is pivotal. Whereas E2 increases tryptophan hydroxylase (the rate-limiting enzyme in serotonin synthesis) and progesterone has no modifying effect, MPA blocks this estrogen effect. MPA may potentiate stress and depression.

Table 20.7. Differential impact of ERT versus HRT

Clinical event	WHI estrogen + progestin	WHI estrogen alone
CHD events	1.29 (1.02–1.63)	0.91 (0.75–1.12) ← MPA
Pulmonary embolism	2.13 (1.39–3.25)	1.34 (0.87–2.06) ← MPA
Breast cancer	1.26 (1.00–1.59)	0.77 (0.59–1.01) ← MPA
Hip fracture	0.66 (0.45–0.98)	0.61 (0.41–0.91) ← CEE, MPA
Stroke	1.41 (1.07–1.85)	1.39 (1.10–1.77) ← CEE, MPA

In every instance, MPA either worsens or does not add benefit.

Taken together, the clinician must conclude that alternatives to MPA should be chosen. However, norethisterone has been shown to induce an even higher risk of breast cancer than MPA. High-frequency administration of oral micronized progesterone (100 mg twice or three times daily) for 10 days aside from its impracticality delivers incomplete endometrial protection. The use of continuous CEE plus progestin regimens for 3 years or more reduces endometrial cancer by 76% (95% CI, 6–60). Sequential therapies are not as efficacious. Use of a progestin every third month increases the risk of endometrial cancer by nearly 300%.

These data raise the important management dilemma alluded to earlier; if sequential or cyclic therapy increases the risk of endometrial cancer but has less adverse effect on breast cancer: How should the clinician resolve this conflict? What is the solution?

The increase in endometrial cancer, a cancer in which cure rates are high and early diagnosis feasible (ultrasound or office biopsy) and that may not even occur let alone be as aggressive with lower doses of estrogen, must be balanced against the greater adverse effect of sequential MPA on breast cancer. For this author, this is a non-issue; any increased risk of breast cancer must be avoided. Unlike cardiovascular risk, no stratification of potential breast cancer risk is available. Given the available alternatives to oral MPA and in all respects heavier burdens of breast cancer compared with endometrial disease, breast cancer risk avoidance takes precedence.

How?

The WHI trials made a valuable contribution by drawing attention to the risk associated with administration of CEE plus MPA in some post-menopausal women. Unfortunately, it generated considerable controversy in the field because it was interpreted as an indictment of post-menopausal hormone replacement when it did not study either. It did not use the natural human ovarian secretions of estradiol and progesterone. As noted above, MPA is not the same as progesterone. Simply put, to achieve a biologically plausible simulation of ovarian secretion, transdermal estradiol is the closest approximation currently possible.

Although women and their physicians prefer the ease and convenience of oral therapy, burdens accrue from oral administration as a result of portal absorption and "first-pass" hepatic clearance. Although application of transdermal E2 has not been studied as rigorously as oral therapy, that is, in large prospective randomized trials, Turgeon [166] has summarized these effects (Table 20.8). By avoidance of first-pass hepatic clearance and thus estrogen stimulation of the synthesis of a number of liver proteins, transdermal estradiol avoids the orally induced effects leading to sodium retention, increased inflammatory cytokines, decreased lean body mass, change in hormonal bioavailability, and increased thrombogenicity. Only

Table 20.8. Attributable risks of hormone content, duration, dosage, and portal of entry: the burden of oral administration and "first-pass" hepatic clearance

Potential liver targets in estrogen replacement	Transdermal	Oral	Potential effects with oral dosing
Angiotensin precursor	No change	↑	Sodium retention, vasoconstriction
C-reactive protein	No change	↑	Risk for atherosclerosis, ischemic stroke
GH-induced IGF-1	No change	↓	Decrease in lean body mass
Serum binding protein	No change	↑	Change in hormone bioavailability
Activated protein C	No change	↑ Resistance	Increased blood coagulation

From Turgeon et al. [166].

holesterol metabolism (increased HDL cholesterol) is improved y oral estrogen administration.

How to apply progesterone is less an issue of efficacy than atient compliance. The argument that oral progesterone is qually beneficial and less detrimental than MPA is not in ispute. But to expect patients to observe the dose and fre-uency required (2 weeks of every month) is unrealistic. For omen who will forego all progestins and accept periodic ultra-ound assessments (measuring endometrial stripe) and/or ffice aspiration biopsies, the solution is straight forward. For thers who are willing, the levonorgestrel progestin-eluting ntra-uterine device is the optimal solution. It provides local ndometrial inhibition without systemic absorption. Accordingly, it allows sufficient estrogen (oral CEE or E2 by atch) for target organ support (vascular, skeletal, and meta-olic) without the risk of endometrial cancer or the MPA-ssociated increase in breast cancer.

How much?

n almost all instances, control of the VMS symptoms of the arly post-menopause requires CEE intake of 0.625 mg per day. However, this is greater than the CEE doses needed to support nost estrogen-dependent systems. For example, skeletal stabil-ty is maintained on micro doses (0.025 μg and lower) of trans-ermal estrogen. There is emerging evidence that endothelial upport is achieved by low-dose replenishment (CEE 0.3 mg) or coronary and carotid arteries. The dose needed to control VMS should not be renewed continually past the phase of asomotor acclimation to lower estrogen concentrations. Once VMS control is established and sustained (several months r longer) on higher dose CEE or E2, slow, step-wise tapering of ormone will wean the patient from the now unnecessary (and otentially excess mammary gland stimulation) hormone levels o the lowest dose which maintains at once reasonable comfort, arget organ support and fewer concerns of safety – a well alanced benefit/risk ratio realized.

How long?

Two studies provide some guidance on the safest length of pplication of hormone therapy. However, each has cautionary mitations so that hard and fast rules cannot be fixed. The uthoritative reviews of the multiple WHI trials and re-analyses an provide only 5-year "risk" estimates for CEE + MPA and ossibly 7 years for CEE alone given the early termination of oth arms of the principal WHI RCTs. On the other hand, NHS has longer term data (20+ years) but as an observational study of a fairly homogeneous group of women, both concerns about the inherent confounding bias of an observational study and possible non-applicability to the ethnic and racial diversity of the general female population limits the value of the NHS findings in regard to duration of therapy.

These reservations aside, and adhering to the provisos regarding timing of initiation (closest to the start of menopause in women age 50 to 59) a reasonable strategy can be outlined (Fig. 20.17). In women with low Framingham coronary heart disease risk scores and less than a 10% risk of stroke by the Framingham Stroke Score (or alternatively by the Berry criteria of the presence of only one risk factor among smoking and the elements of the MetS), healthy women may use hormone ther-apy for up to 10 years. As new information evolves perhaps through the results of the KRONOS and ELITE (www.kronosin-stitute.org/keeps.html) and the Elite trial (http://clin-icaltrials.gov/show/NCT00114517) studies currently under way, these guidelines may be revised and refined and the dura-tion of use possibly extended.

Conclusion

An important aspect of management decisions is that the utility of hormone therapy of any type, dose, duration, or route of administration only applies to women with serious symptoms caused by moderate to severe VMS (hot flashes, intense sweating, and sleep deprivation) that diminish quality of life. Hormone therapy carries potential health risks, some of them serious. If there is either any hint of occult metabolic dysfunction or any identifiable risk factors requiring specific medical management, estrogen cannot be used as the primary therapy.

On the other hand, healthy young women proximal to meno-pause with none or one risk factor should not be discouraged from seeking quality of life enhancement with peri-menopausal or early menopause therapy.

Final notes

The WHI taught valuable lessons in management of meno-pause. Perhaps most important and provocative, it challenged scientists and clinicians to examine this central question: why would endogenous hormones, essential to health, when admin-istered exogenously not only fail to protect but cause harm?

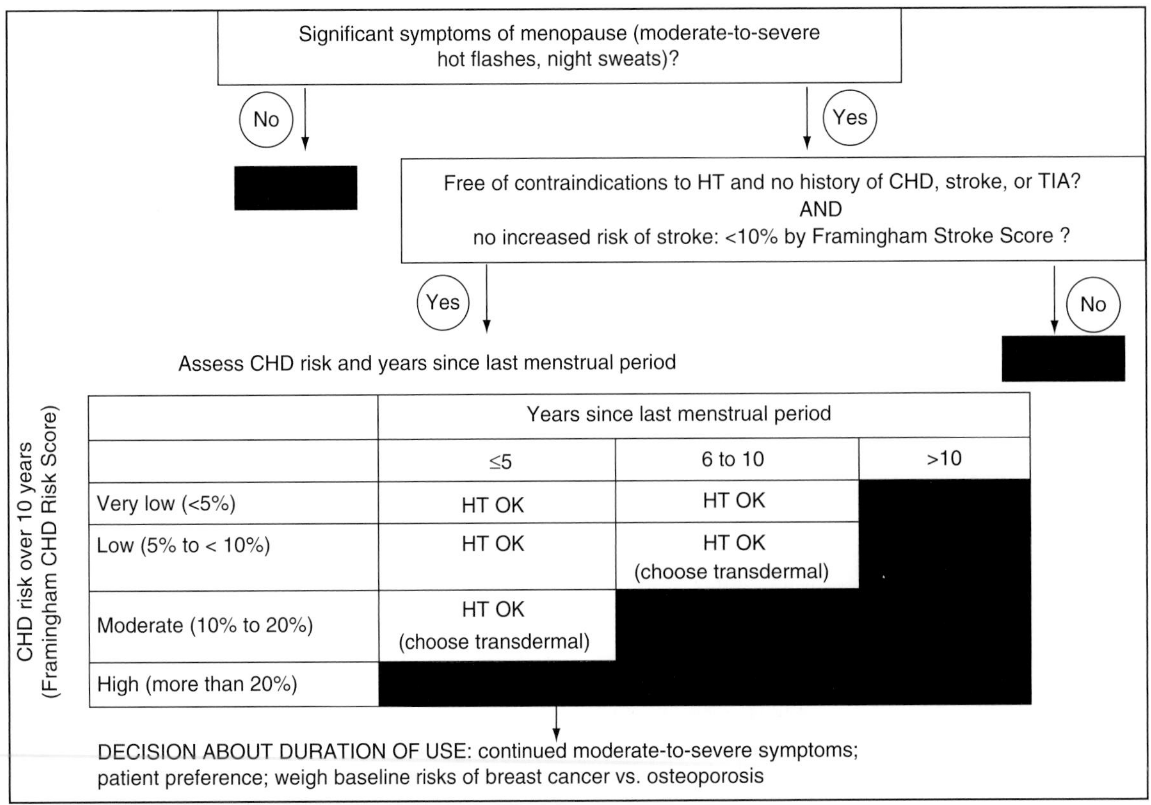

Fig. 20.17. Approach to the patient with menopausal symptoms. A suggested algorithm for maximal clinical benefit/risk hormone therapy (HT) management of the symptomatic young post-menopausal woman. CHD, coronary heart disease; TIA, transient ischemic attack. Adapted from Manson and Bassuk [167].

One answer must be emphasized: it is not that the importance of physiologic estradiol and periodic progesterone to the general health of all women is incorrect, but attempts to reproduce these salutary effects by current therapeutic modalities and strategies are imperfect, and may be hazardous to incompletely identified high-risk recipients.

In addition, clinical diagnostic and management decisions undertaken to support a woman's healthcare needs at any age, but particularly in the mid-life transition, must be organized to yield the maximal balance of efficacy and safety. Achieving this goal requires recognition and integration of the diverse, complex, and dynamic processes which initiate and accelerate disease. Furthermore, these decisions also derive from an understanding that pathogenetic mechanisms evolve silently over a substantial period of time and in variable patterns for populations, groups within populations, and between individuals. Prompt recognition of the earliest signs of emerging dysfunction and application of effective therapeutic reaction leads to stabilization, possible reversal, and hopefully avoidance of otherwise relentless progression of dysfunction and disease.

In this regard, clinical judgment cannot be the product of simple distillation of a list of digital facts that are either present or absent. It is ultimately a thinking process that is flexible, synthetic, and integrative. In short, the essence of effective clinical practice requires patient-specific pattern recognition in the clinical context, not just prevalence in the statistical context.

References

1. Fritz M, Speroff L. Menopause and the perimenopause. Chapter 17. In: Clinical Gynecologic Endocrinology and Infertility, 8th edition. Philadelphia: Wolters Klower; 2011. p 674–748.
2. Fritz M, Speroff L. Post menopausal hormone therapy. CHapter 18. In: Clinical Gynecologic Endocrinology and Infertility, 8th edition. Philadelphia: Wolters Klower: 2011. p 749–857.
3. Santen RJ, Allred DC, Ardoin SP, et al. Postmenopausal hormone therapy: an Endocrine Society scientific statement. J Clin Endocrinol Metab. 2010;**95**(7 Suppl 1):s1–s66.
4. American Association of Clinical Endocrinologists (AACE). In: Cobin RH, Petak SM (Eds.). Position Statement on Hormone Replacement Therapy (HRT) and Cardiovascular Risk. 2011 www.aace.com/.
5. Harlow SD, Gass M, Hall JE, et al. STRAW+10 Collaborative Group. Executive summary of the Stages of Reproductive Aging Workshop addressing the unfinished agenda of stages of reproductive aging. Fertil Steril. 2012;**97**(4):843–51.
6. Taylor HS, Manson JE. Update in hormone therapy use in menopause. J Clin Endocrinol Metab. 2011;**96**(2):255–64.

7. US Census Bureau Report. Table 2. www.census.gov/prof/cen2010/docsf1
8. Oktem O, Urman B. Understanding follicle growth in vivo. Hum Reprod. 2010;**25**(12):2944–54.
9. Voorhuis M, Broekmans FJ, Fauser BC, et al. Genes involved in initial follicle recruitment may be associated with age at menopause. J Clin Endocrinol Metab. 2011;**96**(3):E473–9.
10. Gold EB, Bromberger J, Crawford S, et al. Factors associated with age at natural menopause in a multiethnic sample of midlife women. Am J Epidemiol. 2001;**153**(9):865–74.
11. Snieder H, MacGregor AJ, Spector TD. Genes control the cessation of a woman's reproductive life: a twin study of hysterectomy and age at menopause. J Clin Endocrinol Metab. 1998;**83**:1875–80.
12. Therman E, Laxova R, Susman B. The critical region on the human Xq. Hum Genet. 1990;**85**(5):455–61.
13. Sala C, Arrigo G, Torri G, et al. Eleven X chromosome breakpoints associated with premature ovarian failure (POF) map to a 15-Mb YAC contig spanning Xq21. Genomics. 1997;**40**(1):123–31.
14. Stolk L, Perry JR, Chasman DI, et al. Meta-analyses identify 13 loci associated with age at menopause and highlight DNA repair and immune pathways. Nat Genet. 2012;**44**(3):260–8.
15. McKinlay SM, Bifano NL, McKinlay JB. Smoking and age at menopause in women. Ann Intern Med. 1985;**103**(3):350–6.
16. Tylavsky FA, Anderson JJ. Dietary factors in bone health of elderly lactoovovegetarian and omnivorous women. Am J Clin Nutr. 1988;**48** (3 Suppl):842–9.
17. McKinlay SM, Bifano NL, McKinlay JB. The normal menopause transition. Maturitas. 1992;**14**(2):103–15.
18. Treloar AE. Menarche, menopause, and intervening fecundability. Hum Biol. 1974;**46**(1):89–107.
19. Luborsky JL, Meyer P, Sowers MF, et al. Premature menopause in a multi-ethnic population study of the menopause transition. Hum Reprod. 2003;**18** (1):199–206.
20. Gosden RG, Faddy MJ. Ovarian aging, follicular depletion, and steroidogenesis. Exp Gerontol. 1994;**29**(3–4):265–74.
21. McGee EA, Hsueh AJ. Initial and cyclic recruitment of ovarian follicles. Endocr Rev. 2000;**21**(2):200–14.
22. WHO Scientific Group: Research on the menopause in the 1990s. Report of a WHO Scientific Group. World Health Organ Tech Rep Ser. 1996;**866**:1–79. Geneva, Switzerland: World Health Organization.
23. Randolph JF Jr, Zheng H, Sowers MR, et al. Change in follicle-stimulating hormone and estradiol across the menopausal transition: effect of age at the final menstrual period. J Clin Endocrinol Metab. 2011;**96**(3):746–54.
24. Faddy MJ, Gosden RG, Gougeon A, et al. Accelerated disappearance of ovarian follicles in mid-life: implications for forecasting menopause. Hum Reprod. 1992;**7**(10):1342–6.
25. Randolph JF Jr, Crawford S, Dennerstein L, et al. The value of follicle-stimulating hormone concentration and clinical findings as markers of the late menopausal transition. J Clin Endocrinol Metab. 2006;**91**(8):3034–40.
26. Neugarten BL, Kraines RJ. Menopausal symptoms in women of various ages. Psychosom Med. 1965;**27**:266–73.
27. Ballinger CB, Browning MC, Smith AH. Hormone profiles and psychological symptoms in peri-menopausal women. Maturitas. 1987;**9**(3):235–51.
28. Kronenberg F. Hot flashes: epidemiology and physiology. Ann N Y Acad Sci. 1990;**592**:52–86; discussion 123–33.
29. Iqbal J, Blair HC, Zallone A, Sun L, Zaidi M. Further evidence that FSH causes bone loss independently of low estrogen. Endocrine. 2012;**41**(2):171–5.
30. Sowers M, Crutchfield M, Bandekar R, et al. Bone mineral density and its change in pre-and perimenopausal white women: the Michigan Bone Health Study. J Bone Miner Res. 1998;**13**(7):1134–40.
31. Barbieri RL. Managing the Perimenopause. Washington DC: APGO; 2001.
32. Kase NG. Impact of hormone therapy for women aged 35 to 65 years, from contraception to hormone replacement. Gend Med. 2009;**6**(Suppl 1):37–59.
33. Longcope C, Franz C, Morello C, et al. Steroid and gonadotropin levels in women during the peri-menopausal years. Maturitas. 1986;**8**(3):189–96.
34. Longcope C, Jaffee W, Griffing G. Production rates of androgens and oestrogens in post-menopausal women. Maturitas. 1981;**3**(3–4):215–23.
35. Burger HG, Dudley EC, Cui J, et al. A prospective longitudinal study of serum testosterone, dehydroepiandrosterone sulfate, and sex hormone-binding globulin levels through the menopause transition. J Clin Endocrinol Metab. 2000;**85**(8):2832–8.
36. Adashi EY. The climacteric ovary as a functional gonadotropin-driven androgen-producing gland. Fertil Steril. 1994;**62**(1):20–7.
37. Janssen I, Powell LH, Crawford S, et al. Menopause and the metabolic syndrome: the Study of Women's Health Across the Nation. Arch Intern Med. 2008;**168**(14):1568–75.
38. Feldman S, Shapter A, Welch WR, et al. Two-year follow-up of 263 patients with post/perimenopausal vaginal bleeding and negative initial biopsy. Gynecol Oncol. 1994;**55**(1):56–9.
39. Kroon E, Andolf E. Diagnosis and follow-up of simple ovarian cysts detected by ultrasound in postmenopausal women. Obstet Gynecol. 1995;**85**(2):211–14.
40. Rossouw JE, Anderson GL, Prentice RL, et al. Risks and benefits of estrogen plus progestin in healthy postmenopausal women: principal results from the Women's Health Initiative randomized controlled trial. JAMA. 2002;**288**(3):321–33.
41. Williams RE, Kalilani L, DiBenedetti DB, et al. Frequency and severity of vasomotor symptoms among peri- and postmenopausal women in the United States. Climacteric. 2008;**11**(1):32–43.
42. Col NF, Guthrie JR, Politi M, et al. Duration of vasomotor symptoms in middle-aged women: a longitudinal study. Menopause. 2009;**16**(3):453–7.
43. Mohyi D, Tabassi K, Simon J. Differential diagnosis of hot flashes. Maturitas. 1997;**27**(3):203–14.
44. Sator PG, Sator MO, Schmidt JB, et al. A prospective, randomized, double-blind, placebo-controlled study on the influence of a hormone replacement therapy on skin aging in postmenopausal women. Climacteric. 2007;**10**(4):320–34.

45. Holland EF, Studd JW, Mansell JP, et al. Changes in collagen composition and cross-links in bone and skin of osteoporotic postmenopausal women treated with percutaneous estradiol implants. Obstet Gynecol. 1994;**83**(2):180–3.

46. Avis NE, Brambilla D, McKinlay SM, et al. A longitudinal analysis of the association between menopause and depression. Results from the Massachusetts Women's Health Study. Ann Epidemiol. 1994;**4**(3):214–20.

47. Busch CM, Zonderman AP, Costa PT. Menopausal transition and psychological distress in a nationally representative sample: Is menopause associated with psychological distress? J Aging Health. 1994;**6**:209–28.

48. Freeman EW, Sammel MD, Lin H, et al. Associations of hormones and menopausal status with depressed mood in women with no history of depression. Arch Gen Psychiatry. 2006;**63**(4):375–82.

49. Cohen LS, Soares CN, Vitonis AF, et al. Risk for new onset of depression during the menopausal transition: the Harvard study of moods and cycles. Arch Gen Psychiatry. 2006;**63**(4):385–90.

50. Bromberger JT, Kravitz HM, Matthews K, et al. Predictors of first lifetime episodes of major depression in midlife women. Psychol Med. 2009;**39** (1):55–64.

51. Osterlund MK. Underlying mechanisms mediating the antidepressant effects of estrogens. Biochim Biophys Acta. 2010;**1800**(10):1136–44.

52. Kawai M, Mödder UI, Khosla S, et al. Emerging therapeutic opportunities for skeletal restoration. Nat Rev Drug Discov. 2011;**10**(2):141–56.

53. National Osteoporosis Foundation. http://www.nof.org/prof/ 2009.

54. Holick MF. Vitamin D deficiency. N Engl J Med. 2007;**357**(3):266–81.

55. Wells G, Tugwell P, Shea B, et al. Meta-analyses of therapies for postmenopausal osteoporosis. V. Meta-analysis of the efficacy of hormone replacement therapy in treating and preventing osteoporosis in postmenopausal women. Endocr Rev. 2002;**23**(4):529–39.

56. Trémollieres FA, Pouilles JM, Ribot C. Withdrawal of hormone replacement therapy is associated with significant vertebral bone loss in postmenopausal women. Osteoporos Int. 2001;**12** (5):385–96.

57. Ettinger B, Ensrud KE, Wallace R, et al. Effects of ultralow-dose transdermal estradiol on bone mineral density: a randomized clinical trial. Obstet Gynecol. 2004;**104**(3):443–51.

58. Cummings SR, San Martin J, McClung MR, et al. Denosumab for prevention of fractures in postmenopausal women with osteoporosis. N Engl J Med. 2009;**361**(8):756–65.

59. Eghbali-Fatourechi G, Khosla S, Sanyal A, et al. Role of RANK ligand in mediating increased bone resorption in early postmenopausal women. J Clin Invest. 2003;**111**(8):1221–30.

60. Brown JP, Prince RL, Deal C, et al. Comparison of the effect of denosumab and alendronate on BMD and biochemical markers of bone turnover in postmenopausal women with low bone mass: a randomized, blinded, phase 3 trial. J Bone Miner Res. 2009;**24**(1):153–61.

61. Neer RM, Arnaud CD, Zanchetta JR, et al. Effect of parathyroid hormone (1–34) on fractures and bone mineral density in postmenopausal women with osteoporosis. N Engl J Med. 2001;**344**(19):1434–41.

62. Rosen CJ. The role of parathyroid hormone in the management of osteoporosis. Horm Res. 2005; **64**(Suppl 2):81–5.

63. Black DM, Bilezikian JP, Ensrud KE, et al. One year of alendronate after one year of parathyroid hormone (1–84) for osteoporosis. N Engl J Med. 2005;**353**(6):555–65.

64. Bolton JM, Targownik LE, Leung S, Sareen J, Leslie WD. Risk of low bone mineral density associated with psychotropic medications and mental disorders in postmenopausal women. J Clin Psychopharmacol. 2011;**31**(1):56–60.

65. Tankó LB, Søndergaard BC, Oestergaard S, et al. An update review of cellular mechanisms conferring the indirect and direct effects of estrogen on articular cartilage. Climacteric. 2008;**11**(1):4–16.

66. Cirillo DJ, Wallace RB, Wu L, et al. Effect of hormone therapy on risk of hip and knee joint replacement in the Women's Health Initiative. Arthritis Rheum. 2006;**54**(10):3194–204.

67. Semmens JP, Tsai CC, Semmens EC, et al. Effects of estrogen therapy on vaginal physiology during menopause. Obstet Gynecol. 1985;**66**(1):15–18.

68. Yamaguchi O, Nishizawa O, Takeda M, et al. For the Neurogenic Bladder Society. Clinical guidelines for overactive bladder. Int J Urol. 2009;**16**(2):126–42.

69. Perrotta C, Aznar M, Mejia R, et al. Oestrogens for preventing recurrent urinary tract infection in postmenopausal women. Cochrane Database Syst Rev. 2008;(**2**):CD005131.

70. Preisinger E, Alacamlioglu Y, Saradeth T, et al. Forearm bone density and grip strength in women after menopause, with and without estrogen replacement therapy. Maturitas. 1995;**21**(1):57–63.

71. Naessen T, Lindmark B, Larsen HC. Better postural balance in elderly women receiving estrogens. Am J Obstet Gynecol. 1997;**177**(2):412–6.

72. Meyer PM, Powell LH, Wilson RS, et al. A population-based longitudinal study of cognitive functioning in the menopausal transition. Neurology. 2003;**61**(6):801–16.

73. Smith YR, Giordani B, Lajiness-O'Neill R, et al. Long-term estrogen replacement is associated with improved nonverbal memory and attentional measures in postmenopausal women. Fertil Steril. 2001;**76**(6):1101–7.

74. Maki PM, Zonderman AB, Resnick SM. Enhanced verbal memory in nondemented elderly women receiving hormone-replacement therapy. Am J Psychiatry. 2001;**158**(2):227–33.

75. Yaffe K, Haan M, Byers A, et al. Estrogen use, APOE, and cognitive decline: evidence of gene–environment interaction. Neurology. 2000;**54**(10):1949–54.

76. Kawas C, Resnick S, Morrison A, et al. A prospective study of estrogen replacement therapy and the risk of developing Alzheimer's disease: the Baltimore Longitudinal Study of Aging. Neurology. 1997;**48** (6):1517–21.

77. Baldereschi M, Di Carlo A, Lepore V, et al. Estrogen-replacement therapy and Alzheimer's disease in the Italian Longitudinal Study on Aging. Neurology. 1998;**50**(4):996–1002.

78. Tang MX, Jacobs D, Stern Y, et al. Effect of oestrogen during menopause on risk and age at onset of Alzheimer's

disease. Lancet. 1996;**348**(9025):429–32.

79. Shumaker SA, Legault C, Rapp SR, et al. Estrogen plus progestin and the incidence of dementia and mild cognitive impairment in postmenopausal women: Women's Health Initiative Memory Study: a randomized controlled trial. JAMA. 2003;**289**(20):2651–62.

80. Espeland MA, Rapp SR, Shumaker SA, et al. Conjugated equine estrogens and global cognitive function in postmenopausal women: Women's Health Initiative Memory Study. JAMA. 2004;**291**(24):2959–68.

81. Zandi PP, Carlson MC, Plassman BL, et al. Hormone replacement therapy and incidence of Alzheimer disease in older women: the Cache County Study. JAMA. 2002;**288**(17):2123–9.

82. Crawford SL, Casey VA, Avis NE, et al. A longitudinal study of weight and the menopause transition: results from the Massachusetts Women's Health Study. Menopause. 2000;7(2):96–104.

83. Flegal KM, Carroll MD, Kit BK, Ogden CL. Prevalence of obesity and trends in the distribution of body mass index among US adults, 1999–2010. JAMA. 2012;**307**(5):491–7.

84. Ogden CL, Carroll MD, Kit BK, Flegal KM. Prevalence of obesity and trends in body mass index among US children and adolescents, 1999–2010. JAMA. 2012;**307**(5):483–90.

85. Carr MC. The emergence of the metabolic syndrome with menopause. J Clin Endocrinol Metab. 2003;**88**(6):2404–11.

86. de Luca C, Olefsky JM. Stressed out about obesity and insulin resistance. Nat Med. 2006;**12**(1):41–2; discussion 42.

87. National Health Statistics Reports #13, 2009.

88. St. Onge MP, Janssen I, Heymsfield SB. Metabolic syndrome in normal-weight Americans: new definition of the metabolically obese, normal-weight individual. Diabetes Care. 2004;**27**(9):2222–8.

89. Roger VL, Go AS, Lloyd-Jones DM, et al. Heart disease and stroke statistics – 2012 update: a report from the American Heart Association. Circulation. 2012;**125**(1):e2–220.

90. ADA Statistical Reports. 2011.

91. Berry JD, Dyer A, Cai X, et al. Lifetime risks of cardiovascular disease. N Engl J Med. 2012;**366**(4):321–9.

92. Matthews KA, Meilahn E, Kuller LH, et al. Menopause and risk factors for coronary heart disease. N Engl J Med. 1989;**321**(10):641–6.

93. McGill HC Jr, McMahan CA, Zieske AW, et al. Associations of coronary heart disease risk factors with the intermediate lesion of atherosclerosis in youth. The Pathobiological Determinants of Atherosclerosis in Youth (PDAY) Research Group. Arterioscler Thromb Vasc Biol. 2000;**20**(8):1998–2004.

94. Tirosh A, Shai I, Afek A, et al. Adolescent BMI trajectory and risk of diabetes versus coronary disease. N Engl J Med. 2011;**364**(14):1315–25.

95. Mendelsohn ME, Karas RH. The protective effects of estrogen on the cardiovascular system. N Engl J Med. 1999;**340**(23):1804–11.

96. Mendelsohn ME, Karas RH. Molecular and cellular basis of cardiovascular gender differences. Science. 2005;**308**(5728):1583–7.

97. Anasti JN, Kalantaridou SN, Kimzey LM, et al. Bone loss in young women with karyotypically normal spontaneous premature ovarian failure. Obstet Gynecol. 1998;**91**(1):12–15.

98. Salpeter SR, Walsh JM, Greyber E, et al. Mortality associated with hormone replacement therapy in younger and older women: a meta-analysis. J Gen Intern Med. 2004;**19**(7):791–804.

99. Siegel R, Ward E, Brawley O, et al. Cancer statistics, 2011: the impact of eliminating socioeconomic and racial disparities on premature cancer deaths. CA Cancer J Clin. 2011;**61**(4):212–36.

100. National Cancer Institute. Surveillance Epidemiology and End Results. http://seer cancer.gov/car/1975-2000/. (accessed April 6, 2012).

101. Ravdin PM, Cronin KA, Howlader N, et al. The decrease in breast-cancer incidence in 2003 in the United States. N Engl J Med. 2007;**356**(16):1670–4.

102. Jemal A, Thun MJ, Ries LA, et al. Annual report to the nation on the status of cancer, 1975–2005, featuring trends in lung cancer, tobacco use, and tobacco control. J Natl Cancer Inst. 2008;**100**(23):1672–94.

103. Burstein HJ, Polyak K, Wong JS, et al. Ductal carcinoma in situ of the breast. N Engl J Med. 2004;**350**(14):1430–41.

104. LaCroix AZ, Chlebowski RT, Manson JE, et al. Health outcomes after stopping conjugated equine estrogens among postmenopausal women with prior hysterectomy: a randomized controlled trial. JAMA. 2011;**305**(13):1305–14.

105. Eliassen AH, Colditz GA, Rosner B, et al. Adult weight change and risk of postmenopausal breast cancer. JAMA. 2006;**296**(2):193–201.

106. Hunter DJ, Spiegelman D, Adami HO, et al. Cohort studies of fat intake and the risk of breast cancer – a pooled analysis. N Engl J Med. 1996;**334**(6):356–61.

107. Maruti SS, Willett WC, Feskanich D, et al. A prospective study of age-specific physical activity and premenopausal breast cancer. J Natl Cancer Inst. 2008;**100**(10):728–37.

108. Thiébaut AC, Kipnis V, Chang SC, et al. Dietary fat and postmenopausal invasive breast cancer in the National Institutes of Health-AARP Diet and Health Study cohort. J Natl Cancer Inst. 2007;**99**(6):451–62.

109. McTiernan A, Kooperberg C, White E, et al. Recreational physical activity and the risk of breast cancer in postmenopausal women: the Women's Health Initiative Cohort Study. JAMA. 2003;**290**(10):1331–6.

110. Thune I, Brenn T, Lund E, et al. Physical activity and the risk of breast cancer. N Engl J Med. 1997;**336**(18):1269–75.

111. Brinton LA, Bernstein L, Colditz GA. Summary of the workshop: Workshop on Physical Activity and Breast Cancer, November 13–14, 1997. Cancer. 1998;**83**(3 Suppl):595–9.

112. Friedenreich CM, Bryant HE, Courneya KS. Case-control study of lifetime physical activity and breast cancer risk. Am J Epidemiol. 2001;**154**(4):336–47.

113. Gallagher EJ, LeRoith D. Minireview: IGF, insulin, and cancer. Endocrinology. 2011;**152**(7):2546–51.

114. Calle EE, Rodriguez C, Walker-Thurmond K, et al. Overweight, obesity, and mortality from cancer in a prospectively studied cohort of U.S. adults. N Engl J Med. 2003;**348**(17):1625–38.

115. Hemkens LG, Grouven U, Bender R, et al. Risk of malignancies in patients with diabetes treated with human

insulin or insulin analogues: a cohort study. Diabetologia. 2009;**52**(9):1732–44.

116. Currie CJ, Poole CD, Gale EA. The influence of glucose-lowering therapies on cancer risk in type 2 diabetes. Diabetologia. 2009;**52**(9):1766–77.

117. Wu HK, Squire JA, Catzavelos CG, et al. Relaxation of imprinting of human insulin-like growth factor II gene, IGF2, in sporadic breast carcinomas. Biochem Biophys Res Commun. 1997;**235**(1):123–9.

118. Tamimi RM, Colditz GA, Wang Y, et al. Expression of IGF1R in normal breast tissue and subsequent risk of breast cancer. Breast Cancer Res Treat. 2011;**128**:243–50.

119. Frasca F, Pandini G, Scalia P, et al. Insulin receptor isoform A, a newly recognized, high-affinity insulin-like growth factor II receptor in fetal and cancer cells. Mol Cell Biol. 1999;**19** (5):3278–88.

120. Masur K, Vetter C, Hinz A, et al. Diabetogenic glucose and insulin concentrations modulate transcriptome and protein levels involved in tumour cell migration, adhesion and proliferation. Br J Cancer. 2011;**104** (2):345–52.

121. Alimova IN, Liu B, Fan Z, et al. Metformin inhibits breast cancer cell growth, colony formation and induces cell cycle arrest in vitro. Cell Cycle. 2009;**8**(6):909–15.

122. Libby G, Donnelly LA, Donnan PT, et al. New users of metformin are at low risk of incident cancer: a cohort study among people with type 2 diabetes. Diabetes Care. 2009;**32**(9):1620–5.

123. DuSell CD, Umetani M, Shaul PW, et al. 27-hydroxycholesterol is an endogenous selective estrogen receptor modulator. Mol Endocrinol. 2008;**22**(1):65–77.

124. Asselin-Labat ML, Vaillant F, Sheridan JM, et al. Control of mammary stem cell function by steroid hormone signalling. Nature. 2010;**465**(7299):798–802.

125. Grodstein F, Manson JE, Colditz GA, et al. A prospective, observational study of postmenopausal hormone therapy and primary prevention of cardiovascular disease. Ann Intern Med. 2000;**133**(12):933–41.

126. Manson JE, Allison MA, Rossouw JE, et al. Estrogen therapy and coronary-artery calcification. N Engl J Med. 2007;**356**(25):2591–602.

127. Løkkegaard E, Jovanovic Z, Heitmann BL, et al. Increased risk of stroke in hypertensive women using hormone therapy: analyses based on the Danish Nurse Study. Arch Neurol. 2003;**60** (10):1379–84.

128. Li C, Engström G, Hedblad B, et al. Risk of stroke and hormone replacement therapy. A prospective cohort study. Maturitas. 2006;**54**(1):11–18.

129. Finucane FF, Madans JH, Bush TL, et al. Decreased risk of stroke among postmenopausal hormone users. Results from a national cohort. Arch Intern Med. 1993;**153**(1):73–9.

130. Seely EW, Walsh BW, Gerhard MD, et al. Estradiol with or without progesterone and ambulatory blood pressure in postmenopausal women. Hypertension. 1999;**33** (5):1190–4.

131. Rossouw JE, Anderson GL, Prentice RL, et al. Risks and benefits of estrogen plus progestin in healthy postmenopausal women: principal results from the Women's Health Initiative randomized controlled trial. JAMA. 2002;**288** (3):321–33.

132. Anderson GL, Limacher M, Assaf AR, et al. Effects of conjugated equine estrogen in postmenopausal women with hysterectomy: the Women's Health Initiative randomized controlled trial. JAMA. 2004;**291**(14):1701–12.

133. Manson JE, Hsia J, Johnson KC, et al. Estrogen plus progestin and the risk of coronary heart disease. N Engl J Med. 2003;**349**(6):523–34.

134. Stefanick ML, Cochrane BB, Hsia J, et al. The Women's Health Initiative postmenopausal hormone trials: overview and baseline characteristics of participants. Ann Epidemiol. 2003;**13**(9 Suppl):S78–86.

135. Hays J, Ockene JK, Brunner RL, et al. Effects of estrogen plus progestin on health-related quality of life. N Engl J Med. 2003;**348**(19):1839–54.

136. Appt SE, Clarkson TB, Lees CJ, et al. Low dose estrogens inhibit coronary artery atherosclerosis in postmenopausal monkeys. Maturitas. 2006;**55**(2):187–94.

137. Grodstein F, Manson JE, Colditz GA, et al. A prospective, observational study of postmenopausal hormone therapy and primary prevention of cardiovascular disease. Ann Intern Med. 2000;**133**(12):933–41.

138. Lethbridge-Cejku M, Schiller JS, Bernadel L. Summary health statistics for U.S. adults: National Health Interview Survey, 2002. Vital Health Stat 10. 2004;(222):1–151.

139. Lisabeth LD, Beiser AS, Brown DL, et al. Age at natural menopause and risk of ischemic stroke: the Framingham heart study. Stroke. 2009;**40**(4):1044–9.

140. Lloyd-Jones D, Adams R, Carnethon M, et al. Heart disease and stroke statistics – 2009 update: a report from the American Heart Association Statistics Committee and Stroke Statistics Subcommittee. Circulation. 2009;**119**(3):480–6.

141. Wassertheil-Smoller S, Hendrix SL, Limacher M, et al. Effect of estrogen plus progestin on stroke in postmenopausal women: the Women's Health Initiative: a randomized trial. JAMA. 2003;**289** (20):2673–84.

142. Hendrix SL, Wassertheil-Smoller S, Johnson KC, et al. Effects of conjugated equine estrogen on stroke in the Women's Health Initiative. Circulation. 2006;**113**(20):2425–34.

143. Grodstein F, Manson JE, Stampfer MJ, et al. Postmenopausal hormone therapy and stroke: role of time since menopause and age at initiation of hormone therapy. Arch Intern Med. 2008;**168** (8):861–6.

144. Rossouw JE, Prentice RL, Manson JE, et al. Postmenopausal hormone therapy and risk of cardiovascular disease by age and years since menopause. JAMA. 2007;**297**(13):1465–77.

145. Speroff L. Transdermal hormone therapy and the risk of stroke and venous thrombosis. Climacteric. 2010;**13**(5):429–32.

146. Harman SM, Vittinghoff E, Brinton EA, et al. Timing and duration of menopausal hormone treatment may affect cardiovascular outcomes. Am J Med. 2011;**124**(3):199–205.

147. Santen RJ, Allred DC. The estrogen paradox. Nat Clin Pract Endocrinol Metab. 2007;**3**:496–7.

148. Stefanick ML, Anderson GL, Margolis KL, et al. Effects of conjugated equine estrogens on breast cancer and mammography screening in postmenopausal women with hysterectomy. JAMA. 2006;**295** (14):1647–57.

149. Chen WY, Manson JE, Hankinson SE, et al. Unopposed estrogen therapy and the risk of invasive breast cancer.

Arch Intern Med. 2006;**166**(9):1027–32.

150. Greiser CM, Greiser EM, Dören M. Menopausal hormone therapy and risk of breast cancer: a meta-analysis of epidemiological studies and randomized controlled trials. Hum Reprod Update. 2005;**11**(6):561–73.

151. Welch HG, Black WC, Welch HE. Using autopsy series to estimate the disease "reservoir" for ductal carcinoma in situ of the breast: how much more breast cancer can we find? Ann Intern Med. 1997;**127**(11):1023–8.

152. Song RX, Mor G, Naftolin F, et al. Effect of long-term estrogen deprivation on apoptotic responses of breast cancer cells to 17 beta-estradiol. J Natl Cancer Inst. 2001;**93**(22):1714–23.

153. Schairer C, Gail M, Byrne C, et al. Estrogen replacement therapy and breast cancer survival in a large screening study. J Natl Cancer Inst. 1999;**91**(3):264–70.

154. Jernström H, Frenander J, Fernö M, et al. Hormone replacement therapy before breast cancer diagnosis significantly reduces the overall death rate compared with never-use among 984 breast cancer patients. Br J Cancer. 1999;**80**(9):1453–8.

155. Christante D, Pommier S, Garreau J, et al. Improved breast cancer survival among hormone replacement therapy users is durable after 5 years of additional follow-up. Am J Surg. 2008;**196**(4):505–11.

156. Anderson GL, Judd HL, Kaunitz AM, et al. Effects of estrogen plus progestin on gynecologic cancers and associated diagnostic procedures: the Women's Health Initiative randomized trial. JAMA. 2003;**290** (13):1739–48.

157. Jaakkola S, Lyytinen H, Pukkala E, et al. Endometrial cancer in postmenopausal women using estradiol-progestin therapy. Obstet Gynecol. 2009;**114** (6):1197–204.

158. Lyytinen H, Pukkala E, Ylikorkala O. Breast cancer risk in postmenopausal women using estradiol-progestogen therapy. Obstet Gynecol. 2009;**113** (1):65–73.

159. Mørch LS, Løkkegaard E, Andreasen AH, et al. Hormone therapy and ovarian cancer. JAMA. 2009;**302** (3):298–305.

160. Rossing MA, Cushing-Haugen KL, Wicklund KG, et al. Menopausal hormone therapy and risk of epithelial ovarian cancer. Cancer Epidemiol Biomarkers Prev. 2007;**16**(12):2548–56.

161. Chlebowski RT, Schwartz AG, Wakelee H, et al. Oestrogen plus progestin and lung cancer in postmenopausal women (Women's Health Initiative trial): a post-hoc analysis of a randomised controlled trial. Lancet. 2009;**374** (9697):1243–51.

162. Grodstein F, Newcomb PA, Stampfer MJ. Postmenopausal hormone therapy and the risk of colorectal cancer: a review and meta-analysis. Am J Med. 1999;**106**(5):574–82.

163. Ritenbaugh C, Stanford JL, Wu L, et al. Conjugated equine estrogens and colorectal cancer incidence and survival: the Women's Health Initiative randomized clinical trial. Cancer Epidemiol Biomarkers Prev. 2008;**17** (10):2609–18.

164. Irwin RW, Yao J, Ahmed SS, et al. Medroxyprogesterone acetate antagonizes estrogen up-regulation of brain mitochondrial function. Endocrinology. 2011;**152**(2):556–67.

165. Bethea CL. MPA: medroxy-progesterone acetate contributes to much poor advice for women. Endocrinology. 2011;**152**(2): 343–5.

166. Turgeon JL, McDonnell DP, Martin KA, et al. Hormone therapy: physiological complexity belies therapeutic simplicity. Science. 2004;**304**(5675):1269–73.

167. Manson J, Bassuk S. The menopause transition and postmenopausal hormone therapy. In: Kasper DL, Braunwald E, Fauci AS, et al. (Eds.). Harrison's Principles of Internal Medicine, 17th edition. New York: McGraw-Hill, 2005, pp. 3040–5.

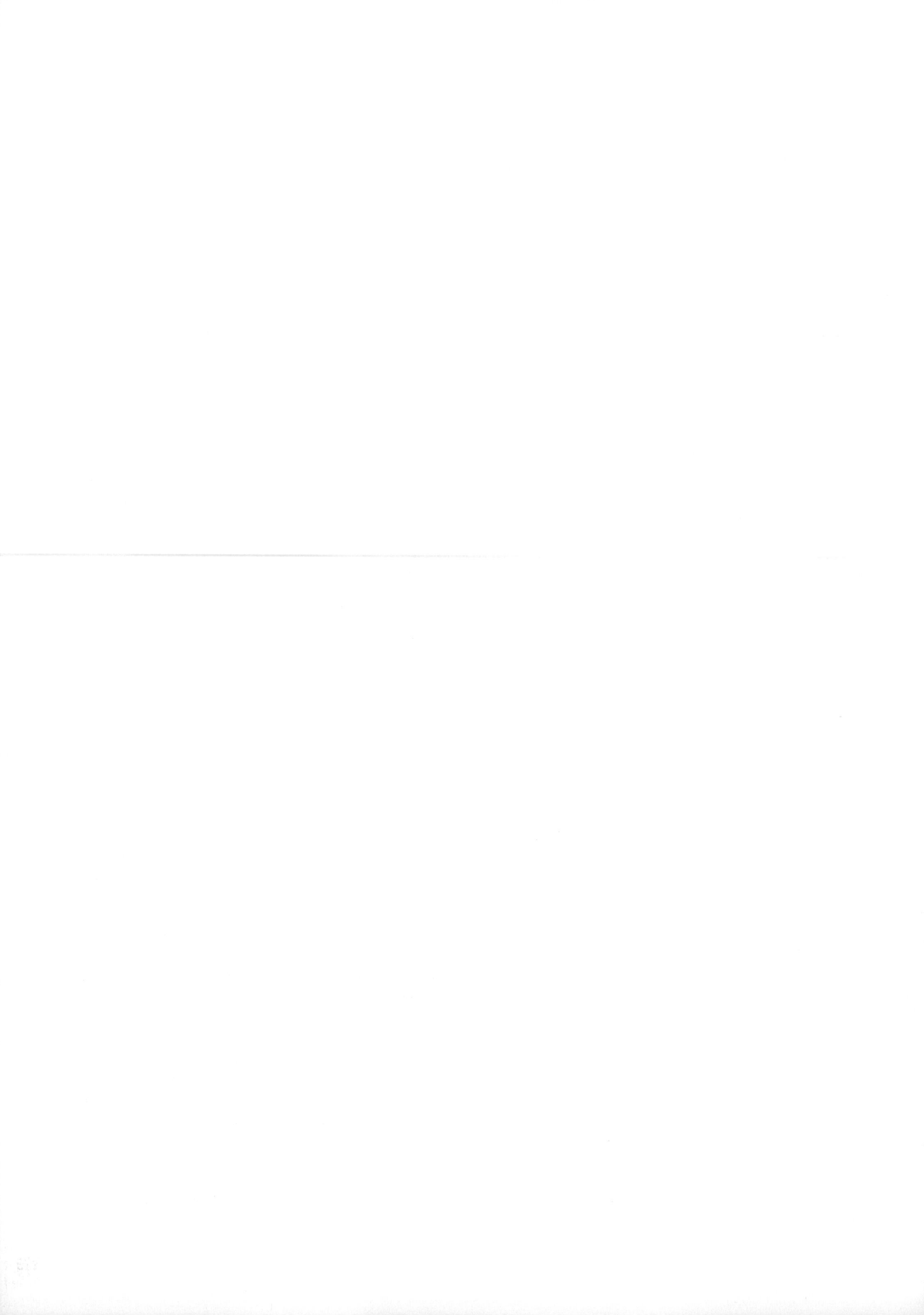

Chapter 21

Clues to ovarian tumors: new concepts of symptoms, signs, syndromes, and paraneoplastic syndromes

Albert Altchek, MD, FACS, FACOG, and David Fishman, MD

Introduction

Early detection of early rather than advanced stage ovarian cancer is emphasized for its correlation to significantly improved patient outcome. Despite improvements in median survival through surgical advances and new chemotherapeutic regimens, the overall survival for women with stage III/IV EOC has remained poor. However, women diagnosed with disease confined to the ovary (stage I) require less morbid surgical intervention, may not require adjuvant chemotherapy, have a significantly improved quality of life, and most importantly, have an overall 5-year survival rate approximating 90%. Enhanced understanding of ovarian cancer molecular biology, etiology, and associated risk factors and pathologies are important in identifying clinically validated tools to save women's lives.

Symptoms: new advancements and discoveries

Within the past decade, the concept of ovarian cancer as a "silent killer" has been challenged by numerous investigators. An important study by Goff et al. identified symptoms presenting before the diagnosis of ovarian cancer, in an effort to minimize delay in detection [1]. Of the 1,725 women with ovarian cancer surveyed, 95% recalled experiencing symptoms before their diagnosis. Of those women, 30% had symptoms within 2 months of diagnosis, 35% had symptoms between 3 and 6 months prior, and 35% reported having symptoms for more than 6 months before discovering the cancer. Although patients with late stage disease were more likely to be symptomatic versus those with early stage disease, women with the latter were only asymptomatic 11% of the time. The specific symptoms were mostly abdominal (77%), gastrointestinal (70%), constitutional (50%), urinary (34%), and pelvic (26%) [1].

These symptoms were further evaluated in an effort to create an epithelial ovarian cancer symptom index. Ovarian cancer patients (n=147) were surveyed as to the characteristics, frequency, and duration of their symptoms before diagnosis. A logistic regression analysis was used to determine independent associations of the symptoms with ovarian cancer. These associations were considered significant when they occurred more frequently than 12 days per month and presented within 1 year of the diagnosis. The symptoms which met these criteria were: pelvic/abdominal pain, increased abdominal size/bloating, difficulty eating/feeling full [2]. In testing the clinical validity of the symptom index, the proportion of ovarian patients with a positive symptom index was compared with those with benign cysts and controls. A total of 65.5% of the patients had a positive index, and the relevant symptoms were significantly more prevalent as compared to the control group. The only symptoms not significantly more common in ovarian cancer patients than those with benign cysts were pelvic/abdominal pain [3].

The number of symptoms a patient may experience before diagnosis continues to be investigated. One study found that women with ovarian cancer reported between one and nine symptoms before diagnosis, with a median number of three [4]. Another study of the general female population in Australia determined that 13% of the women reported three symptoms associated with ovarian cancer [5].

Although the categories of symptoms proposed by the symptom index are constructive, it should be noted that many studies have used slightly different definitions to investigate the symptoms in their respective sample populations.

Pelvic/abdominal pain

The most frequently reported symptoms of ovarian cancer are abdominal in nature [6–11]. When further specified, pain in this area most commonly preceded ovarian cancer diagnosis [4,12–16]. The percentage of women reporting these symptoms varied somewhat with stage of cancer and other factors, but studies have found that "cramping symptoms" were reported by more than 70% [6]. Women with endometrioid epithelial ovarian cancer presented with these symptoms an average of 3 months before diagnosis; 52.9% reported pelvic pain, and 10% upper abdominal pain [17].

The FIGO (International Federation of Gynecology and Obstetrics) stage of ovarian cancer also reflects a difference in the respective prevalence of these symptoms. In one study, abdominal pain was reported by 55% of women with stage I/II and by 66% with stage III/IV [18]. When "pelvic or abdominal pain" was the parameter used to define symptoms starting within 1 year of diagnosis, 48.8% of patients with "borderline"

Altchek's Diagnosis and Management of Ovarian Disorders, ed. Liane Deligdisch, Nathan G. Kase, and Carmel J. Cohen. Published by Cambridge University Press.

cancer experienced these symptoms, compared with 60.9% of those with "invasive" cancer [19].

Although pelvic pain may not be as common as abdominal pain, one study found that patients with ovarian cancer presenting with gastrointestinal symptoms more frequently had a later-stage disease than those with gynecologic symptoms such as pelvic pain. Despite this outcome, women with gynecologic symptoms were more likely to have a shorter delay in diagnostic testing than those with gastrointestinal ailments [20].

Increased abdominal size/bloating

Distention has been experienced by ovarian cancer patients with a frequency between 22% and 36% [12,18]. In a study of 82 women who were fully insured for at least a year before diagnosis of ovarian cancer, an insurance claim associated with bloating was more frequent than comparable controls [21]. In another, population-based case–control study, bloating was found to be "significantly predictive" of localized ovarian carcinoma [22].

The pattern of these complaints may differ with the correlated stage of cancer. Symptoms of bloating and increased abdominal size are approximately three times more commonly associated with late (III and IV) rather than early stage disease [16,23]. There is evidence that mucinous tumors are more likely to be associated with abdominal swelling than other ovarian histologies [10].

This category may be complicated by the fact that while bloating and distention are often thought of as synonymous symptoms among patients, they may be associated with significant differences in clinical predictors [24]. Although women may often present with symptoms of bloating in their primary care visits, persistent abdominal distention is a much less frequent complaint. Therefore, questioning the duration and frequency of symptoms may aid in clarifying risk [25]. A multivariate analysis revealed that the simultaneous coupling of abdominal distention with bloating was more commonly experienced by women with ovarian cancer than controls. However, the controls were significantly more likely to experience sole abdominal distention (without bloating) than those patients with ovarian malignancies [23].

Persistent abdominal distention is more frequently presented with ovarian cancer [26] whereas fluctuating distention/discomfort may not even be significantly associated with the disease [23].

Difficulty eating/feeling full

This parameter does not always provide a significant odds ratio for ovarian cancer patients versus healthy women [21]. In advanced stages, however, women were more likely to experience bloating and loss of appetite [22]. One study found that, according to participants' primary care records, patients with late-stage ovarian cancer were 14 times more likely to experience loss of appetite as compared with controls [18]. Additionally, women with ovarian cancer may be more likely to report feeling full when they are within 6 months of diagnosis [2].

Among women with invasive epithelial ovarian cancer, 57.5% with late-stage disease and 44.1% with early stage disease experienced symptoms of bloating or feeling full. Fewer than 20% of these patients consulted a doctor for their symptoms, and there was no significant difference based on staging [19].

Other symptoms

In addition to the symptoms discussed above, urinary symptoms (usually urgency or frequency) are often reported to occur more commonly among women with ovarian cancer as compared to women in the general population [11,15,16,18,19,25]. These symptoms may be intermittent [26] and/or more significantly associated with early stage cancer [10].

Bowel changes (usually diarrhea or constipation) may be more common in cancer patients than control groups [15,19,26] or than those with benign tumors [27]. They may also occur more frequently among patients with advanced forms of the disease [16,20,22].

Other possible significant symptoms include unexplained weight changes, abnormal or post-menopausal vaginal bleeding [18,22,23] or discharge [12], lack of energy/feelings of fatigue [8,18,26], nausea [19], and lower back pain.

The clinical implications of these studies and consequential translation into gynecological practice have not been determined. Because of the broad and imprecise nature of the symptoms, it would be difficult for physicians to recognize them as related to ovarian cancer until the disease had reached an advanced stage. Furthermore, the low prevalence of ovarian cancer would necessitate a very high sensitivity/specificity to achieve a positive predictive value (PPV) of 10%, high enough to warrant widespread screening [28]. However during the evaluation for persistent (greater than 5 day duration) abdominal/pelvic discomfort, an evaluation of the reproductive tract is critical.

Signs

Most cases of epithelial ovarian cancer are discovered following palpation of an adnexal mass during a pelvic examination. True positive malignant adnexal masses are usually nodular, irregular, fixed, and solid [29]. The differential diagnosis for these masses must also include benign entities such as endometriomas, leiomyomas, and tubo-ovarian abscesses, as well as carcinoma. When masses of this character are found associated with an upper abdominal mass/ascites, an ovarian malignancy should be suspected.

Abdominal distention may be due to ascites or a large tumor. Ascites gives a fluid wave, shifting dullness, umbilical hernia enlargement, and a bowel tympany in the anterior midline in the supine position. There may be umbilical lymph node involvement (Sister Mary Joseph's node). A large ovarian cyst may give a fluid wave (especially if mucinous), no shifting dullness or umbilical enlargement, and bowel tympany laterally. Upper abdominal omental metastases ("omental cake") may have a solid irregular feel. There may also be a partial bowel obstruction or ileus. There may be pleural effusion if ascites is present.

Although the pelvic examination remains the first sign in the eventual detection of ovarian tumors for most women, many present with a "normal" pelvic exam. Therefore, the efficacy of this test as a primary screening tool is questioned. The positive predictive value (PPV) of an adnexal mass found on exam has been estimated at 0.4%. This number is slightly higher when looking at a population of post-menopausal women or of those with presentations consistent with the ovarian cancer symptom index [29].

An ovarian cancer may also be a metastatic lesion from a primary malignancy originating from the gastrointestinal tract, breast, and uterus. Rarely, acute leukemia and lymphoma may metastasize to the ovary presenting as an enlarged ovarian mass. Secondary ovarian tumors are more likely to be solid and less likely to coexist with ascites than those found in patients with a primary malignancy [30,31]. Additionally, some patients with ovarian involvement by metastatic colorectal adenocarcinoma have elevated serum CA125 levels [32].

Following detection of a suspicious pelvic (or abdominal) mass, the transvaginal ultrasound (TVUS) remains the most useful diagnostic imaging modality to evaluate the adnexa. Although conventional sonography is the most widely used method for diagnosing ovarian tumors, it demonstrates limited diagnostic ability to detect EOC at early stages and to differentiate benign from malignant lesions [33–35]. New technological developments, such as three-dimensional transvaginal gray-scale volume imaging (3D TVS) and three-dimensional transvaginal power Doppler imaging (PD3D TVS), provide improvement in the ability to detect early stages of EOC [36–39]. However, recent studies using contrast agents have suggested improved discrimination of benign from malignant ovarian lesions leading to sensitivity estimates between 96% and 100% and specificity between 83% and 98% [40,41]. The existence of a "complex" ovarian mass (cystic and solid makeup), sometimes concurrent with internal septations/echoes, is a significant diagnostic clue suggesting malignancy [42]. Doppler techniques are used to detect tumor neovascularity within solid masses and the complex areas of cystic masses. The spectral trace showing low impedance arterial flow is suggestive of malignancy. A combination of ultrasound and Doppler improves sensitivity and specificity of diagnosis [43].The discovery of, or suspicion of, a pelvic and/or abdominal mass requires an ultrasound. Transvaginal ultrasound has higher specificity than transabdominal ultrasounds in ovarian cancer detection; however, the former may not be optimal when enlarged uterine fibroids coincide with discovery of an adnexal mass.

Recent technologic developments significantly enhance sonographic depiction of vascularity and flow [44]. These include power or amplitude color Doppler sonography, the use of harmonics to improve signal-to-noise ratio and structural conspicuity, as well as the use of intravenous contrast agents to detect and quantitate vascularity and flow [45,46]. Contrast agents may significantly improve the diagnostic ability of ultrasound to identify early microvascular changes that are known to be associated with early stage ovarian cancer [41,47–49]. Currently, contrast agents play a pivotal role in the imaging modalities of computed tomography (CT) and magnetic resonance imaging (MRI). By increasing the density or signal intensity of a particular organ and thus, the signal-to-noise ratio, contrast agents help to detect and characterize parenchymal lesions. Indeed, contrast agents have received such widespread acceptance, that a CT exam performed without intravenous contrast for many indications is now considered limited. Similarly, the use of intravenous contrast agents in ultrasound holds great promise in a multitude of potential clinical applications, especially in identifying aberrant vascular changes associated with malignancy. These contrast techniques have recently been applied to evaluate lesions in the liver, kidneys, and breast [41,47–51].

Ultrasound contrast agents for intravenous use consist of small, stabilized microbubbles usually on the order of 1–10 microns in diameter [52]. These bubbles cause increased echogenicity and are thus termed "echoenhancers." The agents create this effect by causing an acoustic impedance mismatch with the adjacent red blood cells in the vessels. This, in turn, causes increased scattering and reflection of the sound beam, thereby leading to increased sonographic signal and increased echogenicity. The degree of echoenhancement depends on a multitude of factors including the size of the microbubble, the density of the contrast agent, and the compressibility of the bubbles as well as the interrogating ultrasound frequency. The greater the size, density, and compressibility of the agent, the more reflection and echogenicity is elicited by the agent [53,54].

Other signs

In premenarchal girls, an adnexal mass of 2 cm is viewed with suspicion, and a solid 2-cm mass associated with endocrine-related symptoms such as sexual precocity and irregular bleeding from the endometrium usually require surgery [58]. With use of ultrasound, physiological simple unilocular asymptomatic cysts of the ovary in premenarchal girls are not unusual and generally spontaneously disappear. They may be associated with a transient spurt of precocious puberty.

Sudden severe abdominopelvic pain may be due to a biologic accident such as torsion of an ovarian mass and/or fallopian tube. The child/adolescent is at increased risk because of a long pedicle from the infundibulopelvic ligament. Such torsion can occur even from a benign hemorrhagic corpus luteum or dermoid cyst. Prompt diagnosis and surgical detorsion may salvage the ovary. This might require resection of the cyst to reduce the ovarian size and stabilizing the ovarian ligament to prevent repeated torsion. Another acute surgical problem is spontaneous rupture of a malignant ovarian tumor with bleeding.

For the young adult postmenarchal woman, a simple asymptomatic ovarian cyst, as determined by ultrasound criteria, up to 8 cm in diameter with negative tumor markers, may be observed with a repeat transvaginal ultrasound in 6–8 weeks or may be given a 2-month trial of hormonal (oral contraceptive) suppression for two cycles. With decreasing tumor size, the patient may be continued to be observed. This may occur with hemorrhagic corpus luteum cysts, which may show a high-volume, low-pressure flow erroneously suggestive of malignancy with color Doppler flow study. Such physiological angiogenesis means that such a study is best done in the proliferative phase. Ectopic pregnancy or endometrioma may also give a false positive study. If after two cycles there is an increase or persistence in size, surgery is considered. If the cyst is over 8 cm, is complex, has suspicious ultrasound appearance, is symptomatic, or has positive tumor markers, then prompt surgery is advised. As the majority of these malignancies are unilateral, comprehensive surgical staging is critical for optimal management. As the majority of these patients desire future fertility, every attempt to retain fertility should be a priority. Therefore unilateral salpingo-oophorectomy with preservation of the uterus and contralateral ovary can be performed in most cases.

Syndromes

Syndromes have potential value: (1) remembering the syndrome facilitates recognition; (2) identifying those as increased risk for ovarian tumors; (3) the possibility of discovering overlapping or associated gene mutations with predisposition to ovarian tumors; and (4) the possibility of discovering metabolic pathways leading to tumors and chemoprevention.

Residual ovarian syndrome

Following hysterectomy without removal of ovaries, a patient may develop the pathology of residual ovarian syndrome (ROS). ROS may consist of several symptoms, appearing either as a single finding, or as a cluster. In descending order of frequency, symptoms of ROS may include recurrent or chronic pelvic pain, urinary tract disturbances, dyspareunia, and pelvic mass on bimanual examination [60]. There is a 0.33–4.30% incidence of second operation for non-malignant conditions of retained ovaries, but it most likely reaches a 4–5% likelihood with lifetime follow-up [59].

A 20-year study investigated 2,651 patients who underwent (non-malignancy related) hysterectomies with either one or both ovaries left intact. A total of 2.85% of patients were eventually diagnosed with ROS. Of those who required re-exploration, 71.3% (52 cases) were due to chronic pelvic pain, and an asymptomatic pelvic mass was the reason for 24.6% of the explorations. At the end of 5 years, 46.6% re-explorations had been done and within 10 years, 75.4% had been done. Functional cysts were found in 50.7%, benign neoplasms in 42.6%, and ovarian carcinoma in 12.3% [61].

Ovarian remnant syndrome

Ovarian remnant syndrome (ORS) includes symptoms from residual ovarian tissue left in women who have undergone a bilateral salpingo-oophorectomy, independent of hysterectomy status. ORS usually presents with pelvic pain or a pelvic mass resulting from the remnant tissue [62].

Risk factors for ORS during laparoscopic oophorectomy include improper application of surgical loops, linear staples, or bipolar electrocoagulation to the infundibulopelvic ligaments. Prior multiple pelvic surgeries, adhesions, and endc metriosis increase these risks [62].

With prophylactic laparoscopic salpingo-oophorectomy t prevent ovarian cancer, there is the possibility of incomplet removal of the ovary by transection close to the ovary to avoi the ureter as it goes through the base of the infundibulopelvi ligament containing the ovarian blood vessels. Because th patient has hereditary ovarian cancer predisposition, the ovar ian remnant can form an ovarian cancer [63].

Meigs' syndrome

Meigs' syndrome is a benign solid ovarian tumor necessaril accompanied by ascites and/or pleural effusion [64]. A tumo resection characteristically results in complete resolution of th two symptoms. The ovarian tumor is most often a fibroma, bu may be a thecoma, granulosa cell tumor, or Brenner tumor. Al other gynecological tumors with accompanying ascites an hydrothorax are considered "pseudo-Meigs' syndrome" [65] These syndromes must be differentiated from "pseudo-pseud Meigs' syndrome," which is associated with ascites, pleura effusions, and enlarged ovaries caused by SLE [66].

Meigs' syndrome is rare, with an association to 1% of al ovarian fibromas. There is only one case of sudden death fron Meigs' syndrome reported in the literature [67]. There is recen evidence to suggest that fluid accumulation in pseudo-Meigs syndrome may be related to VEGF overproduction in ovaria tissues [65].

Struma ovarii rarely presents as pseudo-Meigs' syndrome (5% incidence). Pseudo-Meigs' syndrome also occurs with benign cyst of the ovary, leiomyomas of the uterus, and teratomas. In at leas 10 cases reported in the literature, CA125 levels were elevated in struma-ovarii causing pseudo-Meigs' syndrome. Levels of CA125 exceeding those typically observed in benign ascites, along with ar ovarian mass, are suggestive of malignancy [68].

The precise cause of ascites and pleural effusion in thes syndromes is still unknown, although several theories hav been proposed. Possibilities for the etiology of ascites includ the stimulation of peritoneal fluid following hard tumor mediated irritation of peritoneal surfaces. Direct pressur from the tumor is thought to affect stimulation of cytokine and other lymphatics [69], as well as pushing fluid to escap from the lymphatic channels [70]. Another clue may com from resolution of increased levels of the anti-inflammatory cytokines IL-6, IL-1β, and IL-8 levels after resection of th ovarian tumor (TNF-α remained elevated) [69].

The pleural effusion is likely a secondary result of the ascites transferred through the lymphatic system [69].

Pseudo-Meigs' syndrome has been associated with gastrointestinal malignancies, ovarian metastasis from colorectal cancer, one case of breast cancer [69], and two cases of uterin leiomyosarcoma [70].

Polycystic ovary syndrome

Polycystic ovary syndrome (PCOS) is defined by two features (1) Excess androgen production, and (2) ovarian dysfunctior (oligo-anovulation and/or polycystic ovaries). Although there is some disagreement within the literature as to which feature (or sub-category) is absolutely necessary to confirm a PCOS diagnosis, all agree on some combination of the criteria. A woman is considered to have polycystic ovarian morphology (PCOM) if she has 12 or more follicles measuring between 2 and 9 mm and/or an ovarian volume of more than 10 mL (this volume may not be appropriate for young women). However, PCOM is present in 16–25% of normal women with regular menstrual cycles and no PCOS [71] and polycystic ovaries in general occur in 20–30% of all women.

Total free circulating testosterone and DHEAS levels are elevated in 50–75% of women with PCOS [72]. Diagnosis of PCOS necessitates excluding other syndromes with similar clinical presentations. HAIR-AN syndrome affects as many as 3% of androgen excess patients and idiopathic hirsutism accounts for 5–7% of all hirsute patients. The 21-hydroxylase-deficient NC-CAH can be determined and excluded from the differential with basal 17-hydroxyprogesterone level screening [73].

Hyperandrogenemia may manifest as excessive hair growth in women, acne vulgaris, male-pattern alopecia, seborrhea, hyperhidrosis, and hidradenitis suppurativa. In an estimated 50% of patients with subsequent PCOS diagnosis, their initial complaint was obesity. In fact, even women with normal BMIs have been found to have a body fat content significantly greater than normal [74]. Insulin resistance is characteristic of women with PCOS, even beyond what would be predicted with the high prevalence of obesity and adiposity. This may be due to defects in glucose transport, GLUT4 production specifically, paracrine signaling, or altered adipose tissue morphology [73]. Women with PCOS are reported to have a five-fold increase in developing type II DM than their age- and weight-matched counterparts [72].

PCOS is associated with elevated risks of endometrial abnormalities, including carcinomas, particularly as a result of hyperinsulinemia and hyperestrogenemia in patients. There are some reports of PCOS representing an increased risk of breast and ovarian cancer, but this has not been systematically substantiated to date [72]. Recent studies have also suggested that mood disorders should be assessed in all PCOS patients [75].

Future genome-wide association studies will hopefully revolutionize the diagnostic (and eventual therapeutic) approach to PCOS.

Metabolic and endocrine syndromes

Metabolic syndrome (MS) is defined by the presence of at least three of the following metabolic abnormalities: (1) central obesity with a waist circumference > 88 cm (35 in.); (2) fasting serum triglyceride ≥ 150 mg/dL (1.7 mmol/L); (3) serum high density lipoprotein (HDL) cholesterol < 50 mg/dL (1.3 mmol/L); (4) blood pressure ≥ 135/85 mmHg; or (5) type II diabetes mellitus (DM) [76]. Because of the overlapping risk factors (CVD and obesity-related) and definition including insulin resistance, there is some debate as to whether or not PCOS is a subset of MS or a similar condition. At a minimum, it is clinically important to be aware of the association, as a recent report indicated that there is 42% prevalence of metabolic syndrome in PCOS [77]. In addition to type II DM and CVD-related risk factors common to many PCOS patients, MS also has reported associations with non-alcoholic fatty liver disease (NAFLD) and certain cancers [78].

In patients with virilization (those with severe masculinization, hirsutism, etc.), the symptomology suggests mutations in the insulin receptor gene, androgen-secreting tumors, and/or androgenic substance abuse [13].

Hyperandrogenism, insulin resistance, and acanthosis nigricans (HAIR-AN) syndrome "represents a series of usually inherited syndromes that are distinct from PCOS and are associated with the overwhelming feature of abnormal insulin/glucose metabolism to a much greater degree than patients with PCOS. Patients with HAIR-AN syndrome tend to have a greater degree of associated morbidity, including type II diabetes, hypertension, and cardiovascular disease. The pathogenesis is thought to be related to an insulin receptor and/or postreceptor defect resulting in the compensatory increases in circulating insulin and luteinizing hormone (LH). These hormones stimulate excess ovarian androgen secretion. The clinical signs of hyperandrogenemia in these patients can be marked and signs and symptoms of virilization mimicking an androgen-secreting tumor are common. The syndrome has overlapping features with PCOS and ovarian hyperthecosis"[79].

Wener's syndrome may be associated with early onset hyperandrogenism caused by ovarian hyperthecosis, ancanthosis nigricans, and peripheral neuropathy [80].

Berardinelli–Seip syndrome (congenital generalized lipodystrophy) is a hereditary autosomal recessive generalized deficiency of adipose tissue, muscular hypertrophy, tall stature, acromegaly, encephalopathy, hyperpigmentation, acanthosis nigricans, generalized hypertrichosis, clitoris hypertrophy, polycystic ovaries, extremes insulin resistance due to insulin receptor defect, hyperlipidemia, and non-ketonic DM in the second decade of life [81].

Patients with *familial partial lipodystrophy (Dunnigan variety)* develop hirsutism, menstrual abnormalities, and polycystic-appearing ovaries approximately 20–33% of the time. Although FPLD is rare, it is important to consider in lean-body PCOS women [82].

The Rabson–Mendenhall syndrome is characterized by extreme insulin resistance and polycystic ovaries. Common to this syndrome are also symptoms of hirsutism and acanthosis nigricans [83].

Cancer anorexia–cachexia syndrome (CACS) is a common and crippling consequence of cancer. It is characterized by anorexia, tissue wasting, involuntary weight loss, and eventual death [144]. In ovarian cancer patients, the symptoms are caused by the metabolic effects of the advanced course of the disease including growing tumor and bowel obstruction. "Mechanisms involved in the pathogenesis of obstruction may include extrinsic occlusion of the bowel due to pelvic, mesenteric omental masses, or intestinal motility disorders due to infiltration of the mesentery or bowel muscle and nerves. The relief of malnutrition and cachexia may be attempted through nutritional support, pharmacological approach (megestrol acetate, cyclooxygenase inhibitors) and palliative treatment of bowel obstruction" [145].

Ataxia-telangiectasia syndrome (A-T); (*Louis Bar syndrome*) is an autosomal recessive disorder of cerebellar ataxia, oculo-cutaneous telangiectasis, and immune deficiency. Immune-compromised status results in sinopulmonary infections and malignant tumors (mainly leukemias and lymphomas). A variety of ovarian malignancies include dysgerminoma, yolk sac (endodermal sinus) tumor, gonadoblastoma, and carcinoma [105].

Muir–Torre syndrome has recently been reclassified as a variant of Lynch syndrome. The most frequent mutations are found in MMR genes *MSH2* and *MLH1*. This condition is often discovered concurrent with cutaneous sebaceous adenoma. One case was recently reported in an ovarian mature cystic teratoma [146].

Sweet syndrome, also known as febrile neutrophilic dermatosis, presents with fever, leukocytosis, and erythematous plaques infiltrated by neutrophils. There have been rare reported associations with ovarian carcinoma [147].

Leser-Trélat signs are often associated with malignant acanthosis nigricans. It is a rare paraneoplastic syndrome involving an acute onset and rapid enlargement of seborrheic keratosis. In no more than a few cases, these signs presented with ovarian cancer [148].

Trousseau syndrome is characterized by cancer-associated migratory thromboembolitic events, including disseminated intravascular coagulopathy (DIC). Ovarian cancer patients are among those at risk for Trousseau's [149].

Blepharophimosis syndrome is a rare, congenital, ophthalmic condition affecting the eyelids. Type I is associated with premature ovarian failure. There have also been reported cases of patients developing ovarian and endometrial cancer [150].

Malignant acanthosis nigricans (MAN) is associated with a variety of internal malignancies. MAN has been reported to coincide with, and even predate, ovarian cancer diagnoses. One recent case study suggests that sudden-onset MAN coinciding with tripe palms should alert the physician for possible ovarian and other gynecological malignancies [84].

Ovarian hyperstimulation syndrome (OHSS) is an iatrogenic complication of ovulation induction. Severe OHSS is characterized by massive ovarian enlargement, ascites, pleural effusion, oliguria, hemoconcentration, and potentially life-threatening thromboembolic phenomena [85]. Women with PCOS undergoing assisted reproduction have a significantly elevated incidence of OHSS. Even women without PCOS per se but with a high LH:FSH ratio, hyperandrogenism, or a high number of resting hormones also exhibit a higher level of OHSS. This is most likely due to the fact that these women are more sensitive to exogenous FSH and gonadotropin stimulation. Patients with PCOS have increased expression of VEGF within the ovarian stroma, a potential cause of the increased susceptibility to development of OHSS [86].

A prospective study of women who underwent IVF-ICSI cycles after ovarian stimulation with GnRH antagonist–recombinant FSH protocol determined that a minimum of 18 follicles or E2 concentrations of >5,000 ng/L was able to achieve a 83% sensitivity rate/(up to) 84% specificity rate for severe cases of OHSS. Late OHSS was always related to pregnancy and to a high incidence of multiple pregnancies. Early OHSS patients had significantly elevated E2 concentrations as compared with those diagnosed with late OHSS (± SEM; 2,970 ± 233 vs. 2,127 ± 219) [87].

Women with OHSS are at a significant risk of thrombosis compared with their non-pregnant and pregnant counterparts. Venous thromboembolism (mostly in the upper limb, head, and neck) is estimated to be three times more common than arterial thrombosis (mostly related to cerebrovascular accidents and occurs with the onset of the syndrome). These patients may have a slightly elevated risk of developing a PE. Hemoconcentration anomalies almost certainly lead to this elevated risk; another theory is that there is drainage of ascetic fluid into the upper lymphatics [88]. Immobilization, hyperestrogenemia, and pelvic pressure (from enlarged ovaries or ascites) are considered risk factors for thromboembolism in severe cases of OHSS [85]. The women with severe OHSS who later had thromboembolism have had elevated concentration of leukocytes, plasmin inhibitor, D-dimers, and other markers of the fibrolytic system. High concentrations of these markers may signal imminent thromboembolism in these patients [89]. Because of the frequency and severity of venous thrombosis in OHSS, whenever a risk is determined, preventative heparin should be administered [25].

The MR scan in OHSS patients typically shows bilaterally enlarged ovaries with multiple cysts. Although the images may be similar to cystic ovarian neoplasms with septations (e.g., mucinous cystic and granulosa cell tumors), the cysts in OHSS scans should be uniformly sized [90].

The lack of clarity regarding the etiology of OHSS has led to the continued evolution of prevention practices. If OHSS is considered a risk for a woman (if she has PCOS or had OHSS before), a physician may alter the ovulation strategy (such as the use of metformin, in vitro maturation, GnRH antagonist and low-dose FSH protocol, GnRH antagonist protocol). During stimulation, preventive therapies include coasting, GnRH antagonist administration, IV fluids (albumin, hydroxyethyl starch, 3.5% colloidal intravenous infusion solution, and dextran). New modalities of prevention may include the use of IV calcium infusion [91] and dopamine agonists [92].

Luteinized unruptured follicle (LUF) *syndrome* is a cause of female infertility in which LH and progesterone levels mimic those of ovulation, even though there is no follicular rupture or release of the oocyte. Incidence and recurrence rates of LUF syndrome are increased when infertile women are treated with clomiphene citrate during consecutive cycles [93].

Resistant ovary syndrome is a cause of infertility in which the patients appear to have normal follicles on ultrasound, but are completely resistant to normal stimulation by gonadotropins [94]. It may be associated with autoimmune endocrinopathy and a benign thymoma.

Empty follicle syndrome (EFS) is diagnosed when no oocytes are retrieved after a seemingly successful ovarian stimulation during IVG. Reported incidence ranges from 0.2% to 7%. Recently, EFS was subdivided into two distinct categories: false and genuine. False EFS is considered in a case of low β-HCG level. In contrast, genuine EFS (GEFS) is defined as futile retrieval on days of optimal β-HCG levels and otherwise apparently normal follicular development. Furthermore, many authors believe that failure to retrieve oocytes should be considered as a "sporadic event" rather than a syndrome. The risk of recurrence of GEFS increased with age, increasing to 57% for women older than 40 [95].

Primary empty sella syndrome is a neuroanatomical–radiological entity with variable endocrine implications. There may be multiple endocrine abnormalities due to panhypopituitarism including lack of response to GnRH and posterior pituitary deficiency (diabetes insipidus). It may result from trauma, tumor, or meningioencephalitis.

In *Bardet–Biedl syndrome*, CT scanning shows empty sella associated with obesity and primary hypogonadism [96]. A 10-year-old female with Bardet-Biedl was found with hypoplastic fallopian tubes and uterus, and bilateral ovarian cysts on ultrasound [97].

McCune–Albright syndrome (MAS) (Albright syndrome, Weil–Albright syndrome, osteitis fibrous dysplasia) refers to rare disease with a characteristic clinical triad of polyostotic fibrous dysplasia of bone, café-au-lait skin pigmentation, and precocious puberty. Endocrinopathies including hyperthyroidism, elevated growth hormone levels, and Cushing syndrome are often associated with the clinical presentation. Scoliosis and renal involvement are seen in many MAS patients. MAS rarely results in malignant transformation of fibrous lesions. The mechanism for the syndrome is somatic mutations of the GNAS gene, encoding for a cAMP-regulating protein, Gsα.

Clinicians must distinguish between MAS and an ovarian neoplasm (as well as idiopathic causes) when a patient presents with precocious puberty. When MAS is the diagnosis, these symptoms are a result of high levels of serum estradiol resulting from "intermittent autonomous activation of ovarian tissue" [98].

Other syndromes

Ovarian vein syndrome (OVS) includes a variety of non-specific and variable symptoms, including abdominal pain (frequently presenting in the iliac fossae, flanks and hypochondrium). Women often experience the pain most intensely when right before menstruation or when lying down, particularly on the affected side. Many cases of OVS have been diagnosed during or immediately after pregnancy. There are a few theories as to the pathophysiology of OVS. One postulate is that malformed ovarian vein may crown or compress a ureter. Another is that a web of dilated veins entraps the ureter. OVS most often involves the right ureter. The broad characteristics of OVS necessitate its differentiation from endometriosis, pelvic inflammatory disease, salpingitis, ovarian vein thrombophlebitis, and pelvic condition syndrome [99].

Pelvic congestion syndrome (PCS) is a common, underdiagnosed condition in which women present with pelvic pain/aching that existed for more than 6 months. Signs of inflammatory disease preclude diagnosis. The pain is most acute on one side, when the patient stands for prolonged periods of time, during menstruation, pregnancy, and post-coitus. On physical examination, vulval varices may extend on to the medial thigh and long saphenous area. Tenderness may be elicited by deep palpation at the ovarian point (the point where the upper third meets the lower two-thirds of an imaginary line from the anterior superior iliac spine to the umbilicus). A combination of ovarian point tenderness and postcoital ache was reported to be 94% of this syndrome. Minimally invasive treatments are now available [100].

PCS may be clinically differentiated from OVS by the infrequent complaint of urinary symptoms [99].

Acute pelvic pain syndrome is a common emergency syndrome in women and is usually due to gynecologic problems such as ectopic pregnancy, miscarriage, and pelvic inflammatory disease. It may also be due to appendicitis, sigmoid diverticulitis, urinary tract infection, and renal colic [101].

Munchausen syndrome is a psychological disorder in which a patient imagines, pretends, or self-induces an illness and seeks care for their "illness." A 40-year-old single woman feigned a diagnosis of stage IV ovarian cancer. She had a daughter with a confirmed diagnosis of leukemia [102].

Sotos syndrome (cerebral gigantism) "is a pleiotropic syndrome of multiple congenital anomalies, developmental delay, and overgrowth characterized by macrocephaly, prominent forehead (dolichocephalic), variable mental deficiency, hypotonia, hyperreflexia, prenatal onset of excessive size, large hands and feet, advanced bone age, down-slanting palpebral fissures, a high hairline, a prominent jaw, a high narrow palate, generalized overgrowth, and psychomotor developmental delay."

"Sotos syndrome belongs to overgrowth syndromes, which have an increased risk of neoplasms, including Wilms tumor, adrenal carcinoma, gonadoblastoma, hepatoblastoma in Beckwith-Wiedemann syndrome, mesodermal hamartomas in Ruvalcaba-Myhre-Smith syndrome, neuroblastoma in Weaver syndrome, neurofibromas, astrocytomas, cutaneous angiomas, subcutaneous leiomyomas, carcinoid tumors, xanthogranulomas, acoustic neuromas in neurofibromatosis, subcutaneous hamartomas and fibroadenomas in Proteus syndrome, and cavernous hemangiomas in Klippel–Trenaunay–Weber syndrome." Neoplasms found with Sotos syndrome include Wilms tumor, hepatocarcinoma, vaginal epidermoid carcinoma, osteochondroma, neuroectodermal tumor, giant cell granuloma of mandible, neuroblastoma, multiple hemangiomas, non-Hodgkin lymphoma, acute lymphocytic leukemia, small cell lung carcinoma, testicular yolk sac tumor, sacrococcygeal teratoma, mixed parotid tumor, and cardiac fibroma of the left ventricle.

A 26-year-old woman with Sotos syndrome had a left 8-cm and a right 3-cm ovarian fibroma with extensive foci of calcification and occasional ossification. This is similar to young women with basal cell nevus syndrome. Since Sotos syndrome and bilateral calcified ovarian fibromas in young women are rare it "… suggests the effects of overgrowth in Sotos syndrome on ovarian tumorigenesis" [103].

Nevoid basal cell carcinoma syndrome (NBCS) (basal cell nevus syndrome, Gorlin's syndrome) is an autosomal dominant inherited disorder with high penetrance but variable presentation increasing with age. They include multiple nevoid basal cell carcinomas, multiple jaw keratocysts, skeletal developmental defects (rib, vertebral, craniofacial), palmar and plantar skin pits, epidermal inclusion cysts, milia, ectopic calcification (falx cerebri diaphragm sellae), and a variety of extra-cutaneous neoplasms especially of the ovary, brain (meduloblastoma, meningioma), and fibroma of the heart.

Approximately 75% of women with NBCS have ovarian fibromas, usually bilateral and multinodular, or multifocal and calcified. They are usually found in young adults, adolescents, and even children, and may recur after excision [104]. Rarely, an ovarian fibrosarcoma may develop secondarily. Gestational hypertension may develop from renin secretion from the ovarian tumor. One case of NBCS had a bilateral sclerosing stromal tumor found during pregnancy.

In the general population, ovarian fibromyomas cause 4% of ovarian neoplasms, develop at an average age of 48, are usually unilateral, not calcified, are single, and unusual under age 30 [105].

Gorlin syndrome is associated with mutations in the tumor suppressor gene *PTCH*, located on chromosome band 9q22.3. An estimated 20–30% of NBCS cases arise from de novo mutations [106]. Despite the risk of recurrence in young women, the ovarian fibroma should be removed but the normal ovary should be preserved whenever possible [104].

Two recent cases of NBCS were reported: a 15-year-old female patient [106,107] and a 22-year-old woman with this syndrome and past history of multiple keratocysts of the maxillary bone, who was discovered to have bilateral and calcified ovarian fibromas [108].

Proteus syndrome is a rare, sporadic, and complex overgrowth disorder. Clinically, it is highly variable with patients who exhibit (among other symptoms) disproportionate tissue overgrowth, lipomatosis, vascular malformations, and visceral hamartomatous tumors. There have been a small number of cases reported with ovarian cysts. One case did involve sexual precocity, one was associated with multiple meningiomas, and one involved a case of a unilateral ovarian dermoid cyst accompanied by an ipsilateral paratubal cyst in a 5-year-old female patient [109].

The *Townes syndrome* (Townes–Brocks syndrome), including anomalies of the ears, thumbs, anus, kidneys, and cystic ovaries, is an autosomal dominant disease [110].

The *Rudiger syndrome* of developmental failure of limbs and diaphragm with coarse facial features and autosomal recessive inheritance also includes ovarian cysts [111].

Fraser and associated syndromes include autosomal recessive cryptophthalmos, fused eyelids, anomalies of the head and nose, and syndactyly [112].

Von Hippel–Lindau syndrome is an autosomal dominant disease that manifests as any number of benign and malignant vascular tumors in many organs. Retinal angiomas and cerebellar hemangioblastomas are the most common presentations, and renal cell carcinomas or pheochromocytomas may also develop. Recently, the first two cases of testosterone-secreting lipid cell tumors of the ovary in VHL were reported [113]. Von Hippel–Lindau syndrome may be associated with poor prognosis of ovarian clear cell carcinoma" [114].

Weaver syndrome of macrosomia, accelerated skeleton maturation, camptodactyly, and unusual facies has been found to have cardiovascular anomalies and neoplasia with an ovarian endodermal sinus tumor reported [115].

Sclerosing peritonitis is considered a subtype of luteinized thecoma. There is fibroblastic and myofibroblastic cell proliferation. Sclerosing peritonitis is most often attributed to chronic ambulatory peritoneal dialysis and practolol therapy. Presenting symptoms may include abdominal pain/distention, palpable mass, weight loss, ascites, and intestinal obstruction. There have been a few cases of luteinized thecoma with sclerosing peritonitis concurrent with elevated serum CA125 [116]. A case of idiopathic sclerosing peritonitis appeared in a 39-year-old woman with associated ovarian cysts and keratoconjunctivitis sicca syndrome [117]. In a recent analysis of sclerosing peritonitis, 24 of the 27 patients had clinically bilateral ovarian lesions, often with "striking cerebriform aspect." Three of these patients died of the syndrome, and 30 had no evidence of spread of their lesions [118].

Lymphangioleiomyomatosis syndrome is a rare disease occurring only in women, primarily during their menstrual life. It is a systemic disorder that involves proliferation of atypical pulmonary interstitial smooth muscle and by the formation of cysts within the lung. Uncommonly, lymphangioleiomyomatosis may arise without pulmonary symptoms. One 30-year-old woman in Japan initially presented with an accumulation of chylous ascites, erroneously suggesting advanced ovarian cancer [119].

Peutz–Jeghers syndrome (PJS) is an autosomal dominantly inherited syndrome that exhibits an increased susceptibility to tumors, including, but not limited to, benign ovarian sex cord tumors, cervical cancer, breast cancer, gastrointestinal cancer, thyroid cancer, pancreatic cancer, and endometrial cancer. Most PJS patients present with hamartomatous polyps and mucosal hyperpigmentation. Brown–blue macules are often found on the border of the lips, palms, soles, eyes, nose, and peri-anal region. Characteristically, the macules progressively lose the boldness of pigmentation over time [120].

"A definitive diagnosis after identification of a histologically confirmed hamartoma is made when two of the following are present: family history of PJS, mucocutaneous hyperpigmentation, or small bowel polyposis" [121].

A systematic review, culminating in 2009, collected data on cancer and PJS. The most frequent malignancy was colorectal cancer, followed by breast, small bowel, gastric, and pancreatic cancers. The lifetime risk of cancer was reported between 37% and 93%. Women with PJS have been shown to develop ovarian carcinomas, mucinous neoplasms of the ovary, and ovarian sex-cord tumors with annular tubules (SCATs). SCATs are generally benign at the outset, and are characterized by the risk of inducing sexual precocity and infertility [122]. Over one-third of patients with SCTAT also have PJS [123].

Most patients with SCTATs and PJS exhibit gastrointestinal polyposis and mucocutaneous melanin pigmentation. Some of these patients may present with menstrual irregularity, abdominal/pelvic pain, and fewer than 10% may have sexual precocity [124].

SCTATs have distinct features when associated with PJS. The tumors themselves are typically benign, bilateral, small, and "multifocal with tumorlets scattered in the ovarian stroma." When SCTATs appear in patients without PJS, they are most often unilateral, large, and relatively more likely to be malignant [121].

In rare instances, patients with PJS had SCATs that underwent malignant change. A 54-year-old woman with PJS had SCATs with aggressive, recurrent, malignant change. This is only one of three cases reported in the literature. The patient had a missense mutation in the LKB1 gene [121].

Inactivation of the tumor suppressor gene STK11 has been implicated in up to 91% of PJS cases [125]. Although PJS is generally considered an inherited disorder, between 10% and 20% of cases are results of spontaneous germline mutations in *LKB1* (which encodes for STK11) [121].

When Sertoli–Leydig cell tumors (SLCTs) are discovered in patients with PJS, they are most often benign. In one 2-year-old patient, a presentation of precocious puberty led to a diagnosis of SLCT of the ovary; this led to a confirmation that the girl was suffering from PJS. Both patient and father were found to have the same *STK11* gene deletion [125].

A 52-year-old woman with PJS developed ovarian mucinous cystadenoma, minimal deviation adenocarcinoma of the cervix, and areas of mucinous metaplasia of the endometrium and tubal mucosa. The initial pap-smear produced a false-negative result due to the well-differentiated character of the malignancy. After investigation, hard palate pigmentation and hamartomatous polyps of the colon were discovered [123].

A 53-year-old female patient with PJS acquired mucinous glandular lesions in the bladder, lobular endocervical glandular hyperplasia in the uterine cervix, mucinous metaplasia in the right fallopian tube, and mucinous adenoma in the left ovary. The lesions were all associated with pyloric gland metaplasia [126].

Several other reports of PJS in association with ovarian tumors have been published recently. One woman with PJS was diagnosed with unilateral ovarian gonadoblastoma, unilateral breast cancer, and cervical adenocarcinoma [127]. Another was discovered to have ovarian serous cystadenoma [128].

Ruvalcaba–Myhre-Smith or Bannayan–Zonnana syndrome (BRRS), and *Cowden disease* (CD) have recently been grouped together after identification of mutation in the tumor suppressor gene PTEN (10q22–q23) in up to 80% of CD patients and up to 60% of BRRS patients. These conditions will likely all be considered subsets of "PTEN hamartoma tumor syndromes" (PHTS). These mutations are associated with an elevated incidence of multiple hamartomas in various organ systems, although ovarian incidence is rare [120]. One patient with CD developed thyroid, ovarian, stomach, and colon carcinomas, as well as other cancers (and a benign meningioma) over the course of 23 years [129]. A 23-year-old woman with CD and a germline *PTEN* missense mutation was found to have a mucinous cystadenoma of the left ovary. Clinically, her manifestations mimicked Proteus syndrome [130].

BRRS patients typically experience delays in motor skills, macrocephaly, lipomatosis, and lentigines on the glans penis. The syndrome is associated with an elevated risk of follicular thyroid cancer and several gynecological cancers [120].

Carney complex (CNC) is an autosomal dominantly inherited neoplastic syndrome and lentiginosis. It involves spotty skin pigmentation, myxomas, schwannomas, and endocrine over-activity. A variety of endocrine tumors are associated with CNS, including primary pigmented nodular adrenal cortical disease (PPNAD), growth hormone-secreting pituitary adenomas, large-cell calcifying Sertoli cell tumors, Leydig cell tumors, and thyroid neoplasms [120].

"In the context of CNC, frequent female reproductive organ manifestations include ovarian benign or malignant tumors (such as serus cystadenomas, cystic teratomas, mucinous adenocarcinomas, endometrioid carcinomas) and myxoid uterine leiomyomas, while an atypical mesenchymal neoplasm of the uterine cervix has also been reported"[131].

Isolated mucocutaneous melanotic pigmentation (IMMP) is a related PJS syndrome without intestinal polyposis. Of 26 cases reviewed at the Mayo Clinic, 10 developed malignancies, with an RR = 7.8 for an increase of breast and gynecological cancers. Additional malignancies were in the cervix, endometrium, kidney, lung, colon, and lymphatics. Of interest is that there were no LKB1 mutations found which is common with PJS. Thus, IMMP is another lentiginosis with cancer predisposition [132].

Ollier's and Malfucci syndromes also occur. *Juvenile granulosa cell tumor* (JGCT) and SLCT of the ovary occur with Ollier's or Malfucci's syndromes in the first or second decades as part of generalized mesodermal dysplasia [133]. They are generally considered to be non-familial syndromes, possibly arising from a germline mutation associated with a somatic mosaic mutation [134]. JGCT can cause isosexual precocious puberty, and sometimes presents with acute symptoms due to hemorrhage and necrosis. For the usually unilateral stage I, JGCT unilateral saplingo-oophorectomy "... is almost always curative." Recurrences, if they develop, usually appear within 3 years, unlike the adult GCT with late recurrences [105]. In a recent literature review, JGCT was associated with Ollier's disease in eight patients, and four with Maffucci syndrome. Ten of these patients exhibited characteristics of hyperestrogenism [134].

Bilateral JCGT may occur with other congenital syndromes or abnormalities such as Goldenlar's syndrome of craniofacial and skeletal abnormalities, and Potter's syndrome. Phenotypically normal females with unilateral JGCT may have bone or soft tissue tumors [105]. Ovarian granulosa cell tumor has been associated with tamoxifen therapy and leprechaunism.

Ollier's syndrome or disease is a rare congenital but non-hereditary sporadic disorder of asymmetric, multiple sporadic enchondromas and and association with enchondrosarcomas. There may be a rare ovarian fibroma or fibrosarcoma. There is also an association with ovarian JGCT [133] with isosexual precocious puberty in the first or second decade. Enchondrosarcomas usually occur after the second decade [105]. A novel case of an adult (36-year-old) woman with

Ollier's syndrome and JCGT was recently recorded. In older patients, malignant transformation is common [134].

Malfucci's syndrome is enchondromal (like Ollier's) but with soft tissue hemangiomatosis. Ovarian JGCT may occur, and there have been single cases with ovarian fibroma and fibrosarcoma [105].

Association of SLCTs and thyroid adenomas, an unnamed syndrome, is a familial inherited autosomal dominant with a variable degree of expressivity. Occasionally, there is an additional ovarian mucinous cystadenoma or cystadenocarcinoma. Even those under 30 with sporadic SLCTs have an increase in thyroid masses. The usual thyroid masses in familial and sporadic SLCTs are solitary or multiple adenomas or nodular goiter, but also there has been hyperthyroidism and carcinoma [105].

Ovarian size syndromes: With *ovulation induction* in fertility cases, there may be an ovarian hyperstimulation syndrome with huge tender ovaries and ascites. This usually responds with time and support.

A recent concern is the question of persistent ovulation induction inducing carcinoma. This is complicated by the fact that with carcinoma or a predisposition to it, there is reduced fertility and with hereditary ovarian carcinoma each generation tends to have an earlier onset of carcinoma [105]. Several subsequent reports from various national studies showed no excess risk of ovarian cancer among ever users of fertility drugs/induced ovulation. However, certain selected drugs on particular subsets of women warrant further investigation. These include women with increased baseline risks [135].

Palpable post-menopausal ovary

In former years, it was thought that the post-menopausal ovary was always small, quiescent, and non-palpable. The palpable firm ovary of the size of menstruating ovary in a post-menopausal woman might be a sign of early cancer, but it is usually benign.

In recent years, it has been found that approximately 14% of normal asymptomatic post-menopausal women have small, unilocular ovarian cysts, many of which spontaneously disappear or recur after a few months. Among women with one simple ovarian cyst at their first screen, 32% had complete resolution of the cyst by their next annual exam. These simple cysts did not increase risk of subsequent invasive ovarian cancer. If simple ovarian cysts are discovered in post-menopausal women, intervention is not recommended [42].

A post-menopausal woman may have a pelvic mass that is suspicious for a malignant ovarian neoplasm if one of the following indicators is present: elevated CA125 level, ascites, a nodular or fixed pelvic mass, evidence of abdominal or distant metastasis, or a relevant family history [29].

The *post-menopausal ovary syndrome* (PPOS) is the palpation of what is a normal sized ovary for the pre-menopausal woman, but is indicative of an enlargement in the post-menopausal woman. It refers to size and consistence. It does not refer to small cysts reported on ultrasound [136]. In clinical practice, approximately 15% of normal women may have a small asymptomatic, thin-walled, unilocular cyst on transvaginal ultrasound which may persist or disappear, and may or may not occur. It is usually not palpable, apparently benign, and in the general population patient, it is usually observed by repeated ultrasound. In high-risk cases for ovarian cancer, especially after menopause, there is concern for malignancy.

Growing teratoma syndrome (GTS) is defined as an unresected mature teratoma enlarging/persistent during or after chemotherapy for germ cell tumors. GTS is rare in cases of ovarian germ cell tumors. Teratomas result from compression of the adjacent anatomic structures [137]. GTS may arise from malignant cell differentiation into mature teratoma or "chemotherapy induced destruction of immature elements." It is essential to completely excise the mass to avoid possible malignant transformation or physical complications including vascular thrombosis, ureteral obstruction, bowel obstruction, bile duct obstruction, and fecal fistula [138].

A recent review found that the median age at onset of primary GTS of the ovary is 21 years and the median time of the onset was 8 months (ranging from 3 to 156) after the chemotherapy [139]. All reported GTS cases of the ovary arose after surgical and chemotherapy treatments for malignant ovarian cell tumors. Most often, the primary histology was immature teratroma [138].

A GTS was discovered in a 36-year-old woman during the follow-up after chemotherapy and the primary surgical resection of a malignant immature teratoma of the ovary [139]. One case reported a GTS following laparoscopic surgery for germ cell tumor of ovary [138] and another noted the development of a secondary tumor, a trabecular carcinoid, arising from a peritoneal nodule of mature teratoma in a patient with a GTS of the ovary [137].

Tumor lysis syndrome describes the development of a range of metabolic abnormalities following cytotoxic therapy for malignancy. It is characterized by hyperuricemia, hyperkalemia, hyperphosphatemia, hypocalcemia, and increased levels of serum lactate dehydrogenase. Often, it leads to renal insufficiency or failure. It is rarely reported with cases of solid tumors and very few have been reported in connection with ovarian cancer [140]. One case developed in a 14-year-old adolescent with a locally disseminated ovarian anaplastic large-cell lymphoma [141].

Pseudomyxoma peritonei syndrome (PMP) is clinically distinguished by progressive abdominal distention caused by the accumulation of mucinous fluid in the peritoneal cavity. It most commonly appears in middle-aged women, presenting with an ovarian mass [142]. An ovarian origin of PMP is very rare (3–8%) and thought to only develop from mature cystic teratoma of the ovary. The origin is most often in the appendix and can be distinguished histoimmunologically [143].

Possible unnamed syndromes also occur: the autosomal dominant variable expressivity hereditary association of ovarian *SLCTs with thyroid adenomas*, nodular goiter, Grave's disease and carcinoma [105].

Cases of ovarian cancer among women with Down syndrome/trisomy 21 are infrequent, at most. There have been reports suggesting a connection between ovarian dysgerminoma and Down syndrome. Although ovarian dysgerminoma is rare, there have been five cases reported in concurrence with Down syndrome. The most recent report suggests that the presence of trisomy 21 may be directly responsible for the increased risk of development of an ovarian germ cell tumor, especially dysgerminoma [151].

Cutaneous melanosis has been found with stromal carcinoid tumor [105].

Benign peritoneal melanosis is a rare condition, sometimes associated with ovarian dermoid cysts, ovarian serous cystadenoma, and ovarian mucinous cystadenoma (concurrent with colonic adenocarcinoma). Because this syndrome is characterized by melanin pigment deposition in the peritoneum, one must be careful to distinguish its presence from metastatic malignant melanoma, peritoneal endometriosis, and peritoneal lipofuscinosis [152].

Ovarian non-Hodgkin lymphoma and HIV

The increasing length and frequency of survival in patients with HIV/AIDS provides increasing likelihood of the concurrence of the disease with ovarian cancer. One recent case reported HIV-associated primary non-Hodgkin's lymphoma of ovary. If proper diagnosis is made following differential diagnosis of ovarian mass, prognosis (with subsequent appropriate treatment) is assumed to be very favorable [153].

Paraneoplastic syndromes

Neurologic

Paraneoplastic cerebellar degeneration (PCD) occurs mainly in patients with cancer of the ovary, uterus, fallopian tube, breast, and lung. It is immunologically induced by effects of a distant underlying cancer [154]. PCD is a rare form of neurological paraneoplastic syndrome, distinguished in part by lack of neuropathological inflammation. Middle-aged women are most commonly the cohort diagnosed with PCD. Patients with PCD may exhibit limb, trunk, stance, or gait ataxia, dysarthria, or optomotor dysfunction [155]. Symptoms of diplopia and vertigo may also exist [156].

There is a strong association among neuronal paraneoplastic syndromes of anti-Yo antibodies with ovarian and other gynecological cancers [157].

Among 557 patients with ovarian cancer, Yo antibodies were less prevalent in the group of patients where blood samples were obtained before or after surgery (ovary group I) compared with the group where all samples were obtained before tumor resection (ovary group II) [158]. Patients with PCD without anti-Yo antibodies may be positive for anti-Hu, anti-Ri, or anti-Tr antibodies [156].

In up to 60% of patients with PCD, cerebellar symptoms appear before discovery of the cancer [167]. PCD is often fatal between 2 and 3 years after the first manifestations are noted. A 63-year-old woman with symptoms of PCD developed brain metastases and ovarian cancer; she died nearly 3 years after initial presentation [157].

Two patients were diagnosed with delayed onset of PCD associated with high titer of CSF anti-Yo and elevated CA125 at 6 months and 1 year before discovery of ovarian carcinoma. Approximately 4 months after treatment with IVIG, chemotherapy, and surgical resection of the tumor, both patients experience various degrees of relief from their neurological deficits [159].

PCD may also follow a presentation of ovarian carcinoma. One study described a case of PCD 2 years post-diagnosis [160] and another described one 6 years later [161]. Three years after an ovarian cancer diagnosis, a 56-year-old woman was discovered to have PCD. Although her carcinoma improved, her neurologic symptoms endured [162].

PCD and non-bacterial thrombotic endocarditis may coexist as a presenting paraneoplastic symptom of an underlying ovarian malignancy [163]. One case of a recurrent ovarian carcinoma presented with PCD and myasthenia gravis [156].

Immature ovarian teratomas can manifest as paraneoplastic encephalitis. NMDAR antibodies may be associated with the syndrome [164].

Patients with ovarian teratoma-associated encephalitis (OTE) may display acute prominent psychiatric symptoms, seizures, central hypoventilation, hypersalivation, and problems with cardiac conduction. On average, tumor diagnosis was 4 months after the onset of symptoms. With IVIG, it is possible for OTE patients to have complete neurological remission [165].

A 32-year-old woman with an initial diagnosis of psychosis and panic disorders was subsequently discovered to have ovarian teratoma-induced paraneoplastic limbic encephalitis. Her symptoms were ultimately attributed to the paraneoplastic syndrome [166].

A 59-year-old woman presented with acquired neuromyotonia 2 years before diagnosis of clear cell ovarian adenocarcinoma. The symptoms of the hyperexcitability syndrome resolved after tumor resection [167].

One study found epilepsy to be a paraneoplastic syndrome associated with a 30 × 28 × 15 cm primary ovarian leiomyoma. After resection of the tumor, the patient did not return with any neurological symptoms [168].

Ovarian cancer infrequently spreads to the spinal cord. One case of a 65-year-old woman had confirmed metastases to the high cervical spinal cord [169].

The incidence of central nervous system metastases in epithelial ovarian cancer is increasing. It has recently been reported at 5%, among 400 patients with ovarian cancer. Prognosis is most often poor [170].

Skin dermatomyositis

Patients with dermatomyositis (DM), and to a lesser extent, polymyositis (PM) have exhibited significant risk of malignancy. The risk is highest within 1 year of myositis diagnosis. In Western countries, DM has been associated with ovarian, gastrointestinal, and lung cancers [171]. Dermatomyositis typically presents with a heliotrope rash on the upper eyelids and proximal muscle weakness. Patients may also have an erythematous rash or Gottron papules. An estimated 10 to 25% of cases are paraneoplastic [172].

Since the association of DM with ovarian cancer, it has been seen as the initial presentation [173]. In one study, seven patients with dermatomyositis were later diagnosed with ovarian cancer. Three of those women had an elevated CA125 [174]. PM is rarely associated with malignancy. It is an inflammatory myopathy without associated dermatological findings [172].

Recently, few cases of PM and ovarian cancer without evidence of DM have been reported. One case documented PM as the presenting symptom of a woman with stage IV ovarian carcinoma [175]. Another case of ovarian cancer (clear cell stage IIIc) was discovered 4 years after diagnosis of PM. The patient is in remission following surgical resection of the malignancy and eight cycles of chemotherapy [176]. Both women were in their 50s at the time of cancer diagnosis.

Other skin syndromes

Many cancers exhibit cutaneous manifestations, often providing the first clue to underlying malignancy. These may include skin markers of inherited syndromes that are associated with an increased incidence of internal malignancy, dermatological changes due to hormone-secreting tumors, and many proliferative/inflammatory dermatoses with associations to many forms of cancer [177].

Cutaneous metastatic ovarian cancer is most often discovered 2 years after diagnosis of the underlying malignancy. The most common presentation is one or more (grouped) nodules on the abdominal wall. If it occurs on the umbilicus, it is usually purple; when painful, ulcerated, or suppurative, it is associated with poor prognosis [178].

Skin metastastes from ovarian cancer may also appear on the chest wall, breast, and buttocks. Rare presentations may also include the scalp [179].

Tripe palms, when concurrent with malignant acanthosis nigricans, may be indicative of underlying ovarian cancer. This is characterized by velvety thickening of the palms and exaggeration of normal skin markings [84]. A recent study reported the first occurrence of malignant acanthosis nigricans, tripe palms, and the sign of Leser–Trélat in a patient with ovarian cancer [180].

Cowden syndrome may present with small popular lesions and kerotic plaques on the upper/lower extremities. It may coexist with ovarian cystadenoma or ovarian dysgerminoma [181].

Ovarian cancer has also presented with cutaneous angiogenesis, digital necrosis, edema, palmar fasciitis, and polyarthritis (PFPA), Raynaud's phenomenon, scleroderma [178], and disseminated superficial porokeratosis [182].

Hematologic

The association between coagulation disorders and various malignancies has been well documented since the 19th century. VTE includes deep venous thrombosis (DVT), pulmonary embolism (PE), superficial vein thrombosis (SVT), and thrombosis in vena cavae, pelvis, and other ports [183]. In particular, there is an established relation between ovarian cancer and VTE. Of 253 women with epithelial ovarian cancer, there were 4 with a pulmonary embolism (PE) and 38 with DVT [184]. A recent meta-analysis revealed that the relative risk for VTE among women with ovarian cancer compared with controls is greater than six [185]. Among patients with ovarian cancer, preoperative DVT was significantly more frequent when the women presented with massive ascites. One possible rationale for this is the ascites-induced dehydration increased the viscosity of blood [186]. In another study, women with clear cell carcinoma have been found to have a significantly higher frequency of VTE than other subtypes of ovarian carcinoma [187].

It has been suggested that VTE may be the earliest sign of cancer: an estimated 10% of patients with "unprovoked" VTE are diagnosed with malignancy within 2 years. Ovarian cancer exhibits a high prevalence of metastatic-stage disease at the time of diagnosis [188]. Recently, a woman with a GCT presented with DIC as the first symptom of malignancy [189].

Postoperative DVT has declined as a complication for gynecologic malignancies (from one-third of all surgeries to consistently below 10%). However, PEs remain the leading cause of death postoperatively for gynecological cancers [190].

Recently, a case of a primary non-Hodgkin's lymphoma (NHL) of both ovaries was preceded by an internal jugular vein thrombosis (IJVT) as paraneoplastic syndrome [191].

Paradoxical embolisms are considered a risk among patients with patent foramen ovale. Ovarian malignancies have been discovered subsequent to paradoxical embolism as the initial symptom. On occasion, these cases result in stroke [192,193].

Thrombosis and disseminated intravascular coagulation (DIC) are most likely due to the ability of most cancer cells to activate the coagulation system. The tumor's production of tissue factor and inflammatory cytokines, as well as its interaction with blood and endothelial cells is an assumed cause of its ability to induce coagulation [194].

On occasion, ovarian tumors have been associated with idiopathic thrombocytopenic purpura; combination chemotherapy was found useful for the ovarian malignancy [195]. Other reported associations include pancytopenia [196], systemic mastocytosis [197], and thrombocytosis [198].

Autoimmune hemolytic anemia has been reported in association with mature cystic teratromas (dermoid cysts). AIHA should resolve completely and immediately after surgical excision of the cyst [199].

Ocular

Bilateral diffuse uveal melanocytic proliferation (BDUMP) is a rare paraneoplastic syndrome associated with rapid and irreversible blindness. It often appears with exudative retinal detachment and progressive cataract formation [200]. Often, the symptoms mimicking metastatic disease to the eye develop in patients before their underlying malignancy is discovered [201].

Among women, BDUMP is most commonly associated with ovarian cancer. Six of 14 women with this syndrome had ovarian carcinoma [202]. Mean age of diagnosis is in the 50s, with a mean number of 11.6 months between appearance of ocular symptoms and patient death [203].

BDUMP is not generally thought likely to metastasize. There is one case reported of a patient with a history of ovarian cancer (not recurred) and BDUMP who developed skin lesions consistent with metastatic amelanotic malignant melanoma [203].

Autoimmune hemolytic anemia syndrome

Autoimmune hemolytic anemia (AIHA) *syndrome* is a rare condition in which the blood has a lower than normal amount of red blood cells. The red blood cells are destroyed and removed from the bloodstream before their normal lifespan. AIHA as a manifestation of ovarian dermoid cysts (ODC) is a rare syndrome with an unknown pathogenesis. Rarely, dermoid cysts may cause a Coombs positive autoimmune hemolytic anemia.

Paraendocrine syndromes

Hypercalcemia

Small cell ovarian cancer is a rare type of epithelial cancer that originates in the tissues that line the organs and cavities of the body. Hypercalcemia is a metabolic disorder associated with neoplastic diseases that accounts for two-thirds of small cell carcinoma of the ovary [215,216]. Small cell carcinoma of the ovary, hypercalcemic type (SCCOHT), is a rare and poorly characterized tumor that is usually unilateral. Ninety-nine percent of cases are unilateral, but bilateral familial cases have been reported [205,207].

SCCOHT is an aggressive neoplasm that does not have a clear histology or pathological characterization due to its scarcity, unknown etiology, and resemblance to other ovarian neoplasms, which opens the door to a wide range of potential differential diagnoses. Upon examination, SCCOHT is presented as a large, mostly solid mass (mean diameter, 15 cm) made up of a sheet-like arrangement of small, closely packed epithelial cells [206]. SCCOHT can easily be misinterpreted as highly malignant germ cell tumors of the ovary, specifically dysgerminoma, ovarian lymphoma, or granulosa cell tumors.

To date, 400 patients have been diagnosed with SCCOHT [207,208] and fewer than 250 cases have been reported in the literature [204]. Small cell carcinoma of the ovary, hypercalcemic type generally occurs in women between the ages of 10 and 40, with a peak incidence observed in 23-year-old women (range, 1–55) [204,205,208]. The youngest patient to date has been 14 months [205]. The most common presenting symptoms of SCCOHT are non-specific. Symptoms include abdominal pain and distention, nausea, anorexia, weight loss, and vomiting [209]. Some of these symptoms can be associated with hypercalcemia and may require immediate treatment for hypercalcemia.

Commonly, germ-cell or sex-cord tumors make up the majority of ovarian tumors in young women while SCCOHT represents a minority [204]. Although it is rare, SCCOHT is the most common form of undifferentiated ovarian carcinoma in women younger than 40 years of age. Less than 30% of SCCOHT cases develop in women younger than 20 years and less than 1% develops in children [206]. At the time of diagnosis, SCCOHT is usually in FIGO stage III, where the one-year survival rate is approximately 50% and the 5-year survival rate is approximately 10% [204]. Women diagnosed with stage IA small cell carcinoma of the ovary have a postoperative disease-free survival rate of approximately 33% over a range of 1 to 13 years [205]. Despite the 33% chance of survival, more than 50% of patients die of the disease.

Humoral hypercalcemia of malignancy

Hypercalcemia occurs in less than 5% of female genital tract malignancies and in virtually all of those cases (an estimated 95%), it is humoral hypercalcemia of malignancy (HHM) [212].

HHM is caused by the secretion of tumor hormones produced by tumor cells into the systemic circulation, which causes bone resorption. Gynecologic malignancies complicated by HHM include neoplasms of the uterus, cervix, ovary, vulva, and the vagina. Among these neoplasms, ovarian cancer is the most common gynecologic malignancy associated with HHM. Reportedly, HHM occurs in a relatively high percentage of rare ovarian tumors such as small cell carcinoma of the ovary and clear cell carcinoma of the ovary. Small cell carcinoma of the ovary makes up approximately 1% of ovarian cases (66% of which are associated with HHM) while the latter makes up approximately 5% of ovarian cancers (5–10% are associated with HHM) [212].

Humoral hypercalcemia of malignancy is marked by the absence of skeletal metastasis, low PTH, and elevated PHTrP serum levels. Approximately 80% of gynecologic malignancies of the HHM type are caused by parathyroid hormone-related protein (PTHrP) [212]. Increased levels of PTHrP produced at high levels by the malignant cells circulate and cause an increase in bone resorption and in renal calcium that ultimately leads to hypercalcemia.

Parathyroid hormone receptor

PTHrP is expressed in a wide variety of normal fetal and adult tissues and organs, playing an important role in normal growth and development [213]. When functioning normally, PTHrP is thought to act as an autocrine or paracrine hormone that regulates calcium metabolism [214]. PTHrP shares the same N-terminal end as parathyroid hormone (PTH), and can, therefore, simulate most of the actions of PTH, including increases in bone resorption and renal calcium resorption which leads to hypercalcemia [215]. An editorial comment suggests a molecular heterogeneity of PTHrP. It also points out the intriguing unknown roles of PTHrP. It is an endothelium-derived vascular smooth muscle relaxing factor. Its synthesis increases with distention of hollow organs to relax the smooth muscle walls in the rat urinary bladder and uterus. "It is present in human amniotic fluid at high concentrations; and is important for maintaining the placental calcium gradient in experimental animal models." In addition, there are "mild increases or PTHrP associated with normal pregnancy and lactation ..."

[216]. Obviously this is a fascinating unexplored aspect of pregnancy physiology.

Most HHM cases are caused by PTHR1 (parathyroid hormone 1 receptor), which functions as a receptor for the parathyroid hormone (PTH) and PTHrP. PTHrP mRNA was documented in tumors associated with humoral hypercalcemia of malignancy. This finding determined that PTHrP is a main factor that causes HHM. Up-regulated PTHrP expression is often found in tumors with skeletal metastasis [217].

Renin

Renin is a proteolytic enzyme that is released into the bloodstream in response to reduced salt levels or low blood volume. The ovarian renin-angiotensin system plays a crucial role in reproductive functions such as folliculogenesis, oocyte maturation, ovulation, steroid synthesis, and the formation of the corpus luteum [218]. The majority of renin-secreting tumors originate in the kidney. Renin-producing ovarian epithelial carcinoma is extremely rare. Rarely ovarian tumors, especially sex cord-stromal tumors, may cause hypertension by secretion of renin and secondary hyperaldosteronism.

There may be an overlap with Gorlin's syndrome with ovarian fibromas. Gorlin's syndrome, also known as nevoid basal cell carcinoma syndrome (NBCCS), is a rare inherited multisystem disorder. Fifteen to 25% of women with Gorlin syndrome develop ovarian fibromas that are often calcified, multinodular, and bilateral [108]. Sometimes there may be an aldosterone-secreting tumor with low or normal plasma renin. Rarely there may also be isosexual pseudoprecocious puberty with elevated estradiol and testosterone.

Although clinical signs of hypereninism are rare with ovarian tumors, "... subclinical secretion of renin by some ovarian tumors may be relatively common. "Possibly 50% of sex cord-stromal tumors may be immuno-reactive for renin without hypertension of hypokalemia." The occurrence of renin-secreting ovarian tumors is consistent with recent observations that a complete renin-angiotension system exists in the follicular apparatus of the normal ovary" [105].

Carcinoid

Carcinoid tumors are marked by excessive amounts of secretion of the hormone serotonin (5-hydroxytryptamine), which helps nerves communicate with each other in the human body. Carcinoid of the ovary is extremely uncommon; less than 1% of all carcinoid tumors involve the ovary [219]. Carcinoid tumors of the ovary can be categorized into two groups: primary ovarian carcinoid tumors and metastatic ovarian carcinoid tumors.

Primary ovarian carcinoid syndrome is more common than the metastatic type. Primary ovarian carcinoid tumors make up less than 0.1% of all ovarian tumors [220]. Whereas primary ovarian carcinoid is usually benign in character (less than 2% are malignant), patients diagnosed with metastatic ovarian carcinoid have a 75% chance at survival after 3 years.

Primary ovarian carcinoid tumors have other teratomatous components in 85–90% of cases, usually dermoid cyst, strumal carcinoid, mature solid teratoma, or a cystic mucinous tumor. The primary ovarian carcinoid tumors can be further divided into insular (or islet carcinoid), trabecular and strumal carcinoid. The most common type of primary ovarian carcinoid is the insular type. Strumal carcinoid tumor is composed of a mixture of thyroid tissue and carcinoid.

Primary ovarian carcinoid syndromes originate from neuroendocrine tissue. Carcinoid tumors may be associated with the carcinoid spectrum, ectopic ACTA syndrome, or other polypeptide hormone-secreting syndromes, including MSH like peptide, glucagon, gastrin, vasoactive intestinal peptide, insulin calcitonin, and anti-diuretic hormone.

Cushing's syndrome

Cushing's syndrome is a rare endocrine disease characterized by excess exposure, use, or production of cortisol. Cortisol is a hormone produced in the adrenal glands which helps the body respond to stress and change. Symptoms of Cushing's syndrome include: truncal obesity, facial fullness, diabetes, amenorrhea, hypertension, proximal myopathy, skin atrophy and bruising, and osteoporosis [221]. Causes of Cushing's syndrome include exogenous glucocorticoid administration and endogenous hypercortisolism. Currently, the use of exogenous glucocorticoids (use of oral corticosteroid medication) is the most common cause of Cushing's syndrome [222]. Glucocorticoids are naturally produced steroid hormones that inhibit the process of inflammation. Endogenous Cushing's syndrome is caused by either excessive adrenocorticotropic hormone (ACTH) production or by autonomous adrenal cortisol production. The ectopic ACTH-producing syndrome (Cushing's syndrome with hyperpigmentation) is one of the most common nonendocrine tumor syndromes causing a humoral syndrome. When due to a malignant tumor, it is the most common unrecognized type of Cushing's syndrome [223].

Polycystic ovaries (PCO) and polycystic ovarian syndrome (PCOS) is common among women with Cushing's syndrome. PCOS is a common heterogeneous disorder in women that affects an estimated 6–10% of reproductive-aged women [223]. The exact etiology of PCOS remains uncertain, but it is thought that the pathogenesis of PCOS is associated with genetics and environmental influences.

Zollinger–Ellison syndrome

Zollinger–Ellison syndrome (ZES) is a rare disorder that arises from tumors or ulcers in the digestive system. ZES is typically characterized by the presence of hypergastrinemia secondary to gastrin-secreting tumor, also known as gastrinoma [224]. A pancreatic islet usually stimulates excessive gastrin production but excessive gastrin may be produced by cystadenoma of the ovary in ectopic sites. If benign or malignant mucinous ovarian tumors produce gastrin within the cyst wall, an individual may present with ZES [225]. In addition, Zollinger–Ellison syndrome can present with borderline tumors and cystadenocarcicnomas which have neuroendocrine intestinal-type gastrin-containing cells and clinically active elevated plasma gastrin.

Multiple endocrine neoplasia type 1

Multiple endocrine neoplasia, type 1 (MEN-1) is characterized by the co-occurrence of parathyroid hyperplasia with pancreatic endocrine tumors and/or pituitary adenoma. MEN-1 is caused by a germline mutation in the tumor suppressor protein, menin. In 2000, a very rare case of ovarian gastrinoma in the context of MEN-1, including hyperparathyroidism and Zollinger–Ellison syndrome, was reported [226].

Hyperthyroidism

Hyperthyroidism is a condition in which the thyroid gland overproduces thyroid hormones. In 2000, a study indicated that a woman diagnosed with hyperthyroidism has an 80% high risk of developing ovarian cancer. This was the first study conducted in attempt to characterize the relationship between hyperthyroidism and ovarian cancer.

Struma ovarii is a teratoma with predominant thyroid tissue; the thyroid tissue comprises more than 50% of the overall mass. Although careful history reveals thyroid tissue in 20% of dermoids, clinical hyperthyroidism occurs in only 5% of struma ovarii. Approximately 5–10% of strumas are malignant and less than half of these have spread beyond the ovary.

A rare case of Hashimoto thyroiditis arising in the ovary was reported. The patient was a 38-year-old woman who presented with clinical symptoms of hyperthyroidism [227]. A diagnostic oophorectomy revealed thyroid tissue in ovarian masses with all the features of Hashimoto thyroiditis in the right ovary. Following the surgery, all signs of hyperthyroidism diminished and the patient's thyroid levels were normal after 1 month.

In pure form, the thyroid tissue in the ovary appears as a brownish, solid gelatinous tissue, occasionally mixed with a dermoid cyst or with a solid carcinoid tumor (strumal carcinoid). Infrequently, the opposite ovary has a dermoid cyst or another struma ovarii. Hyperthyroidism may result from hydatidiform mole or choriocarcinoma because of the thyrotropic stimulation of human chorionic gonadotropin.

Ovarian tumors with functioning stroma

Ovarian tumors with functioning stroma (OTFS) are separate from sex cord-stromal and steroid cell tumors. OFTS are ovarian tumors whose stroma are consistent with steroid hormone secretion, and are associated with estrogenic, androgenic, or progestagenic manifestations. Ovarian tumors with functioning stroma typically present with either hyperestrogenism or hyperandrogenism. Clues to OTFS include estrogenic vaginal cytology and endometrial hyperplasia.

In OFTS, steroid hormones are secreted by ovarian stroma cells, under the stimulus of tumor cells instead of being directly produced by tumor cells. Functioning stroma mostly occurs in metastatic ovarian tumors, especially mucinous and endometrioid surface epithelial-stromal carcinomas, and large intestine metastatic tumors. Metastatic ovarian tumors can appear as multilocular cystic masses or mainly as solid masses. OFTS can be characterized into three groups: (1) tumors that contain syncytiotrophoblastic cells that produce human chorionic gonadotropin (hCG) and stimulate the ovarian stroma; (2) tumors occurring during pregnancy; and (3) tumors that do not contain syncytiotrophoblastic cells and do not occur during pregnancy [228]. The final group is by far the most common case of OTFS.

Chorionic gonadotropin secretion

Human chorionic gonadotropin (hCG) is a glycoprotein hormone secreted by the blastocyst immediately after fertilization and has chemoattractant properties. Clinical signs of hCG production are usually due to germ cell tumors containing syncytiotrophoblastic cells. Steroid hormones may be stimulated by luteinized tumor, stromal cells, or in the adjacent ovarian stroma. hCG may activate the stroma of primary and secondary ovarian tumors. Subclinical serum hCG has been reported with various ovarian tumors and in 10 to 40% of surface epithelial benign and malignant tumors associated with "active stroma."

Inappropriate antidiuresis syndrome

Inappropriate secretion of antidiuretic hormone (SIADH) is the most common cause of hyponatremia, an electrolyte disorder. There was a case report of ovarian serous carcinoma with a component of small cell carcinoma of pulmonary type with neuroendocrine granules containing anti-diuretic hormone.

Hyperprolactinemia

Hyperprolactinemia occurs when there is an abnormally high level of prolactin, a hormone secreted by the pituitary gland, in the blood. Rarely, dermoid cysts may contain a small prolactinoma, which may cause amenorrhea, galactorrhea, and hyperprolactinemia.

Hypoglycemia

Hypoglycemia is a condition characterized by abnormally low levels of glucose in the blood. It may occur with various malignant and benign neoplasms because of insulin and proinsulin secretion. In addition, carcinoid ovarian tumors may cause cutaneous melanosis due to secretion of alpha-melanocytic-stimulating hormone, and rarely there is an association with parathyroid adenoma and pituitary hyperplasia as part of the type 1 multiple endocrine neoplasia syndrome.

Amylase secretion

Amylase is secreted from the pancreas into the duodenum. High-stage serous surface epithelial carcinomas may contain amylase and secrete it into cystic, ascitic, and pleural fluid, as well as serum and urine. Ovarian neoplasm amylase is similar to salivary amylase and has a different electrophoretic pattern than pancreatic amylase.

Chromosomal abnormalities

Turner's syndrome

Turner's syndrome (TS) is a genetic condition that occurs when a phenotypical female infant is born with a missing or changed X chromosome. TS may be referred to as chromosome XO syndrome, Turner–Albright, Morgagni–Turner, Shereschevskii–Turner, Bonnevie–Ullrich, Ullrich–Turner, genital dwarfism, gonadal dysgenesis, ovarian dwarfism, and ovarian short stature syndrome. Turner syndrome affects approximately one in 2,500 live-birth females. While it is one of the most common chromosomal abnormalities, there is not a clear explanation as to why TS occurs: any female can be born with TS.

The most common features of TS include short stature and ovaries that do not produce hormones or ova, which can lead to premature ovarian failure and infertility. The ovaries are characterized by fibrous streaks ("streak ovaries") without ovulation and do not produce estrogen resulting in primary amenorrhea due to ovarian failure. Further symptoms include an exceptionally wide neck (webbed neck), a broad chest, minor eye problems, prominent auricles, and a narrow palate. The chance of mortality is increased throughout the lifespan of a patient with TS. Reduced bone mass is present in adults with Turner's syndrome and 24 to 40% of adults with TS are at risk of hypertension. Cardiovascular disease is the most common cause of death of adulthood TS. In 10% of patients, TS diagnosis may be delayed until adulthood.

Turner's syndrome is diagnosed through a karyotype, a specific blood test that looks at chromosomes. TS is characterized by X chromosome monosomy, the presence of an abnormal X chromosome, or mosaicism of a 45,X chromosome, in which only one X chromosome is present. Mosaicism of a 45,X cell line may be 46,XX, 46,XY or have an abnormal sex chromosome rearrangement [229]. In these mosaic cases, there may be some ovarian function with 10 to 20% having spontaneous puberty and 2 to 5% transient spontaneous menses and rarely pregnancy. The most common karyotype result is 45,X monosomy.

Women with 45,X/ 46,XY mosaicism have a 6% increased risk of developing ovarian gonadoblastoma. A gonadoblastoma is a rare neoplasm that develops almost exclusively in the dysgenetic gonads of women with Y chromosome mosaicism. Most pure gonad dysgenesis and Turner's syndrome patients do not have Y chromosomes and, therefore, do not have a predisposition to gonadoblastomas or germ cell tumors. If there is a 46,XY karyotype with pure gonadal dysgenesis or a 45,X/46,XY or mosaic karyotype in mixed gonadal dysgenesis, there is an increased risk of gonadoblastoma and dysgerminoma (which is malignant).

Androgen-insensitivity syndrome (testicular feminization)

Androgen insensitivity syndrome (AIS) is a sex development disorder caused by mutations in the androgen receptor gene, which leads to a variety of phenotypic abnormalities. The usual mechanism is an abnormality of the androgen receptor gene in the long arm of the X chromosome. AIS may be sporadic or familial. It occurs in approximately 1 of 20,400 male live births. Genetically, a child with AIS is born a male, but they exhibit complete female or partial female and male genitalia. Furthermore, AIS patients have a normal feminine psyche and are reared as females. AIS is typically characterized by feminization of the external genitalia at birth, abnormal secondary development in puberty, and infertility in individuals with a 46,XYY karyotype [230].

Androgen-insensitivity syndrome can be categorized into two main subgroups: complete androgen insensitivity syndrome (CAIS) and partial androgen insensitivity syndrome (PAIS). CAIS, formerly referred to as testicular feminization syndrome, is characterized by the complete absence of virilization of the internal and external male genitalia. Externally, the patient looks like a female, but internally there is typically a short vagina and no uterus, fallopian tubes, or ovaries. The testes secrete Mullerian-inhibiting substance, which prevents the development of the uterus and fallopian tubes. CAIS occurs in approximately 1 of 20,000 live births. PAIS, also known as Reifenstein syndrome, is when the body is unable to respond appropriately to male sex hormones. Individuals born with PAIS can have normal female sex characteristics, both male and female characteristics, or normal male characteristics. Externally, an individual with PAIS may look male or female. The genitalia are characterized by either a slightly enlarged clitoris or a small penis; hypospadias is very common.

Both subgroups of androgen insensitivity syndrome have little medical morbidity or mortality. However, over time untreated patients may be at an increased risk of malignant degeneration and development of gonadoblastoma of the testes. After puberty, there is a tendency for benign and malignant hamartomas and neoplasms to occur. The most common are benign hamartomas and often bilateral. Sertoli cell adenomas may develop and may be confused with the malignant Sertoli cell tumor, which does not form frequently. Approximately 8% of adults develop GCTs, usually seminomas.

It is generally agreed that the testes should be removed, but there are differences of opinion regarding timing. Pediatric surgeons advise surgery in childhood for the small chance of early development of tumors and to avoid emotional trauma. Gynecologists often wait until after puberty to allow spontaneous puberty development. Psychological aspects are important with the testes being referred to as "abnormal gonads."

Tumors associated with abnormal sexual development

Gonadoblastoma

Gonadoblastoma is a rare benign germ cell–sex cord stromal tumor. It has the potential to become malignant and 30% of all patients with gonadoblastoma develop germ cell tumors, mainly dysgerminoma/seminoma [231]. Gonadoblastoma is observed in younger patients, typically in the second decade of life. About one-third of the cases are in children under 15 years of age. The majority of gonadoblastoma cases occur in patients with an underlying gonadal disorder. Gonadoblastoma accounts for approximately two-thirds of gonadal tumors in women with abnormal gonadal development. Patients with TS are at an increased risk for the development of gonadoblastoma. The tumor is more common in phenotypic females than in phenotypic males [232].

Gonadoblastoma is usually typically small in size, normally less than 8 cm, and partially calcified. It can increase in size if the tumor is overgrown by dysgerminoma or other malignant germ cell elements. Fifty percent may develop into dysgerminomas and 10% develop into other malignant germ cell neoplasms. Patients usually present with primary amenorrhea, virilization, or abnormal genitalia. It is often more common in the right gonad than the left gonad. On the microscopic level, gonadoblastoma is composed of collections of cellular nests surrounded by connective tissue stroma [232].

Pure gonadoblastomas do not metastasize and can regress spontaneously. They may secrete estrogen or testosterone. Gonadoblastomas themselves are benign but have a high frequency of developing into a malignant germ cell tumor. Dysgerminomas are malignant and may develop from benign gonadoblastomas in phenotypic females with gonadal dysgenesis with 46,XY pure gonadal dysgenesis or with mixed gonadal dysgenesis with 45,XY/46,XY mosaicism.

References

1. Goff BA, Mandel L, Muntz HG, Melancon CH. Ovarian carcinoma diagnosis. Cancer. 2000;**89**:2068–75.
2. Goff BA, Mandel LS, Drescher CW, et al. Development of an ovarian cancer symptom index: possibilities for earlier detection. Cancer. 2007;**109**:221–7.
3. Kim Y. A hospital-based case-control study of identifying ovarian cancer using symptom index. J Gynecol Oncol. 2010;**21**:65.
4. Rufford BD, Jacobs IJ, Menon U. Feasibility of screening for ovarian cancer using symptoms as selection criteria. BJOG. 2007;**114**:59–64.
5. Pitts MK, Heywood W, Ryall R, et al. High prevalence of symptoms associated with ovarian cancer among Australian women. Aust N Z J Obstet Gynaecol. 2011;**51**:71–8.
6. Bankhead CR, Kehow ST, Austoker J. Symptoms associated with diagnosis of ovarian cancer: a systematic review. BJOG. 2005;**112**:857–65.
7. Chan YM, Ng TY, Lee PW, Ngan HY, Wong LC. Symptoms, coping strategies, and timing of presentations in patients with newly diagnosed ovarian cancer. Gynecol Oncol. 2003;**90**:651–6.
8. Ferrell B, Smith S, Cullinane C, Melancon C. Symptom concerns of women with ovarian cancer. J Pain Symptom Manag. 2003;**25**:528–38.
9. Smith LH, Morris CR, Yasmeen S, et al. Ovarian cancer: can we make the clinical diagnosis earlier? Cancer. 2005;**104**:1398–407.
10. Webb PM, Purdie DM, Grover S, et al. Symptoms and diagnosis of borderline, early and advanced epithelial ovarian cancer. Gynecol Oncol. 2004;**92**(1):232–9.
11. Wynn ML. Temporal patterns of conditions and symptoms potentially associated with ovarian cancer. J Womens Health (Larchmt). 2007;**16**:971–86.
12. Khan A, Sultana K. Presenting signs and symptoms of ovarian cancer at a tertiary care hospital. J Pak Med Assoc. 2010;**60**:260–2.
13. Behtash N, Ghayouri Azar E, Fakhrejahani F. Symptoms of ovarian cancer in young patients 2 years before diagnosis, a case–control study. Eur J Cancer Care. 2008;**17**:483–7.
14. Friedman G, Skilling JS, Udaltsova NV, Smith LH. Early symptoms of ovarian cancer: a case–control study without recall bias. Fam Pract. 2005;**22**:548–53.
15. Yawn BP, Barrette BA, Wollan PC. Ovarian cancer: the neglected diagnosis. Mayo Clin Proc. 2004;**79**:1277–82.
16. Lataifeh I, Marsden DE, Robertson G, et al. Presenting symptoms of epithelial ovarian cancer. Aust N Z J Obstet Gynaecol. 2005;**45**:211–14.
17. Lim MC, Chun KC, Shin SJ, et al. Clinical presentation of endometrioid epithelial ovarian cancer with concurrent endometriosis: a multicenter retrospective study. Cancer Epidemiol Biomarkers Prev. 2010;**19**:398–404.
18. Hamilton W, Peters TJ, Bankhead C, Sharp D. Risk of ovarian cancer in women with symptoms in primary care: population based case-control study. BMJ. 2009;**339**:b2998.
19. Rossing MA, Wicklund KG, Cushing-Haugen KL, Weiss NS. Predictive value of symptoms for early detection of ovarian cancer. J Nat Cancer Inst. 2010;**102**:222–9.
20. Ryerson AB, Eheman C, Burton J, et al. Symptoms, diagnoses, and time to key diagnostic procedures among older U.S. women with ovarian cancer. Obstet Gynecol. 2007;**109**:1053–61.
21. Devlin S, Diehr PH, Andersen MR, et al. Identification of ovarian cancer symptoms in health insurance claims data. J Womens Health (Larchmt). 2010;**19**:381–9.
22. Lurie G, Thompson PJ, McDuffie KE, Carney ME, Goodman MT. Prediagnostic symptoms of ovarian carcinoma: a case-control study. Gynecol Oncol. 2009;**114**:231–6.
23. Bankhead C, Collins C, Stokes-Lampard H, et al. Identifying symptoms of ovarian cancer: a qualitative and quantitative study. BJOG. 2008;**115**:1008–14.
24. Jayde V, White K, Blomfield P. Symptoms and diagnostic delay in ovarian cancer: a summary of the literature. Contemp Nurse. 2009;**34**:55–65.
25. Goff BA, Mandel LS, Melancon CH, Muntz HG. Frequency of symptoms of ovarian cancer in women presenting to primary care clinics. JAMA. 2004;**291**:2705–12.
26. Olson SH, Mignone L, Nakraseive C, et al. Symptoms of ovarian cancer. Obstet Gynecol. 2001;**98**:212–7.
27. Olsen C, Cnossen J, Green AC, Webb PM. Comparison of symptoms and presentation of women with benign, low malignant potential and invasive ovarian tumors. Eur J Gynaecol Oncol. 2007;**28**:376–80.
28. Clarke-Pearson DL. Screening for ovarian cancer. N Engl J Med. 2009;**361**:170–7.
29. Liu JH. Management of the adnexal mass. Obstet Gynecol. 2011;**117**:1413–28.
30. Skírnisdóttir I, Garmo H, Holmberg L. Non-genital tract metastases to the ovaries presented as ovarian tumors in Sweden 1990–2003: occurrence, origin

and survival compared to ovarian cancer. Gynecol Oncol. 2007;**105**:166–71.

31. Antila R, Jalkanen J, Heikinheimo O. Comparison of secondary and primary ovarian malignancies reveals differences in their pre- and perioperative characteristics. Gynecol Oncol. 2006;**101**:97–101.
32. Lewis MR, Euscher ED, Deavers MT, Silva EG, Malpica A. Metastatic colorectal adenocarcinoma involving the ovary with elevated serum CA125: A potential diagnostic pitfall. Gynecol Oncol. 2007;**105**:395–8.
33. Fishman DA, Cohen LS. Is transvaginal ultrasound effective for screening asymptomatic women for the detection of early-stage epithelial ovarian carcinoma? Gynecol Oncol. 2000;**77**:347–9.
34. Fishman DA, Cohen L, Blank SV, et al. The role of ultrasound evaluation in the detection of early-stage epithelial ovarian cancer. Am J Obstet Gynecol. 2005;**192**:1214–21.
35. Cohen L, Fishman DA. Ultrasound and ovarian cancer. Cancer Treat Res. 2002;**107**:119–32.
36. Buy JN, Ghossain MA, Sciot C, et al. Epithelial tumors of the ovary: CT findings and correlation with US. Radiology. 1991;**178**:811–18.
37. Jain KA, Friedman DL, Pettinger TW, et al. Adnexal masses: comparison of specificity of endovaginal US and pelvic MR imaging. Radiology. 1993;**186**:697–704.
38. Hamper UM, Sheth S, Abbas FM, et al. Transvaginal color Doppler sonography of adnexal masses: differences in blood flow impedance in benign and malignant lesions. AJR Am J Roentgenol. 1993;**160**:1225–8.
39. Reles A, Wein U, Lichtenegger W. Transvaginal color Doppler sonography and conventional sonography in the preoperative assessment of adnexal masses. J Clin Ultrasound. 1997;**25**:217–25.
40. Marret H, Sauget S, Giraudeau B, et al. Contrast-enhanced sonography helps in discrimination of benign from malignant adnexal masses. J Ultrasound Med. 2004;**23**:1629–39.
41. Ordén MR, Jurvelin JS, Kirkinen PP. Kinetics of a US contrast agent in benign and malignant adnexal tumors. Radiology. 2003;**226**:405–10.
42. Aletti GD, Gallenberg MM, Cliby WA, Jatoi A, Hartmann LC. Current management strategies for ovarian cancer. Mayo Clin Proc. 2007;**82**:751–70.
43. Bharwani N, Reznek RH, Rockall AG. Ovarian cancer management: the role of imaging and diagnostic challenges. Eur J Radiol. 2011;**78**:41–51.
44. Fleischer AC. Recent advances in the sonographic assessment of vascularity and blood flow in gynecologic conditions. Am J Obstet Gynecol. 2005;**193**:294–301.
45. Goldberg BB. Contrast agents. Ultrasound Med Biol. 2000;**26**(Suppl 1):S33–4.
46. Burns PN, Hope Simpson D, Averkiou MA. Nonlinear imaging. Ultrasound Med Biol. 2000;**26**(Suppl 1):S19–22.
47. Brasch R. MRI characterization of tumors and grading angiogenesis using macromolecular contrast media: status report. Eur J Radiol. 2000;**34**:148–55.
48. Leen E. Ultrasound contrast harmonic imaging of abdominal organs. Semin Ultrasound CT MRI. 2001;**22**:11–24.
49. Ferrara KW, Merritt CR, Burns PN, et al. Evaluation of tumor angiogenesis with US: imaging, Doppler, and contrast agents. Acad Radiol. 2000;**7**:824–39.
50. Hall GH. Use of dynamic contrast-enhanced MRI to assess the functional vascular pharmacokinetic parameters of normal human ovaries. J Reprod Med. 2002;**47**:107–14.
51. Huber S, Helbich T, Kettenbach J, et al. Effects of a microbubble contrast agent on breast tumors: computer-assisted quantitative assessment with color Doppler US – early experience. Radiology. 1998;**208**:485–9.
52. Furlow B. Contrast-enhanced ultrasound. Radiol Technol. 2009;**80**:547S–61S.
53. Eckersley RJ, Sedelaar JP, Blomley MJ, et al. Quantitative microbubble enhanced transrectal ultrasound as a tool for monitoring hormonal treatment of prostate carcinoma. Prostate. 2002;**51**:256–67.
54. Krix M, Kiessling F, Vosseler S, et al. Comparison of intermittent-bolus contrast imaging with conventional power Doppler sonography: quantification of tumour perfusion in small animals. Ultrasound Med Biol. 2003;**29**:1093–103.
55. Weinberg LE, Lurain JR, Singh DK, Schink JC. Survival and reproductive outcomes in women treated for malignant ovarian germ cell tumors. Gynecol Oncol. 2011;**121**:285–9.
56. Schorge JO, Williams JW. Williams's Gynecology. New York: McGraw-Hill Medical; 2008.
57. Gershenson DM. Management of ovarian germ cell tumors. J Clin Oncol. 2007;**25**:2938–43.
58. Berek JS, Hacker NF. Practical Gynecologic Oncology. Baltimore: Lippincott Williams & Wilkins; 2000.
59. Madsen EM. Oophorectomy in the prevention of ovarian cancer. Acta Obstet Gynecol Scand. 1993;**72**:599–600.
60. Pastore M, Manci N, Marchetti C, et al. Late aortic lymphocele and residual ovary syndrome after gynecological surgery. World J Surg Oncol. 2007;**5**:146.
61. Dekel A, Efrat Z, Orvieto R, et al. The residual ovary syndrome: a 20-year experience. Eur J Obstet Gynecol Reprod Biol. 1996;**68**:159–64.
62. Magtibay PM, Magrina JF. Ovarian remnant syndrome. Clin Obstet Gynecol. 2006;**49**:526–34.
63. Narayansingh G, Cumming G, Parkin D, Miller I. Ovarian cancer developing in the ovarian remnant syndrome. A case report and literature review. Aust N Z J Obstet Gynaecol. 2000;**40**:221–3.
64. Brun JL. Demons syndrome revisited: a review of the literature. Gynecol Oncol. 2007;**105**:796–800.
65. Okuchi Y, Nagayama S, Mori Y, et al. VEGF hypersecretion as a plausible mechanism for pseudo-Meigs' syndrome in advanced colorectal cancer. Jpn J Clin Oncol. 2010;**40**:476–81.
66. Cheng MH, Yen MS, Chao KC, Sheu BC, Wang PH. Differential diagnosis of gynecologic organ-related diseases in women presenting with ascites. Taiwanese J Obstet Gynecol. 2008;**47**:384–90.
67. Hlaise KK, Shingange SM. Sudden death associated with Meigs syndrome: an autopsy case report. Am J Forensic Med Pathol. 2012;**33**:58–60.
68. Jiang W, Lu X, Zhu ZL, Liu XS, Xu CJ. Struma ovarii associated with pseudo-Meigs' syndrome and elevated serum CA 125: a case report and review of the literature. J Ovarian Res. 2010;**3**:18.
69. Kawakubo N, Okido M, Tanaka R, et al. Pseudo-Meigs' syndrome associated

with breast cancer metastasis to both ovaries: report of a case. Surg Today. 2010;**40**:1148–51.

70. Marci R, Giugliano E, Carboni S, Martinello R, Patella A. Pseudo-Meigs' syndrome caused by a uterine leiomyosarcoma: a new clinical condition. Gynecol Obstet Invest. 2011;**72**:68–72.
71. Alsamarai S, Adams JM, Murphy MK, et al. Criteria for polycystic ovarian morphology in polycystic ovary syndrome as a function of age. J Clin Endocrinol Metab. 2009;**94**:4961–70.
72. Goodarzi MO, Dumesic DA, Chazenbalk G, Azziz R. Polycystic ovary syndrome: etiology, pathogenesis and diagnosis. Nat Rev Endocrinol. 2011;7:219–31.
73. Azziz R, Carmina E, Dewailly D, et al. The Androgen Excess and PCOS Society criteria for the polycystic ovary syndrome: the complete task force report. Fertil Steril. 2009;**91**:456–88.
74. Bartoszek MP. Recognizing polycystic ovary syndrome in the primary care setting. Nurse Pract. 2009;**34**:22–9.
75. Wild RA. Assessment of cardiovascular risk and prevention of cardiovascular disease in women with the polycystic ovary syndrome: a consensus statement by the Androgen Excess and Polycystic Ovary Syndrome (AE-PCOS) Society. J Clin Endocrinol Metab. 2010;**95**:2038–49.
76. Pesant MH, Baillargeon JP. Polycystic ovary syndrome and metabolic syndrome. In: Zeitler PS, Nadeau KJ (Eds.). Insulin Resistance. New York: Humana Press; 2009. p 245–61.
77. Dey R, Fleming R, Sattar N, Greer IA, Wallace AM. Association of metabolic syndrome in polycystic ovarian syndrome: an observational study. J Obst Gynecol India. 2011;**61**:176–81.
78. Pothiwala P, Jain SK, Yaturu S. Metabolic syndrome and cancer. Metab Syndr Relat Disord. 2009;7:279–88.
79. Somani N, Harrison S, Bergfeld WF. The clinical evaluation of hirsutism. Dermatol Ther. 2008;**21**:376–91.
80. Blanc F. [Werner's syndrome with early onset with hyperandrogenism caused by ovarian hyperthecosis, acanthosis nigricans and peripheral neuropathy]. Ann Dermatol Venereol. 1990;**117**:785–6.
81. Wiedemann HR, Kunze J, Grosse FR. Clinical Syndromes. London: Mosby-Wolfe; 1997.
82. Keller J, Subramanyam L, Simha V, et al. Lipodystrophy: an unusual diagnosis in a case of oligomenorrhea and hirsutism. Obstet Gynecol. 2009;**114**(Pt 2):427–31.
83. Grunberger G, Alfonso B. Syndromes of extreme insulin resistance. In: Poretsky L (Ed.). Principles of Diabetes Mellitus. New York: Springer; 2010. p 259–77.
84. Oh CW, Yoon J, Kim CY. Malignant acanthosis nigricans associated with ovarian cancer. Case Rep Dermatol. 2010;**2**:103–9.
85. Mathur R, Evbuomwan I, Jenkins J. Prevention and management of ovarian hyperstimulation syndrome. 2005;**15**:132–8.
86. Zivi E. Ovarian hyperstimulation syndrome: definition, incidence, and classification. Semin Reprod Med. 2010;**28**:441–7.
87. Papanikolaou EG, Pozzobon C, Kolibianakis EM, et al. Incidence and prediction of ovarian hyperstimulation syndrome in women undergoing gonadotropin-releasing hormone antagonist in vitro fertilization cycles. Fertil Steril. 2006;**85**:112–20.
88. Zimmerman C. Ovarian hyperstimulation syndrome and development of pulmonary embolism in pregnancy: case report. Obstet Gynecol. 2010;**1**:1.
89. Aboulghar M. Treatment of ovarian hyperstimulation syndrome. Sem Reprod Med. 2010;**28**:532–9.
90. Tamai K, Koyama T, Saga T, et al. MR features of physiologic and benign conditions of the ovary. Eur Radiol. 2006;**16**:2700–11.
91. Gurgan T. Intravenous calcium infusion as a novel preventive therapy of ovarian hyperstimulation syndrome for patients with polycystic ovarian syndrome. Fertil Steril. 2011;**96**:53–7.
92. Spitzer D, Woqatzky J, Murtinger M, et al. Dopamine agonist bromocriptine for the prevention of ovarian hyperstimulation syndrome. Fertil Steril. 2011;**95**:2742–4.
93. Qublan H, Amarin Z, Nawasreh M, et al. Luteinized unruptured follicle syndrome: incidence and recurrence rate in infertile women with unexplained infertility undergoing intrauterine insemination. Hum Reprod. 2006;**21**:2110–3.
94. Shelling AN. Premature ovarian failure. Reproduction. 2010;**140**:633–41.
95. Vutyavanich T, Piromlertamorn W, Ellis J. Immature oocytes in "apparent empty follicle syndrome": a case report. Case Report Med. 2010;**2010**:367505.
96. Soliman AT. Empty sellae, impaired testosterone secretion, and defective hypothalamic-pituitary growth and gonadal axes in children with Bardet-Biedl syndrome. Metab Clin Exp. 1996;**45**:1230–4.
97. Karaman A. Bardet-Biedl syndrome: a case report. Dermatology Online J. 2008;**14**:9.
98. Dumitrescu CE, Collins MT. McCune-Albright syndrome. Orphanet J Rare Dis. 2008;**3**:12.
99. Bhutta HY, Walsh SR, Tang TY, Walsh CA, Clarke JM. Ovarian vein syndrome: a review. Int J Surg. 2009;**7**:516–20.
100. Freedman J, Ganeshan A, Crowe PM. Pelvic congestion syndrome: the role of interventional radiology in the treatment of chronic pelvic pain. Postgrad Med J. 2010;**86**:704–10.
101. Burlet G, Judlin P. [Acute pelvic pain syndrome. Diagnostic and therapeutic approach in women]. Rev Fr Gynecol Obstet. 1994;**89**:537–42.
102. Cunningham JM, Feldman MD. Munchausen by internet: current perspectives and three new cases. Psychosomatics. 2011;**52**:185–9.
103. Chen CP, et al. Bilateral calcified ovarian fibromas in a patient with Sotos syndrome. Fertil Steril. 2002;**77**:1285–7.
104. Seracchioli R. Conservative treatment of recurrent ovarian fibromas in a young patient affected by Gorlin syndrome. Hum Reprod (Oxford). 2001;**16** (6):1261–3.
105. Scully RE, Young RH, Clement PB (Eds.). Tumors of the Ovary, Maldeveloped Gonads, Fallopian Tube, and Broad Ligament. Atlas of Tumor Pathology. Third Series, Fascicle 23. Washington, DC: Armed Forces Institute of Pathology. 1998.
106. Morse CB, McLaren JF, Roy D, et al. Ovarian preservation in a young patient with Gorlin syndrome and multiple bilateral ovarian masses. Fertil Steril. 2011;**96**(1):e47–50.
107. Ball A, Wenning J, Van Eyk N. Ovarian fibromas in pediatric patients with basal cell nevus (Gorlin) syndrome. J Pediatr Adolesc Gynecol. 2011;**24**(1):e5–7.

108. Aram S. Bilateral ovarian fibroma associated with Gorlin syndrome. J Res Med Sci. 2009;**14**(1):57–61.
109. Hong JH. Unilateral ovarian dermoid cyst accompanied by an ipsilateral paratubal cyst in a girl with Proteus syndrome discovered by laparoscopic surgery. J Pediatr Adolesc Gynecol. 2010;**23**(3):107–10.
110. Jones KL, Smith DW. Smith's Recognizable Patterns of Human Malformation. Philadelphia: Saunders; 1997.
111. Winter RM, Baraitser M. Multiple Congenital Anomalies: A Diagnostic Compendium: First Supplement. New York: Chapman & Hall Medical; 1993.
112. Mena W. Fused eyelids, airway anomalies, ovarian cysts, and digital abnormalities in siblings: a new autosomal recessive syndrome or a variant of Fraser syndrome? Am J Med Genet. 1991;**40**(3):377–82.
113. Wagner M, et al. Lipid cell tumors in two women with von Hippel-Lindau syndrome. Obstet Gynecol. 2010;**116**(Suppl 2):535–9.
114. Lee S. Over-expression of hypoxia-inducible factor 1 alpha in ovarian clear cell carcinoma. Gynecol Oncol. 2007;**106**(2):311–17.
115. Huffman C. Weaver syndrome with neuroblastoma and cardiovascular anomalies. Am J Med Genet. 2001;**99**(3):252–5.
116. Vieira SC, et al. Sclerosing peritonitis associated with luteinized thecoma and elevated serum CA 125 levels: case report. Sao Paulo Med J. 2008;**126**(2):123–5.
117. Koak Y. Idiopathic sclerosing peritonitis. Eur J Gastroenterol Hepatol. 2008;**20**(2):148–50.
118. Staats PN. Luteinized thecomas (thecomatosis) of the type typically associated with sclerosing peritonitis: a clinical, histopathologic, and immunohistochemical analysis of 27 cases. Am J Surg Pathol. 2008;**32**(9):1273–90.
119. Yamashita S, et al., Lymphangioleiomyomatosis suspected to be a gynecologic disease. J Obstet Gynecol Res. 2011;**37**(3):267–9.
120. Lodish MB. The differential diagnosis of familial lentiginosis syndromes. Fam Cancer. 2011;**10**:481–90.
121. Barker D. An unusual case of sex cord tumor with annular tubules with malignant transformation in a patient with Peutz-Jeghers syndrome. Int J Gynecol Pathol. 2010;**29**(1):27–32.
122. van Lier MGF, et al. High cancer risk in Peutz-Jeghers syndrome: a systematic review and surveillance recommendations. Am J Gastroenterol. 2010;**105**(6):1258–64.
123. Tantipalakorn C, et al. Female genital tract tumors and gastrointestinal lesions in the Peutz-Jeghers syndrome. J Med Assoc Thai. 2009;**92**(12):1686–90.
124. Swanger RS. Ultrasound of ovarian sex-cord tumor with annular tubules. Ped Radiol. 2007;**37**(12):1270–1.
125. Howell L. Sertoli Leydig cell ovarian tumour and gastric polyps as presenting features of Peutz-Jeghers syndrome. Pediatr Blood Cancer. 2010;**55**(1):206–7.
126. Kato N, et al. Pyloric gland metaplasia/differentiation in multiple organ systems in a patient with Peutz-Jegher's syndrome. Pathol Int. 2011;**61**(6):369–72.
127. Kilic-Okman T. Breast cancer, ovarian gonadoblastoma and cervical cancer in a patient with Peutz-Jeghers syndrome. Arch Gynecol Obstet. 2008;**278**(1):75–7.
128. D'costa GF, et al. Peutz-Jegher's syndrome with ovarian serous cystadenoma: an unusual association. Indian J Pathol Microbiol. 2007;**50**(4):768–70.
129. Vasovcak P, et al. Multiple primary malignancies and subtle mucocutaneous lesions associated with a novel PTEN gene mutation in a patient with Cowden syndrome: case report. BMC Med Genet. 2011;**12**(1):38.
130. Babovic N, et al. Mucinous cystadenoma of ovary in a patient with juvenile polyposis due to 10q23 microdeletion: expansion of phenotype. Am J Med Genet A. 2010;**152A**(10):2623–7.
131. Lytras A, Tolis G. Reproductive disturbances in multiple neuroendocrine tumor syndromes. Endocr Relat Cancer. 2009;**16**(4):1125–38.
132. Boardman L, et al. Association of Peutz-Jeghers-like mucocutaneous pigmentation with breast and gynecologic carcinomas in women. Medicine (Baltimore). 2000;**79**(5):293–8.
133. Gell JS. Juvenile granulosa cell tumor in a 13-year-old girl with enchondromatosis (Ollier's disease): a case report. J Pediatr Adolesc Gynecol. 1998;**11**(3):147–50.
134. Rietveld L, et al. First case of juvenile granulosa cell tumor in an adult with Ollier disease. Int J Gynecol Pathol. 2009;**28**(5):464–7.
135. La Vecchia C. Infertility, ovulation, induced ovulation, and female cancers. Eur J Cancer Prev. 2011;**20**(3):147–9.
136. Barber HR, Graber EA. The PMPO syndrome (postmenopausal palpable ovary syndrome). CA Cancer J Clin. 1972;**22**(6):357–9.
137. Djordjevic B. Growing teratoma syndrome of the ovary: review of literature and first report of a carcinoid tumor arising in a growing teratoma of the ovary. Am J Surg Pathol. 2007;**31**(12):1913–18.
138. Sengar AR, Kulkarni JN. Growing teratoma syndrome in a post laparoscopic excision of ovarian immature teratoma. J Gynecol Oncol. 2010;**21**(2):129–31.
139. Kikawa S, et al. Growing teratoma syndrome of the ovary: a case report with FDG -PET findings. J Obstet Gynecol Res. 2011;**37**(7):926–32.
140. Yahata T, et al. Tumor lysis syndrome associated with weekly paclitaxel treatment in a case with ovarian cancer Gynecol Oncol. 2006;**103**(2):752–4.
141. Chong AL. Anaplastic large cell lymphoma of the ovary in a pediatric patient. J Pediatr Hematol Oncol. 2009;**31**(9):702–4.
142. Saluja M, Kenwright DN, Keating JP. Pseudomyxoma peritonei arising from a mucinous borderline ovarian tumour: case report and literature review. Aust N Z J Obstet Gynaecol. 2010;**50**(4):399–403.
143. Hwang JH, et al. Borderline-like mucinous tumor arising in mature cystic teratoma of the ovary associated with pseudomyxoma peritonei. Int J Gynecol Pathol. 2009;**28**(4):376–80.
144. Inui A. Cancer anorexia-cachexia syndrome: current issues in research and management. CA Cancer J Clin. 2002;**52**(2):72–91.
145. Gadducci A, et al. Malnutrition and cachexia in ovarian cancer patients: pathophysiology and management. Anticancer Res. 2001;**21**(4B):2941–7.
146. Smith J, Crowe K, McGaughran J, Robertson T. Sebaceous adenoma arising within an ovarian mature cystic teratoma in Muir–Torre syndrome. Ann Diagn Pathol. 2012;**16**:485–8.

147. Ehrsam EPJ, et al. Sweet's syndrome associated with ovarian carcinoma. J Eur Acad Dermatol Venereol. 1993;**2**(3):235–8.
148. Bolke E, et al. Leser-Trelat sign presenting in a patient with ovarian cancer: a case report. J Med Case Reports. 2009;**3**:8583.
149. Veras E. Metastatic HPV-related cervical adenocarcinomas presenting with thromboembolic events (Trousseau syndrome): clinicopathologic characteristics of 2 cases. Int J Gynecol Pathol. 2009;**28**(2):134–9.
150. Athappilly GK, Braverman RS. Congenital alacrima in a patient with blepharophimosis syndrome. Ophthalmic Genet. 2009;**30**(1):37–9.
151. Satgé D, et al. An ovarian dysgerminoma in Down syndrome. Hypothesis about the association. Int J Gynecol Cancer. 2006;**16**(S1):375–9.
152. Kim SS. Peritoneal melanosis associated with mucinous cystadenoma of the ovary and adenocarcinoma of the colon. Int J Gynecol Pathol. 2010;**29**(2):113–16.
153. Lanjewar DN, Dongaonkar DD. HIV-associated primary non-Hodgkin's lymphoma of ovary: A case report. Gynecol Oncol. 2006;**102**(3):590–2.
154. Santillan A, Bristow R. Paraneoplastic cerebellar degeneration in a woman with ovarian cancer. Nat Clin Pract Oncol. 2006;**3**(2):108–12; quiz.
155. Finsterer J, Voigtländer T, Grisold W. Deterioration of anti-Yo-associated paraneoplastic cerebellar degeneration. Neurol Sci. 2011;**308**:139–41.
156. Caliandro P, et al. Cerebellar degeneration and ocular myasthenia gravis in a patient with recurring ovarian carcinoma. Neurol Sci. 2010;**31**(1):79–81.
157. Stepanic V, et al. Ovarian cancer: PCD and brain metastases. Coll Antropol. 2007;**31**(2):633–6.
158. Monstad SE, et al. Yo antibodies in ovarian and breast cancer patients detected by a sensitive immunoprecipitation technique. Clin Exp Immunol. 2006;**144**(1):53–8.
159. Phuphanich S, Brock C. Neurologic improvement after high-dose intravenous immunoglobulin therapy in patients with paraneoplastic cerebellar degeneration associated with anti-Purkinje cell antibody. J Neurooncol. 2007;**81**(1):67–9.
160. Goldstein B, et al. Ovarian cancer and late onset paraneoplastic cerebellar degeneration. Arch Gynecol Obstet. 2009;**280**(1):99–101.
161. Bonakis A, et al. Acute onset paraneoplastic cerebellar degeneration. J Neurooncol. 2007;**84**(3):329–30.
162. Bradley W, Dottino P, Rahaman J. Paraneoplastic cerebellar degeneration in ovarian carcinoma: case report with review of immune modulation. Int J Gynecol Cancer. 2008;**18**(6):1364–7.
163. Singh V, Bhat I, Havlin K. Marantic endocarditis (NBTE) with systemic emboli and paraneoplastic cerebellar degeneration: uncommon presentation of ovarian cancer. J Neurooncol. 2007;**83**(1):81–3.
164. Fitzpatrick AS, et al. Opsoclonus-myoclonus syndrome associated with benign ovarian teratoma. Neurology. 2008;**70**(15):1292–3.
165. Tonomura Y, et al. Clinical analysis of paraneoplastic encephalitis associated with ovarian teratoma. J Neurooncol. 2007;**84**(3):287–92.
166. de Bot ST, et al. [From psychiatric symptoms to paraneoplastic syndrome]. Tijdschr Psychiatr. 2008;**50**(9):603–9.
167. Issa SS, Herskovitz S, Lipton RB. Acquired neuromyotonia as a paraneoplastic manifestation of ovarian cancer. Neurology. 2011;**76**(1):100–1.
168. Yumru A, et al. The relation between the presence of a giant primary ovarian leiomyoma and the occurrence of epilepsy as a paraneoplastic syndrome. Arch Gynecol Obstet. 2010;**281**(3):531–4.
169. Miranpuri AS, et al. Upper cervical intramedullary spinal metastasis of ovarian carcinoma: a case report and review of the literature. J Med Case Rep. 2011;**5**(1):311.
170. Cormio G, et al. Central nervous system metastases from epithelial ovarian cancer: prognostic factors and outcomes. Int J Gynecol Cancer. 2011;**21**(5):816–21.
171. Zahr Z, Baer A. Malignancy in myositis. Curr Rheumatol Rep. 2011;**13**(3):208–15.
172. Pelosof LC, Gerber DE. Paraneoplastic syndromes: an approach to diagnosis and treatment. Mayo Clin Proc. 2010;**85**(9):838–54.
173. Venhuizen AC, Martens JE, Van Der Linden PJQ. Dermatomyositis as first presentation of ovarian cancer. Acta Obstet Gynecol Scand. 2006;**85**(10):1271–2.
174. Zhang W, Jiang SP, Huang L. Dermatomyositis and malignancy: a retrospective study of 115 cases. Eur Rev Med Pharmacol Sci. 2009;**13**(2):77–80.
175. Ghosh A, Malak T, Pool A. Polymyositis and ovarian carcinoma: a case report. Arch Gynecol Obstet. 2007;**275**(3):195–7.
176. Kalogiannidis I, et al. Clear cell ovarian carcinoma following polymyositis diagnosis: a case report and review of the literature. Hippokratia. 2008;**12**(3):181–5.
177. Thiers BH, Sahn RE, Callen JP. Cutaneous manifestations of internal malignancy. CA Cancer J Clin. 2009;**59**(2):73–98.
178. Scheinfeld N. A review of the cutaneous paraneoplastic associations and metastatic presentations of ovarian carcinoma. Clin Exp Dermatol. 2008;**33**(1):10–15.
179. Yilmaz Z, et al. Skin metastasis in ovarian carcinoma. Int J Gynecol Cancer. 2006;**16**(S1):414–8.
180. Kebria MM, et al. Malignant acanthosis nigricans, tripe palms and the sign of Leser-Tre'lat, a hint to the diagnosis of early stage ovarian cancer: a case report and review of the literature. Gynecol Oncol. 2006;**101**(2):353–5.
181. Cho M-Y. First report of ovarian dysgerminoma in Cowden syndrome with germline PTEN mutation and PTEN-related 10q loss of tumor heterozygosity. Am J Surg Pathol. 2008;**32**(8):1258–64.
182. Cannavó SP, et al. Simultaneous development and parallel course of disseminated superficial porokeratosis and ovarian cancer: coincidental association or true paraneoplastic syndrome? J Am Acad Dermatol. 2008;**58**(4):657–60.
183. Streiff MB, et al. Venous thromboembolic disease. J Natl Compr Canc Netw. 2011;**9**(7):714–77.
184. Tateo S, et al. Ovarian cancer and venous thromboembolic risk. Gynecol Oncol. 2005;**99**(1):119–25.
185. Iodice S, et al. Venous thromboembolic events and organ-specific occult cancers: a review and meta-analysis. J Thromb Haemost. 2008;**6**(5):781–8.

186. Satoh T, et al. High incidence of silent venous thromboembolism before treatment in ovarian cancer. Br J Cancer. 2007;**97**(8):1053–7.

187. Uno K, et al. Tissue factor expression as a possible determinant of thromboembolism in ovarian cancer. Br J Cancer. 2007;**96**(2):290–5.

188. White RH, et al. Incidence of venous thromboembolism in the year before the diagnosis of cancer in 528 693 adults. Arch Intern Med. 2005;**165**(15):1782–7.

189. Mehta S. A rare paraneoplastic presentation of a functional ovarian tumor. J Pelvic Med Surg. 2008;**14**(5):405–7.

190. Peedicayil A, et al. Incidence and timing of venous thromboembolism after surgery for gynecological cancer. Gynecol Oncol. 2011;**121**(1):64–9.

191. Snijders MP, Morsink M, van Spronsen DJ, de Kievit-van der Heijden IM. Internal jugular vein thrombosis as paraneoplastic syndrome of primary ovarian non-Hodgkin's lymphoma. Eur J Gynaecol Oncol. 2010;**31**:675–8.

192. Wada Y, et al. Paradoxical cerebral embolism as the initial symptom in a patient with ovarian cancer. J Stroke Cerebrovasc Dis. 2007;**16**(2):88–90.

193. Holthouse DJ, Robbins P, Watson P. Paradoxical embolism secondary to ovarian carcinoma resulting in stroke. J Clin Neurosci. 2004;**11**(2):194–6.

194. De Cicco M. The prothrombotic state in cancer: pathogenic mechanisms. Crit Rev Oncol Hematol. 2004;**50**(3):187–96.

195. Wakana K, Yasugi T, Nako Y, et al. Successful surgical treatment and chemotherapy for ovarian cancer in a patient with idiopathic thrombocytopenic purpura. Int J Clin Oncol. 2011;**16**:447–9.

196. Shimura K, Shimazaki C, Okano A, et al. [Therapy-related myeloid leukemia following platinum-based chemotherapy for ovarian cancer.] Rinsho Ketsueki. 2001;**42**(2):99–103.

197. Lee JW, Yang WS, Chung SY, et al. Aggressive systemic mastocytosis after germ cell tumor of the ovary: C-KIT mutation documentation in both disease states. J Pediatr Hematol Oncol. 2007;**29**(6):412–15.

198. Haddad LB, Laufer MR. Thrombocytosis associated with malignant ovarian lesions within a pediatric/adolescent population. J Pediatr Adolesc Gynecol. 2008;**21**(5):243–6.

199. Shanbhogue AKP, et al. Clinical syndromes associated with ovarian neoplasms: a comprehensive review. Radiographics. 2010;**30**(4):903–19.

200. Alabduljalil T. Paraneoplastic syndromes in neuro-ophthalmology. Curr Opin Ophthalmol. 2007;**18**(6):463–9.

201. Prefontaine M, Gragoudas ES. Blindness as a consequence of a paraneoplastic syndrome in a woman with clear cell carcinoma of the ovary. Gynecol Oncol. 1999;**73**(3):424–9.

202. O'Neal KD, et al. Bilateral diffuse uveal melanocytic proliferation associated with pancreatic carcinoma: a case report and literature review of this paraneoplastic syndrome. Survey Ophthalmol. 2003;**48**(6):613–25.

203. Duong HVQ, McLean IW, Beahm DE. Bilateral diffuse melanocytic proliferation associated with ovarian carcinoma and metastatic malignant amelanotic melanoma. Am J Ophthalmol. 2006;**142**(4):693–5.

204. Dykgraaf RHM, et al. Clinical management of ovarian small-cell carcinoma of the hypercalcemic type: a proposal for conservative surgery in an advanced stage of disease. Int J Gynecol Cancer. 2009;**19**(3):348–53.

205. Rovithi M, et al. Small cell ovarian cancer in adolescents: report of two cases and review of the literature. Case Report Med. 2011;2011:749516.

206. Clement PB. Selected miscellaneous ovarian lesions: small cell carcinomas, mesothelial lesions, mesenchymal and mixed neoplasms, and non-neoplastic lesions. Mod Pathol. 2005;**18**(Suppl 2):113–29.

207. Pressey JG. The treatment of small cell carcinoma of the ovary hypercalcemic type. Oncol Rev. 2010: 1–6 [published online: 17 September 2010].

208. Young RH, Goodman A, Penson RT, et al. Case records of the Massachusetts General Hospital. Case 8-2010. A 22-year-old woman with hypercalcemia and a pelvic mass. N Engl J Med. 2010;**362**(11):1031–40.

209. Wynn D, Everett GD, Boothby RA. Small cell carcinoma of the ovary with hypercalcemia causes severe pancreatitis and altered mental status. Gynecol Oncol. 2004;**95**(3):716–18.

210. Montalto SA, et al. Small cell carcinoma of the ovary: hypercalcaemic type. J Obstet Gynaecol. 2011;**31**(2):199–200.

211. Harrison M, et al. Small cell of the ovary, hypercalcemic type – Analysis of combined experience and recommendation for management. A GCIG study. Gynecol Oncol. 2006;**100**(2):233–8.

212. Piura B. [Hypercalcemia in malignancies of the female genital tract]. Harefuah. 2008;**147**(3):229–34.

213. Wysolmerski JJ, Broadus AE. Hypercalcemia of malignancy: the central role of parathyroid hormone-related protein. Ann Rev Med. 1994;**45**(1):189–200.

214. Klein M, Weryha G, Dousset B, et al. [Physiological role of PTHrP]. Ann Endocrinol (Paris). 1995;**56**:193–204.

215. Datta NS, Abou-Samra AB. PTH and PTHrP signaling in osteoblasts. Cell Signal. 2009;**21**(8):1245–54.

216. Bruns D. Parathyroid hormone-related protein in benign lesions. Am J Clin Pathol. 1996;**105**(4):377–9.

217. Suwaki N, et al. Parathyroid hormone related protein as a potential tumor marker: a case report of ovarian clear cell carcinoma. J Obstet Gynecol Res. 2006;**32**(1):94–8.

218. De Nuccio I, et al. Physiopathology of the renin-angiotensin system in the ovary. Minerva Endocrinol. 1999;**24**(2):77–81.

219. Rabban JT, et al. Primary ovarian carcinoid tumors may express CDX-2: a potential pitfall in distinction from metastatic intestinal carcinoid tumors involving the ovary. Int J Gynecol Pathol. 2009;**28**(1):41–8.

220. Cafà E, Angioli R, Scollo P. Ovarian carcinoid tumor with nodal metastases: case report. J Cancer Sci Ther. 2010;**2**:120–1.

221. Baldwin D. Cushing's syndrome. In: Myers JA, Millikan KW, Saclarides TJ (Eds.). Common Surgical Diseases. New York: Springer; 2008. p 107–9.

222. Newell-Price J. Etiologies of Cushing's syndrome. In: Bronstein MD (Ed.). Contemporary Endocrinology: Cushing's Syndrome: Pathophysiology, Diagnosis and Treatment. Springer Science+Business Media. 2011. p 21–29.

223. Nieman LK, Biller BM, Findling JW, et al. The diagnosis of Cushing's syndrome: an endocrine society clinical

practice guideline. J Clin Endocrinol Metab. 2008;**93**(5):1526–40.

224. Kim AW, Richter HM. Zollinger Ellison syndrome. In: Myers JA, Millikan KW, Saclarides TJ (Eds.). Common Surgical Diseases: An Algorithmic Approach to Problem Solving. Springer, 2008. p 123–6.

225. Hamm B, Forstner R, Beinder E. MRI and CT of the Female Pelvis. New York: Springer Verlag; 2007.

226. Abboud P, Bart H, Namsour G, et al. Ovarian gastrinoma in multiple endocrine neoplasia type I: a case report. Am J Obstet Gynecol. 2001;**184**(2):237–8.

227. D'Antonio A, et al. Hashimoto Thyroiditis as a manifestation of struma ovarii. Endocrinologist. 2010;**20**(5):220.

228. Lloyd RV. Endocrine Pathology: Differential Diagnosis and Molecular Advances. Totowa, NJ: Humana Press Inc; 2004.

229. Elsheikh M, Dunger DB, Conway GS, Wass JA. Turner's syndrome in adulthood. Endocr Rev. 2002;**23**(1):120–40.

230. Gottlieb B, Beitel LK, Trifiro MA. Androgen Insensitivity Syndrome. Seattle, WA: University of Washington; 2007.

231. Peña-Alonso R, Nieto K, Alvarez R, et al. Distribution of Y-chromosome-bearing cells in gonadoblastoma and dysgenetic testis in 45, X/46, XY infants. Mod Pathol. 2004;**18**(3):439–45.

232. Blaustein A, Kurman RJ. Blaustein's Pathology of the Female Genital Tract. New York: Springer Verlag; 2002.

Chapter 22

When is ovarian carcinoma discovered in stage I?

Liane Deligdisch, MD, and Albert Altchek, MD, FACS, FACOG

Introduction

Only a minority of ovarian cancers of epithelial origin are diagnosed in early stages, when confined to the ovaries. This is the main reason for the high mortality due to this elusive neoplasm, the most lethal of all gynecologic cancers. The 5-year survival of patients diagnosed with stage I ovarian cancer, confined to the ovaries is 80–90%, as compared to the 5-year survival rate of 19–32% for late stages of the disease, when extended to other pelvic and/or abdominal sites. The majority of patients (80–85%) are diagnosed in stage III–IV [1].

Early detection of ovarian carcinoma represents a major challenge for the women healthcare community. Absence or paucity of specific symptoms and of reliable tumor markers are considered the main obstacles to unmask this "silent killer" at its inception.

Histopathology and classification

The vast majority of ovarian carcinomas (OC), tumors originating in the ovarian epithelium which represents an extension of the peritoneal mesothelium, are serous papillary carcinomas. According to recent histopathologic studies based on molecular biology, the serous carcinomas involving most ovarian cancers, more often than previously thought, involve the fallopian tube and the pelvic peritoneum. Actually, for many late stage ovarian cancers, it is difficult if not impossible to establish the anatomic origin of the neoplasms; therefore, it was suggested to include ovarian, fallopian tube, and peritoneal tumors in the term "pelvic serous carcinoma" [2]. They represent about 68–87% of all ovarian cancers. They are associated with BRCA1 and 2 mutations more often than the non-serous carcinomas. Also included in this group are malignant mixed Mullerian tumors (MMMT), many of which were proven by immuno-histochemistry to be poorly differentiated carcinomas, occasionally admixed with malignant stromal elements. OC histologically diagnosed as "non-serous" include endometrioid, mucinous, and clear cell carcinomas, and are by far less numerous.

A subclassification based on both histological and immuno-phenotypical criteria divides the ovarian carcinomas in high-grade and low-grade tumors according to the biological behavior and related to the prognosis [3,4].

Unfortunately, the high-grade tumors are the most numerous and are characterized by a rapid and aggressive growth with early spread to the neighboring anatomic structures, and high lethality.

Obviously, the high-grade tumors are more likely to be diagnosed in late stages (Fig. 22.1). They are mostly clinically "silent" being only occasionally detected in early stages either in patients who are followed very closely because of the patients' high-risk factors, or incidentally when the patients are seeking medical attention for other reasons.

The low-grade serous OC are histologically and biologically different from the common large group of high-grade serous carcinomas. They include a relatively small, still controversial group of serous papillary invasive, but low-grade micropapillary carcinoma, probably arising in borderline (low malignant potential) serous papillary tumors. Most low-grade OC are non-serous and include the more common endometrioid, and the less common clear cell adenocarcinomas, both often associated with ovarian and/or pelvic endometriosis. They are of low-grade malignancy in many cases, especially in younger patients, but high-grade endometrioid ovarian cancers are not unusual and their biological behavior when diagnosed late can be as aggressive as that of serous high-grade tumors.

Other non-serous OC are mucinous adenocarcinomas which seem in recent studies [5] to be rarely primary ovarian in origin. Most are metastatic from the gastrointestinal tract, often from the appendix, especially when bilateral. The rather few primary and unilateral ovarian mucinous carcinomas are in their majority borderline or well differentiated, therefore considered low-grade.

What is the relationship between histo-immunologic phenotype and the clinical stage the tumor is detected?

The most common OC as mentioned, those that represent the vast majority of all ovarian cancers, are the least often detected in stage I, when confined to the ovaries. The less common, non-serous histologic variants: endometrioid, clear cell, and mucinous carcinomas are the malignancies of epithelial origin most often diagnosed in stage I, when confined to the ovary(ies). The histologic distribution of OC is therefore different for stage I from that of OC in all stages. The immunophenotype of the two categories of OC is different as well: low-grade OC are associated with mutations of *KRAS*, *BRAF*, *PTEN*, and the gene for betacatenin, while high-grade OC, including serous and high-grade endometrioid OC are frequently associated with perturbations in the p53 pathway

Altchek's Diagnosis and Management of Ovarian Disorders, ed. Liane Deligdisch, Nathan G. Kase, and Carmel J. Cohen. Published by Cambridge University Press.

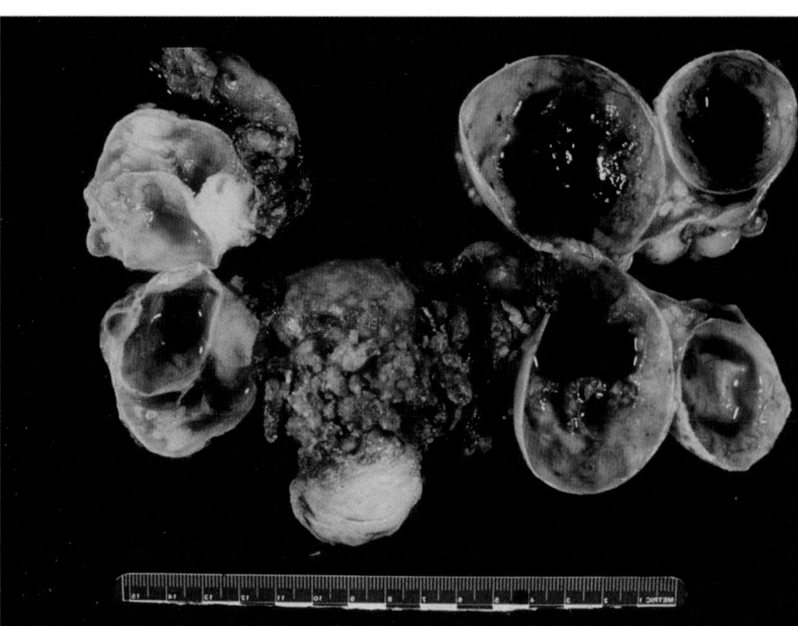

Fig. 22.1. Ovarian stage III high-grade serous papillary adenocarcinoma. Bilateral ovarian and pelvic serosal involvement by tumor. Patient is 68 years old, was asymptomatic until 2 weeks before presenting with ascites.

resulting in p53 overexpression [6]. The genetic alterations are also quite different, with microsatellite instability being more frequent in the high-grade OC [3].

Clinical correlations

Historically, ovarian carcinoma was called the "silent killer" because symptoms generally occur late in the course of the disease when most patients seek medical attention because of abdominal distention, nausea, early satiety, and urinary frequency.

Studies have found that symptoms occur in many women even at the early stages of the disease but these are non-specific, non-gynecologic, and often go unreported [7].

The symptoms that were most commonly reported were abdominal pain/discomfort and abdominal swelling/bloating recurring more frequently and becoming more severe before the diagnosis of ovarian carcinoma, often associated with urinary urgency [8].

Use of symptoms recognition may potentially identify women with early stage disease. The symptoms, however, are less frequent in early stage disease than in late stage disease. Age and family history contribute to risk assessment for ovarian cancer [9].

Evaluation of symptoms (symptom index) is the first step in the sequential process that will include abnormal serum CA125 concentration and imaging studies consisting of pelvic and vaginal ultrasound.

Paraneoplastic gastrointestinal motor dysfunction has also been reported in a study of the Mayo Clinic [10].

Other symptoms are fatigue, back pain, pain with intercourse, constipation, and menstrual irregularity, all non-specific and often present in the general female population. The retrospective histories of those non-specific, often vague histories are characterized by their persistency and frequency during the months preceding the diagnosis of OC.

As mentioned, the histopathologic variant of the majority of ovarian carcinomas considered "clinically silent" or preceded by the above described rather non-specific symptoms, is the serous papillary (high-grade) cystadenocarcinoma, or as recently designated the pelvic serous carcinoma also including peritoneal and fallopian tube malignancy.

For the non-serous ovarian cancers that represent a smaller but still considerable group of ovarian cancer, the early symptomatology is by far more significant and conducive to an earlier diagnosis. Most but not all of the non-serous ovarian carcinomas are now classified as low-grade cancers, arising from known benign or borderline precursor tumors [11]. These include the endometrioid and clear cell carcinomas often associated with atypical endometriosis, the mucinous carcinomas arising in borderline mucinous tumors, and the small group of invasive low-grade serous micropapillary carcinomas arising in borderline serous carcinomas.

The endometrioid OC are the most common in this group. They are often (about 15–20%) associated with endometriosis ovarian and extra-ovarian, in patients frequently presenting with infertility, irregular menses, and dyspareunia. They are also associated with uterine pathology in 30%, of patients, of whom about 14% have endometrial carcinoma. Frequently associated extra-ovarian pathology includes adenomyosis, leiomyomas, endometrial polyps, as well as endometrial hyperplasia ranging from benign glandular and cystic to complex atypical and endometrial carcinoma. Ovarian endometriosis and cyst adenofibromas are benign lesions with a potential risk to become ovarian carcinomas.

Endometrioid OC is diagnosed in FIGO stage I–II in 52% of cases and represents about 10–15% of all ovarian carcinomas [12]. These neoplasms are mostly unilateral, by difference from the serous OC which are mostly bilateral. Clear cell carcinomas are the OC most commonly associated with endometriosis, and are also diagnosed more often in stage I–II than serous ırcinomas. Non-serous carcinomas of the ovary are usually iagnosed in patients younger, on average, by 10–15 years, than ıe serous OC.

Vhy are the non-serous ovarian carcinomas liagnosed at an earlier stage than the erous carcinomas?

'he prognosis of ovarian non-serous carcinomas is evidently ıore favorable in most cases than that of serous carcinomas, lthough, if compared stage by stage, there would not be any gnificant difference. So why are most non-serous carcinomas iagnosed in earlier stages? Is it because they are slower growıg tumors, different histologically, genetically, and immunoɔgically from the high-grade serous carcinomas? Or is it ecause they are associated with symptomatic pathological hanges that bring the patients earlier to medical attention?

A study of 76 cases of stage I ovarian carcinoma has emonstrated that more than two-thirds of stage I ovarian arcinomas were non-serous OC [13]. In this group, most arcinomas were endometrioid (40 of 54 [71%]), 10 clear cell arcinomas and four mixed endometrioid and clear cell carciomas (Table 22.1).

The patients diagnosed with non-serous OC had associated athologic changes of the uterus consisting of endometrial olyps, endometrial hyperplasia (11 cases), and endometrial rimary carcinoma (19 cases), and of the ovaries such as endoıetriosis and cystadenofibromas. In the majority of patients ıese changes manifested clinically as painful pelvic masses nd/or vaginal bleeding. Only one patient presented with astrointestinal symptoms and one had a history of breast arcinoma. Five patients had clinically "silent" OC, of which ɔur endometrioid and one clear cell OC were detected during ysterectomy performed for uterine pathology. The average age ı this group of patients with non-serous OC was 54 years.

Patients with serous OC were diagnosed in less than onehird of the cases (22 [29%]) in stage I of the disease. Thirteen of hese 22 patients were completely asymptomatic and their pelvic ıasses were detected fortuitously, on routine examination. Eight ad a history of previous breast cancers and had been on close urveillance with transvaginal sonograms. Four of them had ermline BRCA1 mutations and four were not tested. Only two resented with pelvic pain and one with vaginal bleeding. This atient had a history of breast carcinoma treated with tamoxifen nd subsequently developed endometrial carcinoma detected ue to vaginal bleeding. At hysterectomy for the endometrial ancer an otherwise symptomless ovarian carcinoma was emoved. Two patients complained of upper gastrointestinal ymptoms (bloating, nausea) and two had abnormal pap smears, nrelated to the ovarian tumor. The average age of the patients in he group of serous ovarian carcinoma was 61 years.

This study confirmed that the histologic distribution of tage I ovarian epithelial cancers is very different from that een in all stages, where the serous carcinomas are by far the ıost frequent, endometrioid carcinomas are about 15%, and lear cell carcinomas less than 6% [14].

Table 22.1. Stage I ovarian carcinoma: 76 cases

Pathology	OSPC[1]	OEC[2]	OCCC[3]	MC[4]
Total	22	40	10	4
Well differentiated (G1)	4	12	6	–
Moderately differentiated (G2)	5	22	3	2
Poorly differentiated (G3)	13	3	1	2
Ovarian endometriotic cyst	1	26	7	3
Pelvic endometriosis	1	12	1	1
Ovarian adenofibroma	1	4	2	–
Endometrial adenocarcinoma	1	19	1	–
Bilateral ovarian tumors	11	3	1	1
EC well differentiated (G1)	–	1	–	–
EC moderately differentiated (G2)	–	7	1	–
EC poorly differentiated (G3)	1	4	–	–
Endometrial polyps/ hyperplasia	3	11	2	2
Clinical data				
Pelvic mass, asymptomatic	13	2	0	1
Pelvic mass, symptomatic	2	19	10	4
Vaginal bleeding	1	16	3	1
Hx breast cancer	8	–	1	–
Ovarian cancer dx at hysterectomy for endometrial neoplasm	–	4	1	–
Ascites	2	–	1	–
GI symptoms	2	–	1	–
Abnormal Pap smear	2	–	–	–
Previously dx endometriosis	–	16	–	–
Average age	61	52.9	58.6	52.2

[1] Ovarian serous papillary carcinoma.
[2] Ovarian endometrioid carcinoma.
[3] Ovarian clear cell carcinoma.
[4] Mixed endometrioid/clear cell carcinoma.

It could, therefore, be assumed that patients with non-serous OC have a better prognosis because of their more common association with symptomatic pathology, while the serous OC tend to be clinically silent, or only vaguely and non-specifically symptomatic [15]. This is also confirmed by a study reporting rather disappointing early symptomatic findings for OC [7]. Early-stage ovarian patients were less likely to have symptoms (except nausea) than those with late stage cancer, and the estimated "positive predictive value" of the symptoms was very low (0.6–1.1%) overall and less than 0.5% for early stage disease.

These conclusions were reported without specifying the histologic pattern of the ovarian tumors.

Endometrioid, clear cell, and mucinous ovarian carcinomas are considered as having a better prognosis and being more often diagnosed in early stages. This is generally thought to be due to their slower, less aggressive growth as compared with most serous carcinomas. However, both endometrioid and clear cell carcinomas when diagnosed late, in stage III–IV, have a similar dismal prognosis as the serous carcinomas.

The difference in the outcome of these tumors lies in great part in the fact that the patients seek medical attention due to symptoms elicited by the accompanying pathologic changes such as pelvic and abdominal masses creating adhesions to the gastrointestinal tract due to endometriosis. Endometriotic cysts can reach large volume and produce symptoms of compression and adhesion to neighboring organs. While endometriosis is a very common affliction, fortunately endometrioid OC is relatively rare. However, it is now considered that atypical histologic changes of the endometrioid lining of endometriotic cysts, mostly ovarian but occasionally also extra-ovarian, are potential precursors of neoplastic changes [12,16]. These atypical changes of the histologic phenotype as well as the immuno-cytologic and genetic abnormalities of this epithelium have been demonstrated adjacent to the overt OC, sometimes at the transition between benign endometriotic lining and OC. A somehow analogous situation is that of dysplastic changes of the ovarian epithelium identified adjacent to serous carcinomas, as well as incidentally, on prophylactic salpingo-oophorectomy specimens removed from patients at genetic risk (see Chapter 6). The precursor changes are perhaps more subtle and more difficult to identify in serous OC because of the aggressive and clinically silent proliferation of serous high-grade pelvic carcinomas, rapidly overgrowing the dysplastic changes. These tumors, statistically the most numerous and most lethal of all ovarian cancers, have recently been described as associated with frequent fallopian tube involvement, where precursor, non-invasive (dysplastic, in-situ) changes have been identified in the fimbrial portion of the fallopian tube. Molecular abnormalities may precede the phenotypical expression of these changes, such as the "p53 signature" (see Chapter 7).

Is early diagnosis of ovarian cancer possible?

In comparison with other gynecologic malignancies the prognosis of which has dramatically improved during the past decades such as cervical and endometrial cancer often detected in their precursor or early clinical stages, ovarian cancer is still diagnosed late in the vast majority of cases despite the abundance of clinical and biological research. The identification of histological potential precursors and early stages of the cancer is highly significant representing the changes to be sought after. The major problem is the access to the organ. The ovaries have a secluded location in the pelvis/abdomen. They became more accessible with radiologic visualization techniques (transvaginal ultrasound, MRI) and new laparoscopic techniques. Serum markers, the most common being CA125 as well as proteomic (see Chapter 27) are promising but so far, unfulfilling method to detect early OC, being neither specific enough (especially in younger women) nor sensitive enough in the early stages of the disease.

Prophylactic salpingo-oophorectomies performed on women with high risk for ovarian carcinoma due to genetic mutations and/or family history of breast cancer, or Lynch syndrome may reveal clinically "silent" stage I ovarian carcinoma. This may also occur occasionally sporadically, at TAH BSO performed for unrelated diseases of the uterus or adnexae.

Non-serous OC usually occur in a different clinical setting involving younger patients, often with a history of infertility, hyperestrogenic lesions such as endometriosis, adenomyosis, leiomyomas, endometrial polyps, and hyperplasia/neoplasia. The coexistent ovarian tumor may not be manifested clinically and is detected due to the symptomatic associated lesions benign or malignant: endometrial changes manifested by vaginal bleeding, pelvic pain, and urinary or intestinal symptoms due to the presence of endometriotic cystic or solid masses in the ovary, pelvis or abdomen, or both. Patients with persistent symptoms of hyperestrogenism, infertility, or endometriosis may be considered at risk for OC [17] and associated endometrial carcinoma [18].

In conclusion, the diagnosis of stage I OC is rare for high grade serous OC requiring major efforts directed at identifying early malignant lesions in this large group of tumors. The less common low-grade, non-serous OC are more likely to be diagnosed in earlier stages due both to their slower growth and frequent associated symptomatic lesions.

Confocal optical biopsy

Most ovarian epithelial neoplasms arise from the ovarian surface epithelium and its invaginations, often creating cystic structures in the ovarian cortex.

The detection of precancerous and early malignant changes in the uterine cervix, which resulted in a spectacular decrease in the morbidity and mortality due to cervical cancer, was possible because of the easy visualization of the cervical lesions and the minutious description of their microscopic structure detected by colposcopy and correlated with cytologic and virologic studies.

The ovaries became visually accessible by laparoscopic techniques. A recent technique opened new horizons to the access of microscopic visualization in real time mode. Already widely used in the gastrointestinal tract, optic confocal endoscopy visualizes lesions in a manner similar to histologic sections seen "from above" though, while histologic sections are perpendicular. This method has been applied to the human ovary ex-vivo and has the potential of screening the ovarian surface up to 250 μm in depth [19]. Because most ovarian tumors arise from the ovarian surface epithelium, it seems that the ovary is suitable for this technique that would benefit from additional improvements adding depth to the obtained images.

This technique could be used for early diagnosis of asymptomatic ovarian cancer and for preinvasive dysplastic lesions as described by histology, computerized image analysis (morphometry) and immuno-histochemistry, especially in women at risk for ovarian cancer (see Chapter 6).

Because the optic biopsies make real-time diagnosis possible, further surgery in case of positive findings could be performed and unneeded surgery, especially in young women desiring to preserve fertility, could be avoided. Initially, this method may be used to locate unusual regions for guided biopsies: the in longer term, traditional biopsies may be replaced by "optical" real-time biopsies.

At the present time no valid screening method for early ovarian epithelial cancer is implemented. Tumor markers are neither sensitive nor specific enough for localized tumors and pelvic examination, symptom recognition, and radiologic imaging detect only a small percentage of stage I ovarian carcinoma. Further studies of serologic markers (proteomics [20]), are promising (see Chapter 27). Improved laparoscopic techniques including confocal optic biopsies may help early detection of OC perhaps in a similar way as colposcopy did with cervical cancer precursors.

References

1. Jemal A, Siegel R, Ward E, et al. Cancer statistics, 2008. CA Cancer J Clin. 2008; **58**(2):71–96.
2. Crum CP. Intercepting pelvic cancer in the distal fallopian tube: theories and realities. Mol Oncol. 2009;**3**(2):165–70.
3. Shih IeM, Kurman RJ. Ovarian tumorigenesis: a proposed model based on morphological and molecular genetic analysis. Am J Pathol. 2004;**164**(5):1511–8.
4. McCluggage WG. My approach to and thoughts on the typing of ovarian carcinomas. J Clin Pathol. 2008;**61**(2):152–63.
5. Seidman JD, Cho KR, Ronnett BM, et al. In: Blaustein's pathology of the female genital tract, 6th edition. In: Kurman RJ, Hedrick Ellenson L, Ronnett BM (Eds.). Mucinous Tumors. New York: Springer; 2011. p 735.
6. Comes CP, Andrade L. PTEN and P53 expression in primary ovarian carcinomas: immunohistochemical study and discussion of pathogenetic mechanisms. Int J Gynecol Cancer. 2006;**16**:254–8.
7. Mulcahy N. Symptoms of ovarian cancer not much help in detecting disease. Medscape Medical News. 2010. http://www.medscape.org/viewarticle/716656.
8. Goff BA, Mandel LS, Drescher CW, et al. Development of an ovarian cancer symptom index: possibilities for earlier detection. Cancer. 2007;**109**(2):221–7.
9. Goff B, Muntz H. Ovarian cancer: recognizing early symptoms can make a difference. Contemp Ob Gyn. 2008;**53**:26.
10. Lee HR, Lennon VA, Camilleri M, et al. Paraneoplastic gastrointestinal motor dysfunction: clinical and laboratory characteristics. Am J Gastroenterol. 2001;**96**(2):373–9.
11. Vang R, Shih IM, Kurman RJ. Ovarian low-grade and high-grade serous carcinoma: pathogenesis, clinicopathologic and molecular biologic features, and diagnostic problems. Adv Anat Pathol. 2009;**16**(5):267–82.
12. Seidman JD, Cho KR, Ronnett BM, et al. In: Blaustein's pathology of the female genital tract, 6th edition. In: Kurman RJ, Hedrick Ellenson L, Ronnett BM (Eds.). Endometrioid Adenocarcinoma. New York: Springer; 2011. p 751.
13. Deligdisch L, Pénault-Llorca F, Schlosshauer P, et al. Stage I ovarian carcinoma: different clinical pathologic patterns. Fertil Steril. 2007;**88**(4):906–10.
14. Seidman JD, Cho KR, Ronnett BM, et al. In: Blaustein's pathology of the female genital tract, 6th edition. In: Kurman RJ, Hedrick Ellenson L, Ronnett BM (Eds.). Clear Cell Carcinoma. New York: Springer; 2011. p 759.
15. Cass I, Karlan BY. Ovarian cancer symptoms speak out – but what are they really saying? J Natl Cancer Inst. 2010;**102**(4):211–2.
16. Ogawa S, Kaku T, Amada S, et al. Ovarian endometriosis associated with ovarian carcinoma: a clinicopathological and immunohistochemical study. Gynecol Oncol. 2000;77(2):298–304.
17. Walsh C, Holschneider C, Hoang Y, et al. Coexisting ovarian malignancy in young women with endometrial cancer. Obstet Gynecol. 2005;**106**(4):693–9.
18. Catasús L, Bussaglia E, Rodrguez I, et al. Molecular genetic alterations in endometrioid carcinomas of the ovary: similar frequency of beta-catenin abnormalities but lower rate of microsatellite instability and PTEN alterations than in uterine endometrioid carcinomas. Hum Pathol. 2004;**35**(11):1360–8.
19. Tanbakuchi AA, Udovich JA, Rouse AR, et al. In vivo imaging of ovarian tissue using a novel confocal microlaparoscope. Am J Obstet Gynecol. 2010;**202**(1):90.e1–9.
20. Tchagang AB, Tewfik AH, DeRycke MS, et al. Early detection of ovarian cancer using group biomarkers. Mol Cancer Ther. 2008;7(1):27–37.

Chapter

23

Early detection of ovarian cancer

Christina E. Curtin, Pierre S. Gordon, MD, and David A. Fishman, MD

Introduction

Incidence, prevalence, mortality rates, and natural history

Ovarian cancer is a heterogeneous and rapidly progressive disease of low prevalence and poor survival. In developed countries, the number of deaths attributed to ovarian cancer approximates all other gynecologic malignancies combined [1]. Globally, approximately 225,000 women are diagnosed with ovarian cancer with 140,000 deaths annually [2]. Within the United States, ovarian cancer is the most lethal of all gynecologic malignancies and is the fifth leading cause of cancer-related deaths and ninth most common malignancy [3]. An estimated 21,880 new cases of ovarian cancer were diagnosed in 2010 within the United States with the expectation of 13,850 women dying from this disease [4]. The lifetime risk of developing ovarian cancer in the general population, without any risk factors, is 1 in 72 (1.39%) [5,6]. The lifetime risk of dying from ovarian cancer for women living in the United States is 1 in 96 (1.04%) [5]. In the postmenopausal population the incidence is 1 in 2,300. Ovarian cancer carries a high case-to-fatality ratio. Compared with breast cancer, it is more lethal by a factor of 3.

Unfortunately, the majority of ovarian carcinoma cases are diagnosed at advanced stages (stages III and IV), when the disease has already metastasized to the peritoneal cavity or other surrounding organs, such as the liver or lungs [4]. Less than 20% of ovarian cancers are detected when the cancer is still confined to the ovary (stage I). Women who are diagnosed with early stage ovarian cancer (stages I to II) have 5-year survival rates that range from 57 to 90% [7]. In contrast, the 5-year survival rates for patients who are diagnosed with advanced stage disease range from 18 to 45% [7]. Despite advances in surgery and platinum-based chemotherapy the mortality rates of individuals with ovarian cancer remain poor. In the past 40 years, the median 5-year survival rate for women with advanced-stage cancer has increased from 37 to 46% [8,9]. Ovarian cancer is rarely seen in women under 40. The average age at diagnosis is 58 years and the highest incidence occurs from 65 to 75 years of age.

While all cancer patients could potentially benefit from earlier detection methods the development of new screening methods for epithelial ovarian cancer (EOC) is unique in the promise of clinical and public health benefits from earlier diagnosis. EOC is the fifth leading cause of death in American women due to the continued inability to detect early stage (I) disease. Early detection and reduced mortality efforts have been unsuccessful thus far because the pathogenesis of ovarian cancer is poorly understood. Until recently, ovarian cancer has been considered a 'silent killer' because its symptoms were thought to develop only after the disease had progressed to an advanced stage [10]. Evidence suggests that early detection and inhibition of ovarian carcinoma will require the development of strategies based on the molecular, genetic, and biochemical events that regulate carcinogenesis, invasion, and metastatic dissemination. Because of the low prevalence of ovarian cancer in the general population, current screening methods focus on asymptomatic women who are at increased risk of developing ovarian cancer. Current studies are investigating the use and effectiveness of genetic counseling, state-of-the-art imaging techniques, and serum tumor markers in detecting early stage ovarian cancers in high-risk asymptomatic women. Additionally, new powerful technologies using genomics and proteomics are also used to detect early stage ovarian cancer.

Classification and staging of ovarian carcinoma

Etiology

A clear etiology of ovarian cancer has yet to be identified. The ovary is surrounded by a single-cell layer of coelomic epithelium that has the potential to undergo malignant transformation and differentiate into a variety of cell types resembling those found in the fallopian tube, uterus, cervix, and ovarian stroma [9]. Carcinomas of the ovary, fallopian tube, and peritoneal cavity have been regarded as separate disease entities, each with a distinct site of origin [11]. Ovarian cancer is due to the accumulation of genetic mutations. These mutations occur in genes involved in cell senescence, apoptosis, and proliferation. Several theories exist regarding the mechanism by which these mutations come into existence. These include incessant ovulation whereby uninterrupted ovulatory cycles results in a chance for malignant transformation of

Altchek's Diagnosis and Management of Ovarian Disorders, ed. Liane Deligdisch, Nathan G. Kase, and Carmel J. Cohen. Published by Cambridge University Press.

invaginated surface epithelium when under oncogenic influence. Another theory involves malignant transformation of the epithelium as a result of exposure to continued elevated concentrations of pituitary gonadotropins. An alternate theory is the retrograde menstruation hypothesis where carcinogens are carried from the vagina and/or uterus to the ovary at menses.

Until recently, it was widely accepted that ovarian cancer progressed on either the epithelial layer surrounding the ovary or within postovulatory inclusion cysts [12]. Current dogma has been challenged as it is currently suggested that a higher percentage of ovarian cancers originate in the fimbriated end of the fallopian tube with metastasis to the ovary [13]. Other ovarian cancers are believed to originate from components of the secondary Mullerian system, which includes paraovarian and paratubal cysts [14].

Ovarian cancer is a heterogeneous and rapidly progressive disease of low prevalence and poor survival. This heterogeneity is not only due to the cells from which these tumors arise but also to their biologic behavior. Ovarian neoplasms are classified according to the type of cell from which they arise: epithelial, germ cell, and stromal tumors [15]. Epithelial tumors constitute 90% of ovarian cancers and were thought to develop within the thin layer of surface epithelium that covers the ovaries. This group is composed of serous, endometrioid, mucinous, clear cell, Brenner, mixed, and undifferentiated tumors. The most common of the epithelial ovarian cancers is of the serous type, responsible for 60% of cases. Endometrioid and mucinous tumors follow, accounting for 15% and 10%, respectively. In addition to their cell of origin, ovarian cancers can be categorized according to their pathogenesis using a classification system devised by Shih and Kurman. Type I ovarian cancers are the well-differentiated serous, mucinous, malignant Brenner, clear cell, and endometrioid tumors. Low-grade tumors (type 1 tumors) are slowly developing tumors that progress through a stepwise mutation process and are less responsive to chemotherapy in the recurrent setting than high-grade ovarian cancers [9]. Type I tumors also exhibit slow progression through the different stages. Type II ovarian cancers include malignant mixed mesodermal tumors, carcinosarcomas, undifferentiated carcinomas, and serous carcinomas of the moderately or poorly differentiated variety. Type II tumors are more aggressive in that they have a rapid onset, early metastasis, and demonstrate higher genetic instability [16].

Germ cell and stromal tumors both constitute approximately 5% of ovarian cancer cases, and arise in the cells that form eggs and the connective tissue, respectively. The germ cell tumors are subdivided into dysgerminomas and nondysgerminomas. The nondysgerminoma group is made up of yolk sac tumors also known as endodermal sinus tumors, teratomas, both mature and immature, embryonal carcinoma, and ovarian choriocarcinoma, not to be confused with the gestational trophoblastic uterine choriocarcinoma. Finally, the gonadal-stromal ovarian tumors include the Sertoli–Leydig tumors, granulosa cell tumors, thecoma-fibromas, and gonadoblastomas.

Table 23.1. AJCC classifications for ovarian cancer *

	Stages	Description
T	TX	Primary tumor cannot be assessed
	T0	No evidence of primary tumor
	T1	Tumor confined to the ovaries (one or both)
	T1a	Tumor confined to one ovary; capsules intact, no tumor on ovarian surface, no malignant cell in ascites of peritoneal washings
	T1b	Tumor limited to both ovaries; capsules intact, no tumor on ovarian surface, no malignant cell in ascites or peritoneal washings
	T1c	Tumor limited to one or both ovaries with any of the following: capsule ruptured, tumor on ovarian surface, malignant cells in ascites or peritoneal washings
	T2	Tumor involves one or both ovaries with pelvic extension
	T2a	Extension and/or implants on the uterus and/or tube(s); no malignant cells in ascites or peritoneal washings
	T2b	Extension to other pelvic tissues; no malignant cells in ascites or peritoneal washings
	T2c	Pelvic extension (2a or 2b) with malignant cells in ascites or peritoneal washings
	T3	Tumor involves one or both ovaries with microscopically confirmed peritoneal metastasis outside the pelvis and/or regional lymph nodes metastasis
	T3a	Microscopic peritoneal metastasis beyond the pelvis
	T3b	Macroscopic peritoneal metastasis beyond the pelvis (≤ 2 cm in the greatest dimension)
	T3c	Peritoneal metastasis beyond the pelvis (≥2 cm in the greatest dimension)
	NX	Regional lymph nodes cannot be assessed
N	N0	No regional lymph node metastasis
	N1	Regional lymph node metastasis
	MX	Presence of distant metastasis cannot be assessed
M	M0	No distant metastasis
	M1	Distant metastasis (excludes peritoneal metastasis)

* Data taken from American Joint Committee on Cancer (18).
The International Federation of Gynecology and Obstetrics (FIGO) stages ovarian cancer stages I to IV. Both the AJCC and FIGO further divide stages 1 to 3 into subgroups (a to c).

Staging and grading of ovarian cancer is crucial for prognosis and treatment recommendations. Ovarian cancer is categorized into four stages: stages I to IV. The American Joint Committee on Cancer (AJCC) first stages the primary tumor (denoted as TX, T0, T1, T2, T3) and then stages the lymph node involvement (N) [17,18]. The final staging determines whether the cancer has metastasized (M) [18] (Table 23.1 and 23.2).

Staging for ovarian cancer is based on operative findings confirmed by pathological assessment. The factors that determine ovarian cancer staging include: the size of the tumor,

Table 23.2. AJCC TNM classification in relation to FIGO stages*

AJCC classifications	FIGO stages
T1a, N0, M0	IA
T1b, N0, M0	IB
T1c, N0, M0	IC
T2a, N0, M0	IIA
T2b, N0, M0	IIB
T2c, N0, M0	IIC
T3a, N0, M0	IIIA
T3b, N0, M0	IIIB
T3c, N0, M0 Or: Any T, N1, M0	IIIC
Any T, Any N, M1	IV

* Data taken from NYU Medical Center, Health wise (17).

whether the tumor has grown into other tissues or has metastasized to other areas of the body, and whether the lymph nodes have cancer [17]. The staging and sub-grouping of ovarian cancer enables a physician to recommend optimal treatment plans and discuss the expected future outcome (prognosis) with the patient, based on the stage, tumor histology, and grade and the patient's co-morbid medical condition [17].

Controversy exists regarding the biology of early versus advanced disease. The transition time from stage I to stage III is unclear, because it is unknown whether there is a natural progression from an early to advanced stage or whether the disease may initially arise as a stage III cancer in the peritoneal cavity [16].

Presentation of ovarian cancer: history, signs, and symptoms

Ovarian cancer in the past has been dubbed a silent killer due to the fact that it has been thought to be relatively asymptomatic until the later stages. In fact approximately 75% of women are diagnosed with advanced stage disease. Efforts to find early, specific, and sensitive symptoms in the screening of ovarian cancer have been met with varying success. Obstacles to creating a symptom index include lack of specificity (probability of the test being negative in those without the disease) and low prevalence. A high specificity is required to avoid unnecessary surgery.

Currently, symptoms such as pelvic and abdominal pain, changes in urination, bloating, and early satiety are used when evaluating patients for ovarian cancer. Additionally, as a consequence of disease progression patients may present with abnormal uterine bleeding, shortness of breath and dullness to percussion, and palpable inguinal lymph nodes. Furthermore, the least common of all symptoms are gynecologic. In fact, one large study showed that 95% of patients had symptoms 3 months before presenting to their physician. In studies evaluating symptom frequency and duration, it has been found that the interval from symptom onset to diagnosis was short no matter the stage of disease. Other modalities must be pursued to achieve early diagnosis of ovarian cancer in the general population. The sensitivity (probability of the test being positive in individuals with the disease) of these symptoms in detecting women with ovarian cancer is likely to be higher in those patients with genetic predisposition (such as *BRCA* and *HNPCC*). Those patients with higher than average risk presenting with the above mentioned symptoms should be evaluated for a gynecologic malignancy which should include a pelvic exam and transvaginal ultrasound.

Clinical symptom index

In 2007, the Society of Gynecologic Oncologists and the American Cancer Society released a statement noting precise symptoms to be sought out when screening for ovarian cancer after the publication of the symptom index developed by Goff et al. A positive symptom index was defined as persistent symptoms for more than 12 days in a month, but lasting less than 1 year. Goff et al. reported sensitivities of the symptom index for early and late stage ovarian cancer as 60 and 79% respectively. Rossing et al. reported 60% and 79.1% in a larger study. Furthermore, the specificities and positive predictive values for stage I and II cancers were 94.9% and 0.17–0.49% while stage III and IV were 94.9% and 0.56–0.62% when using Goff's symptom index. Due to the low prevalence of ovarian cancer, the low specificity and consequently low positive predictive value of symptoms in screening for the disease, most women with symptoms will not have ovarian cancer [19]. When comparing performance of the symptom index between women younger and older than 50 years, the specificity was 86% for the former and 90% for the latter.

Comparing symptoms in cases and controls

Many studies in the past have reported that women more often than not will have and complain of at least one symptom months before establishing the diagnosis of ovarian cancer. Those studies also reported that these women have more symptoms, but for a shorter duration than those without cancer. Finally, women with ovarian cancer had more frequent, persistent, and/or severe symptoms than those without [19].

Comparing symptoms in early and late stage ovarian cancer

Rossing et al. reported that, when comparing various symptoms found in early and late stage ovarian cancers, women with early stage disease reported more nausea than those with advanced. Note that there is an overlap between early and late stage disease with regard to the types of symptoms experienced. Symptoms that are more associated with late instead of early stage disease include abdominal distention, swelling, ascites, diarrhea, constipation, and abdominal pain [19]. No studies have shown longer duration of symptoms in those diagnosed at later stages.

Comparing symptoms in type I versus type II ovarian cancer

Women with type II tumors are more likely to seek evaluation by a physician than type I tumors. This may be due to more severe symptoms in these tumors that are known to progress rapidly.

Impediments to symptoms being adequate for diagnosis or screening

One barrier to the use of symptoms to detect ovarian cancer in its early stage is that there is a short time from the onset of symptoms to the time of diagnosis. This suggests rapid progression between stages thereby mitigating the ability to diagnose these tumors earlier [20]. This theory is not consistent with the fact that the majority of ovarian cancers are of epithelial origin, specifically the serous origin which are classified as type I according to Shih and Kurman and therefore should progress at a slower rate. Therefore, if serous tumors do progress at a slower rate, even these tumors are still too fast to be detected before widespread dissemination. Rossing et al. found that the length of time that symptoms persisted in women with a positive symptom index was not as long as originally proposed (i.e., for more than 12 days in a month but lasting less than 1 year) but longer than that proposed for the consensus criteria (i.e., nearly every day for more than a few weeks). Another potential barrier is that of unrecognized metastases. Recent theories in the pathogenesis of high-grade serous ovarian cancers propose that it represents metastasis from a fallopian tube primary. Other type II tumors are thought to metastasize early in the disease process [20]; these reduce the possibility of detection of early stage cancer.

Symptoms appear to have a low sensitivity and specificity for detecting early stage ovarian cancer as it is not well characterized by unique symptoms even though they may be unique to the patient. As the majority of ovarian cancers continue to be diagnosed as late-stage disease, there is relatively little information regarding the prevalence in this group. Additionally, Goff et al. reported that women with advanced stage ovarian cancer are more likely to have a positive symptom index resulting in a lower percent being diagnosed with low stage disease [20].

Screening/risk assessment

Cancer risk assessment is a process by which individuals are identified who are at increased risk for a hereditary or familial cancer and can be offered a different approach to prevention and screening than individuals in the general population [21]. The goal of cancer screening is to detect precancerous or early disease so that treatment will significantly reduce disease morbidity and mortality. An ideal screening method should be noninvasive and inexpensive to achieve widespread acceptance and applicability.

Although new technologies, advances in imaging, and discoveries of new biomarkers offer hope for an effective screening method, the majority of women are still diagnosed with advanced stage ovarian cancer. An ideal screening test must be: accurate, reliable, cost effective, and widely acceptable. The disease should be readily and successfully treatable [24]. An ideal screening test for ovarian cancer will have a high sensitivity to correctly diagnos all women with the disease and a high specificity to avoid false-positive results.

To be clinically useful, an effective screening test must have a sensitivity greater than 75% and a specificity greater than 99.6% to achieve a positive predictive value (PPV) of 10% [12,16,25]. A positive predictive value determines how likely it is an individual has the disease if one tests positive for it. On the other hand, a negative predictive value determines how likely it is that an individual actually does not have the disease. For ovarian cancer, false-positive or false-negative results can lead to an inaccurate diagnosis or an unnecessary operation.

In order for a screening test to be clinically effective, it must also meet several other requirements: the disease being addressed should have significant prevalence, cause significant mortality, have a long latent, precursor, or preinvasive stage and there should be effective and available treatment [26,27]. Ovarian cancer is presumed to meet all of these requirements except a significant prevalence. Within the United States, the prevalence rate of ovarian cancer is so low (approximately one in 2,500) that it significantly affects the strategies and tests that may be of any use in the detection of ovarian cancer in its early stages [12]. Ideally, an effective screening method would consist of a simple blood or urine test that has a high sensitivity and a high specificity. Unfortunately, studies to date do not exhibit high sensitivities with low specificities, or vice versa [28].

A handful of symptoms reported by women have been associated with ovarian cancer. These symptoms include: bloating, pelvic or abdominal pain, difficulty eating or feeling full quickly, and urinary frequency and urgency [29]. While these symptoms may help to detect more early stage ovarian carcinomas, the symptoms are not useful in differentiating early stage ovarian cancer from late-stage ovarian cancer. Furthermore, in a majority of cases (~75%), the first physician consulted by women with these symptoms may not immediately suspect the diagnosis [9]. Rather, these symptoms are often associated with menopause, aging, dietary changes, stress and depression [9]. Aside from the symptoms index, current screening programs to detect ovarian cancer use pelvic examinations, serum tumor markers (most commonly CA125), ultrasonography, proteomic approaches, or a multimodal method which is a combination of all of these tests [12,26].

Risk factors

Many risk factors have been associated with an increased prevalence of ovarian cancer. Risks include a personal history of disease, family history, genetics, age, and low parity [9]. Factors associated with a decrease in risk include higher parity, use of oral contraception, and gynecologic procedures such as hysterectomy and tubal ligation [30]. In fact, oral contraceptive use is one of the most significant methods for decreasing the risk of ovarian cancer.

The most important risk factor is a family history of breast or ovarian cancer. Women who have had breast cancer are a greater risk of developing ovarian cancer. The risk of ovarian cancer after breast cancer is highest in women who have a family history of breast cancer. In contrast to the 1.8% general population at risk for ovarian cancer, a family history of ovarian cancer in a first-degree relative (mother, daughter, sister) triples a woman's lifetime risk of developing ovarian cancer [9]. The risks further increase with two or more afflicted first-degree relatives (~7%). Up to 10% of ovarian cancers result from an inherited tendency to develop the disease. While 90% of diagnosed epithelial ovarian cancers occur sporadically, 10% are associated with the inheritance of an autosomal dominant genetic aberration [29]. Women who have inherited high-penetrance cancer susceptibility genes, such as mutated BRCA1 or BRCA2 genes or those constituents of Lynch syndrome (hereditary nonpolyposis colorectal cancer, HNPCC), are at a greatly increased risk of developing ovarian cancer. Women who have had breast cancer are at greater risk of developing ovarian cancer. A woman with BRCA1 mutation has a lifetime risk of 39 to 70% of developing ovarian cancer and a risk of 11 to 25% for BRCA2 carriers [6]. The NIH consensus statement concluded that women at increased risk should have at least an annual comprehensive gynecological examination (pelvic and rectovaginal), serum marker CA125, and transvaginal/abdominal ultrasound [31]. To reduce the morbidity and mortality from ovarian cancer one must identify early rather than advanced stage disease.

Genetic testing/counseling

A woman who is concerned about or is suspected to have a hereditary predisposition to ovarian cancer should undergo an initial risk evaluation. If determined necessary by the initial evaluation, the patient will then undergo a formal risk assessment. Genetic testing identifies increased risk of developing ovarian cancer. While genetic counseling can also help an individual know more about risks for additional cancers, it is only recommended for individuals with a family history of cancer and/or genetic mutations.

In the primary assessment, the patient's family history and personal history with respect to cancers are evaluated [30]. Testing is usually carried out if an individual meets certain criteria identified in The National Comprehensive Cancer Network (NCCN) guideline. Some of the criteria listed by the NCCN include: an individual from a family with a known *BRCA1/BRCA2* mutation, a personal history of epithelial ovarian/fallopian tube/primary peritoneal cancer, a personal history of breast and/or ovarian cancer at any age with two close blood relatives (first-, second-, and third-degree relatives) with pancreatic cancer at any age, and a family history of breast and/or ovarian/fallopian tube/primary peritoneal cancer as criteria for a hereditary ovarian cancer syndrome testing [30]. If an individual meets any of the criteria presented by the NCCN, a referral for genetic assessment is recommended.

Cancer screening tests and genetic counseling is a multi-step process. A detailed family history is essential. Cancer diagnoses in the family are verified by medical records, pathology reports, and death certificates whenever possible [30]. The collected family history of an individual is then documented on a pedigree diagram to illustrate family relationships (first-, second-, third-degree relatives) and disease information [30].

Following family history, medical and surgical information from the patient's personal history is collected. The collection of an individual's personal medical history allows a counselor to evaluate the likelihood that other risk factors may exist. These other risk factors may associate with inherited syndromes to affect a patient's risk of ovarian cancer. In some cases, a physical examination may be included in a risk assessment. If involved, the physical examination primarily focuses on the specific organs of a patient that can be affected by a particular hereditary cancer syndrome.

The purpose of genetic counseling is to inform at-risk individuals about the relevant genetic, biological, and environmental risk factors related to the individual's inherited syndrome or cancer. Genetic counseling includes pre-test and post-test counseling. Pre-test counseling focuses on informed consent, why the test is being offered, and the possible outcomes and accuracy of a test. Post-test counseling reports test results, the significance of the results, and follow-up plans for the patient [30].

Genetic testing should be performed by an officially qualified genetic counselor who should be able to explain how family history and laboratory testing provide an adjusted risk for developing cancer, and provide a clear explanation of the risk for cancer development along with the preventative, screening, and diagnostic processes that are available to the patient based on the adjusted risk [20].

In our National Ovarian Cancer Early Detection Program (NOCEDP) women upon entry receive such care with follow-up every 6 months. Screening is intense: women are also followed by their healthcare provider(s) in the interim for routine healthcare. The NOCEDP offers high-risk individuals formal genetic evaluation (including individualized genetic analysis), ultrasonography and a thorough gynecologic examination every 6 months.

Approximately 5–10% of epithelial ovarian cancers (EOC) are attributable to the inheritance of highly penetrant mutations in the breast/ovarian cancer susceptibility genes BRCA-1 and -2 [32]. Ovarian cancer is a component of the autosomal dominant hereditary breast-ovarian cancer syndrome, and may be due to a mutation in either *BRCA1* or *BRCA2*. Two mutations in *BRCA1* (185delAG and 5382insC) and one mutation in *BRCA2* (6174delT) are common in the Ashkenazi Jewish population. Each mutation is associated with an increased risk of ovarian cancer, and it is expected that a significant proportion of Jewish women with ovarian cancer will carry one of these mutations.

Since 1994, we have evaluated over 8,000 women deemed at increased risk for EOC based on formal genetic pedigree assessment and genetic testing. We identified a total of 87 mutations among 230 women, including 58 in *BRCA1* and 29 in *BRCA2*. The frequency of mutations varied by age of onset: a *BRCA1* mutation was found in 37.3% of women diagnosed between the ages of 30 and 60 and in 11.1% of those diagnosed above age 60 ($P < 0.0001$ for difference). A *BRCA2* mutation was found in

8.7% of women diagnosed between 30 and 60 and in 18.2% of women diagnosed after age 60 (P = 0.045). There were no mutations found among the five cases diagnosed below the age of 30. Women with *BRCA1* mutations were diagnosed with ovarian cancer at a younger age than cases for whom no mutation was detected (50.6 years and 57.9 years, respectively; P = 0.0004). In contrast, women with *BRCA2* mutations were older at diagnosis than cases for whom no mutation was detected (62.1 years vs. 57.9 years; P = 0.08). *BRCA2* mutations were more numerous than *BRCA1* mutations in women diagnosed with ovarian cancer after age 60 (18 cases vs. 11 cases, respectively). Those women at increased risk form the cohort who might benefit from a combination of non-invasive and minimally invasive tests to detect early stage ovarian cancer. Increased risk is assigned to those women with either a personal history of breast cancer (4× increase), a family history of affected first-degree relatives (2–7× increase), membership within a recognized inherited malignancy syndrome (40–60% increase), or the presence of an inherited BRCA mutation (16–100%) [33].

To estimate the proportion of ovarian cancers attributable to founding mutations in *BRCA1* and *BRCA2* in the Jewish population, and the familial cancer risks associated with each, Narod et al. interviewed 238 Jewish women with ovarian cancer at eleven medical centers in North America and Israel, and offered genetic testing for the three founder mutations. They obtained a detailed family history on all cases and on a control population of 386 Ashkenazi Jewish women without ovarian or breast cancer. The cumulative incidence of ovarian cancer to age 75 was found to be 6.3% for female first-degree relatives of the ovarian cancer cases, compared with 2.0% for the female relatives of healthy controls (relative risk, 3.1; 95% confidence interval [CI], 1.4–6.5; P = 0.003). The relative risk to age 75 for breast cancer among the female first-degree relatives was 2.0 (95%CI: 1.4–2.9; P = 0.0002). A *BRCA1* or *BRCA2* mutation was present in 37.8% of the cases; the three founding mutations accounted for almost all of the observed excess risk of ovarian and breast cancer in relatives. Overall, a greater proportion of ovarian cancers were attributable to *BRCA1* mutations (25.2%) than to the *BRCA2* mutation (12.6%). However, the cumulative incidence of ovarian cancer in the relatives of the *BRCA2* carriers (12.3% to age 75) exceeded that for the first-degree relatives of the *BRCA1* carriers (8.2% to age 75). This unexpectedly high risk is due to the high prevalence of *BRCA2* mutations among elderly Jewish patients with ovarian cancer; among patients diagnosed above age 70, *BRCA2* mutations outnumbered *BRCA1* mutations by four to one.

We performed surgical procedures on 847 women with recognized *BRCA* mutations (56% *BRCA1*, 44% *BRCA2*), and 68 *BRCA*$^-$ women with a pedigree analysis consistent with an inherited cancer syndrome all received prophylactic operations. These women all had a normal physical and ultrasound examination before surgery. Those individuals with known masses were excluded. Of the 915 bilateral salpingo-oophorectomies performed, 897 were benign and 18 unexpected malignancies: 3 ovary, 2 stage IA and IIIA; 5 primary peritoneal, all stage III; 4 fallopian tube, 3 stage I and I stage IIIA); and 6 metastatic cancers (breast, colon) were detected. To date, none of the women receiving prophylactic surgery has developed primary peritoneal cancer and four developed stage I grade 1 endometrial adenocarcinoma.

We reported that approximately 2% of our high-risk population were found to have an unexpected malignancy at the time of prophylactic surgery. Interestingly all fallopian tube carcinomas were distal and all peritoneal cancers were advanced stage. Comprehensive evaluation of the abdominal cavity with washings and peritoneal biopsies in conjunction with a thorough pathologic inspection are critical for the optimal management of this patient population.

Women with a *BRCA* mutation not desirous of prophylactic surgery may be at significantly increased risk for the development of ovarian cancer (40%) as well as breast cancer (60%) by age 70 and therefore require more intensive clinical surveillance. Those women with family histories consistent with a genetic predisposition of hereditary cancers require more intensive evaluations when presenting with abdominal/pelvic complaints even if they are vague. The early diagnosis of EOC is a complex task and therefore most effective when performed within the context of a multidisciplinary team approach. The American College of Obstetrics and Gynecology committee opinion has stated that women with a documented familial history of an inherited malignancy syndrome that increases their risk for the development of ovarian cancer who do not wish to retain fertility may be offered a prophylactic bilateral salpingo-oophorectomy (BSO), after age 35 [32]. It is our clinical practice to offer women who have inherited BRCA mutations, after formal genetic counseling, prophylactic surgery for both breast and ovarian cancer. As gynecologic oncologists we routinely perform a laparoscopic BSO, which is an outpatient procedure. Accordingly the challenge is not only to identify those women at high-risk, by either family history or genetic testing, but also to offer a comprehensive multidisciplinary program combining expertise in the clinical and basic sciences to optimize healthcare.

Syndromes associated with ovarian cancer

Hereditary breast and ovarian cancer syndrome (HBOC) is an inherited condition that significantly increases an individual's risk of certain cancers. HBOC syndrome is caused by deleterious mutations on the BRCA1 and BRCA2 genes. Because BRCA mutations are inherited in an autosomal dominant pattern, there is a 50% chance that the mutation will be passed from a parent who carries the mutation to each child.

BRCA1 and *BRCA2* are responsible for 85% of all cases of hereditary breast and epithelial ovarian cancer [24]. *BRCA1*, located on chromosome 17q, and *BRCA2*, located on chromosome 13q, are tumor suppressor genes that function as essential parts of the normal mechanisms that repair double-strand DNA breaks through recombination with undamaged, homologous DNA strands [30]. *BRCA1* and *BRCA2* produce proteins that are involved in the repair of damaged DNA and the prevention of abnormal cell proliferation [34]. Mutations of *BRCA1* and *BRCA2* associated with the development of both malignancies are found throughout the coding regions and at splice sites, with most of these mutations being small insertions or deletions that lead to frameshift mutations, nonsense mutations, or splice site alterations [36].

Women who inherit *BRCA1* mutations have a 35 to 70% chance of being diagnosed with ovarian cancer, while the lifetime ovarian risk for women who are *BRCA2* positive is estimated to be between 10% and 30% [20]. The mean age of onset of ovarian cancer is significantly earlier in women with a *BRCA1* mutation, 45 years, compared with over 60 years of age for those with a *BRCA2* mutation [22].

Some populations and communities have a higher frequency of certain *BRCA1/BRCA2* mutations than is found in the general population. Women of Eastern European, or Ashkenazi Jewish descent, are at higher risks of being positive carriers of *BRCA1* or *BRCA2* mutations. Of patients diagnosed with ovarian cancer, 35–40% of Ashkenzai women have a *BRCA1* or *BRCA2* mutation, compared with the 10% of the general population [37]. What also distinguishes this community is that three mutations (185delAG and 5382insC in *BRCA1* and 6174delT in *BRCA2*) account for approximately 98% of mutations detected [36,38,39].

When functioning properly, *BRCA1* prevents random bursts of cell growth and division that could threaten an individual's health by increasing the chances of the development of abnormal tissue. BRCA1 plays a role in all phases of the cell cycle and is an essential component of cell-cycle checkpoints by inhibiting progression through the cell cycle when DNA damage is detected. In response to DNA damage, BRCA1 becomes hyperphosphorylated during the G_1 and S phases of the cell cycle. The central region of BRCA1 interacts with the DNA repair protein complex Mre11-Rad50-NBS1 (M/R/N) and the transcriptional repressor ZBRK1 [40]. The Mre11-Rad50-NBS1 complex binds to and processes DNA double stranded breaks.

When BRCA1 is mutated, cell-cycle checkpoints suffer from the inability to respond appropriately to genomic damage. Without the necessary mechanisms to repair DNA damage, mutant cells are able to enter the M phase and pass damaged DNA to daughter cells, which leads to genetic instability. Abnormal and random cell reproduction significantly increases an individual's potential of developing a tumor. Various studies have shown that hypermethylation of *BRCA1* strongly associates with the loss of BRCA1 protein and RNA [41]. Consequently, immense amounts of hypermethylation of *BRCA1* are correlated with ovarian tumors.

While *BRCA1* mutations are primarily associated with breast and ovarian cancers, *BRCA2* mutations are associated with a large spectrum of cancers. Similar to *BRCA1*, *BRCA2* provides instructions for making a protein that is directly involved in the repair of damaged DNA. In the nucleus of many types of normal cells, the BRCA2 protein interacts with several other proteins, including the proteins produced from the *RAD51* and *PALB2* to mend breaks in DNA [42].

BRCA2 mutations are usually caused by insertions or deletions of a small number of DNA base pairs in the gene. As a result of these mutations, the protein product of *BRCA2* is abnormal and does not function properly. Similar to *BRCA1* mutations, mutations in the BRCA2 gene build up and can cause cells to divide in an uncontrolled way that may lead to tumorigenesis.

Cowden's disease

Cowden disease, or multiple hamartoma syndrome, is an autosomal dominant condition characterized by the formation of multiple hamartomas in any organ of the body. Individuals affected by Cowden's disease primarily experience thyroid problems, thyroid cancer, and breast cancer, but women also have an increased risk of developing ovarian cancer. Approximately 80% of Cowden disease cases are caused by mutations in *PTEN* (phosphate and tensin homolog) tumor suppressor gene [43]. PTEN tumor is a dual specificity phosphatase with multiple and as yet incompletely understood roles in cellular regulation [44]. As a tumor suppressor gene, the *PTEN* product plays a role in a chemical pathway by signaling abnormal cells to stop dividing and triggering apoptosis. Normal *PTEN* prevents uncontrolled cell growth that could possibly lead to the formation of malignant tumors.

HNPCC (Lynch syndrome)

In addition to *BRCA1* or *BRCA2* mutations, familial cancer syndromes, such as Lynch syndrome or Cowden's syndrome, also significantly increase a woman's lifetime risk of developing ovarian cancer. Women with hereditary non-polyposis colorectal carcinoma (HNPC), also known as Lynch syndrome, have a high risk of developing colon cancer and an increased risk of developing endometrial and ovarian cancer. Women who are affected by Lynch syndrome have a 9 to 12% lifetime risk of developing ovarian cancer and 40% risk for endometrial cancer [8]. Lynch syndrome is the most common inherited colon cancer predisposition syndrome and is responsible for 2 to 3% of all colorectal cancer (CRC) diagnoses annually [45]. Lynch syndrome is an autosomal dominant syndrome caused by germline mutations in the DNA multistep mismatch repair (MMR) system. The majority (~90%) of Lynch syndrome cases are caused by variations in *MLH1* and *MSH2* [23, 46]. *MSH6* and *PMS2* also increase an individual's risk of developing Lynch syndrome. When functioning properly, these genes are involved in the repair of mistakes made when DNA is copied in preparation for cell division. Mutations in any of these genes prevent the proper repair of DNA replication mistakes.

Despite the high risk for developing EOC among women with or at risk for Lynch syndrome, these mutations account for a relatively small proportion of all cases of ovarian cancer [36]. While most cases of ovarian cancer in HNPCC families are malignant epithelial tumors, most are well or moderately differentiated and present as International Federation of Gynecology and Obstetrics (FIGO) stage I or II disease at the time of diagnosis. This is in sharp contrast to BRCA mutation-associated tumors, which tend to present in a more advanced stage and be more poorly differentiated [36].

Li Fraumeni syndrome (LFS), p53 signature, and ovarian cancer

In serous carcinomas of the pelvis, especially ovarian, there is a short interval from symptom onset to diagnosis of advanced disease. It was thought that serous cancers were due to pathology of the ovarian surface epithelium because it grows rapidly and often involves surfaces of the ovary and peritoneum [35]. Recent findings allude to the fallopian tube as a potential source of serous cancers, such as ovarian papillary serous carcinoma. The reason for this hypothesis is the finding of serous carcinomas confined to the distal epithelium of fallopian tubes in surgical specimens from *BRCA* mutation carriers, as well as those with ovarian and peritoneal serous cancers [47].

p53 signature, which is a *p53* mutation in normal-appearing tissue, is thought to be a precursor to serous carcinoma. Among the evidence to support the hypothesis that this premalignant lesion is tied to the origin of serous pelvic cancers is the fact that both p53 signatures and tubal intra-epithelial carcinoma (A) are often found in the fimbriae of the fallopian tube, (B) show a response to DNA damage that is confirmed by H2AX immune staining in these p53 signatures, (C) both entities share low parity and body mass index as risk factors, (D) Li Fraumeni syndrome (LFS) is a disorder involving germline mutation in p53. This mutation increases the risk of various malignancies in affected individuals and families by 50-fold. This risk may be increased even more when ionizing radiation becomes a factor. Although LFS involves p53 mutation it has not yet been shown to increase the risk of developing ovarian cancer, yet 90% of pelvic serous carcinomas have to explain mutant p53 [47]. Theories the late presentation of serous cancers involve a fast change of the surface or ovarian cortex epithelium from benign to malignant [47].

While to this point there has been no association of ovarian cancer and LFS, Xian et al. were able to demonstrate the same p53 signatures in fallopian epithelium and women with LFS and ovarian cancer cases from the general population and BRCA mutation carriers. The difference lies in the number of p53 signatures where a higher number is found in women with LFS [47].

In addition to inherited genetic mutations and syndromes, other factors such as age and reproductive history affect a woman's risk of developing ovarian cancer. All women are at some risk of developing ovarian cancer, but two-thirds of ovarian cancers are diagnosed in women who are over the age of 55 years [28]. The median age at diagnosis is 58 years [48]. Most ovarian cancer cases are diagnosed after menopause, when the ovaries have a limited physiological role and consequently abnormal ovarian function causes no symptoms [8]. The incidence rates of ovarian cancer increase throughout a woman's late 70s, before slightly declining among women beyond 80 years [6,9].

Furthermore, unintentionally nulliparous women have an increased risk of being diagnosed with ovarian cancer unless they were on oral contraceptives for greater than 5 years when their risk is decreased [9]. Conversely, women who have given birth have a lower chance of developing ovarian cancer; in general, the lifetime risk of developing ovarian cancer decreases with each live birth [9]. Statistically, a woman is at increased risk of developing ovarian cancer if she started menstruating at an early age (commonly before 12 years), has not given birth to any children, had her first child after 30, experienced menopause after 50, and has never taken oral contraceptives [15]. A study involving over 110,000 women from 21 countries showed that women who took oral contraceptives for 5 years had a 50% decreased risk of developing ovarian cancer [49]. The same study noted the risk for ovarian cancer in women who continued taking oral contraceptives for approximately 15 years was almost halved and was decreasing with continual use [49].

How to achieve the detection of early stage ovarian cancer

Clinical evaluation

Pelvic examination, transvaginal ultrasound, and serum CA125 level is the current standard in screening for ovarian cancer. As this multimodal method is not without flaws, efforts are under way to strengthen its screening ability, or find better methods altogether.

Pelvic examination

Unfortunately, pelvic examinations are not efficient in distinguishing an early or premalignant lesion from a normal ovary based on palpation [50]. Evidence from a screening study at the Duke Evidence-based Practice Center (EPC) under contract to the Agency for Healthcare Research and Quality (AHRQ), demonstrated that the sensitivity and specificity of detecting a pelvic mass based solely on a pelvic examination is 40% and 90%, respectively [51]. The same study reported that a pelvic examination is able to distinguish between a benign and malignant mass with 58% sensitivity and 98% specificity [51].

The low sensitivity percentages of 40% and 58% illustrate that a pelvic examination may very likely produce a false negative with serious medical consequences. This false negative result may overlook a pelvic mass or it may incorrectly diagnose an individual as not having a malignant tumor. Similarly, the specificity rates of 90% and 98%, which are below the required specificity for an effective screening test, are inefficient because of the likelihood of a false-positive result being produced. A false-positive result may either suggest a pelvic mass that does not actually exist, or diagnose an individual as having a malignant tumor when in actuality the tumor is benign.

Diagnostic imaging

Preoperative evaluation of adnexal masses has been performed by several methods. Notable among these are the noninvasive diagnostic radiologic modalities such as transabdominal and transvaginal gray scale sonography, three-dimensional sonography, color and power Doppler sonography, computed tomography (CT), magnetic resonance imaging (MRI), and positron emission tomography (PET).

CT and MRI have not been clinically useful for characterization of the adnexa. They may be used to locate large solid masses and distinguish benign from frankly malignant ovarian tumors, with overall accuracy of 88 to 93% [52]. However, cross-sectional imaging appears less accurate for borderline ovarian tumors and small adnexal masses. A recent study using PET/CT showed that detection of the areas of abnormal increased metabolic activity considered highly suspicious for malignant tumors in preoperative discrimination of benign versus malignant ovarian diseases had a sensitivity of 100% and specificity of 92.5% [53]. However, because of relative expense and limited availability as well as possible delays in referral and surgery, routine use of PET/CT is not recommended in this setting.

Transvaginal sonography (TVS) is the initial radiographic diagnostic modality of choice for the evaluation of most pelvic masses. However, the sensitivity and specificity of TVS for the definitive diagnosis of ovarian cancer are limited. Because of this, the differential diagnosis of morphologically suspicious adnexal masses, especially in post-menopausal women, typically includes ovarian cancer. Conventional sonographic criteria for diagnosing ovarian cancer, are based on the morphological classification of ovarian masses. Malignancy is unlikely in those simple cysts with smooth walls, but the presence of a solid mass or solid projections into the cyst cavity significantly increases the risk of malignancy.

Sonography often fails to differentiate between benign and malignant lesions [54]. The accuracies of gray scale sonography and color Doppler imaging for distinguishing malignant from benign tumors are 80 to 83% and 35 to 88%, respectively [55,56]. As the result of these studies, many morphological sonographic scoring systems have been developed, including features such as the presence of papillary projections or irregular or thick septae [57,58]. However, results of a meta-analysis provide scientific evidence that sonographic techniques that combine gray scale morphologic assessment with tumor vascularity imaging information in a diagnostic system are significantly better in ovarian lesion characterization than Doppler arterial resistance measurements, color Doppler flow imaging, or gray scale morphologic information alone [59].

Detection of early stage EOC is difficult. In multiple studies, sonography has not been proven to decrease mortality from ovarian cancer, although newer large ongoing studies show promise [60,61]. The reason for this is likely multifactorial; however, any means of improving visualization of the ovary may be helpful in the detection of early lesions. The following innovative sonographic techniques are currently used to improve identification of early stage EOC.

Ultrasound contrast imaging

Contrast-enhanced sonography is a great tool for detection and characterization of angiogenesis. Ultrasound contrast agents for intravenous use consist of small, stabilized microbubbles usually on the order of 1–10 microns in diameter [62]. These bubbles cause increased echogenicity and are thus termed echoenhancers. The agents create this effect by causing an acoustic impedance mismatch with the adjacent tissues. This, in turn, causes increased scattering and reflection of the sound beam, thereby leading to increased sonographic signal and increased echogenicity. The degree of echo-enhancement depends on a multitude of factors including the size of the microbubble, the concentration of contrast agent, and the compressibility of the bubbles as well as the interrogating ultrasound frequency [62].

Pulse inversion harmonic imaging

In pulse inversion harmonic imaging two pulses are transmitted down each ray line. The first is a normal pulse, the second is an inverted replica of the first so that wherever there was a positive pressure on the first pulse there is an equal negative pressure on the second. Any linear target such as soft tissues responds equally to positive and negative pressures and will reflect back to the transducer equal but opposite echoes. Microbubbles respond in a non-linear manner and do not reflect identical inverted waveforms. This allows the separation of the fundamental component of the bubble echoes from the background, improving resolution, and increasing sensitivity to contrast agents.

Microvascular imaging

Pulse inversion harmonic imaging has led to the ability to image individual bubbles in small vessels within and adjacent to tumors with very low blood flow rates. Microvascular imaging allows the capture and tracking of the bubbles as they go around and through these small leaky vessels, providing improved visualization of slowly perfused tumors. This technique involves selection of maximum pixel values throughout consecutive pulse inversion harmonic images as the bubbles replenish the imaging plane. A composite image showing the vascular architecture is constructed and can be used to improve our ability to detect areas of abnormal vascularity.

Flash contrast imaging

While the ability to visualize microvascular blood flow in real-time is a significant advancement, the ability to destroy contrast at will also has diagnostic potential. By destroying the contrast within the scanplane, a "negative bolus" of contrast is created locally. Then, the time it takes for contrast to refill the scan plane and the amount of the contrast in the region of interest may be used for estimation of microvessel cross-sectional area, blood flow velocity, and tumor perfusion [63].

Contrast-enhanced sonography may significantly improve the diagnostic ability of ultrasound to identify early microvascular changes that are known to be associated with early stage ovarian cancer [62,64]. Currently, contrast agents play a pivotal role in the imaging modalities of CT and MRI by increasing image conspicuity. By increasing the density or signal intensity of a particular organ and thus, the signal-to-noise ratio, contrast agents help to detect and characterize parenchymal lesions. Indeed, contrast agents have received such widespread acceptance that a CT examination performed without intravenous contrast for many indications is now considered limited. Our preclinical studies demonstrated that the intravenous contrast agents in ultrasound hold great promise in a multitude of potential clinical applications, especially in identifying aberrant vascular changes associated with malignancy [62,65–69].

Previous studies have addressed the use of contrast-enhanced sonography for benign and malignant tumors by showing greater enhancement of malignant tumors on Doppler imaging. According to Kupesic et al. the use of a contrast agent with three-dimensional power Doppler sonography showed diagnostic efficiency (95.6%) that was superior to that of nonenhanced three-dimensional power Doppler sonography (86.7%) [69]. However, simple documentation of tumor enhancement may not be sufficient because some benign tumors show detectable contrast enhancement. This limitation can be addressed by assessment of the contrast enhancement kinetics. Only two studies have been published that used kinetic parameters of the contrast agent to compare benign with malignant tumors in the power Doppler mode. Ordén et al. demonstrated that, after microbubble contrast agent injection, malignant and benign adnexal lesions behave differently in degree, onset, and duration of Doppler US enhancement. Doppler CEUS parameters in that study had a sensitivity of 79–100% and 77–92% specificity [70]. Marret et al. reported that washout times and areas under the curves were significantly greater in ovarian malignancies than in other benign tumors ($P < 0.001$), leading to sensitivity estimates between 96% and 100% and specificity estimates between 83% and 98%. They concluded that Doppler CEUS parameters had slightly higher sensitivity and slightly lower specificity when compared with transvaginal sonographic variables of the resistive index and serum CA125 levels [71].

Our clinical studies explored differences in enhancement parameters in benign versus malignant ovarian masses using the new method of CEUS using pulse inversion harmonic imaging [71,72]. This method produces more reliable estimates of tumor microvascular perfusion and provides more consistent results compared with Doppler CEUS. We reported that all malignant tumors and 50% of benign ones showed detectable contrast enhancement (image intensity >10% above the baseline) after contrast injection. When contrast enhancement dynamics were assessed, we found that malignant lesions had a similar time to peak (26.2 ± 5.9 vs. 29.8 ± 13.4 seconds; $P = 0.4$), greater peak enhancement (21.3 ± 4.7 vs. 8.3 ± 5.7 dB; $P < 0.001$), a longer half wash-out time (104.2 ± 48.1 vs. 32.2 ± 18.9 seconds; $P < 0.001$), and a greater AUC (1,807.2 ± 588.3 vs. 413.8 ± 294.8 seconds^{-1}; $P < 0.001$) when compared with enhancing benign lesions.

Our data suggest that, except for the wash-in time, contrast enhancement parameters are significantly different in benign versus malignant ovarian masses. The wash-in time probably reflects intrinsic circulation depending on cardiac contraction, blood pressure, and overall vascular tone. Once blood circulates through the tumor, however, differences may reflect the unique branching patterns and vessel morphologic characteristics in the microvascularity of the tumors. The area under the enhancement curve greater than 787 seconds^{-1} was the most accurate diagnostic criterion for ovarian cancer, with 100.0% sensitivity and 96.2% specificity. Additionally, peak contrast enhancement of greater than 17.2 dB (90.0% sensitivity and 98.3% specificity) and a half wash-out time of greater than 41.0 seconds (100.0% sensitivity and 92.3% specificity) proved to be useful. These results show that contrast-enhanced PIH sonography is a more appropriate method for characterizing blood flow dynamics in ovarian tumors, and it can provide an important tool to aid differential diagnoses between benign and malignant ovarian tumors.

In summary, contrast enhancement patterns significantly differ between benign and malignant ovarian masses. The addition of a vascular ultrasound contrast agent allows a more complete delineation of the vascular anatomy through enhancement of the signal strength from small vessels and provides an entirely new opportunity to time the transit of an injected bolus. Contrast sonography has higher sensitivity and specificity to differentiate between benign and malignant lesions than conventional TV-US and for discriminating between endometriosis and detecting occult stage I disease.

CA125 serum tumor marker

While dozens of potential serum markers have been identified, CA125 is the most thoroughly assessed and most frequently used biomarker. CA125, which was first developed in 1981, is a high-molecular-weight glycoprotein originally detected by a murine monoclonal antibody (OC125). CA125 is a coelomic epithelial antigen produced by mesothelial cells that line the peritoneum, pleural cavity, and pericardium [73]. The 1970s marked the discovery of CA125. Monoclonal antibodies to that protein were created by immunizing mice with human ovarian cancer cells, known as AVCA433, resecting their spleens, and creating hybridomas. The appropriate antibody clones produced by these immunized mice were selected according to their affinity for ovarian cancer cells and lack thereof for B-lymphocytes that were made immortal by infection with Epstein Barr Virus. The 125th antibody clone was interesting in that it showed specificity to the endometrium and fallopian tube, in addition to ovarian cancer cells, but would not bind to normal ovarian epithelium. This antibody was named ovarian cancer 125 (OC125), and the target it recognized was cancer antigen 125 (CA125) [74].

Structurally, CA125 is a mucin-like high-molecular weight glycoprotein with a molecular weight ranging from 2.5 to 5 million Dalton [74,75]. It is a type I protein and is like other mucins in that the molecule spans the cell membrane. CA125 has an N-terminal extracellular domain made up of more than 12,000 amino acids that is greatly glycosylated. This domain has a tandem repeat portion. The C-terminal domain of CA125 is a cytoplasmic tail accepted as having the potential to be phosphorylated during signal transduction [75]. It is encoded by the MUC16 gene found on chromosome 19p13.2 [74]. CA125 is expressed in 80% of ovarian cancers; it is amplified in only 5% and mutated in 4.7% of high-grade ovarian cancers [74].

Because of this, it is thought that CA125 expression is regulated at a transcriptional or post-transcriptional level

74]. Shedding and/or expression of CA125 is highly regulated nd expression is modestly increased by inhibition of PKC beta, yrosine phosphatase, and EGFR as well as by stimulation of KA. Expression is moderately decreased by decreased levels of GF and LPA while glucocorticoids cause a significant drop. gents not shown to have any effect on CA125 expression or hedding include IGF, estrogen, IFN-alpha and gamma, TNF, EGF, M-CSF, and IL-6 [74].

The function of CA125 is suggested by its interaction with ther proteins. For example CA125 selectively binds to meso- helin and possibly leads to peritoneal adhesion of ovarian ancer cells [74,75]. By virtue of its glycosylated portion A125 can also bind to galectin which allows cancer cell adhe- ion to other tissues [74]. Various genetic experiments have ontributed to the understanding of CA125's function. In emale mice MUC16 is thought to occupy the same locations s in humans. This being the case, genetically altered mice have een used to better understand the function of CA125/MUC16. KOv3 ovarian cancer cells with the genes for cell surface IUC16 knocked out were constructed and have decreased nterval stationary growth, a decrease in clonogenic growth, nd inhibition of xenographic growth.

On the other hand, adding the MUC16 construct that was reviously knocked-down creates an aggressive line of cancer ells as it leads to enhancement of anchorage-dependent cell rowth, cell migration, colony formation independent of nchorage, invasion, and metastasis [74]. In addition, these ells showed evidence of transition from epithelial to mesen- hymal tissue types by means of up-regulation of N-cadherin nd vimentin expression and down-regulation of E-cadherin xpression [74]. Further evidence of CA125's function comes rom a reduction in the potential for invasion and adhesion when CA125 RNAi is knocked-down in SKOV-8 cells [74]. astly, CA125 may inhibit the activity of natural killer cells by recluding the synapse with ovarian cancer cells. As the above bservations would support, poor outcomes are associated with levated CA125 levels. This may not be dependent on tumor urden. Additionally, lack of CA125 expression at higher stages s a poor prognostic sign.

CA125 is physiologically expressed in epithelial tissues. xamples of these tissues include those of Mullerian origin uch as endometrium, endocervix, and fallopian tubes, those f coelomic origin such as pleural mesothelium, pericardial, nd peritoneal. CA125 has also been found in conjunctiva 25,74]. It is elevated in various conditions including endome- riosis, pregnancy, uterine leiomyomas, benign and malignant varian tumors, liver disease, and cancers of the stomach, ancrease, colon, uterus, and fallopian tubes [62]. Free CA125 s found after the extracellular domain is cleaved near the cell urface membrane [74]. The antigen was also found outside the ell, in body fluids like seminal fluid, and culture media. One uthor quoted CA125's sensitivity for ovarian cancer as being 2% [76]. A study by Nakae et al. demonstrated 66.3% specific- ty and 84.4% sensitivity for CA125. As this has been the oldest nd one of the best performing biomarkers, it is likely that a iomarker panel used to detect ovarian cancer in its early stage will include CA125 [77].

The issue with CA125 as a tumor marker is that changes in its serum levels are not specific to ovarian cancer. Elevations may be physiologic as in ovulation or pathophysiologic as in fibroids and endometriosis in addition to ovarian cancer [76]. In screening for ovarian cancer the specificity of serum CA125 level is higher in post-menopausal women. In screening for early stage ovarian cancer, CA125 has been found to be less useful due to a decrease in sensitivity with that stage of disease. CA125 may often be used as a component for the evaluation of a pelvic mass, but it is non-specific to ovarian cancer.

CA125 is elevated in many disease states, benign diseases, and physiological conditions [22,27]. It has been noted that because CA125 levels are naturally elevated due to ovulation, endometriosis, and other benign conditions, CA125 as a tumor marker is more effective in post-menopausal women [78]. CA125 is only elevated in 47% of women with early stage ovarian cancer, while CA125 levels are elevated in 80 to 90% of advanced-stage ovarian cancers [25,27]. Furthermore, CA125 has a sensitivity of only 50 to 60% for early stage diagnosis in post-menopausal women, when specificity is set at 99% [78]. Clinically, CA125 is useful to follow women diagnosed with ovarian cancer for prognosis, surveillance, and optimization of care.

Tools and techniques to develop ovarian cancer-specific biomarkers

Despite the urgent need for biomarkers to improve cancer clinical outcome through early detection, relatively few new cancer biomarkers have been advanced to routine clinical use [62,79]. The poor yield of clinically useful biomarkers is not for lack of trying by thousands of scientists worldwide. Unfortunately, discovery of cancer-specific markers is much harder than was initially anticipated. The three major impediments are: (1) molecular heterogeneity between tumors, (2) prevalence of non-cancer diseases that reduce biomarker specificity for cancer, and (3) low biomarker concentrations, especially for early stage disease, thus reducing sensitivity. Gene and protein array data have revealed that each cancer may have a different molecular portrait [80]. Consequently, a single given biomarker may only work for a subset of tumors within a group being tested. In the general population, cancer will be in low prevalence compared with hundreds of other more prevalent conditions. Shared pathophysiologic events between cancer and prevalent non-cancer conditions will confound biomarker specificity. Finally, early stage cancer lesions are small in tissue volume, thus limiting the biomarker production rate to a level well below the threshold of detection by most diagnostic platforms.

To improve the clinical sensitivity and specificity of cancer biomarkers, we may have to abandon the assumption that a single cancer biomarker exists for one or multiple types of cancer. Cancer cells are genetically deranged normal cells, not exogenous infectious agents. Consequently, biomarkers associated with cancer are logically expected to be quantitatively, but not qualitatively, different from normal cellular molecules. Indeed all clinically used circulating cancer biomarkers to date appear to be present in both malignant and non-malignant conditions [81].

In an attempt to improve specificity and sensitivity, investigators have been evaluating the use of multiple panels of (1) identified markers [62], or (2) panels of unidentified and uncharacterized molecules. The rationale for this approach is based on a new appreciation of the tumor microenvironment. Tumor cells participate in complex interactions with surrounding organ parenchyma, local stroma, vasculature, and immune cell populations. This biochemical cross-talk is hypothesized to generate a cascade of specific and sensitive biomarkers elaborated directly from the tumor cell population, indirectly from the interacting non-tumor cells or extracellular molecules, or a specific product of the microenvironment. The most specific cancer biomarkers may turn out to be clipped or enzymatically modified molecules, derived from this latter category.

Molecules that normally play a non-malignant role in physiology may be cleaved, phosphorylated, glycosylated, or otherwise chemically altered in a manner that provides an ongoing and specific biomarker record of the pathophysiology in the tumor-host microenvironment and blood [62]. Larger proteins that may be unable to cross the endothelial vascular wall due to their size and are excluded from the circulatory proteome may in fact be represented in the blood by smaller clipped isoforms. Thus, fragments in the circulatory proteome (host macroenvironment) may indeed provide a fountainhead of new diagnostic information of the tissue-specific host microenvironment.

While the ultimate cause of EOC is underpinned by mutational changes at the genetic level, the resulting protein defects (non-functional, hyperfunctional, under- or over-abundant expression) ultimately dictate the aberrant biological state [62]. The advent of recent technologic advances has enabled the analysis of the entire protein complement, or proteome, of a cell. Serum tumor markers have been evaluated for their ability in detecting ovarian cancer at early stages. Currently, there are no clinically validated biomarkers for the accurate detection of early stage ovarian carcinoma [62].

Tumor microenvironment

A discussion of tumor biomarkers emerges from the concept of a tumor microenvironment. This suggests that, in addition to the neoplastic mass itself causing measurable changes, the surrounding parenchymal cells also contribute. The microenvironment constitutes interactions of tumor cells, leukocytes, and stromal fibroblasts that in some instances promote tumor development and progression [82]. For example, matrix metalloproteinases (MMP), which are enzymes involved in tumor invasion, represent one class of factors that is produced by cells other than the tumor. Within the peritoneal cavity, initial ovarian cancer metastasis occurs by detachment of cells from the ovary and then adhesion of cancer cells to the mesothelial lined peritoneum and serosa of distant organs followed by extracellular matrix degradation and then invasion into the normal host stroma [83]. This stromal invasion is facilitated by MMPs. Hundreds of other circulating factors also play a role in adhesion and invasion and as such have potential as biomarkers of ovarian cancer. Many of these have shown promising results for clinical use in early ovarian cancer detection.

Among the novel biomarkers is human epididymal protein 4 (HE4), which is over-expressed in ovarian cancer. HE4, combined with CA125 is used to monitor the progression and recurrence of disease. Similarly kallikreins, which are serine proteases have been shown to be involved in angiogenesis, tissue invasion and cell growth. Kallikreins have also been used in combination with CA125 [25]. Other potential biomarkers include VCAM-1 insulin-like growth factor-2 (IGF-2), vascular endothelial growth factor (VEGF), epidermal growth factor (EGF), and epidermal growth factor receptor (EGF-R). Inflammatory molecules such as cytokines such as IL-8, IL-6, and M-CSF facilitate communication between these cells of the tumor microenvironment [84]. Additional biomarkers include prolactin, osteopontin, leptin lysophosphatidic acid, apoliprotein A1 transthyretin, COOH osteopontin fragments, and eosinophil-derived neurotoxin. Some of these factors have shown elevations in specificity and sensitivity for detection of ovarian cancer [76].

Techniques for discovery

Currently, useful research techniques for biomarker discovery can be placed into three major categories; transcriptomics, genomics, proteomics, and others.

Transcriptomics studies the expression of genes. Examples are cDNA and oligonucleotide microarrays and SAGE. Serial analysis of gene expression (SAGE) is used to quantify gene expression by measuring mRNA transcripts and creating a profile of the genes expressed physiologically and in disease states. One advantage of this technology over microarrays is that it can detect previously unknown genes [85]. Among the biomarkers most commonly identified as being overexpressed in ovarian cancer by transcriptomic studies is VEGF. A glycosylated state is found for 55% of biomarkers found [86]. Such being the case, one of the next areas likely to emerge is glycomics, the characterization of glycan interactions and roles in biology.

Genomics: Genomics is a branch of biotechnology that focuses on DNA sequencing and genetic mapping of a specific organism using high-speed genetics and molecular biology techniques. In ovarian cancer research genomics seeks to determine the presence of single gene products or genetic mutations conferring increased risk of developing malignancy, whether inherited or acquired. Genomics may quantitatively evaluate genetic expression for example using antibody micro-array [87]. It also seeks polymorphisms that may be associated with differential response to therapy (e.g., *BRCA1* or *BRCA2*).

DNA sequencing is a genomic tool used in cancer research. It facilitates discovery of new biomarkers with potential in disease diagnosis as well as characterization of mutations in genes of interest. Furthermore, sequencing of diagnostic markers is part of clinical patient management in finding variants in DNA sequences, as well as gene insertions or deletions that are specific to the tumor [88]. Others include single nucleotide polymorphism (SNP) arrays, differential methylation

Table 23.3. Tools and techniques in ovarian cancer research

Standard of care	Pelvic examination, CA125, TVUS
Transcriptomics/ genomics	cDNA and oligonucleotide microarrays, SAGE
Proteomics	2D PAGE with mass spectrometry, protein microarrays, SEREX, ELISA, multiplex bead arrays, nanoparticle proteomics
Others	SNP arrays, DMH, CGH

Note: PAGE, polyacrylamide gel electrophoresis; SEREX, serologic analysis of recombinant cDNA expression; SNP, single nucleotide polymorphism; DMH, differential methylation hybridization; ELISA, enzyme-linked immunosorbant assay.

hybridization (DMH), and CGH. DMH is a tool that uses methylation-sensitive restriction enzymes to evaluate methylated fragments of DNA by binding them to CpG island microarrays [89]. Tools evaluating gene expression profiles, specifically cDNA microarrays and oligonucleotide arrays, have been the preferred method of studying ovarian cancer of late stages [90] (Table 23.3).

Profiling studies have led to the recognition that ovarian cancer represents a group of different diseases. This has been supported by the finding of a separate genomic background for endometrioid, mucinous, and clear cell ovarian cancers compared with serous cancers of the ovary. Additionally, serous borderline tumors have a different genetic origin from late stage, high-grade serous ovarian cancers. Possible lesions of origin to ovarian cancer include inclusion cysts, fimbriae of the fallopian tubes, tubal epithelium, or just the surface epithelium of the ovary [90].

Microarrays: A myriad of genes have been evaluated by microarrays. A microarray is a physical platform such as a slide made of glass or plastic, minute beads (with diameters of 5 μm for example), or a microchip upon which nucleic acid probes, or proteins are chemically attached in a regular pattern. When DNA is used it may have a known nucleotide sequence, which will allow identification and sequencing of genes or DNA in the cell or tissue samples being evaluated [87]. Both diagnostic and prognostic information has been obtained by this method. For example, one author identified hundreds of genes that are associated with cisplatin resistance in ovarian cancer, another found genes encoding secretory proteins that are overexpressed in ovarian cancer cell lines using cDNA microarrays, a third reported finding 285 different expressions of genes using cDNA-DASL from formalin-fixed paraffin-embedded samples [91].

Proteomics: is a branch of biotechnology that evaluates the structure, interactions, and function of proteins using techniques of molecular biology, biochemistry, and genetics while creating databases from the information obtained. Tools used in proteomic analysis of ovarian cancer include mass spectrometry, enzyme-linked immunosorbent assay (ELISA), and multiplex bead arrays. Cancer is a disease that has its roots in protein pathways [92]. Proteomics may be used to determine differences in protein profiles in different states, and it can determine the roles of proteins in signaling pathways, their interactions and their activation states [92].

Mass spectrometry: Mass spectrometry evaluates the "mass spectrum" of the sample of interest, and detects changes in this molecular profile related to disease states. Matrix-assisted laser desorption and ionization time-of-flight (MALDI-TOF) and its offshoot surface-enhanced laser desorption and ionization time-of-flight (SELDI-TOF) are two techniques commonly used with mass spectrometry. In these techniques ultraviolet light-absorbing compounds are crystallized with proteins in the sample. The crystals are vaporized using an ultraviolet laser beam. The proteins, now ionized, are accelerated in an electric field.

A time of flight analyzer will calculate the ion's mass-to-charge ratio by the amount of time the ion takes to reach a detector [93]. The mass-to-charge ratio is obtained by dividing the molecular weight by the elementary charge and is provided for all components of the sample being studied. Using a mass spectrometer, proteins within a sample can be identified [94]. Refinements to the proteomic approach of biomarker discovery include quantitative isotopic labeling, and new mass spectrometry algorithms [88,90].

Nanoparticle proteomics

Nanotechnology is a recent addition to the emergence of proteomic tools. This involves a hydrogel core-shell nanoparticle. The hydrogel particles are three-dimensional cross-linked polymers. Different surface properties can be given and diverse proteins or other entities may be used as bait. A number of materials can be linked to *N*-isopropylacrylamide, which makes a good hydrogel. While the gels tend to be stable and uniform, the number of pores and the gel's size can be manipulated by changing temperature. Furthermore, the addition of an affinity bait can increase the gel's specificity.

For example, anions may be sequestered by allyamine while saccharides can be attracted by boronate. Once introduced into the medium to be analyzed, the nanoparticles facilitate capture and concentration of low-abundance and low molecular weight proteins. Capture is achieved by the nanoparticles' selectivity for specific substances by means of the charge, chemical groups and surface topology given to it. Capture allows proteins to be unbound to albumin carriers, be purified, and be kept from degradation. Once the proteins of interest are bound, affinity and molecular sieve chromatographies are simultaneously performed by the nanoparticles [92]. The particles are recovered and washed to take away unwanted proteins. An eluent is used to remove the molecules of interest that are then analyzed [92].

Immunoassay: An immunoassay is a test that qualitatively or quantitatively determines the presence of a substance (e.g., a protein) that is caused to react as an antibody or an antigen. An ELISA is an example of an immunoassay. In performing an ELISA, undetermined amounts of antigen are captured onto a polystyrene microtiter plate. The antigen is then detected by binding of a secondary antibody that itself is conjugated to an enzyme. That enzyme brings about a reaction leading to a chromogenic or fluorometric signal [87].

If an enzyme is used as a label and attached to the antibody or antigen, the test is then referred to as an enzyme immunoassay. Multiplex bead-based immunoassays offer the capability of concurrently determining the concentrations of antibodies to many different antigens [95]. In a bead-based immunoassay, microbeads with antibodies bound to them are mixed with the sample of interest and detector antibodies. Antibodies (the capture antibody) covalently bound to the beads (spectrally addressed carboxylated polystyrene microspheres) will bind to antigens in the sample. Detector antibodies (secondary antibodies) will then bind to already bead-antibody bound antigens. The mix is washed and then fluorescence of the secondary antibody is analyzed using a flow cytometer.

Multiplex bead-based immunoassays have been used in studying ovarian cancer as Nolen et al. have done to analyze over 60 proteins found in the circulation of women with adnexal masses. Gorelik et al. used this technology to evaluate CA125 and 24 cytokines as potential markers for early stage ovarian cancer. Among the findings of their study were elevations in circulating levels of CA125, VEGF, IL-6, and IL-8 and decreases in EGF and, MCP-1 levels. These findings are comparable to those obtained from ELISA.

Another study reported the multiplex bead array was able to reproduce analysis of four markers (Prolactin, leptin, osteopontin (OPN), and IGF-2) with sensitivities and specificities once similar to those found using ELISA. When CA125 and macrophage migration inhibitory factor (MIF) were added there was 95.3% sensitivity and 99.4% specificity [87]. It should be noted that the positive predictive values of the test from the first two studies were not sufficient to warrant use of the array in the general population. As a result changes are being made to refine the technique.

Autoantibodies: The immune system has been shown to play a role in cancer with the existence of autoantibodies to proteins related to the disease state. It appears that overexpression of tumor protein or the presence of mutant proteins leads to a response by the humoral immune system. For example, antibodies to HER2 protein have been found but only in 5–10% of cancer patients [88]. Antibodies to p53 have also been found. Discovery of autoantibodies is accomplished by means of serologic identification of antigens by recombinant expression technology (SEREX). It works by using serum from a patient to screen a cDNA library made from a tumor from the same patient. The issue with autoantibodies in diagnosing cancer at this time is their low sensitivity. This problem plagues antibodies for HER2 as well as p53 missense mutants.

As stated earlier autoantibodies are made in response to the development of ovarian cancer. The antibody to interleukin-8 (IL-8) has been evaluated by Lokshin et al. [92]. They reported elevated levels of anti-IL-8 in early stage ovarian cancer when compared with controls. The specificity for this antibody as a biomarker of ovarian cancer was 98% with a sensitivity of 65% [92]. Similarly, another study took advantage of this concept of immunity in cancer and showed a complete remission in chemotherapy-resistant advanced ovarian cancer when trastuzumab was added to the carboplatin plus paclitaxel regimen [96].

Novel ovarian cancer biomarkers

Biomarkers are defined as cellular, biochemical, and molecular (including genetic and epigenetic) characteristics by which normal and/or abnormal processes can be recognized and/or monitored. They are measurable in biological materials, such as in tissues, cells, and/or bodily fluids. Recognition of these characteristics may be used in screening, early diagnosis, prognosis, tracking treatment response, or recurrence of disease [77]. As clinical methods do not have the requisite positive predictive value to screen for ovarian cancer in its early stage, the focus has turned to other modalities like biomarkers with and without combined imaging techniques (Table 23.4).

After finding novel biomarkers, the genes or proteins need to be sequenced. Then appropriate assays are developed to measure protein concentrations. In clinical practice once a positive test is obtained from the biomarker panel this information would have to be confirmed by imaging to increase the sensitivity and specificity of the positive results [62].

There is currently no single biomarker with a high enough positive predictive value to detect ovarian cancer. One barrier to finding this one biomarker includes a lack of homogeneity in the molecular makeup between tumors [62,87]. In addition, shared pathophysiology between malignant and benign processes leading to a decrease in biomarker specificity, and low biomarker serum levels especially early in the course of malignancy also make it difficult to find a single suitable biomarker [62]. A panel of biomarkers may be necessary at the moment. The hope is that with each additional biomarker the sensitivity and specificity of the screening method increases [87].

With this panel one can add contrast-enhanced ultrasonography, not unlike the screening protocol currently used in obstetrics for neural tube defects, trisomy 13, 18, and 21. In attempting to find this panel, proteomics have been used to identify other molecules that may be expressed during the disease process as a result of effects and response of different organ parenchyma, stroma, vasculature, and immune cells on and to each other [62].

Additionally, physiologic molecules may play a pathophysiologic role after being modified by phosphorylation, cleavage, or glycosylation. These altered proteins with resulting alterations in function (over- or under-expression and hyper-, hypo-, or non-functional) may be the disease markers that provide the PPV and specificity needed to screen for ovarian cancer [62].

MUC16

Increasing and decreasing levels of MUC16 are associated with disease progression and regression. This then allows the use of MUC16 levels in following patients with a diagnosis of cancer [75]. It has been theorized that MUC16 promotes invasion of endometriosis by acting as a chemo-attractant when found in the peritoneal fluid. MUC16's role in ovarian cancer metastasis has been suggested by mediating

Table 23.4. Screening for ovarian cancer

Tumor markers		
Marker	**Physiology**	**Significance in cancer detection**
CA125	MUC16 product; protein found in endometrium, fallopian tube, and ovarian cancer cells	Expressed in 80% of non-mucinous epithelial ovarian cancer
HE4	Product of WAP-type four disulfide-core gene (*WFDC*); found in the distal epididymis and ovarian cancers	Higher levels seen in serous and endometrioid ovarian cancers; less false positives and comparable sensitivity to CA125
MCSF (CSF1)	Proto-oncogene c-*FMS* product; Involved in mononuclear cell differentiation and growth	Expression correlates with tumor aggressiveness, decreased recurrence interval, poor prognosis, and worsened outcome
uPAR:	Receptor involved in cell signaling and tissue remodeling	Elevated levels carry a poor prognosis; Has the ability to discriminate benign from early malignant adnexal processes
Transthyretin (TTR)/Prealbumin	Indicator of nutritional status; Acute Phase reactant	Involved in tumor development
Transferin	Iron transport; anti-apoptotic effects	Promotes tumor development and survival
OVX1	An ovarian- or breast cancer-related antigen	Included in > 70% of ovarian cancers; in 59% of ovarian cancers with nl CA125; 76% sensitivity; unstable
Osteopontin	Bone remodeling, immune function	Involved in metastasis and tumor progression; useful to monitor recurrence
Mesthelin	Protein expressed by mesothelial cells	Elevated in mesothelioma, pancreatic and ovarian cancers
B7-H4	Immune modulator	May promote malignant transformation; expressed in endometrioid, clear cell, and serous ovarian cancers
Prostain	Trypsin-like serine protease; found physiologically in prostate and semen	Elevated in nonmucinous epithelial ovarian cancers
EGF-R	Member of the tyrosine kinase growth factor receptor family	Repair of post-ovulation ruptured follicle; linked to MMP synthesis; causes ovarian surface epithelium to shift and exhibit characteristics resembling immature, regenerating or neoplastic epithelia
VEGF	Angiogenesis mediator	Linked to malignant ascites; potential role in monitoring response to therapy
MMP	Tissue remodeling	Involved in angiogenesis, stromal invasion, possibly tumor growth
IGF	Regulating cell proliferation and survival	Possible role in carcinogenesis and tumor progression
IGFBP-3	Suppress mitogenesis and regulation of apoptosis	Decreased serum levels in 44% of epithelial ovarian cancer
VCAM	Secreted by endothelial cells; promotes WBC attachment and extravasation	Possibly involved in metastasis of ovarian cancer; possible role in detecting early or pre-clinical ovarian cancer
Serologic factors and acute-phase proteins		
CRP	Marker of inflammation	Weak association ovarian cancer
SAA		No significant improvement in ovarian cancer detection
Apolipoprotein A1	Part of HDL	Protective factor
Cytokines and other inflammatory mediators		
IL-6	Promotes inflammation	Poor prognosis and clinical outcome
IL-8	Recruiting leukocytes	Poor prognosis and clinical outcome
Anti-tumor antibody		
IgG	Immunoglobulin	Distinguishes between early and late-stage disease
Panels		
OVA1	Panel of CA125, beta2-microglobulin, transferrin, apolipoprotein A1, transthyretin	For triage; if pre-menopausal with score of 5.0 or greater or post-menopausal with score of 4.4 or greater then increased likelihood of cancer

IGF-2, insulin-like growth factor 2; MIF, macrophage inhibitory factor.

heterotypic cell adhesion when interacting with mesothelin. Among the reported properties of MUC16 are the ability to dampen natural killer cell activity and prevention of apoptosis from genotoxic drugs [75].

MUC 16 has a role in cancer pathogenesis. The amino terminal domain is involved in cell–cell interactions by working with mesothelin and forms the basis for the hypothesis that MUC16 is involved in the cancer metastasis. Additional evidence suggesting MUC16's role in cancer pathogenesis is that it shows resemblance to MUC1 and MUC4 proteins that have been proven to be involved in tumorigenesis [75]. Being able to migrate and invade through tissues enhances the metastatic ability of cancer cells, which is associated with changes at the molecular and cellular level where there is new expression of N-cadherin and vimentin with corresponding lack of E-cadherin expression.

Interaction of cancer cells with the stroma is promoted by this replacement of E-cadherin by N-cadherin at the cell surface. RNA interference-mediated loss of E-cadherin expression has been shown to increase the likelihood of metastasis in ovarian cancer while an increase in N-cadherin expression leads to invasion in breast cancer. Theriault et al. showed that cell-density-dependent tumor cell growth arrest could be induced by knocking-down the MUC16 protein.

The converse is also true. When cells containing the MUC16 C-terminal domains are created, there is no cell-density-dependent arrest and more tumors form both in vitro and in vivo. Thieriault et al. cloned MUC16 C-terminal domain gene into SKOV3 cells to evaluate the function of the genes presence; SKOV3-MUC16TMU cells had the transmembrane domain and the extracellular unique portion of the protein but lacked the majority of the cytoplasmic region. These mutant cells were used in experiments to evaluate tumor cell growth in vitro, wound healing, colony formation, tumorigenicity, migration, and invasion assays. SKOV3-EV cells, which are ovarian cancer cells, were used as controls.

MUC16 knockout did not affect proliferation at low cell density, yet growth was arrested upon confluence. It must be noted that an effect of on cell proliferation rate or apoptotic pathway does not explain the decreased cell growth rate seen in MUC16 knockdown cells [75]. Regional dissemination within the peritoneum is the classic spread pattern of ovarian cancer. Knocking down *MUC16* abolished the cell's ability to form tumors. MUC16CTD has effects on cell growth rate in that it is associated with cells' ability to form high-density islets by piling up on one another [75]. It enhances tumorigenicity as larger tumor formation, higher tumor burden, and decreased survival interval have been seen with the presence of MUC16. MUC16 may be associated with increased cell motility and more sites of metastases than controls, which can translate into more aggressive tumors.

Western blot analysis has confirmed lower expression of E-cadherin and associated increased expression of N-cadherin and vimentin in the presence of MUC16. This finding suggests that the presence of MUC16 promotes tumor metastasis.

HE4

HE4 is a protein that was first discovered in the distal epithelium of the epididymis. The protein has a WAP-type four disulfide-core (WFDC) and is encoded by *WFDC2* found on chromosome 20q1213.1 [97]. It is found to be elevated in ovarian cancer as there is evidence of increased HE4 mRNA expression in different types of EOC [90]. HE4 shows differential expression, where levels are found to be higher in serous and endometrioid types compared with other ovarian cancers. HE4 is said to have fewer false positives and comparable sensitivity to CA125.

Alone, the sensitivity of this marker has been reported to be 90% with a specificity of 77.6% [76]. When combined with CA125 the sensitivity is 94%. An HE4–CA125 panel is currently used to identify cancers before surgery [76]. HE4 has recently obtained FDA approval for disease monitoring only at this time. In cases where women with ovarian tumors have normal CA125 levels, HE4 levels may be obtained. If elevated one may decide to use this protein level to monitor treatment response as is done with CA125 (NILM).

Moore et al. reported a sensitivity of 76.5% and specificity of 95% when CA125 and HE4 were combined to differentiate benign from malignant lesions in a retrospective study [98,99]. Prospectively, this panel correctly identified 93.8% of high- and low-risk malignancies. The serum levels of mesothelin, CA125, and HE4 were measured in symptomatic patients and individuals 0 to 3 years before diagnosis. Elevated levels for all three markers were found to be optimal at 1 year before diagnosis. Another study evaluated the ability of different biomarker panels to detect undiagnosed disease at different time intervals. No panel was able to outperform CA125 alone, which itself showed optimal results at 0–6 months before diagnosis. This is to say that to diagnose new disease there is no marker better than CA125 from 0 to 6 months before diagnosis. The use of CA125, HE4, and Symptom Index to prospectively differentiate benign from malignant lesions showed a sensitivity of 84% and specificity of 98.5% [100].

The scoring systems

The risk of malignancy index (RMI) is a tool currently being used in women who have no symptoms of ovarian cancer [101]. It allows patients who are more likely to have epithelial ovarian cancer to be triaged into a group that would be seen by a gynecologic oncologist compared with patients with a lower probability of malignancy. Those patients would be managed by a practitioner without advanced training [101]. RMI is obtained by multiplying serum CA125 levels in units per milliliter by a score given for specific pelvic ultrasound findings, and by a score given for menopausal status.

Ultrasound results are scored on a scale of 0, 1, and 3, where findings of metastases in the abdomen, multilocular, solid, cystic, or bilateral lesions each earn 1 point. The points are added and incorporated into the formula accordingly. The exception is that any ultrasound total greater than or equal to 2 has an ultrasound score of 3 incorporated into the formula [102]. Menopausal state is scored as a 1 for pre-menopausal and 2 for post-menopausal states [90]. RMI score of 200 is used as the cut-off with sensitivity of 90%, specificity of 89%, PPV of 96%, and NPV of 78% [102].

ROMA is a risk of malignancy algorithm that uses a patient's menopausal status and her HE4 levels manipulated by a logarithmic formula. ROMA uses the coefficient for the log of serum values and incorporates that into one of two logistic regression formulas, depending on menopausal status.

If pre-menopausal, the formula is predictive index (PI)= −12.0 +2.38*LN (HE4) + 0.0626*LN(CA125). If post-menopausal, the formula becomes PI = − 8.09+1.04*LN(HE4) + 0.732LN (CA125) (102). When (ROMA) incorporated HE4 and CA125 to detect malignancy, it showed a sensitivity of 94.3% and specificity of 75% (104). These rates were higher than those obtained by the RMI. HE4 with CA125 were also found to be able to discriminate endometriotic cysts from ovarian cancer [103].

Comparing HE4 and CA125

As RMI originally used CA125 levels as the marker incorporated into the formula, the emergence of HE4 as a comparative tumor marker has prompted its incorporation into RMI and the comparison of the two markers as was done by Jacobs et al. In studies comparing diagnostic ability of HE4, CA125, HE4, and CA125 incorporated into RMI alone and together, and HE4 and CA125 incorporated into ROMA alone and together, the following results were obtained. HE4 was superior to CA125 in finding ovarian borderline tumors, cancers of the fallopian tubes as well as early staged EOC.

However, combining HE4 and CA125 and attempting to detect early-stage EOC with and without incorporating the tumor markers into RMI and ROMA did not show any improvement because the expression profile of CA125 and HE4 are similar [90]. There was better specificity calculated from combined HE4 and ROMA when they were used to compare the borderline/cancer group to benign disease as opposed to the healthy group. The ability to differentiate cancer from endometriosis was shown best by ROMA with an area under the curve (AUC) of 0.89, specificity of 80%, and sensitivity of 85.4% [90].

To differentiate borderline tumors from the healthy controls/benign disease group, HE4 alone was the best test with AUC of 0.81 and 0.83, specificities of 81.8% and 85.9%, and sensitivities of 62.5% and 62.5%, respectively [86]. When evaluating each test's ability to differentiate members of the healthy controls and benign disease group from those of the peritoneal cancer group, sensitivities were 80% for all modalities. However, the highest values for AUC and test specificity were obtained by the RMI-CA125*HE4 modality at 0.97 for healthy or benign and 0.94 for peritoneal cancer and specificities of 97% for healthy control or benign disease or and 95.8% for peritoneal cancer [90]. When detection of FIGO stage I and II borderline tumors was compared with healthy or benign disease the best AUCs were 0.85 and 0.87, respectively, when using ROMA, and 0.86 and 0.86, respectively, when HE4 was used [90].

Serologic factors and acute-phase proteins

Acute phase reactants are also associated with ovarian cancer. It has long been shown that there is a relationship between cancer and chronic inflammation that involves continued injury to tissue with repair and accumulation of damage to DNA. One study had findings that were weakly suggestive of an elevated ovarian cancer risk in patients with elevated C-reactive protein (CRP) levels [104]. An acute phase reactant known as SAA has been found. Although the addition of SAA levels combined with CA125 levels yielded the classification rate when attempting to differentiate between patients with benign versus malignant process. SAA did not significantly ameliorate CA125's detection ability. Accuracy rates were 95.2% for combined SAA and CA125 and 86.2% for CA125 alone [105].

Certain cytokines and chemokines have been found to be significantly higher in cancer patients compared with controls. This underscores the need to evaluate the entire tumor microenvironment in the search for biomarkers. Incorporated into some of the better biomarker panels are growth factors, acute-phase reactants, serologic factors, hormones, stromal cell adhesion molecules and matrix metalloproteinases.

Apolipoprotein A1 (Apo-A1) is one of the constituents of the cholesterol-removing high-density lipoprotein. A total of 70% of circulating Apo A1 is made by the liver, and 30% by the small intestines. It is made up of 243 amino acid residues. The protein's structure entails eight segments of 22 amino acid residues each arranged into an alpha helix, of 2–11 residues, long repeats and an N-terminal region of 44 residues. The molecular weight is 28 kDa. It is accepted that Apo-A1 has a polar end that is in contact with the aqueous phase and a hydrophobic surface that is in contact with lipids (lipid library). Research has shown that exogenous Apo-A1 prevents tumor development in mice while lowered Apo-A1 levels are associated with ovarian cancer [106].

Apo-A1 has been shown to have anti-inflammatory and anti-oxidant capabilities in addition to counteracting atherogenesis. This is important as other factors known to be associated with tumorigenesis and cancer progression have been found to be elevated in several cancers including ovarian. Additionally, these factors may be produced by the tumors and/or the tumor microenvironment.

Macrophage colony-stimulating factor

Macrophage colony-stimulating factor (M-CSF), also known as CSF-1, is a cytokine that is associated with placental implantation as well as being involved in differentiation and growth of mononuclear cells (macrophages and monocytes). Along with its receptor CSF-1R, M-CSF is the product of c-fms, a proto-oncogen [107]. This factor is produced by osteoclasts, stromal cells, and macrophages and, therefore, has autocrine and paracrine activity.

CSF-1 has some clinical value. Its expression correlates with tumor aggressiveness, decreased recurrence interval, poor prognosis, and worsened outcome. CSF-1 is found at low levels in normal ovarian tissue and benign ovarian lesions. It is overexpressed in ovarian epithelial cancers and their metastases [108]. Furthermore metastases of ovarian cancer express CSF-1 and CSF-1R whereas the coexpresion is not seen in benign and non-invasive borderline lesions [107]. CSF-1 levels complement CA125. Furthermore, M-CSF levels have been shown to be elevated in 56% of patients with tumors who have normal CA125 [88]. Specificity is 98% with CA125; the sensitivity is 90% [76].

uPAR

uPAR is urokinase-type plasminogen activator receptor. Its truncated forms have been evaluated with regard to differentiating malignant from benign adnexal masses and therefore as a potential biomarker in ovarian cancer. Urokinase plasminogen activator (uPA) has been found to be involved in tumor angiogenesis, development, inflammation, and metastasis. The enzyme cleaves plasminogen into plasmin that in turn breaks down extracellular matrices and basement membranes or promotes metastasis by activating other zymogens (e.g., procollagenase) [110]. The receptor, being found on the cell membrane, allows localization of the enzyme itself. The receptor may be found in three forms. First in its full-length form uPAR I-III, as the cleaved uPAR II–III, or uPAR I [110].

One study evaluated the serum levels of CA125 and soluble uPAR forms to find statistically different levels of all four markers of invasive cancer as well as malignant and benign masses of the adnexa [77]. The combination of CA125 with suPARI-III + suPAR II–III showed a specificity of 85%, sensitivity not stated [110]. There were no differences found between serum levels of patients with endometriosis and other benign ovarian cysts. Serum levels in these benign cases, including endometriosis, are low in comparison to that seen in ovarian cancer. Therefore this panel shows the ability to discriminate benign from early malignant adnexal processes [110]. Further evaluation is needed. uPARI levels have prognostic value, in that elevated levels carry a poor prognosis [110].

Cytokines and other inflammatory mediators

IL-6 promotes inflammation while IL-8 functions as a chemokine by recruiting leukocytes. Proposed sources of both include the tumor, infiltrating macrophages, and other white blood cells. In vitro, chemoresistance has been mediated by IL-6. Cancer proliferation, invasion, as well as poor prognosis and clinical outcome have been associated with these interleukins [111].

Anti-tumor antibody

Another point of interest is the anti-tumor antibody. Here, the presence and concentration of IgG would be used not only to identify disease but also distinguishes between early and late stage disease. They are also relatively more specific than the biomarkers investigated in the past.

Transthyretin (TTR), also known as pre-albumin, is an acute-phase protein with a role in tumor development in addition to being an indicator of nutritional status [112].

Transferin, involved in iron transport in the body, has been described to act as a promoter of tumor development and survival by means of anti-apoptotic effects [112].

OVX1

OVX1 refers to either the ovarian or breast cancer-related antigen on a high molecular weight mucin-like glycoprotein or the monoclonal murine antibody that recognizes it. OVX1 has been reported to be elevated (>7.2 U/mL) in 70% of patients with ovarian tumors. Increased levels of OVX1 can be found in 59% of patients with ovarian tumors and normal CA125 levels [88]. There is a 76% sensitivity when OVX1 is combined with M-CSF and CA125II [76]. Evidence suggests that OVX1 may be unstable, which makes shipping samples to be evaluated at outside facilities difficult [88]. This is one limitation to its routine clinical use.

Osteopontin

Osteopontin is an adhesive glycoprotein that has been found to be involved in tumor metastasis and progression. Osteopontin has a role in bone remodeling as well as certain immune functions [113]. This biomarker is made by osteoblasts and endothelial cells. There is evidence that osteopontin is made by macrophages in the ovarian tumor microenvironment [113]. Increased levels of osteopontin are associated with tumor metastasis as one of the functions of this protein is the inhibition of apoptosis. It has been shown to be involved in survival and cell proliferation as well as invasion [113].

After surgical intervention for ovarian cancer, OPN has been used to monitor for disease recurrence. Higher levels of OPN are associated with poorer prognosis. OPN as a sole biomarker has a sensitivity of 81.3%. When combined with CA125 there is a 33.7% specificity and 93.8% sensitivity [76]. A potential use of OPN is in early noninvasive detection of ovarian cancer as levels may be measured in urine.

Mesothelin

Mesothelial cells that cover body cavities express mesothelin. Its interaction with CA125 is reported to be essential in cancer pathogenesis. Elevated levels of this protein are found in malignancies of the pancreas and ovarian as well as mesothelioma. Mesothelin has a potential role in diagnosis of early ovarian cancers for high-risk individuals, as its stability is time dependent. Specificity and sensitivity have been shown to be similar to that of CA125 [76]. Testing for this protein is noninvasive as levels can be measured in urine.

B7-H4

B7-H4 is an immune-modulator found in ovarian cancer as well as T cells. Specific tumors expressing this protein are endometrioid, serous, and clear cell ovarian cancers. There is evidence that epithelial cell malignant transformation is promoted by B7-H4. Alone, this protein's specificity has been reported as 97% with sensitivity of 45%. When combined with CA125, the sensitivity of both markers increases to 65% [76].

Prostasin

Prostasin is a trypsin-like serine protease with a molecular weight of 40 kDa. It is physiologically found at its highest levels in the prostate and semen. Lower levels are expressed by the bronchi, lungs, liver, kidneys, colon, and salivary glands. Prostasin is found at elevated levels in ovarian cancers, especially those of nonmucinous epithelial origin. The sensitivity is 92% and specificity is 94% for this marker [76]. Real-time PCR has been used to show that ovarian cancers produce more prostasin than normal ovarian tissue by a factor of 120 to 410. Prostasin levels are decreased following surgical intervention [114].

Epidermal growth factor receptor

Among the tyrosine kinase growth factor receptor family is the epidermal growth factor receptor (EGFR). Receptor homo- and hetero-dimerization is promoted by binding of a ligand to the receptor. This then leads to activation of the tyrosine kinase domain within the cell and subsequent steps related to cell survival, proliferation, differentiation of both benign and malignant ovarian tissue, angiogenesis, and metastasis. EGFR is involved in ovarian follicular growth, development, and differentiation. As the receptor is expressed on the gonadal surface epithelium, it is thought to be involved in repair of the ruptured follicle after ovulation by means of epithelial–mesenchymal transition. Inclusion cysts are thought to be the result of malfunction in this repair mechanism and thereby increase the likelihood of malignancy at that site.

Upon provocation from the EGFR, the OSE exhibits characteristics resembling immature, regenerating, or neoplastic epithelia, by shifting its phenotype from epithelial to fibroblastic. Abnormal expression of EGF receptors and/or ligands have been shown to exist in ovarian cancer. Ovarian tumors overexpress EGFR. *EGFR* is estimated to be overexpressed in 10–20% of ovarian cancers while minimal increases are seen in 43% of cases [115]. It is thought that the factor that determines overall and disease-free survival is the EGFR. Increased expression of EGFR is associated with poorer outcomes as this is seen with more aggressive entities. This observation has been supported by meta-analysis and worse outcomes seen in other epithelial cancers with overexpressed EGFR [115].

A study done by Zeineldin showed the behavior of ovarian tumors is driven by EGFR. Activation of EGFR has the effect of inducing mitosis within the cell. Studies have shown that growth of ovarian tumor cells is promoted by EGFR and that blocking of the EGFR precludes such growth. E-cadherin-mediated intercellular junctions are broken and proteinases able to degrade extracellular matrix are synthesized as part of the epithelial–mesenchymal transition induced by EGFR. It is thought that the transition may promote cell survival when in suspension as in ascites, help in chemoresistance, and anchoring of intra-peritoneal metastases [115]. Conversely, there is evidence that down-regulation of EGFR by alpha-TEA promotes apoptosis in ovarian cancer cells even in tumors that are resistant to cisplatin [116]. Additionally, synthesis of MMPs, which are involved in metastases, has been linked to EGF/EGFR signaling by means of oncogene c-fos and c-jun induction within the nucleus.

Higher levels of EGFR in tissues have been associated with higher tumor grades, later disease stage, presence of metastases, and post-operative residual disease. Lastly, lower levels of this protein's soluble form are found in the sera of ovarian cancer patients. This is likely due to increased renal clearance of EGFR.

Vascular endothelial growth factor

Vascular endothelial growth factor (VEGF) is a mediator of angiogenesis by promoting novel capillaries to form. It is constantly produced in both physiologic and pathophysiologic conditions. The production of malignant ascites seen in ovarian cancer has been associated with VEGF activity. Both metastatic and benign ovarian tumors have been shown to express elevated levels of VEGF. Higher levels are also found in stage I ovarian cancer when compared with nonmalignant disease. Levels were higher still in late staged disease in comparison to early staged. When combined with CA125 the specificity is low but sensitivity is 96% [76].

As lower levels of VEGF are found in postoperative patients compared with preoperative individuals, monitoring of response to treatment could be a potential role of this protein, that is, if it is possible to overcome the low specificity obtained when VEGF is added to biomarker panels. In addition higher levels are found in patients with metastatic versus locally restricted disease. This suggests a potential role of VEGF in determining prognosis.

Hormones

Several hormones have been implicated in ovarian cancer. Prolactin has been found to be a risk factor for breast and prostate cancer [117]. Not only do ovarian cancer cells express prolactin, but women with a family history of ovarian cancer have been shown to have elevated levels as prolactin has been shown to induce cancer cell growth and transcription factors, as well as promote transformation of normal ovarian epithelial cells to become immortalized and cancerous [118].

Growth hormone is thought to play a role in tumorigenicity by means of its interactions with IGF-1. Ovarian cancer has been linked to changes in circadian rhythms and high nocturnal cortisol levels. It is likely that overexpression of hydroxysteroid dehydrogenase leads to increase conversion of cortisone to cortisol yielding this high cortisol level. Adipokine leptin is a protein hormone with the ability to stimulate growth of ovarian cancer by means of MAP kinase activation. It also has value as a prognostic indicator.

OvaSure: One of the multimarker panels that was made commercially available is OvaSure. It is made of CA125, prolactin, leptin, IGF-2, macrophage inhibitory factor, and osteopontin. Sensitivity has been reported to be 95.3% and specificity 99.4% (50). This panel was available commercially until it was found that an inaccurate ovarian cancer prevalence rate was used to calculate the PPV of the test.

OVA1

The immunoassay OVA1 is a new test approved by the FDA in 2009 as a method of triaging women with masses. This is not a screening test but one that is intended to be used to further characterize pelvic masses found clinically or on imaging. The sensitivity of the test is reported to be greater than 90% with a negative predictive value of 90%. The test itself is not unlike a prostate-specific antigen (PSA) test used in the evaluation of prostate cancer. Here, the result is an OVA1 score ranging from 0 to 10, with cut-offs set as 5.0 for pre-menopausal women and 4.4 for post-menopausal women. Patients with scores higher than these thresholds are to be evaluated by a gynecologic oncologist due to the higher likelihood of the pelvic mass being cancerous [119]. The test itself is composed of five proteins: CA125, beta2-microglobulin, transferrin, apolipoprotein A1, and transthyretin (prealbumin). In addition to these proteins, there is proprietary software involved in calculating the OVA1 score [119].

In addition to OvaSure and Ova1, other panels have been evaluated. Among them is one comprised of CA125, HE4, vascular cell adhesion molecule, and carcino-embryonic antigen showing sensitivity of 86% and specificity of 91.3% for detection of early disease. Another panel reported 94.1% sensitivity and 91.3% specificity when IL-6, IL-8, CA125, C-reactive protein, and serum amyloid A were combined [120].

Implementation of biomarker-based screening

There are currently two different approaches being implemented in developing multi-marker panels. The first is attempting to make tools to be used in screening the general population better, as screening in that group is not currently recommended due to poor performance of available techniques. It should be noted that the search for new biomarkers does continue with the hope of being useful in conjunction with transvaginal ultrasound or other imaging as second line in certain high-risk groups.

The second approach involves using biomarkers as part of a triage algorithm in women with a pelvic mass where benign disease can be treated with less invasive methods while malignancies can be referred appropriately and thereby benefit from lower overall morbidity and increased overall survival [57].

Before any panels may be used in the clinical setting, these marker combinations must be evaluated by means of prospective randomized controlled trials and validated by evaluating the panel in samples from undiagnosed ovarian cancer. Previous authors have described a roadmap to be implemented in attempts to find a suitable screening or diagnotic test for early ovarian cancer. This "roadmap" involves discovery, verification/validation, and clinical implementation phases. Various screening steps, sample sources, and validation techniques are used in obtaining the final test [87].

Challenges of screening

To be acceptable, a screening method for early detection of ovarian cancer should have a specificity of at least 99.6%, sensitivity of at least 75%, and PPV of at least 10% [12,16,24]. A screening method relying on biomarkers as first-line and transvaginal ultrasound as second line would provide a slightly lower specificity of 98% according to previous studies [121]. Identification of a premalignant lesion, with adequate sensitivity and specificity, is the goal of an ideal screening tool. Recent studies suggest that finding such a premalignant lesion, one which accumulates genetic mutations, is on the horizon. High-risk individuals being targeted for screening are likely to help make this goal into reality.

In early stage ovarian cancer as well as in all pre-menopausal women, CA125 has a lower sensitivity. For this reason, CA125 alone is not meant to be used in screening the general population. While CA125 alone is not useful in assessing the prognosis or diagnosis of ovarian cancer, it is useful in monitoring response to treatment as well as monitoring for recurrence surveillance. It is thought that, to achieve a higher sensitivity and specificity, a multimodal method of screening should be used. At this time, screening of high-risk individuals involves transvaginal ultrasound and CA125 levels. This approach includes tumor marker levels at certain times along with ultrasound evaluation.

Evaluating screening on mortality

The value of screening is a question yet to be answered. Overall survival benefit using combined CA125 and transvaginal ultrasound screening methods, in healthy post-menopausal women is being evaluated by two randomized control trials known as the Prostate, Lung, Colorectal, and Ovarian (PLCO) screening and the United Kingdom Collaborative Trial of Ovarian Cancer Screening (UKCTOCS). Preliminary reports indicate a PPV of 1–1.3% by PLCO and 35.1% by UKCTOCS [122,123].

The United Kingdom Collaborative Trial of Ovarian Cancer Screening (UKCTOCS) is the largest trial of its kind to date, randomizing 202,638 post-menopausal women to no treatment (control), annual multimodal screening by serum CA125 assay and transvaginal ultrasound known as multimodality screening (MMS), and transvaginal ultrasound screening alone. According to these results, the sensitivity, specificity, and positive-predictive values for all primary ovarian and tubal cancers were 89.4%, 99.8%, and 43.3% for MMS, and 84.9%, 98.2%, and 5.3% for ultrasound, respectively. For primary invasive epithelial ovarian and tubal cancers, the sensitivity, specificity, and positive-predictive values were 89.5%, 99.8%, and 35.1% for MMS, and 75.0%, 98.2%, and 2.8% for USS, respectively. Results of the study showed in the ultrasound group that 845 of 48,230 had surgery while this corresponded to only 97 of the 50,078 in the ultrasound with CA125 group (multimodalitiy screening). Specificity, sensitivity, and PPVs were 99.8%, 89.5%, and 35.1%, respectively, for the multimodality group.

The study reported to have diagnosed 48% of malignancies as stage I or II [76]. There was a significant difference in specificity ($P < 0.0001$) but not sensitivity between the two screening groups for both primary ovarian and tubal cancers as well as primary epithelial invasive ovarian and tubal cancers.

The authors concluded that the sensitivity of the multimodality and ultrasound alone screening strategies is encouraging. Moreover, the multimodality screening approach had higher specificity than ultrasound alone, resulting in lower rates of repeat testing and surgery. The prevalence screen has established that the screening strategies are feasible. It should be noted that according to the UKCTOCS protocol, the decision to operate was made by clinicians acting on the basis of their clinical assessment. Furthermore, in the UKCTOCS, it appears that no guidelines were given to the clinicians with regard to the level of risk above which surgical intervention had to be warranted.

Epigenetics

Epigenetics is another area of focus. Here, changes that affect gene expression, such as chromatin remodeling, as well as post-translational modification of proteins are evaluated.

dditionally, micro-RNAs have also been shown to be subject) epigenetic modifications.

Chromatin remodeling and post-translational modification ome in the form of histone acetylation and DNA methylation. pigenetic changes have been found to be associated in some varian cancers. Both hyper- and hypo-methalation leading to oss of heterozygosity have been observed. Methylation hen occurring in the promoter region of a tumor suppressor ene inhibits expression of that gene and in effect allows tumorgenicity [88]. These methylation events can be detected using olymerase chain reaction (PCR).

Enzymes that facilitate methylation are DNA methyltranserases (DNMT), of which three have been well described. DNMT3a and DNMT3 work to initiate methylation of DNA while DNMT1 works to maintain the methylated state [88]. Among the tumor suppressor genes that have been silenced this way are *BRCA1*, *p16*$^{\mathrm{INK4a}}$, *p15*$^{\mathrm{INK4b}}$, *p14*^{ARF}, *p73*, and *APC*. Hypermethylation can be reversed by DNMT inhibitors like 5-azadeoxycytidine (5-aza-dc), which is a cytosine analog. DNMTs covalently bind to 5-aza-dc which cannot be methylated, leading to depletion of the enzyme [88].

MicroRNA (miRNA) are small ribonucleic acids of about 22 nucleotides. These miRNAs are the products of RNA polymerase II or III, and Drosha and Dicer, which are RNAse III-related enzymes. miRNA is a component of an RNA-induced silencing complex (RISC) which functions to repress the translation of or just destabilize specific mRNAs by targeting that mRNA's 3′ untranslated region. In cancer down-regulation of miRNAs by means of epigenetic mechanisms have been seen [88]. When miRNAs are down-regulated the functioning of the silencing complex is altered. miRNAs may be used as biomarkers as a result of their small size which allows detection in body fluids and tumors [88].

Hypomethylation

Metastasis-related gene synuclein gamma

Metastasis-related gene synuclein gamma (MRGSG) is a pathophysiologic product of chromosome 10. The protein is found in aggressive and late staged ovarian epithelial cancers. When the gene is hypomethylated, it functions to promote cell multiplication and differentiation. It has been found that 75 to 100% of the gene may not be methylated. This is also expressed in breast cancer [76].

Satellite 2 and satellite alpha

Hypomethylation of satellite 2 DNA (30%) and satellite alpha (33%) of chromosome 1 has been found in ovarian cancer. This finding may help in identifying ovarian endometrioid and serous tumors. There may be a correlation between the degree of satellite 2 methylation and tumor stage [76].

MCJ

MCJ is found on chromosome 13q14.1 and has potential as a determinant of prognosis. It is methylated and therefore silenced physiologically. When hypomethylated in ovarian tumors this gene has been reported to increase tumor sensitivity to cisplatin and paclitaxel. Hypermethylation, specifically >90%, is associated with poorer prognosis and resistance to chemotherapy [76].

P53

P53 is a tumor suppressor gene found to be mutated leading to loss of the allele in 50% of ovarian cancers across all stages. This marker is useful in differentiating high-grade serous ovarian tumors from other cancers of the ovary as well as determining potential for metastasis [76].

ARID1a

Evidence exists that *ARID1a* may encode a tumor suppressor involved in unwinding of DNA during the process of chromatin remodeling. It is suggested that mutations in this gene allow cancer formation as 46% of clear cell and 30% of endometrioid carcinomas have been shown to carry this inactivated gene [76].

IGF-2 mediates gonadotropin activity and is the primary IGF in the ovary. Prolactin regulates ovarian follicular synthesis of steroids. Specifically, prolactin blocks the secretion of progesterone early in the follicular growth and enhances the luteal phase [87]. Leptin is thought to be associated with gondotropin releasing hormone and involved in the hypothalamic–pituitary–ovarian axis. Osteopontin is overexpressed in various cancers including ovarian. CA125 is discussed elsewhere in this chapter. MIF is an inflammatory mediator.

It is proposed that disruption of the microecology by the presence of aberrant cells leads to overexpression of the biomarkers evaluated. It is thought that protein expression is a result of balance between ovarian components [87]. Further propositions include inability to detect tumor molecular products till late in disease, but detection of the body's response to the presence of tumor is possible in its early stages [87].

One author suggested that screening the general population may not be the best approach in detecting early staged ovarian cancer and that efforts should be turned to high-risk groups where prevalence will be higher and the test specificities are more likely to meet the minimum requirements. Furthermore, to best use screening modalities within high-risk groups, PPV, sensitivity, and specificity may have to be calculated for these different groups, for example, *HNPCC* versus *BRCA1/BRCA2* versus positive family histories.

A total of 75% of ovarian cancers are diagnosed at late stages. That is to say that they have invaded the peritoneal cavity or at least show evidence of local spread. At these stages, the possibility of curing disease is minimal [110].

Numerous genes have been found to have their protein products overexpressed in ovarian cancer using cDNA and oligonucleotide microarrays. HE4 is one of these genes. It is found on chromosome 20q12–13.1. Immunohistochemical experiments have found HE4 in the epididymal duct with an apical granular pattern. It is also found in the endocervix, the fallopian tubes, endometrium, trachea, and other epithelia. Studies have shown that serous and endometrioid ovarian cancer tissues exhibited staining in the cell membranes, cytoplasm, and in the perinuclear area. In contrast, mucinous ovarian tumors do not stain positive for HE4. Therefore, HE4 may hold promise in differentiating between various types of epithelial ovarian cancer [110].

One of the theories regarding the development of ovarian carcinoma involves Mullerian epithelium in cortical inclusion cysts [109]. The proposed mechanism for this calls for the loss of the basement membrane in the cortical inclusion cyst allowing contact of the CIC epithelia with the stroma which induces metaplasia of the epithelial cells. Evidence that supports the progenitor cortical inclusion cyst theory includes the following: (1) patients with unilateral ovarian cancer have more cortical inclusion cysts in the contralateral normal-appearing ovary than patients without ovarian cancer; (2) women with family histories of ovarian cancer have more cortical inclusion cysts upon prophylactic removal than those without the family history; (3) the epithelial cells lining the cortical inclusion cyst have been shown to harbor p53 mutations; (4) reports exist of inclusion cyst epithelium showing intra-epithelial neoplasia [110].

A common finding in neoplasia is a modification in glycosylation of proteins. The same is seen here with ovarian cancer. Drapkin et al. showed that HE4 is secreted in a glycosylated form by ovarian cancer. This glycosylated form was larger than that predicted using recombinant HE4 and HE4 expressed by High Five insect cells. Hellstrom et al. reported HE4 to be found in the circulation of ovarian cancer patients and not in individuals without ovarian cancer. They also showed that the sensitivity and specificity of HE4 is similar to that of CA125 [110].

Even in the glycosylated form, HE4 is a relatively small protein. On sodium dodecyl sulfate-polyacrylamide gel electrophoresis (SDS-PAGE) its molecular weight appeared to be no more than 25 kDa. This being the case, it is possible that this protein may be filtered by the kidneys. If this is proven to be the case, then a noninvasive urine-based assay may be in the realm of possibilities [110].

Conclusion

Unfortunately, 70–75% of women continue to be diagnosed with stage III or IV epithelial ovarian carcinoma and these stages have a predicted 5-year survival of 15–40%. In contrast, if detected when confined to the ovary (stage I), the 5-year survival approaches 90%, women require less radical and morbid operations, and may not require adjuvant chemotherapy [4]. This suggests that novel strategies for detection of early stage EOC will have a great impact on the survival of women with this disease. Whereas all cancer patients can potentially benefit from early detection, the development of new strategies based upon the molecular, genetic, and biochemical events that regulate carcinogenesis, invasion, and metastatic dissemination are critical for the detection of early stage EOC.

Globally, hundreds of clinically relevant serum/plasma/urine markers have been identified that are based on the molecular biology of ovarian metastases. These markers require validation and interfacing with newly developed diagnostic technologies (e.g., ovarian Pap test, contrast enhanced sonography) to achieve the goal of detection of early stage disease. Ultimately, the optimal screening program depends upon an integrated, multidisciplinary collaboration of clinicians, scientists, institutions, and industry partners having complementary expertise unifying to facilitate the detection of early stage EOC in asymptomatic high-risk women.

References

1. Jamal A, Bray F, Center MM, et al. Global Cancer Statistics 2011. CA Cancer J Clin. 2011;**61**(2):69–90.
2. National Cancer Institute. PDQ® Genetics of Breast and Ovarian Cancer. Bethesda, MD: National Cancer Institute. Date last modified: 06/02/2011. Available at: http://cancer.gov/cancertopics/pdq/genetics/breast-and-ovarian/HealthProfessional (accessed June 6, 2011).
3. National Cancer Society. Cancer Facts & Figures 2010. Atlanta, American Cancer Society; 2010.
4. Jelovac D, Armstrong DK. Recent progress in the diagnosis and treatment of ovarian cancer. CA Cancer J Clin. 2011;**61**(3):183–203.
5. Rock JA, Jones HW III. TeLinde's Operative Gynecology, 10th edition. Philadephia: Lippincott Williams & Wilkins; 2008. p 1307–12.
6. American Cancer Society. Ovarian Cancer. Atlanta, American Cancer Society. Date last modified: 10/13/2010. Available at: http://www.cancer.org/cancer/ovariancancer/detailedguide/ovarian-cancer-survival-rates (accessed June 6, 2011).
7. American Cancer Society. Early detection, diagnosis, and staging topics. Available at: http://www.cancer.org/cancer/ovariancancer/detailedguide/ovarian-cancer-survival-rates.
8. Schorge JO, Modesitt SC, Coleman RL, et al. SGO White paper on ovarian cancer: etiology, screening and surveillance. Gynecol Oncol. 2010;**119**(1);7–17.
9. Anderson MR, Goff BA, Lowe KA, et al. Combining a symptoms index with CA125 to improve detection of ovarian cancer. Cancer. 2008;**113**(3):484–9.
10. Joyner AB, Runowicz CD. Ovarian cancer screening and early detection. Women's Health (Lond Engl). 2009;**5**(6):693–9.
11. Ricciardelli C, Oehler MK. Diverse molecular pathways in ovarian cancer and their clinical significance. Maturitas. 2009;**62**(3):270–5.
12. Kindelberger DW, Lee Y, Miron A, et al. Intraepithelial carcinoma of the fimbria and pelvic serous carcinoma: evidence for a casual relationship. Am J Surg Pathol. 2007;**31**(2):161–9.

13. Cho KR, Shih IM. Ovarian cancer. Annu Rev Pathol. 2009;**4**:287–313.
14. Ovarian Cancer National Alliance. Overview. Available at: http://www.ovariancancer.org/about-ovarian-cancer/introduction/ (accessed June 10, 2011).
15. Kurman RJ, Shih IM. The origin and pathogenesis of epithelial ovarian cancer: a proposed unifying theory. Am J Surg Pathol. 2010;**34**(3):433–43.
16. Healthwise. Stage and grade of ovarian cancer. Boise, ID, Healthwise. Date last modified: 06/15/2009. Available at: http://www.med.nyu.edu/healthwise/article.html?hwid=tw9761#tw9761-sec (accessed June 10, 2011).
17. Protocol Information Management System Gynecologic: AJCC Stage Information. Available at: https://www.protocols.fccc. edu/fccc/pims/staging/ajcc/ovary_ajcc.html#Primaryformation. Fox Chase Cancer Center (accessed June 10, 2011).
18. Rossing MA, Wicklyn KG, Cushing-Haugen KL, et al. Predictive value of symptoms for early detection of ovarian cancer. J Natl Cancer Inst. 2010;**102**:222–9.
19. Russo A, Calo V, Bruno L, et al. Hereditary ovarian cancer. Crit Rev Oncol Hematol. 2009;**69**(1):28–44.
20. Pavlik EJ, Saunders BA, Doran S, et al. The search for meaning-symptoms and transvaginal sonography screening for ovarian cancer. Cancer. 2009;**115** (16):3689–98.
21. Cass L, Karlan BY. Ovarian cancer: speak out – but what are they really saying? J Natl Cancer Inst. 2010;**102**(4):211–2.
22. Wilson JMG, Junger G. Principles and Practice of Screening for Disease. World Health Organization. 1968; Public Health Papers No. 34. Available at: http://whqlibdoc.who.int/php/WHO_PHP_34.pdf (accessed June 6, 2011).
23. Lynch HT, Casey MJ, Snyder CL, et al. Hereditary ovarian carcinoma: heterogeneity, molecular genetics, pathology, and management. Mol Oncol. 2009;**3**(2):97–137.
24. Dutta S, Wang FQ, Fishman DA. The dire need to develop a clinically validated screening method for the detection of early-stage ovarian cancer. Biomark Med. 2010;**4**(3):437–9.
25. Bast RC. Status of tumor markers in ovarian cancer screening. J Clin Oncol. 2003;**21**:200s–5s.
26. Dutta S, Wang FQ, Phalen A, et al. Biomarkers for ovarian cancer detection and therapy. Cancer Biol Ther. 2010;**9**(9):668–77.
27. Goff BA, Mandel LS, Drescher CW, et al. Development of an ovarian cancer symptom index. Cancer. 2007;**109**(20):221–7.
28. Clarke-Pearson DL. Screening for ovarian cancer. N Engl J Med. 2009;**361**(2):170–7.
29. Rein BJD, Gupta S, Dada R, et al. (Review Article) Potential markers for detection and monitoring of ovarian cancer. J Oncol. 2011;**2011**:475983.
30. Ovarian Cancer: Screening, Treatment, and Followup. NIH Consens US Statement. 1994;**12**(3):1–30.
31. Hartikainen JM, Kataja V, Pirskanen M, et al. Stack MS. Screening for BRCA1 and BRCA2 mutations in Eastern Finnish breast/ovarian cancer families. Clin Genet. 2007;**74**:311–20.
32. Fishman DA, Cohen L, Maihle N, Baron E, Stack SM. The National Ovarian Cancer Early Detection Program. Chicago: Northwestern University; 2003.
33. NCCN Clinical Practice Guidelines in Oncology (NCCN Guidelines). Ovarian Cancer Including Fallopian Tube Cancer and Primary Peritoneal Cancer. Date last modified: 11/15/2010. Available at: http://www.nccn.org/professionals/physician_gls/pdf/genetics_screening.pdf. (assessed June 13, 2011).
34. Venkitaraman AR. Cancer susceptibility and the functions of BRCA1 and BRCA2. Annu Rev Pathol. 2009;**4**:461–87.
35. Shulman LP. Hereditary breast and ovarian cancer (HBOC): clinical features and counseling for BRCA1 and BRCA2, Lynch syndrome, Cowden syndrome, and Li-Fraumeni syndrome. Obstet Gynecol Clin North Am. 2010;**37**(1):109–33.
36. Rodabaugh K, Brewer MA, Chalas E, et al. Hereditary breast and ovarian cancer. Am Col Obstet Gynecol. 2008;1–39.
37. Stadler ZK, Salo-Mullen E, Patil SM, et al. Prevelance of BRCA1 and BRCA2 mutations in Ashkenazi Jewish families with breast and pancreatic cancer. Cancer. 2012;**118**:493–9.
38. Metcalfe KA, Poll A, Royer A, et al. Screening for founder mutations in BRCA1 and BRCA2 in unselected Jewish women. J Clin Oncol. 2010;**28**(3):387–91.
39. Lee EYHP, Muller WJ. Oncogenes and tumor suppressor genes. Cold Spring Harbor: Cold Spring Harbor Laboratory Press; 2010.
40. Press JZ, De Luca A, Boyd N, et al. Ovarian carcinomas with genetic and epigenetic BRCA1 loss have distinct molecular abnormalities. BMC Cancer. 2008;**8**:17.
41. Genetics Home Reference: BRCA2. U.S. National Library of Medicine. Date last modified: 08/2007. Available at: http://ghr.nlm.nih.gov/gene/BRCA2 (accessed June 13, 2011).
42. Farooq A, Walker LJ, Bowling J, Audisio RA. Cowden syndrome. Cancer Treat Rev. 2010;**36**(8):577–83.
43. Pilarski R. Cowden syndrome: a critical review of the clinical literature. J Genet Counsel. 2009;**18**:13–27.
44. Koehler-Santos P, Izetti P, Abud J, et al. Identification of patients at-risk for Lynch syndrome in a hospital – based colorectal surgery clinic. World J Gastroenterol. 2011;**17**(6):766–73.
45. The University of Texas M.D. Anderson Cancer Center: Lynch Syndrome Hereditary Nonpolyposis Colorectal Cancer Syndrome or HNPCC. Last modified 12/17/2008, http://www2.mdanderson.org/app/pe/index.cfm?pageName=opendoc&docid=2133 (accessed June 13, 2011).
46. Xian W, Miron A, Roh, M, et al. The li fraumeni syndrome (lfs): a model for the initiation of p53 signatures in the distal fallopian tube. J Pathol. 2010;**220**(1):17–23.
47. Altekruse SF, Kosary CL, Krapcho M, et al. (Eds.). SEER Cancer Statistics Review, 1975–2007. Bethesda, MD: National Cancer Institute, http://seer.cancer.gov/csr/1975_2007/. (accessed June 6, 2011).
48. Grimbizis GF, Tarlatzis BC. The use of hormonal contraception and its protective role against endometrial and ovarian cancer. Best Pract Res Clin Obstet Gynaecol. 2010;**24**(1):29–38.

49. Cragun JM. Screening for ovarian cancer. Cancer Control. 2011;**18**(1):16–21.

50. Myers ER, Bastian LA, Havrilesky LJ, et al. Management of Adnexal Mass. Evidence Report/Technology Assessment No. 130 (Prepared by the Duke Evidence-based Practice Center under Contract No. 290–02–0025.) AHRQ Publication No. 06-E004. Rockville, MD: Agency for Healthcare Research and Quality. February 2006.

51. Bazot M, Daraï E, Nassar-Slaba J, et al. Value of magnetic resonance imaging for the diagnosis of ovarian tumors: a review. J Comput Assist Tomogr. 2008;**32**:712–23.

52. Risum S, Hogdall C, Loft A, et al. The diagnostic value of PET/CT for primary ovarian cancer: a prospective study. Gynecol Oncol. 2007;**105**:145–9.

53. Roman LD, Muderspach LI, Stein SM, et al. Pelvic examination, tumor marker level, and gray-scale and Doppler sonography in the prediction of pelvic cancer. Obstet Gynecol. 1997;**89**:493–500.

54. Reles A, Wein U, Lichtenegger W. Transvaginal color Doppler sonography and conventional sonography in the preoperative assessment of adnexal masses. J Clin Ultrasound. 1997;**25**:217–25.

55. Hamper UM, Sheth S, Abbas FM, et al. Transvaginal color Doppler sonography of adnexal masses: differences in blood flow impedance in benign and malignant lesions. AJR Am J Roentgenol. 1993;**160**:1225–8.

56. Liu JH, Zanotti KM. Management of the adnexal mass. Obstet Gynecol. 2011;**117**:1413–28.

57. Hassen K, Ghossain MA, Rousset P, et al. Characterization of papillary projections in benign versus borderline and malignant ovarian masses on conventional and color Doppler ultrasound. AJR Am J Roentgenol. 2011;**196**:1444–9.

58. Kinkel K, Hricak H, Lu Y, et al. US characterization of ovarian masses: a meta-analysis. Radiology. 2000;**217**:803–11.

59. Fishman DA, Cohen L, Blank SV, et al. The role of ultrasound evaluation in the detection of early-stage epithelial ovarian cancer. Am J Obstet Gynecol. 2005;**192**:1214–21; discussion, 1221–2.

60. Cohen L, Fishman DA. Ultrasound and ovarian cancer. Cancer Treat Res. 2002;**107**:119–32.

61. Dutta S, Wang FQ, Fleischer AC, et al. New frontiers for ovarian cancer risk evaluation: proteomics and contrast-enhanced ultrasound. AJR Am J Roentgenol. 2010;**194**:349–54.

62. Yankeelov TE, Niermann KJ, Huamani J, et al. Correlation between estimates of tumor perfusion from microbubble contrast-enhanced sonography and dynamic contrast-enhanced magnetic resonance imaging. J Ultrasound. 2006;**25**:487–97.

63. Marret H, Sauget S, Brewer M, et al. Contrast-enhanced sonography helps in discrimination of benign from malignant adnexal masses. J Ultrasound Med. 2004;**23**:1629–39.

64. Brasch R, Turetschek K. MRI characterization of tumors and grading angiogenesis using macromolecular contrast media: status report. Eur J Radiol. 2000;**34**:148–55.

65. Leen E. Ultrasound contrast harmonic imaging of abdominal organs. Semin Ultrasound CT MR. 2001;**22**:11–24.

66. Orden MR, Jurvelin JS, Kirkinen PP. Kinetics of a US contrast agent in benign and malignant adnexal tumors. Radiology. 2003;**226**:405–10.

67. Ferrara KW, Merritt CR, Burns PN, et al. Evaluation of tumor angiogenesis with US: imaging, Doppler, and contrast agents. Acad Radiol. 2000;**7**:824–39.

68. Hall GH, Atkin SL, Turnbull LW. Use of dynamic contrast-enhanced MRI to assess the functional vascular pharmacokinetic parameters of normal human ovaries. J Reprod Med. 2002;**47**:107–14.

69. Kupesic S, Kurjak A. Contrast-enhanced, three-dimensional power Doppler sonography for differentiation of adnexal masses. Obstet Gynecol. 2000;**96**:452–8.

70. Marret H, Sauget S, Giraudeau B, et al. Contrast-enhanced sonography helps in discrimination of benign from malignant adnexal masses. J Ultrasound Med. 2004;**23**:1629–39.

71. Fleisher AC, Lyshchik AP, Jones HW, et al. Early detection of ovarian cancer with contrast enhanced transvaginal sonography. J Oncol. 2009;**53**:49–54.

72. Moore RG, MacLaughlan S. Current clinical use of biomarkers for epithelial ovarian cancer. Curr Opin Oncol. 2010;**22**:492–7.

73. Bast RC, Spriggs, DR. (Editorial) More than a biomarker: CA125 may contribute to ovarian cancer pathogenesis. Gynecol Oncol. 2011;**121**:429–30.

74. Theriault C, Pinard M, Comamala M, et al. MUC16 (CA125) regulates epithelial ovarian cancer cell growth, tumorigenesis and metastasis. Gynecol Oncol. 2011;**121**:434–43.

75. Rein BJD, Gupta S, Dada R, et al. (Review Article) Potential markers for detection and monitoring of ovarian cancer. J Oncol. 2011;**2011**:475983.

76. Drapkin D, Adam C, Skates S. uPar: a beacon of malignancy? Clin Cancer Res. 2008;**14**:5643–5.

77. Yurkovetsky Z, Skates S, Lomakin A, et al. Development of a multimarker assay for early detection of ovarian cancer. J Clin Oncol. 2010;**28**:2159–66.

78. Petricoin EF, Calvo KR, Wulfkuhle J, Liotta LA. Mass spectrometry-based profiling of the circulatory proteome for cancer detection and stratification. In: Rockett JC, Burczynski ME (Ed.). Surrogate Tissue Analysis: Genomic, Proteomic, and Metabolomic Approaches. Informa Healthcare; 2005. p 93–107.

79. Kulasingam V, Diamandis EP. Strategies for discovering novel cancer biomarkers through utilization of emerging technologies. Nat Clin Pract Oncol. 2008;**5**:588–99.

80. Burczynski ME, Rockett JC. Surrogate Tissue Analysis: Genomic, Proteomic and Metabolomic Approaches. Boca Raton: CRC; 2006.

81. Barnas JL, Simpson-Abelson MR, Yokota SJ, et al. T cells and stromal fibroblasts in human tumor microenvironments represent potential therapeutic targets. Cancer Microenviron. 2010;**3**:29–47.

82. Tan DSP, Agarwal R, Kaye SB. Mechanisms of transcoelomic metastasis in ovarian cancer. Lancet Oncol. 2006;**7**:925–34.

83. Iijima J, Konno K, Itano N. Inflammatory alterations of the

extracellular matrix in the tumor microenvironment. Cancers (Basel). 2011;**3**:3189–205.

84. Horan MP. Application of serial analysis of gene expression to the study of human genetic disease. Hum Genet. 2009;**126**:605–14.
85. Jacob F, Meier M, Caduff R, et al. No benefit from combining HE4 and CA125 as ovarian tumor markers in a clinical setting. Gynecol Oncol. 2011;**121**:487–91.
86. Kim K, Visintin I, Alvero AB, et al. Development and validation of a protein based signature for the detection of ovarian cancer. Clin Lab Med. 2009(**1**):47–55.
87. Tainsky MA. Genomic and proteomic biomarkers for cancer: a multitude of opportunities. Biochim Biophys Acta. 2009;**1796**:176–93.
88. Yan PS, Potter D, Deatherage DE, et al. Differential methylation hybridization: profiling DNA methylation with a high-density CpG island microarray. Methods Mol Biol. 2009;**507**:89–106.
89. Jacob F, Goldstein DR, Fink D, et al. Proteogenomic studies in epithelial ovarian cancer: established knowledge and future needs. 2009;**3**:743–56.
90. Chon HS, Lancaster JM. Microarray-based gene expression studies in ovarian cancer. Cancer Control. 2010;**18**:8–15.
91. Meani F, Pecorelli S, Liotta L, et al. Clinical application of proteomics in ovarian cancer prevention and treatment. Mol Diagn Ther. 2009;**13**:297–311.
92. Ceccarelli M, d'Acierno A, Facchiano A. A scale space approach for unsupervised feature selection in mass spectra classification for ovarian cancer detection. BMC Bioinformatics. 2009;**10**(Suppl 12):S9.
93. Lowenthal MS, Mehta AI, Frogale K, et al. Analysis of albumin-associated peptides and proteins from ovarian cancer patients. Clin Chem. 2005;**51**:1933–45.
94. Elberse KE, Tcherniaeva I, Berber GA, et al. Optimization and application of a multiplex bead based assay to quantify serotype-specific IgG against *Streptococcus pneumoniae* polysaccharides: response to the booster vaccine after immunization with the pneumococcal 7-valent conjugate vaccine. Clin Vaccine Immunol. 2010;**17**:674–82.
95. Ray-Coquard I, Guastalla JP, Allouache D, et al. HER2 overexpression/ amplification and trastuzumab treatment in advanced ovarian cancer: a GINECO phase II study. Clin Ovarian Cancer. 2008;54–9.
96. Galgano MT, Hampton GM, Frierson HF Jr. Comprehensive analysis of he4 expression in normal and malignant human tissue. Mod Pathol. 2006;**19**:847–53.
97. Moore RG, McMeekin DS, Brown AK, et al. A novel multiple marker bioassay utilizing HE4 and CA125 for the prediction of ovarian cancer in patients with a pelvic mass. Gynecol Oncol. 2009;**112**:40–6.
98. Moore RG, Brown AK, Miller MC, et al. The use of multiple novel tumor biomarkers for the detection of ovarian carcinoma in patients with a pelvic mass. Gynecol Oncol. 2008;**108**:402–8.
99. Andersen MR, Goff BA, Lowe KA, et al. Use of S symptom index, CA125, and HE4 to predict ovarian cancer. Gynecol Oncol. 2010;**116**:378–83.
100. Jacobs I, Oram D, Fairbanks J, et al. A risk of malignancy index incorporating CA 125, ultrasound and menopausal status for the accurate preoperative diagnosis of ovarian cancer. Br J Obstet Gynecol. 1990;**97**:922–9.
101. Obeidat BR, Amarin ZO, Latimer JA, et al. Risk of malignancy index in the preoperative evaluation of pelvic masses. Int J Gynaecol Obstet. 2004;**85**:255–8.
102. Moore RG, Jabre-Raughley M, Brown AK, et al. Comparison of a novel multiple marker assay vs. the risk of malignancy index for the prediction of epithelial ovarian cancer in patients with a pelvic mass. Am J Obstet Gynecol. 2010;**203**:1–6.
103. Lundin E, Dossus L, Clendenen T, et al. C-reactive protein and ovarian cancer: a prospective study nested in three cohorts (Sweden, USA, Italy). Cancer Causes Control. 2009;**20**(7):1151–9.
104. Moshkovskii SA, Vlasova MA, Pyatnitskiy MA, et al. Acute phase serum amyloid A in ovarian cancer as an important component of proteome diagnostic profiling. Proteomics Clin Appl. 2007;**1**:107–17.
105. Li H, Li C, Wu H, et al. Identification of Apo-A1 as a biomarker for early diagnosis of bladder transitional cell carcinoma. Proteome Sci. 2011;**9**:21.
106. Toy EP, Azodi M, Folk NL, et al. Enhanced ovarian cancer tumorigenesis and metastasis by the macrophage colony-stimulating factor. Neoplasia. 2009;**11**:136–44.
107. Chambers SK. Role of CSF-1 in progression of epithelial ovarian cancer. Future Oncol. 2010;**5**:1429–40.
108. Su F, Kozak KR, Imaizumi S, et al. Apolipoprotein A-I (apoA-I) and apoA-I mimetic peptides inhibit tumor development in a mouse model of ovarian cancer. Proc Natl Acad Sci USA. 2010;**107**:19997–20002.
109. Drapkin R, Von Hosten HH, Lin Y. Human epididymis protein 4 (he4) is a secreted gycoprotein that is overexpressed by serous and endometrioid ovarian carcinomas. Cancer Res. 2005;**65**:2162–9.
110. Lee CC, Liu KJ, Huang TS. Tumor-associated macrophage: its role in tumor angiogenesis. J Cancer Mol. 2006;**2**:135–40.
111. Park JW, Lee MH, Choi JO, et al. Tissue-specific activation of mitogen-activated protein kinases for expression of transthyretin by phenylalanine and its metabolite, phenylpyruvic acid. Exp Mol Med. 2010;**28**:105–15.
112. Courter D, Cao H, Kwok, Kong C, et al. The RGD domain of human osteopontin promotes growth and metastasis through activation of survival pathways. PLos One. 2010;**5**:e9633.
113. Costa FP, Junior EL, Zelmanowicz A, et al. Prostasin, a potential tumor marker in ovarian cancer: a pilot study. Clinics (Sao Paulo). 2009;**64**:641–4.
114. Zeineldin R, Muller CY, Stack MS, et al. Targeting the EGF receptor for ovarian cancer therapy. J Oncol. 2010;**2010**:1–11.
115. Shun MC, Yu W, Park SK, et al. Downregulation of epidermal growth factor receptor expression contributes to alpha-TEA's proapoptotic effects in human ovarian cancer cell lines. J Oncol. 2010;**2010**:824571.
116. Huang GS, Brouwer-Visser J, Ramirez MJ, et al. Insulin-like growth factor

2 expression modulates Taxol resistance and is a candidate biomarker for reduced disease-free survival in ovarian cancer. Clin Cancer Res. 2010;**16**:2999–3010.

117. Levina VV, Nolen B, Su Y, et al. Biological significance of prolactin in gynecological cancers. Cancer Res. 2009;**69**:5226.

118. Fung ET. A recipe for proteomics diagnostic test development: the OVA1 test from the biomarker discovery to FDA clearance. Clin Chem. 2010;**56**;327–9.

119. Edgell T, Martin-Rousset G, Barker G, et al. Phase II biomarker trial of a multimarker diagnostic for ovarian cancer. J Cancer Res Clin Oncol. 2010;**136**:1079–88.

120. Skates SJ, Horick N, Yu Y, et al. Preoperative sensitivity and specificity for early-stage ovarian cancer when combining cancer antigen CA-125II, CA15–3, Ca72–4, and macrophage colony stimulating factor using mixtures of multivariate normal distributions. J Clin Oncol. 2004;**22**:4059–66.

121. Menon U, Gentry-Maharaj A, Hallett R, et al. Sensitivity and specificity of multimodal and ultrasound screening for ovarian cancer, and stage distribution of detected cancers: results of the prevalence screen of the UK Collaborative Trial of Ovarian Cancer Screening (UKCTOCS). Lancet Oncol. 2009;**10**:327–40.

122. Patridge E, Kreimer AR, Greenlee RT, et al. Results from four rounds of ovarian cancer screening in a randomized trial. 2009;**113**:775–82.

123. Katz VL, Lobo RA, Lentz G, Gershenson D. Comprehensive Gynecology, 5th edition. Philadelphia: Mosby Elsevier; 2007.

Chapter 24

Laparoscopic evaluation and management of adnexal masses and ovarian cancer

Farr R. Nezhat, MD, FACOG, FACS, Jason Sternchos, MD, Tamara Finger, MD, and Tanja Pejovic, MD, PhD

Introduction

The American Cancer Society estimates that 21,990 women will be diagnosed with ovarian cancer and 15,460 will die of the disease in 2011 [1]. Of these 21,990 patients, 20% will have stage I disease, for which 5-year survival rates approach 90%. However, numerous studies have shown that a significant percentage of patients with apparent early stage (stage I) ovarian cancer actually harbor microscopic metastatic disease. Consequently, the benefits of surgical staging for epithelial ovarian carcinoma have been well established.

Traditionally, it has been recommended that a comprehensive surgical staging procedure for epithelial ovarian and fallopian tube cancers include a total abdominal hysterectomy, bilateral salpingo-oophorectomy, peritoneal cytologic washings, biopsies of adhesions and peritoneal surfaces, omentectomy, and retroperitoneal lymph node sampling from the pelvic and para-aortic regions through a generous vertical midline laparotomy incision [2]. With the advent of minimally invasive surgical techniques, surgeons are now able to perform all of the necessary procedures for comprehensive surgical staging, including pelvic and para-aortic lymphadenectomies and omentectomies, using conventional videolaparoscopy or robotic-assisted videolaparoscopy in selected patients.

Laparoscopy offers multiple advantages over laparotomy such as better visualization, smaller incisions, shorter hospital stays, decreased estimated blood loss, less need for analgesics, more rapid recovery, and shorter interval to chemotherapy if indicated. In the assessment of an adnexal mass and early stage ovarian cancer, laparoscopy can be both diagnostic and therapeutic. The combination of laparoscopic visualization and frozen section analysis is the most reliable method for the detection of malignancy [3]. Laparoscopy can not only be used to rule out or rule in malignancy but can be used as a tool to relieve pain and compressive symptoms of an adnexal mass whether benign or malignant. Once malignancy is diagnosed, comprehensive surgical staging can be performed laparoscopically which has been shown to be not only feasible, but safe and accurate in borderline and invasive early stage disease. In select cases of localized disease, laparoscopy can also be used to perform fertility-sparing surgical staging [4].

The first study to show feasibility of staging in early stage invasive ovarian cancer was reported in 1994. Querleu and Leblanc reported complete laparoscopic surgical staging procedures for ovarian or fallopian tube cancer [5]. Eight referred patients with ovarian and fallopian tube cancers underwent complete laparoscopic staging after inadequate initial surgical staging. Since this initial series, others have confirmed the feasibility of comprehensive laparoscopic surgical staging of ovarian or fallopian tube cancers [6–9].

Although there is limited published data regarding laparoscopy in advanced ovarian cancer, multiple applications of laparoscopy have thus far emerged in the literature. This includes a triage tool for resectability, primary and secondary cytoreduction, second-look evaluation, and placement of intraperitoneal catheters.

Adnexal masses

The most common adnexal masses in reproductive-age women are benign functional cysts of the ovaries. These include follicular cysts, corpus luteum cysts, theca lutein cysts, and polycystic ovaries. Functional ovarian cysts are usually asymptomatic and tend to resolve spontaneously in 4 to 6 weeks. Occasionally, they may be accompanied by some degree of pelvic discomfort, pain, or dyspareunia. In addition, the rupture of one of these cysts leads to peritoneal irritation and possibly hemoperitoneum. A functional cyst may also be complicated by torsion, resulting in severe pain. Other related benign conditions include endometriosis (with ovarian endometriotic cysts) (Figs. 24.1 and 24.2), inflammatory enlargement of the fallopian tubes and ovaries (hydrosalpinges, tubo-ovarian abscess) due to pelvic infection, ectopic pregnancy, and trophoblastic disease.

True benign ovarian neoplasms could cause adnexal enlargement. These include most frequently serous or mucinous cystadenomas and benign cystic teratomas (Fig. 24.3). Cystic teratomas make up 70% of benign neoplasms in women younger than 30 and are made of the three germ cell layers. Mucinous and serous cystadenomas (Fig. 24.4) are usually multiloculated, with thin walls. It is unlikely that these are precursors of malignant neoplasms, although some changes may represent true ovarian intra-epithelial neoplasia. Other common adnexal masses and neoplastic processes include para-ovarian cysts and ovarian (Fig. 24.5) and fallopian tube cancers. See Table 24.1 for differential diagnosis of adnexal masses.

Altchek's Diagnosis and Management of Ovarian Disorders, ed. Liane Deligdisch, Nathan G. Kase, and Carmel J. Cohen. Published by Cambridge University Press.

Table 24.1 Differential diagnosis of an adnexal mass.

Organ	Cystic	Solid
Ovary	Functional cyst Endometriosis Cystic neoplasm Benign Malignant	Benign Malignant
Fallopian tube	Tubo-ovarian abscess or hydrosalpinx Paratubal cyst	Ectopic pregnancy Tubo-ovarian abscess Neoplasm
Uterus	Intra-uterine pregnancy	Myoma
Bowel	Distended colon with gas and/or feces	Appendicitis Diverticulitis Diverticular abscess Colon cancer

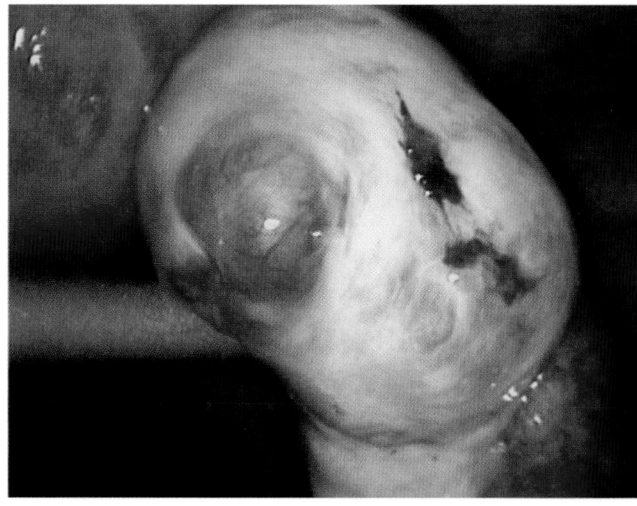

Fig. 24.1. Ovary with corpus luteum and superficial endometriosis.

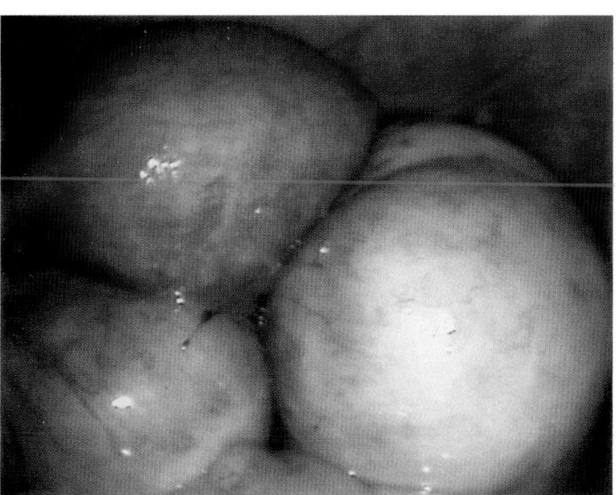

Fig. 24.2. Bilateral endometriomas.

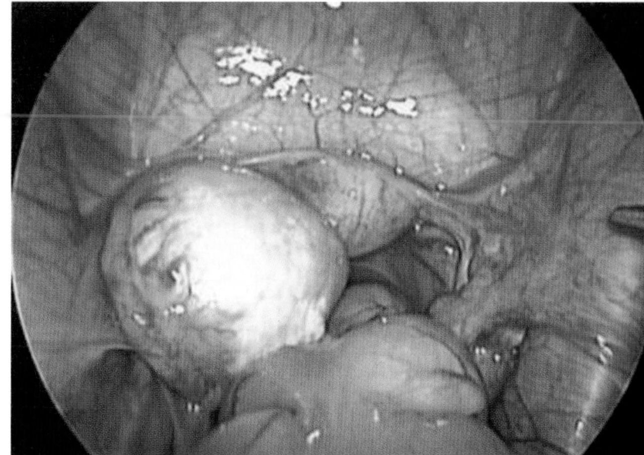

Figure 24.3. Benign cystic teratoma.

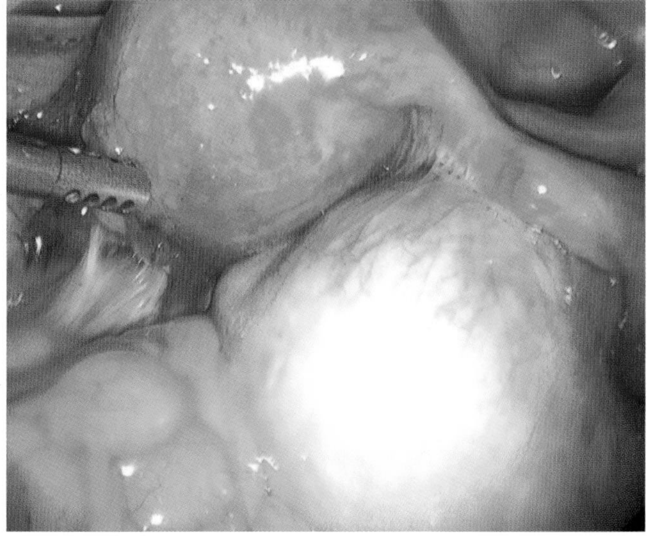

Fig. 24.4. Serous cystadenoma.

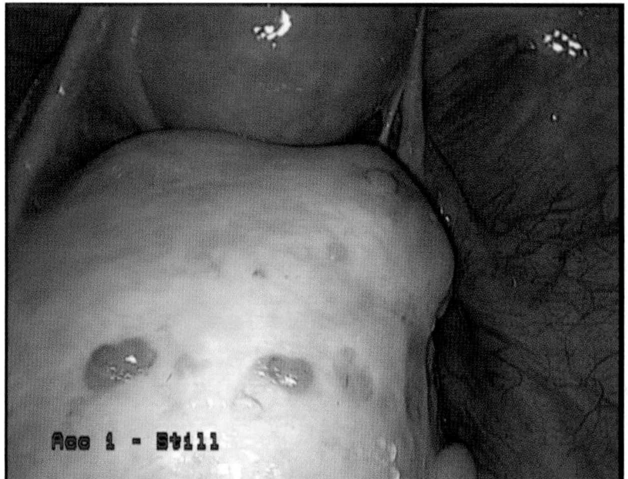

Fig. 24.5. Surface excrescences on malignant neoplasm of left ovary.

Table 24.2 Clinical signs of a malignant versus benign adnexal mass

Malignant	Benign
Prepubertal or post-menopausal	Reproductive age
Personal history of nongynecologic cancer	
Family history of ovarian, breast, or colon cancer	
Rapid growth	No growth
Ascites	No ascites
Fixed	Mobile
Nodularity of rectovaginal septum	Smooth rectovaginal septum
Bilateral	Unilateral
Solid or complex	Cystic
Irregular	Smooth

Any enlargement of the ovary is abnormal in the post-menopausal women and should be considered malignant until proven otherwise. The post-menopausal ovary atrophies to 1.5 × 1.0. × 0.5 cm in size and should not be palpable on pelvic examination. Ovaries that are palpable must alert the physician to possible malignancy. The risk of malignancy is increased from 13% in pre-menopausal to 45% in post-menopausal women [10]. Still, 55% of post-menopausal women with palpable ovaries do have a benign tumor.

Surgical exploration is the gold standard for diagnosis; however, much can be discerned about the diagnosis of an adnexal mass from a careful history, exam, and imaging. The majority of patients present with symptoms related to compression of the local pelvic organs due to the adnexal mass. Less commonly, an ovarian mass is discovered during a routine pelvic examination in an asymptomatic patient.

Once a mass is identified, onset and quality of pain, menstrual associations, and bowel and bladder involvement may help develop an index of suspicion (Table 24.2). Patients with a personal or family history of colon, ovarian, or breast cancer are at higher risk for malignancy than others. Mutations in the *BRCA-1* and *BRCA-2* genes confer a higher risk for ovarian cancer, and testing is available.

A seminal work by Sassone et al. evaluated an ultrasound scoring system to predict ovarian malignancy [11]. Transvaginal sonographic pelvic images of 143 patients were correlated with surgicopathologic findings. The variables in the scoring system included the inner wall structure of the adnexal cyst, wall thickness, presence and thickness of septa, and echogenicity. The scoring system was useful in distinguishing benign from malignant masses, with a specificity of 83%, sensitivity of 100%, and positive and negative predictive values of 37% and 100%, respectively. Subsequently, Alcazar and Jurado developed a logistic model to predict malignancy based on menopausal status, ultrasound morphology, and color Doppler findings in 79 adnexal masses [12]. The authors derived a mathematical formula to estimate preoperatively the risk of malignancy (or benignity) of a given adnexal mass in a simple and reproducible way. When this formula was applied prospectively, 56 of 58 (96.5%) adnexal masses were correctly classified. Although following a model would make management decisions more concrete, most clinicians base their decisions on the full clinical picture.

In general, CT is not routinely indicated for the evaluation of the adnexal mass, as it is not sensitive to lesions less than 2 cm in size. It is, therefore, not a good tool for the early detection of ovarian cancer. However, in cases in which malignancy is suspected, a CT scan may be used to further evaluate a patient with a hard fixed lateralized mass, ascites, abnormal liver function tests, or palpable abdominopelvic mass.

Once surgery is decided on, accurate diagnosis at surgery is essential in the management of adnexal masses. The ability to identify a malignancy during laparoscopy has been well studied. In the largest series of laparoscopically managed adnexal masses in reproductive-age women, Nezhat et al. reported that the most reliable indicators of malignancy were the combination of laparoscopic visualization of the whole peritoneal cavity and frozen section analysis [3].

Overall, the combined accuracy of laparoscopic visualization and intra-operative frozen section is an excellent tool for the identification of malignancies. The two important exceptions are in very large tumors or tumors with borderline characteristics. The accuracy in these instances depends on the relative sample bias. The solution to this problem should be in removing the entire adnexa and allowing pathologic rather than surgical sampling. If a malignant ovarian neoplasm is discovered at the time of laparoscopy, the current standard of care is the performance of a comprehensive surgical staging procedure.

Borderline ovarian tumors

Borderline ovarian tumors (BOTs) do not invade the basal membrane but may spread widely across peritoneal surfaces. They represent 10–20% of epithelial ovarian tumors and usually have an excellent prognosis [13]. They tend to occur in patients younger than those with invasive epithelial ovarian cancer, and their prognosis is better than the latter. Fifteen percent to 40% of serous BOTs are associated with peritoneal disease. The prognosis for such patients with advanced-stage disease is perceptibly different from those with stage I disease. The most important prognostic factor is the type of peritoneal implants (invasive or noninvasive). Prognosis of patients with noninvasive implants remains good if the totality of peritoneal implants is removed. The treatment is exclusively surgical, without adjuvant treatment. In selected cases of young patients with advanced-stage disease, conservative surgery could be proposed to maintain fertility [14].

Laparoscopic staging in BOTs is increasingly common with advances in endoscopic techniques and instruments. In one of the first case reports of laparoscopic treatment of BOTs, Nezhat et al. described the surgical staging technique which included a laparoscopic hysterectomy, bilateral adnexectomy, peritoneal sampling, peritoneal cytology, and partial omentectomy [15]. Subsequently, multiple case series studies emerged to further

Table 24.3 Laparoscopic management of borderline ovarian tumors

Author	No. of patients	Complications	Conversions to laparotomy	Mean follow-up (mo)	Recurrence	Survival
Darai et al. [16]	25	0	7 (Presumption of cancer and failure of laparoscopic procedure)	41	3	23[a]
Seracchioli et al. [17]	19[b]	0	0	42	1	19
Querleu et al. [78]	30[c]	3	0	29	1	30
Desfeux et al. [79]	14	–	16	29	1	47 ANED 1 DOD
	34[b]					
Fauvet et al. [18]	107	0	42 (For suggested cancer of large tumor volume)	27.5	13	103 ANED 4 AWED
Romagnolo et al. [80]	52	–	0	47	7	51 ANED 1 DOD
Brosi et al. [81]	21	0	0	78	0	35 ANED[a]
	20[b]					

ANED, alive with no evidence of disease; AWED, alive with evidence of disease.
[a] Missing patients were lost to follow-up.
[b] Conservative treatment (cystectomy or unilateral adnexectomy).
[c] Restaging cases.

evaluate the clinical outcomes and feasibility of laparoscopic treatment of BOTs [13,16,17]. In the largest case series to date, 107 patients underwent laparoscopic treatment of BOTs. The mean follow-up was 27.5 months with 100% survival and only four with evidence of disease [18]. A retrospective review was subsequently conducted of 113 patients diagnosed with BOTs, of whom 52 underwent laparoscopy and 61 underwent laparotomy. No difference occurred in progression-free survival between the two groups with a mean 44-month follow-up [13]. The longest documented follow-up (78 months) reports a survival of at least 83% and the remaining patients lost to follow-up [18]. A summary of the current literature on laparoscopic treatment of BOTs is provided in Table 24.3, yielding an overall survival of 98%.

Early stage invasive ovarian cancer

An estimated 20% of women with epithelial ovarian cancer have early stage disease at diagnosis. In these patients, complete surgical staging is required to obtain important prognostic information and to plan treatment options.

The first study to show feasibility of staging in early stage invasive ovarian cancer was reported in 1994 [5]. This case series included complete pelvic and para-aortic lymph node dissection in nine patients undergoing restaging procedures for either ovarian or fallopian tube cancers.

Since then, several prospective, retrospective and case series reports have demonstrated the feasibility and safety of a laparoscopic approach to the management of early stage ovarian cancers. These studies are summarized in Table 24.4 and show laparoscopy to be associated with decreased estimated blood loss and shorter hospital stay without compromising safety.

Because of the rarity of early stage ovarian cancer diagnoses, as well as challenges associated with preoperative diagnoses, a randomized controlled trial has not been feasible. Alternative evaluations of accuracy can be inferred by comparing upstaging rates and nodal yields between laparoscopic and laparotomy cases. In restaging procedures, the current literature suggests the rate of upstaging among complete laparoscopic staging procedures ranges from 11 to 19% [19]. The upstaging rate among patients who had complete laparotomy restaging procedures was reported as 30 to 36% [20]. The feasibility of laparoscopic completion of surgical staging in patients with incompletely staged ovarian, fallopian tube, endometrial, and primary peritoneal cancers was shown in Gynecologic Oncology Group (GOG) protocols 9302 and 9402 [7]. A total of 84 patients were eligible, of whom 74 had ovarian, fallopian tube, or primary peritoneal cancers. All patients with evidence of metastatic disease or in whom laparoscopy was contraindicated were excluded. In all, 58 (69%) patients underwent complete laparoscopic staging, confirmed with photographic documentation. Nine (10%) patients were incompletely staged laparoscopically because of lack of peritoneal biopsies, cytology, or bilateral lymph nodes. Seventeen patients (20%) required conversion to laparotomy: 13 because of lack of exposure from adhesions, 3 because of complications, and 1 because of metastatic macroscopic disease. Complications associated with laparoscopically treated patients included five bowel injuries, one cystotomy, one small bowel obstruction, one venotomy, and two with extensive blood loss requiring transfusion. In comparing patients treated laparoscopically with those treated

Table 24.4 Summary of laparoscopic staging of apparent early stage ovarian cancer.

Author	No. of patients	Operative time (min)	PLN (n)	PALN (n)	Blood loss (mL)	Length of stay (days)	Upstaged (%)	Follow-up (months)	Current status
Querleu et al. [5]	9	227	n/a	8.6	<300	2.8	11.1	n/a	n/a
Pomel et al. [82]	8	313	7.5	8.5	n/a	4.75	10	n/a	8 ANED
Childers et al. [6]	14	149–196	n/a	n/a	n/a	1.6	35.7	n/a	n/a
Amara et al. [39]	4	215	n/a	n/a	193	n/a	n/a	n/a	3 ANED 1 Died
LeBlanc et al. [19]	42	238	14	20	n/a	3.1	18	54	4 Died
Tozzi et al. [8]	24	166–182	19.4	19.6	n/a	7	20.8	46.4	36 ANED
Chi et al. [83]	20	312	12.3	6.7	235	3.1	10	n/a	n/a
Spirtos et al. [7]	73	187.9	18.6	10.3	171.9	3.35	11	n/a	n/a
Ghezzi et al. [84]	15	377	25.2	6.5	n/a	3	26.6	16	20 ANED
Park et al. [85]	17	303.8	13.7	8.9	231.2	9.4	5.9	19	1 Died 16 ANED
Park et al. [21]	19	220	27.2	6.6	240	8.9	21.1	17	19 ANED
Nezhat et al. [22]	36	229	14.8	12.2	195	2.3	17.6	55.9	36 ANED
Colomer et al. [86]	20	223	18	11.3	n/a	3	20	24.7	19 ANED 1 Recurrence

ANED, alive with no evidence of disease; AWED, alive with evidence of disease; DOD, died of disease; n/a, not available.

with laparotomy, the laparoscopic group showed a significantly shorter blood loss, hospital stay, and Quetlet index along with comparable nodal yields. In patients undergoing laparoscopy, six apparent early stage ovarian cancers were found to have advanced disease. Hospital stay was significantly shorter with laparoscopy alone (3 vs. 6 days, $P = 0.04$). The investigators concluded that interval laparoscopic staging of gynecologic malignancies can be successfully undertaken in selected patients, but laparotomy for adhesions or metastatic disease and risk of visceral injury should be anticipated [7]. Lack of experience in advanced operative laparoscopy may have played a role in the higher incidence of conversion to laparotomy and complications in this study compared with other groups.

In another comparison between laparoscopy and laparotomy, Park et al. compared 52 consecutive patients undergoing complete surgical staging of apparent stage I ovarian or fallopian tube cancer [21]. They did not find any significant differences in the upstage rate, nodal yield, or omental size resected at time of completion of surgery. Laparoscopy was also associated with quicker return of bowel function as well as with the ability to administer adjuvant chemotherapy in a shorter interval compared with after laparotomy. Time to adjuvant chemotherapy was significantly shorter in the laparoscopy group (12.8 vs. 17.6 days, respectively). Seventy-nine percent of patients in each group received combination chemotherapy and after a median follow-up time of 17 and 23 months, respectively, there was no recurrence or death in either group.

Recently, Nezhat et al. published one of the largest retrospective case series of laparoscopic staging for apparent early stage ovarian cancer [22]. Any patient found to have disease beyond the ovary during laparoscopic evaluation was excluded. A total of 36 patients who underwent laparoscopic staging for apparent early stage disease were included. Nine patients had been referred for restaging after occult cancer was found on final pathology following cystectomy or adnexectomy. The remaining 27 patients had presented with an adnexal mass. Twenty had invasive epithelial tumors, 11 borderline tumors, and the remaining 5 non-epithelial tumors (3 granulosa cells, 1 sertoli cell, and 1 dysgerminoma). Of 11 patients who underwent fertility-sparing operations, 6 had borderline tumors, 3 had mucinous carcinomas, and 1 had papillary serous carcinoma. Mean estimated blood loss was 195 mL. There were no major intra-operative complications. Three patients had lymphocele develop: two were managed conservatively and one required drainage. A mean of six peritoneal biopsies as well as 12.2 para-aortic nodes and 14.8 pelvic nodes were obtained. Eighty-three percent of patients underwent omentectomies. Seven patients were upstaged. During a mean follow-up of 55.9 months, three patients had recurrences:

two with borderline tumors in the remaining ovary and one with clear cell carcinoma in the pelvis. All three recurrences had originally undergone fertility-sparing procedures and had their recurrences subsequently resected with the recurrent clear cell carcinoma managed with adjuvant chemotherapy as well. At the time of publication, all patients were alive with no evidence of disease.

As suggested, these studies support the concept that laparoscopy may offer an advantage in the management of early stage ovarian cancer by allowing better visualization of difficult areas such as the subdiaphragmatic areas, peritoneal surfaces, obturator spaces, and anterior and posterior cul-de-sacs, as well as magnification and detection of smaller lesions that may be missed on laparotomy. They also suggest superior perioperative outcomes in terms of decreased blood loss, hospital stay, and complication rates while not compromising accuracy. Thus, comprehensive surgical staging of early stage ovarian cancer is not only feasible but evidence shows it is at least as safe as laparotomy while offering multiple perioperative and postoperative advantages with comparable recurrence rates and survival outcomes.

Advanced-stage invasive ovarian cancer

Most patients who are diagnosed with ovarian, fallopian tube, and primary peritoneal epithelial cancer present at advanced stages. Risk factors that contribute to a poor prognosis include FIGO stage, volume of residual disease, CA125 levels, histologic subtype and grade, and other surgical observational factors such as malignant ascites and capsular penetration [23]. The mainstay of treatment for advanced-stage invasive epithelial ovarian cancer is optimal cytoreduction followed by platinum-based combination chemotherapy [24]. Optimal cytoreduction, preferably to microscopic disease, is associated with increased survival [25–28]. However, not all patients are able to be optimally cytoreduced at time of initial surgery.

Laparoscopy is an important tool in triaging patients with ovarian cancer and in cytoreductive surgery (Figure 24.6). It also plays a role in placing intra-peritoneal ports for the purpose of IP chemotherapy and in second-look procedures. Thus, four applications of laparoscopy in advanced ovarian cancer have emerged thus far in the literature: a triage tool for resectability, placement of intra-peritoneal catheters for IP chemotherapy, second-look evaluation, and primary or recurrent cytoreduction in select cases [4].

Assessment of the feasibility of laparoscopic optimal cytoreductive surgery in ovarian cancer

Residual disease after surgery is one of the most important prognostic factors for patients with advanced ovarian cancer and the complete excision of all measurable disease has been shown to provide better survival compared with small 1- to 2-cm residual tumor [29]. In fact, a meta-analysis including 6,885 patients found that maximal cytoreduction is among the most powerful determinants of cohort survival among stage III and IV ovarian cancer patients. For every 10% increase in maximal cytoreduction in these patients, there was an associated 5.5% increase in median survival time. However, depending on individual institutions, surgical skills, and aggressiveness, the percentage of patients with no measurable tumor following debulking surgery ranges from 8 to 85% [25]. Furthermore, some patients originally selected for debulking treatment will be able to undergo only explorative laparotomy because of extremely advanced disease.

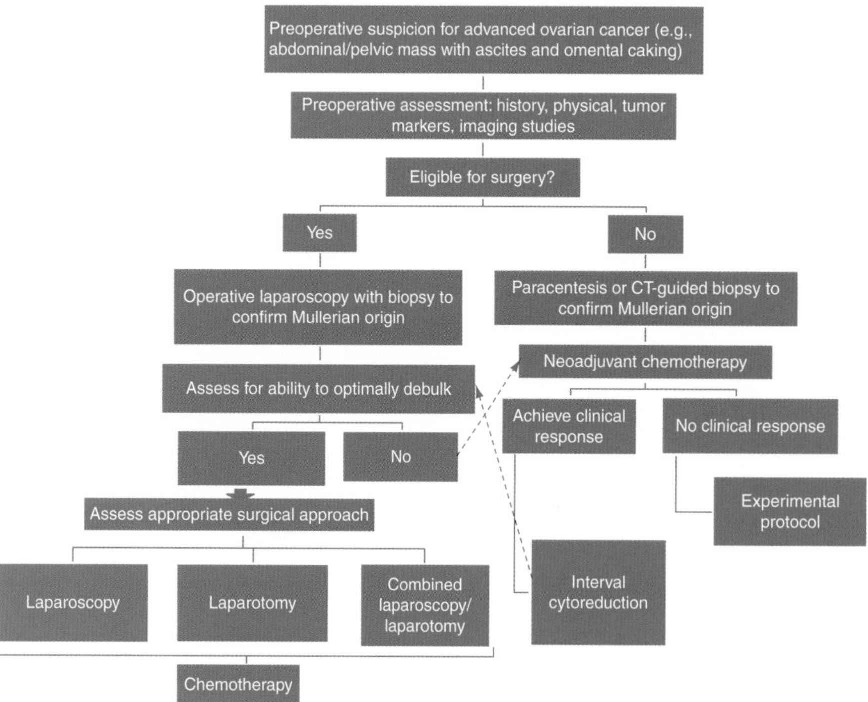

Fig. 24.6. Treatment algorithm for patients with preoperative suspicion for advanced ovarian cancer.

An accurate and reliable method should be pursued to avoid unnecessary explorative laparotomies and to better select patients for surgical and/or medical specific treatments. Bristow et al. elaborated a "predictive index model" based on preoperative CT scanning, which is highly accurate in recognizing patients with advanced epithelial ovarian carcinoma unlikely to undergo optimal primary cytoreductive surgery [30]. However, the study did not address the appropriateness of extensive open surgical staging, a keystone in the management of patients with advanced ovarian cancer.

Although certain imaging, like CT scanning, can accurately recognize patients unlikely to undergo optimal cytoreduction, such as those with bulky retroperitoneal disease and disease involving the liver parenchyma or porta hepatis, it is not as accurate in recognizing patients likely to be optimally debulked [30]. By adding the power of laparoscopy to imaging, the accuracy of predicting the probability that a patient can undergo optimal cytoreduction is increased. Also, not all patients with advanced disease are the same and as such survival data on these patients have been variable likely due to different inclusion criteria [31]. Laparoscopy can aid in differentiating FIGO stage IIIC patients who are likely to undergo primary optimal cytoreduction from those who are unlikely to undergo optimal cytoreduction and would thus benefit from neoadjuvant chemotherapy.

Fagotti et al. compared the power of laparoscopy with the standard explorative laparotomy in predicting optimal cytoreduction in the same group of advanced ovarian cancer patients [32]. The few well-known indicators of unresectability (i.e., extensive bulky carcinomatosis, agglutinated bowel/mesentery, diaphragm bulky disease, and unresectable upper abdominal metastases) were investigated by laparoscopy. The accuracy rate of laparoscopy in predicting the laparotomic probability of each one of these parameters ranged from 80 to 100%. In particular, all cases with peritoneal and/or diaphragmatic carcinomatosis and/or mesentery disease were correctly identified by laparoscopy (positive predictive value [PPV] = 100%, 82%, and 100%, respectively), resulting in an overall predictive judgment of unresectability, or negative predictive value (NPV) of 100%. In this context, NPV represents a very important clinical parameter, that is, the rate of inappropriate nonexploration or the ratio of patients thought to have unresectable disease but who will in fact undergo optimal surgery if operated on. This measure corresponds to the false-negative rate and in this study was zero, because in no case was the laparoscopic decision changed by the immediately following laparotomy. In this study, an optimal debulking was achievable in 34 of 39 patients (87%) selected as completely resectable by explorative laparoscopy. In another series, open laparoscopy was used in 285 patients to determine whether the patient could be optimally debulked and they found a 96% accuracy of resectability [33].

Feasability of neoadjuvant chemotherapy

There is recent compelling data showing the feasibility of neoadjuvant chemotherapy followed by debulking surgery in treatment of advanced stage ovarian cancer. In 2010, in a prospective randomized control trial of 632 eligible patients, Vergote et al. showed that in patients with bulky stage IIIC or IV ovarian carcinoma, neoadjuvant chemotherapy (platinum-based) followed by interval debulking was not inferior to primary debulking surgery followed by platinum-based chemotherapy [34]. Median overall survival was 29 months in the primary surgery group compared with 30 months in the primary neoadjuvant chemotherapy group. Median progression-free survival was 12 months in both groups. This study also confirmed the importance of complete resection of all macroscopic disease. Complete resection was the best independent predictor of overall survival in both the primary debulking group and the primary neoadjuvant followed by interval debulking group. When analyzed with respect to residual tumor, both groups showed that overall survival was inversely proportional to the amount of residual tumor after surgery regardless of whether the patient received primary surgery or primary neoadjuvant chemotherapy followed by interval cytoreduction. The overall survival in women who underwent primary debulking surgery followed by chemotherapy with no residual tumor, those with residual tumor 1 to 10 mm, and those with residual tumor larger than 10 mm was 45, 32, and 26 months, respectively. The overall survival in women who underwent neoadjuvant chemotherapy was 38, 27, and 25 months, respectively. Thus, this trial confirms the significance of optimal surgical cytoreduction regardless of whether surgery is performed before or after neoadjuvant chemotherapy.

Triage of resectability

One of the first roles of laparoscopy as a triage tool is to rule in or rule out malignancy. Even if malignancy is found it is not always of primary Mullerian origin. Laparoscopy affords the surgeon the opportunity to diagnose a non-gynecologic malignancy and to triage/refer the patient accordingly to the appropriate surgeon/oncologist whether the tumor is GI, breast, lung, or of any other primary. However, once a gynecologic malignancy is confirmed the question then becomes whether the tumor can be optimally cytoreduced.

Laparoscopy can be used to identify those patients who are candidates for upfront primary cytoreductive surgery and those patients that might benefit from neoadjuvant chemotherapy (Figs. 24.6–24.8) followed by cytoreduction. Thus, laparoscopy is a triage tool in an attempt to increase the rate of patients who can be optimally cytoreduced, because these patients have significant survival benefit in the setting of primary advanced-stage ovarian cancer [35]. It can also be used to assess patients with recurrent disease who are candidates for cytoreductive surgery (Fig. 24.9). The sequence of cytoreductive surgery and chemotherapy is determined at the time of diagnostic videolaparoscopy. Once primary Mullerian malignancy is confirmed through tissue biopsies, the decision whether the patient can be optimally surgically cytoreduced is then made. If optimal primary cytoreduction can be accomplished then it is immediately performed by means of

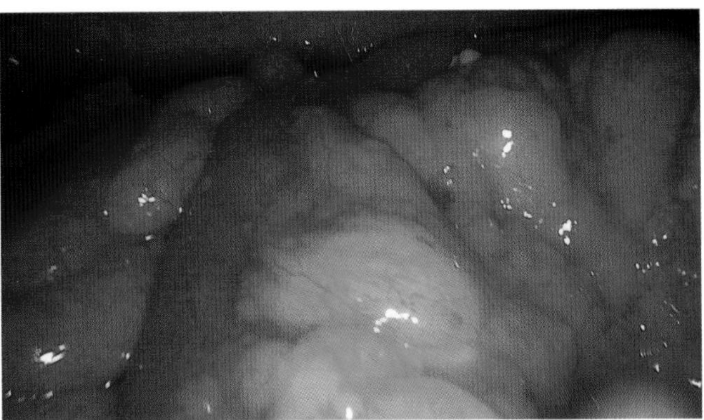

Fig. 24.7. Diffuse bowel and mesenteric metastases before neoadjuvant chemotherapy.

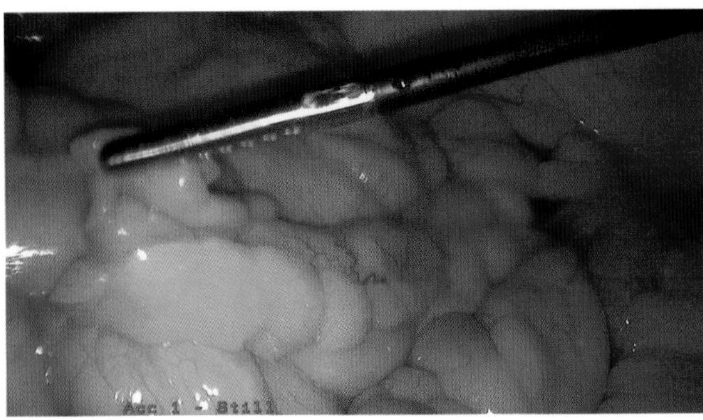

Fig. 24.8. Bowel and mesentery in the same patient after neoadjuvant chemotherapy.

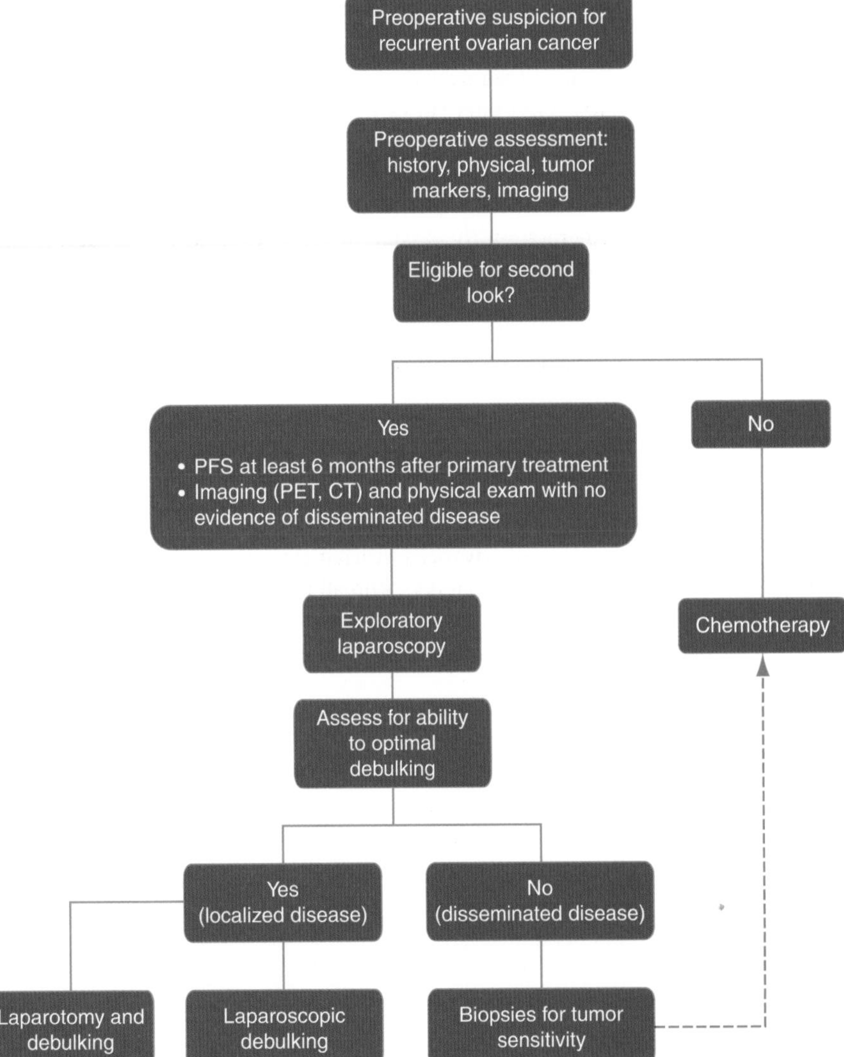

Fig. 24.9. Treatment algorithm for patients with preoperative suspicion for recurrent ovarian cancer.

laparoscopy (videolaparoscopy or robotic-assisted videolaparoscopy), laparotomy or a combination of laparoscopy and mini-laparotomy. In this situation, we have achieved the benefits of diagnostic videolaparoscopy for better visualization and assessment of disease in the abdominal-pelvic cavity, especially the upper abdomen, while decreasing the morbidity associated with a large vertical incision. If at the time of initial videolaparoscopy the patient is deemed to likely have a sub-optimal cytoreduction due to advanced disease or medical comorbidities, then the decision is made to terminate the procedure after appropriate biopsies are performed and to administer neoadjuvant chemotherapy in a timely manner. Such patients would then benefit from having only undergone diagnostic videolaparoscopy as opposed to laparotomy because there would be less morbidity, quicker recovery time, and shorter interval to administration of neoadjuvant chemotherapy [4]. Select patients may even begin chemotherapy the day after diagnostic laparoscopy [36]. Neoadjuvant chemotherapy would then be followed by interval cytoreduction either by laparoscopy or by laparotomy based on the response to chemotherapy.

Second-look laparoscopy and insertion of intra-peritoneal catheters

The role of second-look surgery in the management of advanced epithelial ovarian cancer is controversial. High recurrence rates after negative histologic findings, the lack of consistently effective salvage therapy, and the absence of data showing improved survival benefits have diminished acceptance of the routine use of second-look surgery. Nevertheless, patients with suboptimal initial cytoreductive surgery for stage III ovarian cancer who have had a complete clinical response to platinum-based combination chemotherapy appear to achieve a distinct survival benefit from second-look surgical procedures [37].

The management of advanced epithelial ovarian cancer includes surgical staging and aggressive debulking by laparotomy followed by intravenous chemotherapy. Nevertheless, even in cases of a good response after optimal debulking surgery and intravenous chemotherapy, 50% of the patients with no clinical evidence of residual disease will suffer a recurrence because of the presence of microscopic peritoneal implants. In those patients, the failure of second-line intravenous chemotherapy to control residual disease has led to the use of intra-peritoneal chemotherapies for small microscopic residual disease.

Until recently, second-look procedures and insertion of intra-peritoneal catheters were almost always carried out by laparotomy or "blind" surgical technique. With the improvement of instrumentation and surgical techniques, we are now able to perform these procedures by laparoscopy.

Considering that all patients were previously operated on by laparotomy, we prefer to introduce the trocar in the left upper quadrant as previously discussed. Three 5- or 10-mm trocars are then inserted in places free of any adhesion. The sites of the trocars are chosen according to the site of planned adhesiolysis.

Peritoneal washings are performed for cytologic evaluation. Subsequently, adhesiolysis between the small or large bowel and the abdominal wall is first performed with the help of laparoscopic scissors and harmonic shears. Every aspect of the abdominal cavity, the entire surface of the parietal peritoneum, and the surfaces of the intra-peritoneal organs are observed. Biopsies from the pelvic side walls, the pelvic cul-de-sac, the bladder, the paracolic gutters, and the diaphragm are taken. Small peritoneal tumors may also be resected and put into an intra-peritoneal bag for abdominal extraction. A 5-mm polyurethane catheter (Sims Deltec, Inc., St Paul, MN) is then inserted into the abdomen by means of a 5-mm trocar transfixing the left rectus abdominis muscle. A laparoscopic forceps holds the intra-peritoneal part of the catheter, and the 5-mm trocar is then withdrawn.

The laparoscopic entry incision is then prolonged vertically and cranially over the ninth and eighth ribs on the mid-clavicular line. The laparoscope entry site is closed layer by layer and carefully flushed. A peritoneal pocket is then created by dissecting the tissue over the eighth and ninth ribs. A laparoscopic forceps is introduced through this incision, running on the aponeurosis toward the catheter entry. The extra-peritoneal extremity of the catheter is grasped with this forceps and brought to the portal. The catheter is cut to the required length and connected to the portal chamber. The portal chamber and the catheter are then flushed with heparinized saline (50 IU/mL). The four corners of the portal are sutured to the underlying fascia using permanent sutures (Silk O; Sherwood, Davis & Geck St. Louis, MO, USA). After disinfection of the sites, the subcutaneous tissue and the skin are closed over the catheter entry site and the portal. The other trocar entry sites are then closed.

Using this technique, Anaf et al. showed that laparoscopy was possible in all of their eight patients and the catheters were easily inserted [38]. All patients received intra-peritoneal chemotherapy on the second postoperative day. The authors did not observe any complication after a mean follow-up of 12 months.

Cytoreductive surgery for primary advanced or recurrent ovarian cancer

There is a paucity of published studies describing laparoscopic debulking of recurrent or primary advanced ovarian cancer (see Table 24.5). The first report of successful laparoscopic cytoreduction of advanced ovarian cancer was a case series which included three patients who all underwent successful total laparoscopic primary or secondary cytoreduction [39].

In 2004, Trinh et al. retrospectively assessed 36 asymptomatic patients with recurrent chemosensitive stage III or IV ovarian cancer who previously underwent laparotomic debulking followed by chemotherapy [40]. These patients were asymptomatic with elevated CA125 and had no radiologic evidence of disease. They subsequently underwent laparoscopic secondary cytoreduction using an electrosurgical loop excision procedure and argon beam coagulator. Of the 36 patients, only 2 were converted to laparotomy, while 34 patients underwent successful laparoscopic debulking and, of those, 32 patients had all visible disease resected. Of the two cases converted to laparotomy one was converted for repair of enterotomies and the other for repair of an obstructed small bowel loop. Of the 34 patients, the pathology reports of 2 patients did not show recurrent disease. Of the 34 patients successfully resected using laparoscopy, 2 had surgical complications including an epigastric hematoma and a cystotomy that was repaired laparoscopically. None of the patients had port-site metastases.

Nezhat et al. retrospectively analyzed their experience with 23 patients who underwent attempted laparoscopic cytoreduction

Table 24.5. Summary of laparoscopic staging of primary or recurrent advanced stage ovarian cancer

Author	Patients (n)	Laparoscopic	Robotic	Conversions to laparotomy	Operative time (min)	Blood loss (mL)	Length of stay (days)	Optimally debulked	Complications	Follow-up (months)	Current status
Amara et al. [39]	3	3	n/a	0	196.7	281.7	3	n/a	1 postop	5	3 ANED
Trinh et al. [40]	36	36	n/a	2	156	70	1	32(microscopic)	3 intra-op	24	22 ANED 7 AWD 7 DOD
Nezhat et al. [42]	17	17	0	0	241.3	247.6	6.1(all LSC) 3.8 (LSC excluding 2 suboptimally debulked)	15 (<0.5 cm) 4 (microscopic)	1 intra-op 6 postop	19.7	9 ANED 6 AWD 2 DOD
	11	11	n/a	11	307.0	609.0	8.2	8 (<1 cm)	2 intra-op 7 postop	25.8	3 ANED 5 AWD 3 DOD
Fanning et al. [43]	25	25	n/a	2	138	340	1	23 (<0.5 cm) 9 (microscopic)	6 postop	19.2	19 ANED 4 AWED 2 DOD 8 recurrences

ANED, alive with no evidence of disease; AWED, alive with evidence of disease; DOD, died of disease; LSC, laparoscopy.

for recurrent ovarian, fallopian tube, or primary peritoneal cancer [41]. There was one conversion to laparotomy due to extensive intra-abdominal and pelvic adhesions. The remaining 22 patients underwent laparoscopic cytoreduction with 18 (81.8%) patients optimally cytoreduced to less than 1 cm. Median blood loss, operative time, and hospital stay was 75 mL, 200 minutes, and 2 days, respectively. There were no intra-operative complications and one (4.5%) patient had a postoperative ileus which was successfully managed conservatively with bowel rest. After a median follow-up of 14 months, 12 patients were alive with no evidence of disease (ANED), 6 were alive with evidence of disease (AWD), and 4 had died of disease (DOD).

In another retrospective analysis of a prospective case series, Nezhat et al. analyzed their experience with 32 patients with presumed advanced (FIGO stage IIC or greater) ovarian, fallopian tube, or primary peritoneal cancer who underwent laparoscopic triage for resectability [42]. These patients were divided into three groups: (1) diagnostic laparoscopy and biopsies, (2) primary cytoreduction and interval debulking by means of laparoscopy, and (3) diagnostic laparoscopy followed by primary cytoreduction and debulking by means of laparotomy. Of the 32 patients, 4 underwent diagnostic laparoscopy and biopsies only. Of these, two were diagnosed with primary GI malignancies and were referred to medical oncologists, one had primary peritoneal cancer but declined debulking due to advanced age and medical comorbidities, and the last one was diagnosed with benign disease. Seventeen patients (all stage ≥ IIIA with two stage IV), thought to be debulkable laparascopically, underwent primary or interval cytoreduction by laparoscopy with no conversions to laparotomy. Of the 17 patients, 15 were optimally debulked to <0.5 cm (88.2%). Four of these optimally debulked patients were cytoreduced to microscopic disease. Of the 15 optimally debulked patients, 4 underwent interval cytoreduction with 2 patients debulked to microscopic disease. Two of the 17 patients were not optimally debulked secondary to medical conditions (one patient who had stage IV disease and bowel obstruction declined aggressive management preoperatively and the other patient could not tolerate prolonged surgery due to multiple pulmonary emboli preoperatively). Of note, 9 of 17 patients had upper abdominal disease in addition to pelvic disease. Of these 9 patients, only one patient was suboptimally debulked because of her other medical conditions such that she preoperatively declined aggressive management. Of the 17 patients who underwent total laparoscopic cytoreduction, there was one intra-operative complication which was a right ureteral transection in a patient with extensive endometriosis and distorted anatomy. The complication was identified intra-operatively and repaired laparoscopically with a ureteroneocystotomy. Of the 17 patients, 4 had seven postoperative complications. Of the 32 total patients, 11 underwent diagnostic laparoscopy followed by primary cytoreduction by means of laparotomy due to the extent of disease. All 11 patients had stage IIIB and 8 were optimally debulked to <1 cm (72.7%) with 1 to microscopic disease. All but one of these 11 patients had upper abdominal disease in addition to pelvic disease. There were two intra-operative complications which included a cystotomy repaired intra-operatively as well as a patient who required transfusion of 4 units of packed red blood cells due to 1.5 L of blood loss. Five of these laparotomy patients had seven postoperative complications. Although there were more complications in the laparotomy group these did not reach significance. Also, there was no significant difference in OR time between the two groups. The laparoscopy group had significantly less estimated blood loss (247.6 vs. 609.1 mL, P = 0.008) and shorter hospital stay compared with the laparotomy group (6.1 vs. 8.2 days, P = 0.03; 3.8 [if excluding two from laparoscopy group] vs. 8.2 days, P = 0.003, respectively). In the laparoscopy group, nine patients were ANED, six were AWD, two were DOD, and a 31.7-month median time to recurrence with a 19.7-month mean follow-up time. In the laparotomy group, three patients were ANED, five were AWD, three were DOD, and a 21.5-month median time to recurrence with a 25.8-month mean follow-up time. There were no port-site metastases in any of these patients. The authors concluded that in advanced ovarian, fallopian, and primary peritoneal cancer, laparoscopy is a technically effective and feasible tool to diagnose, triage, and/or debulk, even with upper abdominal disease, in a well selected population. However, this study is limited in that it was not randomized which may account for the high optimal debulking rate.

In another retrospective analysis of a prospective case series, Fanning et al. evaluated the feasibility and survivability of patients with presumed stage III/IV primary ovarian cancer undergoing laparoscopic-assisted cytoreduction [43]. Twenty-five patients were included with a median age of 63, median BMI of 25 kg/m^2, and 60% of them had prior abdominal surgery. The surgical technique included a supracervical hysterectomy and the use of a 6-cm periumbilical Maylard incision to aid in the extraction of the uterus, adnexae, and omentum and to manipulate the bowel when necessary during omentectomy, lysis of adhesions, repair of bowel, or bowel resection and reanastomosis. Of the 25 patients, 23 were successfully cytoreduced laparoscopically (92%) without conversion to laparotomy. Of the two cases converted to laparotomy, one was converted due to extensive omental disease and the second case due to bulky metastasis surrounding the rectosigmoid. All 25 patients were cytoreduced to less than 2 cm and 36% had no residual disease. Median operative time and blood loss was 2.3 hours and 340 mL, respectively. Median length of stay was 1 day. Six patients had postoperative complications: including one with acute tubular necrosis which spontaneously resolved, one had developed pneumonia requiring hospitalization, three had ileuses managed conservatively, and one developed a skin infection.

The remaining literature involving laparoscopy in the treatment of advanced ovarian cancer involves hand-assisted laparoscopic surgery. This modality will be discussed in greater depth below.

Surgical technique

A multipuncture operative laparoscopic approach is used as previously described [44]. Closed transumbilical or left upper quadrant (Palmer's point) entry using a Veress needle is used most often. A 0° 5- or 10-mm transumbilical videolaparoscope is used. Pelvic washings are collected for cytology, and parietal and visceral peritoneal surfaces of the deep pelvis and middle and upper abdominal cavities are thoroughly inspected (Fig. 24.10). Any suspicious growth is biopsied. In the case of normal visual exploration, 8 to 10 random peritoneal biopsies are performed in the Douglas pouch, pelvic and abdominal parietal peritoneum, paracolic gutters, hemidiaphragms, and mesentery. Small and large bowel can also be carefully inspected laparoscopically. "Running" the small bowel can be accomplished from the ileocecal valve to the ligament of Treitz using two atraumatic bowel graspers (Figure 24.11). When conservative treatment is considered, biopsy of the contralateral ovary is performed only in the case of suspicious growth. In this context, dilatation and curettage are performed so as not to miss a possible endometrial spread or a synchronous tumor. Every attempt should be made to avoid the rupture of a suspicious adnexal mass in the abdomen, including choosing unilateral adnexectomy over ovarian cystectomy, limited manipulation of the mass, use of nontraumatic graspers, and preventive coagulation to avoid bleeding, which may obscure the identification of the cleavage planes. Additional safety measures are the removal of the specimen exclusively by means of a laparoscopic bag and control of the bag integrity once extracted (Fig. 24.12). Laparoscopy is intrinsically limited by the size of the trocar incisions. Even when the incision is enlarged, a puncture is required to remove large masses. If the puncture can be located within an Endobag (United States Surgical), and the Endobag's integrity is preserved, the procedure is safe according to previous findings.

To achieve an infracolic omentectomy, the patient is placed in dorsal lithotomy position in reverse Trendelenburg and the bowel is directed toward the pelvis. The primary surgeon stands in between the patient's legs with the first and second assistant standing on each side of the patient. The position of the primary surgeon can be changed depending on port placement and the tissue being manipulated or resected. In patients with extensive upper abdominal disease, it is our practice to place a 5- or 10-mm port in the mid to upper right abdomen and a 5-mm port in the left upper abdomen. The omentum is excised from the inferior margin of the transverse colon using a Harmonic Scalpel (Ethicon Endo-Surgery, Cincinnati, OH, USA), a bipolar forceps, Endoshears (United States Surgical), a linear stapler, endoligature, or sutures. The Harmonic Scalpel and endoligature are superior for omentectomy because of minimal plume formation, ease and speed of use, and lack of protruding staple edges (Fig. 24.13). The omentum specimen can also be removed with an Endobag (Fig. 24.14).

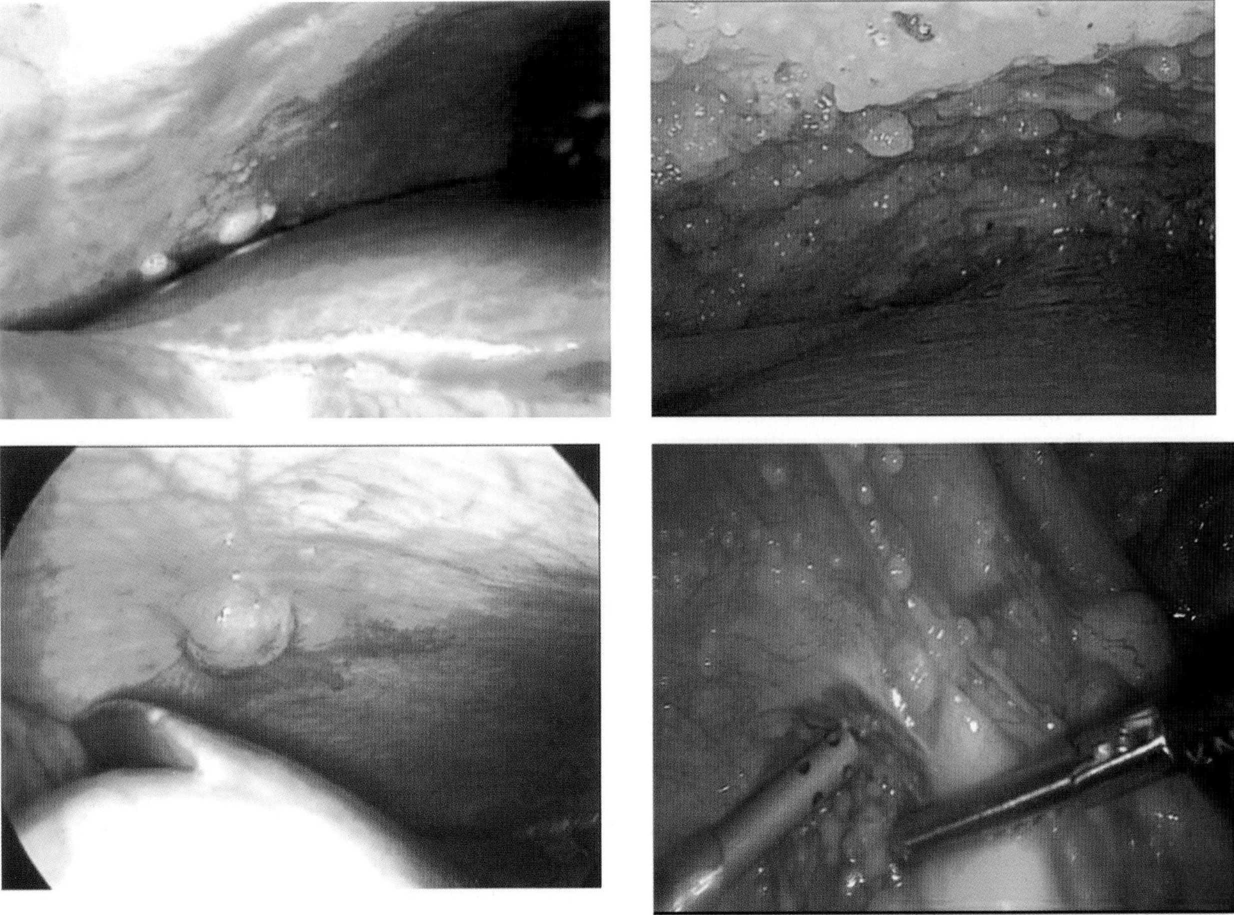

Fig. 24.10. Metastatic lesions of the right hemidiaphragm and pelvis are noted in the upper abdomen and deep pelvis upon initial inspection.

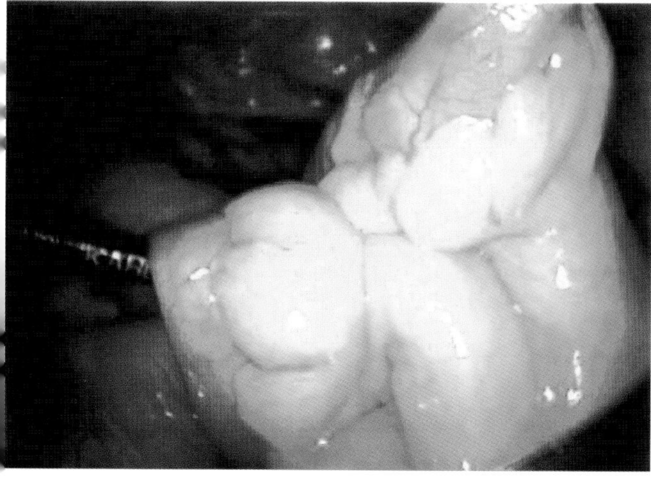

Fig. 24.11. "Running" the small bowel using atraumatic bowel graspers.

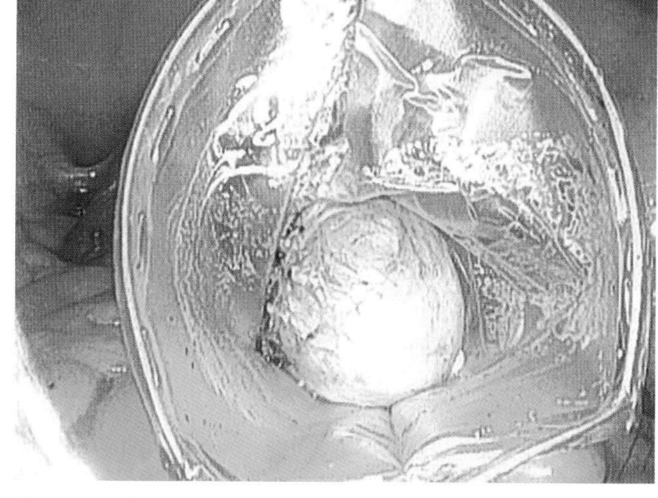

Fig. 24.12. A specimen is removed using a laparoscopic bag.

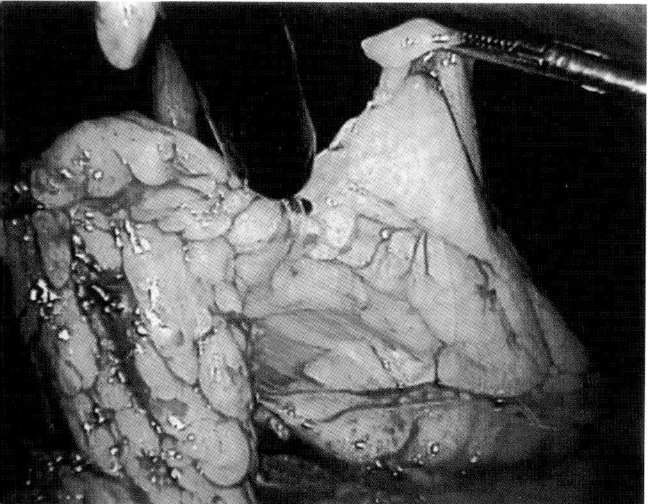

Fig. 24.13. Laparoscopic omentectomy using the Harmonic Scalpel (Ethicon Endo-Surgery).

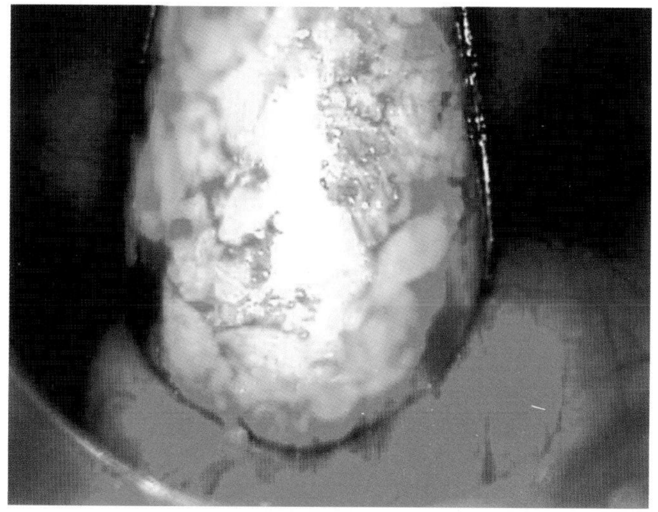

Fig. 24.14. The omentum specimen is removed using an endoscopic specimen bag.

This position is also optimal for diaphragmatic ablation and stripping, supracolic omentectomy, as well as resection of further upper abdominal disease. Diaphragmatic ablation can be performed using CO_2 laser, PlasmaJet (Plasma Surgical Limited, UK), and argon beam coagulator. From this position, the patient can be rotated to the right for better visualization of the spleen or for further dissection or mobilization of the transverse or descending colon near the splenic flexure. This position is also optimal for dissection near the stomach, in the lesser sac, during a splenectomy, and near the pancreas. If a splenectomy is indicated, the short gastric vessels can be secured using ultrasonic shears, an endoligature, surgical clips, and/or stapler while gaining access to the lesser sac (Fig. 24.15). The spleen can then be mobilized from its attachments and ligaments. The splenic vessels can then be cut and the spleen removed using the laparoscopic stapling device (Ethicon Endo-Surgery) (Fig. 24.16). The patient can be rotated to the left for further dissection near the liver, porta hepatis, and ascending colon. The position can be further manipulated to aid in small and large bowel resections.

Transperitoneal pelvic and/or para-aortic lymph node dissection is performed as previously described while the patient is in Trendelenburg position [18]. For pelvic lymph node retrievals, the primary surgeon stands on either side of the patient facing the monitors, which are positioned on both sides of the patient's legs. The first assistant stands across from the surgeon while the second assistant is at the bottom of the table, between the patient's legs. The peritoneum overlying the psoas muscle is incised from the round ligament to the base of the infundibular pelvic ligament. External and internal iliac vessels, their major branches, and the ureter are delineated and the avascular spaces developed. Following delineation of the anatomy of the pelvic side wall, sampling or complete removal of all nodal packets along the external and internal iliac vessels and the obturator fossa is performed

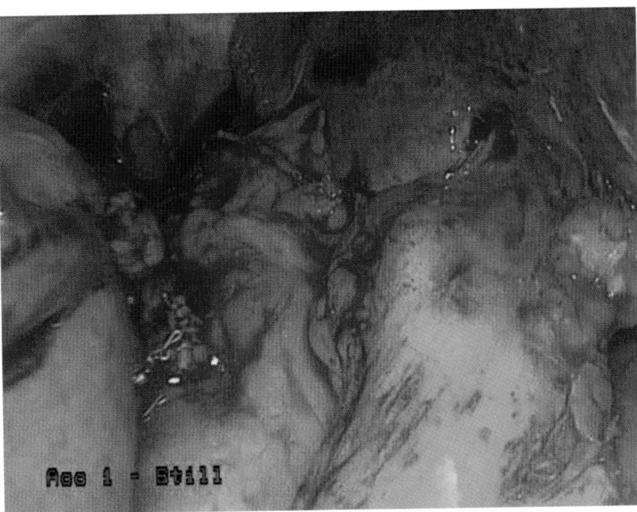

Fig. 24.15. The short gastric vessels are secure using the laparoscopic stapler while gaining access to the lesser sac.

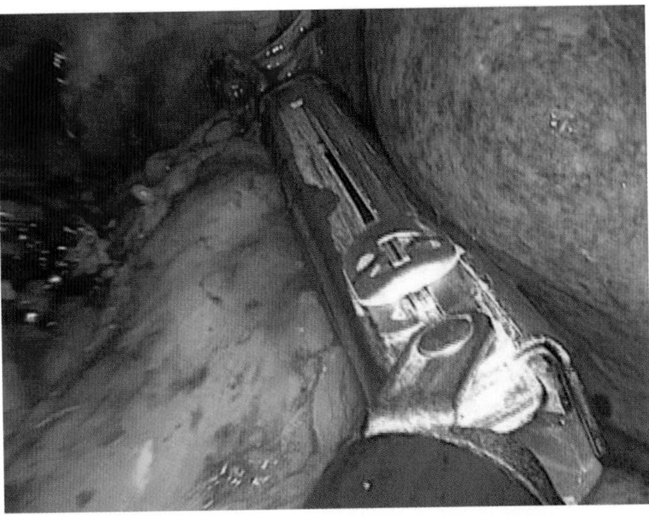

Fig. 24.16. The spleen is removed with the stapling device.

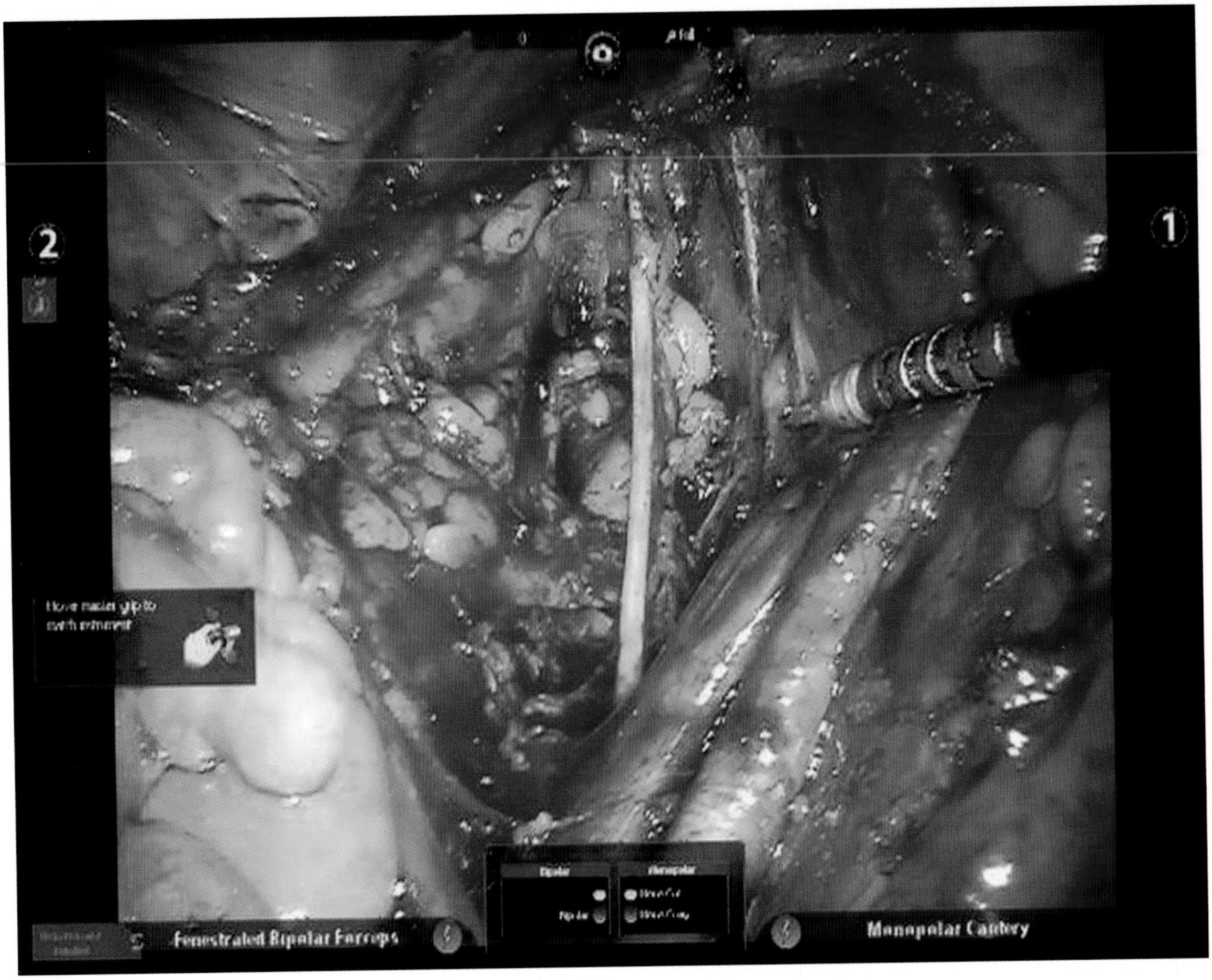

Fig. 24.17 Robotic dissection of the right pelvic sidewall exposing the iliac vessels and obturator fossa.

(Figs. 24.17 and 24.18a). While held with a grasper, the lymphatic tissue is teased off the underlying vessels using either a suction–irrigator probe or ultrasonic shears. The feeding lymphatic and vascular channels are isolated and then coagulated and divided using low and high ultrasonic power, respectively. Lymph nodes are retrieved through the suprapubic trocar sleeve (10- to 12-mm) avoiding contamination of the abdominal wall.

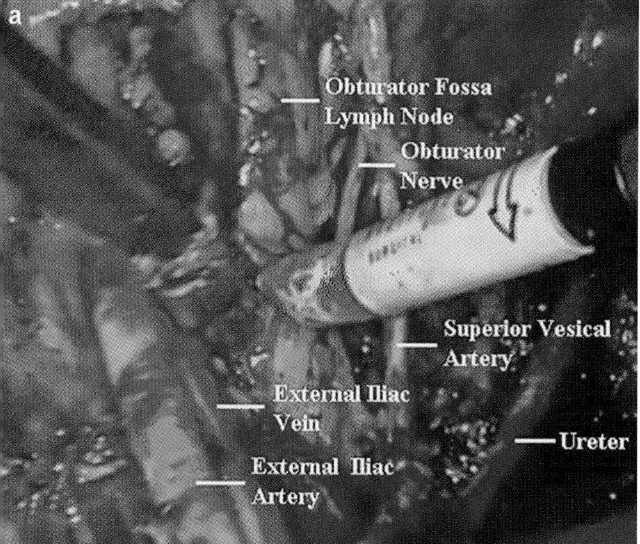

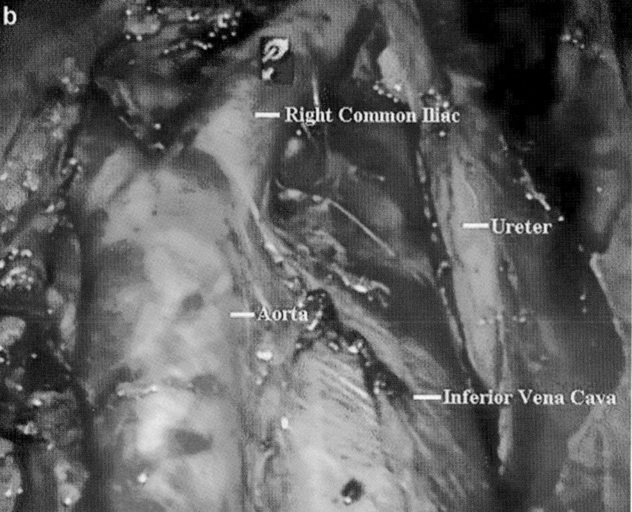

ig. 24.18. (a). Robotic pelvic lymphadenectomy (b). Robotic para-aortic mphadenectomy.

For para-aortic lymph node dissection, the room setup and rocar placement is similar to that for pelvic lymphadenectomy ith the laparoscope introduced through the umbilical port. An dditional 5-mm port is placed in the left or right mid-abdomen iteral to the rectus muscle for introduction of the ultrasonic hears. When para-aortic lymphadenectomy is extended to the vel of the left renal vein, the camera is moved from the ransumbilical port to another port placed approximately 3 to cm higher in the midline. If robotic-assisted videolaparo-copic para-aortic lymphadenectomy is performed, then the nitial port placement of the camera would be supraumbilical facilitate this dissection (Fig. 24.19). The patient is placed in teep Trendelenburg position; the bowel is directed toward ne upper abdomen and is held in that position with a grasper r laparoscopic fan. The peritoneum is incised over the right ommon iliac artery, and the incision is extended cephalad ver the inferior vena cava and lower abdominal aorta to the vel of the duodenum, exposing the ureters (Figs. 24.18b, 24.20), ovarian vessels, and inferior mesenteric artery. The nodal packets are removed using the technique described for the pelvic lymphadenectomy using the ultrasonic shears. All precaval and para-aortic nodes are removed from the bifurcation of the common iliac arteries up to the level of the renal vein. Following the procedure, no drains are placed and all retroperitoneal spaces are left open.

By placing two upper abdominal ports along with an umbilical/supraumbilical port and two 5-mm or 8-mm robotic ports in the lower abdomen, the ability to perform videolaparoscopic cytoreduction of the upper abdomen along with robotic-assisted laparoscopic cytoreduction of the pelvis is feasible. Videolaparoscopic hysterectomy, bilateral adnexectomy, and pelvic cytoreduction can also be performed with these port placements. Once pneumoperitoneum is obtained, the anatomy is inspected and appropriate biopsies are obtained. The patient can then be placed in reverse Trendelenburg position and videolaparoscopy can be used to obtain biopsies and resect the omentum and further upper abdominal disease. Once the upper abdomen has been cytoreduced, the patient is placed in steep Trendelenburg and the robot can be docked. At this point, pelvic and para-aortic lymph node dissections can be performed along with the hysterectomy, bilateral adnexectomy, and cytoreduction of pelvic disease. All specimens can then be removed through the vagina and the vaginal cuff can be reapproximated intra-corporeally or vaginally.

Bowel resections can also be performed laparoscopically using the appropriate port placement. This is especially true for a bulky lesion involving the rectosigmoid colon. Using a laparoscopic 60-mm GIA stapler, a rectosigmoid resection can be performed proximally and distally. Once the proximal sigmoid colon is appropriately mobilized, this end can be brought out through a widened incision in the left lower quadrant or lower middle incision along with the specimen. An anvil can then be placed and secured with a purse string suture. The anvil and proximal sigmoid colon is then brought back into the pelvis and an end-to-end anastomosis can be performed with an EEA stapler passed through the rectum. Once the device is properly activated, it is important to test the integrity of the anastomosis. This can be accomplished by clamping the proximal colon with a bowel grasper, filling the pelvis with lactated Ringer's, and insufflating the rectum with air while observing laparoscopically. The anastomosis can be alternatively or additionally examined by filling the rectum with indigo carmine and observing for leakage [41].

Hand-assisted laparoscopy in ovarian cancer

Hand-assisted laparoscopic surgery (HALS) is a unique surgical approach that combines traditional laparoscopy with the ability to place a hand intra-peritoneally. The potential benefits include those associated with laparoscopy, including decreased EBL, hospital stay, postoperative pain, as well as superior visualization. The addition of the hand port also allows for retaining tactile sensation for the surgeon and the ability for specimen removal through the port without morcellation or rupture. However, the potential disadvantages include pain and

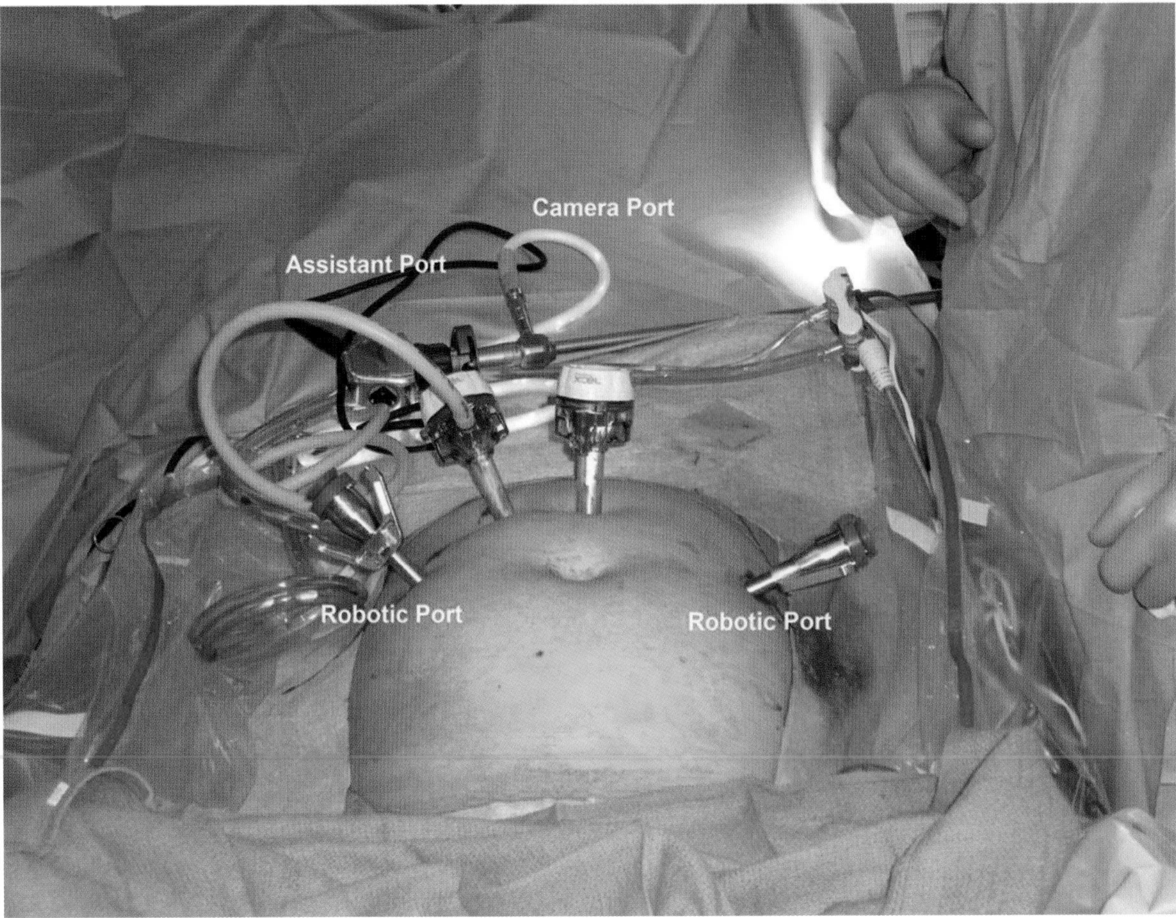

Fig. 24.19. Supraumbilical placement of the camera port to facilitate robotic para-aortic dissection.

morbidity (i.e., wound infection and risk of hernia) associated with the incision. Other potential disadvantages include the loss of intra-abdominal and pelvic operating space due to the size of the hand as well as loss of pneumoperitoneum due to leaky devices [45].

General surgeons and urologists already use hand-assisted laparoscopy for a wide range of surgical procedures on a variety of organ systems, including the kidney, spleen, liver, prostate, and gastrointestinal tract [46]. The surgical literature supports the role of HALS as a safe and effective technique with multiple advantages over conventional laparotomy. Compared with laparotomy, HALS has been shown to be associated with decreased blood loss, hospital stay, and morbidity [47].

There are few reports to date using HALS in gynecologic oncology. The first report using this surgical approach for treating patients with gynecologic malignancies was by Klingler et al. [48]. The authors reported using HALS to perform a splenectomy in a patient with an isolated ovarian cancer recurrence. Pelosi et al. used HALS to stage two patients: one with an ovarian dysgerminoma and the other with a grade 3 endometrial adenocarcinoma [49]. The authors also used HALS to repair a small bowel herniation through the vaginal cuff after a cytoreductive procedure.

Spannuth et al., using a retrospective chart review, compared HALS with open surgery for the surgical evaluation of women with pelvic masses [50]. Twenty-nine patients underwent HALS, and 41 patients underwent exploratory laparotomies. Both groups were comparable in terms of age, mas size, and BMI. Similar procedures were also performed betwee the two groups ranging from salpingo-oophorectomy to hysterectomy, staging, and adhesiolysis. Only one HALS patien (3%) was converted to laparotomy and no intra-peritoneal mas ruptures were noted in either group. Seven HALS patients wer found to have invasive disease on final pathology: one ha diffuse B-cell lymphoma, one had stage IIC dysgerminoma and five had advanced epithelial ovarian adenocarcinoma. O the five patients with advance stage epithelial ovarian carcinoma, four underwent debulking procedures with residual disease <2 cm at the end of the HALS procedure. HALS wa associated with significantly decreased blood loss (108 vs. 20 mL; $P = 0.004$), shorter hospital stay (2.8 vs. 4.2 days; $P = 0.03$) and fewer postoperative complications (4 vs. 11; $P = 0.05$). O note, there were no intra-operative complications in the HAL group. Operative time was similar between the two groups (9 vs. 72 min; $P = 0.9$).

Krivak et al. recently managed 25 ovarian cancer patient with HALS. Six patients had apparent advanced-stage ovaria cancer at the time of referral, and 19 patients had apparen early stage ovarian cancer [46]. Of the 19 patients with presumed early stage disease, 5 patients were upstaged base on retroperitoneal lymph node involvement, 3 had disease i

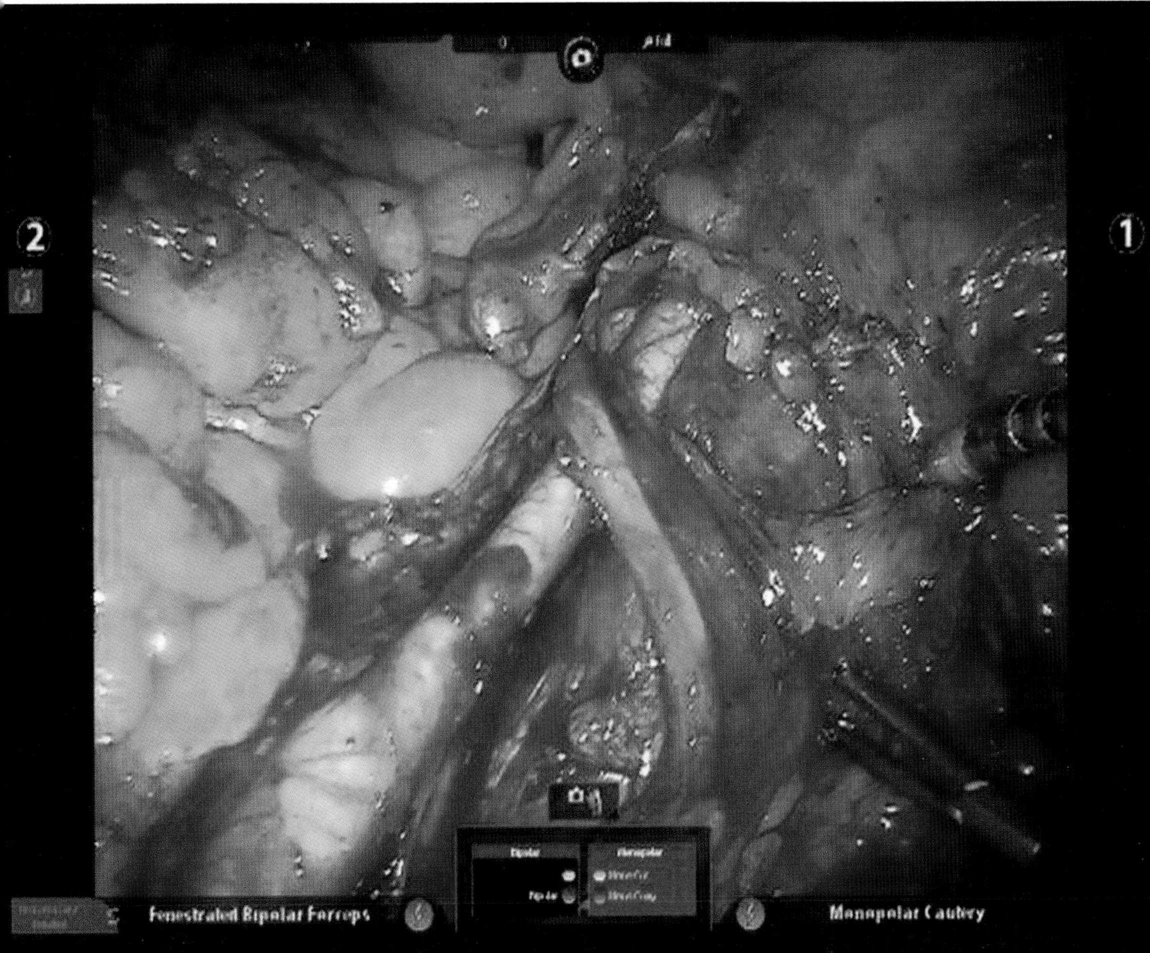

Fig. 24.20. Robotic dissection exposing the bifurcation of the common iliac and mobilizing right ureter laterally for nodal dissection.

other pelvic structures, and 2 had microscopic disease in the omentum. Twenty-two patients had their surgeries completed by means of HALS, and three required conversion to laparotomy for completion of debulking surgery. Complication rates were low, with three complications requiring reoperation or hospitalization. The mean hospital stay was 1.8 days for the 22 patients who underwent a complete HALS procedure. Operating times were variable and ranged from 81 to 365 minutes.

As noted above, HALS has been shown to be effective in the resection of recurrent ovarian carcinoma. In a review of the role of minimally invasive surgery in gynecologic oncology, Schlaerth and Abu-Rustum describe the ideal surgical candidate for HALS as one who is platinum-sensitive with an isolated recurrence that appears resectable on imaging [51]. Chi et al. report successful splenectomies being performed using HALS in three patients with presumed persistent or recurrent ovarian cancer isolated to the spleen [52]. All three had no residual disease after splenectomy. There were no significant complications and all three were ANED from the time of splenectomy (2–24 month follow-up).

For HALS, all patients are consented for laparoscopy as well as laparotomy and are admitted on the day of surgery following mechanical bowel prep. In patients with suspected early stage disease, a 10-mm laparoscopic intra-umbilical trocar is placed intra-peritoneally using a direct-entry technique. A pneumoperitoneum is obtained and a thorough review of the abdomen and pelvis performed. Two 5-mm lateral ports and a 5- or 10-mm suprapubic midline port are placed under direct visualization. If HALS is deemed necessary for completion of the surgery, a 6-to 7-cm periumbilical or suprapubic vertical midline incision is made depending on the site of disease. The length of the hand port incision is equal to the surgeon's glove size (e.g., 7 cm for glove size 7). A hand-assisted device (Lap Disc; Ethicon Endo-Surgery) is placed to permit free insertion and withdrawal of the surgeon's hand from the abdomen while maintaining an intact pneumoperitoneum. After the hand port is placed, and with the assistance of the laparoscope, the surgeon has the ability to visualize and palpate all peritoneal surfaces and retroperitoneal structures. Staging biopsies and washings are performed as indicated. If an extensive dissection and resection are necessary, standard minimally invasive techniques are augmented with the hand placed intra-peritoneally. Small bowel, colon, or omentum can be elevated out of the peritoneal cavity and the dissection performed extra-corporeally using standard techniques [46].

Although the role of HALS in the primary surgical management of gynecologic malignancies requires further investigation, it appears that select patients with pelvic masses as well as early and advanced-stage ovarian cancer may be treated appropriately and successfully with HALS. Patients treated by means of this approach appear to benefit from the advantages associated with traditional minimally invasive surgery.

Robotics and ovarian cancer

Over the past decade, the use of robotic-assisted laparoscopic surgery for gynecologic malignancies has increased. There are data to show more favorable perioperative outcomes when comparing a robotic approach to laparotomy for the treatment of endometrial and cervical cancer as well as comparable data to that of a laparoscopic approach [53].

Recently, Magrina et al. compared perioperative and survival outcomes for patients undergoing primary surgical treatment of epithelial ovarian cancer by all three surgical approaches [54]. In their retrospective case–control analysis, they compared 25 patients with ovarian cancer undergoing a robotic approach to similar patients undergoing a laparoscopic approach (27 patients) and laparotomic approach (119 patients). Sixty percent, 75%, and 87% of the patients in each respective group were found to have FIGO stage III–IV disease. The remaining patients had FIGO stage I–II disease. Mean EBL (164 vs. 267 vs. 1307 mL; $P < 0.001$) and length of hospital stay (4 vs. 3 vs. 9 days, $P < 0.001$) were significantly less in the robotic and laparoscopic group compared with the laparotomy group. Node counts were similar in all three groups. The robotic group had a significantly longer operating time compared with the other modalities (315 vs. 254 vs. 261 minutes, $P = 0.009$). Overall survival was similar for all three groups (67.1% vs. 75.6% vs. 66.0%; $P = 0.08$). A strength to this study is that patients were also subdivided and compared according to the extent and number of major procedures. The rate of intra-operative complications was similar in all three groups undergoing type 1 debulking (primary tumor excision defined as routine ovarian cancer staging procedure) and type 2 debulking (primary tumor excision + one major procedure, i.e., resection of intestines, liver, spleen or diaphragm). However, in type 3 debulking (primary tumor excision + two or more major procedures) there were only two patients in the robotic arm (0 complications), no laparoscopic patients, and, out of 32 laparotomy patients, 7 (22%) had intra-operative complications. Postoperative complications were similar in all three groups undergoing type 1 debulking, lower for the robotic and laparoscopy patients undergoing type 2 debulking, and similar between robotic and laparotomy patients undergoing type 3 debulking (no laparoscopy patients to compare in this group). Magrina et al. concluded that for patients undergoing primary tumor excision of epithelial ovarian cancer alone or with one additional major surgery that robotics and laparoscopy is preferable to laparotomy. They also concluded that overall survival is not influenced by the type of surgical approach but by the extent of debulking (complete vs. incomplete debulking). None of the robotic or laparoscopy patients had port-site metastases. The authors hypothesize that the lack of port-site metastases is likely, in part, due to early initiation of chemotherapy.

Concerns about laparoscopy and ovarian cancer

There are presently several concerns regarding the widespread implementation of laparoscopy in ovarian cancer. These concerns include the potential for port-site metastases, inadequate resection and staging, tumor cell peritoneal dissemination with CO_2 pneumoperitoneum, and a possibly higher incidence of iatrogenic cyst rupture [4].

Port-site metastases

The occurrence of port-site metastases has raised significant concern about the use of laparoscopic surgery for procedures associated with malignant disease. The exact etiology is unknown; however, there have been several hypotheses to explain this phenomenon. These include direct spread from the instrumentation and/or sheaths where the instruments are exchanged, tumor cell entrapment, and the chimney effect. The tumor cell entrapment theory theorizes that free-floating tumor cells implant on the raw incisional surfaces that are created during the introduction of needles, trocars, and/or instruments during laparoscopy. These implanted tumor cells are then protected by the fibrinous exudates formed during normal tissue healing which can then lead to port-site metastases. The chimney effect theory posits that tumor cells are dispersed or aerosolized with the leaking gas along the sheaths of the trocars although studies have been inconclusive. Direct contamination cannot explain why port-site metastases occur where instruments are not exchanged or tissue is not manipulated such as Veress needle puncture sites or the laparoscope trocar sites [55,56]. Questions still remain regarding these hypotheses because they do not explain all incidents.

Regardless of the etiology, port-site metastases have been well documented in the literature including borderline and invasive ovarian cancer. A small number of cases of port-site metastases have been reported after laparoscopic treatment of borderline ovarian cancer. Morice et al. reports nine cases for which overall survival was 100% after surgical excision with 6 to 72 months of follow-up [57]. The actual incidence of port-site metastases is unknown; however, estimates range from 0 to 2.3%. The overall incidence of port-site metastases in gynecologic cancers in a study by Nagarsheth et al. was 2.3%. The risk of port-site metastases was highest (5%) in patients with recurrence of ovarian or primary peritoneal malignancies undergoing procedures in the presence of ascites [58]. Vergote et al. demonstrated that in a study of 173 patients undergoing diagnostic laparoscopy for ovarian masses, ascites, and/or carcinomatosis, port-site metastases were seen in 5% of patients [59]. The overall prognosis was not affected as these patients tend to respond to chemotherapy without relapse. However, tumor cells can remain dormant for multiple years and can persist even after chemotherapy [23]. Huang et al. reported that port-site metastases that occur during or after chemotherapy are associated with a poor prognosis [60]. Possible techniques to reduce the risk of these metastases include removal of an intact specimen and layered closure of trocar sites [61]. Other techniques, such as deflation of the abdomen with trocars in place, irrigation of the trocar site with 5% povidone – iodine, and closure of the peritoneal trocar sites (10- to 12-mm trocars), have been suggested to decrease the risk of port-site metastases; however, their effectiveness has not been shown in clinical studies.

Inadequate resection and staging

Inadequate resection and staging is a major concern regarding the implementation of laparoscopy in ovarian cancer, especially in advanced cases. Certain factors can lead to inadequate staging such as inaccurate frozen section tumor evaluation, limited institutional gynecologic oncology support, and low intra-operative suggestion of malignancy [4]. Adequacy of staging can be measured by assessing nodal yields and/or upstage rate. Numerous studies have shown comparable upstaging rates in early ovarian cancer staging procedures (see Table 24.4) as well as comparable nodal yields [21,54]. As mentioned above, Magrina et al. concluded that, for patients undergoing primary tumor excision alone for epithelial ovarian cancer (or with one additional major surgery), robotics and laparoscopy are preferable to laparotomy [54]. In select patients, complete and adequate laparoscopic staging should be possible in the hands of an experienced gynecologic oncologist.

Tumor cell peritoneal dissemination with carbon-dioxide (CO_2) pneumoperitoneum

Secondary to the natural progression and peritoneal spread of ovarian cancer, the effects of carbon-dioxide pneumoperitoneum on malignant tissue are of particular concern. The question of whether CO_2 can promote significant growth or spread of ovarian cancer in humans has not been answered. There have been several in vitro and animal studies but very few human studies on this matter. CO_2 has been shown to promote in vitro growth of the ovarian epithelial carcinoma cell line SKOV-3 [62]. However, when compared with laparotomy or gasless laparoscopy, some animal studies suggest no deleterious effect [63].

A retrospective review by Abu-Rustum et al. evaluating the survival of 289 patients with FIGO stage III–IV invasive ovarian cancer found to have persistent disease during second-look operation demonstrated that those who underwent laparoscopic second look did not have reduced overall survival [64]. The median overall survival for the 45% of patients who underwent laparoscopy was 41.1 months which was statistically similar to the 38.8 month overall survival rate in the laparotomy group. Thus, overall survival appeared to be independent of laparoscopy with CO_2 pneumoperitoneum.

Iatrogenic cyst rupture

There are conflicting data regarding the rate of cyst rupture when comparing laparoscopy to laparotomy. There are some studies which show a difference in rupture rates between the two groups yet there are others showing no difference [4]. In general, rupture rates range from 10.5 to 41.8% [18,21]. Park et al. found no statistical difference in intra-operative rupture rates between the two groups undergoing surgical staging of early ovarian and fallopian tube cancer [21]. Intra-operative rupture occurred in two patients (10.5%) undergoing laparoscopy and four patients (12.1%) undergoing laparotomy.

Regardless of the rate of tumor rupture or whether there is a difference in rupture rate between laparoscopy and laparotomy, there is no consensus on whether iatrogenic tumor spillage has any significant impact on prognosis and/or survival. To date, the available retrospective data are conflicting, and there are no prospective clinical trials showing that intra-operative cyst rupture in early stage ovarian cancer will worsen prognosis. However, if spillage of cyst contents occurs, massive irrigation and immediate surgical treatment and staging are prudent because there is also no evidence to support the safety of delayed definitive management after capsular rupture [65].

When intra-operative cyst rupture and spillage of tumor cells occur with the resulting upstaging from stage IA to stage IC, there are no compelling data to answer the question of whether adjuvant chemotherapy should be administered. Should a patient be treated postoperatively with chemotherapy based on cyst rupture if she otherwise would have not been recommended for any postoperative adjuvant therapy? Although many experts would recommend treatment for such patients, there are no good studies that address the problem [65]. A confounding variable in this already uncertain area is the role of iatrogenic controlled cyst decompression which may include an endoscopic bag to prevent spillage and a laparoscopic syringe. This being said, there is no substitute for avoiding tumor spillage and maintaining oncologic principle.

Surgical training and patient referral

Although videolaparoscopy and robotic-assisted videolaparoscopy provide excellent outcomes, its integration into gynecologic cancer surgery is hampered by a significant learning curve and lack of training at the subspecialty level. Because large prospective trials are lacking, the route used to perform staging or restaging will mainly depend on the surgeon's training. As shown in a series on other gynecologic malignancies, all patients undergoing laparoscopy have a better surgical outcome in terms of morbidity when compared with patients undergoing laparotomy [66]. A group of patients with ovarian cancer most likely to benefit from a laparoscopic approach is young patients with early stage disease wishing to retain their fertility. In fact, laparoscopy has been shown to be associated with a lower rate of adhesion formation than laparotomy and therefore may impinge less on a patient's fertility. When a physician is confronted with this latter situation, referral to oncologic centers with adequate skills in laparoscopic management of ovarian cancer would probably be in the best interest of the patient. There is a growing data supporting the safety and efficacy of the use of laparoscopy in BOTs and early stage ovarian cancer and appropriate patients should be counseled and referred accordingly. Although there is a paucity of literature involving laparoscopic cytoreduction of recurrent and advanced ovarian cancer, the limited data do support the use of laparoscopy in multiple roles in a select population.

Pathophysiology and future direction of ovarian cancers

There has been growing data that suggests that there are two distinct subgroups of epithelial ovarian cancers developing along two distinct pathways. These two groups are divided based on shared genetic mutations and observed progression from precursor lesions. Type 1 tumors include low-grade serous carcinomas, clear cell, endometrioid, and mucinous tumors as well as BOTs (serous, mucinous, endometrioid). The mutations involved in these tumors involve an assortment of pathways including mismatch repair genes, *BRAF*, *KRAS*, *PTEN*, and *CTNNB1* (encoding beta-catenin) [67,68]. This subset has historically been associated with a precursor lesion. An example would be endometrioid tumors of the ovary which usually arise from the substance of the ovary and are strongly associated with endometriosis, cystadenofibromas, or BOTs [69].

Type 2 tumors, on the other hand, are high-grade serous carcinomas which typically are discovered at an advanced stage and thus associated with a poorer prognosis. Unfortunately, they are the most common type of ovarian epithelial malignancy accounting for 60–70% of all cases [70,71]. These tumors commonly have p53 mutations and are not associated with BOTs. There is evidence that points toward a histologic precursor lesion that precedes a large percentage of high-grade serous carcinomas, which had been unknown until recently. This precursor is thought to be serous tubal intra-epithelial carcinoma (STIC) which arises from the distal end of the fallopian tube at the fimbria. An important feature of STICs is that they usually stain for p53. This concept suggests that it is the epithelium of the fallopian tube not the ovary that is the source for many high-grade serous carcinomas.

Examination of the fallopian tubes in women with *BRCA1*/*BRCA2* mutations who underwent risk-reducing bilateral salpingo-oophorectomies has shown that many occult serous carcinomas involved the fallopian tubes either as intra-epithelial or invasive carcinoma [67]. In fact, 57–100% of cases of occult serous carcinomas involve the tube based on the presence of STIC or invasive carcinoma [72–75]. This phenomenon of a precursor lesion has also been well demonstrated in unselected women with sporadic pelvic serous carcinomas [69,76,77].

Roh et al. analyzed 87 consecutive non-uterine pelvic serous carcinomas at their institution and used 37 consecutive pure pelvic endometrioid carcinomas as a control group to determine if dominant ovarian mass (DOM), fimbrial mucosal involvement, and tubal intra-epithelial carcinoma could be used to identify exclusive subsets of pelvic serous carcinomas and aid in assigning malignant origin [69]. They found that there were no STICs found in any of the controls and that 87% of these patients had a DOM which supports the notion that endometrioid tumors (a type 1 tumor) usually arise from the substance of the ovary. The authors suggest that patients that fit into this category who have a DOM and do not have STIC likely have primary serous ovarian carcinoma. On the other hand, STIC was found in a significant proportion of the pelvic serous carcinomas and there was a strong inverse relationship between the presence of a DOM and STIC. Fifty-four percent of the pelvic serous carcinomas fell into the category of not having a DOM while at the same time having fimbrial mucosal involvement. Fifty-seven percent of this category had STIC. The authors suggest that patients that fit into this category likely have primary serous tubal carcinoma.

Although this concept of a precursor lesion answers some questions involving advanced ovarian cancer, many more questions still remain unanswered. Further elucidating molecular pathogenesis of ovarian cancer and assessing genetic determinants of ovarian cancer risk still hold promise for an effective screening technique for diagnosing ovarian cancer and reducing its high mortality rate.

Until now, surgery followed by chemotherapy has been the standard treatment of advanced-stage ovarian cancers. However, this has not significantly improved survival and prognosis in these women. The future depends on finding the different developmental pathways of this disease, finding appropriate chemotherapy and biological agents, targeting specific tumor cell types, and individualizing therapies.

References

1. American Cancer Society. Cancer Facts & Figures, 2011. Atlanta, GA: ACS; 2011.
2. Moore DH. Primary surgical management of early epithelial ovarian carcinoma. In: Rubin SC, Sutton GP (Eds.). Ovarian Cancer. 2nd edition. Philadelphia: Lippincott Williams & Wilkins; 2001. p 201–18.
3. Nezhat F, Nezhat C, Welander CE, et al. Four ovarian cancers diagnosed during laparoscopic management of 1011 women with adnexal masses. Am J Obstet Gynecol. 1992;**167**:790–6.
4. Liu CS, Nagarsheth NP, Nezhat FR. Laparoscopy and ovarian cancer: a paradigm change in the management of ovarian cancer? J Minim Invasive Gynecol. 2009;**16**:250–62.
5. Querleu D, Leblanc E. Laparoscopic infrarenal para-aortic lymph node dissection for restaging of carcinoma of the ovary or fallopian tube. Cancer. 1994;**73**:1467–71.
6. Childers JM, Lang J, Surwit EA, et al. Laparoscopic surgical staging of ovarian cancer. Gynecol Oncol. 1995;**59**:25–33.
7. Spirtos NM, Eisekop SM, Boike G, et al. Laparoscopic staging in patients with incompletely staged cancers of the uterus, ovary, fallopian tube, and primary peritoneum: a Gynecologic Oncology Group (GOG) study. Am J Obstet Gynecol. 2005;**193**:1645–9.
8. Tozzi R, Kohler C, Ferrara A, et al. Laparoscopic treatment of early ovarian

cancer: surgical and survival outcomes. Gynecol Oncol. 2004;**93**:199–203.

9. Tozzi R, Schneider A. Laparoscopic treatment of early ovarian cancer. Curr Opin Obstet Gynecol. 2005;**17**:354–8.
10. Curtin JP. Management of the adnexal mass. Gynecol Oncol. 1994;**55**: S42–6.
11. Sassone A, Timor-Tritch I, Artner A, et al. Transvaginal sonographic characterization of ovarian disease: evaluation of a new scoring system to predict ovarian malignancy. Obstet Gynecol. 1991;**78**:7–11.
12. Alcazar JL, Jurado M. Prospective evaluation of a logistic model based on sonographic morphologic and color Doppler findings developed to predict adnexal malignancy. J Ultrasound Med. 1999;**18**:837–43.
13. Romagnolo C, Gadducci A, Sartori E, et al. Management of borderline ovarian tumors: results of an Italian multicenter study. Gynecol Oncol. 2006;**101**:255–60.
14. Camatte S, Morice P, Pautier P, et al. Fertility results after conservative treatment of advanced stage serous borderline tumors of the ovary. BJOG. 2002;**109**:373–80.
15. Nezhat F, Nezhat C, Burrell M. Laparoscopically assisted hysterectomy for the management of a borderline ovarian tumor: a case report. J Laparoendosc Surg. 1992;**2**:167–9.
16. Darai E, Teboul J, Fauconnier A, et al. Management and outcome of borderline ovarian tumors incidentally discovered at or after laparoscopy. Acta Obstet Gynecol Scand. 1998;**77**:451–7.
17. Seracchioli S, Venturoli FM, Colombo F, et al. Fertility and tumor recurrence rate after conservative laparoscopic management of young women with early-stage borderline ovarian tumors. Fertil Steril. 2001;**76**:999–1004.
18. Fauvet J, Boccara C, Dufournet C, et al. Laparoscopic management of borderline ovarian tumors: results of a French multicenter study. Ann Oncol. 2005;**16**:403–10.
19. LeBlanc E, Querleu D, Narducci F, et al. Laparoscopic restaging of early stage invasive adnexal tumors: a 10-year experience. Gynecol Oncol. 2004;**94**:624–9.
20. Le T, Adolph A, Krepart GV, et al. The benefits of comprehensive surgical staging in the management of early stage epithelial ovarian carcinoma. Gynecol Oncol. 2002;**85**:351–5.
21. Park JY, Kim DY, Suh DS, et al. Comparison of laparoscopy and laparotomy in surgical staging of early-stage ovarian and fallopian tubal cancer. Ann Surg Oncol. 2008;**15**:2012–19.
22. Nezhat F, Ezzati M, Rahaman J, et al. Laparoscopic management of early ovarian and fallopian tube cancers: surgical and survival outcome. Am J Obstet Gynecol. 2009;**83**:e1–6.
23. Barakat RR, Markman M, Randall ME. Principles and Practice of Gynecologic Oncology, 5th edition. Philadelphia: Lippincott Williams & Wilkins; 2009.
24. Katz VL, Lentz GM, Lobo RA, Gershenson DM. Comprehensive Gynecology, 5th edition. Philadelphia: Mosby Elsevier; 2007.
25. Bristow RE, Tomacruz SR, Armstrong DK, et al. Survival effect of maximal cytoreductive surgery for advanced ovarian carcinoma during the platino-era: a meta analysis. J Clin Oncol. 2002;**20**:1248–59.
26. Winter WE III, Maxwell GL, Tian C, et al. Gynecologic Oncology Group Study. Prognostic factors for stage III epithelial ovarian cancer: a Gynecologic Oncology Group Study. J Clin Oncol. 2007;**25**:3621–7.
27. Winter WE III, Maxwell GL, Tian C, et al. Tumor residual after surgical cytoreduction in prediction of clinical outcome in stage IV epithelial ovarian cancer: a Gynecologic Oncology Group Study. J Clin Oncol. 2008;**26**:83–9.
28. Du Bois A, Reuss A, Pujade-Lauraine E, et al. Role of surgical outcome as prognostic factor in advanced epithelial ovarian cancer: a combined exploratory analysis of 3 prospectively randomized phase 3 multicenter trials: by the Arbeitsgemeinschaft Gynaekologische Onkologie Studiengruppe Ovarialkarzinom (AGO-OVAR) and the Groupe d' Investigateurs Nationaux Pour les Etudes des Cancers l'Ovaire (GINECO). Cancer. 2009;**115**:1234–44.
29. Hoskins WJ, Bundy BN, Thigpen JT, et al. The influence of cytoreductive surgery on recurrence-free survival in small volume stage III epithelial ovarian cancer: a gynecologic oncology group study. Gynecol Oncol. 1992;**47**:159–66.
30. Bristow RE, Duska LR, Lambrou NC, et al. A model for predicting surgical outcome in patient with advanced ovarian carcinoma using computed tomography. Cancer. 2000;**89**:1532–40.
31. Vergote I, Trope CG, Amant F, et al. Neoadjuvant chemotherapy is the better treatment option in some patients with stage IIIc to IV ovarian cancer. J Clin Oncol. 2011;**29**:4076–8.
32. Fagotti A, Fanfani F, Ludovisi M, et al. Role of laparoscopy to assess the chance of optimal cytoreductive surgery in advanced ovarian cancer: a pilot study. Gynecol Oncol. 2005;**96**:729–35.
33. Vergote I, De Wever I, Tjalma W, et al. Neoadjuvant chemotherapy or primary debulking surgery in advanced ovarian carcinoma: a retrospective analysis of 285 patients. Gynecol Oncol. 1998;**71**:431–6.
34. Vergote I, Trope CG, Amant F, et al. Neoadjuvant chemotherapy or primary surgery in stage IIIC or IV ovarian cancer. N Engl J Med. 2010;**363**:943–53.
35. Bristow RE, Montz FJ, Lagasse LD, et al. Survival impact of surgical cytoreduction in stage IV epithelial ovarian cancer. Gynecol Oncol. 1999;**72**:278.
36. Angioli R, Palaia I, Zullo MA, et al. Diagnostic open laparoscopy in the management of advanced ovarian cancer. Gynecol Oncol. 2006;**100**:455–61.
37. Rahaman J, Dottino P, Jennings TS, et al. The second-look operation improves survival in suboptimally debulked stage III ovarian cancer patients. Int J Gynecol Cancer. 2005;**15**:19–25.
38. Anaf V, Gangji D, Simon P, et al. Laparoscopical insertion of intraperitoneal catheters for intraperitoneal chemotherapy. Acta Obstet Gynecol Scand. 2003;**82**:1140–5.
39. Amara DP, Nezhat C, Teng N, et al. Operative laparoscopy in the management of ovarian cancer. Surg Laparosc Endosc. 1996;**6**:38–45.
40. Trinh H, Ott C, Fanning J. Feasibility of laparoscopic debulking with electrosurgical loop excision procedure and argon beam coagulator at recurrence in patients with previous laparotomy debulking. Am J Obstet Gynecol. 2004;**190**:1394–7.
41. Nezhat F, DeNoble S, Brown D, et al. The safety and efficacy of laparoscopic cytoreduction of recurrent ovarian, fallopian tube, and primary peritoneal cancers". 19th Annual Meeting and

Endo Expo of the Society of Laparoendoscopic Surgeons, New York, New York, September 1–4, 2010.

42. Nezhat FR, DeNoble, SM, Liu CS, et al. The safety and efficacy of laparoscopic surgical staging and debulking of apparent advanced stage ovarian, fallopian tube, and primary peritoneal cancers. JSLS. 2010;**14**:155–68.
43. Fanning J, Yacoub E, Hojat R. Laparoscopic-assisted cytoreduction for primary ovarian cancer: success, morbidity and survival. Gynecol Oncol. 2011;**123**:47–9.
44. Nezhat F, Yadav J, Rahaman J, et al. Laparoscopic lymphadenectomy for gynecologic malignancies using ultrasonically activated shears: analysis of first 100 cases. Gynecol Oncol. 2005;**97**:813–19.
45. Brotherton J, McCarus S, Redan J, et al. Hand-assisted laparoscopic surgery for the gynecologic surgeon. JSLS. 2009;**13**:484–8.
46. Krivak TC, Elkas JC, Rose GS, et al. The utility of hand-assisted laparoscopy in ovarian cancer. Gynecol Oncol. 2005;**96**:72–6.
47. Spannuth WA, Rocconi RP, Huh WK, et al. A comparison of hand-assisted laparoscopy and conventional laparotomy for the surgical evaluation of pelvic masses. Gynecol Oncol. 2005;**99**:443–6.
48. Klingler PJ, Smith SL, Abendstein BJ, et al. Hand assisted laparoscopic splenectomy for isolated splenic metastasis from an ovarian carcinoma. Surg Laparosc Endosc. 1997;**8**: 49–54.
49. Pelosi MA, Pelsoi MA III, Eim J. Hand assisted laparoscopy for pelvic malignancy. J Laparoendosc Adv Surg Tech. 2000;**10**:143–50.
50. Spannuth WA, Rocconi RP, Huh WK, et al. A comparison of hand-assisted laparoscopy and conventional laparotomy for the surgical evaluation of pelvic masses. Gynecol Oncol. 2005;**99**:443–6.
51. Schlaerth AC, Abu-Rustum NR. Role of minimally invasive surgery in gynecologic cancers. Oncologist. 2006;**11**:895–901.
52. Chi DS, Abu-Rustum NR, Sonoda Y, et al. Laparoscopic and hand-assisted laparoscopic splenectomy for recurrent and persistent ovarian cancer. Gynecol Oncol. 2006;**101**:224–7.
53. Cho JE, Shamshirsaz AHA, Nezhat C, et al. New technologies for reproductive medicine: laparoscopy, endoscopy, robotic surgery and gynecology. A review of the literature. Minerva Ginecol. 2010;**62**:137–67.
54. Magrina JF, Zanagnolo V, Noble BN, et al. Robotic approach for ovarian cancer: perioperative and survival results and comparison with laparoscopy and laparotomy. Gynecol Oncol. 2011;**121**:100–5.
55. Childers JM, Aqua KA, Surwit EA, et al. Abdominal-wall tumor implantation after laparoscopy for malignant conditions. Obstet Gynecol. 1994;**84**:765–9.
56. Ramirez PT, Wolf JK, Leveback C. Laparoscopic port-site metastases: etiology and prevention. Gynecol Oncol. 2003;**91**:179–89.
57. Morice P, Camatte S, Larregain-Fournier D, et al. Port-site implantation after laparoscopic treatment of borderline ovarian tumors. Obstet Gynecol. 2004;**104**:1167–70.
58. Nagarsheth NP, Rahaman J, Cohen CJ, et al. The incidence of port-site metastases in gynecologic cancers. JSLS. 2004;**8**:133–9.
59. Vergote I, Marquette S, Arnant F, et al. Port-site metastases after open laparoscopy: a study in 173 patients with advanced ovarian carcinoma. Int J Gynecol Cancer. 2005;**15**: 776–9.
60. Huang KG, Wang CJ, Chang TC, et al. Management of port-site metastases after laparoscopic surgery for ovarian cancer. Am J Obstet Gynecol. 2003;**189**:16–21.
61. Morice P, Camatte S, Larregain-Fournier D, et al. Port-site implantation after laparoscopic treatment of borderline ovarian tumors. Obstet Gynecol. 2004;**104**:1167–70.
62. Smidt VJ, Singh DM, Hurteau JA, et al. Effect of carbon dioxide on human ovarian carcinoma cell growth. Am J Obstet Gynecol. 2001:**185**:1314–17.
63. Dorrance HR, Oien K, O'Dwyer PJ. Effects of laparoscopy on intraperitoneal tumor growth and distant metastases in an animal model. Surgery. 1990;**125**:35–40.
64. Abu-Rustum NR, Sonoda Y, Chi DS, et al. The effects of CO_2 pneumoperitoneum on the survival of women with persistent metastatic ovarian cancer. Gynecol Oncol. 2003;**90**:431–4.
65. Vaisbuch E, Dgani R, Ben-Arie A, et al. The role of laparoscopy in ovarian tumors of low malignant potential and early-stage ovarian cancer. Obstet Gynecol Surv. 2005;**60**:326–30.
66. Chi DS, Curtin JP. Gynecologic cancer and laparoscopy. Obstet Gynecol Clin North Am. 1999;**26**:201–15.
67. Folkins AK, Jarobe EA, Roh MH, et al. Precursors to pelvic serous carcinoma and their clinical implications. Gynecol Oncol. 2009;**113**:391–6.
68. Pejovic T, Nezhat F. Missing link: inflammation and ovarian cancer. Lancet Oncol. 2011;**12**:833–4.
69. Roh MH, Kindelberger D, Crum CP. Serous tubal intraepithelial carcinoma and the dominant ovarian mass. Am J Surg Pathol. 2009;**33**:376–83.
70. Shaw PA, Rouzbahman M, Pizer ES, et al. Candidate serous cancer precursors in fallopian tube epithelium of BRCA 1/2 mutation carriers. Mod Pathol. 2009;**22**:1133–8.
71. Nezhat F, Datta M, Hanson V, et al. The relationship of endometriosis and ovarian malignancy: a review. Fertil Steril. 2008;**90**:1559–70.
72. Powell CB, Kenley E, Chen LM, et al. Risk-reducing salpingo-oophorectomy in BRCA mutation carriers: role of serial sectioning in the detection of occult malignancy. J Clin Oncol. 2005;**23**:127–32.
73. Finch A, Shaw P, Rosen B, et al. Clinical and pathologic findings of prophylactic salpingo-oophorectomies in 159 BRCA1 and BRCA2 carriers. Gynecol Oncol. 2006;**100**:58–64.
74. Callahan MJ, Crum CP, Medeiros F, et al. Primary fallopian tube malignancies in BRCA-positive women undergoing surgery for ovarian cancer risk reduction. J Clin Oncol. 2007;**25**:3985–90.
75. Leeper K, Garcia R, Swisher E, et al. Pathologic findings in prophylactic oophorectomy specimens in high-risk women. Gynecol Oncol. 2002;**87**:52–6.
76. Kindelberger DW, Lee Y, Miron A, et al. Intraepithelial carcinoma of the fimbria and pelvic serous carcinoma: evidence for a causal relationship. Am J Surg Pathol. 2007;**31**:161–9.
77. Carlson JW, Miron A, Jarboe EA, et al. Serous tubal intraepithelial carcinoma: its

potential role in primary peritoneal serous carcinoma and serous cancer prevention. J Clin Oncol. 2008;**26**:4160–5.

78. Querleu D, Papageorgiou T, Lambaudie E, et al. Laparoscopic restaging of borderline ovarian tumors: results of 30 cases initially presumed as stage IA borderline ovarian tumors. BJOG. 2003;**110**:201–4.

79. Desfeux P, Camatte S, Chatellier G, et al. Impact of surgical approach on the management of macroscopic early ovarian borderline tumors. Gynecol Oncol. 2005;**98**:390–5.

80. Romagnolo C, Gadducci A, Sartori E, et al. Management of borderline ovarian tumors: results of an Italian multicenter study. Gynecol Oncol. 2006;**101**:255–60.

81. Brosi N, Deckardt R. Endoscopic surgery in patients with borderline tumor of the ovary: a follow-up study of thirty-five patients. J Minim Invasive Gynecol. 2007;**14**:606–9.

82. Pomel C, Provencher D, Dauplat J, et al. Laparoscopic staging of early ovarian cancer. Gynecol Oncol. 1995;**58**:301–6.

83. Chi DS, Abu-Rustum NR, Sonoda Y, et al. The safety and efficacy of laparoscopic surgical staging of apparent stage I ovarian and fallopian tube cancers. Am J Obstet Gynecol. 2005;**192**:1614–19.

84. Ghezzi F, Cromi A, Uccella S, et al. Laparoscopy versus laparotomy for the surgical management of apparent early stage ovarian cancer. Gynecol Oncol. 2007;**105**:409–13.

85. Park JY, Bae J, Lim MC, et al. Laparoscopic and laparotomic staging in stage I epithelial ovarian cancer: a comparison of feasibility and safety. Int J Gynecol Cancer. 2008;**15**:2012–19.

86. Colomer AT, Jimenez AM, Bover Barcelo M. Laparoscopic treatment and staging of early ovarian cancer. J Minim Invasive Gynecol. 2008;**15**:414–9.

Chapter 25

Ovarian cancer: the initial laparotomy

Jamal Rahaman, MD, DGO, FACS, FACOG,
Valentin Kolev, MD, and Carmel J. Cohen, MD

Introduction

Surgical assessment and histologic evaluation are the only means by which a neoplasm can be classified as benign or malignant, primary, or metastatic. When an early primary ovarian cancer is diagnosed, the next goal is determining the extent of disease or stage. Surgical staging is required to define those patients in whom surgery alone may be curative and those who will require adjuvant therapy, and to determine the modality, intensity, and duration of such treatment. Accurate surgical staging also permits assignment of prognosis, allows comparison of cure rates, and defines subsequent surveillance. In the 70 to 75% of patients who present with advanced ovarian cancer, the goal of laparotomy is also to remove as much tumor as possible through a process of surgical "cytoreduction" to maximize response to chemotherapy, and improve survival. We offer epithelial ovarian cancer as a model; the principles of treatment also apply to ovarian germ-cell tumors, stromal tumors, and other primary ovarian cancers.

Preoperative preparation

A thorough history is obtained, including age, parity, history of medication use (including oral contraception and ovulation induction drugs), and treatment for endometriosis.

Patients with a family history or personal history of ovarian, breast, or colon cancer are at increased risk for developing ovarian cancer, although only 5 to 10% of patients with ovarian cancers have such histories [1]. The risk of developing ovarian cancer in the general female population is approximately 1 in 70 after the age of 40 years. A woman with two or more first-degree relatives with the disease has been assumed to have up to a 50% lifetime risk of developing ovarian cancer [2]. Current detection of *BRCA1* and *BRCA2* adds precision to risk estimation [3–5].

Complete physical examination determines suitability for extensive surgery and may reveal the extent of disease. A fixed pelvic mass, cul-de-sac nodularity or upper abdominal mass requires appropriate preoperative planning for resection of bowel. Occult fecal blood should be explained by colonoscopy. Any woman over 40 who has not had previous colonoscopy should have this procedure before treatment for ovarian cancer.

Patients should have a thorough assessment of intercurrent medical illnesses, and deficits must be corrected preoperatively. Preoperative assessment of hemogram, electrolytes, and liver and renal function should be made. Serum markers for cancer should be measured.

Preoperative computerized (CT) scanning of the chest, abdomen, and pelvis is essential in identifying disease in the chest and abdominal retroperitoneal compartment, especially in the lymph nodes and along the ureters whose normal position might be distorted by disease. In addition, it allows assessment of the probability of achieving optimal cytoreduction in the epigastrium. When successful cytoreduction seems unlikely, or the patient is a poor surgical risk, neo-adjuvant chemotherapy before attempted cytoreduction might have utility [7]. CT scan criteria predicting inability to achieve optimal cytoreduction have been published [8,9].

All patients with a suspicion of advanced ovarian cancer should have complete bowel preparation as resection is often necessary [10,11]; and lack of adequate mechanical preparation is associated with higher infectious morbidity [12]. Ambulatory bowel preparation using a combination of clear liquid diet with oral laxatives and enemas with or without antibiotics is an alternative to preoperative hospitalization [13]. Liquid electrolyte solutions (Go-lytely) may be used to empty the bowel; however, these preparations are sometimes poorly tolerated by patients with ascites or upper abdominal disease. Currently, we prefer the use of magnesium citrate, which is better tolerated and provides an equivalent mechanical effect.

Detailed explanation of the anticipated surgical procedure, its risks, and the probability of finding cancer should be offered to the patient and her family [14]. Younger patients wishing to maintain child-bearing ability should be counseled about the possibilities and limitation of preserving fertility based on the operative findings and the current range of conservative options with the expanded role of artificial reproductive technologies including oocyte cryopreservation. Patients at low risk of having ovarian cancer undergoing laparoscopic removal of an adnexal mass should also be warned that a laparotomy may be necessary if unexpected cancer is found. Intra-operative discovery of cancer in an uninformed and uncounselled patient can have tragic consequences.

Altchek's Diagnosis and Management of Ovarian Disorders, ed. Liane Deligdisch, Nathan G. Kase, and Carmel J. Cohen. Published by Cambridge University Press.

Table 25.1. FIGO staging classification of epithelial ovarian cancer

Stage	Description
Stage I	Growth limited to the ovaries
Stage Ia	Growth limited to one ovary; no ascites containing malignant cells present; no tumor on the external surfaces; capsule intact
Stage Ib	Growth limited to both ovaries; no ascites containing malignant cells present; no tumor on the external surfaces; capsule intact
Stage Ic*	Tumor either stage 1a or 1b but with tumor on the surface of one or both ovaries; or with the capsule ruptured; or with ascites present containing malignant cells or with positive peritoneal washings
Stage II	Growth involving one or both ovaries with pelvic extension
Stage IIa	Extension and/or metastasis to the uterus and/or tubes
Stage IIb	Extension to other pelvic tissues
Stage IIc	Tumor either stage IIa or IIb but with tumor on the surface of one or both ovaries; or with capsule(s) ruptures; or with ascites present containing malignant cells or with positive peritoneal washings
Stage III	Tumor involving one or both ovaries with peritoneal implants outside the pelvis and/or positive retroperitoneal or inguinal nodes; superficial liver metastasis equals stage III; tumor is limited to the true pelvis but with histologically verified malignant extension to small bowel or omentum
Stage IIIa	Tumor grossly limited to the true pelvis with negative nodes but with histologically confirmed microscopic seeding of abdominal peritoneal surfaces
Stage IIIb	Tumor of one or both ovaries; histologically confirmed implants of abdominal peritoneal surfaces, none exceeding 2 cm in diameter; nodes negative
Stage IIIc	Abnormal implants 2 cm in diameter and/or positive retroperitoneal or inguinal nodes
Stage IV	Growth involving one or both ovaries with distant metastasis; if pleural effusion is present, there must be positive cytologic test results to allot a case to stage IV; parenchymal liver metastasis equals stage IV

*To evaluate the impact on prognosis of the different criteria for allotting patients to stage Ic or IIc, it would be of value to know if rupture of the capsule was (1) spontaneous or (2) caused by the surgeon and if the source of the malignant cells detected was (1) peritoneal washings or (2) ascites.

Early ovarian cancer

Staging laparotomy

Ovarian cancer is a surgically staged disease by mandate of The International Federation of Gynecology and Obstetrics (FIGO) (Table 25.1). Understanding the three main mechanisms of spread is important in staging of ovarian cancer (Table 25.2). Tumor may spread by direct extension to adjacent pelvic structures. Abdominal structures that come in contact with pelvic tumor may also be involved with disease. When the tumor is no longer confined by the ovarian capsule, tumor cells exfoliate into the peritoneal cavity and circulate with peritoneal fluid, flowing through the abdominal cavity, implanting on omentum, undersurfaces of the diaphragm, and mesenteric surfaces of the large and small bowel. The third mechanism of tumor spread is endo-lymphatic. Tumor cells travel through the rich lymphatic channels in the broad ligament to the iliac vessels and then ascend into the para-aortic lymph node chain. Para-aortic lymph nodes may also be the site of direct lymphatic spread by way of the infundibulopelvic ligaments [15,16]. Surgical staging requires a meticulous examination of all peritoneal and retroperitoneal surfaces and structures at risk for tumor spread. Table 25.3 outlines the procedures necessary for a thorough staging laparotomy. An incision large enough to remove the pelvic mass and organs and to adequately assess and/or treat the upper abdomen is necessary. We prefer a vertical midline

Table 25.2. Mechanisms of spread in ovarian cancer

Direct extension
Exfoliation of malignant cells
Lymphatic spread

Table 25.3. Surgical staging procedure for apparent early ovarian cancer

Total abdominal hysterectomy*
Bilateral salpingo-oophorectomy*
Peritoneal washings
Pelvic Paracolic gutters Subdiaphragmatic surfaces
Pelvic biopsies
Pelvic sidewall peritoneum Anterior and posterior peritoneum Bladder and rectal serosa
Infracolic omentectomy
Bilateral pelvic lymph node biopsy
Para-aortic lymph node biopsy

*Unilateral salpingo-oophorectomy may be performed in selected patients wishing to preserve fertility.

incision. On entering the peritoneal cavity, pelvic fluid should be collected for cytology. If no fluid is present, pelvic washings should be obtained. The pelvis is then closely examined. The size of pelvic tumor masses should be recorded as should the presence of tumor on the surface of the ovarian capsule, adhesions and direct extension to adjacent pelvic structures as well as pre-operative or intra-operative cyst rupture. Several of these factors affect prognosis in stage I cancers [17–19]. The upper abdomen, bowel serosa, mesenteric surfaces, and retroperitoneal structures are palpated. Removal of the uterus, both tubes, and ovaries should be completed unless the patient has an apparent early stage tumor and is a candidate for fertility conservation [20]. Para-aortic lymph node sampling should extend to the renal vessels as illustrated in Figure 25.1 (Table 25.4).

Table 25.4. Site of metastatic disease in apparent early ovarian cancer

Site	Positive (%)	References
Cytology	17/92 (18)	22,81,82
Omentum	16/225 (6)	22, 81–85
Diaphragm	22/241 (9)	22,81,82,84,86
Pelvic tissue	16/112 (14)	22,81,82
Abdominal tissue	10/122 (8)	22,81,82,86
Pelvic nodes	16/203 (8)	22,82,83,85,87
Para-aortic nodes	30/263 (11)	22,82–85,88

There have been several reports of inappropriate incisions and inadequate staging [21–25]. Young et al. reported a 31% rate of upstaging of ovarian cancer patients presumed to have stage I or II at initial inadequate surgery. A total of 77% of upstaged patients actually had stage III disease when properly staged. The importance of stage at presentation can be inferred by inspecting the 5-year survivals for patients with ovarian cancer in Table 25.5 [26]. Overall 5-year survival for stage I disease approaches 89%, but when disease is found outside the pelvis it drops to less than 24% [26]. When patients are treated for presumed early stage disease when in fact their disease is advanced, cure is prevented.

Disease confined to the ovary and with low histologic grade requires no further therapy to achieve survival [27]. Patients with poor prognosis stage I tumors have been shown to benefit from thorough surgical staging and platinum-based chemotherapy with improved disease-free intervals and extended survival [28–30]. The role of platinum-based chemotherapy in advanced disease has been documented [31–33], and the current standard uses a taxane/platinum combination [34–37]. The negative prognostic implications of an inadequate staging

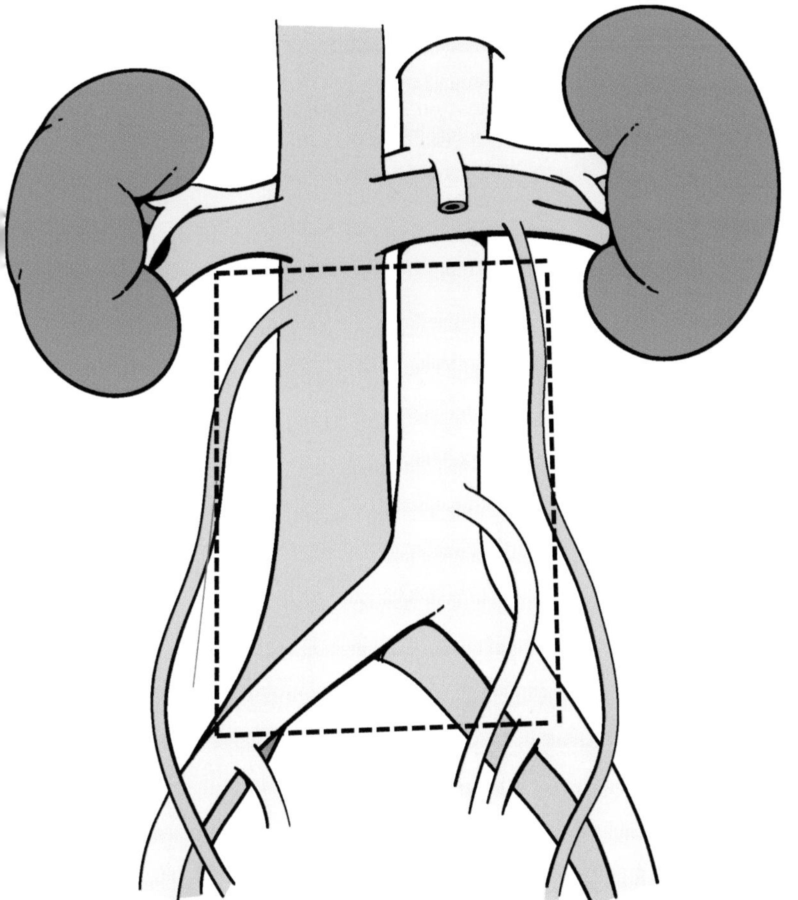

Fig. 25.1. The para-aortic lymph node sampling extending to the renal vessels.

Table 25.5. Five-year survival in ovarian cancer by stage

Stage	5-year survival (%)
Ia	92.1
Ib	84.9
Ic	82.4
IIa	69.0
IIb	56.4
IIc	51.4
IIIa	39.3
IIIb	25.5
IIIc	17.1
IV	11.6

operation can therefore be appreciated. The magnitude of this problem is reflected in a recent report using the NCI/SEER database, which indicated that only 10% of American women with apparent early stage ovarian cancer had appropriate surgical staging [38]. Increased intra-operative consultation with gynecologic oncologists for remedy of this deficiency after intra-operative histologic analysis of the removed specimen is recommended.

Ovarian tumors of borderline or low malignant potential

Ovarian tumors of borderline or low malignant potential (LMP) are a group of epithelial ovarian tumors having histologic features of cancer, but biologic features that do not show invasion. At presentation, approximately 80% of such cancers are confined to the pelvis. Conservative surgery to preserve fertility is an option in patients with disease confined to the ovaries. Patients with tumors of LMP, even those with widespread disease, can look forward to long disease-free intervals if left with no residual tumor. Adjuvant chemotherapy and radiotherapy have not been found to impact on disease-free interval and survival in most centers [39,40]. In advanced disease, the presence of invasive implants (22% of cases) is the most important prognostic indicator and such patients should be treated for invasive disease with adjuvant therapy. While survival of stage I tumors is virtually 100%, in advanced disease after 7.4 years of follow-up, patients with non-invasive implants have a 95.3% survival rate compared with only 66% in those with invasive implants [41].

Advanced ovarian cancer

Role of cytoreduction

The aim of the first surgery in patients with early epithelial ovarian cancer is staging. The goal of laparotomy in advanced disease is removal of all visible cancer so as to maximize the patient's response to adjuvant chemotherapy and improve survival. This is not always possible. Removal of all tumors greater than 1.0–1.5 cm results in improved survival after adjuvant treatment [42,43]. While there are no prospective randomized data, there are abundant data to identify optimal cytoreduction as the most consistent independent prognostic variable affecting survival. The large series of reports studying the effect of cytoreduction is typified by the Danish Ovarian Cancer Group report on 361 advanced ovarian cancer patients which found a 10% risk of progression during chemotherapy and a 46% 5-year survival in optimally cytoreduced patients [44]. Suboptimally cytoreduced patients had a 40% risk of progression and a 5-year survival of only 14%. At Mount Sinai, between 1985 and 1994, 230 stage III primary ovarian cancer patients underwent primary cytoreductive surgery and platinum-based chemotherapy (no paclitaxel was used in this era). Patients achieving optimal primary cytoreduction to < 1 cm (64.2%) had significantly improved survival ($P < 0.0001$) with Kaplan-Meier 2-, 3-, and 5-year survivals of 82.5%, 73.6%, and 59.2%, respectively, versus 59.8%, 38.8%, and 18.8% in those with sup-optimal primary cytoreduction [45]. Furthermore, a recent meta-analysis of 6,848 patients with advanced ovarian cancer during the platinum era has identifed maximal cytoreduction as one of the most powerful determinants of cohort survival [46]. The ability optimally to cytoreduce is therefore critical, and the Mount Sinai Group has recently demonstrated that elderly patients with advanced disease who can be optimally cytoreduced enjoy similar survival benefits as their younger counterparts, and therefore should not be denied access to curative management options [47].

While cytoreductive surgery is important, the biology of the disease itself has independent importance. Cancers that present as small-volume disease or can be successfully cytoreduced to small-volume may be biologically different from those that cannot [48]. Cytoreduction may improve overall survival; however, it may not provide survival benefit equivalent to that of small-volume abdominal disease at presentation. These differences may reflect differences in the biologic activity of the tumor or a difference in the duration of disease. Tumors with more aggressive biologic behavior or those which have had more time to become entrenched may have a poorer prognosis regardless of the surgeon's ability to remove them. These notions still await scientific proof.

Cytoreduction techniques

Primary cancer of pancreas, colon, and stomach may present with findings which are clinically indistinguishable from those of ovarian cancer, yet the value of cytoreduction is unproven for non-ovarian cancer. Accurate histologic evaluation early in the surgery may avoid an unnecessary, lengthy surgical procedure when a palliative procedure is indicated instead. Thus, obtaining early intra-operative histologic analysis is essential.

An initial assessment should be made to determine resectability of the tumor. Disease may be considered unresectable when it involves the porta hepatis, extensive involvement of the base of the small bowel mesentery, and multiple liver parenchymal lesions [49]. However, cytoreduction of solitary accessible intra-parenchymal liver lesions is feasible and should be attempted if it renders the patient surgically disease-free. In fact, the ability to achieve optimal cytoreduction of the hepatic involvement has independent prognostic value in improving survival [50]. Once the upper abdominal disease has been thoroughly evaluated and considered resectable, attention is turned to the pelvic disease. Extensive involvement of pelvic organs is usual in advanced ovarian cancer. The so-called "frozen pelvis" is often prematurely deemed inoperable, but with care and persistence cytoreduction is usually possible [49,51,52]. It is therefore important for patients to be cared for by specially trained clinicians.

Fortunately, ovarian cancer tends to spread over peritoneal surfaces allowing removal of large tumors by approaching avascular retroperitoneal planes and identifiable retroperitoneal structures. This requires complete understanding of retroperitoneal anatomy. By incising the peritoneum lateral to the external iliac vessels and the psoas muscles, access to the retroperitoneal space is gained. The round ligament can usually be identified in its retroperitoneal location and is ligated and cut. The peritoneal incision continues inferiorly over the bladder peritoneum, outside any peritoneal implants to remove as much tumor as possible. Using sharp dissection, the peritoneum of the anterior cul-de-sac is dissected away from the bladder until it connects with the uterine serosa thus removing all of the involved anterior cul-de-sac peritoneum effecting an "anterior cul-dectomy." The bladder is then sharply dissected away from the lower uterine segment, anterior cervix, and vagina. The lateral peritoneal incision is extended superiorly to the level of the infundibulopelvic (IP) ligament. The ureter is identified on the medial leaf of the pelvic peritoneum and then the IP ligament can be safely ligated and divided. By dissecting the ureter off of the peritoneum and following it, the uterine artery is identified, ligated and divided. If there is no rectosigmoid involvement a subtotal hysterectomy then completes the pelvic resection.

If the rectosigmoid colon is extensively involved with the pelvic tumor it can all be removed as an en bloc specimen by using the avascular presacral space. The sigmoid colon is transected proximal to any disease with a mechanical stapler. Care should be taken to preserve as much colon as possible to allow a tension-free anastamosis. Sigmoid mesenteric vessels are individually identified and ligated. At the base of the sigmoid mesentery the presacral space can be entered and developed with blunt dissection. Care should be taken to avoid the anterior surface of the sacrum where trauma to perforating veins can produce tremendous blood loss. The rectal pillars and the lateral rectosigmoid attachments are clipped or ligated until the distal margin of the sigmoid resection is identified.

A subtotal hysterectomy or total hysterectomy is performed, and the posterior cul-de-sac is mobilized with the specimen and the rectovaginal space is entered. The distal margin of the rectal resection is then transected with a mechanical stapler. Bowel continuity is re-established with an end-to-end stapler, allowing low-rectal reanastomosis without need for a protective colostomy.

The omentum is a common site of bulky upper abdominal disease [43,49,51]. A total (supracolic) or partial (infracolic) omentectomy should be performed so that no gross residual disease remains. Routine lymphadenectomy in obvious, advanced disease is not performed. The pelvic and para-aortic retroperitoneal lymph nodes should be palpated and palpable nodes removed, especially if such a maneuver results in complete cytoreduction.

The data suggesting that cytoreduction ("debulking") has a favorable impact on survival has influenced gynecologic surgeons to use more radical surgical procedures to remove as much disease from adjacent pelvic structures as possible [52]. Mechanical stapling devices now commonly used to perform bowel resection and reanastomosis seem to have a lower complication rate than suture anastomosis and certainly save operative time, blood loss, and length of hospital stay [53]. Many authors have confirmed that bowel resection in ovarian cancer cytoreduction is feasible with acceptable postoperative morbidity [52–57]. Mechanical stapling devices allow en bloc resection of extensive pelvic disease with low anterior rectal resection and re-establishment of bowel continuity virtually eliminating the need for colostomy in most patients.

Most well-trained gynecologic oncologists can perform these radical procedures to remove bulky tumor; however, the impact on overall survival of ovarian cancer patients is still being debated [58,59]. Randomized trials to investigate the impact on survival of optimal cytoreduction with bowel resection or other radical debulking procedures are almost impossible to perform. In addition, bowel involvement with cancer may reflect a tumor biology that is different.

The importance of resecting other organs invaded by ovarian cancer to achieve optimal cytoreduction is less well defined. Splenectomy [60,61], lower urinary tract resection [62], and liver resection and diaphragmatic [50,63] resection are now more often performed in attempts to maximize patient response to postoperative chemotherapy.

Role of the gynecologic oncologist

Women with ovarian masses who have been identified preoperatively as having a significant risk of ovarian cancer should be given the option of having their surgery performed by a gynecologic oncologist (NIH Consensus Statement, 1994) [64]. The importance is demonstrated in the report by McGowan et al. which evaluated 291 women with ovarian cancer and found that 97% of patients staged by gynecologic oncologists were properly staged, compared with only 52% and 35% of those cases operated on by obstetrician/gynecologists and general surgeons, respectively [65]. In addition, there are substantial data to indicate that patients operated upon by a gynecologic oncologist had a better prognosis than those treated by other surgeons [66–68].

Conclusion

The initial surgical approach to patients with epithelial ovarian cancer is a critical first step. The principles of management include assessment of preoperative risk of cancer, meticulous surgical staging to determine extent of disease and the need for further therapy in early disease, and removal of all tumor in patients with advanced disease. The adherence to these principles provides patients with the best chance for successful treatment.

The future of surgical management of primary ovarian cancer may already have arrived, as new, minimally invasive technologies have emerged. Laparoscopic staging of an apparent stage I ovarian cancer has been reported [69]. Since that report, several highly skilled laparoscopic surgeons have described the technique of para-aortic lymph node dissection and have reported its feasibility and associated morbidity [70–75]. At present, surgical staging of early ovarian cancer by laparoscopy should be considered an evolving technique, and should be restricted to selected cases performed by appropriately trained surgeons [76-89]. More recently, robotic-assisted laparoscopy has been increasingly used for selected cases of early stage ovarian cancer staging. The initial surgical management of advanced ovarian cancer involves maximal cytoreduction [76–80]. Radical surgical techniques are now being used to achieve optimal surgical debulking. Well-trained surgical subspecialists who understand the biology of ovarian cancer and possess the training and experience necessary to perform these procedures play an important role in ovarian cancer management [65–68]. However, all physicians caring for women should understand the importance of proper surgical management of ovarian cancer.

Prophylactic oophorectomy

Approximately 10–13% of all women with invasive ovarian cancer carry a *BRCA1* or *BRCA2* mutation [90]. The prevalence of these mutations is significantly higher in some ethnic groups. For example, approximately 30–40% of Ashkenazi Jewish women with ovarian cancer carry a *BRCA* mutation [91]. Patients with *BRCA* mutation have a high lifetime risk of developing ovarian or breast cancer. Carriers of *BRCA1* mutation have an estimated 87% lifetime risk of developing breast cancer and a 28–44% risk of developing ovarian cancer; *BRCA2* mutation carriers have an estimated 84% risk of breast cancer and a 20–27% risk of ovarian cancer [92–95]. Because genetic counseling and testing has become widely available for high-risk patients, preventive measures are a choice for many of these women. The proportion of women who tested positive for a *BRCA* mutation and opted for a risk-reducing salpingo-ophorectomy (RRSO), which addresses the risk of not only developing ovarian cancer but also hormone positive breast cancer, is as high as 49% [96].

No current screening techniques, including frequent pelvic examinations, pelvic ultrasound or other imaging, and serum CA125 level, have been shown to decrease the risk of death from ovarian cancer in women who are carriers of *BRCA1* or *BRCA2* mutation. A consensus panel of the National Institute of Health (NIH) recommended prophylactic oophorectomy for high-risk women at age 35 years, or after childbearing is complete [97]. RRSO has been shown to effectively reduce the risk of ovarian cancer by 71–96%, and reduces the risk of breast cancer by 50% [98,99]. Furthermore an age-matched case–control study suggests that RRSO leads to a 90% reduction in breast cancer-specific mortality, a 95% reduction in ovarian cancer-specific mortality, and a 76% reduction in overall mortality [100]. In light of these data, RRSO is highly recommended to all patients who are carriers of *BRCA1* or *BRCA2* mutation.

After completing the RRSO, there is still some risk of developing primary peritoneal cancer. A large study by Finch including 1,828 known carriers of *BRCA1* or *BRCA2* mutation who underwent RRSO found an estimated cumulative incidence of peritoneal cancer of 4.3% at 20 years after oophorectomy [101].

RRSO is performed laparoscopically in the majority of cases unless a laparotomy is performed for other indications. At the beginning of the procedure, all peritoneal surfaces and the upper abdomen should be carefully evaluated for any evidence of nodularity or implants. Pelvic washings need to be obtained for cytological evaluation. Any suspicious lesions should be biopsied and sent for pathologic examination. The surgeon should make an effort to avoid contact with the surface of the ovary and the fimbriated end of the fallopian tube, so that the delicate surface epithelium is not abraded. Microscopic occult carcinomas have been identified in RRSO specimens in approximately 2% of the *BRCA* mutation carriers [101].

Patients who are undergoing a laparoscopic RRSO should be counseled on the probability of discovering cancer at the time of the surgery. If this occurs, the appropriate staging procedures need to be performed.

A growing body of literature suggests that a large proportion of ovarian high-grade serous carcinoma may actually arise from fallopian tube secretory epithelial cells. Many young females carriers of *BRCA1* or *BRCA2* mutation are reluctant to undergo RRSO because of post-RRSO-induced menopause. While the risk of hotmone replacement is less than the risk of retaining the ovaries and fallopian tubes, bilateral salpingo-oophorectomy with ovarian retention until menopause may be offered to patients who refuse oophorectomy before menopause [102].

References

1. Piver MS, Baker TR, Jishi MF, et al. Familial ovarian cancer: a report of 658 families from the Gilda Radner Familial Ovarian Cancer Registry - 1981–1991. Cancer. 1993;**71**(Suppl 2):582–8.
2. Perez R, Godwin A, Hamilton T, et al. Ovarian cancer biology. Semin Oncol. 1991;**15**:186–204.
3. Frank TS. Testing for hereditary risk for ovarian cancer. Cancer Control. 1999;**6**:327–34.
4. Struewing JP, Hartge P, Wacholder S, et al. The risk of cancer associated with specific mutations of *BRCA1* and *BRCA2* among Ashkenazi Jews. N Engl J Med. 1997;**336**:1401–8.
5. Boyd J, Sonodo Y, Federeci MG, et al. Clinicopathological features of BRCA-linked and sporadic ovarian cancer. JAMA. 2000;**283**:2260–5.
6. Guidozzi F, Sonnendecker E. Evaluation of preoperative investigations in patients admitted for ovarian primary cytoreductive

surgery. Gynecol Oncol. 1991;**40**:244–7.

7. Van der Burg MEL, van Lent M, Buyse M, et al. The effect of debulking surgery after induction chemotherapy on the prognosis in advanced epithelial ovarian cancer. N Engl J Med. 1995;**332**:629–34.
8. Nelson BE, Rosenfield AT, Schwartz PE. Preoperative abdominal computed tomographic prediction of optimal cytoreduction in epithelial ovarian carcinoma. J Clin Oncol. 1993;**11**:166–72.
9. Bristow RE, Duska LR, Lambrou NC, et al. A model for predicting surgical outcome in patients with advanced ovarian carcinoma using computed tomography. Cancer. 2000;**89**:1532–40.
10. Hammond R, Houghton C. The role of bowel surgery in the primary treatment of epithelial ovarian cancer. Aust N Z J Obstet Gynaecol. 1990;**30**:166–9.
11. Burghardt E, Lahousen M, Stettner H. The surgical treatment of ovarian cancer. Geburtshilfe-Frauenheilkd. 1990;**50**:670–7.
12. Donato D, Angelides A, Penalver M, et al. Infectious complications after gastrointestinal surgery in patients with ovarian carcinoma and malignant ascites. Gynecol Oncol. 1992;**44**:40–7.
13. Handelsman JC, Zeiler S, Coleman J, et al. Experience with ambulatory preoperative bowel preparation at the Johns Hopkins Hospital. Arch Surg 1993;**128**:441–4.
14. Helewa ME, Krepart GV, Lotocki R. Staging laparotomy in early epithelial ovarian carcinoma. Am J Obstet Gynecol. 1986;**154**:282–6.
15. Eichner E, Bove E. In vivo studies on the lymphatic drainage of the ovary. Obstet Gynecol 1954;**3**:287–97.
16. Feldman G, Knapp R. Lymphatic drainage of the peritoneal cavity and its significance in ovarian cancer. Am J Obstet Gynecol. 1994;**119**:991–4.
17. Vergote I, De Brabanter J, Fyles A, et al. Prognostic importance of degree of differentiation and cyst rupture in stage I invasive epithelial ovarian carcinoma. Lancet. 2001;**357**:176–82.
18. Ahmed FY, Wiltshaw E, A'Hern B, et al. Natural history and prognosis of untreated stage I epithelial ovarian carcinoma. J Clin Oncol. 1996;**14**:2968–75.
19. Dembo AJ, Day M, Stenwig AE, et al. Prognostic factors in patients with stage I epithelial ovarian cancer. Obstet Gynecol. 1990;**75**:263–73.
20. Navot D, Fox JH, Williams M, et al. The concept of uterine preservation with ovarian malignancies. Obstet Gynecol. 1991;**78**(Pt 2):566–8.
21. Piver MS, Lele S, Barlow JJ. Preoperative and intraoperative evaluation in ovarian malignancy. Obstet Gynecol. 1975;**48**:312–15.
22. Young RC, Decker DG, Wharton JT, et al. Staging laparotomy in early ovarian cancer. JAMA. 1983;**250**:3072–6.
23. Hand R, Fremgen A, Chmiel JS, et al. Staging procedures, clinical management, and survival outcome for ovarian carcinoma. JAMA. 1993;**269**:1119–22.
24. Helewa ME, Krepart GV, Lotocki R. Staging laparotomy in early epithelial ovarian carcinoma. Am J Obstet Gynecol. 1986;**154**:282–6.
25. Trimbos JB, Schueler JA, van Lent M, et al. Reasons for incomplete surgical staging in early ovarian carcinoma. Gynecol Oncol. 1990;**37**:374–7.
26. Nguyen HN, Averette HE, Hoskins W, et al. National survey of ovarian carcinoma VI: critical assessment of current International Federation of Gynecologic and Obstetrics staging system. Cancer. 1993;**72**:3007–11.
27. Young RC, Walton LA, Ellenberg SS, et al. Adjuvant therapy in stage I and stage II epithelial ovarian cancer: results of two prospective randomized trials. N Engl J Med 1990;**322**:1021–7.
28. Dottino PR, Plaxe SC, Cohen CJ. A phase II trial of adjuvant cisplatin and duxorubicin in stage I epithelial ovarian cancer. Gynecol Oncol. 1991;**43**:203–5.
29. Bolis G, Colombo N, Pecorelli S, et al. Randomized multicenter clinical trial in stage I epithelial cancer. Ann Oncol. 1995;**9**:887–93.
30. Colombo N, Chari S, Maggioni A, et al. Controversial issues in the management of early epithelial ovarian cancer: conservative surgery and the role of adjuvant therapy. Gynecol Oncol. 1994;**55**:S47–51.
31. Cohen CJ, Goldberg J, Holland JF, et al. Improved therapy with cis-platin regimens for patients with ovarian carcinoma (FIGO stages III and IV) as measured by surgical end-staging (second look operation). Am J Obstet Gynecol Oncol. 1983;**145**:955.
32. Advanced Ovarian Cancer Trialists' Group. Chemotherapy in advanced ovarian cancer: an overview of randomised clinical trials. Br Med J. 1991:**303**:884–93.
33. Advanced Ovarian Cancer Trialists' Group. Chemotherapy in advanced ovarian cancer: four systematic meta-analyses of individual patient data from 37 randomized trials. Br J Cancer. 1998;**78**:1479–87.
34. McGuire WP, Hoskins WJ, Brady MF, et al. Cyclophosphamide and cisplatin compared with paclitaxel and cisplatin in patients with stage III and stage IV ovarian cancer. N Engl J Med. 1996;**334**:1–6.
35. Stuart G, Bertelsen K, Mangioni C, et al. Updated analysis shows highly significant improved overall survival (OS) for cisplatin-paclitaxel as first-line treatment of advanced ovarian cancer: mature results of the EORTC-GCCG, NOCOVA, NCIC, CTG, and Scottish intergroup trial. Proc Am Soc Clin Oncol. 1998;**17**:361.
36. Ozols RF, Bundy BN, Clarke-Pearson D, et al. Randomized phase III study of cisplatin(CIS)/paclitaxel(PAC) versus carboplatin (CARBO)/PAC in optimal stage III epithelial ovarian cancer (OC) Gynecologic Oncology Group Trial (GOG 158). Proc Am Soc Clin Oncol. 1999;**18**:356a.
37. du Bois A, Lueck HJ, Meier W, et al. Cisplatin/paclitaxel vs. carboplatin/paclitaxel in ovarian cancer: update of an Arbeitsgemeinschaft Gynaekologische Onkologie (AGO) Study Group Trial. Proc Am Soc Clin Oncol. 1999;**8**:356a.
38. Munoz KA, Harlan LC, Trimble EL. Patterns of care for women with ovarian cancer in the United States. J Clin Oncol. 1997;**15**:3408–15.
39. Fort M, Pierce V, Saigo P, et al. Evidence for the efficacy of adjuvant therapy in epithelial ovarian tumors of low malignant potential. Gynecol Oncol. 1988;**32**:69–72.
40. Koern J, Trope CG, Abeler VM. A retrospective study 370 borderline tumors of the tumor treated at the Norwegian Radium Hospital from 1970 to 1982. Cancer. 1993;**71**:1810–20.

41. Seidman JD, Kurman RJ. Ovarian serous borderline tumors: A critical review of the literature with emphasis on prognostic indicators. Hum Pathol. 2000;**31**:539–57.
42. Griffiths CT. Surgical resection of tumor bulk in the primary treatment of ovarian carcinoma. Nat Cancer Inst Monogr. 1975;**42**:101–4.
43. Hacker NF, Jonathan SB, Lagasse LD, et al. Primary cytoreductive surgery for epithelial ovarian cancer. Obstet Gynecol. 1983;**61**:413–20.
44. Bertelsen K. Tumor reduction and long-term survival in advanced ovarian cancer: a DACOVA study. Gynecol Oncol. 1990;**38**:203–9.
45. Rahaman J, Dottino P, Jennings TS, et al. Second look operation improves survival in stage III ovarian cancer patients. Int J Gynecol Cancer. 1999;**9**:22.
46. Bristow RE, Tomacruz RS, Armstrong DK, et al. Survival impact of maximum cytoreductive surgery for advanced ovarian carcinoma during the platinum-era: a meta-analysis. J Clin Oncol. 2002;**20**:1248–59.
47. Rahaman J, Jennings TS, Dottino P, et al. Impact of age on survival in advanced ovarian cancer: a re-examination. J Clin Oncol. 2001;**20**:217a.
48. Hoskins WJ, Bundy BN, Thigpen JT, et al. The influence of cytoreductive surgery on recurrence free interval and survival in small-volume stage III epithelial ovarian cancer: a Gynecologic Oncology Group study. Gynecol Oncol. 1992;**47**:159–66.
49. Heintz AP, Hacker NF, Berek JS, et al. Cytoreductive surgery in ovarian carcinoma: feasibility and morbidity. Obstet Gynecol. 1986;**67**:783–8.
50. Bristow RE, Montz FJ, Lagasse LD, et al. Survival impact of surgical cytoreduction in stage IV epithelial ovarian cancer. Gynecol Oncol. 1999;**72**:278–87.
51. Piver MS, Baker T. The potential for optimal (≤ 2 cm) cytoreductive surgery in advanced ovarian carcinoma at a tertiary medical center: a prospective study. Gynecol Oncol. 1986;**24**:1–8.
52. Berek JS, Hacker NF, Lagasse LD. Rectosigmoid colectomy and reanastomosis to facilitate resection of primary and recurrent gynecologic cancer. Obstet Gynecol. 1984;**64**:715–20.
53. Penalver M, Averette H, Sevin B-U, et al. Gastrointestinal surgery in gynecologic oncology: evaluation of surgical techniques. Gynecol Oncol. 1987;**28**:74–82.
54. Castaldo TW, Petrilli ES, Ballon SC, et al. Intestinal operations in patients with ovarian carcinoma. Gynecol Oncol. 1981;**139**:80–4.
55. Soper JT, Couchman G, Berchuck A, et al. The role of partial sigmoid colectomy for debulking epithelial ovarian carcinoma. Gynecol Oncol. 1991;**41**:239–44.
56. Eisenkop SM, Nalick RH, Teng NNH. Modified posterior exenteration for ovarian cancer. Obstet Gynecol. 1991;**78**:879–85.
57. Tamussino K, Lim PC, Webb MJ, et al. Gastrointestinal surgery in patients with ovarian cancer. Gynecol Oncol. 2001;**80**:79–84.
58. Potter ME, Partridge EE, Hatch KD, et al. Primary surgical therapy of ovarian cancer: how much and when. Gynecol Oncol. 1991;**40**:195–200.
59. Partridge EE, Gunter BC, Gelder MS, et al. The validity and significance of substages of advanced ovarian cancer. Gynecol Oncol. 1993;**48**:236–41.
60. Deppe G, Zbella EA, Skogerson K, et al. The rare indication of splenectomy as part of cytoreductive surgery in ovarian cancer. Gynecol Oncol. 1983;**16**:282–7.
61. Sonnendecker EWW, Guidozzi F, Margolius K. Splenectomy during primary maximal cytoreductive surgery for epithelial ovarian cancer. Gynecol Oncol. 1989;**35**:301–6.
62. Berek JS, Hacker NF, Lagasse LD, et al. Lower urinary tract resection as part of cytoreductive surgery for ovarian cancer. Gynecol Oncol. 1982;**13**:87–92.
63. Kapnick S, Griffiths C, Finkler N. Occult pleural involvement in stage III ovarian carcinoma: role of diaphragm resection. Gynecol Oncol. 1990;**39**:135–8.
64. National Institutes of Health. Consensus Development Conference Statement. Gynecol Oncol. 1994;**55**:S4–14.
65. McGowan L, Lesher LP, Norris HJ, et al. Mistaging of ovarian cancer. Obstet Gynecol. 1985;**65**:568–72.
66. Mayer AR, Chambers SK, Graves, et al. Ovarian cancer staging: does it require a gynecologic oncologist? Gynecol Oncol. 1992;**47**:223–7.
67. Eisenkop SM, Spirtos NM, Montag TG, et al. The impact of subspeciality training on the management of advanced ovarian cancer. Gynecol Oncol. 1992;**47**:203–9.
68. Nguyen HM, Averette H, Hoskins W, et al. National survey of ovarian carcinoma part V: the impact of physician's specialty on patients survival. Cancer. 1993;**72**:3663–70.
69. Reich H, McGlynn F, Wilkie W. Laparoscopic management of stage I ovarian cancer: a case report. J Reprod Med. 1990;**35**:601–4.
70. Herd J, Fowler J, Shenson D, et al. Laparoscopic para-aortic lymph node sampling: development of a technique. Gynecol Oncol. 1992;**44**:271–6.
71. Querleu D. Laparoscopic paraaortic node sampling in gynecologic oncology: a preliminary experience. Gynecol Oncol. 1993;**49**:24–9.
72. Querleu D, Leblanc E. Laparoscopic infrarenal para aortic lymph node dissection for restaging of carcinoma of the ovary or fallopian tube. Cancer. 1994;**73**:1467–71.
73. Childers JM, Lang J, Surwit EA. Laparoscopic staging of ovarian cancer. Gynecol Oncol. 1995;**59**:25–33.
74. Possover M, Krause N, Plaul K, Kuhne-Heid R, Schneider A. Laparoscopic para-aortic and pelvic lymphadenectomy: experience with 150 patients and review of the literature. Gynecol Oncol. 1998;**71**:19–28.
75. Dottino PR, Tobias DH, Beddoe AM, Golden AL, Cohen CJ. Laparoscopic lymphadenectomy for gynecologic malignancies. Gynecol Oncol. 1999;**73**:383–8.
76. Bagley CM, Young RC, Schein PS, Chabner BA, DeVita V. Ovarian carcinoma metastatic to the diaphragm frequently undiagnosed at laparotomy. Am J Obstet Gynecol. 1973;**116**:397–400.
77. Rosenoff SH, Young RC, Anderson T, et al. Peritoneoscopy: a valuable staging tool in ovarian carcinoma. Ann Intern Med. 1975;**83**:37–41.
78. Ozols RF, Fisher RI, Anderson T, Makuch R, Young R. Peritoneoscopy in the management of ovarian cancer. Am J Obstet Gynecol. 1981;**140**:611–19.

79. Aburustum NR, Barakat RR, Siegel PL, et al. Second-look operation for epithelial ovarian cancer: laparoscopy or laparotomy? Obstet Gynecol. 1996;**88**:549–53.

80. Rahaman J, Nezhat F, Dottino P, et al. The impact of second-look laparoscopy compared to standard second-look laparotomy on recurrence and survival in advanced stage ovarian cancer. Gynecol Oncol. 2001;**80**:326.

81. Staging of gynecologic malignancies. In: "SGO Handbook". Chicago: Society of Gynecologic Oncologists; 1994. p 29.

82. Piver M, Barlow J, Lele S. Incidence of subclinical metastasis in stage I and II ovarian carcinoma. Obstet Gynecol. 1978;**52**:100–2.

83. Soper JT, Johnson P, Johnson V, et al. Comprehensive restaging laparotomy in women with apparent early ovarian carcinoma. Obstet Gynecol. 1992;**80**:949–53.

84. Knapp R, Friedman E. Aortic lymph node metastasis in early ovarian cancer. Am J Obstet Gynecol. 1974;**119**:1013–17.

85. Delgado G, Chun B, Caglar H, et al. Paraaortic lymphadenectomy in gynecologic malignancies confined to the pelvis. Obstet Gynecol. 1977;**50**:418–23.

86. Buschbaum HJ, Brady MF, Delgado G, et al. Surgical staging of carcinoma of the ovaries. Surg Gynecol Obstet. 1989;**169**:226–32.

87. Rosenoff SH, DeVita VT, Hubbard S, et al. Peritoneoscopy in the staging and follow-up of ovarian cancer. Semin Oncol. 1975;**2**:223–8.

88. Burghardt E, Pickel H, Lahousen M, et al. Pelvic lymphadenectomy in operative treatment of ovarian cancer. Am J Obstet Gynecol. 1986;**155**:315–19.

89. Knipscheer RJ. Para-aortic lymph nodes dissection in 20 cases of primary epithelial ovarian carcinoma stage I (FIGO): influence on staging. Eur J Obstet Gynecol Reprod Biol. 1982;**13**:303–7.

90. Pal T, Permuth-Wey J, Betts JA, et al. *BRCA1* and *BRCA2* mutations account for a large proportion of ovarian carcinoma cases. Cancer. 2005;**104**:2807–16.

91. Moslehi R, Chu W, Karlan B, et al. *BRCA1* and *BRCA2* mutation analysis of 208 Ashkenazi Jewish women with ovarian cancer. Am J Hum Genet. 2000;**66**:1259–72.

92. Ford D, Easton DF, Stratton M, et al. Genetic heterogeneity and penetrance analysis of the *BRCA1* and *BRCA2* genes in breast cancer families. Am J Hum Genet. 1998;**62**:676–89.

93. Struewing JP, Hartge P, Wacholder S, et al. The risk of cancer associated with specific mutations of *BRCA1* and *BRCA2* among Ashkenazi Jews. N Engl J Med. 1997;**336**:1401–8.

94. Easton DF, Ford D, Bishop DT, and the Breast Cancer Linkage Consortium. Breast and ovarian cancer incidence in *BRCA1*-mutation carriers. Am J Hum Genet. 1995;**56**:265–71.

95. Ford D, Easton DF, Bishop DT, et al. Risks of cancer in *BRCA1*-mutation carriers. Lancet. 1994;**343**:692–5.

96. Meijers-Heijboer H, Brekelmans CT, Menke-Pluymers M, et al. Use of genetic testing and prophylactic oophorectomy in women with breast or ovarian cancer from families with a *BRCA1* or *BRCA2* mutation. J Clin Oncol. 2003;**21**:1675–81.

97. NIH Consensus Development Panel on Ovarian Cancer. Ovarian cancer: screening, treatment and follow-up. JAMA. 1995;**273**:491–7.

98. Finch A, Beiner M, Lubinski J, et al. Hereditary Ovarian Cancer Clinical Study Group. Salpingo-oophorectomy and the risk of ovarian, fallopian tube, and peritoneal cancers in women with a *BRCA1* or *BRCA2* mutation. JAMA. 2006;**296**:185–92.

99. Eisen A, Lubinski J, Klijn J, et al. Breast cancer risk following bilateral oophorectomy in *BRCA1* and *BRCA2* mutation carriers: an international case-control study. J Clin Oncol. 2005;**23**:7491–6.

100. Domchek SM, Friebel TM, Neuhausen SL, et al. Mortality after bilateral salpingo-oophorectomy in *BRCA1* and *BRCA2* mutation carriers: a prospective cohort study. Lancet Oncol. 2006;**7**:223–9.

101. Finch A, Beiner M, Lubinski J, et al. Salpingo-oophorectomy and the risk of ovarian, fallopian tube, and peritoneal cancers in women with a *BRCA1* or *BRCA2* mutation. JAMA. 2006;**296**:185–92.

102. Greene MH, Mai PL, Schwartz PE. Does bilateral salpingectomy with ovarian retention warrant consideration as a temporary bridge to risk-reducing bilateral oophorectomy in *BRCA1/2* mutation carriers? Am J Obstet Gynecol. 2011;**204**(1):19.e1–6.

Chapter 26

Chemotherapy of ovarian cancer

Ramez N. Eskander, MD, and Philip J. Di Saia, MD

Introduction

Ovarian cancer accounts for approximately 25% of all malignancies affecting the female genital tract and is the most lethal gynecologic malignancy. According to Cancer Statistics 2010, a projected 21,880 new cases will be diagnosed, with 13,850 deaths [1]. Primary ovarian malignancies can be divided into epithelial ovarian cancers (EOC), including fallopian tube and primary peritoneal cancer, borderline tumors of the ovary, germ cell tumors, and sex cord stromal tumors. Non-epithelial malignancies account for nearly 10% of all ovarian cancer. Despite some similarities in presentation, the management of these tumors both surgically and in the adjuvant setting, with chemotherapy, differs.

Advanced stage epithelial ovarian cancer is traditionally managed with surgery, followed by chemotherapy consisting currently of platinum drugs and a taxane [2]. Patients with advanced stage disease who undergo successful cytoreductive surgery unfortunately have a significant rate of recurrence, and further chemotherapy is required for the treatment of relapse [3]. Some patients will develop chemotherapy resistant clones, with progressive disease, affording an opportunity for research and exploration of alternate therapies [4]. Conversely, the majority of patients with ovarian germ cell tumors are diagnosed at early stages of the disease, have excellent responses to chemotherapy, and are highly curable [5].

Epithelial ovarian cancer

The classic management of epithelial ovarian cancer is based on the integration of surgery and chemotherapy. An evaluation of several clinical, prognostic, and pathologic variables guides management decisions as they apply to adjuvant treatment. Specifically, surgical stage as defined by the International Federation of Gynecologic Oncology (FIGO), tumor grade, histologic type, and the amount of residual disease after primary surgery all impact chemotherapy strategies and survival outcomes.

Early stage high-risk epithelial ovarian cancer

Due to a lack of effective screening, epithelial ovarian cancer is currently diagnosed at an early stage (FIGO stages I–IIA) in only 20% of patients. More recently, a large collaborative trial conducted in the United Kingdom using serial CA125, as well as trans-vaginal ultrasound (MMS) or trans-vaginal ultrasound alone (USS), detected early stage ovarian cancer (stage I–II) in 48.3% of enrolled patients [6]. However, the positive predictive values of MMS and USS were 35.1% and 2.8%, respectively. Despite increased cure rates in these early stage patients, approximately 25% will experience disease recurrence [1].

The benefit of chemotherapy in the management of patients with early stage, high-risk disease, has been studied in three large clinical trials. These patients are defined as having stage Ia and Ib grades II–III tumors, all grades of Ic–IIa and all clear cell carcinomas.

The International Collaborative Ovarian Neoplasm Trial 1 (ICON1), and the Adjuvant Chemotherapy Trial in Ovarian Neoplasia (ACTION) were two large, parallel, randomized phase III clinical trials that compared platinum-based adjuvant chemotherapy with observation alone in patients with early stage epithelial ovarian cancer [7]. Between November 1990 and January 2000, 925 patients (477 in ICON1 and 448 in ACTION) who had surgery for early stage ovarian cancer were randomly assigned to receive platinum-based adjuvant chemotherapy (n = 465) or observation (n = 460) until chemotherapy was indicated.

Overall survival at 5 years was 82% in the chemotherapy arm and 74% in the observation arm (difference = 8%; 95% confidence interval [CI], 2–12; hazard ratio [HR] = 0.67; 95% CI, 0.50–0.90; P = 0.008). Recurrence-free survival at 5 years was also better in the adjuvant chemotherapy arm than it was in the observation arm (76% versus 65%, difference = 11%; 95% CI, 5–16; HR = 0.64, 95% CI, 0.50–0.82; P = 0.001). Importantly, however, surgical staging was not required in the ICON1 trial, and thus a proportion of these women likely had occult disease making them stage III. Furthermore, in the ACTION trial, only one-third of the total group was optimally staged. Within the optimally staged population, no benefit was seen in those treated with adjuvant chemotherapy. These findings suggest that platinum-based adjuvant chemotherapy should be considered in patients with early high-risk disease, not optimally staged surgically. Notably, 57% of patients in the combined studies were treated with single agent carboplatin in the adjuvant setting, with a remaining 27% treated with cisplatin.

The trials initiated by the Gynecologic Oncology Group (GOG) included protocol 157, a randomized trial comparing

Altchek's Diagnosis and Management of Ovarian Disorders, ed. Liane Deligdisch, Nathan G. Kase, and Carmel J. Cohen. Published by Cambridge University Press.

three to six cycles of adjuvant carboplatin and paclitaxel in surgically staged patients with stage IA grade 3, IB grade 3, clear cell, IC, and completely resected stage II EOC [8]. Of 457 patients, 427 (93%) were histologically and medically eligible, with 29% of patients having incomplete or inadequately documented surgical staging. The recurrence rate after six cycles was 24% lower (HR, 0.761; 95% CI, 0.51–1.13; P = 0.18), although this did not reach statistical significance. The estimated probability of recurrence within 5 years was 20.1% (six cycles) versus 25.4% (three cycles). The overall death rate was similar for the two regimens (HR, 1.02; 95% CI, 0.662–1.57). The authors concluded that compared with three cycles, six cycles did not significantly alter the recurrence rate in high-risk early stage EOC.

Most recently, the GOG completed protocol 175, which compared the recurrence-free interval (RFI) and safety profile in patients with completely resected high-risk early stage ovarian cancer treated with intravenous carboplatin and paclitaxel with or without maintenance low-dose paclitaxel for 24 weeks [9]. A total of 571 patients were enrolled onto this study. The 5-year recurrence risk was 20% in the maintenance paclitaxel arm, versus 23% in the observation arm (HR, 0.807; 95% CI, 0.565–1.15). The probability of surviving 5 years was 85.4% and 86.2%, respectively. In addition, the rates of neurologic, dermatologic, and infectious toxicities were significantly more common in the maintenance arm. The authors concluded that maintenance paclitaxel for 24 weeks in addition to three cycles of carboplatin and paclitaxel was not warranted.

Avoidance of overly aggressive therapy in patients with early stage epithelial cancers is important, because of the possibility of chemotherapy-associated leukemia [10]. Travis et al. conducted a case–control study of secondary leukemia in a population-based cohort of 28,971 women in North America and Europe, findings a relative risk of leukemia of 4.0 (95% CI, 1.4–11.4) in women who received platinum-based combination chemotherapy for ovarian cancer. Furthermore, a dose–response relationship was shown with RR of 7.6 in patients receiving 1,000 mg or more of a platinum agent (Table 26.1).

Table 26.1. Randomized clinical trials evaluating adjuvant treatment of early stage EOC

First-line adjuvant therapy		
Study	Trial design	Status
ICON 1 [11]	477 patients randomized: adjuvant chemotherapy vs. observation after surgery	HR 0.66 favoring adjuvant chemotherapy **(surgical staging not required)**
ACTION [12]	448 patients randomized: Ia and Ib grade II–III, all grades of Ic–IIa and all clear cell carcinomas – adjuvant chemotherapy vs. observation	Recurrence-free interval HR 0.63 favoring adjuvant chemotherapy arm. No difference in overall survival (only 1/3 of group optimally staged)
GOG 157[8]	457 patients with stage Ia and Ib grade 3, Ic all grades, clear cell, and completely resected stage II, randomized to 3 vs. 6 cycles of CT	No difference in HR for recurrence or death (29% inadequately staged)
GOG 175[9]	542 patients with Ia/Ib grade 3, clear cell, all Ic and stage II EOC randomized to CT + maintenance T vs. CT followed by observation	No difference in recurrence or 5-year survival

CT, carboplatin/paclitaxel; T, paclitaxel; GOG, Gynecologic Oncology Group; ICON, International Collaborative Ovarian Neoplasm; ACTION, Adjuvant Chemotherapy Trial in Ovarian Neoplasia; HR, hazard ratio.

Advanced stage epithelial ovarian cancer

Currently, patients presenting with advanced stage ovarian cancer are usually managed with maximal surgical resection followed by adjuvant platinum- and taxane-based chemotherapy. These patients can expect 5-year survival rates approaching 40% [1].

Before the discovery and introduction of cisplatin in the treatment of ovarian cancer in the latter half of the 1970s, patients were treated with the alkylating agents melphalan, thiotepa, cyclophosphamide, or chlorambucil as single agents [13]. Following the introduction of cisplatin, platinum-based combination chemotherapy became the cornerstone of treatment, with improved survival when platinum-containing regimens were used instead of non-platinum-containing chemotherapy [14]. Initially, the combination of cyclophosphamide and cisplatin was compared with cyclophosphamide, cisplatin, and doxorubicin in several studies, with similar survival rates [15–18]. Although two meta-analyses showed a slight survival advantage in the doxorubicin-containing arms, the survival curves appeared to converge 8 years out. In addition, the doxorubicin-containing arms had an increased dose intensity, which may have contributed to the observed differences.

The introduction of paclitaxel, isolated initially from the Pacific yew tree, led to a paradigm shift in the treatment of ovarian cancer. Our understanding of the therapeutic benefits of regimens containing cisplatin and paclitaxel originated following the results of the GOG protocol 111 [19]. In GOG 111, 386 women with stage III sub-optimally debulked or stage IV disease were randomly assigned to receive six cycles of cisplatin (75 mg/m^2) plus paclitaxel (135 mg/m^2 over 24 hours) or cisplatin (75 mg/m^2) plus cyclophosphamide (750 mg/m^2). The paclitaxel-containing regimen showed a statistically significant improvement in overall response, clinical complete response (CR), progression-free survival (PFS), and overall survival (OS) (PFS 18 vs. 13 months, OS 38 vs. 24 months, respectively). OV-10, a European-Canadian trial, studied 680 patients treated with cisplatin (75 mg/m^2) and paclitaxel (175 mg/m^2 over 3 hours) or cisplatin (75 mg/m^2) plus cyclophosphamide (750 mg/m^2). The paclitaxel-containing arm showed an improvement in overall response, clinical CR, PFS (16 months vs. 12 months), and OS (36 months vs. 26 months) [20].

Following completion of GOG 111, the GOG opened protocol 158 [3]. This was designed as a non-inferiority trial comparing carboplatin (AUC 7.5) and paclitaxel (175 mg/m^2 over 3 hours) to cisplatin (75 mg/m^2) and paclitaxel (135 mg/m^2 over 24 hours). In previous non-randomized trials, the combination of carboplatin and paclitaxel was shown to be a less toxic and highly active combination regimen in the treatment of ovarian cancer. The GOG enrolled 792 eligible patients, showing decreased gastrointestinal, renal, and metabolic toxicities as well as decreased grade 4 leukopenia in the carboplatin-containing arm. Median PFS (20.7 vs. 19.4 months for carboplatin and cisplatin, respectively) and overall survival (57.4 vs. 48.7 months, respectively) were not significantly different between study groups. The authors thus concluded that the combination of carboplatin and paclitaxel was less toxic, easier to administer, and not inferior to the previous standard of cisplatin and paclitaxel. Furthermore, in patients who were optimally cytoreduced (residual disease at completion of surgery < 1.0 cm) the median survival was nearly 5 years in the carboplatin-containing arm.

The combination of carboplatin and paclitaxel was then studied with gemcitabine, topotecan, or liposomal doxorubicin in sequential doublets or triplets in GOG 182/ICON5. This large international trial recruited more than 4,000 women with advanced stage epithelial ovarian cancer [21]. There was no improvement in either PFS or OS associated with any experimental regimen. Survival analyses of groups defined by size of residual disease also failed to show benefit in any subgroup. The authors concluded that compared with standard paclitaxel and carboplatin, addition of a third cytotoxic agent provided no benefit in PFS or OS after optimal or suboptimal cytoreduction.

In addition to intravenous (IV) therapy, the GOG also investigated intra-peritoneal (IP) treatment options. Following completion of two randomized phase III intergroup trials comparing IV to IV+IP therapy that showed positive results, the GOG opened protocol 172, which compared IV paclitaxel (135 mg/m^2) over 24 hours with IV cisplatin (75 mg/m^2) on day 2, versus IV paclitaxel (135 mg/m^2) over 24 hours, followed by IP cisplatin (100 mg/m^2) on day 2 and IP paclitaxel (60 mg/m^2) on day 8. A total of six courses were administered every 3 weeks [22]. All patients had optimally resected disease with residual tumor limited to less than or equal to 1 cm in size. The median survival for the IV and IP arms was 49.5 and 66.9 months, respectively. The RR of death was 0.71 in the IP group ($P = 0.0076$). The authors noted that tolerability for IP chemo was a concern as grades 3 and 4 hematologic, metabolic, and gastrointestinal toxicities were significantly more common in the IP arm. In fact, only 42% of patients allocated to the IP arm completed six cycles of chemotherapy. The results of the above study, in combination with previous positive studies exploring intra-peritoneal chemotherapy, resulted in a National Cancer Institute (NCI) clinical announcement recommending that women with optimally cytoreduced stage III ovarian cancer be considered for IV+IP therapy.

Neoadjuvant chemotherapy in epithelial ovarian cancer

In some cases, chemotherapy administered before surgery may be indicated. Specifically, neoadjuvant chemotherapy may be appropriate in patients whose pre-operative imaging and exam make optimal cytoreduction by an experienced gynecologic oncologist unlikely and in those cases where patients are at high risk for major abdominal surgery due to medical comorbidities. Bristow et al. conducted a systematic review summarizing the existing data on neoadjuvant chemotherapy as an alternative treatment strategy for patients with advanced stage ovarian cancer [23]. Twenty-six studies, including a total of 1,336 patients, reporting on neoadjuvant chemotherapy administered in lieu of primary cytoreductive surgery were analyzed. The authors concluded that the data suggested that the survival outcome achievable with initial chemotherapy is inferior to successful up-front cytoreductive surgery realizing that the two groups may not include comparable disease states. Additional research is needed to devise universal selection criteria for neoadjuvant chemotherapy, determine the most efficacious treatment program, and characterize the appropriate proportion of patients in which an attempt at primary surgery should be abandoned in favor of initial chemotherapy.

Recently, however, a phase III randomized clinical trial comparing primary cytoreductive surgery followed by chemotherapy to neoadjuvant chemotherapy followed by interval cytoreductive surgery in women with advanced stage ovarian cancer was completed [24]. Of the 670 patients randomly assigned to a study treatment, 632 were deemed eligible and began treatment. The majority of these patients had stage IIC or IV disease at the time of primary surgery. The largest residual tumor was 1 cm or less in diameter in 41.6% of patients after primary debulking and in 80.6% of patients after interval debulking. The rate of post-operative adverse events and mortality was higher after primary debulking than after interval debulking. In addition, the hazard ratio for death (intention-to-treat analysis) in the group assigned to neoadjuvant chemotherapy followed by interval debulking, as compared with the group assigned to primary debulking surgery followed by chemotherapy, was 0.98 (90% CI, 0.84–1.13; $P = 0.01$ for non-inferiority), and the hazard ratio for progressive disease was 1.01 (90% CI, 0.89–1.15). Despite the above findings, Vergote et al. discussed the limited use of neoadjuvant chemotherapy by United States Gynecologic Oncologists [25]. In a survey of 1,137 gynecologic oncologists, of which 339 responded, 60% of practitioners reported using neoadjuvant chemotherapy in less than 10% of their patients with advanced stage ovarian cancer.

Unfortunately, disease recurrence continues to be a major problem in patients diagnosed with epithelial ovarian cancer. Patients with recurrent disease are uncommonly cured, and thus comprise a population of patients for whom clinical trials and investigations into alternative therapies may be beneficial. Patients with disease recurrence 6 months after first-line therapy are termed "platinum sensitive," and have response rates in the range of 30–40% to second-line agents [26]. These patients typically receive a platinum-based regimen, often in combination with paclitaxel, gemcitabine, or pegylated liposomal doxorubicin [27]. On the other hand, patients with disease recurrence within 6 months of primary therapy, termed platinum resistant, and those with disease persistence/progression while on first-line platinum therapy, termed platinum refractory, are typically treated with non-platinum-based regimens [26]. Agents that can be considered in this setting include liposomal doxorubicin, topotecan, gemcitabine, and oral etoposide [28]. Given overall poor response rates within this patient population, enrollment in open clinical trials should be assigned priority and encouraged.

Anti-angiogenic and targeted therapy in ovarian cancer

More recently, targeted therapies have been explored in the treatment of ovarian cancer based on various potential therapeutic pathways, and biologic therapies have emerged. Specifically, anti-angiogenic agents have been the most studied and found to be the most effective targeted therapy in the treatment of ovarian cancer. Angiogenesis is essential for tumor invasion and metastasis, and is required for tumor growth beyond 1–2 mm, through recruitment of vasculature and pro-angiogenic mediators including vascular endothelial growth factor (VEGF) [29]. Ovarian cancer patients with elevated VEGF levels have been shown to have poorer overall prognosis, with VEGF levels being independent indicators of survival.

To date, bevacizumab, a recombinant human monoclonal antibody to the VEGF ligand, has been the most studied anti-angiogenic agent. The immediate mechanism of action of bevacizumab is to bind and inactivate VEGF, thereby inhibiting endothelial, and possibly tumor, cell activation and proliferation [30,31].

Before its investigation in EOC, bevacizumab was studied in patients with clear cell renal, colon, prostate, lung, and breast cancers [32]. The utility of VEGF inhibitors in the treatment of ovarian carcinoma was initially explored in animal models, where VEGF blockade was shown to inhibit ascites formation and slow tumor growth [33]. These were followed by two, single-agent, phase 2 bevacizumab trials exploring its utility in the treatment of recurrent ovarian cancer, the majority of which was platinum-resistant disease. The first, GOG 170D, the largest single agent study, explored the use of bevacizumab at a dose of 15 mg/kg in patients with persistent or recurrent epithelial ovarian cancer or primary peritoneal cancer after one to two prior cytotoxic regimens [34]. The study consisted of 62 eligible and assessable patients. Of these, 66.1% had received two prior cytotoxic chemotherapy regimens, and 41.9% were considered platinum resistant. Thirteen patients (21.0%) experienced clinical responses (two complete, 11 partial; median response duration, 10 months), and 25 (40.3%) survived progression free for at least 6 months. Median PFS and overall survival were 4.7 and 17 months, respectively. The second was an industry-sponsored trial evaluating the efficacy and safety of bevacizumab in patients with platinum-resistant epithelial ovarian carcinoma (EOC) or peritoneal serous carcinoma (PSC) who had experienced disease progression during, or within 3 months of discontinuing topotecan or liposomal doxorubicin [35]. Enrolled patients received single agent bevacizumab 15 mg/kg every 3 weeks, and nearly 84% were platinum resistant. Partial responses were observed in 15.9% with median progression-free survival of 4.4 months (95% CI, 3.1–5.5), and a median survival duration of 10.7 months at study termination. This was followed by two trials combining cytotoxic chemotherapy with bevacizumab in the treatment of recurrent disease. The trials showed response rates of 24% each and 6-month progression-free rates of 50% and 56%, respectively [36].

The above phase II trials were followed by four randomized phase 3 trials, evaluating bevacizumab as a first-line agent and in disease recurrence [37]. Three of these trials have completed accrual, namely GOG 218, International Collaborative Ovarian Neoplasm (ICON) 7, and OCEANS. GOG 218 was a three-arm placebo-controlled study, with all patients receiving carboplatin and paclitaxel. In the first experimental arm, patients were treated with concurrent bevacizumab followed by placebo maintenance, while in the third experimental arm, patients received concurrent and maintenance bevacizumab (15 mg/kg every 3 weeks) for up to 16 doses [38]. A total of 1,873 patients were enrolled. Of these patients, 34% were optimally cytoreduced, with 40% sub-optimally debulked, and 26% being stage 4. Preliminary data, as presented at the 2010 meeting for the American Society of Clinical Oncology (ASCO), showed a significant improvement in PFS in patients treated with concurrent and maintenance bevacizumab, 14.1 months versus 10.3 months in the placebo arm. Relative to arm 1 of the trial, the hazard ratio for first progression in the maintenance arm of the trial was 0.717 (95% CI, 0.625–0.824; $P < 0.0001$). The overall survival data are not yet mature.

ICON-7 was a two armed trial comparing carboplatin and paclitaxel (six cycles) against carboplatin + paclitaxel + bevacizumab (7.5 mg/kg) every 3 weeks for six cycles, followed by 12 cycles of maintenance bevacizumab or disease progression, whichever occurred earlier. Data from this trial were presented in abstract form at the 2010 meeting of the European Society of Medical Oncology (ESMO). A total of 1,528 women were randomized from 263 centers. The reported rate of adverse events was consistent with previous bevacizumab trials. More importantly, relative to arm 1 of the trial, the hazard ratio for disease progression in the bevacizumab arm was 0.81 (95% CI, 0.70–0.94; $P < 0.0041$).

The remaining phase III trials target patients with recurrent disease. GOG 213 is a randomized trial comparing carboplatin and paclitaxel with or without bevacizumab in platinum-sensitive relapsed ovarian cancer patients. It also includes a study of secondary cytoreductive surgery in eligible patients. OCEANS, an industry sponsored study, is a randomized placebo controlled trial, comparing carboplatin and gemcitabine with or without bevacizumab in the treatment of recurrent disease [31]. This trial has completed accrual, with preliminary results presented at the 2011 American Society of Clinical Oncology Meeting. Two hundred and forty-two women were

Table 26.2. Randomized clinical trials evaluating bevacizumab in ovarian cancer

Study	Trial design	Status
First-line adjuvant therapy		
GOG 218	Randomized, placebo-controlled, three-arm, CT ±bev with 18-cycle bev maintenance	Completed accrual: HR 0.717 favoring the concurrent and maintenance bevacizumab arm.
ICON-7	Randomized, two-arm, CT ±bev with 12-cycle bev maintenance	Completed accrual: HR 0.80 favoring the concurrent and maintenance bevacizumab arm.
Second-line therapy		
GOG 213	Randomized, CT ± bev	Open to accrual
OCEANS	Randomized, placebo-controlled, CG ± bev	Completed accrual July 2010. 4 month improvement in the bevacizumab-containing arm (12.4 vs. 8.4 months; HR 0.484 favoring bevacizumab arm)

CT, carboplatin/paclitaxel; CG, carboplatin/gemcitabine; GOG, Gynecologic Oncology Group; ICON, International Collaborative Ovarian Neoplasm; bev, bevacizumab.

Table 26.3. Adverse events associated with bevacizumab

Adverse events	
Common (mild)	Rare (serious)
Headache Hypertension Proteinuria	Non-gastrointestinal fistula formation Arterial thromboembolic events (myocardial infarction, cerebrovascular accident) Gastrointestinal perforation Wound healing complications Reversible posterior leukoencephalopathy syndrome

allocated to each arm of the study, with a median follow-up of 24 months. The median number of chemotherapy cycles was six for each group, and a median of 11 cycles of bevacizumab or placebo was given. PFS was significantly longer for women given bevacizumab (12.4 months vs. 8.4 months in placebo-treated group; HR 0.484; 95% CI, 0.388–0.605; $P < 0.0001$) (Table 26.2).

As with any new antitumor agent, the benefits of bevacizumab in the treatment of patients with ovarian cancer must be weighed against the side effects. Overall, bevacizumab is well tolerated, with a side effect profile unique to its mode of action. In a comprehensive review, Randall et al. investigated the toxicities of bevacizumab in ovarian cancer patients, and their management [31]. Table 26.3 lists the adverse effects that were included in the U.S. Food and Drug Administration (FDA)-approved bevacizumab package insert [39].

The most common toxicities include hypertension (grade 3–4 ranging from 0.3% to 14.8% of patients), and proteinuria (usually grade 1–2). Hemorrhage, arterial and venous thrombotic events, impaired wound healing, and gastrointestinal perforation are less common but serious complications [30,40]. Ultimately, patient-directed decision making, weighing drug efficacy, toxicity, and goals of therapy should be undertaken.

In addition to bevacizumab, multi-targeted anti-angiogenic agents, with effects on platelet derived growth factor (PDGF) and fibroblast growth factor (FGF) are also under investigation. Pre-clinical models point to an interconnection between PDGF/VEGF signaling, with PDGF promoting VEGF resistance through recruitment of pericytes. Sorafenib and sunitinib, both approved for the treatment of advanced renal cell cancer, are currently under development for ovarian cancer. Two phase II trials illustrated partial response rates of approximately 3%. When combined with VEGF, sorafenib showed a 46% partial response rate (6 of 13 patients). In addition, combined VEGF/PDGF/FGF pathway inhibition was hypothesized to increase anti-angiogenic activity. Cediranib, pazopanib, and BIBF 1120 have been evaluated in several phase II clinical trials. Partial response rates in platinum-sensitive recurrent patients ranged from 18–31%. The most commonly reported adverse events included diarrhea, fatigue, and hypertension.

Targeted therapies, specifically the poly-ADP ribose polymerase (PARP) inhibitors, have also been investigated in the treatment of ovarian cancer. PARP-1 and PARP-2 normally play an essential role in base excision repair of damaged DNA. An estimated 10–15% of EOC are hereditary, resulting from *BRCA1/2* mutations. Cancer cells in patients with germline mutations in *BRCA1/2* lose the second allele through mutations and thus have complete loss of BRCA function. These patients comprise a unique group, where one mechanism of cellular DNA repair, homologous recombination, is compromised. By disrupting the alternate pathway by means of PARP inhibitors, these cells can no longer repair damaged DNA, and a phenomenon termed "synthetic lethality" results in cell death.

The PARP inhibitor olaparib has been studied in phase I and II trials in women with known *BRCA1/2* mutations, with a reported 52–63% clinical benefit (RECIST complete response/partial response/stable disease for ≥8 weeks). Currently, phase II trials are exploring the potential use of PARP inhibitors in sporadic cases of serous ovarian cancer, where functional loss of homologous recombination, defined as BRCAness, has been demonstrated.

Borderline ovarian tumors

Borderline ovarian tumors are distinct from invasive epithelial ovarian malignancies. These tumors account for 15% of all epithelial ovarian cancers and, on average, are diagnosed at a younger age than their malignant counterparts. More than 80% of women with borderline ovarian tumors present with stage I disease and can expect significantly better overall survival stage-for-stage in comparison to EOC.

The recommended management of clinically apparent early stage borderline ovarian tumors, in women who have completed childbearing, includes bilateral salpingo-oophorectomy with hysterectomy and surgical staging. For young patients with apparent early stage disease who desire fertility preservation, unilateral oophorectomy or ovarian cystectomy with a staging procedure is an acceptable alternative, although this approach may predispose to a higher risk of recurrence. For advanced-stage and recurrent disease, cytoreductive surgery is the cornerstone of treatment, while adjuvant chemotherapy is reserved for selected cases only (e.g., unresectable disease, invasive metastatic implants, rapid growth rate with progressive symptomatology).

Adjuvant therapy

For patients with disease apparently confined to the ovaries, adjuvant chemotherapy is not recommended. Barnhill et al. reported a GOG prospective study in which 146 patients with stage I serous borderline ovarian tumors were observed without adjuvant therapy [41]. With a median follow-up of 42.2 months, no patient developed recurrent disease. For most patients with stage I tumors, long-term disease-free survival can be expected. To underscore this point, a large meta-analysis demonstrated a disease-free survival rate of 98.2% and a disease-specific survival rate of 99.5% for women with stage I disease [42]. Four prospective randomized trials conducted in Norway showed that for stage I and II disease, the addition of adjuvant therapy did not improve survival and added toxicity, with overall survival rates of 99% and 94% for no adjuvant therapy and adjuvant therapy, respectively [43].

Objective responses to platinum-based chemotherapy among patients with advanced-stage borderline ovarian tumors have been reported at the time of second-look surgery. Gershenson et al. reported complete responses to chemotherapy at second-look laparotomy in 8 of 20 patients with macroscopic residual disease after initial cytoreductive surgery and in 5 of 12 patients with microscopic residual disease after initial surgery [44]. Barakat and colleagues reported that two of seven patients with macroscopic residual borderline ovarian tumors and seven of eight patients with microscopic disease had pathologic complete remissions at second-look laparotomy after platinum-based chemotherapy, with only one death due to progressive disease [45]. Importantly, there was no difference in survival between patients who received chemotherapy and those who did not. Sutton et al. reported the GOG data using a subset of 32 women with advanced-stage borderline ovarian tumors that were optimally cytoreduced [46]. The patients were randomized to treatment with cisplatin and cyclophosphamide with or without adriamycin. Fifteen of 32 patients underwent second-look surgery, and 9 showed evidence of persistent disease. However, at a median follow-up of 31.7 months, 31 of 32 patients were alive. Only one patient died, and this death was unrelated to the ovarian disease process. Due to the low percentage of actively dividing cells that are present in borderline ovarian tumors, these are thought to be relatively resistant to standard cytotoxic agents. Furthermore, adjuvant chemotherapy in patients with ovarian serous borderline tumors with invasive peritoneal implants showed no improvement in time to recurrence or overall survival [47]. However, given the small number of patients and variable follow-up times, it is still possible that a beneficial effect exists. As noted earlier, even patients with advanced stage disease can be expected to have excellent overall survival rates. Therefore, patients must be counseled that the role of adjuvant chemotherapy in advanced stage disease is still unclear.

Ovarian germ cell tumors

Malignant ovarian germ cell tumors are rare and aggressive, but very curable at all presenting stages of disease. They account for only 1–2% of all ovarian cancers, and affect women of reproductive age, with nearly 70% of ovarian germ cell tumors occurring in the first two decades of life [48].

The recommended management of young patients with suspected malignant germ cell tumors of the ovary includes: (1) intact removal of the tumor; (2) sparing of the fallopian tube if not adherent to the tumor; (3) procurement of cytologic washings or harvesting of ascites fluid; (4) examination and palpation of the omentum with removal of suspicious areas; and (5) examination and palpation of the iliac and aortocaval nodes with biopsy of abnormal areas. Following surgical cytoreduction, patients are managed with post-operative systemic chemotherapy, with 90–95% cure rates, except in cases of stage IA, grade I immature teratomas, where observation alone is acceptable.

Our understanding regarding effective chemotherapy for the treatment of ovarian germ cell cancers paralleled advancements in adjuvant therapy for the more common testicular tumors. The combination regimen consisting of vincristine, actinomycin D, and cyclophosphamide (VAC) was the first regimen to reproducibly cure patients with ovarian germ cell tumors. Gershenson et al. studied 80 patients with malignant non-dysgerminomatous germ cell tumors of the ovary who were treated with VAC at the University of Texas M. D. Anderson Hospital and Tumor Institute [49]. Sixty-six patients received VAC as primary postoperative therapy with 46 patients (70%) achieving a sustained remission. This regimen was then modified to include vinblastine, bleomycin, and cisplatin (VBP). In a GOG trial, 97 patients with germ cell tumors were treated with three to four courses of VBP [50]. Of 35 patients with tumors other than dysgerminoma who had clinically measurable disease, 15 (43%; 95% CI, 26–61) had complete responses. Of 56 second-look laparotomies, 40 (71%; 95% CI, 58–83) revealed no tumor or mature glial tissue. The survival rate was 71% (95% CI, 62–89) with a 51% disease-free rate (95% CI, 41–62) at 2 years.

Ultimately, a switch from VBP to combination bleomycin, etoposide, and cisplatin (BEP), resulted from experience with testicular tumors, where the etoposide-containing regimen was shown to have a larger therapeutic index (particularly neurologic and gastrointestinal toxicities) [51]. In a trial randomizing 261 men with disseminated germ cell tumors to VBP versus BEP, 74% of those receiving the regimen including vinblastine and 83% of those receiving the regimen including etoposide became disease-free with or without subsequent surgery.

Among 157 patients with high tumor volume, 61% became disease-free on the regimen that included vinblastine, as compared with 77% on the regimen that included etoposide ($P < 0.05$). Survival among the patients who received etoposide was higher ($P = 0.048$). In addition, the etoposide regimen caused substantially fewer paresthesias ($P = 0.02$), abdominal cramps ($P = 0.0008$), and myalgias ($P = 0.00002$).

Despite the exquisite radiosensitivity of dysgerminomatous germ cell tumors, adjuvant chemotherapy in the form of BEP is preferred given the possible sterilizing effects of radiation in this predominantly young patient population. After adjuvant chemotherapy, Gershenson et al. reported resumption of normal menstrual activity in all 28 enrolled patients treated with the VAC regimen. Importantly, the likelihood of chemotherapy-induced amenorrhea is based on the specific chemotherapy administered as well as the patient's age. The younger the patient at the time of exposure, the larger the oocyte reserve, facilitating recruitment and re-establishment of normal ovulation after completion of chemotherapy [52].

Sex cord-stromal tumors

Given the rare occurrence of these malignancies, information regarding adjuvant chemotherapy for patients with advanced stage or recurrent sex cord-stromal tumors is limited. No prospective trials have been conducted, and it is difficult to draw conclusions regarding optimal therapy due to limitations of retrospective trials, including the small patient numbers, and varying treatment regimens. Nonetheless, several regimens have been explored. Specifically, response rates to combination adriamycin–cisplatin (AP), cyclophosphamide–adriamycin–cisplatin (CAP), PVB and BEP range from 37% to 100% in patients with advanced stage or recurrent disease [53]. More recently, combination carboplatin and paclitaxel has been used. GOG protocol 187 is currently open, investigating the potential benefits of single agent paclitaxel in patients with persistent or recurrent disease after up front therapy. If paclitaxel appears to have an impact in this patient population, its use in primary treatment may be considered further.

Conclusion

In summary, ovarian cancer continues to be an aggressive malignancy; however, with advances in our understanding of the biology of this disease, and discovery of novel chemotherapeutic regimens, there has been an improvement in survival. Five-year survival from ovarian cancer of all stages and histologies has improved in the United States from 37% in 1975–1977 to 46% in 1999–2005 ($P < 0.05$) [1]. In addition, according to 2010 SEER data, the death rate attributed to ovarian cancer per 100,000 females has declined from 10.02 in 1976 to 7.95 in 2008 [54]. Despite these improvements, continued research exploring screening and early detection of disease, improved surgical care, and targeted chemotherapeutic regimens is warranted.

References

1. Jemal A, Siegel R, Xu J, Ward E. Cancer Statistics, 2010. CA Cancer J Clin. 2010;**60**:277–300.
2. Bookman M. Trials with impact on clinical management: first line. Int J Gynecol Cancer. 2009;**19**(Suppl 2): S55–62.
3. Ozols R, Bundy B, Greer B, et al. Phase III trial of carboplatin and paclitaxel compared with cisplatin and paclitaxel in patients with optimally resected stage III ovarian cancer: a Gynecologic Oncology Group study. J Clin Oncol. 2003;**21**:3194–200.
4. Monk B, Choi D, Pugmire G, et al. Activity of bevacizumab (rhuMAB VEGF) in advanced refractory epithelial ovarian cancer. Gynecol Oncol. 2005;**96**:902–5.
5. Williams S, Blessing JA, Liao SY, et al. Adjuvant therapy of ovarian germ cell tumors with cisplatin, etoposide, and bleomycin: a trial of the Gynecologic Oncology Group. J Clin Oncol. 1994;**12**:701–6.
6. Menon U, Gentry Maharaj A, Hallett R, et al. Sensitivity and specificity of multimodal and ultrasound screening for ovarian cancer, and stage distribution of detected cancers: results of the prevalence screen of the UK Collaborative Trial of Ovarian Cancer Screening (UKCTOCS). Lancet Oncol. 2009;**10**;327–40.
7. Trimbos JB, Parmar M, Vergote I, et al. International Collaborative Ovarian Neoplasm trial 1 and Adjuvant ChemoTherapy In Ovarian Neoplasm trial: two parallel randomized phase III trials of adjuvant chemotherapy in patients with early-stage ovarian carcinoma. J Natl Cancer Inst. 2003;**95**:105–12.
8. Bell J, Brady MF, Young RC, et al. Randomized phase III trial of three versus six cycles of adjuvant carboplatin and paclitaxel in early stage epithelial ovarian carcinoma: a Gynecologic Oncology Group study. Gynecol Oncol. 2006;**102**:432–9.
9. Mannel RS, Brady MF, Kohn EC, et al. A randomized phase III trial of IV carboplatin and paclitaxel × 3 courses followed by observation versus weekly maintenance low-dose paclitaxel in patients with early-stage ovarian carcinoma: A Gynecologic Oncology Group Study. Gynecol Oncol. 2011;**122**:89–94.
10. Travis LB, Holowaty EJ, Bergfeldt K, et al. Risk of leukemia after platinum-based chemotherapy for ovarian cancer. N Engl J Med. 1999;**340**:351–7.
11. Colombo N, Guthrie D, Chiari S, et al. International Collaborative Ovarian Neoplasm trial 1: a randomized trial of adjuvant chemotherapy in women with early-stage ovarian cancer. J Natl Cancer Inst. 2003;**95**:125–32.
12. Trimbos JB, Vergote I, Bolis G, et al. Impact of adjuvant chemotherapy and surgical staging in early-stage ovarian carcinoma: European Organisation for Research and Treatment of Cancer-Adjuvant ChemoTherapy in Ovarian Neoplasm trial. J Natl Cancer Inst. 2003;**95**:113–25.
13. Greene MH, Boice JD, Greer BE, et al. Acute nonlymphocytic leukemia after therapy with alkylating agents for ovarian cancer: a study of five

randomized clinical trials. N Engl J Med. 1982;**307**:1416–21.

14. Rose PG, Nerenstone S, Brady MF, et al. Secondary surgical cytoreduction for advanced ovarian carcinoma. N Engl J Med. 2004;**351**:2489–97.
15. Omura GA, Bundy BN, Berek JS, et al. Randomized trial of cyclophosphamide plus cisplatin with or without doxorubicin in ovarian carcinoma: a Gynecologic Oncology Group Study. J Clin Oncol. 1989;**7**:457–65.
16. Long-term results of a randomized trial comparing cisplatin with cisplatin and cyclophosphamide with cisplatin, cyclophosphamide, and adriamycin in advanced ovarian cancer. GICOG (Gruppo Interregionale Cooperativo Oncologico Ginecologia), Italy. Gynecol Oncol. 1992;**45**:115–17.
17. Conte PF, Bruzzone M, Chiara S, et al. A randomized trial comparing cisplatin plus cyclophosphamide versus cisplatin, doxorubicin, and cyclophosphamide in advanced ovarian cancer. J Clin Oncol. 1986;**4**:965–71.
18. Cyclophosphamide plus cisplatin versus cyclophosphamide, doxorubicin, and cisplatin chemotherapy of ovarian carcinoma: a meta-analysis. The Ovarian Cancer Meta-Analysis Project. J Clin Oncol. 1991;**9**:1668–74.
19. McGuire W, Hoskins W, Brady M, et al. Cyclophosphamide and cisplatin compared with paclitaxel and cisplatin in patients with stage III and stage IV ovarian cancer. N Engl J Med. 1996;**334**:1–6.
20. Piccart MJ, Bertelsen K, James K, et al. Randomized intergroup trial of cisplatin-paclitaxel versus cisplatin-cyclophosphamide in women with advanced epithelial ovarian cancer: three-year results. J Natl Cancer Inst. 2000;**92**:699–708.
21. Bookman MA, Brady MF, McGuire WP, et al. Evaluation of new platinum-based treatment regimens in advanced-stage ovarian cancer: a Phase III Trial of the Gynecologic Cancer Intergroup. J Clin Oncol. 2009;**27**:1419–25.
22. Markman M, Bundy B, Alberts D, et al. Phase III trial of standard-dose intravenous cisplatin plus paclitaxel versus moderately high-dose carboplatin followed by intravenous paclitaxel and intraperitoneal cisplatin in small-volume stage III ovarian carcinoma: an intergroup study of the Gynecologic Oncology Group, Southwestern Oncology Group, and Eastern Cooperative Oncology Group. J Clin Oncol. 2001;**19**:1001–7.
23. Bristow RE, Eisenhauer EL, Santillan A, et al. Delaying the primary surgical effort for advanced ovarian cancer: a systematic review of neoadjuvant chemotherapy and interval cytoreduction. Gynecol Oncol. 2007;**104**:480–90.
24. Vergote I, Tropé CG, Amant F, et al. Neoadjuvant chemotherapy or primary surgery in stage IIIC or IV ovarian cancer. N Engl J Med. 2010;**363**:943–53.
25. Vergote I, Amant F, Leunen K. Neoadjuvant chemotherapy in advanced ovarian cancer: what kind of evidence is needed to convince US gynaecological oncologists? Gynecol Oncol. 2010;**119**:1–2.
26. Cannistra S. Evaluating new regimens in recurrent ovarian cancer: how much evidence is good enough? J Clin Oncol. 2010;**28**:3101–3.
27. Pujade-Lauraine E, Wagner U, Aavall-Lundqvist E, et al. Pegylated liposomal doxorubicin and carboplatin compared with paclitaxel and carboplatin for patients with platinum-sensitive ovarian cancer in late relapse. J Clin Oncol. 2010;**28**:3323–9.
28. Cannistra S. Is there a "best" choice of second-line agent in the treatment of recurrent, potentially platinum-sensitive ovarian cancer? J Clin Oncol. 2002;**20**:1158–60.
29. Folkman J. Tumor angiogenesis: therapeutic implications. N Engl J Med. 1971;**285**:1182–6.
30. Burger R. Experience with bevacizumab in the management of epithelial ovarian cancer. J Clin Oncol. 2007;**25**:2902–8.
31. Randall L, Monk B. Bevacizumab toxicities and their management in ovarian cancer. Gynecol Oncol. 2010;**117**:497–504.
32. Ferrara N, Hillan K, Gerber H, et al. Discovery and development of bevacizumab, an anti-VEGF antibody for treating cancer. Nat Rev Drug Discov. 2004;**3**:391–400.
33. Byrne A, Ross L, Holash J, et al. Vascular endothelial growth factor-trap decreases tumor burden, inhibits ascites, and causes dramatic vascular remodeling in an ovarian cancer model. Clin Cancer Res. 2003;**9**:5721–8.
34. Burger R, Sill M, Monk B, et al. Phase II trial of bevacizumab in persistent or recurrent epithelial ovarian cancer or primary peritoneal cancer: a Gynecologic Oncology Group Study. J Clin Oncol. 2007;**25**:5165–71.
35. Cannistra S, Matulonis U, Penson R, et al. Phase II study of bevacizumab in patients with platinum-resistant ovarian cancer or peritoneal serous cancer. J Clin Oncol. 2007;**5**:5180–6.
36. Garcia A, Hirte H, Fleming G, et al. Phase II clinical trial of bevacizumab and low-dose metronomic oral cyclophosphamide in recurrent ovarian cancer: a trial of the California, Chicago, and Princess Margaret Hospital phase II consortia. J Clin Oncol. 2008;**6**:76–82.
37. Nimeiri H, Oza A, Morgan R, et al. Efficacy and safety of bevacizumab plus erlotinib for patients with recurrent ovarian, primary peritoneal, and fallopian tube cancer: a trial of the Chicago, PMH, and California Phase II Consortia. Gynecol Oncol. 2008;**110**:49–55.
38. Auranen A, Grénman S. Radiation therapy and biological compounds for consolidation therapy in advanced ovarian cancer. Int J Gynecol Cancer. 2008;**18**(Suppl 1):44–6.
39. Zhu X, Wu S, Dahut W, et al. Risks of proteinuria and hypertension with bevacizumab, an antibody against vascular endothelial growth factor: systematic review and meta-analysis. Am J Kidney Dis. 2007;**49**:186–93.
40. Kumaran G, Jayson G, Clamp A. Antiangiogenic drugs in ovarian cancer. Br J Cancer. 2009;**100**:1–7.
41. Barnhill DR, Kurman RJ, Brady MF, et al. Preliminary analysis of the behavior of stage I ovarian serous tumors of low malignant potential: a Gynecologic Oncology Group study. J Clin Oncol. 1995;**3**:2752–6.
42. Seidman JD, Kurman RJ. Ovarian serous borderline tumors: a critical review of the literature with emphasis on prognostic indicators. Hum Pathol. 2000;**31**:539–57.
43. Tropé C, Kaern J, Vergote IB, et al. Are borderline tumors of the ovary overtreated both surgically and systemically? A review of four prospective randomized trials including 253 patients with borderline tumors. Gynecol Oncol. 1993;**51**:236–43.

44. Gershenson DM, Silva EG. Serous ovarian tumors of low malignant potential with peritoneal implants. Cancer. 1990;**65**:578–85.

45. Barakat RR, Benjamin I, Lewis JL, et al. Platinum-based chemotherapy for advanced-stage serous ovarian carcinoma of low malignant potential. Gynecol Oncol. 1995;**59**:390–3.

46. Sutton GP, Bundy BN, Omura GA, et al. Stage III ovarian tumors of low malignant potential treated with cisplatin combination therapy (a Gynecologic Oncology Group study). Gynecol Oncol. 1991;**41**:230–3.

47. Gershenson D. Menstrual and reproductive function after treatment with combination chemotherapy for malignant ovarian germ cell tumors. J Clin Oncol. 1988;**6**:270–5.

48. Quirk JT, Natarajan N, Mettlin CJ. Age-specific ovarian cancer incidence rate patterns in the United States. Gynecol Oncol. 2005;**99**:248–50.

49. Gershenson DM, Copeland LJ, Kavanagh JJ, et al. Treatment of malignant nondysgerminomatous germ cell tumors of the ovary with vincristine, dactinomycin, and cyclophosphamide. Cancer. 1985;**56**:2756–61.

50. Williams SD, Blessing JA, Moore DH, et al. Cisplatin, vinblastine, and bleomycin in advanced and recurrent ovarian germ-cell tumors. A trial of the Gynecologic Oncology Group. Ann Intern Med. 1989;**111**:22–7.

51. Williams SD, Birch R, Einhorn LH, et al. Treatment of disseminated germ-cell tumors with cisplatin, bleomycin, and either vinblastine or etoposide. N Engl J Med. 1987;**316**:1435–40.

52. Tewari K, Di Saia P. Ovulatory failure, fertility preservation and reproductive strategies in the setting of gynecologic and non-gynecologic malignancies. Eur J Gynaecol Oncol. 2006;**27**:449–61.

53. Colombo N, Parma G, Zanagnolo V, et al. Management of ovarian stromal cell tumors. J Clin Oncol. 2007;**25**:2944–51.

54. Howlader N, Noone AM, Krapcho M, et al. SEER Cancer Statistics Review, 1975–2008, National Cancer Institute. Bethesda, MD, http://seer.cancer.gov/csr/1975_2008/, based on November 2010 SEER data submission, posted to the SEER web site, 2011.

Chapter 27

Intra-peritoneal chemotherapy

Maurie Markman, MD

Introduction

In early 2006, a third "positive" phase 3 randomized trial examining intra-peritoneal cisplatin-based chemotherapy as primary treatment of small-volume residual advanced ovarian cancer was reported [1]. This outcome led the United States National Cancer Institute to issue a "Clinical Announcement" describing the impact of this management strategy on outcome in this malignancy [2]. Since that time, several favorable and unfavorable critiques regarding this strategy have been published [3–7], revealing the controversy surrounding this novel management strategy. This chapter will review the basic biological foundation supporting intra-peritoneal chemotherapy in the management of ovarian cancer, clinical trial data supporting its routine use, and possible strategies to improve both the efficacy and toxicity associated with regional drug delivery in this setting.

Rationale for intra-peritoneal chemotherapy and early phase clinical trials

The theoretical rationale for delivering regional chemotherapy as treatment of ovarian cancer has previously been described in detail [8–12]. In brief, the arguments include the following considerations: (a) anatomic localization and natural history of the malignancy [9,10]; (b) pharmacokinetic advantage associated with the intra-peritoneal delivery of anti-neoplastic agents with known activity in ovarian cancer [11], and pre-clinical evidence for the impact of a clinically relevant "dose–response" effect for specific cytotoxic drugs against ovarian cancer at concentrations that are potentially achievable with regional delivery, but not after systemic administration [12].

It is particularly notable that, despite the fact it is common to discover extensive intra-abdominal disease at initial presentation of the malignancy, ovarian cancer remains principally confined (at least from the perspective of clinical manifestations) to the peritoneal cavity in most patients [9,10]. It is also relevant to acknowledge that a major attempt at optimal surgical cytoreduction to leave the patient with very small volume or preferably no residual macroscopic cancer before the initiation of cytotoxic chemotherapy has long been accepted as a standard management approach in ovarian cancer.

Phase 1 studies conducted over a period of more than 20 years confirmed both the pharmacokinetic advantage associated with the intra-peritoneal administration of several anti-neoplastic drugs (e.g., cisplatin, carboplatin, paclitaxel) [11,13–19] as well as any unique local toxicities associated with this class of agents when delivered by the intra-peritoneal route [20,21].

It is relevant to specifically comment here on the truly impressive differences in overall tumor exposure to anti-neoplastic drugs documented in these phase 1 trials following intra-peritoneal administration compared with the measured systemic concentrations of the agents when delivered by this route. For example, for cisplatin and carboplatin there was a 10- to 20-fold increase in both the peak concentration and the AUC (area under the concentration vs. time curve, AUC) between the two body compartments [14–17]. For paclitaxel, the peritoneal cavity exposure (peak and AUC) was shown to be 1,000-fold greater in the cavity compared with the systemic compartment with this route of drug delivery [18,19].

However, it is critical to also acknowledge that, because the actual depth of *direct penetration* of such drugs into malignant or normal tissue is quite limited (maximum of several millimeters) [22–24], it is highly likely that only the most superficial layers of cancer cells are actually exposed to the extremely high concentrations of these cytotoxic agents attainable following regional drug delivery [25].

Phase 2 trial of platinum-based intra-peritoneal chemotherapy in ovarian cancer

Based on these intriguing data, phase 2 intra-peritoneal trials, exploring both single agent and combination chemotherapy programs, were initiated in epithelial ovarian cancer [11,13]. These studies were conducted principally in the second-line setting, following the administration of front-line systemic platinum-based programs. The majority of these non-randomized trials were cisplatin-based, although both carboplatin-based and non-platinum-containing programs have been examined in this clinical setting.

In the phase 2 ovarian cancer regional treatment studies, responses were frequently determined by surgical assessment, because patients often began the regional treatment program

Altchek's Diagnosis and Management of Ovarian Disorders, ed. Liane Deligdisch, Nathan G. Kase, and Carmel J. Cohen. Published by Cambridge University Press.

with microscopic residual disease only or small tumor nodules not evident on radiographic evaluation. Of considerable interest and potentially substantial clinical relevance, several series reported complete response rates (surgically defined) to cisplatin-based intra-peritoneal treatment in the 20–40% range, despite the fact that in most circumstances these same patients had previously failed to achieve this clinical state following the administration of platinum-based intra-venous therapy [26].

Phase 3 randomized trials of primary cisplatin-based intra-peritoneal chemotherapy of advanced ovarian cancer

The provocative biological activity observed in the phase 2 setting as well as the reported prolonged survival of a sub-set of ovarian cancer patients treated with this strategy generated considerable interest in the gynecologic cancer community [27–29]. However, despite the existence of these data, it remained unknown if what was being observed was a unique and highly clinically relevant effect of the route of drug delivery, or simply the natural history of the cancers in a "selected" (superior prognostic clinical features) patient population.

Therefore, to directly address this important issue, randomized phase 3 trials comparing intra-peritoneal to intravenous drug delivery in ovarian cancer were initiated by several individual cancer centers and multi-institution cooperative groups. Unfortunately, several of these early attempts at evidence-based studies either failed to meet their original accrual goals or were seriously underpowered in their actual design to provide any meaningful answers to this question.

Fortunately, three well-designed and conducted phase 3 randomized trials undertaken by several cooperative groups in the United States (Gynecologic Oncology Group [GOG], Southwest Oncology Group [SWOG], Eastern Cooperative Oncology Group [ECOG]), have now been reported that directly address the utility of cisplatin-based chemotherapy in the primary management of small volume residual advanced ovarian cancer [1,30,31]. In addition, as previously noted, the impressive results of these trials led the National Cancer Institute (U.S.) to issue a "Clinical Announcement" to inform physicians, patients, and the public of the impact of this strategy on survival when used as primary treatment of small volume residual advanced (stage III) ovarian cancer [2].

The schema for these trials, and their reported results (Table 27.1), are briefly summarized below.

The initial study, conducted by the GOG and SWOG, was designed to compare intravenous cisplatin and cyclophosphamide (the "standard of care" in the management of advanced ovarian cancer at the time of initiation of this study) to a regimen of intra-peritoneal cisplatin plus intravenous cyclophosphamide [30]. Of note, the cisplatin dose was identical in each study arm (100 mg/m^2), and the size of the largest residual tumor mass permitted for trial entry following surgical cytoreduction was 2 cm.

The trial demonstrated reduced neutropenia and tinnitus associated with the regional treatment regimen (presumably due to modified pharmacokinetics and a slightly reduced total concentration of cisplatin present within the systemic circulation), but a somewhat greater risk of abdominal discomfort (mild to moderate in severity). There was no difference in mortality or the overall rate of severe toxicity between the arms. Of greatest importance, the study revealed a statistically significant improvement in survival associated with regional cisplatin administration (Table 27.1) [30].

Because the "standard of care" in the management of ovarian cancer had actually changed since the initiation of this landmark study until its conclusion, with the substitution of paclitaxel for cyclophosphamide [32], some investigators suggested that any documented benefits resulting from intra-peritoneal cisplatin-based treatment would be nullified by simply using the taxane (rather than the alkylating agent).

As a result, a second phase 3 randomized, intra-peritoneal chemotherapy trial was initiated to formally address this important issue [31]. The "control arm" in this study was the "new" GOG standard of intravenous cisplatin (75 mg/m^2) plus intravenous paclitaxel (135 mg^2 over 24 hours) [32].

This second study, conducted by the GOG, SWOG, and ECOG, only permitted patient entry if the largest remaining tumor mass after surgery was < 1 cm in maximum diameter.

It is also relevant to note that this particular study attempted to address an additional experimental question. Because

Table 27.1. Phase 3 trials examining front-line cisplatin-based regional versus systemic chemotherapy for small volume residual advanced epithelial ovarian cancer

	Progression-free survival (median)	Overall survival (median)
IP versus IV cisplatin (plus IV cyclophosphamide)[a] [30]	–	49 versus 41 months ($P=0.02$); HR 0.76
IP versus IV cisplatin (plus IV paclitaxel)[b] [31]	28 versus 22 months ($P=0.01$); HR 0.78	63 versus 52 months ($P=0.05$); HR 0.81
IP cisplatin/paclitaxel versus IV cisplatin (plus IV paclitaxel)[c] [1]	23.8 versus 18.3 months ($P=0.05$); HR 0.77	65.6 versus 49.7 months ($P=0.03$); HR 0.73

IP = intra-peritoneal
IV = intravenous
HR = hazard ratio

[a] Cisplatin dose in both arms 100 mg/m^2; all patients (both study arms) also received IV cyclophosphamide (600 mg/m^2) × 6 cycles.
[b] Control arm: IV cisplatin (75 mg/m^2) plus IV paclitaxel (135 mg/m^2 over 24-hours) × 6 cycles; "experimental arm": IV carboplatin (AUC 9 × 2 cycles) followed by cisplatin (100 mg/m^2) plus IV paclitaxel (135 mg/m^2 over 24-hours) × 6 cycles.
[c] Control arm: IV cisplatin (75 mg/m^2) plus IV paclitaxel (135 mg/m^2 over 24-hours) × 6 cycles; "experimental arm": IP cisplatin (100 mg/m^2) plus IV paclitaxel (135 mg/m^2 over 24-hours) plus IP paclitaxel (60 m/m^2; day 8) × 6 cycles.

previously published pre-clinical data had strongly suggested that regional treatment would be most effective in the setting of the smallest volume of residual cancer volume [22–24], in this phase 3 trial, individuals randomized to the intra-peritoneal treatment regimen were also given two cycles of moderately high dose carboplatin (AUC 9, every 28 days schedule) before the administration of the regional cisplatin (and intravenous paclitaxel) in a specific effort to "chemically debulk" the residual cancer volume before intra-peritoneal drug delivery [33].

Unfortunately, the addition of the systemic carboplatin cycles produced unexpected and excessive toxicity (principally prolonged severe thrombocytopenia). As a result, almost 20% of patients in the experimental study arm were unable to receive more than two courses of the planned regional therapy largely due to the persistent bone marrow abnormalities. However, despite this observation and using an appropriate prospectively defined intention-to-treat analysis, management with the regional treatment regimen/program was found to be associated with a statistically significant improvement in both progression-free and overall survival (Table 27.1) [31].

Of considerable importance, this study while confirming the favorable impact on outcome resulting from the regional administration of cisplatin also revealed the benefit of intra-peritoneal delivery was *additive* to that of the use of intravenous paclitaxel.

Finally, it is notable this phase 3 trial was the first randomized study in advanced ovarian cancer to report a median overall survival in one study arm of greater than 5 years [31].

The most recently reported phase 3 randomized intra-peritoneal trial was designed to more fully take advantage of the regional delivery of two cytotoxic agents, by adding *intra-peritoneal paclitaxel* to the therapeutic regimen.

This decision was based on the results of two previously conducted phase 1 studies which demonstrated a rather profound increase in tumor exposure to intra-peritoneal paclitaxel which resulted from the regional delivery of this agent (>1,000-fold compared with the systemic compartment) [18,19]. Furthermore, in a subsequently conducted second-line single agent paclitaxel phase 2 trial a high surgically documented complete response rate in the presence of only microscopic residual cancer was documented [25].

In the phase 3 study, conducted by the GOG, the "control arm" was again intravenous cisplatin and paclitaxel [32]. In the experimental study arm, paclitaxel was administered by both the intra-peritoneal and intravenous routes.

As might have been anticipated, the study revealed added toxicity associated with intra-peritoneal cisplatin, including both systemic (neutropenia, emesis, neurotoxicity) and local (abdominal pain, catheter-related) side effects [1]. With regard to the observed systemic toxicity for the experimental regimen, it should be noted the dose of intra-peritoneal cisplatin was 100 mg/m^2, while intravenous cisplatin was delivered at a dose of 75 mg/m^2 in the "control" regimen. However, of considerable relevance to the issue of the toxicity of the regional program, there was no difference in treatment-related mortality between the study arms [1].

It is important to also acknowledge that a formal quality-of-life analysis was conducted as a prospective component of this particular phase 3 randomized regional treatment trial. Based on the toxicity profile of the study and control regimens it is not surprising that during treatment the quality-of-life was reduced in the intra-peritoneal study arm compared with the intravenous regimen. However, there was no difference between the regimens in this measured clinical parameter 1 year following the completion of therapy.

Again, treatment with the regionally delivered cisplatin and paclitaxel was associated with an improvement in both progression-free and overall survival (Table 27.1), the third major randomized phase 3 trial to reach this identical conclusion.

Concerns with the results of these evidence-based trials and the toxicity of intra-peritoneal chemotherapy in the management of ovarian cancer

Despite the favorable reported outcomes of these now published phase 3 trials several objections have been raised regarding the study results and the routine use of regional platinum-based chemotherapy outside the setting of a clinical trial. These concerns will be summarized below, with brief corresponding responses:

Intra-peritoneal chemotherapy is too toxic

As previously noted, the administration of intra-peritoneal cisplatin is clearly associated with a greater risk of both systemic and local toxicity, compared with intravenous delivery of cisplatin (particularly at a dose of 100 mg/m^2) or carboplatin-based regimens [1]. However, it must be clearly acknowledged that there was *no increase* in therapy-related mortality in any of the three previously discussed phase 3 intra-peritoneal chemotherapy trials [1,30,31]. Furthermore, a quality-of-life analysis in the third study revealed no statistically significant differences in overall quality-of-life between the intravenous versus intra-peritoneal regimens 1 year after the completion of therapy [1].

Finally, it is quite relevant to specifically state that these three studies were actually conducted in the cooperative group setting (not necessarily "tertiary care") and there is surely a "learning curve" associated with the use of this (or any other) new management strategy. As a result, it is reasonable to speculate that, as a particular center attains greater experience with intra-peritoneal drug delivery, the ability to successfully manage the side effects of such treatment (e.g., dealing with complications of indwelling intra-peritoneal catheters; management of persistent abdominal discomfort due to infused treatment volume) will improve substantially.

Also, as will be discussed below, it is highly likely that quite modest modifications in the intra-peritoneal regimen (e.g., reduced dose of cisplatin) will substantially decrease the toxicity and inconvenience associated with regional therapy.

The favorable survival outcome was the direct result of a greater concentration of cisplatin reaching the systemic circulation with the higher dose of intra-peritoneal cisplatin (100 mg/m^2) compared with intravenous cisplatin (75 mg/m^2) used in the control arms of the two most recent studies

While it is factually correct that a higher total dose of cisplatin was used in these two studies the results of multiple previously published phase 3 randomized trials have now quite convincingly documented that the truly modest increase in "dose intensity" and slightly higher platinum concentrations within the systemic compartment *do not improve* either the objective response rate or survival in advanced ovarian cancer [34–37].

As a result, there is no existing evidence-based data to suggest that any increase in exposure to tumor through the systemic circulation resulting from the slight increase in platinum reaching that compartment by means of the peritoneal space following regional delivery would enhance efficacy, although these high concentrations could surely *increase toxicity* (as demonstrated in these trials).

The "control arm" of the last intra-peritoneal trial should have been carboplatin plus paclitaxel rather than cisplatin plus paclitaxel to truly evaluate the relative efficacy versus toxicity

It is acknowledged that the current "standard-of-care" for the systemic management of epithelial ovarian cancer includes carboplatin, rather than cisplatin. However, multiple phase 3 randomized trials have clearly shown these two platinum agents are equivalent in efficacy in ovarian cancer [38–42]. In fact, the specific choice to use carboplatin in routine clinical practice is based on its *superior toxicity profile*. As a result, while it is highly likely there would have been an even greater difference in observed side effects between the study arms if the control regimen in the third randomized phase 3 trial had been carboplatin plus paclitaxel, rather than cisplatin with paclitaxel, there is absolutely no justification for the suggestion the improved survival outcome associated with regional drug delivery in this study would have been different.

Suggested strategies to decrease the toxicity of intra-peritoneal therapy and make the approach more acceptable in routine clinical practice

Several reasonable approaches have been proposed to improve both the complexity and side effects associated with the intra-peritoneal treatment of ovarian cancer.

As previously acknowledged there will be an obvious "learning curve" when an individual physician or practice elects to use this novel technique. For example, medical, surgical, and gynecologic oncologists may have no prior experience with indwelling catheters. This will include both their placement and the management of complications (e.g., intra-abdominal infections) [43,44].

It is also reasonable to suggest that it may be most appropriate in certain settings for physicians to refer ovarian cancer patients who present with small volume residual advanced ovarian cancer to other oncologists or centers with both the expertise and personnel to administer intra-peritoneal therapy. However, it is critical to acknowledge that the available data clearly indicate this management approach can be safely and effectively delivered outside the setting of a tertiary medical center [1,3,30,31].

It is also appropriate to strongly suggest that the greatest percentage and severity of the toxicity observed in the intra-peritoneal arm of the most recently reported phase 3 randomized trial was the result of higher concentration of cisplatin within the systemic circulation [1]. And in the absence of data demonstrating the therapeutic benefits of such platinum concentrations [38–42], it is very reasonable to conclude that a modest reduction in the dose of cisplatin delivered by the intra-peritoneal route (e.g., to 75 or 80 mg/m^2) will improve the side effect profile of treatment, without a legitimate concern for impairing the efficacy of this strategy. In fact, following this approach, the concentration of platinum within the peritoneal cavity will still be in the range of 10- to 20-fold higher than that achieved in the systemic circulation [14,15].

Finally, it is also reasonable to anticipate that, with further experience with this strategy by clinical investigators, both within university centers and in the community setting, there will be additional practical suggestions offered to improve the utility of this novel approach to the treatment of women of advanced ovarian cancer. For example, by delivering intra-peritoneal cisplatin on day 1, and intravenous paclitaxel on day 2, this should permit the paclitaxel to be administered as a 3-hour, rather than a 24-hour infusion, possibly preventing the requirement for a hospital admission associated with use of this strategy in many practice settings [3].

Future research directions

While the favorable impact of regional drug delivery has been established, several important questions clearly remain, which should be the subject of future randomized trials.

First, an obvious issue is the clinical utility of carboplatin, versus cisplatin, when administered by the intra-peritoneal route in ovarian cancer. Data from phase 1 pharmacokinetic and safety studies have confirmed the potential for use of this agent by the intra-peritoneal route [16,17], and activity has been confirmed in the phase 2 setting [45]. Considering the documented survival advantage associated with intra-peritoneal cisplatin when used as primary chemotherapy of small volume residual advanced ovarian cancer [1,30,31], it would be inappropriate to simply assume carboplatin can be substituted for cisplatin in this setting. Of note, a randomized phase 3 trial addressing this issue and being conducted by the GOG that directly compares intra-peritoneal cisplatin to intra-peritoneal carboplatin is currently in progress.

Second, it will be important that future research efforts focus on a variety of technical aspects of regional treatment which may improve both the effectiveness and toxicity of this management strategy [44,46]. Specific issues that need to be addressed include the optimal type of indwelling catheter and the timing of catheter placement in specific clinical setting (e.g., the same time as primary bowel resection, or at a subsequent surgery?).

Third, existing data lead to the provocative idea that there are other settings where regional treatment of ovarian cancer may be superior to intravenous therapy. One important example is the patient with very advanced disease who undergoes an interval surgical cytoreduction following an excellent response to neoadjuvant chemotherapy and now has no gross residual cancer. Should further treatment be delivered by the intra-peritoneal route? This question is currently being addressed in an important randomized trial being conducted in Canada and Europe.

It will also be important to explore the use of novel anti-neoplastic agents recently demonstrated to be of clinical value in advanced ovarian cancer (e.g., bevacizumab), either administered by the intra-peritoneal route, or systemically in addition to intra-peritoneal platinum-based treatment [47].

Finally, one of the more interesting observations of the phase 3 intra-peritoneal trials previously discussed is the fact that a major survival benefit was noted despite a substantial percentage of the treated population actually being unable to receive all the planned courses of regional therapy. In fact, in the most recently reported study, only 42% of those randomized to intra-peritoneal cisplatin and paclitaxel completed six cycles, compared with > 80% of women completing six cycles in the systemic treatment arm [1].

The obvious questions to be addressed are:

(1) Is it necessary for ovarian cancer patients to receive the planned six cycles of intra-peritoneal cisplatin to achieve maximal utility from use of this route of drug administration? Would patients do as well with only three or four regional cycles, perhaps following an initial three cycles of systemically delivered drugs?
(2) Conversely, is it possible the survival advantage observed in this trial would have been even greater if a larger percentage of patients were able to complete six cycles of intra-peritoneal therapy? Of course, this assumes it is possible to develop strategies to reduce treatment-related toxicity and permit more regional treatment.

It is reasonable to suggest that a future randomized trial designed to directly address these questions might be beneficial in helping to define the optimal use of regional therapy in the management of advanced epithelial ovarian cancer.

References

1. Armstrong DK, Bundy B, Wenzel, et al. Intraperitoneal cisplatin and paclitaxel in ovarian cancer. N Engl J Med. 2006;**354**:34–43.
2. Trimble EL, Alvarez RD. Intraperitoneal chemotherapy and the NCI clinical announcement. Gynecol Oncol. 2006;**103**:S18–19.
3. Markman M, Walker JL. Intraperitoneal chemotherapy of ovarian cancer: a review with a focus on practical aspects of treatment. J Clin Oncol. 2006;**24**:988–94.
4. Ozols RF, Bookman MA, duBois A, et al. Intraperitoneal cisplatin therapy in ovarian cancer: comparison with standard intravenous carboplatin and paclitaxel. Gynecol Oncol. 2006;**103**:1–6.
5. Gore M, duBois A, Vergote I. Intraperitoneal chemotherapy in ovarian cancer remains experimental. J Clin Oncol. 2006;**24**:4528–30.
6. Armstrong DK, Brady MF. Intraperitoneal therapy for ovarian cancer: a treatment ready for prime time. J Clin Oncol. 2006;**24**:4531–3.
7. Cannistra SA. Intraperitoneal chemotherapy comes of age. N Engl J Med. 2006;**354**:77–9.
8. Dedrick RL, Myers CE, Bungay PM, DeVita VT Jr. Pharmacokinetic rationale for peritoneal drug administration in the treatment of ovarian cancer. Cancer Treat Rep. 1978;**62**:1–9.
9. Bergman F. Carcinoma of the ovary: a clinicopathological study of 86 autopsied cases with special reference to mode of spread. Acta Obstet Gynecol Scand. 1966;**45**:211–31.
10. Dauplat J, Hacker NF, Nieberg RK, et al. Distant metastases in epithelial ovarian carcinoma. Cancer. 1987;**60**:1561–6.
11. Markman M. Intraperitoneal drug delivery of antineoplastics. Drugs. 2001;**61**:1057–65.
12. Alberts DS, Young L, Mason N, Salmon SE. In vitro evaluation of anticancer drugs against ovarian cancer at concentrations achievable by intraperitoneal administration. Semin Oncol. 1985;**12**:38–42.
13. Markman M. Intraperitoneal antineoplastic drug delivery: rationale and results. Lancet Oncol. 2003;**4**:277–83.
14. Howell SB, Pfeifle CL, Wung WE, et al. Intraperitoneal cisplatin with systemic thiosulfate protection. Ann Intern Med. 1982;**97**:845–51.
15. Casper ES, Kelsen DP, Alcock NW, Lewis JL Jr. Ip cisplatin in patients with malignant ascites: pharmacokinetic evaluation and comparison with the iv route. Cancer Treat Rep. 1983;**67**:235–8.
16. Degregorio MW, Lum BL, Holleran WM, et al. Preliminary observations of intraperitoneal carboplatin pharmacokinetics during a phase I study of the Northern California Oncology Group. Cancer Chemother Pharmacol. 1986;**18**:235–8.
17. Elferink F, van der Vijgh WJ, Klein I, et al. Pharmacokinetics of carboplatin after intraperitoneal administration. Cancer Chemother Pharmacol. 1988;**21**:57–60.
18. Markman M, Rowinsky E, Hakes T, et al. Phase I trial of intraperitoneal taxol: a Gynecologic Oncology Group study. J Clin Oncol. 1992;**10**:1485–91.
19. Francis P, Rowinsky E, Schneider J, et al. Phase I feasibility and pharmacologic study of weekly intraperitoneal paclitaxel: a Gynecologic Oncology Group Pilot Study. J Clin Oncol. 1995;**13**:2961–7.
20. Markman M, George M, Hakes T, et al. Phase II trial of intraperitoneal mitoxantrone in the management of refractory ovarian cancer. J Clin Oncol. 1990;**8**:146–50.

21. Ozols RF, Young RC, Speyer JL, et al. Phase I and pharmacological studies of adriamycin administered intraperitoneally to patients with ovarian cancer. Cancer Res. 1982;**42**:4265–9.

22. Ozols RF, Locker GY, Doroshow JH, et al. Pharmacokinetics of adriamycin and tissue penetration in murine ovarian cancer. Cancer Res. 1979;**39**:3209–14.

23. Los G, Mutsaers PHA, van der Vijgh WJF, et al. Direct diffusion of cis-diamminedichloroplatinum(II) in intraperitoneal rat tumors after intraperitoneal chemotherapy: A comparison with systemic chemotherapy. Cancer Res. 1989;**49**:3380–4.

24. Nederman T, Carlsson J. Penetration and binding of vinblastine and 5-fluorouracil in cellular spheroids. Cancer Chemother Pharmacol. 1984;**13**:131–5.

25. Markman M, Brady MF, Spirtos NM, et al. Phase II trial of intraperitoneal paclitaxel in carcinoma of the ovary, tube, and peritoneum: a Gynecologic Oncology Group Study. J Clin Oncol. 1998;**16**:2620–4.

26. Markman M, Reichman B, Hakes T, et al. Responses to second-line cisplatin-based intraperitoneal therapy in ovarian cancer: influence of a prior response to intravenous cisplatin. J Clin Oncol. 1991;**9**:1801–5.

27. Markman M, Reichman B, Hakes T, et al. Impact on survival of surgically defined favorable responses to salvage intraperitoneal chemotherapy in small-volume residual ovarian cancer. J Clin Oncol. 1992;**10**:1479–84.

28. Howell SB, Zimm S, Markman M, et al. Long-term survival of advanced refractory ovarian carcinoma patients with small-volume disease treated with intraperitoneal chemotherapy. J Clin Oncol. 1987;**5**:1607–12.

29. Barakat RR, Sabbatini P, Bhaskaran D, et al. Intraperitoneal chemotherapy for ovarian carcinoma: results of long-term follow-up. J Clin Oncol. 2002;**20**:694–8.

30. Alberts DS, Liu PY, Hannigan EV, et al. Intraperitoneal cisplatin plus intravenous cyclophosphamide versus intravenous cisplatin plus intravenous cyclophosphamide for stage III ovarian cancer. N Engl J Med. 1996;**335**:1950–5.

31. Markman M, Bundy BN, Alberts DS, et al. Phase III trial of standard-dose intravenous cisplatin plus paclitaxel versus moderately high-dose carboplatin followed by intravenous paclitaxel and intraperitoneal cisplatin in small-volume stage III ovarian carcinoma: an intergroup study of the Gynecologic Oncology Group, Southwestern Oncology Group, and Eastern Cooperative Oncology Group. J Clin Oncol. 2001;**19**:1001–7.

32. McGuire WP, Hoskins WJ, Brady MF, et al. Cyclophosphamide and cisplatin compared with paclitaxel and cisplatin in patients with stage III and stage IV ovarian cancer. N Engl J Med. 1996;**334**:1–6.

33. Shapiro F, Schneider J, Markman M, et al. High-intensity intravenous cyclophosphamide and cisplatin, interim surgical debulking, and intraperitoneal cisplatin in advanced ovarian carcinoma: a pilot trial with ten-year follow-up. Gynecol Oncol. 1997;**67**:39–45.

34. McGuire WP, Hoskins WJ, Brady MF, et al. Assessment of dose-intensive therapy in suboptimally debulked ovarian cancer: a Gynecologic Oncology Group study. J Clin Oncol. 1995;**13**:1589–99.

35. Gore M, Mainwaring P, A'Hern R, et al. Randomized trial of dose-intensity with single-agent carboplatin in patients with epithelial ovarian cancer. London Gynaecological Oncology Group. J Clin Oncol. 1998;**16**:2426–34.

36. Conte PF, Bruzzone M, Carnino F, et al. High-dose versus low-dose cisplatin in combination with cyclophosphamide and epidoxorubicin in suboptimal ovarian cancer: a randomized study of the Gruppo Oncologico Nord-Ovest. J Clin Oncol. 1996;**14**:351–6.

37. Jakobsen A, Bertelsen K, Andersen JE, et al. Dose-effect study of carboplatin in ovarian cancer: a Danish Ovarian Cancer Group study. J Clin Oncol. 1997;**15**:193–8.

38. Covens A, Carey M, Bryson P, et al. Systematic review of first-line chemotherapy for newly diagnosed postoperative patients with stage II, III, or IV epithelial ovarian cancer. Gynecol Oncol. 2002;**85**:71–80.

39. Alberts DS, Green S, Hannigan EV, et al. Improved therapeutic index of carboplatin plus cyclophosphamide versus cisplatin plus cyclophosphamide: final report by the Southwest Oncology Group of a phase III randomized trial in stages III and IV ovarian cancer. J Clin Oncol. 1992;**10**:706–17.

40. Swenerton K, Jeffrey J, Stuart G, et al. Cisplatin-cyclophosphamide versus carboplatin-cyclophosphamide in advanced ovarian cancer: a randomized phase III study of the National Cancer Institute of Canada Clinical Trials Group. J Clin Oncol. 1992;**10**:718–26.

41. duBois A, Luck HJ, Meier W, et al. A randomized clinical trial of cisplatin/paclitaxel versus carboplatin/paclitaxel as first-line treatment of ovarian cancer. J Natl Cancer Inst. 2003;**95**:1320–9.

42. Ozols RF, Bundy BN, Greer BE, et al. Phase III trial of carboplatin and paclitaxel compared with cisplatin and paclitaxel in patients with optimally resected stage III ovarian cancer: a Gynecologic Oncology Group study. J Clin Oncol. 2003;**21**:3194–200.

43. Davidson SA, Rubin SC, Markman M, et al. Intraperitoneal chemotherapy: analysis of complications with an implanted subcutaneous port and catheter system. Gynecol Oncol. 1991;**41**:101–6.

44. Walker JL, Armstrong DK, Huang HQ, et al. Intraperitoneal catheter outcomes in a phase III trial of intravenous versus intraperitoneal chemotherapy in optimal stage III ovarian and primary peritoneal cancer: a Gynecologic Oncology Group Study. Gynecol Oncol. 2006;**100**:27–32.

45. Fujiwara K, Markman M, Morgan M, Coleman RL. Intraperitoneal carboplatin-based chemotherapy for epithelial ovarian cancer. Gynecol Oncol. 2005;**97**:10–15.

46. Dizon DS, Sill MW, Gould N, et al. Phase 1 feasibility study of intraperitoneal cisplatin and intravenous paclitaxel followed by intraperitoneal paclitaxel in untreated ovarian, fallopian tube, and primary peritoneal carcinoma: a Gynecologic Oncology Group Study. Gynecol Oncol. 2011;**123**:182–6.

47. Burger RA. Overview of anti-angiogenic agents in development for ovarian cancer. Gynecol Oncol. 2011;**121**:230–8.

Chapter 28

Malignant germ cell tumors and sex cord-stromal tumors in adults and children

Jubilee Brown, MD, and David M. Gershenson, MD

Malignant germ cell tumors

Malignant germ cell tumors of the ovary are rare ovarian tumors which tend to arise in adolescent and young adult females. While benign germ cell tumors, such as mature teratomas, represent approximately 25% of all ovarian neoplasms, less than 5% of these tumors are malignant. These tumors are usually curable due to a combination of early detection and exquisite chemosensitivity [1–3].

Epidemiology and risk factors

The incidence of malignant germ cell tumors is estimated to be 0.34 to 0.41 per 100,000 women in the United States, most commonly occurring in adolescents and young adults, with a median age of 23 years [4]. Rates seem to have declined over the past 30 years, but the reason for this is unclear [1,2]. The racial distribution of germ cell tumors is specific only for dysgerminoma, which occurs twice as often in non-blacks compared with blacks, and teratoma, which occurs more often in non-whites compared with whites [2,9].

Most germ cell tumors do not appear to be related to a hereditary cancer syndrome. There are several case reports of familial clusters of germ cell tumors; therefore, a rare familial gonadal tumor syndrome may exist but as yet is undescribed [6].

Females with gonadal dysgenesis, however, are at high risk for developing a malignant germ cell tumor. This defect in gonadal development could result in "streak gonads," in turn causing abnormal sex steroid production with resultant delayed puberty or primary amenorrhea. Two-thirds of dysgenetic gonads are due to Turner's syndrome, most of whom have a mosaic karyotype with 45X and a partial Y fragment. The remainder occur in 46 XX or 46 XY individuals, or in patients with Swyer's syndrome (complete gonadal dysgenesis with 46 XY but a female phenotype) and may affect over 30% of patients [7]. If streak gonads or Swyer's syndrome is identified, prophylactic removal of both gonads is indicated [7].

Classification and pathology

The World Health Organization (WHO) classifies germ cell tumors into three broad categories that include primitive germ cell tumors, biphasic or triphasic teratomas, and monodermal teratomas (Table 28.1). The distribution of subtypes includes immature teratoma (36%), dysgerminoma (33%), endodermal sinus tumor (15%), mixed non-dysgerminoma types (5%), embryonal (4%), mature teratoma with malignant degeneration (3%), and choriocarcinoma (2%) [2].

Certain characteristics are specific to each histologic subtype. Dysgerminomas are usually solid tumors that are gray or white and have sheets of vesicular cells containing large nuclei with a fibrous stroma on microscopic examination. Immature teratomas are predominantly solid but may contain cystic areas. These tumors may contain hair or sebaceous material and exhibit necrosis and hemorrhage. Immature nervous tissue is required for diagnosis, but glands, bone, and muscle may be present [8]. Endodermal sinus tumors are usually solid and cystic with soft, friable, hemorrhagic, or necrotic tissue. Microscopy reveals the Schiller-Duval body (see Chapter 7).

Diagnosis

Most women with germ cell tumors present during adolescence or early adulthood with a mean age in the early 20s. Approximately 85% of patients will present with pelvic pain and/or a mass. Other presenting symptoms include abdominal distention (30%), fever (10%), vaginal bleeding (10%), and ovarian torsion [1,3]. When a pelvic mass is suspected in a woman of childbearing age, a pelvic and/or transvaginal ultrasound is the preferred initial imaging test, as it details ovarian structure well and avoids radiation. Most malignant germ cell tumors appear predominantly solid, [9,10] and specific characteristics may suggest the histologic diagnosis. Benign cystic teratomas, for example, are predominantly smaller and cystic (77% vs. 18%) compared with immature teratomas which are larger and entirely solid [9,10]. Other methods of preoperative extra-pelvic imaging are often omitted in the diagnostic evaluation of a suspected germ cell tumor because of the low likelihood of malignancy and metastatic spread.

Preoperative laboratory testing should include quantitative human β-chorionic gonadotropin (β-HCG), lactate dehydrogenase (LDH), α-Fetoprotein (AFP), and baseline hematology

Altchek's Diagnosis and Management of Ovarian Disorders, ed. Liane Deligdisch, Nathan G. Kase, and Carmel J. Cohen. Published by Cambridge University Press.

Table 28.1. Classification of ovarian germ cell tumors

I. Primitive germ cell tumors

- Dysgerminoma
- Endodermal sinus tumor (yolk sac tumor)
- Embryonal carcinoma
- Polyembryoma
- Nongestational choriocarcinoma
- Mixed germ cell tumor

II. Biphasic or triphasic teratoma

- Immature teratoma
- Mature teratoma
- Solid
- Cystic (dermoid)
- Fetiform teratoma (homunculus)

III. Monodermal teratoma and somatic-type tumors associated with group II (above)

- Thyroid (struma ovarii)
- Carcinoid
- Neuroectodermal
- Carcinoma
- Melanocytic
- Sarcoma
- Sebaceous
- Pituitary-type
- Other

Adapted from World Health Organization classification of tumors: Tavassoli FA and Deville P. Pathology and Genetics of Tumors of the Breast and Female Genital Organs, Lyon France: International Agency for Research on Cancer, 2003.

Table 28.2. Tumor markers in malignant ovarian germ cell tumors

	Tumor marker		
Tumor	AFP	LDH	β-hCG
Dysgerminoma	Usually normal	Elevated	May be elevated
Immature teratoma	May be elevated	May be elevated	Normal
Endodermal sinus tumor	Elevated	May be elevated	Normal
Embryonal carcinoma	Elevated	May be elevated	Elevated
Choriocarcinoma	Normal	Normal	Elevated

and electrolyte panels [11,12]. Elevations in β-HCG and AFP suggest a malignant germ cell tumor, but patterns of marker elevations may vary (Table 28.2). Additionally, non-epithelial ovarian cancers may be suggested by additional immunoassays, such as CA125, transthyretin, apolipoprotein A1, β_2-microglobulin, and transferrin, with up to a 78% sensitivity, but further characterization of these patterns are needed in rare tumor subtypes [13]. A preoperative karyotype may be warranted if gonadal dysgenesis is suspected to enable preoperative counseling for removal of both ovaries, if warranted based on the karyotype. Definitive diagnosis, however, is made by histologic examination of the tumor removed at the time of surgery. Most malignant germ cell tumors are stage I at the time of diagnosis.

Treatment

Surgery

The definitive diagnosis and initial treatment of patients with malignant germ cell tumors of the ovary is surgery, with an emphasis on preservation of fertility. Fertility-sparing surgery appears to be safe with excellent survival after long-term follow-up equivalent to patients undergoing hysterectomy with bilateral salpingo-oophorectomy [4,14]. Because approximately 60% of these tumors are limited to one ovary at the time of surgery, unilateral salpingo-oophorectomy is recommended in females who desire future fertility, as most of the patients with these tumors are in their reproductive years. Both ovaries are affected in 10–15% of dysgerminomas; in which case bilateral salpingo-oophorectomy may be indicated, but every effort should be made to preserve fertility [3]. The uterus can almost always be preserved, as it is not typically involved. Therefore, assisted reproduction with donor egg may be useful in the future for patients requiring bilateral ovarian removal. In the case of widespread uterine serosal involvement, hysterectomy may be indicated, but this is the rare exception. This approach to conservative surgery, in which the maximum amount of reproductive potential is preserved, does not suggest an ovarian cystectomy, but rather a unilateral salpingo-oophorectomy with conservation of the normal-appearing contralateral ovary, tube, and uterus. When an ovarian cystectomy has been performed for presumed benign ovarian disease and the postoperative diagnosis of immature teratoma is rendered, there may be little utility in excising the remaining ovarian tissue, however, as excellent survival has been reported; most of these patients did receive adjuvant chemotherapy [15]. Of note, in patients who have completed childbearing, a hysterectomy and bilateral salpingo-oophorectomy is warranted.

The necessity and extent of comprehensive surgical staging has received some scrutiny. The recommendation has generally been for comprehensive staging to include peritoneal cytology, peritoneal biopsies, omentectomy, and retroperitoneal lymphadenectomy including bilateral pelvic and para-aortic nodes and removal of any suspicious tissue, with tumor reductive surgery to be performed in the setting of disseminated disease. Evidence exists for the utility of lymphadenectomy, as 18% of patients with any malignant germ cell tumor in a SEER database review did have positive lymph nodes, and 28% of women with dysgerminoma had positive lymph nodes. Lymph node positivity was a negative predictor of survival in this study, although other studies refute this association [16,17]. Lymphadenectomy has also allowed chemotherapy to be avoided in patients with negative nodes. In a recent review in which half of patients with malignant germ cell tumors underwent comprehensive staging, none of the fully staged IA patients recurred during observation without adjuvant chemotherapy, while approximately 40% of unstaged apparent stage I patients did recur [18]. However, germ cell tumors are extremely chemosensitive, so most of these patients can be salvaged with chemotherapy if they do recur, with excellent survival regardless of the extent of initial surgical staging [19]. This has been used as evidence to avoid comprehensive surgical staging with lymphadenectomy, and avoid reoperation solely to perform comprehensive staging in the setting of a diagnosis made postoperatively. Additionally, based on the chemosensitivity of these tumors, extensive tumor reductive surgery may be limited to avoid increased morbidity or a long postoperative recovery with a delay in chemotherapy [19].

Chemotherapy

Postoperative chemotherapy consisting of bleomycin, etoposide, and cisplatin (BEP) is recommended for all patients with malignant germ cell tumors except stage I dysgerminomas and stage IA grade 1 immature teratomas. However, there is a growing body of literature supporting omission of chemotherapy for any patient with stage I immature teratoma. The intent to avoid chemotherapy in low-risk patients stems from the exquisite chemosensitivity of these tumors, as recurrences can almost always be successfully salvaged, thereby avoiding potentially unnecessary morbidity from chemotherapy in the majority of patients who will not recur [1,3,20]. Several cooperative group studies are under way to more closely define patient outcomes in low-risk patients who undergo surveillance rather than chemotherapy. To date, several smaller studies have examined patient outcomes in stage I patients undergoing surveillance rather than chemotherapy. Thirty-seven patients with stage IA germ cell tumors were followed after surgery without chemotherapy; 22% of dysgerminomas recurred, and 36% of non-dysgerminomas recurred. Upon salvage, only one patient failed to respond and the remainder were cured [20]. Other recent groups have reported similar rates of cure over 90% with surveillance and chemotherapy given for relapse [3,21–23]. At present, however, NCCN guidelines recommend chemotherapy for women with all malignant germ cell tumors except stage I dysgerminoma and stage IA grade 1 immature teratomas [11]. Additionally, the presence of other elements, such as endodermal sinus tumor, in these tumors is an indication for chemotherapy.

The 3-day and 5-day regimens for administration of BEP are listed in Table 28.3. Other regimens, including etoposide and cis- or carboplatin have been reported but are not first-line. These may be useful in the setting of toxicity. In the rare setting of refractory disease, alternate regimens may be considered, including cisplatin, vincristine, methotrexate, bleomycin (POMB); vinblastine, bleomycin, and cisplatin (VBP); dactinomycin, cyclophosphamide and etoposide (ACE); or vincristine, ifosfamide and cisplatin (VIP). It should be noted that long-term sequelae of regimens containing etoposide and platinum include a 1% risk of developing a secondary malignancy such as leukemia [24].

Radiation

The role of radiation for the treatment of malignant germ cell tumors is largely historical. Although dysgerminomas are sensitive to the effects of radiation with cure rates approaching 100% for early stage and approximately 60% for advanced disease [24], the development of effective chemotherapy in addition to the adverse effect of radiation on ovarian function has eliminated radiation from the treatment of these tumors.

Survival and prognosis

Five-year survival rates for malignant ovarian germ cell tumors approach 100% for stage I disease and up to 75% for advanced stage disease [3]. Overall 5-year survival rates range from 80% to 97% [2,4,5,16,19,20].

Prognostic factors include stage, lymph node involvement, tumor marker elevation, and histologic subtype. The stage at diagnosis is the most important prognostic factor for recurrence risk and overall survival, with a significant difference in reported overall survival of 98% for stage I and II tumors compared with 86% for stage III and IV patients [4]. The prognostic importance of lymph node involvement, although controversial, may indicate an increased risk of death up to three-fold higher compared with women without lymph node involvement [16]. The elevation of β-HCG and AFP at the time of diagnosis may confer a higher risk of recurrence [24,25]. Additionally, elevated markers should normalize during the course of treatment, and persistent elevation indicates refractory disease. Histologic subtype also predicts recurrence risk, with dysgerminomas having the best 5-year survival (99.5–100%), followed by immature teratomas (94.3–100%), and endodermal sinus tumors (72–85.5%) [4,26,27].

Table 28.3. Protocol for BEP (bleomycin, etoposide, and cisplatin)

1. Maintenance fluids of 5% dextrose in normal saline (NS) with 10 mEq/L potassium chloride and 8 mEq/L magnesium sulfate at 42 mL/hr are initiated on admission and continued during and 24 hours after chemotherapy.
2. Thirty minutes before cisplatin administration each day, prehydration with 1 L normal saline with 20 mEq potassium chloride and 16 mEq magnesium sulfate is given at 250 mL/h for 4 hours. The following premedications are also given:
   Ondansetron 8 mg in 50 mL NS intravenous piggyback (IVPB), and
   dexamethasone 20 mg in 50 mL NS IVPB, and
   diphenhydramine 50 mg in 50 mL NS.

Cisplatin 20 mg/m^2/day in 1 L NS with 50 g mannitol IVPB over 4 hours on days 1–5.

3. Follow cisplatin with 500 mL NS with 10 mEq KCl and 8 mEq magnesium sulfate at 250 mL/h.
4. Etoposide 100 mg/m^2 per day in 500 mL NS IVPB over 2 hours on days 1–5.
5. Bleomycin 10 IU in 1L NS IVPB over 24 hours on days 1–3.
6. Follow with:
   opndansetron 8 mg in 50 mL NS IVPB q8h, and
   albuterol nebulizers 2.5 mg q6h for 24 hours, and
   prochlorperazine 10 mg in 50 mL NS IVPB q6h as needed for nausea.

Regimen repeated every 3 weeks.

Therefore, the presence of endodermal sinus tumor elements in any tumor mandates chemotherapy, even if the tumor is stage IA.

Management of recurrent disease

Following active treatment, patients should undergo surveillance visits, consisting of history, physical, and pelvic examination, and relevant tumor markers. There is no role for routine imaging. Most patients with malignant germ cell tumors are cured, but when patients recur, most do so within 1 year after diagnosis. Recurrent disease is extremely rare after 2 years [1,3,24,25]. Elevated tumor markers are sensitive for recurrent disease and should prompt immediate evaluation with directed imaging. Biopsy or resection must confirm the diagnosis of recurrent disease, as immature teratomas can recur with mature benign elements only or with benign gliosis, neither of which is true malignant recurrences and do not require chemotherapy. Surgical resection may have limited success, and is a consideration in patients with immature teratoma.

When recurrence is documented, chemonaive patients should be treated with bleomycin, etoposide, and cisplatin; cure rates approach 100%. Because most patients who recur, however, are not chemonaive, the overall salvage rate is approximately 50%. In patients previously treated with BEP chemotherapy, other regimens can be attempted, including high dose salvage chemotherapy with stem cell transplant; VIP; PVB; POMB; ACE; paclitaxel, carboplatin, and ifosfamide; gemcitabine; oxaliplatin and paclitaxel; and targeted therapies including bevacizumab and sunitinib, but these remain experimental [28].

Special management issues

Post-treatment sequelae

Between 87% and 100% of women who undergo fertility-sparing surgery followed by chemotherapy will have subsequent normal menstrual function, although delayed puberty, irregular menses, and premature menopause have been reported [29,30]. Additionally, pregnancy appears to be frequent after such treatment, with successful pregnancies reported in about a third of the fertile women in one survey and up to 86% in another survey [29,30].

Quality of life has been investigated in survivors of malignant ovarian germ cell tumors, and most survivors have a quality of life equivalent to controls. However, decreased physical quality of life correlates with neurotoxicity. Better physical functioning appears to be associated with younger age of diagnosis and lack of gynecologic symptoms [31]. Survivors also had a higher incidence of hypertension, hypercholesterolemia, numbness, tinnitus, and nausea [32].

Future directions

Cooperative group trials are currently under way to inform the safety and sequelae of surveillance in patients with low-risk disease, namely stage I germ cell tumors.

Sex cord-stromal tumors

Sex cord-stromal ovarian tumors are rare tumors that comprise only 7% of all ovarian cancers, thus representing a small portion of all ovarian cancers, and an even smaller portion of the overall world cancer burden. However, many of these women are in their reproductive years, and successful fertility-sparing treatment is crucial. Additionally, many of these cancers are curable. There has been substantial progress made in the understanding and treatment of these tumors in the last decade. This chapter will present the patient centered data to direct the optimal treatment for patients with malignant sex cord-stromal tumors of the ovary.

Epidemiology and risk factors

The predicted incidence for all new cases of ovarian cancer in the United States is estimated to be 22,280 with 15,500 deaths anticipated for 2005 [33]. While 90% of ovarian malignancies are epithelial in origin, the remaining 10% are comprised of sex cord-stromal tumors, germ cell tumors, soft tissue tumors not specific to the ovary, unclassified tumors, and metastatic tumors [34]. The exact rates of sex cord-stromal ovarian cancers are not specified in these data, and even the estimates from the SEER database are non-specific for stromal ovarian tumors. In general, stromal tumors of the ovary are thought to account for 7% of ovarian malignancies, many of which occur in adolescent and young adult women [35]. Data from the SEER database between 1975 and 1998 suggest that for each 5-year interval between ages 15 and 40, the incidence of non-germ cell ovarian malignancy increases from 8 per million to 79 per million women per year, some of which are stromal tumors [36]. However, these data remain non-specific for stromal ovarian tumors.

Granulosa cell tumors are the most common histologic subtype of sex cord-stromal ovarian cancers and comprise between 2% and 5% of all ovarian cancers. Granulosa cell tumors represent 90% of stromal ovarian tumors, yielding an incidence of 0.58 to 1.6 cases per 100,000 women [37,38]. Adult- and juvenile granulosa cell tumors occur, but the adult subtype represents 95% of all granulosa cell tumors. The designation of juvenile versus adult granulosa cell tumor is not based on age, but instead on specific pathologic characteristics. That said, most adult granulosa cell tumors occur during the reproductive or peri-menopausal years, whereas most juvenile types occur during childhood and adolescence.

Fertility preservation is a significant concern in the treatment of sex cord-stromal tumors, as many of these tumors occur in adolescent and young women. While the majority of young women with ovarian cancer develop germ cell tumors, 10 to 15% of childhood ovarian tumors are sex cord-stromal tumors with juvenile granulosa cell tumors most often occurring in childhood and Sertoli–Leydig cell tumors and unclassified sex cord-stromal tumors occurring during puberty [39,40]. Neonatal presentations of juvenile granulosa cell tumors have been described [41].

Sertoli–Leydig cell tumors are rare tumors representing less than 1% of all ovarian tumors and may contain only Sertoli cells, only Leydig cells, or both. The mean age at diagnosis is 25 years, but intermediate and poorly differentiated tumors tend to be more aggressive and occur approximately 10 years earlier than well-differentiated tumors. The retiform type is usually diagnosed at an even younger age than intermediate or poorly differentiated types [42]. Fertility preservation is therefore an important consideration in many patients with Sertoli–Leydig cell tumors [43].

Sex cord tumor with annular tubules (SCTAT), first described by Scully in 1970, was identified in association with Peutz–Jeghers syndrome, and approximately 15% are associated with adenoma malignum of the cervix [44]. Although these tumors are uncommon in adolescents, they can present with isosexual precocity [45].

Gynandroblastomas are a rare type of stromal tumor which accounts for less than 1% of all ovarian stromal tumors. These tumors tend to occur during the third to fifth decades of life [46].

Steroid cell tumors not otherwise specified (NOS) represent less than 0.1% of all ovarian tumors. These are the most common type of steroid cell tumor and can be malignant and quite aggressive. These tumors present at a mean age of 43 years.

Knowledge on risk factors is scant for sex cord-stromal tumors of the ovary. In general, these do not appear to be hereditary cancers, although a case report describes two first-degree relatives with granulosa cell tumor of the ovary [47]. However, recent advances in genomic characterization of these tumors suggest that very specific mutations may give rise to adult granulosa cell tumors and Sertoli–Leydig cell tumors, respectively. Adult granulosa cell tumors have been linked to a missense mutation of *FOXL2*, which is a transcription factor linked to estrogen production. A specific mutation of cytosine to guanine at the 402 locus appears to be pathognomonic for the development of adult granulosa cell tumors [48]. Additionally, germline truncating mutations in *DICER1* appear to be linked to the development of non-epithelial ovarian tumors, and specifically Sertoli–Leydig cell tumors, in patients with pleuropulmonary blastoma, a familial syndrome characterized by childhood lung tumors and an increased incidence of sex cord-stromal ovarian cancers [49].

Classification and pathology

Sex cord-stromal tumors of the ovary arise from specialized gonadal stromal cells and their precursors. Typically, these tumors arise as a pelvic mass originating within one or both ovaries. These tumors can occur as an isolated histologic subtype or in combination. The classification is presented in Table 28.4 [34]. Specifically, granulosa cells and Sertoli cells arise from sex cord cells, whereas theca cells, Leydig cells, lipid cells, and fibroblasts arise from stromal cells and their pluripotential mesenchymal precursors. These cells are involved in steroid hormone production, and therefore symptoms and signs of excess estrogen or androgen production may be seen at the time of diagnosis [38].

Table 28.4. World Health Organization classification of stromal tumors of the ovary

I. Granulosa stromal cell tumors
Granulosa cell tumors
Juvenile
Adult
Thecomas/fibromas
Thecoma
Fibroma
Cellular fibroma
Fibrosarcoma
Stromal tumor with minor sex cord elements
Sclerosing luteoma
Unclassified (fibrothecoma)
II. Sertoli-stromal cell tumors androblastomas
Well differentiated
Sertoli cell tumor; androblastoma
Sertoli–Leydig cell tumor
Leydig cell tumor
Intermediate differentiation
Variant, with heterologous elements
Poorly differentiated (sarcomatoid)
Variant, with heterologous elements
Retiform
Mixed
III. Sex cord–stromal with annular tubules (SCTAT)
IV. Gynandroblastoma
V. Steroid (lipid) cell tumor
Stromal luteoma
Leydig cell tumor
VI. Unclassified

Sex cord-stromal ovarian tumors are related but have specific characteristics defining pathology [50]. Adult granulosa cell tumors represent 95% of granulosa cell tumors, whereas juvenile granulosa cell tumors represent 5% of granulosa cell tumors. Gross features are similar, with cystic and solid components. Microscopic examination reveals two characteristics which distinguish juvenile from adult granulosa cell tumors: the nuclei of juvenile granulosa cell tumors are rounded and hyperchromatic with moderate to abundant eosinophilic or vacuolated cytoplasm, and the theca cell component is luteinized in juvenile granulosa cell tumors [51].

Sertoli–Leydig cell tumors are solid and may have cystic components. Size is variable, ranging from microscopic to 25 cm. [52]. Well-differentiated tumors, responsible for 11% of cases, tend to be smaller than poorly differentiated tumors and have a predominantly tubular pattern on light microscopy [42]. Sertoli cells are cuboidal or columnar with round nuclei, but with no prominent nucleoli; atypical nuclei are absent or rare, and few mitotic figures are seen. The stroma consists of nests of Leydig cells. The most common variants show intermediate differentiation (54%) and poor differentiation (13%). These subgroups are characterized by a continuum of different patterns and combinations of cell types, with both Sertoli and Leydig components exhibiting various degrees of maturity.

A retiform component is present in 15% of tumors, demonstrating tubules and cysts arranged in a pattern that resembles the rete testis.

Sex cord tumor with annular tubules (SCTAT) is characterized by simple or complex ring-shaped tubules [51]. Gynandroblastomas are comprised of granulosa cell elements, tubules, and Leydig cells. Most of these tumors are solid and large, measuring between 7 and 10 cm in size, with yellow–white cystic areas present. Microscopically, these tumors show unequivocal granulosa/theca cell elements, must be well differentiated, and must demonstrate intimate mixing of all the constituent cell types [46].

Steroid cell tumors not otherwise specified have an average size of 8.5 cm and are often bilateral. The strongest prognostic factor other than stage is the number of mitotic figures, because over 90% of tumors with over two mitoses per 10 high power fields are malignant [51].

Vascular endothelial growth factor is overexpressed in a majority of stromal ovarian tumors, which may account for the typical tumor vascularity [53]. Inhibin and calretinin are immuno-histochemical stains which may aid in the pathologic diagnosis of sex cord-stromal ovarian tumors [54]. SF-1 is a diagnostically useful immuno-histochemical marker that aids in the differential diagnosis of Sertoli cell tumors [55].

Thecomas, fibromas, fibrothecomas, stromal luteomas, Leydig cell tumors, and sclerosing stromal cell tumors of the ovary will not be specifically discussed, as these tumors are considered to be benign.

Diagnosis

The diagnosis of a stromal tumor of the ovary is made on pathologic review of a surgical specimen. However, the diagnosis can be suggested by the history and physical examination and appropriate imaging techniques. The age of the patient in her adolescent or young adult years may suggest the diagnosis. Presenting symptoms and signs include bloating, pelvic pressure or pain, increase in abdominal girth, gastrointestinal or urinary symptoms, and a palpable pelvic mass. Over 95% of juvenile granulosa cell tumors are unilateral at presentation [56]. Juvenile granulosa cell tumor has also been associated with Ollier disease (enchromatosis) and Maffucci syndrome (enchromatosis and hemangiomatosis), so the unusual case of these findings should prompt consideration of a juvenile granulosa cell tumor [51]. Thirty percent of patients with granulosa cell tumors demonstrate evidence of hemoperitoneum, with abdominal pain and tenderness, peritoneal signs, a fluid wave, and even hemodynamic instability [51].

Because stromal tumors of the ovary arise from steroid-producing cells, these tumors are often hormonally active, producing estrogen, progesterone, and androgens. Therefore, physical manifestations of excess estrogens or androgen production can be the presenting symptoms or signs of a stromal tumor [51]. Patients may report hirsutism or virilism, which is present in half of patients with Sertoli–Leydig cell tumors and steroid cell tumors, and adolescents may describe isosexual precocious puberty. Hormonally related findings are present in 60% of patients with gynandroblastoma [51]. Patients during the reproductive years can present with menorrhagia, irregular menstrual bleeding, and amenorrhea. Post-menopausal patients may have vaginal bleeding, breast enlargement or tenderness, and vaginal cornification [57].

Any abnormal bleeding must be addressed during the diagnostic and/or preoperative evaluation. After excluding pregnancy in women during their reproductive years, an endometrial biopsy should be performed to exclude endometrial hyperplasia or cancer, because excess tumor-derived estrogen can induce these endometrial finding. This should be considered either preoperatively in the office or in the operating room upon the diagnosis of the ovarian stromal tumor [51].

Imaging tests which may prove useful in the diagnosis of the adnexal mass include transvaginal ultrasound, computed tomography (CT), and magnetic resonance imaging (MRI). Of these, the ultrasound is often the best for distinguishing the details of pelvic anatomy and may also identify hemoperitoneum or ascites. Findings are non-specific for stromal ovarian tumors, but certain characteristics do occur. Adult granulosa cell tumors may appear as solid masses, multilocular cystic lesions, or completely cystic tumors, and color flow Doppler usually shows increased vascularity [58]. Sertoli–Leydig cell tumors usually appear as a well-defined solid mass which enhances on CT and appears hypointense with variable-sized cystic areas on MRI. The amount of fibrous stroma determines the low signal intensity on T2-weighted MRI [59].

Tumor markers which may be useful in making the diagnosis preoperatively include inhibin A and B and CA125. These tests may facilitate preoperative diagnosis, but may be more important in following the response of the tumor to therapy in the post-operative setting [54].

Treatment

The treatment of stromal ovarian tumors is determined by many factors, including patient age, parity, desire for future fertility, extent of disease, and comorbid conditions. The surgeon may be faced with a patient with an adnexal mass, the precise histologic classification of which is difficult to determine, and frozen section diagnosis is difficult. The surgeon must then follow general guidelines for nonepithelial ovarian tumors during the initial operative management and re-evaluate the need for adjuvant or additional therapy on the basis of the final pathologic results. With close attention to all details, including histologic type, patient characteristics, and extent of disease, the need for re-exploration and more extensive surgery can be minimized.

Surgical therapy

When a pelvic mass is first diagnosed, the specific histologic diagnosis is unknown. However, using patient characteristics including age, physical diagnosis, and imaging characteristics as noted above, a stromal tumor of the ovary can be suspected. A frank discussion should always be held preoperatively with any woman of childbearing age who has an adnexal mass regarding her wishes for future fertility and her desires for maintaining ovarian and/or uterine function in light of the potential operative findings. Although this is often a difficult conversation for the physician to initiate, it is better discussed preoperatively with the patient than intra-operatively with the next of kin when a malignancy is encountered [43]. The goals of surgical therapy are accurate diagnosis, removal of the mass, comprehensive staging, tumor reduction when disseminated disease is present, and preservation of fertility when desired and feasible in patients of reproductive age.

Laparoscopy is appropriate in the occasional patient with a small solid adnexal mass or complex ovarian cyst [60]. However, any patient with a large, solid adnexal mass or evidence of hemodynamic instability should undergo laparotomy through a vertical skin incision to remove the mass without morcellation and allow for appropriate surgical staging, if necessary [38]. Upon initial inspection, gross characteristics noted above can suggest the diagnosis. Upon entering the peritoneal cavity, the surgeon should obtain pelvic washings and evacuate the hemoperitoneum, if present. The site of hemorrhage is most commonly the mass itself, and therefore surgical removal may stop the bleeding. A unilateral mass in a patient of any age should be removed by unilateral salpingo-oophorectomy – not ovarian cystectomy – and sent for immediate histologic evaluation [43]. Morcellation should be avoided, as this results in the disease being classified as a more advanced stage and may adversely affect survival [37]. In cases using minimally invasive surgery, the mass should be placed into a bag and an extended incision should be made to remove the mass in the bag.

Occasionally, to remove what is thought to be a benign dermoid cyst, an ovarian cystectomy is performed in an attempt to preserve ovarian tissue. In these cases, the tumor should be sent for immediate histologic evaluation, and in the event of a sex cord-stromal tumor, the entire ovary should be removed [38,43]. No support exists in the literature for ovarian cystectomy in pre-menopausal patients with sex cord-stromal tumors. Articles that summarize "conservative management" of these tumors refer to unilateral salpingo-oophorectomy with conservation of the normal contralateral ovary in patients with limited disease. Therefore, unilateral salpingo-oophorectomy is the initial step in the treatment of patients with apparent limited disease [38,43].

Once the diagnosis of a sex cord-stromal tumor is made, the surgical procedure includes exploration of the entire abdominopelvic cavity with attention paid to all peritoneal surfaces and abdominopelvic organs. A complete staging procedure should be performed, including cytologic evaluation of each hemidiaphragm, infracolic omentectomy, and peritoneal biopsies from each paracolic gutter, the vesicouterine fold, and the pouch of Douglas. Any suspicious areas should be biopsied. Pelvic and para-aortic lymph node sampling have historically been recommended for a comprehensive staging procedure, but recent literature suggests that lymph node metastases are so very rare that lymphadenectomy may be omitted from the comprehensive staging procedure. Tumor reductive surgery should be performed in patients with advanced disease to reduce the tumor burden as much as possible, preferably leaving the patient with no macroscopic disease [38,43,61].

Patients who have completed childbearing should undergo total abdominal hysterectomy and bilateral salpingo-oophorectomy regardless of the stage of disease. However, fertility-sparing surgery is an essential consideration in patients of reproductive age [43]. In the unusual circumstance that the contralateral ovary and/or uterine serosa are grossly involved by tumor, the surgeon may have no choice but to remove the uterus and both adnexae. If the contralateral ovary and uterine serosa appear normal, conservative management with preservation of the uterus and contralateral adnexa is appropriate, as 95% of sex cord-stromal tumors are unilateral. It is important to note that staging – without lymphadenectomy – should still be performed. Most juvenile granulosa cell tumors, for example, are stage IA tumors [56]. Staging is essential for treatment planning, as platinum-based chemotherapy is recommended for any patients with disease greater than stage IA. Fertility-sparing surgery does not obviate the need for staging, and refers to the safe preservation of a normal-appearing contralateral ovary and uterus in the setting of apparent limited disease.

The management of patients with Sertoli–Leydig cell tumors follows the same guidelines. Fertility preservation is important for many of these patients, and a unilateral salpingo-oophorectomy and staging is usually appropriate, as 95% of lesions are unilateral [43]. Conversely, a total hysterectomy and bilateral salpingo-oophorectomy with staging procedure should be performed in these patients who have completed childbearing [51].

Ovarian SCTATs occur in two clinical subgroups. The first subgroup, associated with Peutz-Jeghers syndrome, tends to be multifocal, bilateral, small, and is almost always benign. Fifteen percent of these patients have an occult adenoma malignum of the cervix, and hysterectomy should be strongly considered. The second subgroup of ovarian SCTATs, unrelated to Peutz-Jeghers syndrome, typically presents with larger tumors with a high likelihood of malignant behavior. Surgical resection is the mainstay of treatment [44].

Patients with gynandroblastomas and steroid cell tumors not otherwise specified should also be staged and aggressively cytoreduced.

The treatment of patients who have had inadequate staging is a controversial issue. Limited data exist to guide decision making in this circumstance. In the setting of a limited initial attempt at tumor reduction with large amounts of residual disease, repeat exploration for tumor reduction would be reasonable. If the patient has had an inadequate exploration, such as through a small Pfannenstiel incision or through a limited laparoscopy, more information needs to be collected before making a decision about postsurgical treatment. The options are immediate repeat laparoscopic or open exploration with full surgical staging versus a physical examination, CT, and measurement of serum inhibin and serum CA125 levels. If the results of all of these are negative, the decision may be made to observe the patient clinically and avoid chemotherapy.

Adjuvant or nonsurgical therapy

Because stromal tumors of the ovary are relatively rare, controlled clinical trials designed to determine which treatment regimens are best for certain histologic subtypes are not feasible. Most published studies combine most or all subtypes of stromal ovarian tumors, and therefore treatment recommendations are based on limited data, most of which has been gathered from adult granulosa cell tumors and generalized to all stromal tumor types [43,51].

Most patients with surgically staged stage I disease do not require adjuvant treatment [43,51]. Patients with stage IC disease may benefit from some adjuvant therapy, either using platinum-based chemotherapy or hormonal therapy with leuprolide acetate [51].

Patients with more advanced disease are typically treated with combination chemotherapy. The use of platinum-based therapy originated in the 1970s and 1980s, with the publication of several anecdotal reports of complete and partial responses to platinum-containing regimens, including VAC, doxorubicin/cisplatin, CAP, and altretamine/cisplatin [51]. In 1986, the combination of bleomycin, vinblastine, and cisplatin was used in patients treated upfront for advanced disease. Of 11 patients, 9 responded, but toxicity was significant [62]. Subsequent trials substituted etoposide (BEP) for vinblastine to alleviate some of this toxicity. In 1996, Gershenson reported an 83% response rate to BEP in nine patients with advanced disease [63]. Subsequently, in 1999 Homesley reported GOG 115, with 57 evaluable patients with stage II–IV disease. Grade 4 myelotoxicity occurred in 61% of patients, and second-look surgery was negative in 37% of patients following chemotherapy. Thus, 69% of patients with advanced stage primary and 51% of patients with recurrent disease remained progression-free, with a progression-free interval of 24 months. As a result, many patients have been treated with three to four courses of bleomycin, etoposide, and cisplatin (BEP) [64]. However, a recent report has shown paclitaxel and carboplatin to have good results and fewer toxic effects [65]. Confirmation of equivalent outcomes between these two regimens will depend on the results of a larger randomized cooperative group trial, which is currently under way.

The treatment recommendations for Sertoli–Leydig cell tumors differ slightly from those for adult and juvenile granulosa cell tumors. Over 90% of patients with Sertoli–Leydig cell tumors have stage IA disease. Well-differentiated tumors tend to be of early stage, and only one death from disease has been reported in a patient with a well-differentiated tumor. However, 10% of intermediate, 60% of poorly differentiated, and 20% of retiform and heterologous subtypes show malignant behavior. Therefore, patients with Sertoli–Leydig cell tumors stage IC disease or greater, with poorly differentiated tumors of any stage or with heterologous elements, should receive adjuvant therapy with either BEP or paclitaxel and carboplatin 120Mod Radiation and hormone therapy have been described, but this is not first-line 66Mod.

Patients with steroid cell tumors not otherwise specified who have tumors that are pleomorphic, have an increased mitotic count, are large, or are at an advanced stage should also receive adjuvant platinum-based chemotherapy [51].

There are no prospective randomized studies showing the value of radiotherapy in stromal ovarian tumors, but several retrospective studies have demonstrated the utility of radiation therapy in select patients with advanced disease [66].

Survival and prognosis

Survival and prognostic factors have been reported in several large series [37,51]. The overall 20-year survival of sex cord-stromal ovarian tumors approximates 40%. Stage at diagnosis represents the strongest prognostic factor, with the 5- to 10-year survival over 90% for stage I, 55% for stage II, and 25% for stage III tumors. Most sex cord-stromal tumors exhibit an indolent course, with late recurrence as a hallmark, sometimes over a decade after the initial diagnosis. The average time to recurrence is 5–10 years. Poor prognostic factors include tumor size, rupture, and bilaterality. In patients with stage I disease, the recurrence rate is rare in tumors less than 5 cm, 20% in tumors 5–15 cm in size, and over 30% in tumors greater than 15 cm [37].

Patients with juvenile granulosa cell tumor also have a stage-related prognosis, with a 5-year survival for patients with stage IA disease of 99%, which declines to 60% for patients with advanced disease [38]. The prognosis of patients with Sertoli–Leydig cell tumors is also related to grade, stage, and histologic subtype, as noted above. This influences the decision to administer adjuvant therapy.

Unfortunately, if patients recur, the eventual prognosis is poor with an overall mortality of 70% despite treatment [51].

Treatment of recurrent disease

Patients with recurrent disease after a long disease-free interval may undergo secondary cytoreductive surgery with long-term survival. In the case of widespread disease or disease refractory to surgery, chemotherapy and hormonal therapy are options for treatment. Although the response rate is higher earlier in the disease course and declines as the number of prior treatment regimens increases, paclitaxel in combination with carboplatin results in a 60% overall response rate with acceptable toxicity [65]. Other chemotherapeutic agents with demonstrated response include carboplatin; BEP; cisplatin, doxorubicin, and cyclophosphamide; etoposide and cisplatin; VAC; oral etoposide; topotecan; liposomal doxorubicin; paclitaxel; and ifosfamide and etoposide [67,68]. Paclitaxel and carboplatin remain the most commonly used single agents at first and second relapse. Early in the treatment of recurrent disease, leuprolide acetate frequently results in the regression or stabilization of disease. Commonly used dosing schedules are listed in Table 28.5. Radiation therapy is also occasionally used in the treatment of localized or symptomatic disease [38]. Bevacizumab has also been evaluated in the treatment of recurrent disease with responses and long-term stable disease noted [53]. A phase 2 cooperative group trial evaluating bevacizumab in the recurrent setting has been completed and will be

Table 28.5. Common dosing schedules for chemotherapy, hormonal therapy, and targeted agents

Agent	Dose	Route	Interval
Paclitaxel/carboplatin	175 mg/m^2, AUC = 5	IV	Every 3 weeks
Paclitaxel	135–200 mg/m^2	IV	Every 3 weeks
Paclitaxel	80–100 mg/m^2	IV	Weekly
Carboplatin	AUC = 5	IV	Every 4 weeks
BEP	Bevacizumab 15–30 units day 1–3, Etoposide 75–100 mg/m^2 days 1–5, Cisplatin 20 mg m^{-2} days 1–5	IV	Every 3 weeks
PAC	Cisplatin 40–50 mg/m^2, Doxorubicin 40 mg/m^2 Cyclophosphamide 400 mg/m^2	IV	Every 4 weeks
EP	Etoposide 100 mg/m^2 Cisplatin 75 mg/m^2	IV	Every 4 weeks
VAC	Vincristine 1.5 mg/m^2 day 1 Actinomycin D 0.5 mg days 1–5 Cyclophosphamide 150 mg/m^2 days 1–5	IV IV IV	Every 2 weeks Every 4 weeks Every 4 weeks
Oral etoposide	Etoposide 50 mg/m^2 day^{-1} × 21 days	PO	Every 21 days
Topotecan	Topotecan 1.5 mg/m^2 day^{-1} × 5 days	IV	Every 3 weeks
Doxil	Doxil 40 mg m^{-2}	IV	Every 4 weeks
Ifosfamide/ etoposide	Ifosfamide 1.2 g/m^2 day^{-1} × 5 days Etoposide 100 mg/m^2 day^{-1} × 5 days	IV IV	Every 3 weeks Every 3 weeks
Leuprolide acetate	7.5 mg or 22.5 mg	IM IM	Every 4 weeks Every 3 months
Bevacizumab	15 mg/kg	IV	Every 3 weeks

IV, intravenous; IM, intramuscular; AUC, area under the curve.

published in the near future. Responses have also been reported after treatment with gonadotropin-releasing hormone antagonists, progestins, and aromatase inhibitors [69].

Future directions

Research in rare tumors is a difficult issue and is best performed in a cooperative group setting. The current ongoing trials should help to better elucidate the most effective and least toxic adjuvant therapy for sex cord-stromal tumors and determine the role of bevacizumab in recurrent disease.

Perhaps the most interesting areas of recent research involve the recognition of the importance of *FOXL2* and *DICER1* mutations. Further research into these mechanisms and targeted therapy directed against these genes may provide new avenues of understanding and novel therapy for patients with ovarian stromal tumors.

References

1. Patterson DM, Rustin GJ. Controversies in the management of germ cell tumours of the ovary. Curr Opin Oncol. 2006;**18**:500–6.
2. Smith HO, Berwick M, Verschraegen CF, et al. Incidence and survival rates for female malignant germ cell tumors. Obstet Gynecol. 2006;**107**:1075–85.
3. Gershenson DM. Management of ovarian germ cell tumors. J Clin Oncol. 2007;**25**:2938–43.
4. Chan JK, Tewari KS, Waller S, et al. The influence of conservative surgical practices for malignant ovarian germ cell tumors. J Surg Oncol. 2008;**98**:111–6.
5. Bryant CS, Kumar S, Shah JP, et al. Racial disparities in survival among patients with germ cell tumors of the ovary – United States. Gynecol Oncol. 2009;**114**:437–41.
6. Giambartolomei C, Mueller CM, Greene MH, Korde LA. A mini-review of familial ovarian germ cell tumors: an additional manifestation of the familial testicular germ cell tumor syndrome. Cancer Epidemiol. 2009;**33**:31–6.
7. Jonson AL, Geller MA, Dickson EL. Gonadal dysgenesis and gynecologic cancer. Obstet Gynecol. 2010;**116**(Suppl 2):550–2.
8. Crum C. The female genital tract. In: Kumar V, Abbas AK, Fausto N (Eds.). Robbins and Cotran Pathologic Basis of Disease, 4th edition. Philadelphia: Elsevier; 2005.
9. Vaysse C, Delsol M, Carfagna L, et al. Ovarian germ cell tumors in children. Management, survival and ovarian prognosis. A report of 75 cases. J Pediatr Surg. 2010;**45**:1484–90.
10. Alotaibi MOS, Navarro OM. Imaging of ovarian teratomas in children: a 9-year

review. Can Assoc Radiol J. 2010;**61**:23–8.

11. Network NCC. NCCN Clinical Practice Guidelines in Oncology: Ovarian Cancer In: Network NCC, ed. Vol 2.2012: www.nccn.org (accessed February 14, 2012).
12. Sturgeon CM, Duffy MJ, Stenman U-H, et al. National Academy of Clinical Biochemistry Laboratory Medicine practice guidelines for use of tumor markers in testicular, prostate, colorectal, breast, and ovarian cancers. Clin Chem. 2008;**54**:e11–79.
13. Ueland F, DeSimone C, Seamon L, et al. The OVA 1 test improves the preoperative assessment of ovarian tumors. Gynecol Oncol. 2010;**116**(Suppl):S23.
14. Weinberg LE, Lurain JR, Singh DK, Schink JC. Survival and reproductive outcomes in women treated for malignant ovarian germ cell tumors. Gynecol Oncol. 2011;**121**:285–9.
15. Beiner ME, Gotlieb WH, Korach Y, et al. Cystectomy for immature teratoma of the ovary. Gynecol Oncol. 2004;**93**:381–4.
16. Kumar S, Shah JP, Bryant CS, et al. The prevalence and prognostic impact of lymph node metastasis in malignant germ cell tumors of the ovary. Gynecol Oncol. 2008;**110**:125–32.
17. Mahdi H, Swensen RE, Hanna R, et al. Prognostic impact of lymphadenectomy in clinically early stage malignant germ cell tumour of the ovary. Br J Cancer. 2011;**105**:493–7.
18. Palenzuela G, Martin E, Meunier A, et al. Comprehensive staging allows for excellent outcome in patients with localized malignant germ cell tumor of the ovary. Ann Surg. 2008;**248**:836–41.
19. Billmire D, Vinocur C, Rescorla F, et al. Outcome and staging evaluation in malignant germ cell tumors of the ovary in children and adolescents: an intergroup study. J Pediatr Surg. 2004;**39**:424–9.
20. Patterson DM, Murugaesu N, Holden L, Seckl MJ, Rustin GJ. A review of the close surveillance policy for stage I female germ cell tumors of the ovary and other sites. Int J Gynecol Cancer. 2008;**18**:43–50.
21. Cushing B, Giller R, Ablin A, et al. Surgical resection alone is effective treatment for ovarian immature teratoma in children and adolescents: a report of the pediatric oncology group and the children's cancer group. Am J Obstet Gynecol. 1999;**181**:353–8.
22. Marina NM, Cushing B, Giller R, et al. Complete surgical excision is effective treatment for children with immature teratomas with or without malignant elements: a Pediatric Oncology Group/Children's Cancer Group Intergroup Study. J Clin Oncol. 1999;**17**:2137–43.
23. Gobel U, Schneider DT, Calaminus G, et al. Germ-cell tumors in childhood and adolescence. GPOH MAKEI and the MAHO study groups. Ann Oncol. 2000;**11**:263–71.
24. Pectasides D, Pectasides E, Kassanos D. Germ cell tumors of the ovary. Cancer Treat Rev. 2008;**34**:427–41.
25. Murugaesu N, Schmid P, Dancey G, et al. Malignant ovarian germ cell tumors: identification of novel prognostic markers and long-term outcome after multimodality treatment. J Clin Oncol. 2006;**24**:4862–6.
26. de La Motte Rouge T, Pautier P, Duvillard P, et al. Survival and reproductive function of 52 women treated with surgery and bleomycin, etoposide, cisplatin (BEP) chemotherapy for ovarian yolk sac tumor. Ann Oncol. 2008;**19**:1435–41.
27. Shah JP, Kumar S, Bryant CS, et al. A population-based analysis of 788 cases of yolk sac tumors: a comparison of males and females. Int J Cancer. 2008;**123**:2671–5.
28. Lai CH, Chang TC, Hsueh S, et al. Outcome and prognostic factors in ovarian germ cell malignancies. Gynecol Oncol. 2005;**96**:784–91.
29. Gershenson DM, Miller AM, Champion VL, et al. Reproductive and sexual function after platinum-based chemotherapy in long-term ovarian germ cell tumor survivors: a Gynecologic Oncology Group Study. J Clin Oncol. 2007;**25**:2792–7.
30. Tangir J, Zelterman D, Ma W, Schwartz PE. Reproductive function after conservative surgery and chemotherapy for malignant germ cell tumors of the ovary. Obstet Gynecol. 2003;**101**:251–7.
31. Champion V, Williams SD, Miller A, et al. Quality of life in long-term survivors of ovarian germ cell tumors: A Gynecologic Oncology Group Study. Gynecol Oncol. 2007;**105**:687–94.
32. Matei D, Miller AM, Monahan P, et al. Chronic physical effects and health care utilization in long-term ovarian germ cell tumor survivors: a Gynecologic Oncology Group study. J Clin Oncol. 2009;**27**:4142–9.
33. Siegel R, Naishadham D, Jemal A. Cancer statistics, 2012. CA Cancer J Clin. 2012;**62**:10–29.
34. World Health Organization. International Histologic Classification of Tumors, No. 9. Geneva: World Health Organization; 1973.
35. Koonings PP, Campbell K, Mishell DR Jr, et al. Relative frequency of primary ovarian neoplasms: a 10-year review. Obstet Gynecol. 1989;**74**:921–6.
36. Brown J, Olson T, Sencer S. Malignancies of the ovary. In: Bleyer WA, Barr RD (Eds.). Cancer in Adolescents and Young Adults. New York: Springer; 2007. p 219–36.
37. Bjorkholm E, Silfversward C. Granulosa and theca cell tumors: incidence and occurrence of second primary tumors. Acta Radiol Oncol. 1980;**19**:161.
38. Schumer ST, Cannistra SA. Granulosa cell tumor of the ovary. J Clin Oncol. 2003;**21**:1180–9.
39. Schultz KA, Sencer SF, Messinger Y, et al. Pediatric ovarian tumors: a review of 67 cases. Pediatr Blood Cancer. 2005;**44**:167–73.
40. Schneider DR, Calaminus G, Harms D, et al. Ovarian sex cord-stromal tumors in children and adolescents. J Reprod Med. 2005;**50**:439–46.
41. Gribbon M, Ein SH, Mancer K. Pediatric malignant ovarian tumors: a 43-year review. J Pediatr Surg. 1992;**27**:480.
42. Zaloudek C, Norris HJ. Sertoli-Leydig tumors of the ovary: a clinicopathologic study of 64 intermediate and poorly differentiated neoplasms. Am J Surg Pathol. 1984;**8**:405.
43. Gershenson DM. Fertility-sparing surgery for malignancies in women. J Natl Cancer Inst Monographs. 2005;**34**:43–7.
44. Srivasta PJ, Keeney GL, Podratz KC. Disseminated cervical adenoma malignum and bilateral ovarian sex cord tumors with annular tubules associated with Peutz–Jeghers syndrome. Gynecol Oncol. 1994;**53**:256.
45. Nosov V, Park S, Rao J, et al. Non-Peutz-Jeghers syndrome associated ovarian sex cord tumor with annular tubules: a case report. Fertil Steril. 2009;**92**:1497.

46. Anderson MC, Rees DA. Gynandroblastoma of the ovary. Br J Obstet Gynecol. 1975;**82**:68.

47. Stevens TA, Brown J, Zander DS, et al. Adult granulosa cell tumors of the ovary in two first-degree relatives. Gynecol Oncol. 2005;**98**:502–25.

48. Shah SP, Kobel M, Senz J, et al. Mutation of FOXL2 in granulosa-cell tumors of the ovary. N Engl J Med. 2009;**360**:2719–29.

49. Heravi-Moussavi A, Anglesio MS, Cheng SW, et al. Recurrent somatic DICER1 mutations in nonepithelial ovarian cancers. N Engl J Med. 2012;**366**:234–42.

50. Young RH, Scully RE. Endocrine tumors of the ovary. Curr Top Pathol. 1992;**85**:113–64.

51. Brown J, Jhingran A, Deavers M, et al. Stromal tumors of the ovary. In: Raghaven D, Brecher ML, Johnson DH, et al. (Eds.). Textbook of Uncommon Cancer. West Sussex, UK: John Wiley and Sons; 2006.

52. Roth LM, Anderson MC, Govan DT, et al. Sertoli-Leydig cell tumors: a clinicopathologic study of 34 cases. Cancer. 1981;**48**:187.

53. Tao X, Sood AK, Deavers MT, et al. Anti-angiogenesis therapy with bevacizumab for patients with ovarian granulosa cell tumors. Gynecol Oncol. 2009;**114**:431–6.

54. McCluggage WG, Maxwell P, Sloan JM. Immunohistochemical staining of ovarian granulosa cell tumors with monoclonal antibody against inhibin. Hum Pathol. 1997;**28**:1034–8.

55. Zhao C, Barner R, Vinh TN, et al. SF-1 is a diagnostically useful immunohistochemical marker and comparable to other sex cord-stromal tumor markers for the differential diagnosis of ovarian sertoli cell tumor. Int J Gynecol Pathol. 2008;**27**:507–14.

56. Young RH, Dickersin GR, Scully RE. Juvenile granulosa cell tumor of the ovary. Am J Surg Pathol. 1984;**8**:575.

57. Gershenson DM, Hartmann LC, Young RH. Ovarian sex cord-stromal tumors. In: Hoskins WJ, Perez CA, Young RC (Eds.). Principles and Practice of Gynecologic Oncology, 4th edition. Philadelphia, PA: Lippincott Williams & Wilkins; 2004.

58. Van Holsbeke C, Domali E, Holland TK. Imaging of gynecological disease: clinical and ultrasound characteristics of granulosa cell tumors of the ovary. Ultrasound Obstet Gynecol. 2008;**31**:450–6.

59. Jung SE, Rha SE, Lee JM, et al. CT and MRI findings of sex cord-stromal tumor of the ovary. AJR Am J Roentgenol. 2005;**185**:207–15.

60. Mettler L, Semm K, Shive K. Endoscopic management of adnexal masses. J Soc Laparosc Surg. 1997;**2**:103–12.

61. Brown J, Sood AK, Deavers MT, Milojevic L, Gershenson DM. Patterns of metastasis in sex cord-stromal tumors of the ovary: Can routine staging lymphadenectomy be omitted? Gynecol Oncol. 2009;**113**:86–90.

62. Colombo N, Sessa C, Landoni F, et al. Cisplatin, vinblastine, and bleomycin combination chemotherapy in metastatic granulosa cell tumor of the ovary. Obstet Gynecol. 1986;**37**:265–8.

63. Gershenson DM, Morris M, Burke TW, et al. Treatment of poor-prognosis sex cord-stromal tumors of the ovary with the combination of bleomycin, etoposide, and cisplatin. Obstet Gynecol. 1996;**87**:527–31.

64. Homesley HD, Bundy BN, Hurteau JA, Roth LM. Bleomycin, etoposide, and cisplatin combination chemotherapy of ovarian granulosa cell tumors and other stromal malignancies: a Gynecologic Oncology Group study. Gynecol Oncol. 1999;**72**:131–7.

65. Brown J, Shvartsman HS, Deavers MT, et al. The activity of taxanes compared with bleomycin, etoposide, and cisplatin in the treatment of sex cord-stromal ovarian tumors. Gynecol Oncol. 2005;**97**:489–96.

66. Savage P, Constenla D, Fisher C, et al. Granulosa cell tumors of the ovary: demographics, survival, and the management of advanced disease. Clin Oncol (R Coll Radiol). 1998;**10**:242–5.

67. Brown J, Shvartsman HS, Deavers MT, et al. The activity of taxanes in the treatment of sex cord-stromal ovarian tumors. J Clin Oncol. 2004;**22**:3517–23.

68. Powell JL, Connor GP, Henderson GS. Management of recurrent juvenile granulosa cell tumor of the ovary. Gynecol Oncol. 2001;**81**:113–6.

69. Martikainen H, Penttinen J, Huhtaniemi I, et al. Gonadotropin-releasing hormone agonist analog therapy effective in ovarian granulosa cell malignancy. Gynecol Oncol. 1989;**35**:406.

Chapter 29

Palliative care of ovarian cancer

Katharine Batt, MD, and Cardinale B. Smith, MD, MSCR

Introduction

Palliative care is the provision of medical care that focuses on improving the quality of life of patients and families facing serious and life-threatening illness through relief of suffering across physical, psychosocial, emotional, and spiritual dimensions [1]. Palliative medicine specialists are an interdisciplinary team that includes physicians, nurse practitioners, nurses, social workers, chaplains, and nutritionists who focus on assisting patients and families with a variety of care needs including symptom control, psychosocial support, communication, addressing care goals, and transitions in care [2–4].

Palliative care is given simultaneously with other disease-modifying treatments and potentially curative treatments. Patients with ovarian cancer can have significant symptom distress either from the disease or the associated treatments (chemotherapy and/or surgery). As such, it is important to provide palliative care early in the course of illness whether the treatment goals are for cure or for maximizing quality of life. National and international organizations currently have clinical guidelines recommending palliative care be routinely integrated into comprehensive cancer care [5,6].

The role of the palliative care team is to support the gynecologic oncologist/gynecologic specialist in the care of ovarian cancer patients by providing aggressive symptom management; assisting with time-consuming and difficult communication between providers, patients, and families; and facilitating transitions in care when there is a change in goals or disease status. There is an existing clinical practice guideline for quality palliative care that identifies eight domains essential to providing exemplary clinical palliative care. These include: structures and processes of care; physical aspects of care; psychological and psychiatric aspects; social aspects; spiritual, religious, and existential aspects; cultural aspects; care of the imminently dying patient; and ethical and legal aspects of care [7]. In this chapter, we will focus on communication, symptom management, and end-of-life/terminal care.

Communication

Effective communication starts with understanding the patient through a complete understanding of his/her physical, spiritual, psychological, emotional, and socioeconomic situation. The lifeline of palliative care is communication, not only in assessing symptom burden, but also in clarifying medical understanding, treatment preferences, and goals. Breaking bad news or discussing goals of care is an important component of communicating with ovarian cancer patients and their families. Poor communication is associated with decreased patient participation in decision-making and increased likelihood of receiving chemotherapy at the end of life [8]. In contrast, effective communication can improve patient satisfaction and decrease patient distress.

To enhance communication, a six-step strategy (SPIKES), adapted from published research, was proposed by Buckman et al. (Table 29.1) [9]. Intended to be used at all levels of medical training (medical students to oncologists), the SPIKES protocol creates a formula to help improve communication between patients, their families, and providers to achieve four main goals: gather information; provide easily understood and appropriate information; provide support in receiving information; and to develop a treatment strategy in alliance with the patient and/or family. Although proposed for use in situations of breaking bad news and addressing goals of care, the guidelines have great versatility in promoting conversation among providers–patients and helping to build effective relationships.

Symptom management

Pain

The International Association for the Study of Pain defines pain as "an unpleasant sensory and emotional experience associated with actual or potential tissue damage, or described in terms of such damage" [10]. Cancer-related pain is extremely prevalent. In patients with ovarian cancer, cancer pain is present in at least 60% of patients, with >40% of patients suffering functional deficits because of pain [11]. Despite the high prevalence of pain, it is often undertreated in patients with ovarian cancer. There are provider, patient, and system level factors that contribute to undertreatment of pain. Providers often have poor knowledge of adequate pain management, fears of patient addiction, and professional concerns regarding the regulation of controlled substances. Similarly, patients frequently inaccurately report pain complaints, often out of fear of not being seen as a "good" patient or that pain symptoms suggest worsening

Altchek's Diagnosis and Management of Ovarian Disorders, ed. Liane Deligdisch, Nathan G. Kase, and Carmel J. Cohen. Published by Cambridge University Press.

Table 29.1. SPIKES protocol

Recommendation	Comments
Set up the interview	Before the meeting determine the most appropriate participants (family members, and other healthcare providers) Establish privacy Sit down Allow adequate time; manage interruptions Determine what to say before the meeting
Patient perception	Ask the patient's understanding of the situation using open-ended questions: "What have you been told about your medical situation so far?" Establish patient understanding, provide an opportunity to correct misinformation and understand illness perception
Invitation to patient	Discuss information disclosure – how much does the patient want to know? How does the patient want the information delivered?
Knowledge exchange	Warn the patient if bad news is coming; use the vocabulary and comprehension of the patient Avoid technical words Avoid overt bluntness Give information in small pieces and check-in frequently with the patient to ensure understanding
Emotions/empathic responses	Observe emotions Identify emotions Identify reason for the emotion Make a reflective, connecting statement integrating emotion with cause
Strategy/summary	Summarize the plan to ensure concordance in understanding between patient/family and provider(s) Plan follow-up, including contact information for additional questions/concerns Continue to review and revise the plan as needed

disease; patients are often resistant to taking pain medications, particularly out of fears of addiction [12]. Additionally, medication unavailability/unaffordability at local pharmacies, close scrutiny of patients using controlled substances, and lack of awareness of cancer pain are system issues associated with undertreatment [13].

A careful pain assessment is, therefore, critical to an effective intervention. It includes an understanding of the intensity, timing, precipitating factors, and duration of the pain complaint in the context of prior pain symptoms, a psychosocial assessment, and a thorough physical and neurologic exam [14]. Although several assessment tools have been developed to standardize the subjective reporting of pain, no assessment tool has emerged as the gold standard. Instead, the mainstay of pain assessment continues to be patient (or caregiver) self-report.

Two broad categories of pain assessment tools have been defined: uni-dimensional and multi-dimensional. In clinical practice, the most commonly used bedside tool is the uni-dimensional numerical rating scale that uses a linear scale ranging from 0 (no pain) to 10 (worst pain) to grade pain severity [15]. Other clinically useful tools include the visual analog scale, a tool using a continuum of visual cues (i.e., faces) to gauge pain severity, and the verbal rating scale which relies on straightforward descriptions of pain intensity: mild, moderate, and severe [16,17]. Multi-dimensional tools are more commonly found in research settings, given the number of dimensions assessed and the time needed to complete such an evaluation. The Brief Pain Inventory (BPI), developed by the WHO [18], is the most frequently used multi-dimensional tool. Designed as a questionnaire with multiple sub-headings such as pain relief, pain intensity and its impact on quality of life, the patient assigns numerical scores to intensity of pain, both in the moment and in the past 24 hours. Initially validated in 1983, the BPI has subsequently been validated in many countries and in multiple languages [19–24].

Types of pain

Pain can be classified as nociceptive, neuropathic, or idiopathic. Nociceptive pain can be further classified as either somatic (resulting from injury to skin and deep tissue) or visceral pain (resulting from injury to internal organs). Visceral pain is often described as dull, vague, or diffuse, while somatic pain is more likely to be well localized and described as sharp or intense. Traditional pain management uses these classifications to target treatment. Neuropathic pain results from direct injury to nerves, either peripherally or centrally. It is often described as burning, tingling, or "electric shock-like" in nature and can arise from primary direct injury to the nervous system or from secondary tumor infiltration [25]. Unlike somatic pains that often resolve as tissues heal, neuropathic pains often linger and are less responsive to pharmacologic management.

Principles of pain management

The WHO developed a stepwise approach to the management of cancer pain with the initial choice of medication based on pain severity (Fig. 29.1). Using non-opioids (aspirin and acetaminophen) for mild pain, "mild opioids" (codeine or oxycodone with acetaminophen) for mild to moderate pain, and "strong opioids" such as morphine for moderate to severe pain, the pain ladder allows clinicians to escalate analgesia based on a patient's reported pain intensity (Fig. 29.1).

The non-opioid medications, non-steroidal anti-inflammatory drugs (NSAIDs: aspirin, acetaminophen), provide direct and adjuvant analgesia [26]. NSAIDs are considered first-line therapy in bony pain and unlike acetaminophen, provide adjuvant relief in pain involving inflammation. However, NSAIDs and aspirin predispose patients to GI ulceration/bleed and can also worsen renal failure and should, therefore, be used with caution. Similarly, acetaminophen must be dose-reduced in patients with existing liver failure. Morphine is frequently a first-line opioid choice, largely from provider familiarity, multiple modes of administration, and drug inexpense. Morphine undergoes a first-pass metabolism in the liver, is broken down into active metabolites and is renally excreted. Morphine and any opiate metabolized to a morphine derivative (i.e., codeine,) should be avoided in patients with renal insufficiency. Among patients with hepatic

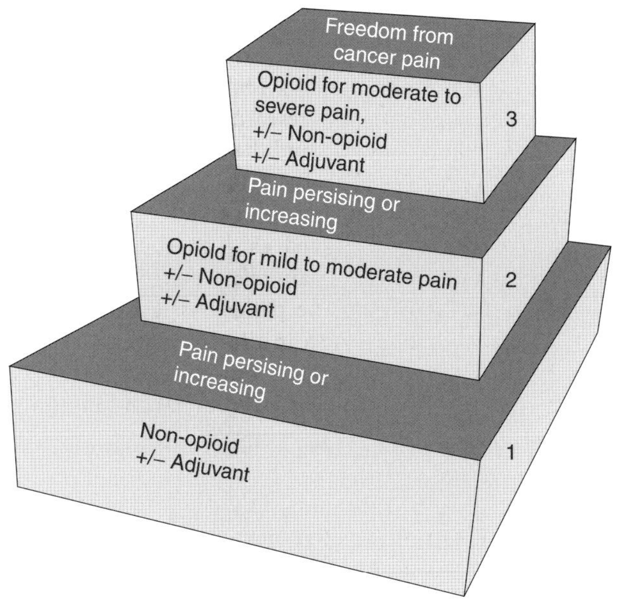

Fig. 29.1. World Health Organization Pain Relief Ladder. http://www.who.int/cancer/palliative/painladder/en/.

Table 29.2. Opioid analgesic equivalences

Opioid agonists	IV/SC/IM (mg)	PO/rectal (mg)	Duration of effect
Morphine	10	30	4 hours
Hydrocodone		30	4 hours
Oxycodone		20	4 hours
Oxymorphone	1	10	4 hours
Hydromorphone (Dilaudid)	1.5	7.5	4 hours
Fentanyl	[a]		1–2 hours
Codeine	130	200	4 hours

[a] Convert morphine PO 3 mg/24 h to fentanyl 1 μg/h transdermal patch; transdermal fentanyl should never be prescribed for an opioid naïve patient. Adapted from Horton, J. R. (in press). Hospital-Based Opioid Analgesia. In: A. Dunn, P. Klotman, & N. Kathuria, (Eds.), *Handbook of Hospital Medicine*. Hackensack, NJ: World Scientific Publishing.

dysfunction, preferred opioid alternatives in patients with liver dysfunction include fentanyl, Dilaudid, and methadone.

Patients with advanced ovarian malignancies can experience pain from multiple causes: tumor progression into soft tissue, nerve or muscle, after chemotherapy administration, or post-surgery. Understanding the disease course and likely etiology of the pain complaint can help target the most appropriate therapy.

Opioid dosing

Several factors must be considered when starting a patient on opioid therapy: severity of pain, end-organ function, patient age, and history of opioid use. Among non-elderly patients who have minimal to no prior exposure to opioids, the initial starting dose of morphine (or its equivalent) is 5–10 mg IV or 15–30 mg orally. For an older or more debilitated patient, one should start at the lower end or below this range (2.5–5 mg IV). Patients should initially be started on short-acting opioids, dosed in 4-hour intervals and given on an as-needed basis. For patients already on opioid therapy, without adequate pain relief, the opioid dose should be titrated to patient comfort. For patients on short-acting opioids requiring more than four doses per day, conversion to longer-acting opioids is appropriate. Patients on long-acting opioids who are still experiencing moderate pain should have the dose increased by 25–50%. Among those with severe pain, the total dose should be increased 50–100%. It is important to note that there is not a maximum ceiling dose to opioids; the only limitations are the side effects. A list of commonly used opioids and their analgesic equivalents can be found in Table 29.2.

Breakthrough pain

Breakthrough pain occurs in up to 50% of patients with cancer-related pain [27]. Unlike the persistent pains that develop gradually over the course of an illness, breakthrough pain is described as a sudden, intense pain, often self-limited but lasting an average of 30 minutes [28]. These pains often arise from movement (voluntary or involuntary), but can also be spontaneous with no clear etiology.

To account for breakthrough pain, additional analgesia needs to be prescribed as part of the overall pain management regimen. Termed “breakthrough dosing,” this additional analgesia is equivalent to 10% of the 24-hour prescribed dose, given at a frequency up to every hour. Use of breakthrough dosing has a slightly different approach depending on the etiology. In cases where pain is anticipated, for example, movement, breakthrough doses are recommended 30 minutes before the expected activity. Otherwise, spontaneous, unexpected pains are treated with analgesia as quickly as possible with re-dosing as often as needed [29].

Adverse effects

The most common opioid-related adverse effects are constipation, nausea and vomiting, drowsiness, pruritus, and delirium. Tolerance develops to all opioid side effects except constipation. A bowel regimen should always be prescribed alongside an opioid-containing pain regimen. Bowel prokinetics (such as senna) is often used as first-line laxative therapy [30,31]. A list of common side effects and potential treatment strategies is provided in Table 29.3.

Other pain dimensions/adjuvant therapy

There is a lack of well-designed randomized controlled clinical trials (RCTs) to support the use of different adjuvant therapies in treating various forms of cancer pain [32,33]. However, the use of NSAIDs in metastatic bony disease associated with breast/prostate cancer has been demonstrated, as has the use of tricyclic anti-depressants/anti-convulsants in neuropathic pain [34,35]. Other factors that affect the experience of pain include anxiety, depression, social isolation, and fatigue. In an initial pain assessment, an evaluation of additional contributing psychological, emotional, spiritual, and socioeconomic factors can facilitate adjuvant therapy. Table 29.4 lists commonly used adjuvant therapeutic medications.

Nausea and vomiting

Nausea is a subjective sensation defined as the need to vomit; vomiting is the forceful expulsion of gastric contents through the mouth. Retching or "dry heaves" involves gastric or esophageal movements without actual vomitus. In women with ovarian cancer, nausea or vomiting can occur in >70% of patients as a complication of disease or while undergoing treatment [36]. The pathophysiology of nausea and vomiting is complex and involves four primary pathways which have been implicated in triggering the regulatory vomiting center, located in the brainstem:

1. *Chemoreceptor trigger zone* (CTZ): Located in a highly vascular area of the medulla, the CTZ lacks a true blood–brain barrier and therefore, responds directly to blood-borne substances such as medications and hormones. The neurotransmitters acetylcholine (ACh), dopamine (D2), histamine (H-1), substance P (NK-1), and serotonin (5HT3) are implicated in CTZ stimulation. In addition, the CTZ receives signals from the GI tract, by means of the vagal afferent nerve (Davis and Hallerberg, 2010).
2. *Vagus nerve*: Peripheral chemo- and mechanoreceptors in the stomach, liver, peritoneum and gut feedback signals by means of the vagus nerve through 5HT3, D2, and Ach/muscarinic receptors.
3. *Vestibular centers*: Input from the vestibulocochlear apparatus, including motion, triggers nausea and vomiting. H-1 and ACh neurotransmitters are involved.
4. *Cortex*: Mediated by psychogenic factors such as anxiety, fear and irritation, primary sensory input (sight, smell, touch), as well as increased intra-cranial pressure and meningeal irritation. ACh and H-1 receptors are thought to be involved.

In ovarian cancer patients, frequent causes of nausea and/or vomiting are chemotherapeutic drugs with known emetogenic potential and radiation therapy, particularly to the gastrointestinal (GI) tract, liver, and brain. Metabolic imbalances (hypercalcemia, hypo/hypernatremia, volume depletion), direct tumor progression (i.e., GI, liver, brain), constipation, and opioids also contribute. Additionally, emotional states, particularly anxiety, can also cause nausea and/or vomiting.

Table 29.3. Opioid side effects

Side effect	Time to tolerance	Treatment strategy
Constipation	N/A	Escalating laxative regimen
Nausea/ vomiting	5–7 days	Anti-emetics: Metoclopramide 5- HT3 antagonist
Drowsiness	3–4 days	Avoid driving, good sleep hygiene
Delirium	At any point	Evaluate cause: untreated pain, infection, electrolyte disturbances, CNS disease, organ failure Antipsychotic: haloperidol
Pruritus	At any point	Opioid rotation; morphine has the highest rate of reported pruritus Anti-histamine: Hydroxyzine

Table 29.4. Common adjuvant therapies

Type of pain	Drug class	Example	Dosing	Comments
Bony/joint pain	NSAIDs	Ibuprofen	400–800 mg PO every 4–6 h	Risk of GI bleed; renal toxicity
	Bisphosphonates	Pamidronate	60–90 mg IV	May worsen renal insufficiency
	Steroids	Dexamethasone	2–8 mg PO/SC in divided doses	Glucose impairment, risk of infection, psychosis
Neuropathic pain	Tricyclic antidepressants	Amitriptyline nortriptyline	10–50 mg at bedtime	Sedating, anticholinergic effects; amitriptyline better studied
	Anticonvulsants	Gabapentin	100–300 mg PO at nighttime, titrated to max dose of 2400 mg daily in divided doses	Sedating, large pills
		Valproate	250 mg PO/PR every 6–8 h	Absorbed rectally
		Carbamazepine	200 mg PO/PR every 6–12 h	Can give rectally (60 mg every 6–8 hours)
		Clonazepam	0.5 mg PO every 6–12 h	Sedating
	Other	Clonidine	0.1–0.3 mg PO every 12 h; transdermal patch 0.1–0.3 mg/24 h	Follow blood pressure, monitor for rebound hypertension
		Baclofen	5–20 mg PO every 8 h	Sedating, dizziness
		Capsaicin	0.025 or 0.075% topical cream every 6–8 h	Burning sensation, thermal hyperalgesia
		Cymbalta	60 mg po daily to max dose of 120 mg daily	Not FDA-approved but used; doses >60 mg rarely effective
Visceral pain	Anticholinergic	Hyoscyamine	0.125 mg PO/SL every 4–8 h	
		Scopolamine	1–2 patches every 72 h	Dry mouth, urinary retention, blurriness
	Steroids	Dexamethasone	4 mg PO/SC every 8–24 h	Discontinue after 5 days if no improvement, particularly with hepatic metastases

Younger patients (<50 years of age) and women often experience worse symptoms [37]; conversely, patients with a significant alcohol history will suffer less nausea/vomiting [38]. The work-up of nausea and vomiting starts with an understanding of the time course of symptoms, recent medication changes, and disease progression. Vital signs, laboratory studies, even imaging if indicated, can help to differentiate infection, electrolyte imbalances, dehydration, or worsening disease as possible etiologies.

Non-pharmacologic management of nausea and/or vomiting range from interventions such as dietary changes (avoid triggering foods/smells), odor-absorbing compounds to wounds, candles/room sprays, and acupressure wrist bands, to more involved techniques such as acupuncture, hypnosis, behavioral therapy, and guided imagery [39].

Pharmacologic treatment is most commonly based on identifying the etiology and administering the most potent antagonist targeted toward the most likely receptor sites [40]. For example, the promotility agent, metoclopramide, has efficacy in symptoms stemming from gastric stasis; however, its promotility properties make it harmful in patients with obstruction. Anticipatory nausea, common in patients undergoing chemotherapy and linked to associated anxiety in conjunction with anti-neoplastic agents, is effectively relieved by low-dose benzodiazepines. Aprepitant, a neuropeptide targeting substance P found in the vomiting center, is an effective agent for highly emetogenic chemotherapy [41].

When selecting the most appropriate anti-emetic agent, selection should also be based on the most appropriate route of administration to ensure greater efficacy. A list of commonly used anti-emetics, routes of administration, and their properties can be found in Table 29.5.

Constipation

Constipation is a serious problem encountered in ovarian cancer patients, often opioid-induced or from functional abnormalities resulting from advanced malignancy. In one study, approximately 18% of patients with ovarian cancer complained of GI disturbances and were also found to have more advanced disease [42].

No single definition for constipation exists in the literature. The consensus definition is a significant change in bowel habits, including a change in frequency of movement (usually fewer than three times weekly), difficulty during defecation (strain with >25% of bowel movements or a sensation of hard stools), or incomplete evacuation [43]. Constipation is present in approximately 2% of the general population but can occur in >50% of patients with ovarian malignancies; bowel obstruction is present in ~10% of patients with progressive disease. Advanced ovarian cancer often causes constipation through tumor mass effect or decreased intestinal motility, particularly from peritoneal carcinomatosis. Additional etiologies include dietary changes (poor fiber consumption, inadequate fluid intake), inactivity, depression, metabolic disorders (hypothyroidism, hypercalcemia, hypokalemia), and medications (antiemetics, opioids, chemotherapy) [36].

An assessment of constipation starts with an understanding of the patient's typical bowel patterns, dietary habits, and medications and how the current situation varies from normal. The physical examination assesses for distention, hypomobility, and fecal impaction. Imaging may be indicated to assess for an obstructed abdomen. Once obstruction is eliminated, therapy can be started.

Non-pharmacologic treatment options include increasing dietary fiber, fluid intake, and physical activity. Initial pharmacologic therapy often uses stool softeners (e.g., docusate sodium) as a single agent or in combination with a stimulant laxative (e.g., senna) [31]. However, data suggest that docusate adds very little to achieving laxation in cancer patients. A Cochrane review in 2006 failed to show the superiority of any laxative regimen due to insufficient randomized controlled trials (RCTs) [44]; however, there are some data supporting the efficacy of polyethylene glycol as an effective measure in the treatment of opioid-induced constipation [45]. Methylnaltrexone, a novel subcutaneous peripheral opioid antagonist, has a growing body of literature showing improved efficacy in opioid-induced constipation after failure of first-line therapy, often within 30 minutes to 4 hours from administration [46]. A list of commonly used laxatives and their properties can be found in Table 29.6.

Diarrhea

Diarrhea can be defined as an alteration in stool consistency from solid to liquid, usually in an amount >300 mL of stool, as well as an increase in frequency of bowel movements (>3 stools in 24 hours). Acute diarrhea extends from 4 days to <2 weeks; diarrhea is chronic when it persists >30 days. Diarrhea more commonly presents in the early stages of ovarian cancer, and can affect 10–24% of patients [47,48]. Conventional causes of diarrhea include chemotherapy, surgery, and radiation therapy [49]; acute changes often result from infections, antibiotic use, and stress. In assessing diarrhea, it is important to evaluate for precipitating events (chemotherapy/radiation, recent travel, contaminated food), to review current and recent medications (antibiotics, laxatives) and to obtain a thorough surgical history (short gut syndrome, partial/total colectomy). In heavily pretreated ovarian cancer patients, bacterial overgrowth syndrome can be seen [50]. Screening for infectious etiologies (*Clostridium difficile*, viral, bacterial, protozoan, parasitic, fungal) through stool cultures and fecal leukocytes is warranted, as well as quantification of the output. A rectal exam can assess for fecal impaction as a potential etiologic factor.

Initial stabilization of a patient with diarrhea includes fluid and electrolyte replacement. Depending on the underlying etiology, a course of antibiotics, anti-diarrheals, or cessation of medications may be indicated. If an infectious etiology is excluded, anti-diarrheals can be started at regularly scheduled intervals. Typically, loperamide is started with diphenoxylate added if no significant effect is seen within 24 hours. Octreotide is added in refractory diarrhea and can be titrated up to a maximum effective dose of 600 μg daily [51]. In all cases of

Table 29.5. Commonly used anti-emetics

Receptor target	Drug name	Site of action	Dosage/route	Adverse effects
Dopamine (D_2)	Prochlorperazine	CTZ, peripherally	10–20 mg PO every 6 h, 5–10 mg IM/IV every 6 h, or 25 mg rectally every 6 h	Extrapyramidal reactions (dystonia, akathisia), less sedation
	Chlorpromazine	CTZ, peripherally	10–25 mg PO every 4 h, 25–50 mg IM/IV every 4 h, or 50–100 mg rectally every 6 h	Sedation, anti-cholinergic effects
	Haldol	Central nervous system	0.5–2 mg PO/IV/SC every 2–6 h (up to 20 mg/day)	Dystonia, akathisia, hypotension, sedation
	Metoclopramide	CTZ, peripherally	10–20 mg PO/IV/SC before meals and at bedtime or every 6 h; IV bolus (up to 6 mg/kg); also comes as ODT 5,10 mg	Dystonia (more common in pts < 30 years old), akathisia (pts > 30 years old), tardive dyskinesia
Histamine (H_1)	Cyclizine	Vomiting center	25–50 mg PO/SC or rectally every 8 h	Dry mouth, sedation, skin irritation at SC sites may occur
	Diphenhydramine		25–50 mg PO/IV/SC every 6 h	Sedation, dry mouth, and urinary retention
Muscarinic/acetylcholine (ACh)	Glycopyrrolate	Peripherally	0.2 mg IV/SC every 4–6 h	Dry mouth, drowsiness, visual changes, urinary retention, fever
	Hyoscine hydrobromide	Centrally, peripherally	1 mg transdermal patch every 72 h	Dry mouth, drowsiness, confusion, ileus
	Scopolamine		1.5 mg transdermal patch every 72 h or 0.1–0.4 mg IV/SC every 4 h	Dry mouth, drowsiness, visual changes, confusion, urinary retention
Serotonin ($5HT_3$)	Dolasetron	CTZ	100 mg PO/IV daily	Headache, diarrhea
	Granisetron		1 mg PO daily or twice a day or 1 mg IV daily	Headache, constipation, weakness
	Ondansetron		4–8 mg PO/IV or dissolvable tablet in divided doses, max dose 32 mg/day; IV every 4–8 h; 24 mg IV bolus (pre-chemotherapy)	Headache, constipation, weakness, maximum dose 8 mg/day in hepatic insufficiency
	Palonosetron	CTZ, GI	0.25 or 0.75 mg IV on day 1 of chemotherapy	Headache, constipation
	Topisetron	CTZ	5 mg PO/IV	Headache. Used internationally not available in the U.S.
Multiple receptors	Olanzapine	CTZ, centrally	5–10 mg PO daily	Extra-pyramidal reactions, sedation, dry mouth, hyperglycemia, postural hypotension, stroke (elderly)
	Promethazine		12.5–25 mg PO/IV every 4–6 h or 2–5 mg rectally every 6 h	Dry mouth, dystonia, akathisia, and sedation
Neurokinin (substance P)	Aprepitant	Vomiting center	125 mg PO followed by 80 mg on day 2–3 of chemotherapy	Headache
	Fosaprepitant		150 mg IV on day 1 of chemotherapy or 115 mg IV on day 1 followed by 80 mg PO on day 2–3	Headache, infusion site pain
Other				
Corticosteroids	Dexamethasone	Cortex	2–10 mg PO/IV daily in divided doses	Hyperglycemia, GI bleeding, insomnia, psychosis
Cannabinoids	Dronabinol		2–20 mg PO daily in divided doses	Dizziness, euphoria in the young and dysphoria in the elderly, hallucinations, somnolence
	Nabilone		1–2 mg PO twice daily	
Benzodiazepines	Lorazepam		0.5–2 mg PO/IV every 4–6 h	Sedation, respiratory depression, ataxia, perceptual disturbances
Somatostatin analog	Octreotide	GI	100 µg every 8–12 h IV/SC or 100 µg/h as continuous IV infusion	Bradycardia, headache, malaise, hyperglycemia

CTZ, chemoreceptor trigger zone; GI, gastrointestinal; IV, intravenous; PO, orally; SC, subcutaneous; PR, per rectum; pts, patients; SL, sublingual; ODT, oral dissolving tablet.

diarrhea, a bland diet (for example, BRAT: bananas, rice, apples, toast) with adequate fluid intake is a gentle reintroduction of solid food and nutrients to the GI tract. Finally, "post-obstructive" diarrhea has been described in ovarian cancer patients with a significant intra-abdominal tumor burden. Debulking or radiation therapy, if appropriate, can provide

Table 29.6. Commonly used laxatives

Type of laxative	Drug name	Onset	Route	Mechanism of action	Comments
Fecal softener	Docusate	24–48 h	PO	Promotes water retention in fecal mass, softening the stool	Use in combination with stimulant laxatives; do not use alone
Lubricant	Mineral oil		PO/PR	Lubricates intestinal mucosa, softens stool allowing for easier passage	Give on an empty stomach at bedtime; interferes with absorption of oil-soluble vitamins and drugs; risk of lipid pneumonitis in elderly patients; avoid use with docusate as it can increase systemic absorption of mineral oil
Stimulant	Senna Bisacodyl	8–12 h	PO/PR	Direct stimulation of intestinal motor activity	Prolonged use can lead to loss of normal bowel motility and laxative dependency; can cause cramping
Saline	Magnesium (magnesium sulfate, milk of magnesia and magnesium citrate), sodium phosphate	0.5–3 h	PO	Pulls water into the intestinal lumen, altering stool consistency, causing bowel distention and inducing peristalsis	Repeated use can result in fluid/electrolyte imbalances; magnesium-based laxatives should be avoided in renal patients; sodium-based laxatives should be avoided in patients with chronic heart failure hypertension, edema
Bulk producers	Methylcellulose psyllium	12–24 h	PO	Hold water in the intestinal tract, soften stool, increase frequency of stool passage	Requires adequate fluid intake (i.e., 240 mL of water), to avoid obstruction; not recommended as bowel regimen with opioids
Osmotic	Lactulose	24–48 h	PO	Not absorbed by the colon; retains water in the GI lumen, increasing osmotic pressure; volume increase leads to peristalsis	Can cause excessive diarrhea with electrolyte imbalance; avoid if obstructed/impacted; causes abdominal distention, cramps
	Polyethylene glycol				Minimal water/sodium loss or gain
Opioid antagonists	Methylnaltrexone	30 min–4 h	SC	Acts on peripheral opioid receptors in the GI tract, displacing opioids and causing laxation	Can only be given by SC injection; long-term side effects unknown

IV, intravenous; PO, orally; SC, subcutaneous; PR, per rectum

Table 29.7. Commonly used anti-diarrheal medications [86,87]

Class	Drug name	Dosage/route	Comments
Opioid agonist	Loperamide	4 mg PO initially, then 2 mg PO after each loose stool; max 16 mg/day	Dizziness, drowsiness, urinary retention, stomach cramping/bloating, vomiting; does not cross blood–brain barrier and has better side effect profile
	Diphenoxylate	10 mg PO initially, then 5 mg PO every 6 h as needed; max	High doses can cause anti-cholinergic side effects
Bulk-forming agent	Kaolin-pectin	4–8 tablespoonfuls PO after each loose bowel movement	May take up to 48 h to be effective; interferes with the absorption of certain other medications
	Psyllium	1–2 tablespoons PO every 8–12 h	Needs adequate fluid intake; can cause abdominal bloating or impaction
Methylcellulose resins	Colestyramine (preferred in radiation enteritis)	4 g PO 3 times daily	Avoid if volume depleted; can cause malabsorption of fat-soluble vitamins
Other	Octreotide	100–600 μg/day IV in divided doses every 8–12 h; 10–80 μg SC every 1 h until symptoms improve	May worsen abdominal cramping

IV, intravenous; PO, orally; SC, subcutaneous; PR, per rectum.

symptom relief in these situations. A list of anti-diarrheal medications and their properties can be found in Table 29.7.

Ascites

Ascites is the excess buildup of fluid in the peritoneal cavity; the presence of cancer cells in ascitic fluid defines malignant ascites. Typically a grave prognostic sign, malignant ascites, occurs in approximately 50% of patient with ovarian cancer [52]. Common associated symptoms include nausea, abdominal fullness, early satiety, and dyspnea. In patients with ovarian cancer, common causes include: tumor-related obstruction, peritoneal carcinomatosis, hepatic dysfunction/cirrhosis, portal vein thrombosis, congestive heart failure, nephritic syndrome, and infections of the peritoneal cavity [53].

A work-up for ascites includes understanding the time course of fluid accumulation, any prior interventions attempted, and a medication review. Radiologic imaging with an ultrasound or CT-scan can confirm the presence of ascites; a diagnostic paracentesis can establish the presence of malignant ascites.

Management of malignant ascites relies primarily on diuretics and therapeutic paracentesis, with paracentesis the preferred modality [54]. Although first-line management is sodium restriction in combination with diuretics, most malignant ascites is resistant to diuretic use. In patients with hepatic metastases however, diuretics have demonstrated greater utility [55]. Large volume paracentesis, with removal of ascitic fluid, is often sufficient to provide symptomatic relief. Older patients are more at risk from fluid shifts and should have smaller amounts of fluid removed. Approximately 90% of patients can be managed with paracentesis [56]. Patients who require frequent paracentesis can be managed using an external drainage catheter (pigtail or tunneled catheter) placed through the abdominal wall and eliminating recurrent needle sticks. Patients and providers can then more easily drain fluid off outside the hospital and clinic setting on an as needed basis [57].

Other modalities such as shunting and intra-peritoneal chemotherapy have also been used to treat malignant ascites associated with ovarian cancer, but are associated with more limitations and are not as effective. A peritovenous shunt system that drains ascitic fluid directly into the venous system (by means of the superior vena cava) may benefit patients with refractory ascites for whom the paracentesis is particularly distressing [58]. However, given the significant risk profile of shunts, they are reserved for patients with a life expectancy of less than 2–3 months [59]. The use of intra-peritoneal chemotherapy for the palliation of malignant ascites and treatment of peritoneal carcinomatosis is currently under investigation but is limited to major cancer centers due to expense and administration requirements [60–62]. Current data suggest that IP therapy has efficacy treating malignant ascites in patients previously responsive to earlier systemic therapy.

Lymphedema

Lymphedema is the swelling that occurs with the accumulation of lymphatic fluid in the interstitium. When lymphedema results from malignancy, it is acquired or "secondary" lymphedema. It can occur from mass effect of the cancer on lymphatics, or from treatment that involves the lymph nodes, particularly surgical excision. Other causes of lymphedema include radiation to the lymph nodes, infection, or trauma. The time course for the development of secondary lymphedema can be immediately post-operatively to weeks or years later [63,64]. Although lower-limb lymphedema has a high prevalence in patients with gynecological cancers, only 5% of ovarian cancer patients will suffer from it [65].

Patients often complain of a feeling of "heaviness" in the affected joint(s), skin "tightening," and limb pain. In physical exam, lymphedema is characteristically a 'nonpitting' edema that most frequently presents in the limbs. In its early stages, lymphedema presents with pitting edema, but as the area fibroses over time, the edema becomes nonpitting. The diagnosis of lymphedema is based on a combination of appropriate history with clinical findings. Lymphoscintigraphy can be used to image the lymphatic system if the diagnosis is unclear; MRI can also be used as a complimentary modality to provide additional anatomical and nodal detail [66].

Non-pharmacologic measures are the mainstay for managing lymphedema. The use of gradient pressure garments (sleeves or stockings), compression bandaging [67], manual lymphatic drainage, and skin stretching/massage have been demonstrated to decrease pain and swelling in patients with lymphedema and to improve functionality [68]. Although all of these modalities may be used with some success, there is no evidence to suggest any modality is significantly better. Exercise, particularly weight-lifting, has been shown to reduce swelling in upper extremities affected by lymphedema but is still under investigation in lower-extremity edema. Finally, preventative techniques focused on maintaining adequate nutrition, maintaining a healthy weight [69], avoiding constrictive clothing or jewelry, and good skin hygiene to evaluate regularly for skin breaks and possible infectious signs are extremely important to managing the chronicity of lymphedema. Clinical trials evaluating pharmacologic interventions have proven largely unrevealing; even diuretics, commonly used to treat edema, are of minimal efficacy given the presence of lymph fluid outside the vascular space.

Dyspnea

Dyspnea or breathlessness is the subjective experience of breathing discomfort that consists of qualitatively distinct sensations that vary in intensity [70]. It is the patient's report of feeling short of breath that defines breathlessness, independent of objective data documenting blood levels of inadequate oxygenation. The pathophysiology of breathlessness is not well-defined but includes physical as well as emotional, psychological, and functional factors; certain states such as fatigue, respiratory muscle weakness, ascites, and anxiety are well-known causes of dyspnea.

The reported frequency of dyspnea in patients with advanced cancer is variable, in part because of physicians' difficulty in recognizing the symptom [71]. However, it is estimated that between 21% and 79% of advanced cancer patients will experience dyspnea [72].

The work-up of dyspnea often includes a measurement of oxygenation (arterial blood gases, oxygen saturation), appropriate laboratory tests (complete blood count), and radiologic studies (chest X-ray, V/Q scan, CT-angiography). Interventions can be targeted once study results reveal possible etiologies. Tracking the intensity of symptoms using the numeric rating scale can help ascertain the efficacy of any attempted interventions. When evaluating dyspnea, it is important to recognize that it is a subjective sensation and objective measurements (oxygen saturation, abg) often do not correlate with a patient's severity of symptoms.

Non-pharmacological means of treating dyspnea will often derive from possible etiologies, for example, repositioning patients with unilateral pleural effusions (lung with pleural effusion placed up), with pulmonary edema or after aspiration (head >30° upright), and breathing/relaxation techniques in anxious patients. Oxygen has efficacy in refractory dyspnea in patients with hypoxia [73]; however, in non-hypoxemic patients, the sensation of air movement from a fan directed at the face is as effective in relieving dyspnea [74].

Acute symptomatic relief of dyspnea usually involves the use of opioids and anxiolytics. Opioids are thought to be effective through both central and peripheral mechanisms, decreasing the central respiratory drive in combination with direct pulmonary relaxation by means of interaction with opioid receptors present throughout the lungs [75]. Anxiolytics, particularly benzodiazepines, are often used in the management of dyspnea. No clear evidence exists to support their routine use if anxiety is not a contributing factor [76,77].

End-of-life/terminal phase

Death is a natural process that will occur for everyone. However, this is a time often fraught with significant distress for both patients and families. The most commonly encountered symptoms in the terminal phase include fatigue, anorexia, delirium, pain, dyspnea, and dry mouth. These symptoms result from a variety of physiologic changes that occur in the last hours to days of life and a summary of these changes can be found in Table 29.8. Delirium can be very upsetting to families and often requires pharmacologic intervention. Neuroleptic agents are the mainstay of pharmacologic treatment and of these agents, haloperidol is the agent of choice. The pharmacologic agents commonly used in the management of delirium can be found in Table 29.9. It is important to prepare patients and families for the typical and normal signs and symptoms of impending death so that they know what is expected to happen. Only medications essential to providing comfort should be continued. The least invasive rate of medication administration should be attempted initially, using the most invasive route only when absolutely necessary.

Table 29.8. Physiologic changes in the terminal phase

Decreased oral intake	• Studies have shown no benefit to parenteral or enteral nutrition in dying patients with metastatic cancer • Most common complaint is dry mouth • Can use lollipop sponges dipped in cold fluids such as water, lemon flavored drink, or sorbet
Respiratory changes	• Breathing becomes shallow and frequent with periods of apnea • This can be a natural part of the dying process and family or caregivers should be prepared for these changes
Loss of ability to swallow	• Manifests as a gurgling noise "the death rattle" • Treat with anti-cholinergic medications; scopolomine (transdermal, IV, SC), glycopyrrolate (IV, SC), atropine (ophthalmic drops given orally)

Hospice

Hospice is a type of palliative care that focuses only on patients at the end-of-life and is not given simultaneously with other forms of life-prolonging or curative therapies. It aims to provide patients with a life expectancy of less than 6 months with the best quality of life and comfort. Hospice services include medications, durable medical equipment, continuous around-the-clock access to care and support, and bereavement services for families. Most hospice care is delivered at home; however, it is also provided in other facilities such as inpatient hospice facilities, nursing homes, assisted living facilities, and hospitals. Approximately 50% of patients with ovarian malignancies will be referred to hospice [78].

Summary

In the patient with ovarian malignancy, palliative care's focus is an interdisciplinary approach to maximizing the patient's quality of life at any point along the disease spectrum – from pursuit of curative treatment to treatment with palliative intent. The extended expertise of palliative care's interdisciplinary providers is designed to coordinate an extended plan of care addressing the multidimensional

Table 29.9. Commonly used agents in delirium

Drug name	Dosage/route	Comments
Haloperidol	0.5–5 mg PO/IV/IM/SC every 6–12 h	Most commonly used agent; can prolong QT interval
Chlorpromazine	12.5–50 mg PO/IV/IM every 8–12 h	Similar efficacy to haloperidol, but more sedating, anti-cholinergic, and hypotensive effects
Lorazepam	0.5–2 mg PO/SL/IV every 4–8 h and titrate as needed	Second most commonly used agent, often in combination with haloperidol; may worsen delirium in the elderly; use with caution in liver failure
Risperidone	Start at 0.5–1 mg/day PO and titrate up to 4–6 mg/day	Only available orally
Olanzapine	5 mg PO at nighttime with titration to effect (max 20 mg/day)	Age > 70, dementia, CNS metastases, hypoxia, and hypoactive delirium indicate poor response
Midazolam	1 mg/h IV with titration to effect	Used for refractory delirium where sedation is needed

needs of both the patient and primary caregivers, and the unique symptom burden experienced by this population.

The beneficial effects of palliative care have been well documented. Most recently, early palliative care integration at time of diagnosis in patients with metastatic lung cancer demonstrated a significant improvement in quality of life, depression, and 2.3-month survival benefit as compared with standard care [79]. Given the global burden of disease represented by ovarian malignancy, palliative care has a significant opportunity to help patients and extended care teams address questions of comfort, autonomy, and dignity in the face of serious and incurable illness. As the number of palliative care programs and specialists continues to increase, it will be important to ensure timely access to this care for patients and their families facing this disease.

References

1. WHO. Cancer: WHO Definition of Palliative Care. Geneva: World Health Organization 2011 (http://www.who.int/cancer/palliative/definition/en/).
2. Bruera E, Michaud M, Vigano A, et al. Multidisciplinary symptom control clinic in a cancer center: a retrospective study. Support Care Cancer. 2001;**9**:162–8.
3. Mancini I, Lossignol D, Obiols M, et al. Supportive and palliative care: experience at the Institut Jules Bordet. Support Care Cancer. 2002;**10**:3–7.
4. Strasser F, Sweeney C, Willey J, et al. Impact of a half-day multidisciplinary symptom control and palliative care outpatient clinic in a comprehensive cancer center on recommendations, symptom intensity, and patient satisfaction: a retrospective descriptive study. J Pain Symptom Manage. 2004;**27**:481–91.
5. Ferris FD, Bruera E, Cherny N, et al. Palliative cancer care a decade later: accomplishments, the need, next steps – from the American Society of Clinical Oncology. J Clin Oncol. 2009;**27**:3052–8.
6. Levy MH, Back A, Benedetti C, et al. NCCN clinical practice guidelines in oncology: palliative care. J Natl Compr Canc Netw. 2009;**7**:436–73.
7. National Consensus Project for Quality Palliative Care. Clinical Practice Guidelines for Quality Palliative Care, 2nd edition. 2009 (http://www.nationalconsensusproject.org).
8. Detmar SB, Muller MJ, Wever LD, et al. The patient–physician relationship. Patient–physician communication during outpatient palliative treatment visits: an observational study. JAMA. 2001;**285**:1351–7.
9. Baile WF, Buckman R, Lenzi R, et al. SPIKES-A six-step protocol for delivering bad news: application to the patient with cancer. Oncologist. 2000;**5**:302–11.
10. Merskey H, Bogduk N. International Association for the Study of Pain. Task Force on Taxonomy. Classification of Chronic Pain: Descriptions of Chronic Pain Syndromes and Definitions of Pain Terms, 2nd edition. 1994, Seattle: IASP Press; xvi.
11. Portenoy RK, Kornblith AB, Wong G, et al. Pain in ovarian cancer patients. Prevalence, characteristics, and associated symptoms. Cancer. 1994;**74**:907–15.
12. Anderson KO, Richman SP, Hurley J, et al. Cancer pain management among underserved minority outpatients: perceived needs and barriers to optimal control. Cancer. 2002;**94**:2295–304.
13. Morrison RS, Wallenstein S, Natale DK, et al. "We don't carry that" – failure of pharmacies in predominantly nonwhite neighborhoods to stock opioid analgesics. N Engl J Med. 2000;**342**:1023–6.
14. Otis-Green S, Sherman R, Perez M, Baird RP. An integrated psychosocial-spiritual model for cancer pain management. Cancer Pract. 2002;**10** (Suppl 1):S58–65.
15. Bruera E, Willey JS, Ewert-Flannagan PA, et al. Pain intensity assessment by bedside nurses and palliative care consultants: a retrospective study. Support Care Cancer. 2005;**13**:228–31.
16. Jensen MP. The validity and reliability of pain measures in adults with cancer. J Pain. 2003;**4**:2–21.
17. Holen JC, Hjermastad MJ, Loge JH, et al. Pain assessment tools: is the content appropriate for use in palliative care? J Pain Symptom Manage. 2006;**32**:567–80.
18. Cleeland CS, Ryan KM. Pain assessment: global use of the Brief Pain Inventory. Ann Acad Med Singapore. 1994;**23**:129–38.
19. Badia X, Muriel C, Gracia A, et al. [Validation of the Spanish version of the Brief Pain Inventory in patients with oncological pain]. Med Clin (Barc). 2003;**120**:52–9.
20. Mystakidou K, Mendoza T, Tsilika E, et al. Greek brief pain inventory: validation and utility in cancer pain. Oncology. 2001;**60**:35–42.
21. Ger LP, Ho ST, Sun WZ, et al. Validation of the Brief Pain Inventory in a Taiwanese population. J Pain Symptom Manage. 1999;**18**:316–22.
22. Radbruch L, Loick G, Kiencke P, et al. Validation of the German version of the Brief Pain Inventory. J Pain Symptom Manage. 1999;**18**:180–7.
23. Saxena A, Mendoza T, Cleeland CS. The assessment of cancer pain in north India: the validation of the Hindi Brief Pain Inventory: BPI-H. J Pain Symptom Manage. 1999;**17**:27–41.
24. Cleeland CS, Nakamura Y, Mendoza TR, et al. Dimensions of the impact of cancer pain in a four country sample: new information from multidimensional scaling. Pain. 1996;**67**:267–73.
25. Paice JA. Mechanisms and management of neuropathic pain in cancer. J Support Oncol. 2003;**1**:107–20.
26. Mercadante S, Fulfaro F, Casuccio A. A randomised controlled study on the use of anti-inflammatory drugs in patients with cancer pain on morphine therapy: effects on dose-escalation and a pharmacoeconomic analysis. Eur J Cancer. 2002;**38**:1358–63.
27. Portenoy RK, Hagen NA. Breakthrough pain: definition, prevalence and characteristics. Pain. 1990;**41**:273–81.
28. Caraceni A, Martini C, Zecca E, et al. Breakthrough pain characteristics and syndromes in patients with cancer pain. An international survey. Palliat Med. 2004;**18**:177–83.

29. Portenoy RK, Hagen NA. Breakthrough pain: definition and management. Oncology (Williston Park). 1989;**3** (Suppl):25–9.

30. Hurdon V, Viola R, Schroder C. How useful is docusate in patients at risk for constipation? A systematic review of the evidence in the chronically ill. J Pain Symptom Manage. 2000;**19**:130–6.

31. Hawley PH, Byeon JJ. A comparison of sennosides-based bowel protocols with and without docusate in hospitalized patients with cancer. J Palliat Med. 2008;**11**:575–81.

32. Carr DB, Goudas LC, Balk EM, et al. Evidence report on the treatment of pain in cancer patients. J Natl Cancer Inst Monogr. 2004;**32**:23–31.

33. Davis MP, Walsh D, Laqman R, LeGrand SB. Controversies in pharmacotherapy of pain management. Lancet Oncol. 2005;**6**:696–704.

34. O'Connor AB, Dworkin RH. Treatment of neuropathic pain: an overview of recent guidelines. Am J Med. 2009;**122**(Suppl):S22–32.

35. Gilron I, Bailey JM, Tu D, et al. Nortriptyline and gabapentin, alone and in combination for neuropathic pain: a double-blind, randomised controlled crossover trial. Lancet. 2009;**374**(9697):1252–61.

36. Herrinton LJ, Neslund-Dudas C, Rolnick SJ, et al. Complications at the end of life in ovarian cancer. J Pain Symptom Manage. 2007;**34**:237–43.

37. Tonato M, Roila F, Del Favero A. Methodology of antiemetic trials: a review. Ann Oncol. 1991;**2**:107–14.

38. Sullivan JR, Leyden MJ, Bell R. Decreased cisplatin-induced nausea and vomiting with chronic alcohol ingestion. N Engl J Med. 1983;**309**:796.

39. Walker J, Lane P. Challenges and choices: an audit of the management of nausea, vomiting and bowel obstruction in metastatic ovarian cancer. Contemp Nurse. 2007;**27**:39–46.

40. Basch E, Hesketh PJ, Kris MG, et al. Antiemetics: American Society of Clinical Oncology Clinical Practice Guideline Update. J Clin Oncol. 2011;**7**:395–8.

41. Jin Y, Wu X, Guan Y, et al. Efficacy and safety of aprepitant in the prevention of chemotherapy-induced nausea and vomiting: a pooled analysis. Support Care Cancer. 2011;**20**:1815–22.

42. Ryerson AB, Eheman C, Burton J, et al. Symptoms, diagnoses, and time to key diagnostic procedures among older U.S. women with ovarian cancer. Obstet Gynecol. 2007;**109**:1053–61.

43. Larkin PJ, Sykes NP, Centeno C, et al. The management of constipation in palliative care: clinical practice recommendations. Palliat Med. 2008;**22**:796–807.

44. Miles CL, Fellowes D, Goodman ML, Wilkinson S. Laxatives for the management of constipation in palliative care patients. Cochrane Database Syst Rev. 2006(4):CD003448.

45. Wirz S, Klaschik E. Management of constipation in palliative care patients undergoing opioid therapy: is polyethylene glycol an option? Am J Hosp Palliat Care. 2005;**22**:375–81.

46. Candy B, Jones L, Goodman ML, et al. Laxatives or methylnaltrexone for the management of constipation in palliative care patients. Cochrane Database Syst Rev. 2011(1):CD003448.

47. Olson SH, Mignone L, Nakraseive C, et al. Symptoms of ovarian cancer. Obstet Gynecol. 2001;**98**:212–17.

48. Goff BA, Mandel LS, Melancon CH, Muntz HG. Frequency of symptoms of ovarian cancer in women presenting to primary care clinics. JAMA. 2004;**291**:2705–12.

49. Engelking C, Rutledge DN, Ippoliti C, Neumann J, Hogan CM. Cancer-related diarrhea: a neglected cause of cancer-related symptom distress. Oncol Nurs Forum. 1998;**25**:859–60.

50. Swan RW. Stagnant loop syndrome resulting from small-bowel irradiation injury and intestinal by-pass. Gynecol Oncol. 1974;**2**:441–5.

51. Currow DC, Cooney NJ. Octreotide in palliative medicine. Palliat Med. 1994;**8**:168.

52. Garrison RN, Kaelin LD, Galloway RH, Heuser LS. Malignant ascites. Clinical and experimental observations. Ann Surg. 1986;**203**:644–51.

53. LeBlanc K, Arnold RM. Evaluation of malignant ascites #176. J Palliat Med. 2010;**13**:1027–8.

54. Lee CW, Bociek G, Faught W. A survey of practice in management of malignant ascites. J Pain Symptom Manage. 1998;**16**:96–101.

55. Saada E, Follana P, Peyrade F, Mari V, Francois E. Pathogenesis and management of refractory malignant ascites. Bull Cancer. 2011;**98**:679–87.

56. Becker G, Galandi D, Blum HE. Malignant ascites: systematic review and guideline for treatment. Eur J Cancer. 2006;**42**:589–97.

57. LeBlanc K, Arnold RM. Palliative treatment of malignant ascites 177. J Palliat Med. 2010;**13**:1028–9.

58. Bieligk SC, Calvo BF, Coit DG. Peritoneovenous shunting for nongynecologic malignant ascites. Cancer. 2001;**91**:1247–55.

59. Chung M, Kozuch P. Treatment of malignant ascites. Curr Treat Options Oncol. 2008;**9**:215–33.

60. Barni S, Cabiddu M, Ghilardi M, Petrelli F. A novel perspective for an orphan problem: old and new drugs for the medical management of malignant ascites. Crit Rev Oncol Hematol. 2011;**79**:144–53.

61. Link KH, Hepp G, Staib L, et al. Intraperitoneal regional chemotherapy with mitroxantrone. Cancer Treat Res. 1996;**81**:31–40.

62. Link KH, Roitman M, Holtappels M, et al. Intraperitoneal chemotherapy with mitoxantrone in malignant ascites. Surg Oncol Clin N Am. 2003;**12**(3):865–72.

63. Lockwood-Rayermann S. Ovarian cancer and lower limb lymphedema. Oncology (Williston Park). 2007;**21**(8 Suppl):20–2.

64. Tada H, Teramukai S, Fukushima M, Sasaki H. Risk factors for lower limb lymphedema after lymph node dissection in patients with ovarian and uterine carcinoma. BMC Cancer. 2009;**9**:47.

65. Beesley V, Janda M, Eakin E, Obermair A, Battistutta D. Lymphedema after gynecological cancer treatment: prevalence, correlates, and supportive care needs. Cancer. 2007;**109**:2607–14.

66. Rockson SG. Lymphedema. Am J Med. 2001;**110**:288–95.

67. Badger CM, Peacock JL, Mortimer PS. A randomized, controlled, parallel-group clinical trial comparing multilayer bandaging followed by hosiery versus hosiery alone in the treatment of patients with lymphedema of the limb. Cancer. 2000;**88**:2832–7.

68. Andersen L, Højris I, Erlandsen M, Andersen J. Treatment of breast-cancer-related lymphedema with or without manual lymphatic drainage – a randomized study. Acta Oncol. 2000;**39**:399–405.

69. Shaw C, Mortimer P, Judd PA. Randomized controlled trial comparing a low-fat diet with a weight-reduction diet in breast cancer-related lymphedema. Cancer. 2007;**109**:1949–56.

70. Ripamonti C, Fulfaro F, Bruera E. Dyspnoea in patients with advanced cancer: incidence, causes and treatments. Cancer Treat Rev. 1998;**24**:69–80.

71. Del Fabbro E, Dalal S, Bruera E. Symptom control in palliative care – Part III: dyspnea and delirium. J Palliat Med. 2006;**9**:422–36.

72. Bruera E, Schmitz B, Pither J, Neumann CM, Hanson J. The frequency and correlates of dyspnea in patients with advanced cancer. J Pain Symptom Manage. 2000;**19**:357–62.

73. Uronis HE, Abernethy AP. Oxygen for relief of dyspnea: what is the evidence? Curr Opin Support Palliat Care. 2008;**2**:89–94.

74. Rousseau P. Nonpain symptom management in terminal care. Clin Geriatr Med. 1996;**12**:313–27.

75. Zebraski SE, Kochenash SM, Raffa RB. Lung opioid receptors: pharmacology and possible target for nebulized morphine in dyspnea. Life Sci. 2000;**66**:2221–31.

76. Clemens KE, Klaschik E. Dyspnoea associated with anxiety-symptomatic therapy with opioids in combination with lorazepam and its effect on ventilation in palliative care patients. Support Care Cancer. 2011;**19**:2027–33.

77. Williams M. Applicability and generalizability of palliative interventions for dyspnoea: one size fits all, some or none? Curr Opin Support Palliat Care. 2011;**5**:92–100.

78. Jackson JM, Rolnick SJ, Coughlin SS, et al. Social support among women who died of ovarian cancer. Support Care Cancer. 2007;**15**:547–56.

79. Temel JS, Greer JA, Admane S, et al. Early palliative care for patients with metastatic non-small-cell lung cancer. N Engl J Med. 2010;**363**:733–42.

Index